# Practical Cardiology

## Principles and Approaches

# Practical Cardiology

## Principles and Approaches

SECOND EDITION

EDITED BY

MAJID MALEKI

AZIN ALIZADEHASL

MAJID HAGHJOO

ELSEVIER

Elsevier
Radarweg 29, PO Box 211, 1000 AE Amsterdam, Netherlands
The Boulevard, Langford Lane, Kidlington, Oxford OX5 1GB, United Kingdom
50 Hampshire Street, 5th Floor, Cambridge, MA 02139, United States

**Notices**

Knowledge and best practice in this field are constantly changing. As new research and experience broaden our
understanding, changes in research methods, professional practices, or medical treatment may become
necessary.

Practitioners and researchers must always rely on their own experience and knowledge in evaluating and using
any information, methods, compounds, or experiments described herein. In using such information or methods
they should be mindful of their own safety and the safety of others, including parties for whom they have a
professional responsibility.

To the fullest extent of the law, neither the Publisher nor the authors, contributors, or editors, assume any liability
for any injury and/or damage to persons or property as a matter of products liability, negligence or otherwise, or
from any use or operation of any methods, products, instructions, or ideas contained in the material herein.

**Library of Congress Cataloging-in-Publication Data**
A catalog record for this book is available from the Library of Congress

**British Library Cataloguing-in-Publication Data**
A catalogue record for this book is available from the British Library

ISBN: 978-0-323-80915-3

For information on all Elsevier publications
visit our website at https://www.elsevier.com/books-and-journals

*Publisher:* Dolores Meloni
*Acquisitions Editor:* Robin R Carter
*Editorial Project Manager:* Tracy I. Tufaga
*Production Project Manager:* Sreejith Viswanathan
*Cover Designer:* Alan Studholme

Typeset by SPi Global, India

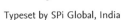

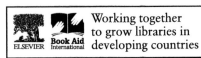

Working together
to grow libraries in
developing countries

www.elsevier.com • www.bookaid.org

# Contents

# Contributors

**Mohammad Javad Alemzadeh-Ansari**
Cardiovascular Intervention Research Center, Rajaie
Cardiovascular, Medical & Research Center, Iran
University of Medical Sciences, Tehran, Iran

**Azin Alizadehasl**
Cardio-Oncology Research Center, Rajaie
Cardiovascular, Medical & Research Center, Iran
University of Medical Sciences, Tehran, Iran

**Ahmad Amin**
Rajaie Cardiovascular, Medical & Research Center, Iran
University of Medical Sciences, Tehran, Iran

**Rasoul Azarfarin**
Rajaie Cardiovascular, Medical & Research Center, Iran
University of Medical Sciences, Tehran, Iran

**Mitra Chitsazan**
Rajaie Cardiovascular, Medical & Research Center, Iran
University of Medical Sciences, Tehran, Iran

**Bahram Fariborz Farsad**
Shaheed Rajaei Cardiovascular, Medical & Research
Center, Iran University of Medical Sciences,
Tehran, Iran

**Amir Farjam Fazelifar**
Department of Cardiac Electrophysiology, Rajaie
Cardiovascular, Medical & Research Center, Iran
University of Medical Sciences, Tehran, Iran;
Cardiac Electrophysiology Research Center, Rajaie
Cardiovascular, Medical & Research Center, Iran
University of Medical Sciences, Tehran, Iran

**Ata Firouzi**
Rajaie Cardiovascular, Medical & Research Center,
Tehran, Iran

**Zahra Ghaemmaghami**
Rajaie Cardiovascular, Medical & Research Center, Iran
University of Medical Sciences, Tehran, Iran

**Samad Ghaffari**
Cardiovascular Research Center, Tabriz University of
Medicine, Tabriz, Iran

**Alireza Alizadeh Ghavidel**
Rajaie Cardiovascular, Medical & Research Center, Iran
University of Medical Sciences, Tehran, Iran

**Majid Haghjoo**
Department of Cardiac Electrophysiology, Rajaie
Cardiovascular, Medical & Research Center, Iran
University of Medical Sciences, Tehran, Iran

**Saeid Hosseini**
Heart Valve Disease Research Center, Rajaie
Cardiovascular, Medical & Research Center, Iran
University of Medical Sciences, Tehran, Iran

**Zahra Hosseini**
Assistant Professor of Interventional Cardiology,
Cardiovascular Intervention Research Center, Rajaie
Cardiovascular, Medical & Research Center, Iran
University of Medical Sciences, Tehran, Iran

**Farzad Kamali**
Department of Cardiac Electrophysiology, Rajaie
Cardiovascular, Medical & Research Center, Iran
University of Medical Sciences, Tehran, Iran

**Zahra Khajali**
Rajaie Cardiovascular, Medical & Research Center, Iran
University of Medical Sciences, Tehran, Iran

**Reza Kiani**
Cardiovascular Intervention Research Center, Rajaei
Cardiovascular, Medical & Research Center, Iran
University of Medical Sciences, Tehran, Iran

**Majid Kyavar**
Cardiovascular Intervention Research Center, Rajaie
Cardiovascular, Medical & Research Center, Iran
University of Medical Sciences, Tehran, Iran

**Shabnam Madadi**
Rajaie Cardiovascular, Medical & Research Center,
Tehran, Iran

**Nejat Mahdieh**
Cardiogenetic Research Center, Rajaie Cardiovascular,
Medical & Research Center, Iran University of Medical
Sciences, Tehran, Iran;
Growth and Development Research Center, Tehran
University of Medical Sciences, Tehran, Iran

**Hadi Malek**
Rajaie Cardiovascular, Medical & Research Center, Iran
University of Medical Sciences, Tehran, Iran

**Alireza Maleki**
Resident of Anesthesiology, Iran University of Medical
Sciences, Tehran, Iran

**Majid Maleki**
Rajaie Cardiovascular, Medical & Research Center, Iran
University of Medical Sciences, Tehran, Iran

**Ali Zahed Mehr**
Cardiovascular Intervention Research Center, Rajaie
Cardiovascular, Medical & Research Center, Iran
University of Medical Sciences, Tehran, Iran

**Bahram Mohebbi**
Cardiovascular Intervention Research Center, Cardio-
Oncology Research Center, Rajaie Cardiovascular,
Medical & Research Center, Iran University of Medical
Sciences, Tehran, Iran

**Hamid Mojibian**
Department of Radiology and Biomedical Imaging, Yale
University School of Medicine, New Haven, CT,
United States

**Jamal Moosavi**
Cardiovascular Intervention Research Center, Rajaie
Cardiovascular, Medical & Research Center, Iran
University of Medical Sciences, Tehran, Iran

**Nasim Naderi**
Rajaie Cardiovascular, Medical & Research Center, Iran
University of Medical Sciences, Tehran, Iran

**Feridoun Noohi**
Rajaie Cardiovascular, Medical & Research Center, Iran
University of Medical Sciences, Tehran, Iran

**Zeinab Norouzi**
Cardiac Rehabilitation Department, Rajaie
Cardiovascular, Medical & Research Center, Tehran,
Iran

**Hamidreza Pouraliakbar**
Rajaie Cardiovascular, Medical & Research Center, Iran
University of Medical Sciences, Tehran, Iran

**Bahareh Rabbani**
Rajaie Cardiovascular, Medical & Research Center, Iran
University of Medical Sciences, Tehran, Iran

**Hasan Allah Sadeghi**
Rajaie Cardiovascular, Medical & Research Center

**Parham Sadeghipour**
Rajaie Cardiovascular, Medical & Research Center, Iran
University of Medical Sciences, Tehran, Iran

**Anita Sadeghpour**
Rajaie Cardiovascular, Medical & Research Center,
Tehran, Iran;
Visiting Research Scholar in Duke Cardiovascular MR
Center, Durham, NC, United States

**Sedigheh Saedi**
Rajaie Cardiovascular, Medical & Research Center,
Tehran, Iran

**Hanieh Salehi**
Shaheed Rajaei Cardiovascular, Medical & Research
Center, Iran University of Medical Sciences, Tehran,
Iran

**Hamidreza Sanati**
Cardiovascular Intervention Research Center,
Rajaei Cardiovascular Research and Medical Center,
Iran University of Medical Sciences,
Tehran, Iran

**Omid Shafe**
Cardiovascular Interventional Research Center, Rajaie
Cardiovascular, Medical & Research Center, Iran
University of Medical Sciences, Tehran, Iran

**Farshad Shakerian**
Cardiovascular Intervention Research Center,
Rajaie Cardiovascular, Medical & Research Center,
Iran University of Medical Sciences,
Tehran, Iran

**Samira Tabiban**
Rajaie Cardiovascular, Medical & Research Center, Iran University of Medical Sciences, Tehran, Iran

**Azita Haj Hossein Talasaz**
Tehran Heart Center, Tehran University of Medical Sciences, Tehran, Iran

**Reza Yousefi-Nooraie**
Department of Public Health Sciences, University of Rochester, Rochester, NY, United States

# Preface

This second edition has been broadly expanded to address changes and provide a more thorough overview of the current extensiveness of the field of cardiology.

We have been extremely grateful for the positive feedback to our first edition of practical cardiology and so we were excited to provide a new edition of this book.

Beyond simply updating the texts, this second edition has given us the opportunity to further explore new topics such as a new challenge of the world with Covid-19 and its impact on the cardiovascular system. Also, new electrophysiology, acute coronary syndrome, and echocardiography chapters have been added. Besides in congenital heart disease and hemodynamic chapters, new figures, modalities, and attractive images have been incorporated for a better and juicy understanding of the issue.

Other changes in the book are more subtle. We have rearranged sections and added headings in some chapters to make them flow better. This book is written for cardiologists, different fellowships, residents, internists, cardiac surgeons, and professionals who wish to understand the principle and applications of information and practical points of technologies in cardiovascular sciences.

It is suitable as a practical textbook for undergraduate and postgraduate training in the clinical aspects of cardiology.

At least for this edition, we think we have managed to keep the book up to date with all necessary practical points and design to be used by all cardiology professionals.

**Majid Maleki, MD, FACC**
*Professor in Cardiology*
**Azin Alizadehasl, MD, FASE**
*Professor in Cardiology*
**Majid Haghjoo, MD, FACC**
*Professor in Cardiology*

# Acknowledgments

We would like to acknowledge those we have added in the preface of the first edition. We should thank all our colleagues for their support and providing their knowledge and expertise for this edition from whom we have learnt a lot.

We are especially grateful for the ongoing encouragement and support of all of our fellows, residents, and fans at the Rajaie Cardiovascular, Medical & Research Center.

Expert secretarial help was provided by Sara Tayebi and Arefeh Ghorbani.

Importantly this edition would not have been possible without invaluable and great help and support of Robin R. Carter and Tracy I. Tufaga from estimable Elsevier Publishing Company.

Last but not least we wish to acknowledge the support and patience of our family without which this book would not have been possible.

**Majid Maleki, MD, FACC**
**Azin Alizadehasl, MD, FACC, FASE**
**Majid Haghjoo, MD, FACC**

# CHAPTER 1

# Evidence-Based Cardiology Practice

Reza Yousefi-Nooraie[a], Parham Sadeghipour[b]
[a]Department of Public Health Sciences, University of Rochester, Rochester, NY, United States, [b]Rajaie Cardiovascular, Medical & Research Center, Iran University of Medical Sciences, Tehran, Iran

---

**KEY POINTS**

- Evidence-based medicine (EBM) is the timely, critical, and systematic use of best research evidence in clinical care.
- EBM relies on three principles:
  - Optimal clinical practice requires knowledge of best evidence.
  - Assessing the quality and the trustworthiness of evidence is crucial.
  - Evidence alone is never enough for making a final decision.
- EBM resources help us to find the best evidence.
- Evidence-based clinical guidelines are valuable EBM resources, which are systematically developed statements aiming to help clinicians and patients making decisions about specific clinical situations.

---

## INTRODUCTION

The prophylactic use of lidocaine to prevent lethal ventricular arrhythmia in patients with acute myocardial infarction (MI) was considered common practice for decades. Lidocaine was shown to suppress arrhythmia. So at that time, it seemed like a rational decision to prescribe lidocaine to patients with heart attack who were at risk of developing life-threatening arrhythmia.[1] During the 1980s, increasing number of randomized controlled trials (RCTs) failed to show any effect for prophylactic lidocaine and even showed some evidence of harm. Clinicians who mainly relied on their own experience and interpretation did not take the research evidence from RCTs seriously, until 1989, when the meta-analyses showed overwhelming evidence for its lack of effectiveness and the possibility of harm.[2] It took 2 decades to convince the clinicians to change their routine practice in light of the available high-quality evidence. In this case, the lack of a conceptual framework for assessing the quality and using available evidence from high-quality research in practice and the lack of methodology to review and summarize the evidence into systematic reviews and to develop recommendations to guide practice resulted in a long-term delay in practice change. This classic example showed *how* and more important *why* evidence-based medicine was created. Proposed by a group of epidemiologists in the early 1990s, the term *evidence-based medicine* (*EBM*) has been itself "critically appraised" through time.

EBM is built on three main principles.[3] First, knowledge of best available evidence is crucial in making sound clinical decisions. EBM and basically the philosophy of science showed that pure reasoning stemming from personal experience might easily miss some aspects of a problem and be affected by various biases. Therefore, each new idea should be empirically tested and evaluated before being adopted for making clinical decisions. Second, researchers should be guided through assessing the quality and trustworthiness of the evidence. This involves development of quality assessment skills. Several tools and guidelines have also been created to assist clinicians through the quality assessment process. And third, evidence alone is never enough to support a final clinical decision.

## EVIDENCE-BASED MEDICINE RESOURCES

The use of research evidence to inform clinical practice requires timely access to high-quality and relevant research. At the early formative years of EBM, this meant a time-consuming process of searching in general medical databases; looking for original studies; appraising their quality; extracting, summarizing, and interpreting their findings; and applying the findings to individual patients. But during the past decade, there have been many efforts to process the huge mass of medical literature and provide the busy clinicians with preappraised and summarized extracts of high-quality and up-to-date research evidence. The 5S model (Fig. 1.1) provides a quick conceptual framework of the hierarchy of preappraised evidence-based resources.[4] It resembles a funnel through which the raw material of original studies is processed and concentrated into digested resources applicable to the clinical process.

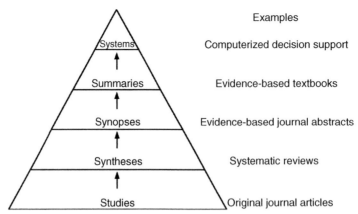

FIG. 1.1 The 5S model. (From Haynes B. Of studies, syntheses, synopses, summaries, and systems: the "5S" evolution of information services for evidence-based healthcare decisions. *Evid Based Nurs*. 2007;10:6–7, with permission.)

Original studies, at the bottom of the funnel, are what you generally find by searching MEDLINE or Google Scholar. The challenge with extracting evidence from original studies is that the quality assessment is the responsibility of the reader. Even though most well-known journals are peer reviewed and there already has been a preliminary assessment of the quality when a study is published, that peer review is not meant to appraise a study for the quality of the evidence, and many other factors, such as the attractiveness of the topic or the findings, may reduce the validity of peer review as the only quality assessment prior to publication.[5]

In addition, because of the ever-increasing pace of proliferation of medical studies, it is very likely that you miss some high-quality studies if you only perform a quick search or only explore the first few pages of your search results, which is a very plausible scenario, given the limited time clinicians can spend on literature review.

Thus, there is a need for systematic reviews (the "synthesis") that follow a predefined and transparent procedure to find virtually all studies relevant to a specific clinical question, appraise their quality using an objective quality assessment framework, extract their finding, and synthesize them using quantitative (meta-analysis) or qualitative (narrative) pooling techniques. Unlike an unstructured review, systematic reviews try to minimize all the biases that may happen in the abovementioned steps.[6] The reviews developed by the Cochrane Collaboration are an example of such studies (http://cochranelibrary.com); however, a high-quality systematic review is not necessarily a Cochrane review, and you can ascertain the validity and comprehensiveness of the review procedure by a quick overview of the Methods section of a review claiming to be systematic.

"Synopses" are predigested excerpts of selected individual studies, which could be an RCT or a systematic review. A few journals (e.g., Evidence-Based Medicine, http://ebm.bmj.com, and ACP Journal Club, http://annals.org/journalclub.aspx) are dedicated to preparing and publishing such predigested synopses. They are more suitable for busy clinicians who do not have the time or motivation to go through a long, detailed systematic review and prefer to rely on the assessments of an EBM expert group.

"Summaries" integrate the best available evidence obtained from lower levels of the funnel into clinical practice by proposing practice recommendations that are easily transferable to the patient's bedside. Evidence-based clinical practice guidelines (CPGs) are in this category. They include a comprehensive synthesis of research evidence, expert opinion, and patient perspective; an assessment of benefits, harms, and alternative care options; and development of recommendations about specific care options in a brief and easily understandable language, which are generally graded according to the strength of recommendation and the validity of underlying evidence.[7]

And at the tip of the funnel there exist "systems" (e.g., computerized decision support systems) that aim to link the high-quality evidence to individual patient characteristics in a dynamic and intelligent way. They require a sophisticated electronic medical record infrastructure that has not been widely implemented but has been shown to moderately improve morbidity outcomes.[8]

## CLINICAL PRACTICE GUIDELINES
We talked about CPGs as a common example of "summaries" in the 5S model. Guidelines are systematically developed statements aiming to help clinicians and patients making decisions about specific clinical situations.

The development of a rigorous CPG usually involves a complex multistep process.[9] A multidisciplinary team including various stakeholders (which usually also includes patient representatives) is formed, which formulates one or more specific clinical questions. The team conducts a systematic literature review to find available research evidence for various strategies and outcomes that are formulated in the well-defined question. The team appraises the quality of obtained studies, summarizes and interprets the findings, and tries to reach consensus on the best ways to formulate the recommendations. The draft recommendations are sent for external review by groups of intended users and stakeholders. The team then prepares an action plan for dissemination and implementation of the final version.

Why does it all matter? Guidelines are meant to inform clinical decisions. Therefore, their statements should be valid, clear, and applicable to clinical situations and should reflect the values and expectations of all involved stakeholders (which could be patients, doctors, policymakers, and others). The process of guideline development should be both methodologically rigorous and socially engaging. In addition, the final recommendations should be informative, clear, and practice oriented. Generally, the recommendations are graded to help the users easily judge the quality of evidence and the strength of recommendations. Traditionally, the recommendations have been graded by assigning A, B, C, and D, which mostly reflected the quality of evidence according to a hierarchy in which RCTs stood at the top and crude clinical speculation at the bottom. This hierarchy has resulted in widespread debate since its creation. Designing and performing an RCT to address a specific clinical problem is sometimes impossible or irrelevant. For example, to study prognosis, we rely mostly on the observational studies reporting on infrequent adverse events. This hierarchical system of evidence quality also confuses the quality of the evidence with the strength of recommendations because, on the one hand, RCTs are not ideal designs for all clinical questions, and on the other hand, a finding from an RCT does not necessarily dictate a strong clinical recommendation.[10]

Among various grading frameworks, the GRADE system (which stands for Grading of Recommendations Assessment, Development and Evaluation; http://gradepro.org) is more systematic and explicit, addressing various shortcomings of existing grading systems. It has been adopted by more than 100 organizations, including the World Health Organization, the Cochrane Collaboration, and the National Institute for Health and Care Excellence (NICE).[11] GRADE scores are calculated for each clinical decision. The supporting evidence is classified into high quality (where further research is very unlikely to change our confidence in the estimate of the effects) to very low quality (any evidence of the effect is uncertain and is very likely to change by further

research). The strength of recommendation is calculated based on the quality of evidence (above), uncertainty about the balance between benefits and harms of the intervention, variability in values and preferences, and uncertainty about the cost effectiveness of the intervention.[12] By integrating all these factors, the GRADE system addresses the methodological quality of supporting evidence, consistency across various studies, generalizability of findings to different clinical contexts, and effectiveness of the treatments in addressing the health problem.

Even though CPGs are created to facilitate the translation of research evidence into clinical practice, not all CPGs are equal in terms of rigor of development and applicability to clinical circumstances. In fact, the majority of the available guidelines fall short of quality.[13] Therefore, users should be equipped with tools to appraise the quality of guidelines. AGREE II (Appraisal of Guidelines for Research and Evaluation; http://www.agreetrust.org) is an internationally recognized tool to assess the quality of guidelines. AGREE II defines quality as the level of confidence to the extent the guideline successfully tackled threats to the rigor of the development, presentation and applicability, and clarity and transparency of the development process.[9,14] The AGREE II instrument consists of 23 items organized in six domains[15]: *Scope and Purpose* (the overall aim of the guideline, the specific health questions, and the target population), *Stakeholder Involvement* (the extent to which the guideline was developed by the appropriate stakeholders and represents the views of its intended users), *Rigor of Development* (the process used to gather and synthesize the evidence, the methods used to formulate the recommendations, and the methods used to update them), *Clarity of Presentation* (the language, structure, and format of the guideline), *Applicability* (the likely barriers to and facilitators of implementation, strategies to improve uptake, and resource implications of applying the guideline), and *Editorial Independence* (the formulation of recommendations not being unduly biased with competing interests). AGREE II has been used internationally and is the most comprehensively validated tool for appraisal of clinical guidelines.[16]

The quality of the development and reporting of a CPG is a necessary but not sufficient condition for implementation in clinical practice. It is not always feasible, cost effective, or necessary to develop localized guidelines in each country and practice environment, and usually it is wise to use already available high-quality guidelines. However, the recommendations of a guideline that has been developed for another context is not always readily applicable to local environments. Sometimes the required skills and equipment do not exist, and sometimes the recommendations are less likely to be adopted by local clinicians and patients because of cultural and economical reasons. So, the recommendations of available guidelines should be adapted to other contexts through systematic and participatory processes, which recognize various local differences while they preserve the quality of recommendations.

The ADAPTE Collaboration (http://www.ADAPTE. org) developed a framework for the adaptation of clinical guidelines to local context in a systematic way that is more likely to be implemented. The ADAPTE framework ascertains that the evidence-based principles of guideline development are respected, the key stakeholders are engaged to promote the sense of ownership, the context

of implementation is recognized, and the process is transparently reported.[17] The process consists of 24 steps, starting with the *setup phase* (the preparatory tasks before starting the adaptation), continuing with the *adaptation phase* (formulating specific health questions; searching for existing guidelines; assessing the consistency, quality, currency, and applicability of evidence; making decisions regarding adaptation; and preparation of the draft adapted guideline), and finishing with the *final phase* (getting feedback from stakeholders, consulting with the developers of source guidelines, planning for the review and update, and creation of the final document).[18] Fig. 1.2 summarizes the ADAPTE process.

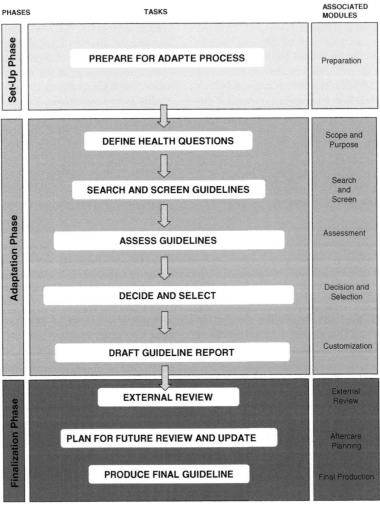

FIG. 1.2 Summary of the ADAPTE process. (From the ADAPTE Collaboration. Guideline Adaptation: A Resource Toolkit. Version 2.0. http://www.g-i-n.net/document-store/working-groups-documents/adaptation/adapte-resource-toolkit-guideline-adaptation-2-0.pdf/view?searchterm=ADAPTE%20resource%20toolkit; 2009, with permission.)

## EVIDENCE IS NOT ENOUGH

Imagine that on a night shift the intensivist has requested a cardiac consult for one of his patients in the emergency department intensive care unit. The patient is a 61-year-old woman with terminal cancer, which has been complicated by an inferior MI. The patient was intubated 30 days ago and was hospitalized initially for palliative management. Best evidence indicates that reperfusion therapies are indicated in acute MI to improve survival. But is this a right therapeutic intervention for this patient?

This example reminds us of the third EBM principle: Evidence alone is never enough to make a clinical decision. Clinical decision-making is a subjective process. We should always balance the objectivity of the evidence with the complexity of the unique clinical condition and values and preferences of the unique patient. Box 1.1 summarizes the required knowledge and skills for an optimal EBM practice.

## REFERENCES

1. Hampton J. Therapeutic fashion and publication bias: the case of anti-arrhythmic drugs in heart attack. *J R Soc Med.* 2015; 108:418–420.
2. Guyatt G. Evidence-based medicine: past, present, and future. *Evid Based Med.* 2003; 1:27–32.
3. Guyatt G, Rennie D, Meade M, Cook D. *Users' Guides to the Medical Literature: A Manual for Evidence-Based Clinical Practice*. Chicago, IL: AMA Press; 2002.
4. Haynes B. Of studies, syntheses, synopses, summaries, and systems: the "5S" evolution of information services for evidence-based healthcare decisions. *Evid Based Nurs.* 2007; 10:6–7.
5. Dwan K, Altman D, Arnaiz J, et al. Systematic review of the empirical evidence of study publication bias and outcome reporting bias. *PLoS One.* 2008; 3:e3081.
6. Cook D, Mulrow C, Haynes R. Systematic reviews: synthesis of best evidence for clinical decisions. *Ann Intern Med.* 1997; 126:376–380.
7. Institute of Medicine. *Clinical Practice Guidelines We Can Trust*; 2011. http://www.nationalacademies.org/hmd/Reports/2011/Clinical-Practice-Guidelines-We-Can-Trust.aspx. Accessed 9 October 2020.
8. Moja L, Kwag K, Lytras T, et al. Effectiveness of computerized decision support systems linked to electronic health records: a systematic review and meta-analysis. *Am J Public Health.* 2014; 104:e12–e22.
9. Brouwers M, Stacey D, O'Connor A. Knowledge creation: synthesis, tools and products. *Can Med Assoc J.* 2010; 182:E68–E72.
10. Thornton J, Alderson P, Tan T, et al. Introducing GRADE across the NICE clinical guideline program. *J Clin Epidemiol.* 2013; 66:124–131.
11. Alonso-Coello P, Schünemann H, Moberg J, et al. GRADE Evidence to Decision (EtD) frameworks: a systematic and transparent approach to making well informed healthcare choices. 1: Introduction. *BMJ.* 2016; 353:i2016.
12. Guyatt G, Oxman A, Vist G, et al. GRADE: an emerging consensus on rating quality of evidence and strength of recommendations. *BMJ.* 2008; 336:924–926.
13. Alonso-Coello P, Irfan A, Solà I, et al. The quality of clinical practice guidelines over the last two decades: a systematic review of guideline appraisal studies. *Qual Saf Health Care.* 2010; 19:1–7.
14. AGREE Collaboration Writing Group. Development and validation of an international appraisal instrument for assessing the quality of clinical practice guidelines: the AGREE project. *Qual Saf Health Care.* 2003; 12:18–21.
15. AGREE Next Steps Consortium. *The AGREE II Instrument [Electronic Version]*; 2009. http://www.agreetrust.org. Accessed 9 October 2020.
16. Siering U, Eikermann M, Hausner E, Hoffmann-Eßer W, Neugebauer E. Appraisal tools for clinical practice guidelines: a systematic review. *PLoS One.* 2013; 8: e82915.
17. Harrison M, Graham I, Fervers B, van den Hoek J. 2 Adapting knowledge to local context. In: Straus S, Tetroe J, Graham I, eds. *Knowledge Translation in Health Care: Moving From Evidence to Practice*. Oxford: John Wiley; 2013:110–120.
18. *The ADAPTE Collaboration. The ADAPTE Process: Resource Toolkit for Guideline Adaptation. Version 2.0*; 2009. http://www.g-i-n.net/document-store/working-groups-documents/adaptation/adapte-resource-toolkit-guideline-adaptation-2-0.pdf/view?searchterm=ADAPTE%20resource%20toolkit. Accessed 9 October 2020.

# CHAPTER 2

# Evaluation of Patient With Cardiovascular Problem

MAJID MALEKI

Rajaie Cardiovascular, Medical & Research Center, Iran University of Medical Sciences, Tehran, Iran

## HISTORY

Like other body systems, ability of cardiologist to diagnose cardiovascular disorders depends on precise history-taking and physical examination. Comprehensive history-taking can also help to understand the reason for cardiovascular signs due to systemic diseases and their effects. History can help to find modifiable risk factors, to order necessary diagnostic tests, and to evaluate the functional capacity of the heart. We have to ask about the past medical history such as childhood rheumatic fever, any addiction hereditary disorders in the family like hypertrophic cardiomyopathy, Marfan syndrome, dyslipidemia, and premature coronary artery disease. Common signs of cardiovascular disorders are chest discomfort, palpitation, dyspnea, syncope, and edema.

**Chest pain:** It is one of the common complaints that can be due to several disorders. It is very important to notice the characteristics of the chest pain such as location, duration, radiation, quality of the pain, precipitating, and relieving factors. Some patients define chest pain as chest discomfort or heavy feeling on the chest during heavy exercise or mental stress.

The reasons for cardiac chest pain and its characteristics are summarized in Table 2.1.

One of the methods that has been suggested for taking history is asking question from the past. Advantage of this kind of approach is that you don't forget the important question. Patients will be surprised how their physicians are accurate. The following lists are some examples of preparing a list of questions regarding the different cardiac problems.

### General Question

It is recommended to consider the quality, quantity, timing, location, and associated symptoms.

When you are taking history from a patient with history of congenital heart disease or cyanosis, it is recommended to ask:

How long the duration of cyanosis has been started?

Is it from birth or since childhood?

Does it have a gradual or sudden start?

Is it congenital or family type?

What are the accompanied symptoms?

Some other helpful questions such as

1. When was the first time you were told you have disease?
2. Why are you in the clinic or hospital?
3. Chief complaint
4. If you have come for consultation what is your main problem?

### Congestive Heart Failure Questions

1. Dyspnea on exertion
2. Orthopnea
3. Paroxysmal nocturnal dyspnea (PND)
4. History of pulmonary edema
5. Drug history
6. Abdominal enlargement
7. Nausea and vomiting
8. Syncope
9. Asthenia and easy fatigability
10. Sweating
11. Hemoptysis

### Ischemic Heart Disease (Questions)

1. Angina pectoris
2. History of myocardial infarction
3. Family history of diabetes mellitus, dyslipidemia, and premature coronary artery disease
4. History of peripheral vascular disease, intermittent claudication, and cerebrovascular accident
5. Smoking
6. Cough

**TABLE 2.1**
**Chest Pain Characteristics and Their Etiology**

| Reason | Duration | Precipitation Factor | Accompanying Symptoms | Quality |
|---|---|---|---|---|
| **CORONARY ARTERY DISEASE** | | | | |
| Angina | 1–10 min | Exercise, mental stress, cold | Dyspnea | Pressure, heaviness dyspepsia |
| Myocardial infarction | More than 30 min | More intense, not relieved by TNG | Dyspnea, vomiting, hypertension | As angina but more intense |
| Aortic dissection | Persistent | Hypertension | Increased blood pressure | Severe pain Anteroposterior of chest |
| Pericarditis | Up to few days | Inspiration | Pericardial rub | Burning, sharp knife |
| Pulmonary emboli | Up to few days | Inspiration | Dyspnea, pleural rub | pressure, burring |
| GI upset cholecystitis | Few days | GI symptoms | | Nonspecific |

## Congenital Heart Disease (Questions)
1. Growth and development history
2. History of viral disease or drug history of the pregnant mother
3. Family history
4. History of cyanosis, clubbing fingers, phlebotomy, or squatting
5. Syncope
6. Headache

## Rheumatic Heart Disease and Endocarditis (Questions)
1. Fever and nocturnal sweating
2. History of dental extraction or surgery
3. History of embolic event
4. History of benzathine penicillin injection
5. Hemoptysis
6. Chorea
7. Arthritis
8. History of sore throat or scarlet fever or history of tonsillectomy
9. History

## Dyspnea (Questions)
1. How far can the patient walk without symptoms?
2. Functional class evaluation
3. Accompanying symptoms such as chest pain, palpitation, chest discomfort, anxiety, excitement, cough, hemoptysis, and sputum
4. Precipitating and relieving factors such as exercise, anxiety, and rest

5. History of lung disease
6. History of smoking
7. Job
8. History of pulmonary function test and their results
9. Duration, interval, and repetition of PND

## Syncope (Questions)
1. When was the first time that syncope happened?
2. Interval, the shortest and longest period of syncopal attack
3. Accompanied symptoms such as preattack symptoms, nausea, vomiting, loss of consciousness, seizure, incontinence, hypotension, and bradycardia
4. History of trauma
5. Does it happen during rest or exercise?
6. Does it happen in special body position?
7. History of diabetes mellitus and antihypertensive drug

## Chest Pain (Questions)
1. Location
2. Radiation
3. When does it happen?
4. Frequency of pain
5. Duration, pain characteristic such as burning, vague, shallow, and sword pain
6. Precipitating factor such as activity, relieving factor such as TNG and rest
7. Effects of different conditions such as activity, cold weather, excitement, food, smoking, and alcohol
8. Accompanying factors such as dyspnea palpitation, pallor, nausea, and vomiting

## PHYSICAL EXAMINATION

The physical examination consists of observation, palpation, and auscultation. Despite advanced diagnostic techniques such as echocardiography, catheterization, angiography, cardiac MR, CT angiography, and nuclear cardiology, physical examination must be routinely performed.

### Patient Observation

Careful observation can help to suspect several cardiac anomalies.

How does the patient look?

Cyanotic, obese, cachectic, and skinny.

It is also noteworthy to consider patient face and look at teeth (Fig. 2.1).

Many conditions can help to conclude cardiovascular abnormalities by observing the patient.
1. Marfan syndrome: arm span more than patient height (aortic insufficiency)
2. Kyphoscoliosis (pulmonary hypertension)
3. Obesity (Cushing)
4. Warm and wet hands (hyperthyroidism)
5. Clubbing fingers and cyanosis (cyanotic congenital heart disease and pulmonary disease)
6. Dry hand and edematous face (hypothyroidism, pericardial effusion, and hyperlipemia)
7. Acromegaly (hypertension and heart failure)
8. Short stature (Turner syndrome, coarctation of aorta, and hypothyroidism)
9. Reversed differential cyanosis (transposition of great arteries with coarctation of aorta)
10. Differential cyanosis [pulmonary artery hypertension (PAH) with reversed patent ductus arteriosus (PDA) shunt]
11. Splinter hemorrhage (infective endocarditis)
12. Xanthoma or xanthelasma (premature atherosclerosis)
13. Hyperflexible joints and multiple scar (Ehlers–Danlos syndrome)
14. Bilateral simian creases (Noonan syndrome, mongolism with ASD, VSD, TF, etc.)

### Arterial Pulse Examination

Palpation and examination of peripheral arteries give useful information about pulse rhythm and rate with its characteristics.

#### Arterial pulse

All major peripheral pulses should be evaluated at both sides for their characteristics. I recommend palpation of both carotid arteries to evaluate cardiac functions because it reflects central aortic pressure. It is also advisable to look at both carotid arteries and venous pulse simultaneously (Table 2.2 and Fig. 2.2).

### Venous Pulse Examination

Clinically, jugular veins evaluations are superior to other body veins. Jugular veins have direct correlation with right atrium (RA) and ventricle (RV) and so are representative of RA and RV pressure.

### Normal Jugular Venous Pulse (JVP)

A wave: atrial contraction

C: due to tricuspid valve closure

X: negative wave due to atrial relaxation

X': continuation of atrial relaxation

V: positive wave due to RA filling at the time of tricuspid valve closure

Y: negative wave due to the rapid filling of RV from RA

There are three positive waves (a, c, v) and two negative (x, y) to evaluate jugular vein precisely. It is needed to note its relation to another phenomenon that occurs during a cardiac cycle such as heart sounds.

#### Increased a wave

A wave amplitude will be increased when there is any obstruction during RA filling to RV such as tricuspid stenosis (TS), right ventricular hypertrophy (RVH), pulmonary stenosis, or some arrhythmia such as complete heart block.

Canon A wave is produced when atrium and ventricle contract simultaneously. It may happen during premature contraction or ventricular tachycardia. During atrial fibrillation A wave, which is due to atrial contraction, disappears.

#### X descent

Disappearance or diminished X descent happens in tricuspid regurgitation (TR). Deeper X descent happens in constrictive pericarditis.

#### V wave

It starts at the end of systole. TR produces prominent V wave, which is premature (CV wave) and makes X descent disappear. High cardiac output states may cause increased amplitude of V wave such as exercise, anemia, and hyperthyroidism. Atrial septal defect can increase V amplitude.

#### Y wave (diastolic collapse)

Deep Y wave occurs during TR, RV dilatation, and RV failure. Tricuspid stenosis makes Y wave less deep. Also, RVH may have the same effects (Table 2.3).

### Palpation and Observation of the Chest

This is one of the most important parts of cardiovascular examination (Table 2.4 and Figs. 2.3–2.15).

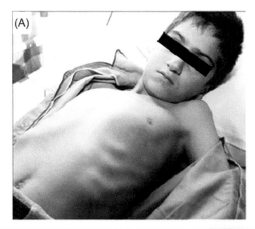

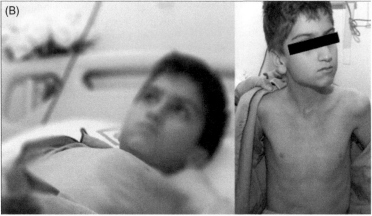

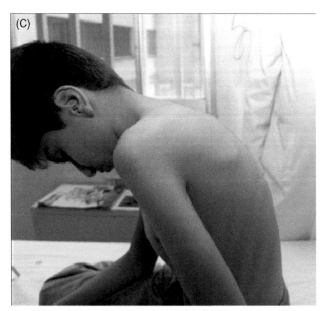

FIG. 2.1 Intercostal retractions in a child with congestive heart failure. (A)–(C) Chest deformity and bulging of left hemithorax in a patient with severe right ventricular enlargement.

**TABLE 2.2**
**Different Cardiac Situation With Their Pulse Characteristic**

| Pulse | Situation |
|---|---|
| Hyperkinetic | Exercise, fever Athletics, PDA, aortic insufficiency "AI" Anemia, pregnancy, hemodialysis |
| Bisferiens (two waves in systole) | Hypertrophic cardiomyopathy, AI, AS +AI, PDA, fever |
| Hypokinetic | Hypovolemia, LV failure, AS or mitral stenosis "MS" |
| Parvus et tardus | AS, severe LV dysfunction |
| Dicrotic One wave in systole, one in diastole | LV dysfunction |
| Paradoxical pulse (amplitude decrease during inspiration) | Tamponade |
| Pulsus alternans | Severe LV dysfunction |

**TABLE 2.3**
**A Wave of JVP**

| A Wave During Arrhythmia | |
|---|---|
| AF | Absent A wave |
| Complete heart block | Irregular canon wave |
| PVC | Irregular large A wave |
| VT | Irregular A wave |
| Atrial flutter | Occasional large A wave |
| 2:1 AV block | Occasional large A |

**TABLE 2.4**
**Observation and Palpation of Heart**

| Pathology | Observation and Palpation |
|---|---|
| AS, hypertension, LVH | Sustained apical impulse, increased apical impulse |
| LV enlargement, aortic insufficiency "AI," mitral regurgitation "MR" | Lateral and downward displacement of apical impulse |
| Ischemic heart disease "IHD," LV aneurysm | Paradoxical bulging of LV impulse |
| Right ventricular hypertrophy "RVH" | Sustained deviation of left lower sternum border during systole |

Hyperkinetic pulse in high output state

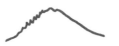

Parvus and tardus pulse in aortic stenosis

Bisferiens pulse in hypertrophic obstructive cardiomyopathy, AI, and AS,AI

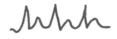

Pulses alternans in heart failure

**SYS   Dias**

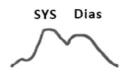

Dicrotic pulse in LV dysfunction

FIG. 2.2 Different arterial pulses contour

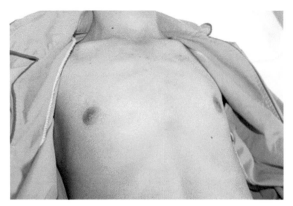

FIG. 2.3 Observation of chest deformity.

## Auscultation

Heart sounds are generated by contraction of the heart and flow across different parts of it. First and second heart sounds are the result of closing of atrioventricular and semilunar valves. It is recommended to listen to the heart sounds from the least intensity focus of the sounds, is right lower sternal border and inching space to reach to the apex, where the sounds are the strongest.

When you report the heart sounds, it is advised to start with this order: heart sounds including $S_1, S_2, S_3, S_4$, additional sounds such as ejection or nonejection click, tumor PLOP, pericardial sound, pacemaker sounds,

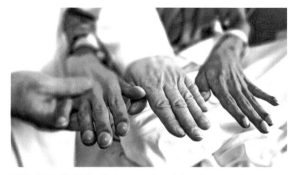

FIG. 2.5 Clubbing fingers and peripheral cyanosis.

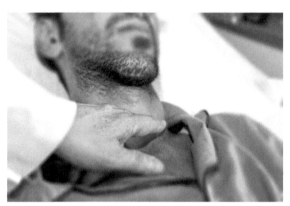

FIG. 2.6 Looking at JVP.

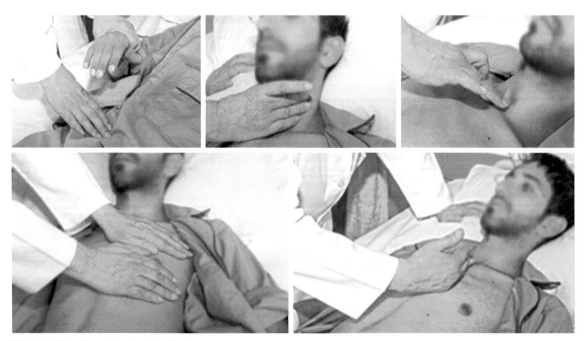

FIG. 2.4 Palpation of the heart and pulses.

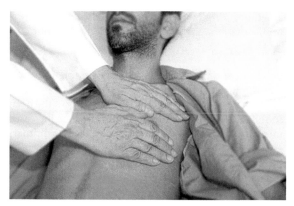

FIG. 2.7 How to palpate the chest.

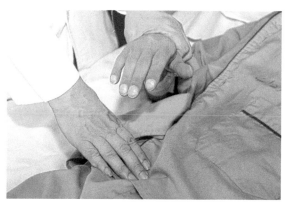

FIG. 2.10 Comparing peripheral pulses in coarctation of aorta.

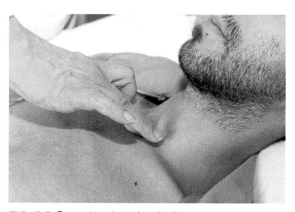

FIG. 2.8 Suprasternal notch palpation.

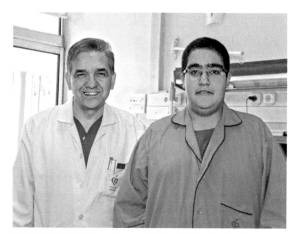

FIG. 2.11 10-Year obese patient with dyslipidemia.

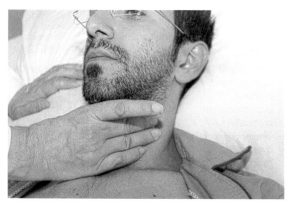

FIG. 2.9 Comparing carotid pulses.

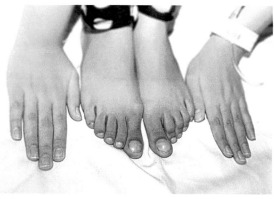

FIG. 2.12 Differential cyanosis.

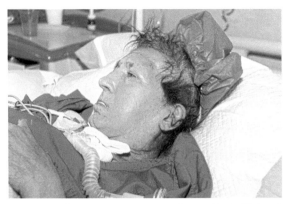

FIG. 2.13 Central venous pressure in a patient with heart failure.

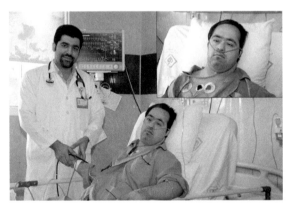

FIG. 2.14 Down syndrome and complex congenital heart disease.

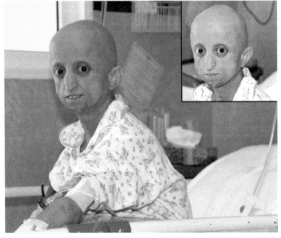

FIG. 2.15 Progeria in a 34-year-old man after coronary artery bypass surgery.

and murmurs. You have to point out the intensity duration, radiation, quality, and timing of the murmur.

## Auscultation of the Heart

Fire heart sound (S1) starts at the beginning of systole and is loudest at the apex.

We have to pay attention to the intensity of the heart sounds if these have normal, diminished, or increased intensity. Heart sounds intensity can lead to primary guidance of different cardiac abnormalities such as increased first heart sound intensity in noncardiac disorders such as young age, fever, hyperthyroidism, pregnancy, or cardiac anomalies such as mitral stenosis with pliable mitral leaflets.

### First Heart Sounds ($S_1$)

This sound consists of two parts including mitral (M) and tricuspid (T) valve closure (Table 2.5).

### Second Heart Sounds ($S_2$)

The second heart sounds include aortic ($A_2$) and pulmonic ($P_2$) valve closure (Table 2.6).

### Third and Fourth Heart Sounds ($S_3$ and $S_4$)

$S_3$ and $S_4$ are low-frequency sounds and heard with the bell of stethoscope at the apex of the heard, while the patient is in left lateral position.

$S_3$ can be heard in young people without any cardiovascular abnormality. Sometimes it can be heard in large left to right shunts in congenital heart abnormality such as large atrial septal defect "ASD" ($S_3$ of right side) or ventricular septal defect ($S_3$ of left side). It can also be heard in valvular regurgitation without congestive heart failure. One of the most common reasons of hearing $S_3$ is heart failure.

**TABLE 2.5**
**First Heart Sound Characteristic ($S_1$)**

| Loud $S_1$ | Soft $S_1$ | Variable $S_1$ |
| --- | --- | --- |
| High output state such as fever, exercise, hyperthyroidism, pregnancy, AV fistula, hyperdynamic heart, mitral stenosis, short P-R interval, atrial myxoma | The calcified mitral valve, first-degree AV block, severe MR dilated cardiomyopathy, myocarditis | AF, complete AV block, ventricular tachycardia |

**TABLE 2.6**
**Second Heart Sound Characteristic ($S_2$)**

| Loud $A_2$ | Loud $P_2$ | Soft $A_2$ | Soft $P_2$ | Wide Split $S_2$ More Than 30 ms | Reversed Split $S_2\downarrow$ |
|---|---|---|---|---|---|
| Hypertension, tachycardia | Pulmonary artery hypertension | Calcified aortic stenosis "Aortic insufficiency" | Pulmonary insufficiency | Atrial septal defect (wide or fixed) pulmonary stenosis RBBB | LBBB, MR |

$S_4$ is also a low-frequency sound that can be heard when there is reduced compliance of left ventricle such as aortic stenosis, ischemia, hypertrophic cardiomyopathy, or systemic arterial hypertension. It may be heard in acute onset mitral regurgitation due to chordae tendineae rupture.

**Clicks:** Clicks consist of ejection and nonejection click. Ejection clicks are early systolic sounds originating from pulmonary or aortic valve halting (Table 2.7).

There are also pericardial and pleural friction rubs. The pericardial rub can have one, two, or three components. It is usually louder during inspiration. It is high frequency, scratchy sound.

The pleural rub has one sound during inspiration and one during expiration. It is also louder during inspiration. Pleural rub is of high frequency as pericardial rub.

*Murmur*

Murmurs should be classified according to their timing (systolic, diastolic, and continuous), intensity (I–VI), location, radiation, and their quality such as holosystolic ejection, etc.

We can simply differentiate the characteristics of several murmurs by their timing (Table 2.8).

These sounds can occur during systole or diastole as a result of turbulence of flow. The etiology of these sounds is commonly due to leakage of flow across the value such as aortic regurgitation or tricuspid regurgitation or it may occur due to flow disturbance across a stenotic valve such as pulmonary or aortic valve stenosis.

There are also flow murmurs that are the result of high output states such as pregnancy. This type of

**TABLE 2.7**
**Additional Heart Sounds[a]**

| | Origin | Respiration | Etiology |
|---|---|---|---|
| Ejection click | Aortic valve | No change | AS, bicuspid aortic valve "BAV," dilated aortic root |
| | Pulmonary valve | Decreased with inspiration | PS, PAH, dilated PA |
| Nonejection click | Mitral and tricuspid valve | Decreased with inspiration | Mitral valve prolapsed |
| Opening snap | Mitral and tricuspid valve | Decreased with inspiration | Mitral stenosis ASD, tricuspid stenosis, atrial myxoma |

Prosthetic valves: depending on the prosthetic valves and their location varies. They usually have opening sounds as opening snap and closing sound coinciding with $S_1$ at mitral position or $S_2$ at aortic position.
[a]Prosthetic valves have some additional sounds depending on their location, they usually have opening and closing clicks (see also Chapter 30).

**TABLE 2.8**
**Causes of Heart Murmur and Their Timing**

| Timing | Cause of Murmur |
|---|---|
| Early systole | Acute MR, VSD, TR |
| Mid-systole | AS (supra, valvular, and subvalvular) PS (supra, valvular, and subvalvular) ASD, dilated PA |
| Late systole | MVP, TVP |
| Holosystole | MR, TR, VSD |
| Early diastolic | AI, PI |
| Mid-diastolic | MS, TS, MR, VSD |
| Late diastolic | Presystolic accentuation of MS Austin flint |
| Continuous | PDA, AV fistula, ruptured sinus of valsalva, venous hum, ASD, coronary artery stenosis |

*AS*, aortic stenosis; *ASD*, atrial septal defect; *MR*, mitral regurgitation; *PS*, pulmonic stenosis; *TR*, tricuspid regurgitation; *VSD*, ventricular septal defect.

murmur which has usually short duration can occur in structurally normal heart. As I mentioned before, we have to note to the quality (loud, soft, harsh, etc.), intensity, and time to first and second heart sound. One of the most important features of murmurs regarding etiology of murmur is timing. To differentiate etiology of the murmur, various maneuvers such as respiration, valsalva, squatting, and handgrip can help.

**Systolic murmurs.** These murmurs may be normal or abnormal. They can be at different parts of systolic cycle as early, mid, late, or holosystolic.

**Ejection murmurs.** These murmurs are produced by the turbulent flow across stenotic pulmonary or aortic valves. Systolic ejection murmur may occur in normal heart because of high output states.

**Regurgitation murmur.** These murmurs are produced due to abnormal flow through insufficient mitral or tricuspid valves or ventricular septal defect into chambers that are at lower pressure. They are usually pansystolic. Mitral valve prolapse or papillary muscle dysfunction can make a late systolic murmur with or without click.

**Diastolic murmurs.** These murmurs are always abnormal. They can be early, mid, or late diastolic. Diastolic rumble is usually due to tricuspid or mitral stenosis. Any kind of left ventricular inflow treat obstruction such as mitral stenosis, ball valve thrombosis, or myxoma may induce diastolic rumble.

On the other hand, diastolic blowing murmur can result from pulmonary or aortic insufficiency.

**Continuous murmurs.** These murmurs occur during all the systolic and diastolic cycle. They are usually abnormal. PDA, aorta pulmonary window, arteriovenous fistula, and severe pulmonary artery branch stenosis can make continuous murmur.

Venous hum is a physiologic finding that heard in the right supraclavicular fossa in children. Mammary soufflé is heard over the breast and usually is louder in systole. It can be heard in pregnancy.

Other cause of continuous murmur includes ruptured aneurysm of sinus of valsalva, bronchial collateral circulation, and coronary cameral fistula.

## DIFFERENTIAL DIAGNOSIS OF MURMURS BY MANEUVERS

As I stated before, maneuver such as respiration, valsalva maneuver, squatting, handgrip, and pharmacological tools such as amyl nitrite can differentiate the etiology of abnormal sounds.

For example, inspiration increases venous return and augments right heart sounds and murmurs of tricuspid stenosis and regurgitation. The phase of release of valsalva can increase volume of the left ventricle and consequence lead to aortic stenosis after a few beats. However, this happens immediately for pulmonary stenosis. Squatting can decrease venous return simultaneously by increasing afterload and thus increasing murmur of aortic regurgitation and mitral regurgitation, however, it usually reduces murmur of hypertrophic obstructive cardiomyopathy and mitral valve prolapse.

In summary, the cardiologist must pay attention on each part of the cardiac cycle and noting each heart sound and murmur. It is recommended to have a look at chest, jugular venous pulse, and to palpate arterial pulse at the same time for better understanding of normal or abnormal auscultatory findings.

## FURTHER READING

Hurst JW, Morrin DC. *The Heart*. New York: McGraw-Hill Publishing Company; 2001;203–273.

Christie Jr. LG. Systemic approach to evaluation of angina like chest pain. *Am Heart J*. 1981;102:897–912.

Vander Belt RJ. History. In: Chiznet M, ed. *Classic Teaching in Clinical Cardiology: A Tribute to W. Harvey*. New York: Laennec; 1996;41–54.

Seth R, Magner P, Matziner F. How far is the sternal angle from the mid-right atrium. *J Gen Intern Med*. 2002;17:852.

Mann DL, Zipes DP, Libby P, Bonow R. *Braunwald's Heart Disease: A Textbook of Cardiovascular Medicine*. 10th ed. Elsevier; 2015;95–112.

Von Beckerath O, Gaa J, et al. Intermittent claudication in a 28-year-old man with pseudoxanthoma elasticum. *Circulation*. 2008;118:102.

Maleki M, Alizadehasl A, Haghjoo M. *Atlas of Cardiology*. JAYPEE; 2016.

Pinsky LE, Wipf JE. *Learning and Teaching at the Bedside*. 2012.

# CHAPTER 3

# Electrocardiography

MOHAMMAD JAVAD ALEMZADEH-ANSARI
Cardiovascular Intervention Research Center, Rajaie Cardiovascular, Medical & Research Center, Iran, University of Medical Sciences, Tehran, Iran

**KEY POINTS**

- Recognition of normal electrocardiography (ECG) findings and normal variants for better interpretation is necessary.
- The ECG is a noninvasive and inexpensive method with acceptable accuracy used for diagnosis of cardiovascular disorders; therefore, recognition of abnormal ECG findings is mandatory.
- Recognition about technical errors and artifacts that may occur during ECG recording is necessary.

## INTRODUCTION

The electrocardiogram (ECG) is the most important and often first diagnostic method in detection of cardiovascular disorders, such as cardiac rhythm disturbances, conduction system abnormalities, myocardial ischemia, cardiomyopathy, and pericarditis. Also, ECG can help physicians in various fields of cardiovascular diseases such as determining the presence and severity of acute myocardial ischemia, localizing sites of myocardial ischemia and determining the culprit coronary artery, localizing sites of origin and distinguishing types of tachyarrhythmias, and identifying and evaluating patients with genetic diseases who are prone to arrhythmias. This chapter describes the principles of normal ECG and then shows common ECG traces that a physician may encounter in routine practice.

## NORMAL ELECTROCARDIOGRAMS

The clinical ECG is performed using 12 leads, including 3 standard limb leads (leads I, II, and III), 6 precordial leads (leads V1 through V6), and 3 augmented limb leads (leads aVR, aVL, and aVF). The right pericardial leads can be used to assess right ventricular abnormalities and left posterior leads to detect acute posterolateral infarctions. The waveforms and intervals of a standard ECG are displayed in Fig. 3.1. Normal values for durations of ECG waves and intervals are presented in Table 3.1. It should be mentioned that significant differences in ECG patterns may occur in the same individual in ECGs recorded days, hours, or even minutes apart.

### The Pattern of Normal Waves and Intervals

**P wave:** A mean axis of the P wave in the frontal plane is approximately 60 degrees. Morphology of the P wave in different leads is presented in Table 3.2. The amplitude of a normal sinus P wave in the limb leads is less than 0.25 mV, and the terminal negative deflection in the right precordial leads is less than 0.1 mV in depth.[1]

**PR segment and interval:** The PR segment is part of the PR interval. The majority of the PR segment represents slow conduction within the atrioventricular (AV) node, but the terminal small part of this segment represents the rapid conduction via the bundle of His and bundle branches. The PR interval is shorter at faster heart rates, secondary to adrenergic enhancement of AV nodal conduction.

**QRS complex:** The initial wave (low amplitude and of brief duration, less than 30 ms) is positive in leads

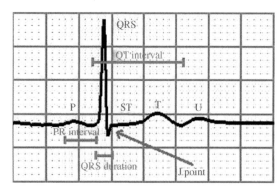

FIG. 3.1 The waves and intervals of a normal electrocardiogram.

**TABLE 3.1**
**Normal Values for Durations of Electrocardiography Waves and Intervals**

|  | Duration (ms) | Comments |
|---|---|---|
| P-wave duration | <120 | In the lead with the widest P wave |
| PR interval | 120–200 | In the lead with the shortest PR interval |
| QRS duration | 60–110 | In the lead with the widest QRS complex |
| QT interval (corrected), men | 390–440 | In the lead with the widest QT interval (most commonly lead V2 or V3) If a prominent U wave is present, use the leads with absent U wave (usually aVR or aVL) |
| QT interval (corrected), women | 390–450 | Same as above |
| JT interval | ≤120 | In the setting of a bundle branch block: JT interval = JT (HR + 100)/518 |

*HR*, heart rate.

**TABLE 3.2**
**Morphology of the Normal Sinus P Wave in Different Leads**

| Lead | Morphology |
|---|---|
| II | Always positive |
| I, aVL, aVF | Usually positive |
| aVL, III | May be upright or downward |
| Right precordial leads (V1 and, occasionally, V2) | Upright or often biphasic (positive–negative deflection) |
| Lateral leads (V3–V6) | Upright |

**TABLE 3.3**
**Axis of QRS Complex**

| Range of QRS Axis (degrees) | |
|---|---|
| Normal | −30 to +90 |
| Right axis deviation | >+90 |
| • Moderate | +90 to +120 |
| • Marked | +120 to +180 |
| Left axis deviation | <−30 |
| • Moderate | −30 to −45 |
| • Marked | −45 to −90 |
| Superior axis deviation | −80 to −90 |
| Extreme axis deviations (right superior axis deviations) | −90 to −180 (+180 to +270) |

aVR and V1 and is negative in leads I, aVL, V5, and V6 (represented as septal q waves). The QRS pattern in inferior leads may be predominantly upright (qR, Rs, or RS pattern complexes) and in lead I may present as an isoelectric RS pattern or a predominantly upright qR pattern. The normal mean QRS axis in adults is between −30 degrees and +90 degrees (Table 3.3). Causes of QRS axis deviation are presented in Table 3.4. In the pericardial leads, the transition zone (in this zone, the QRS complex presents an isoelectric RS pattern) typically occurs in lead V3 or V4. It should be mentioned that men have greater QRS amplitudes and longer QRS durations than women. In contrast to the PR interval, the duration of the QRS complex is not influenced by heart rate.

**J point:** The intersection of the end of the QRS complex and the beginning of the ST segment is termed the *J point*, and it is normally at or near the isoelectric baseline of the ECG. The greatest amplitude of the J point is seen in lead V2 (Table 3.5).

**ST segment:** In normal persons, the ST segment is usually isoelectric and has a slight upward concavity.

**T wave:** This wave normally has the same polarity as that of the QRS complex. Thus, the T wave usually is positive in leads II and aVF and the lateral leads; negative in lead aVR; and variable in leads III, V1, and V2.

**QT and JT intervals:** The JT interval is a more accurate measure of ventricular repolarization, especially in patients with bundle branch block (BBB). The QT interval is rate dependent, decreasing as the heart rate increases (Fig. 3.2).[2]

Formula for measurement of corrected QT interval:
1. Bazett formula (the QT and RR intervals are measured in seconds)[3]: $QTc = QT/RR^{1/2}$
2. Fridericia's formula (the QT and RR intervals are measured in seconds)[4]: $QTc = QT/RR^{1/3}$
3. Formula based on linear model[5] (intervals are measured in milliseconds): QTc = QT + 1.75 (heart rate − 60)

## TABLE 3.4
### Causes of QRS Axis Deviation

| Right Axis Deviation | Left Axis Deviation |
| --- | --- |
| Normal variation (vertical heart with an axis of 90 degrees) | Normal variation (physiologic, often with age) |
| Mechanical shifts, such as inspiration and emphysema | Mechanical shifts, such as expiration, high diaphragm (pregnancy, ascites, abdominal tumor) |
| Right ventricular hypertrophy | Left ventricular hypertrophy |
| Right bundle branch block | Left bundle branch block |
| Left posterior fascicular block | Left anterior fascicular block |
| Dextrocardia | Congenital heart disease (primum atrial septal defect, endocardial cushion defect) |
| Ventricular ectopic rhythms | Emphysema |
| Preexcitation syndrome (Wolff–Parkinson–White syndrome) | Preexcitation syndromes (Wolff–Parkinson–White) |
| Lateral wall myocardial infarction | Inferior wall myocardial infarction |
| Secundum atrial septal defect | Ventricular ectopic rhythms |
| | Hyperkalemia |

## TABLE 3.5
### Upper Limits of Normal J-Point Elevation Based on Various Conditions

| Leads V2 and V3 | |
| --- | --- |
| • Men $\geq$40 years | 0.2 mV |
| • Men <40 years | 0.25 mV |
| • Women | 1.15 mV |
| Leads (except V2 and V3) | 0.1 mV |

Formula for measurement of corrected QT interval in patients with atrial fibrillation:
1. $(QTc_{short} + QTc_{long})/2$
2. Onset of R wave to peak of peak T wave (if this is more than ½ of the R–R interval, then the QTc interval is likely to be above the critical threshold of 500 ms)
3. Average of multiple QTc intervals (up to 10)
4. Measure the QT interval in a beat where the R–R interval is of exactly 1-s duration (because the square root of 1 is 1, in this beat, QTc interval = noncorrected QT interval)

Formula for measurement of corrected JT interval (in the setting of a BBB):
1. Formula based on QT interval[5]: JTc = QTc − QRS
2. JT interval = JT (HR + 100)/518

The JT interval equal to or more than 112 ms identifies a repolarization prolongation (Figs. 3.3 and 3.4).

U wave: A U wave may be seen in some leads, especially the precordial leads V2–V4. The amplitude of the U wave is typically less than 0.2 mV (Figs. 3.5 and 3.6).

### Normal Variants on Electrocardiograms
• T waves can be inverted in the right precordial leads.
• The persistent juvenile pattern (inverted T waves in leads to the left of V1) is more common in women.
• The ST segment can be elevated in the right and midprecordial leads.
• Early repolarization
• J wave syndromes (classic feature: upwardly concave ST-segment elevation, tall precordial R waves, distinctive J waves with slurring or notching of the terminal QRS complex, an early R wave transition in the precordial leads, and asymmetric T waves with a gradual upslope and rapid descent) are most prevalent in young male adults who are athletically active.
• An rSr′ morphology in lead V1 (and sometimes V2) with a narrow QRS duration ($\leq$100 ms) is a common physiologic or positional variant and may normalize when the right precordial electrodes are placed one interspace lower than usual.

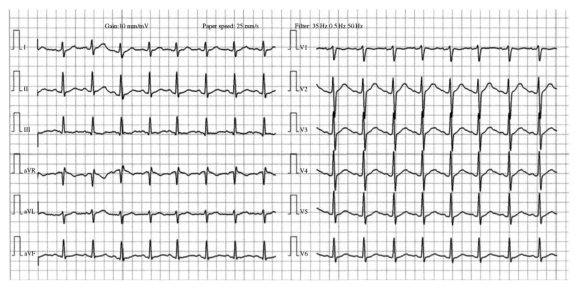

FIG. 3.2 Prolonged QT interval during sinus tachycardia. The corrected QT interval based on the Bazett formula equals 671 ms; based on Fridericia's formula, 617 ms; and based on the linear model, 590 ms.

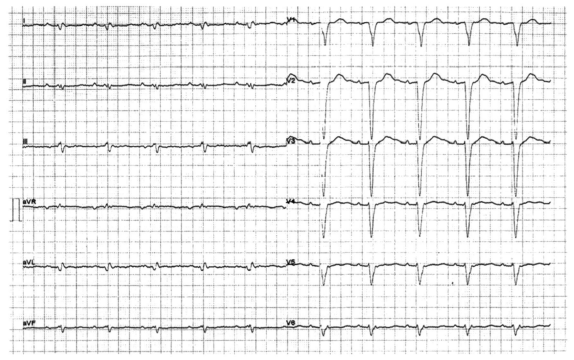

FIG. 3.3 Electrocardiogram from a patient with interventricular conduction delay and prolonged repolarization. The JT interval is about 142 ms.

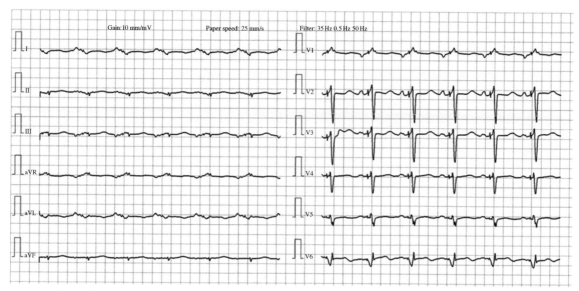

FIG. 3.4 A patient with cardiac resynchronization therapy (CRT) device who treated with amiodarone. Note the long JT interval (132 ms).

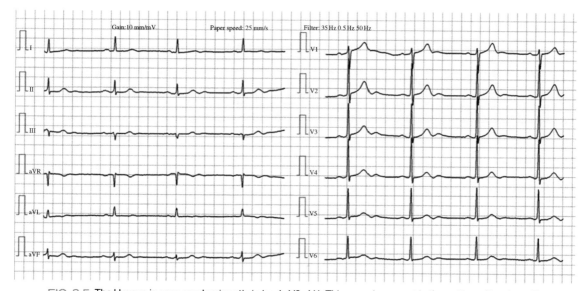

FIG. 3.5 The U wave is seen predominantly in leads V2– V4. This wave is present in the setting of bradycardia with an amplitude less than 0.2 mV.

## Benign Early Repolarization

The ECG pattern of benign early repolarization (BER) is most commonly seen in young, healthy patients younger than 50 years of age (Box 3.1). It produces widespread ST-segment elevation that may mimic pericarditis or acute MI (Figs. 3.7 and 3.8). BER can be difficult to differentiate from pericarditis because both conditions are associated with concave ST elevation. Using the ST-segment elevation (from the end of the PR segment to the J point) compared with the amplitude of the T wave in V6 can distinguish between these two conditions. An ST-segment–T-wave ratio greater than 0.25 suggests pericarditis, but if the ratio is less than 0.25, it is consistent with BER[6–10] (Table 3.6 and Fig. 3.9).

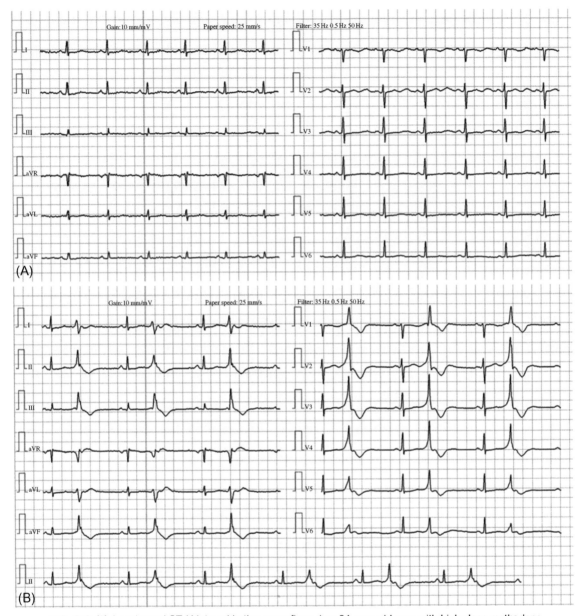

FIG. 3.6 (A) A prolonged QT-U interval in the upper figure in a 24-year-old man with high-dose methadone consumption. The electrolyte levels were in the normal ranges. (B) After some minutes, short-coupled bigeminy premature ventricular contractions (R-on-T phenomenon) were seen. This patient is at risk of the development of torsades de pointes.

Widespread concave ST-segment elevation, most prominent in the mid to left precordial leads (V2–V5)

Concavity of initial upsloping portion of the ST segment

Notching or slurring at the J point

Prominent, slightly asymmetrical T waves that are concordant with the QRS complexes (pointing in the same direction)

The degree of ST-segment elevation is modest compared with the T-wave amplitude (<25% of the T-wave height in V6; against pericarditis)

ST elevation compatible with criteria in Table 3.5

No reciprocal ST depression to suggest STEMI (except in aVR)

ST changes are relatively stable overtime (no progression on serial electrocardiogram tracings).

Reduction in ST-segment elevation with sympathomimetic factors

*STEMI*, ST-segment-elevation myocardial infarction.

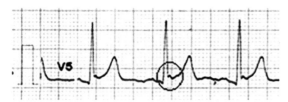

FIG. 3.7 Notching at the J point in the lateral leads in a patient with benign early repolarization.

## ABNORMAL ELECTROCARDIOGRAMS

### Malignant Early Repolarization

This form of early repolarization is associated with increased risk of arrhythmia and also sudden death. In contrast, manifestations of early repolarization in lateral leads, the inferior distribution of J waves has conferred an increased risk of arrhythmic death.[11] The distinguishing malignant early repolarization from benign early repolarization is shown in Fig. 3.10.

### Atrial Abnormality

Three general categories of P waves that can alter atrial activation to produce abnormal P-wave patterns include abnormal patterns of activation and conduction, left atrial abnormalities, and right atrial abnormalities. The common diagnostic criteria for left and right atrial abnormalities are listed in Table 3.7.

**Left atrial abnormality:** Anatomic abnormalities of the left atrium that alter the P waves include atrial dilation, atrial muscular hypertrophy, and elevated intra-atrial pressures (Fig. 3.11). The most common conditions that lead to left atrial enlargement include hypertension, valvular heart diseases, heart failure, and atrial fibrillation.[12]

**Right atrial abnormality:** Right atrial abnormality is a marker of the severity of disease and predicts outcome in some disorders, including tricuspid regurgitation, pulmonary hypertension, congenital heart disease, and right heart failure. Enlargement of the right atrium may result from right atrial volume or pressure load[12] (Fig. 3.12).

**Biatrial abnormality:** ECG pattern findings include large biphasic P waves in lead V1 and tall and broad P waves in leads II, III, and aVF[12] (Fig. 3.13).

### Ventricular Hypertrophy

**Left ventricular hypertrophy (LVH):** LVH causes change in the QRS complex, the ST segment, and the T wave. The most characteristic finding is increased amplitude of the QRS complex. The common diagnostic criteria for LVH are listed in Table 3.8. The most common causes of LVH are hypertension (the leading cause), aortic stenosis or regurgitation, mitral regurgitation, coarctation of the aorta, and hypertrophic cardiomyopathy. The prolongation of intrinsic deflection is a criterion for diagnosis of LVH or BBBs. This deflection represents an estimate of the electrical activation time when an exploratory electrode is placed in direct contact with the myocardium[1,12] (Fig. 3.14).

**Dilated cardiomyopathies (DCMs):** The presence of relatively low limb voltage (QRS voltage <0.8 mV in each of the limb leads) accomplished with relatively prominent QRS voltage in the pericordial leads (SV1 or SV2 + RV5 or RV6 >3.5 mV) and poor R-wave progression in pericardial leads suggests DCM. These changes are relatively specific but not sensitive signs for DCM[13] (Figs. 3.15 and 3.16).

**Hypertrophic cardiomyopathy (HCM):** The presence of LVH with prominent downward ST-segment depression and deep asymmetrical T-wave inversion in pericardial leads suggests apical HCM. However, pseudoinfarction patterns in each territory may be seen. For example, the presence of prominent inferolateral Q waves and tall, right precordial R waves is probably related to increased depolarization forces generated by the markedly hypertrophied septum[13,14] (Fig. 3.17).

**Right ventricular hypertrophy (RVH):** The common diagnostic criteria for RVH and ECG criteria for RVH based on its severity are listed in Box 3.2[15] and Table 3.9. Evidence of true RVH in patients with

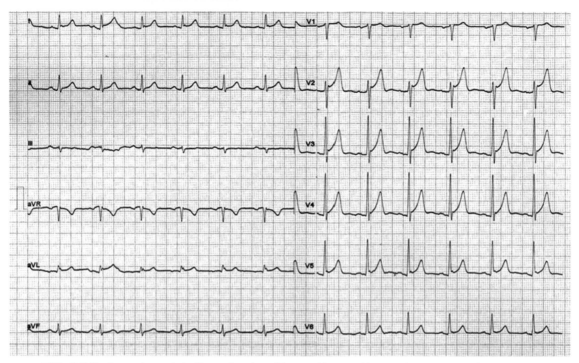

FIG. 3.8 Benign early repolarization pattern in a 47-year-old man with normal coronary arteries. Note the "notching" and "slurring" of the J point and concave upward ST-segment elevation in the precordial leads, especially lead V5.

**TABLE 3.6**
**Criteria for Distinction Benign Early Repolarization from Pericarditis**

| In Favor of BER | In Favor of Pericarditis |
| --- | --- |
| ST elevation limited to the precordial leads | Generalized ST elevation |
| Absence of PR depression | Presence of PR depression |
| Prominent T waves | Normal T-wave amplitude |
| ST-segment/T-wave ratio <0.25 | ST-segment/T-wave ratio >0.25 |
| Characteristic "fish-hook" appearance in V4 | Absence of "fish-hook" appearance in V4 |
| ECG changes relatively stable over time | ECG changes evolve over time |

BER, benign early repolarization; ECG, electrocardiography.

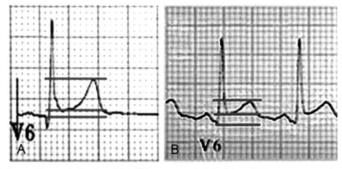

FIG. 3.9 (A) Benign early repolarization. The ST-segment height (1 mm)–T-wave height (6 mm) ratio is 0.16. (B) Pericarditis. The ST-segment height (2 mm)–T-wave height (4 mm) ratio is 0.5.

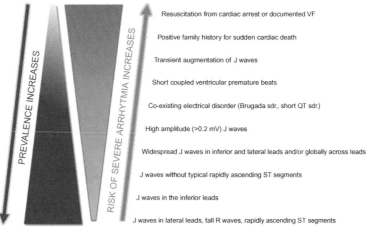

FIG. 3.10 A simplified illustration of the prevalence and risk associated with various electrocardiographic findings in early repolarization pattern. *sdr.*, syndrome; *VF*, ventricular fibrillation. (Data from Tikkanen J, Huikuri H. Characteristics of "malignant" vs. "benign" electrocardiographic patterns of early repolarization. *J Electrocardiol.* 2015;48(3):390–394.)

**TABLE 3.7**
**The Common Diagnostic Criteria for Left and Right Atrial Abnormalities**

| Left Atrial Abnormalities | Right Atrial Abnormalities |
|---|---|
| <ul><li>Prolonged P-wave duration to >120 ms in lead II</li><li>Prominent notching of P wave, usually most obvious in lead II, with the interval between notches of >0.40 ms ("P mitrale")</li><li>Ratio between the duration of the P wave in lead II and duration of the PR segment >1.6</li><li>Increased duration and depth of terminal-negative portion of P wave in lead V1 (P terminal force) so that area subtended by it >0.04 mm s</li><li>Leftward shift of mean P-wave axis to between −30 and −45 degrees</li></ul> | <ul><li>Peaked P waves with amplitudes in lead II to >0.25 mV ("P pulmonale")</li><li>Prominent initial positivity in lead V1 or V2 >0.15 mV (1.5 mm at usual gain)</li><li>Increased area under initial positive portion of the P wave in lead V1 to >0.06 mm s</li><li>Rightward shift of mean P-wave axis to more than +75 degrees</li><li>qR pattern in the right precordial leads without evidence of MI (but especially with other signs of RV overload)</li><li>Low-amplitude (<600 μV = 6mm at usual gain) QRS complexes in lead V1 with a ≥3 increase in lead V2</li></ul> |

*MI*, myocardial infarction; *RV*, right ventricular.
Data from Mann DL, Zipes DP, Libby P, Bonow RO. *Braunwald's Heart Disease: A Textbook of Cardiovascular Medicine*. Philadelphia: Elsevier Health Sciences; 2014.

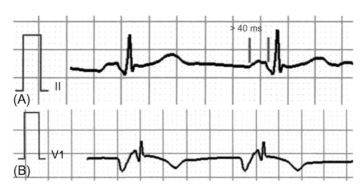

FIG. 3.11 Left atrial abnormality. (A) Note the prolonged P-wave duration in lead II, prominent notching of P wave in lead II and (B) increased duration and depth of terminal negative portion of P wave in lead V1.

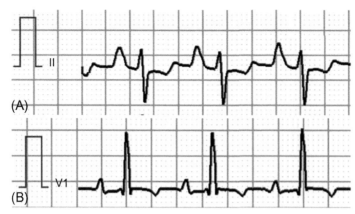

FIG. 3.12 Right atrial abnormality. (A) Note the peaked P waves in lead II and (B) prominent initial positivity in lead V1("P pulmonale").

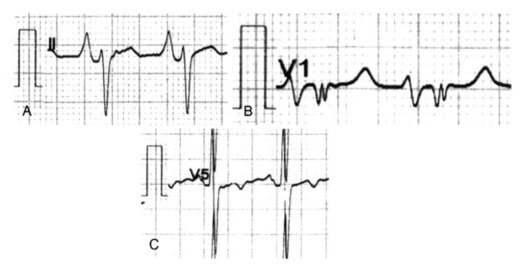

FIG. 3.13 Biatrial abnormality with tall P waves in lead II (right atrial abnormality) (A) and an abnormally large terminal negative component of the P wave in lead V1 (left atrial abnormality) (B). (C) The P wave also is notched in lead V5.

**TABLE 3.8**
**Common Diagnostic Criteria for Left Ventricular Hypertrophy**

| Measurement | Criteria |
|---|---|
| Sokolow–Lyon voltages | SV1 + RV5 >3.5 mV RaVL >1.1 mV |
| Romhilt–Estes point score system (4 points: probable LVH and ≥5 points: definite LVH) | Any limb lead R wave or S wave >2.0 mV (3 points) or SV1 or SV2 ≥3.0 mV (3 points) <br> or RV5 to RV6 ≥3.0 mV (3 points) <br> ST/T-wave abnormality, no digitalis therapy (3 points) ST/T-wave abnormality, digitalis therapy (1 point) Left atrial abnormality (3 points) Left axis deviation ≥−30 degrees (2 points) QRS duration ≥90 ms (1 point) <br> Intrinsicoid deflection in V5 or V6 ≥50 ms (1 point) |
| Cornell voltage criteria | SV3 + RaVL ≥2.8 mV (for men) SV3 + RaVL >2.0 mV (for women) |

LVH, left ventricular hypertrophy.
Data from Mann DL, Zipes DP, Libby P, Bonow RO. *Braunwald's Heart Disease: A Textbook of Cardiovascular Medicine*. Philadelphia: Elsevier Health Sciences; 2014.

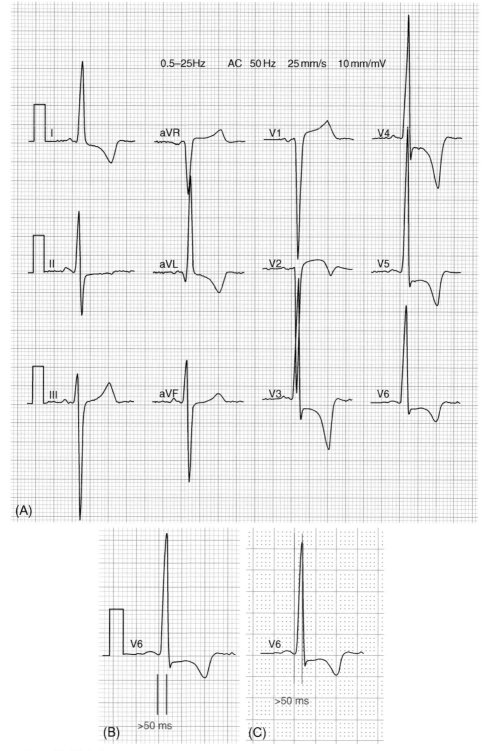

FIG. 3.14 (A)–(C) Left ventricular hypertrophy in a patient with hypertrophic cardiomyopathy. Note the increased left ventricular voltages (S wave in V1 + R wave in V6 >35 mm; R wave in aVL >11 mm), intrinsicoid deflection in V5–V6 greater than 50 ms, and left ventricular secondary change.

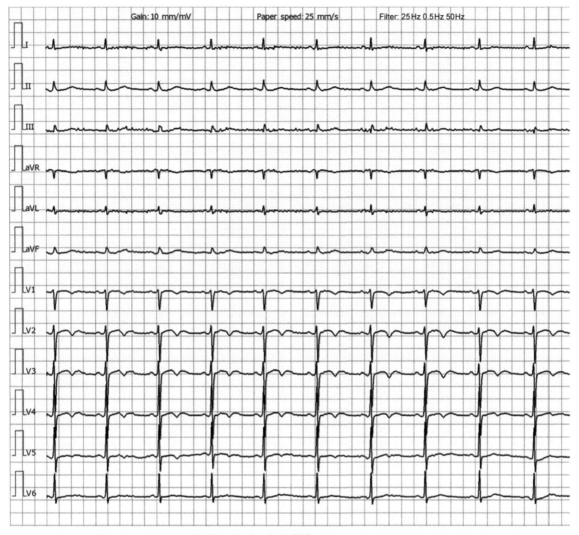

FIG. 3.15 Dilated cardiomyopathy. Note the low limb QRS voltage in the limb leads with relatively prominent QRS voltage in the pericordial leads and poor R-wave progression in pericardial leads.

chronic obstructive pulmonary disease includes right axis deviation more positive than 110 degrees, deep S waves in the lateral precordial leads, and an S1Q3T3 pattern. Hyperinflation of the lungs in these patients could lead to reduced amplitude of the QRS complex, right axis deviation, and delayed transition in the precordial leads even in the absence of RVH (Figs. 3.18 and 3.19).

**Biventricular hypertrophy:** In this condition, specific ECG criteria for either RVH or LVH are seldom observed. In the ECG of these patients, evidence of LVH with the below criteria was seen:

1. Tall R waves in the right and left precordial leads
2. Vertical heart position or right axis deviation
3. Deep S waves in the left precordial leads
4. Shift in the precordial transition zone to the left

In patients with congenital heart defects (e.g., ventriculoseptal defect) and RVH, the presence of combined tall R waves and deep S waves in leads V2–V4 with a combined amplitude greater than 6.0 mV suggests

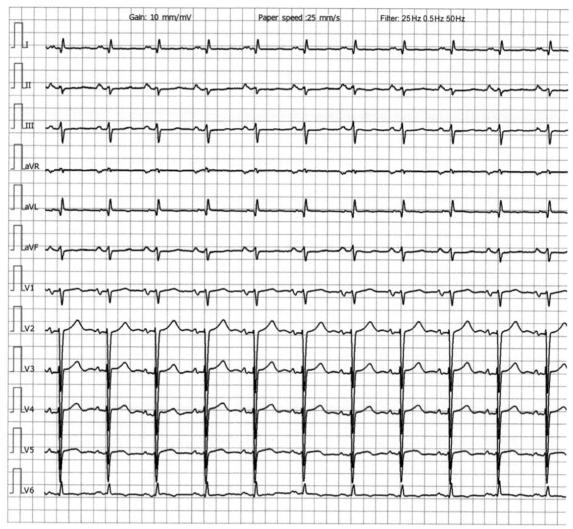

Gain: 10 mm/mV     Paper speed :25 mm/s     Filter: 25 Hz 0.5 Hz 50 Hz

**FIG. 3.16** Dilated cardiomyopathy (DCM). Note the low limb QRS voltage in the limb leads with relatively prominent QRS voltage in the pericordial leads and poor R-wave progression in pericardial leads, suggesting DCM. Also, biatrial enlargement is seen. The presence of low-amplitude QRS complexes in lead V1 with a 3 or greater increase in lead V2 suggests a right atrial abnormality.

the presence of LVH (Katz–Wachtel phenomenon)[12] (Fig. 3.20).

## Intraventricular Conduction Delays

**Left anterior fascicular block (LAFB):** LAFB probably is the most common cause of left axis deviation and is common in persons without overt cardiac disease. The most characteristic finding is marked left axis deviation[16,17] (Fig. 3.21). The common diagnostic criteria are listed in Table 3.10.

**Left posterior fascicular block (LPFB):** LPFB is unusual in healthy persons, and it occurs in patients with any cardiac disease[16,17] (Fig. 3.22). The common diagnostic criteria are listed in Table 3.10.

**Left bundle branch block (LBBB):** The common diagnostic criteria for LBBB are listed in Table 3.11. The mean QRS axis can be normal, deviated to the left, or deviated to the right. In most cases, the ST-T segments are discordant with the QRS complex. LBBB has significant prognostic implications. In persons with or

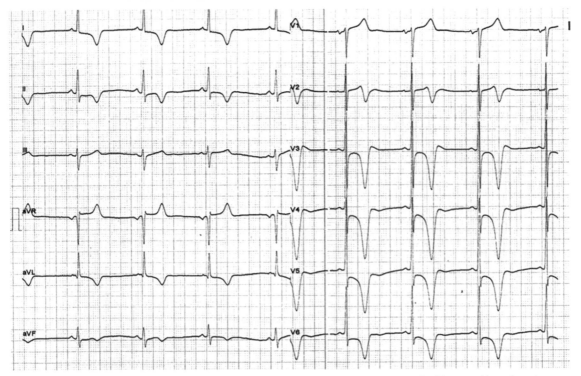

FIG. 3.17 Electrocardiogram from a patient with apical hypertrophic cardiomyopathy (Yamaguchi syndrome) and normal coronary artery. Note the left ventricular hypertrophy with prominent downward ST-segment depression and deep asymmetrical T-wave inversion in pericardial leads.

---

### BOX 3.2
### The Common Diagnostic Criteria for Right Ventricular Hypertrophy

- R in V1 ≥0.7 mV
- QR in V1
- R/S in V1 >1 with R >0.5 mV
- R/S in V5 or V6 <1
- S in V5 or V6 >0.7 mV

- R in V5 or V6 ≥0.4 mV with S in V1 ≤0.2 mV
- Right axis deviation (>90 degrees)
- S1Q3 pattern
- S1S2S3 pattern
- P pulmonale

Data from Murphy ML, Thenabadu PN, de Soyza N, et al. Reevaluation of electrocardiographic criteria for left, right and combined cardiac ventricular hypertrophy. *Am J Cardiol.* 1984;53(8):1140–1147.

---

### TABLE 3.9
### Electrocardiography Criteria for Right Ventricular Hypertrophy Based on Severity

| Moderate to Severe Concentric RVH | Less Severe Hypertrophy (Limited to the Outflow Tract of the Right Ventricle[a]) |
|---|---|
| • Tall R waves in anteriorly and rightward-directed leads (leads aVR, V1, and V2)<br>• Deep S waves and small r waves in leftward-directed leads (I, aVL, and lateral precordial leads)<br>• A reversal of normal R-wave progression in the precordial leads<br>• Shift in the frontal plane QRS axis to the right<br>• Presence of S waves in leads I, II, and III (the S1S2S3 pattern) | • rSr′ pattern in V1<br>• Persistence of s (or S) waves in the left precordial leads |

[a]This pattern is typical of right ventricular volume overload such as that produced by an atrial septal defect.
*RVH,* right ventricular hypertrophy.
Data from Mann DL, Zipes DP, Libby P, et al. *Braunwald's Heart Disease: A Textbook of Cardiovascular Medicine.* Philadelphia: Elsevier Health Sciences; 2014.

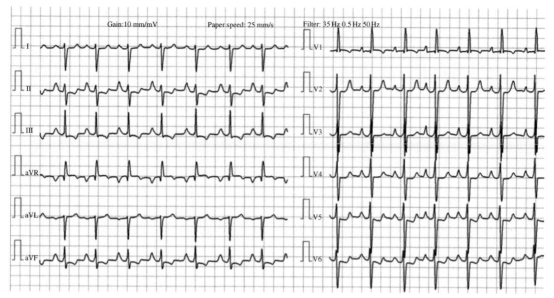

FIG. 3.18 Right ventricular hypertrophy. Note the right axis deviation, right atrial abnormality, dominant R wave in V1 (>7 mm tall), dominant S wave in V6 (>7 mm deep and R/S ratio <1). Also, reversal of normal R-wave progression in the precordial leads is seen.

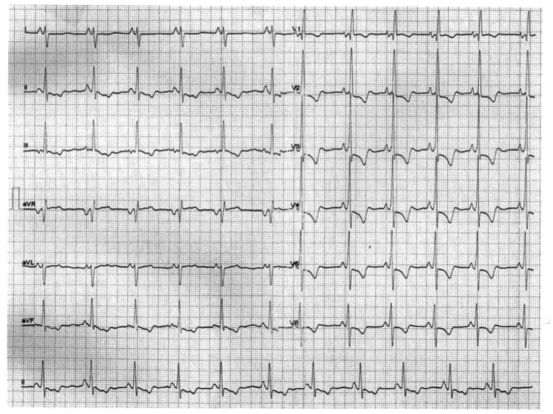

FIG. 3.19 Large atrial septal defect secondum with severe pulmonary artery hypertension (systolic pulmonary arterial pressure, 80 mmHg). Note the LAD, right ventricular hypertrophy, and T-wave inversion in pericardial leads (volume overload).

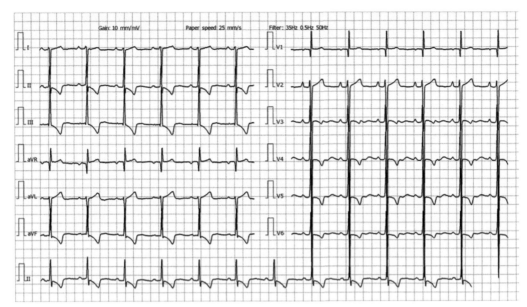

FIG. 3.20 Biventricular hypertrophy in a 35-year-old woman with ventricular septal defect and Eisenmenger syndrome. Note the Katz–Wachtel phenomenon and enormous QRS voltages.

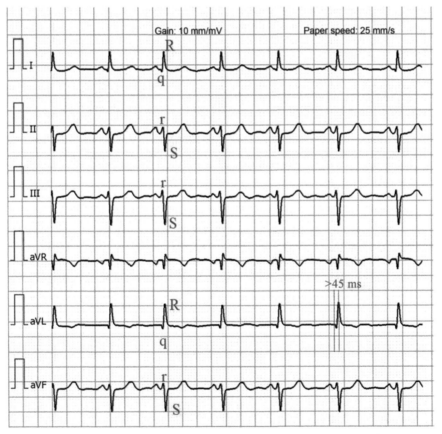

FIG. 3.21 Left anterior fascicular block. Note the qR complexes in leads I and aVL and rS complexes in II, III, and aVF. Also note the prolonged R-wave peak time in aVL (the time from onset of the QRS to the peak of the R wave >45 ms).

## TABLE 3.10
## Common Diagnostic Criteria for Fascicular Blocks

| Left Anterior Fascicular Block | Left Posterior Fascicular Block |
|---|---|
| • Frontal plane mean QRS axis between −45 and −90 degrees<br>• qR pattern in lead aVL<br>• QRS duration <120 ms<br>• Prolonged intrinsicoid deflection (time to peak R wave) in aVL ≥45 ms | • Frontal plane mean QRS axis between +90 and +180 degrees<br>• rS pattern in leads I and aVL with qR patterns in leads III and aVF<br>• QRS duration <120 ms<br>• Prolonged intrinsicoid deflection (time to peak R wave) in aVF ≥45 ms<br>• Exclusion of other factors causing right axis deviation (e.g., right ventricular overload patterns, lateral infarction) |

Data from Mann DL, Zipes DP, Libby P, Bonow RO. *Braunwald's Heart Disease: A Textbook of Cardiovascular Medicine.* Philadelphia: Elsevier Health Sciences; 2014.

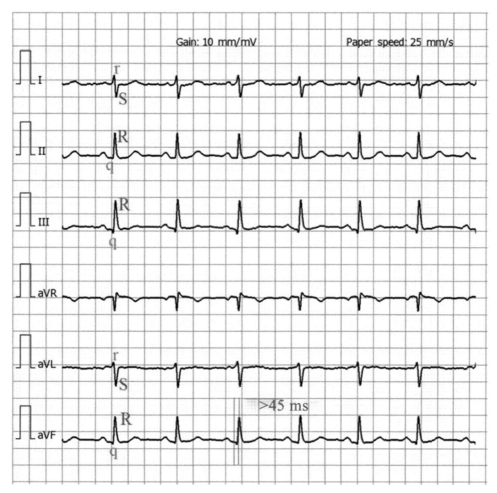

FIG. 3.22 Left posterior fascicular block. Note the rS complexes in leads I and aVL and qR complexes in II, III, and aVF. Also note the prolonged R-wave peak time in aVF (the time from onset of the QRS to the peak of the R wave >45 ms).

**TABLE 3.11**
**Common Diagnostic Criteria for Bundle Branch Blocks**

| Complete Left Bundle Branch Block | Complete Right Bundle Branch Block |
| --- | --- |
| • QRS duration ≥120 ms<br>• Broad, notched, or slurred R waves in leads I, aVL, V5, and V6<br>• Small or absent initial r waves in right precordial leads (V1 and V2) followed by deep S waves<br>• Absent septal q waves in leads I, V5, and V6<br>• Late intrinsicoid (prolonged time to peak R wave) in V5 and V6 >60 ms | • QRS duration ≥120 ms<br>• rsr', rsR', or rSR' patterns in leads V1 and V2<br>• S waves in leads I and V6 ≥40 ms wide<br>• Early intrinsicoid (normal time to peak R wave) in leads V5 and V6<br>• Late intrinsicoid (prolonged time to peak R wave) in V1 >50 ms |

without overt heart disease, LBBB is associated with a higher risk of mortality and morbidity from myocardial infarction, heart failure, and arrhythmias such as high-grade AV block[17–20] (Fig. 3.23).

**Right bundle branch block (RBBB):** The common diagnostic criteria for RBBB are listed in Table 3.11. In contrast to LBBB, RBBB is a common finding in the general population. An RBBB pattern was seen in many persons without overt structural heart disease. In healthy individuals, although RBBB may lead to right ventricular dilation and reduced function, it generally is not associated with an increase in risk of cardiac morbidity or mortality.[20,21] Incomplete RBBB, produced by lesser delays in conduction in the right bundle branch system, may be caused by RVH (especially with a rightward QRS axis) without intrinsic dysfunction of the conduction system (Fig. 3.24).

**Multifascicular blocks:** Bifascicular block refers to RBBB with LAFB, RBBB with LPFB, and LBBB alone (delay in both the anterior and posterior fascicles) (Fig. 3.25).

Trifascicular block refers to conduction delay in the right bundle branch with delay in either the main left bundle branch or both the left anterior and the left posterior fascicles. The ECG patterns can be divided into incomplete and complete trifascicular block. The incomplete (impending) trifascicular block includes bifascicular block with first-degree AV block (the most common form), bifascicular block with second-degree AV block, RBBB plus alternating LAFB and

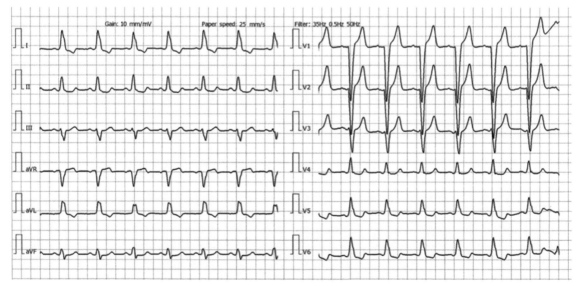

FIG. 3.23 Left bundle branch block. Note the broad and notched R wave in leads I, aVL, V5, and V6; absent initial r wave in V1 followed by deep S waves; and absent septal q waves in leads I, V5, and V6.

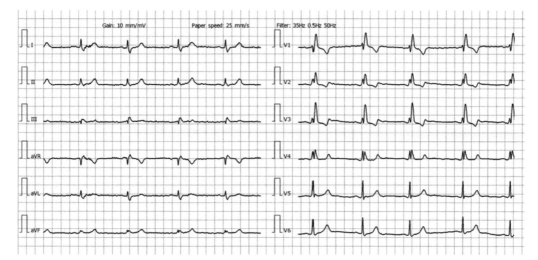

FIG. 3.24 Right bundle branch block. Note the rsR′ patterns in lead V1 and S waves in lead I ≥40 ms wide.

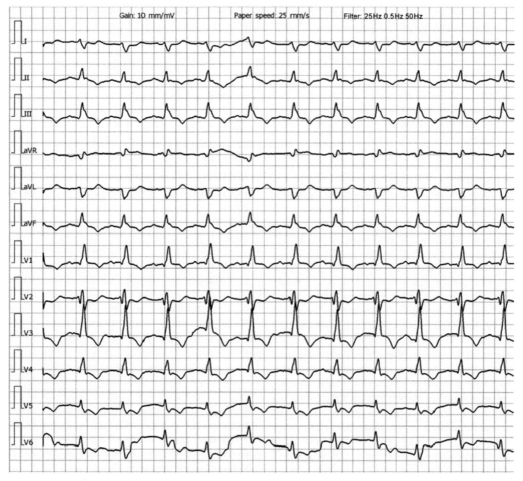

FIG. 3.25 Bifascicular block. Note the presence of right bundle branch block with left posterior fascicular block.

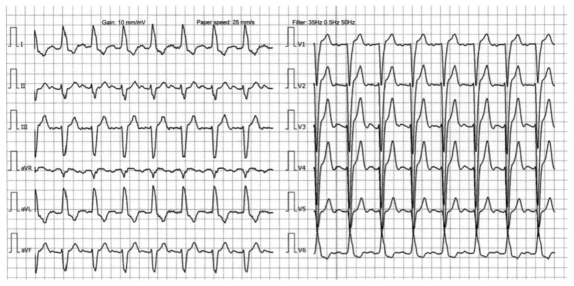

FIG. 3.26 Incomplete trifascicular block. Note the presence of left bundle branch block accomplished with first-degree atrioventricular block. The QRS left axis deviation in this electrocardiogram indicates more severe conduction system disease.

LPFB, and alternating RBBB and LBBB patterns (Fig. 3.26). Complete trifascicular block is referred to bifascicular block plus third-degree AV block (Figs. 3.27 and 3.28).

The main causes of multifascicular blocks include ischemic heart disease (the most common cause); hypertension; aortic stenosis; primary degenerative disease of the conducting system (Lenegre disease); congenital heart disease; digoxin toxicity; and electrolyte imbalance, especially hyperkalemia (which resolves with treatment).[1,22]

**Rate-dependent conduction blocks:** These blocks can be observed at relatively high or low heart rates. In acceleration (tachycardia)-dependent block, conduction delay occurs when the heart rate exceeds a critical value. While deceleration (bradycardia)-dependent block, conduction delay occurs when the heart rate falls below a critical level.

Deceleration-dependent block is less common than acceleration-dependent block and usually is seen only in patients with significant conduction system disease. Other causes of ventricular aberration include concealed conduction in the bundle branches, preexcitation syndromes, depressed myocardial conduction from drugs or hyperkalemia, and the effect of changing cycle length on refractoriness (the Ashman phenomenon)[23] (Fig. 3.29).

## Alternans Patterns on Electrocardiograms

The beat-to-beat total electrical alternans with sinus tachycardia is a specific but not highly sensitive marker of tamponade physiology. This alternans is caused by the heart swinging back and forth within a large fluid-filled pericardium with each contraction. However, in this condition, the reduced ECG voltage may be seen, but this finding is nonspecific (Fig. 3.30). The causes of low-amplitude QRS complexes (<0.5 mV in all frontal plane leads and <1.0 mV in the precordial leads) are shown in Table 3.12. Other mechanical causes such as massive pleural effusion may lead to low-amplitude QRS complexes[24–27] (Fig. 3.31).

Other ECG alternans patterns have primary electrical rather than mechanical causes. The QRS and sometimes R–R alternans may occur in different types of supraventricular tachycardias, especially atrioventricular reentrant tachycardia.[28] In the setting of acute ischemia, ST-T alternans is recognized as a marker of electrical instability, and it may precede ventricular tachyarrhythmia. In chronic heart disease, the presence of microvolt T-wave (or ST-T) alternans is considered as a noninvasive marker for an increased risk of ventricular tachyarrhythmias.[29–31] Also, T-U-wave alternans in the setting of hereditary or acquired long QT syndromes may be a marker of imminent risk of torsades de pointes.

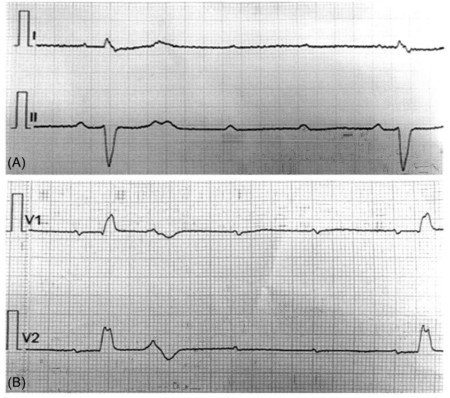

FIG. 3.27 (A) and (B) Complete trifascicular block. Note the right bundle branch block with left axis deviation and third-degree heart block.

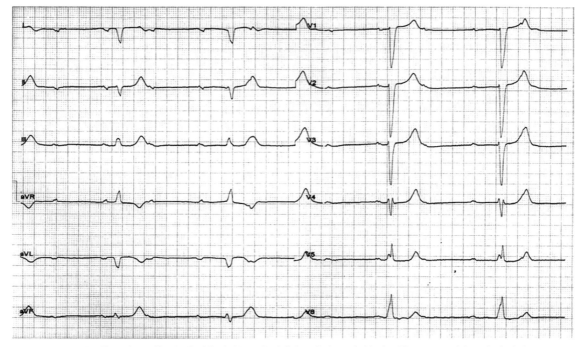

FIG. 3.28 Complete trifascicular block. Note the left bundle branch block with extreme right axis deviation.

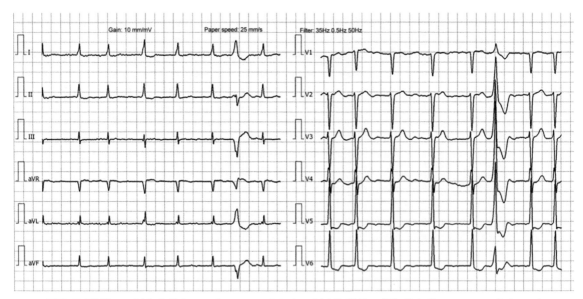

FIG. 3.29 Phase 3 block (Ashman phenomenon) during atrial fibrillation (AF). Note the presence of aberrant atrioventricular conduction with right bundle branch block complex morphology (short cycle) after a long RR cycle in a patient with AF.

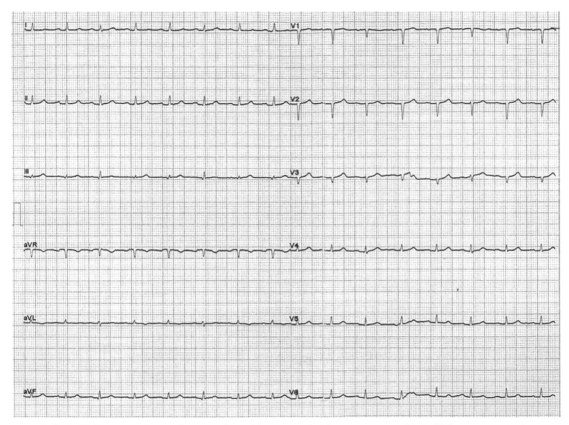

FIG. 3.30 Electrocardiogram from a patient with tamponade. Note the low-amplitude QRS complexes in the limb and pericardial leads with total electrical alternans.

**TABLE 3.12**
**Causes of Low-Amplitude QRS Complexes**

| Normal Variant | |
| --- | --- |
| Cardiac causes | Multiple infarctions Infiltrative cardiomyopathies Myocarditis |
| Extracardiac causes | Pericardial effusion Chronic obstructive pulmonary disease Pneumothorax Pleural effusion |

## Technical Errors and Artifacts

Lead switches are a common mistake when ECGs are made[32]; thus, any right axis or small signal in an extremity lead should be reason enough to check lead positioning (Figs. 3.32–3.40). The switch of the left and right arm is the easiest error to identify in routine clinical practice ECGs, which cause a negative P wave and QRS complex in lead I. But in contrast to dextrocardia (this pattern was recorded normally in these patients), in left-right arm switch, the progression of the R wave in the precordial leads is normal.

The most common errors during ECG recording are placement of the V1 and V2 electrodes in the second

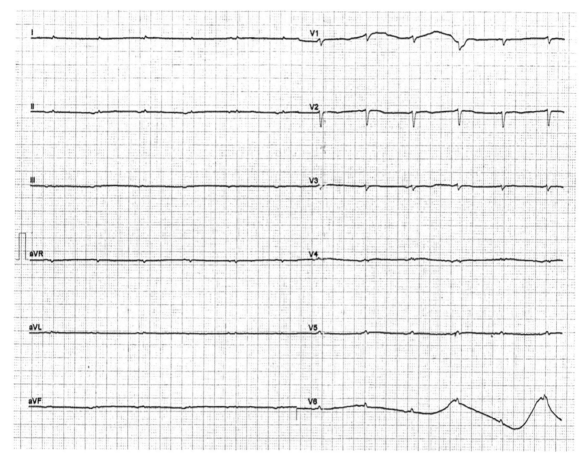

FIG. 3.31 Electrocardiogram from a patient with severe systolic heart failure and massive bilateral pleural effusion. No pericardial effusion was detected by echocardiography. Note the low-amplitude QRS complexes in limb and pericardial leads without total electrical alternans.

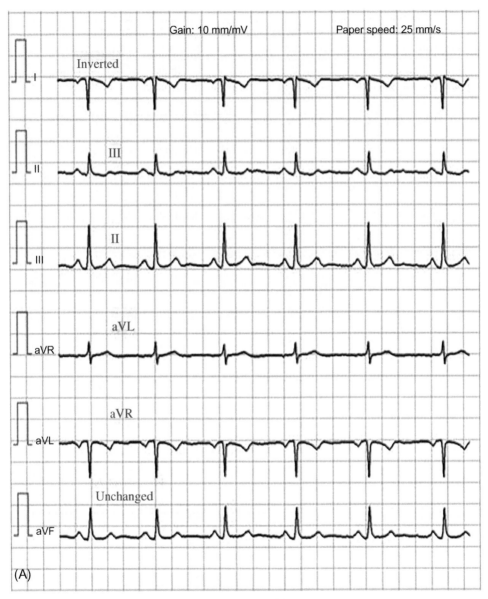

Gain: 10 mm/mV          Paper speed: 25 mm/s

FIG. 3.32 Right (A) and left (B) arm reversal.

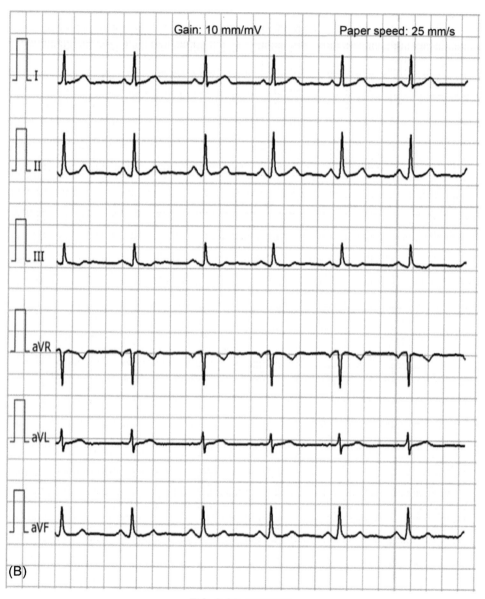

Gain: 10 mm/mV    Paper speed: 25 mm/s

(B)

FIG. 3.32, CONT'D

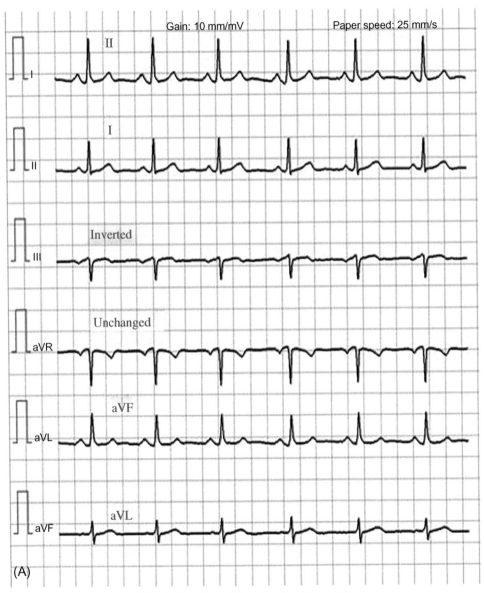

FIG. 3.33 Left arm (A) and left leg (B) reversal.

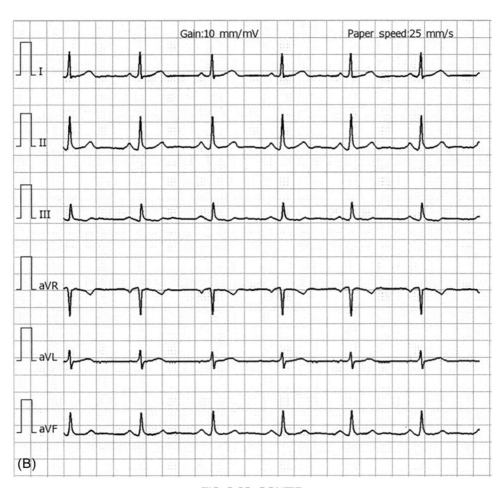

Gain:10 mm/mV    Paper speed:25 mm/s

(B)

FIG. 3.33, CONT'D

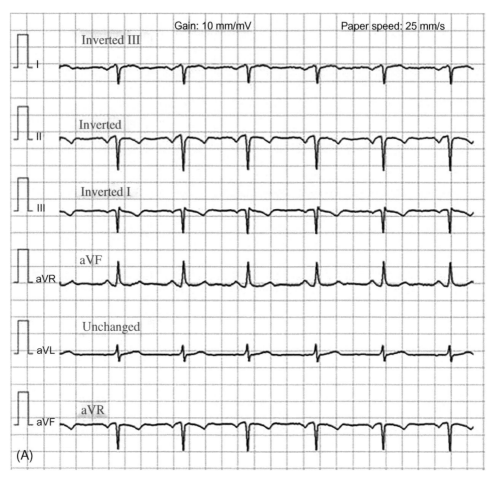

FIG. 3.34 Right arm (A) and left leg (B) reversal.

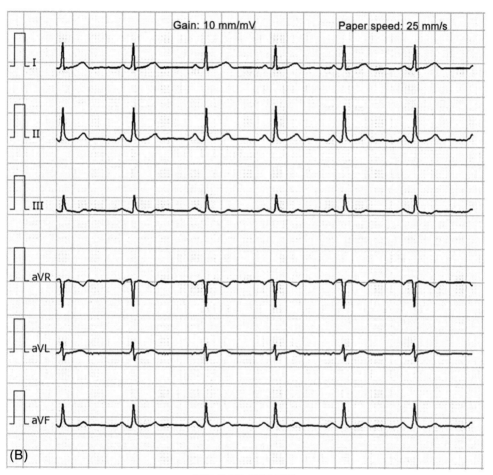

FIG. 3.34, CONT'D

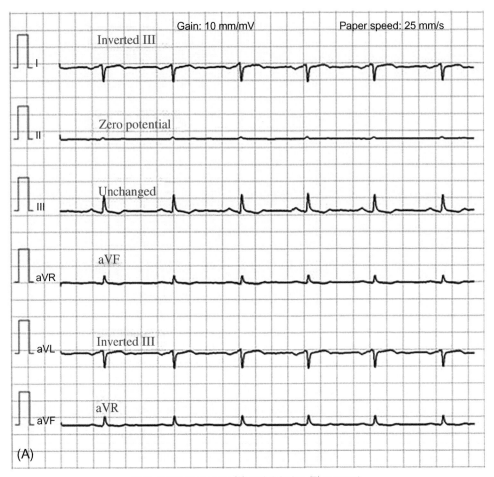

FIG. 3.35 Right arm (A) and right leg (B) reversal.

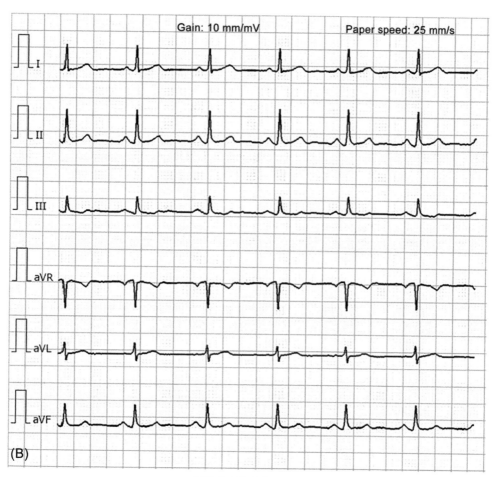

FIG. 3.35, CONT'D

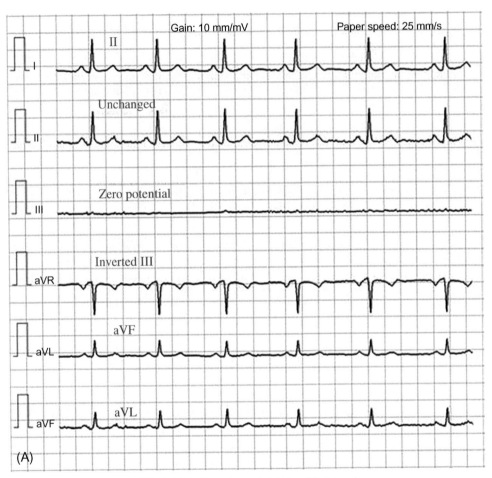

FIG. 3.36 Left arm (A) and right leg (B) reversal.

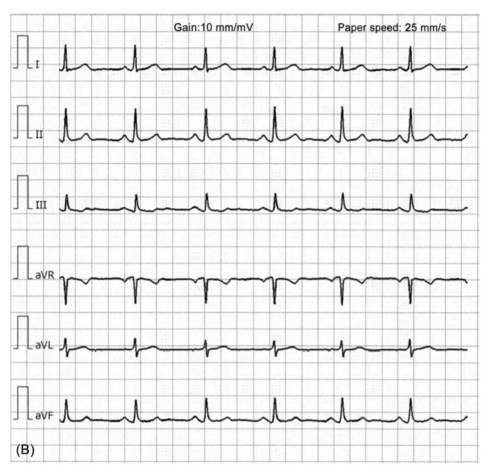

FIG. 3.36, CONT'D

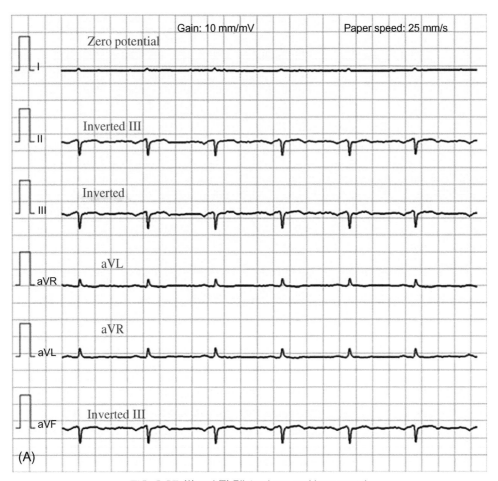

FIG. 3.37 (A) and (B) Bilateral arm and leg reversal.

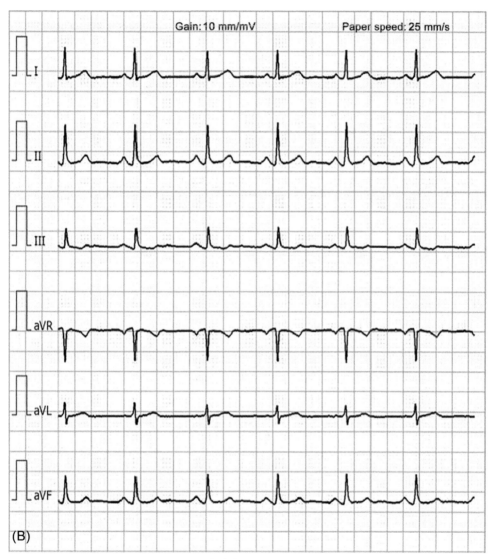

FIG. 3.37, CONT'D

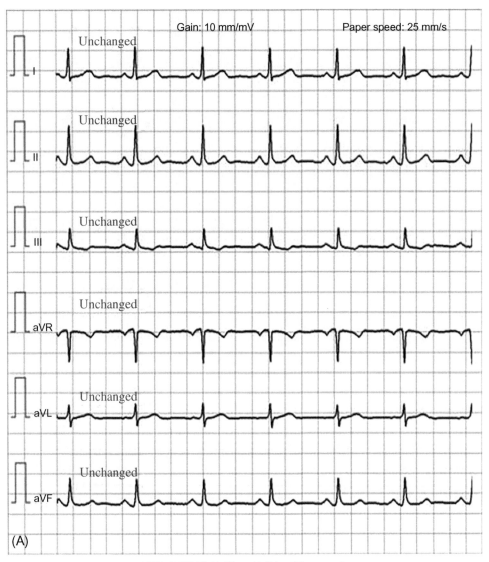

Gain: 10 mm/mV    Paper speed: 25 mm/s

FIG. 3.38 Right (A) and left leg (B) reversal.

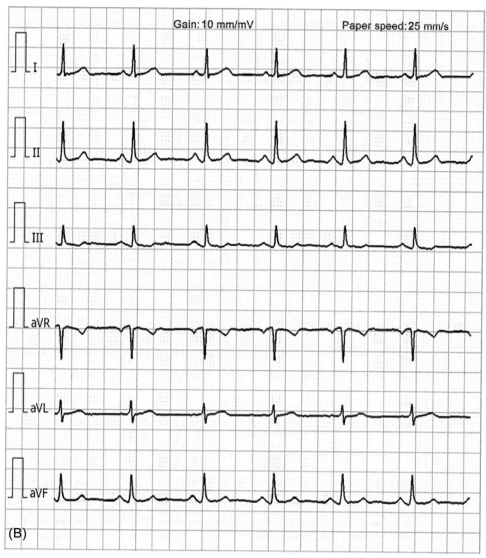

FIG. 3.38, CONT'D

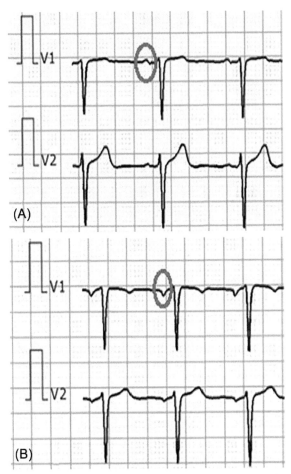

FIG. 3.39 (A) Lead V1 and V2 placed in normal position (fourth intercostal space). (B) After high placement of them (second intercostal space), the P wave becomes negative.

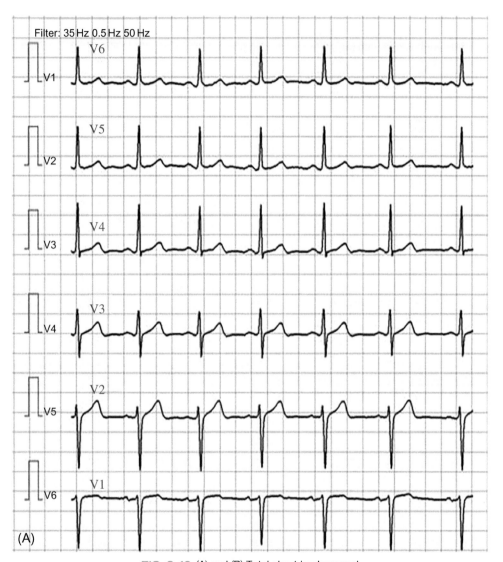

Filter: 35 Hz 0.5 Hz 50 Hz

FIG. 3.40 (A) and (B) Total chest lead reversal.

Continued

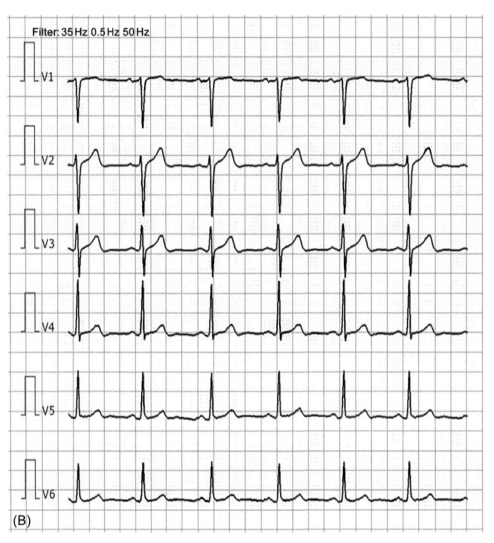

FIG. 3.40, CONT'D

or third rather than in the fourth intercostal space. Another common error is placement of the V4–V6 electrodes too high on the lateral chest. In healthy subjects, the P wave in V1 is positive or biphasic, and if an exclusively negative P wave is seen in V1, this indicates that this lead is recording in highest placement. Also, chest lead reversals lead to inappropriate R-wave progression (which is seen normally in dextrocardia)[33] (Table 3.13).

The presence of tremor, voluntary movements of the patient, or poorly secured electrodes during ECG may simulate clinical pathology. Some of the artifacts can mimic arrhythmia and lead to unnecessary testing and therapy (Fig. 3.41). For example, the presence of involuntary patient tremor in Parkinson disease or diaphragmatic contractions in singultus or hiccups may produce ECG artifacts.[33]

---

**TABLE 3.13**
**Technical Errors During the Acquisition of the Electrocardiogram**

| **INCORRECT PLACEMENT OF LIMB LEADS** | |
| --- | --- |
| Right and left arm | Inversion of lead I<br>Marked right axis deviation<br>Reversal of leads II and III<br>Reversal of leads aVR and aVL<br>Unchanged lead aVF |
| Left arm and left leg | Reversal of leads I and II<br>Reversal of leads aVL and aVF<br>Inversion of lead III<br>Unchanged lead aVR |
| Right arm and left leg | Inversion of leads I, II, and III Reversal of leads I and III<br>Reversal of leads aVR and aVF<br>Unchanged lead aVL |
| Right arm and right leg | Diminished signal (zero potential) in lead II (increases voltage when the right leg electrodes are elevated to the iliac crests)<br>Lead I becomes an inverted lead III<br>Leads aVR and aVF become identical<br>Lead aVL approximates an inverted lead III |
| Left arm and right leg | Lead I becomes identical to lead II<br>Lead II is unchanged<br>Diminished signal (zero potential) in lead III<br>Lead aVR approximates to an inverted lead II<br>Leads aVL and aVF become identical |
| Bilateral arm–leg reversal (left arm and left leg plus right arm and right leg) | Diminished signal (zero potential) in lead I Inversion of leads III<br>Leads aVR and aVL become identical<br>Lead II and aVF becomes approximately an inverted lead III |
| Right and left leg | No change |
| **INCORRECT PLACEMENT OF PRECORDIAL LEADS** | |
| High placement of V1 and V2 | Negative P wave rSr pattern in V1 |
| Chest lead reversals | Inappropriate R-wave progression |

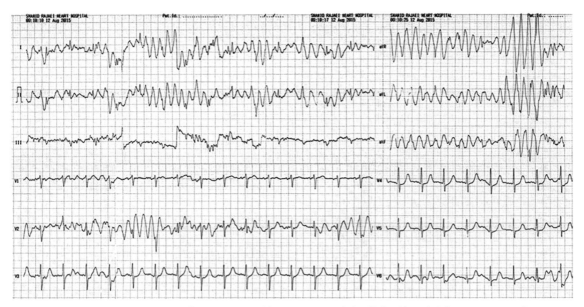

FIG. 3.41 Electrocardiograms from a woman with severe tremor in her limbs. Note that the waves secondary to tremor mimic the ventricular arrhythmia in limb leads, and the pericordial leads show the sinus rhythm with narrow QRS complexes.

## REFERENCES

1. Mann DL, Zipes DP, Libby P, Bonow RO. *Braunwald's Heart Disease: A Textbook of Cardiovascular Medicine*. Philadelphia: Elsevier Health Sciences; 2014.
2. Luo S, Michler K, Johnston P, Macfarlane PW. A comparison of commonly used QT correction formulae: the effect of heart rate on the QTc of normal ECGs. *J Electrocardiol*. 2004;37:81–90.
3. Bazett HC. An analysis of the time-relations of electrocardiograms. *Heart*. 1920;7:353–370.
4. Fridericia LS. The duration of systole in the electrocardiogram of normal subjects and of patients with heart disease. *Acta Med Scand*. 1920;53:469–486.
5. Rautaharju PM, Surawicz B, Gettes LS. AHA/ACCF/HRS recommendations for the standardization and interpretation of the electrocardiogram: part IV: the ST segment, T and U waves, and the QT interval: a scientific statement from the American Heart Association Electrocardiography and Arrhythmias Committee, Council on Clinical Cardiology; the American College of Cardiology Foundation; and the Heart Rhythm Society Endorsed by the International Society for Computerized Electrocardiology. *J Am Coll Cardiol*. 2009;53(11):982–991.
6. Chan TC, Brady WJ, Harrigan RA, Ornato JP, Rosen P. *ECG in Emergency Medicine and Acute Care*. Philadelphia, PA: Elsevier Mosby; 2005.
7. Edhouse J, Brady WJ, Morris F. ABC of clinical electrocardiography: acute myocardial infarction–part II. *BMJ*. 2002;324(7343):963.
8. Surawicz B, Knilans T. *Chou's Electrocardiography in Clinical Practice: Adult and Pediatric*. Philadelphia: Elsevier Health Sciences; 2008.
9. Haïssaguerre M, Derval N, Sacher F, et al. Sudden cardiac arrest associated with early repolarization. *N Engl J Med*. 2008;358(19):2016–2023.
10. Mattu A, Brady WJ. *ECGs for the Emergency Physician 2*. Massachusetts: Blackwell Publishing; 2011.
11. Tikkanen J, Huikuri H. Characteristics of "malignant" vs. "benign" electrocardiographic patterns of early repolarization. *J Electrocardiol*. 2015;48(3):390–394.
12. Hancock EW, Deal BJ, Mirvis DM, Okin P, Kligfield P, Gettes LS. AHA/ACCF/HRS recommendations for the standardization and interpretation of the electrocardiogram: part v: electrocardiogram changes associated with cardiac chamber hypertrophy: a scientific statement from the American Heart Association Electrocardiography and Arrhythmias Committee, Council on Clinical Cardiology; the American College of Cardiology Foundation; and the Heart Rhythm Society endorsed by the International Society for Computerized Electrocardiology. *J Am Coll Cardiol*. 2009;53(11):992–1002.
13. Goldberger AL, Goldberger ZD, Shvilkin A. *Goldberger's Clinical Electrocardiography: A Simplified Approach*. 8th ed. Philadelphia: Saunders; 2012.
14. Goldberger AL. Deep T wave inversions: ischemia, cerebrovascular accident, or something else? *ACC Curr J Rev*. 1996;5(6):28–29.

15. Murphy ML, Thenabadu PN, de Soyza N, et al. Reevaluation of electrocardiographic criteria for left, right and combined cardiac ventricular hypertrophy. *Am J Cardiol.* 1984;53(8):1140–1147.

16. Elizari MV, Acunzo RS, Ferreiro M. Hemiblocks revisited. *Circulation.* 2007;115(9):1154–1163.

17. Surawicz B, Childers R, Deal BJ, Gettes LS. AHA/ACCF/HRS recommendations for the standardization and interpretation of the electrocardiogram: part III: intraventricular conduction disturbances: a scientific statement from the American Heart Association Electrocardiography and Arrhythmias Committee, Council on Clinical Cardiology; the American College of Cardiology Foundation; and the Heart Rhythm Society endorsed by the International Society for Computerized Electrocardiology. *J Am Coll Cardiol.* 2009;53(11):976–981.

18. Varma N, Jia P, Rudy Y. Electrocardiographic imaging of patients with heart failure with left bundle branch block and response to cardiac resynchronization therapy. *J Electrocardiol.* 2007;40(6):S174–S178.

19. Bacharova L, Szathmary V, Mateasik A. Electrocardiographic patterns of left bundle-branch block caused by intraventricular conduction impairment in working myocardium: a model study. *J Electrocardiol.* 2011;44(6):768–778.

20. Aro AL, Anttonen O, Tikkanen JT, et al. Intraventricular conduction delay in a standard 12-lead electrocardiogram as a predictor of mortality in the general population. *Circ Arrhythm Electrophysiol.* 2011;4(5):704–710.

21. Kim JH, Noseworthy PA, McCarty D, et al. Significance of electrocardiographic right bundle branch block in trained athletes. *Am J Cardiol.* 2011;107(7):1083–1089.

22. Fisch C. *Electrocardiography of Arrhythmias.* Philadelphia: Lea & Febiger; 1990.

23. Fisch C, Zipes DP, McHenry PL. Rate dependent aberrancy. *Circulation.* 1973;48(4):714–724.

24. Dudzinski DM, Mak GS, Hung JW. Pericardial diseases. *Curr Probl Cardiol.* 2012;37(3):75–118.

25. Shabetai R. *The Pericardium.* Norwell, MA: Kluwer; 2003.

26. Maisch B, Seferović PM, Ristić AD, et al. Guidelines on the diagnosis and management of pericardial diseases executive summary. *Eur Heart J.* 2004;25(7):587–610.

27. Seferović PM, Ristić AD, Maksimović R, et al. Pericardial syndromes: an update after the ESC guidelines 2004. *Heart Fail Rev.* 2013;18(3):255–266.

28. Maury P, Raczka F, Piot C, DAVY J. QRS and cycle length alternans during paroxysmal supraventricular tachycardia: what is the mechanism? *J Cardiovasc Electrophysiol.* 2002;13(1):92–93.

29. Verrier RL, Klingenheben T, Malik M, et al. Microvolt T-wave alternans: physiological basis, methods of measurement, and clinical utility—consensus guideline by International Society for Holter and Noninvasive Electrocardiology. *J Am Coll Cardiol.* 2011;58(13):1309–1324.

30. Gupta A, Hoang DD, Karliner L, et al. Ability of microvolt T-wave alternans to modify risk assessment of ventricular tachyarrhythmic events: a meta-analysis. *Am Heart J.* 2012;163(3):354–364.

31. Nemati S, Abdala O, Monasterio V, Yim-Yeh S, Malhotra A, Clifford G. A nonparametric surrogate-based test of significance for T-wave alternans detection. *IEEE Trans Biomed Eng.* 2011;58(5):1356–1364.

32. Rowlands DJ. Inadvertent interchange of electrocardiogram limb lead connections. Analysis of predicted consequences. *J Electrocardiol.* 2008;41(2):84–90.

33. García-Niebla J, Llontop-García P, Valle-Racero JI, Serra-Autonell G, Batchvarov VN, De Luna AB. Technical mistakes during the acquisition of the electrocardiogram. *Ann Noninvasive Electrocardiol.* 2009;14(4):389–403.

# CHAPTER 4

# Exercise Stress Testing

SEDIGHEH SAEDI

Rajaie Cardiovascular, Medical & Research Center, Tehran, Iran

## KEY POINTS

- Exercise stress testing is a simple and noninvasive clinical test that helps objectively assess patient's activity-related symptoms of myocardial ischemia in a controlled and monitored environment.
- Exercise test performance and correct interpretation are essential for all cardiologists in clinical practice.

Exercise stress testing (EST) is a readily available and non-invasive tool for evaluating the patient's response to physiologic stress (exercise) and associated increase in myocardial demand. Before proceeding with the exercise test, a focused history of symptoms, risk factors, previous interventions or device implantations, medications, contraindications, and familiarity with treadmill-predicted physical activity level should be taken and a brief physical examination for detection of murmurs, rales, wheezing, and other relevant signs performed.[1,2]

During exercise testing, the electrodes for rhythm recording are placed over the torso to reduce motion artifacts. Therefore the recordings are interpreted differently from the routine 12-lead electrocardiogram (ECG). In a standard EST tracing the QRS axis could shift rightward. If the voltage in the inferior leads is increased, previous Q waves might disappear and a new Q wave might appear in lead aVL.[2]

## INDICATIONS FOR EST

- Evaluation for exertion-induced ischemia, chest pain, ST-T changes, and stratifying patient's cardiovascular risk level
- Evaluation of functional capacity
- Evaluation for arrhythmia induction, suppression, or exacerbation during physical activity and heart rate response in bradyarrhythmias (e.g., congenital complete heart block)
- Evaluation of response to drug therapy (including antiarrhythmic and anti-ischemic drugs)
- Objective evaluation of symptoms related to significant structural and valvular heart disease
- To determine patient prognosis
- Perioperative risk assessment for noncardiac surgery

## CONTRAINDICATIONS[3]
### Absolute
- Acute myocardial infarction (MI) and ongoing ischemia
- Unstable hemodynamics and significant arrhythmias
- Active endocarditis
- Severe and symptomatic aortic stenosis
- Acute pulmonary embolism or deep vein thrombosis
- Endocarditis in its active phase
- Acute pericarditis
- Acute myocarditis
- Aortic dissection

### Relative Contraindications
- Left main coronary artery stenosis
- Complete or advanced congenital heart block
- Hypertrophic obstructive cardiomyopathy with high outflow gradients at rest
- Recent transient ischemic attack or stroke
- Uncooperative patient
- Significant hypertension (resting systolic or diastolic blood pressures >200/110 mmHg)

## EXERCISE STRESS TEST PROTOCOLS
Different exercise test protocols (including Naughton, Bruce, and Ramp protocols) exist and are used based on the patient's underlying condition and ability to exercise.

The most commonly used protocol is the Bruce protocol, which consists of four 3-min stages with an increase in slope and speed at the end of each stage. The modified Bruce protocol is used in those with a more limited function capacity; the first two levels have a lower speed and grade, and then it continues like the Bruce protocol.

EST could be performed in maximal, symptom-limited, and submaximal modes. In symptom-limited EST, the test is continued until the patient asks for the test to be stopped because of symptoms or the indications for termination appear.

Submaximal EST is performed up to a predefined point, for example, reaching 70% of maximum predicted heart rate for age or 5–7 metabolic equivalents (METs) based on the patient's condition. This modality is used to assess for provocable ischemia during daily life activities in a minority of patients who have not undergone coronary angiography after an acute coronary event and have low-risk features, including left ventricular ejection fraction greater than 40% before hospital discharge. It could also be performed to guide future therapies or before starting a cardiac rehabilitation program.[2–4]

## EVALUATION OF FUNCTIONAL CAPACITY

Functional capacity is a strong predictor of prognosis with or without underlying coronary artery disease (CAD) and is expressed based on METs. One MET is the energy used during rest and equals approximately 3.5 mL oxygen/kg body weight/min. Activity-related METs are calculated by dividing the measured respiratory oxygen uptake during the activity in mL oxygen/kg body weight/min by 3.5 mL oxygen/kg body weight/min. Respiratory oxygen uptake and other ventilatory parameters are clinically determined using cardiopulmonary exercise testing, but "estimated METs" could be calculated based on exercise time or other parameters.[1,2]

$$\text{METs(based on exercise time in Bruce protocol)} = 1.11 + 0.016(\text{duration in seconds})^5$$

There are formulas for prediction of the expected functional capacity based on age and to classify the patient's function capacity level from poor to high. Generally, an exercise capacity of more than 10 METs in patients undergoing maximal testing should be achieved to rule out significant CAD.[3]

## HEART RATE RESPONSE

Evaluation of heart rate response in EST is important for determination of adequacy of exercise, patient effort, and prognosis. A commonly used equation to predict the maximum achievable heart rate is 220 − age. However, more precise formulas have been developed according to gender and patient characteristics, including:

$$\text{Women}: \ HR_{max} = 206 - (0.88 \times \text{age})$$

$$\text{Men}: \ HR_{max} = 208 - (0.7 \times \text{age})$$

$$\text{Patients using effective doses of beta} - \text{blockers}: \\ HR_{max} = 164 - (0.7 \times \text{age})$$

For the exercise test to be reliable in detecting underlying ischemia, the patient should achieve at least 85% of maximum predicted heart rate for age. In patients on therapeutic doses of beta-blockers, values of 62% or less could be considered abnormal.[1,3]

If the patient fully accomplishing the EST does not reach 85% of the maximum predicted heart rate for age, the term "chronotropic incompetence" is used. However, some patients do not reach this point because of lack of enough effort (e.g., using hand rails, exercise protocol being too easy) or use of heart rate-lowering medications.

When the patient cannot achieve maximal exercise duration, chronotropic index, or proportional HR reserve used should be considered; this is calculated as the difference between age-predicted maximal heart rate and resting heart rate divided by the observed heart rate reserve. Values below 80% are in favor of chronotropic incompetence.

$$\text{Chronotropic index} = [(HR_{max} - HR_{rest}) \times 100] \\ - [(220 - \text{age}) - HR_{rest}]$$

Early inappropriate acceleration in heart rate could occur and might be attributable to anxiety, anemia, left ventricular dysfunction, physical deconditioning, dehydration, or atrial fibrillation.

After the cessation of the exercise, normal individuals are expected to have an initial faster drop in heart rate followed by a slower return to baseline. In those with abnormal heart rate response, this return is relatively slower and is associated with increased mortality caused by reduced vagal tune independent of other underlying patient factors.

The common method of calculation of heart rate recovery is the peak heart rate minus heart rate after 1 min of termination of exercise. In the first minute of recovery phase, a decrease in heart rate of less than 12 beats/min is abnormal when the patient is standing in the recovery phase or less than 18 beats/min when the recovery is in a supine or sitting position. After 2 min, a decrease of less than 42 beats is an abnormal heart rate recovery.[2,3]

**Double product:** The multiple of peak heart rate and systolic blood pressure at each stage defines the rate–pressure product, which increases with progressive exercise. This is an indicator of myocardial oxygen demand, is affected by cardiac drug therapy, and is often between 20,000 and 35,000. A peak double product minus a resting double product of less than 10,000 (double-product reserve) indicates the possibility of a worse prognosis for cardiovascular events.[2]

## BLOOD PRESSURE RESPONSE
### Hypertensive Response
Blood pressure is expected to increase with progressive exercise to a range of 160–200 mmHg, with the higher limits being more prevalent in older patients. Peak systolic blood pressure above 210 mmHg in men and 190 mmHg in women is considered a hypertensive response. This abnormality could be a sign of propensity to develop hypertension in the future if the patient is currently normotensive.

Diastolic blood pressure is not expected to change much during EST. An increase of more than 10 mmHg above the resting level or a value of 90 mmHg or more is abnormal and increases the likelihood of CAD.

### Hypotensive Response
Hypotensive blood pressure response is generally an indication for exercise termination and indicates significant CAD, cardiomyopathy, or left ventricular outflow tract obstruction. It is defined as a 10-mmHg or greater fall in blood pressure after an initial increase or a fall in blood pressure below baseline resting levels during continuous exercise. An increase of less than 10 mmHg, if not due to poor activity level, is also considered an abnormal response. Some patients with initial anxiety might have a greater baseline blood pressure, which is decreased after the start of the EST but shows a normal rising trend with activity. Other benign causes include a vasovagal reaction or hypovolemia.[2,3]

## ELECTROCARDIOGRAM CHANGES
During progressive exercise, if the patient has myocardial ischemia, the ST segment becomes more and more horizontal. The PQ segment is generally considered for comparing and interpreting the level of ST-segment depression.

ST-segment depression of 1 mm or more compared with the PQ segment occurring 80 ms after the J point (ST80) in three consecutive beats without baseline shifts could be a sign of myocardial ischemia. ST60 point (60 ms after J point) should be used for interpretation in heart rates above 130 beats/min.

If the ST segment has baseline ST depressions, an additional 1-mm ST depression should happen for the test result to be considered abnormal, although if the baseline depression is already more than 1 mm, it is preferred that another imaging modality be used.

If there is baseline J point elevation or early repolarization, ST-segment depression should be measured after the J point has returned to baseline during progressive exercise.

Leads with ST-segment depression do not indicate the coronary artery involved. In contrast, ECG leads with ST-segment elevation could localize the diseased vessel.

Most exercise test machines produce an average beat (i.e., a beat showing the average ST-T changes at each stage and usually to the right of ECG tracings) in addition to momentary patient ECG. These average beats should be considered in interpretation in addition to the three nonaveraged beats with a stable baseline. ST-segment slope measurements at ST80 or ST60 by the computer are other components of the interpretation (Fig. 4.1).

### Normal Response
A normal response to exercise includes progressive shortening of the PR, QRS, and QT intervals; downsloping of the PR segment; and J point depression.

### Rapid Upsloping Response
This is a type of normal response to exercise and is more commonly seen in older patients. The ST60 or ST80 depression is less than 1.5 mm, and the slope is sharply upward and positive (>1 mV/s) (Fig. 4.2).

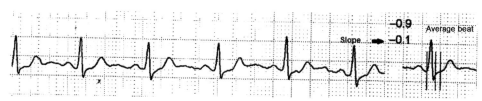

FIG. 4.1  ST-segment deviation and slope is calculated and depicted on the average beat generated by the computer system.

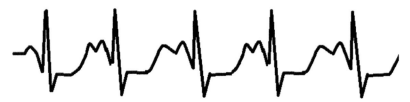

FIG. 4.2 The ST60 point depression is about 1 mm, and the slope is positive. The response is rapid upsloping.

### Slow Upsloping ST Changes

The ST60 or ST80 depression is 1.5 mm or greater, but the slope is upward and positive (>1 mV/s). Slow upsloping changes are considered abnormal, especially in the presence of coronary risk factors or a high pretest probability of CAD in a patient (Fig. 4.3).

### Horizontal ST-Segment Depression

Horizontal ST-segment depression is the classic abnormal response indicating underlying CAD. The ST60 or ST80 depressions is 1 mm or more, and the slope is near zero (Fig. 4.4).

### Minor ST-Segment Changes

When there is horizontal ST-segment depression of less than 1 mm but the exercise has been stopped in less than the maximum predicted workload of the patient,

the response is called minor ST-segment depression and is an abnormal response. For example, ST-segment depression of 0.9 mm with a slope of almost zero in a patient who has exercised only up to 4 METs is considered an abnormal response (Fig. 4.5).

### Downsloping ST-Segment Depression

Downsloping ST-segment depressions also point to the presence of myocardial ischemia. In this setting, there is a ST60 or ST80 depressions of 1 mm or more with a negative and downward slope (Fig. 4.6).

### ST-Segment Elevation

ST-segment elevation during EST occurs as a result of severe myocardial ischemia. ECG shows J point and ST60 or ST80 elevations of 1 mm or more. The test should be stopped immediately (see Fig. 4.7).

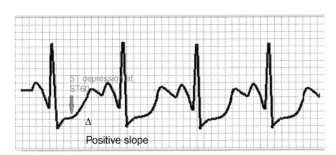

FIG. 4.3 Electrocardiogram showing ST60 depression of about 1.5 mm with an upward slope. The changes are of the slow upsloping type.

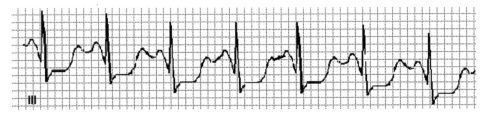

FIG. 4.4 The ST60 depression is about 2 mm, and the slope is near zero, so the changes are the horizontal type.

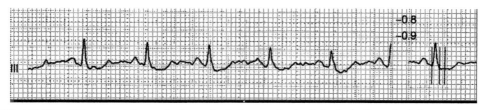

FIG. 4.5 Minor ST-segment depression in a patient who exercised only for 5 min; the patient stopped because of leg pain.

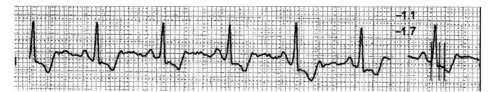

FIG. 4.6 Electrocardiogram changes showing downsloping-type ST depressions.

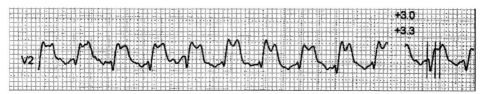

FIG. 4.7 ST-segment elevation during exercise.

### ST-Segment Elevation in Leads With Previous Q Wave

ST-segment elevation in Q wave leads is generally caused by significant myocardial wall motion abnormality in patients with prior MI.[6]

T-wave changes, including inversion or pseudonormalization in patients with low risk of CAD, are not specific findings. However, normalization of baseline ST-segment depression and T inversion could occur in some patients with ischemia. An increase in T-wave height in leads V2–V4 (>2.5 mV) in patients with chest pain during EST has been reported to be indicative of ischemia.[1–3,5]

### ARRHYTHMIAS

- **Right bundle branch block (RBBB):** EST is uninterpretable in leads V1–V4 in RBBB, but changes in II, III, AVF, and V5–V6 could be interpreted (Fig. 4.8).
- **Left bundle branch block (LBBB):** EST is uninterpretable in LBBB. Exercise-induced LBBB might indicate ischemia, particularly in heart rates below 125

beats/min. ST-T changes before and after resolution of LBBB should be reported (Fig. 4.8).
- **Wolff–Parkinson–White syndrome (WPW):** EST is uninterpretable for ischemia. Abrupt disappearance of the delta wave may help identify patients that are at low risk of development of life-threatening rapid ventricular tachycardia if atrial fibrillation occurs.
- **Premature ventricular complexes (PVCs):** These could be suggestive of underlying ischemia. Frequent PVCs occurring during recovery phase probably imply a worse prognosis.
- **Catecholaminergic polymorphic ventricular tachycardia:** In this genetic condition polymorphic or bidirectional ventricular tachycardia appears during maximal exercise. EST is useful in diagnosis and evaluation of response to therapy.
- **Long-QT syndrome:** In long-QT1 (LQT1) the prolonged QT does not shorten or becomes more prolonged during EST. In LQT2 there is normal shortening of QT and in LQT3 there is shortening beyond normal expected level.

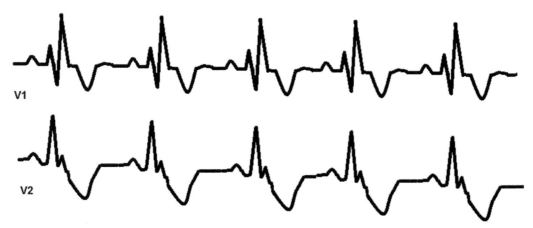

FIG. 4.8 Exercise stress testing in a patient with right bundle branch block and secondary ST-T changes in V1–V2.

- **Pacemakers and implantable cardioverter-defibrillator (ICD):** EST may be used for evaluation of rate-adoptive pacemakers in patients with remarkable levels of physical activity and to correct pacemaker rate response-related exercise intolerance. In patients with an ICD the device should either be deactivated by a magnet or programmed to higher detection rates to avoid discharge during exercise. EST should be terminated at heart rates around 10 beats/min below the detection rate of the device. Paced beats are uninterpretable for ischemia.[2,4]

## RECOVERY

Patients should be kept and monitored after termination of exercise for at least 6 min and until all hemodynamics, ECG changes, and symptoms have returned to the resting state. In some patients, ST-T changes might only occur in the recovery phase, which is notable for myocardial ischemia even in the absence of changes during exercise.[1,2,5,6]

## INDICATIONS FOR TERMINATION OF EXERCISE STRESS TESTING[3]

- ST-segment elevation (in leads other than aVR, aVL, and V1) or significant ST-segment depression (>2–3 mm)

- Significant drop in systolic blood pressure during progressive exercise
- Significant chest pain or central nervous system symptoms (presyncope, dizziness)—e.g., during exercise
- Significant arrhythmias, including sustained ventricular tachycardia or atrioventricular block
- Problems with monitoring system
- Patient asking for the test to terminate
- Severe hypertensive response

## REFERENCES

1. Fuster V, Walsh RA, Harrington RA, eds. *Hurst's the Heart.* 13th ed. New York: McGraw-Hill; 2011.
2. Mann DL, Zipes DP, Libby P, Bonow RO. *Braunwald's Heart Disease: A Textbook of Cardiovascular Medicine.* Elsevier Health Sciences; 2019.
3. Fletcher GF, Ades PA, Kligfield P, et al. Exercise standards for testing and training: a scientific statement from the American Heart Association. *Circulation.* 2013; 128:873.
4. *American College of Sports Medicine Guidelines for Exercise Testing and Prescription.* 9th ed. Philadelphia: Lippincott Williams & Wilkins; 2013.
5. Froelicher VF, Quaglietti S. *Handbook of Exercise Testing.* Little Brown & Company; 1996.
6. Saedi S. Exercise testing. In: *Color Atlas of Cardiology: Challenging Cases.* JP Medical Ltd; 2017:10.

# CHAPTER 5

# Echocardiography

ANITA SADEGHPOUR[a,b], AZIN ALIZADEHASL[c]
[a]Rajaie Cardiovascular, Medical & Research Center, Tehran, Iran, [b]Visiting Research Scholar in Duke Cardiovascular MR Center, Durham, NC, United States, [c]Cardio-Oncology Research Center, Rajaie Cardiovascular, Medical & Research Center, Iran University of Medical Sciences, Tehran, Iran

---

**KEY POINTS**

- Echocardiography is the most common noninvasive imaging modality that provides real-time images of the heart with comprehensive information regarding the structure, function, and hemodynamics of the heart. However, image acquisition and interpretation are operator-dependent skills and need considerable training.
- The principle of image generation is based on the reflection and refraction of the high-frequency sound waves (ultrasound waves with 2–10-MHz frequency) from the heart.

---

Ultrasound waves have the advantages of being directed and focused as a beam and also refracted and reflected when passes through a medium with different acoustic properties, besides being attenuated as the ultrasounds propagate. The major drawback is its poor transmission through the air. For this reason, gel is being used on the transducer. Ultrasound beam should be steered mechanically or electronically. Nowadays, most transducers use electrical steering and called phased-array transducers.

The standard basic transthoracic echocardiography (TTE) includes M-mode, two-dimensional, and Doppler study with the following modes: continuous wave, pulsed wave, color Doppler, and tissue Doppler imaging (TDI).

In M-mode echocardiography, a single scan line is sent from the transducer toward the moving heart and making a one-dimensional image as is shown on the y-axis over the time on the x-axis. M-mode has a high temporal resolution (more than 1000 lines per second in comparison with 25 images per second in 2D study) which makes it a proper mode for recording the detailed motions of the heart (Fig. 5.1).

Also 2D-guided M-mode study still is using for quantitative measurements of the LV size, function, and mass.

2D beam is formed of multiple scan lines, which can be focused and electronically steered and creating a fan-shaped sector. In 2D echo image formation is based on the US waves reflection and refraction off the heart structures. The optimal images are the ones that target and the beam are at right angles, which is contrary to the Doppler mode that the blood flow and beam should be in parallel for providing the best information.

Table 5.1 depicts some common problems encountered in daily practice and their suggested solutions.

## TRANSTHORACIC STUDY

In routine TTE study, a fan-shaped beam of ultrasound waves is directed through a number of selected planes of the heart to record a set of standard views of the cardiac structures for consequent analysis. These views are designed by the location of the transducer, the orientation of the viewing plane in relation to the primary axis of the heart, and the structures encompassed in the image. Each image is defined based on the *window*, which is the position of the transducer, and the *view*, which is the imaging plane (Fig. 5.2).

Sometimes more images from other nonstandard windows are required, including the right parasternal, supraclavicular, and right apical windows for dextrocardia.[1,2]

### Standard Windows

There are four standard windows in routine TTE: left parasternal, apical, suprasternal, and subcostal windows.

### *Left parasternal window*

In adults, TTE begins with left parasternal window by positioning the transducer alongside the left parasternal border at the third or fourth intercostal space in a patient with left lateral position. The transducer marker should be toward the patient's right (Fig. 5.3). From this location, long and short axis images of the heart may be acquired.[1]

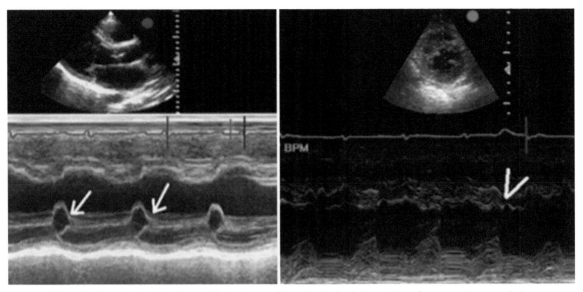

FIG. 5.1 M-mode study. *Left panel*: Early closure of the mitral valve in the setting of acute aortic regurgitation (*white arrow*). *Right panel*: Thickened pericardium and septal bounce in constrictive pericarditis (*arrow head*).

**TABLE 5.1**
**Common Problems in Echocardiography and Possible Solutions for Them**

| Difficulties and Pitfalls | Solutions |
|---|---|
| Obese patients with suboptimal imaging | Decrease ultrasound transmission frequency of the ultrasound beam |
| Potentially two small structures lying along the axis of the beam cannot be differentiated | Increase the transmission frequency of the ultrasound beam |
| In the apical four-chamber projection, the interatrial septum cannot be seen clearly and might mimic a patent foramen ovale or an atrial septal defect | 1. Use modified views. 2. Increase the gain of the received signal. 3. Inject agitated saline as a contrast with the Valsalva maneuver |
| Moving cardiac structures in real-time scanning are aesthetically of rather low quality | Lower the sector width of the display and/or the depth of the field |
| Chronic mitral regurgitation that seems to be severe, though the left ventricle is not dilated | Adjust properly the color gain settings of the machine, using more quantitative data |
| | Decreasing |
| Patients with no history of myocardial infarction and abnormal perfusion of the apex in rest images | The focus button should be adjusted to the level of the interest |

From Sadeghpour A, Alizadehasl A. *Case-Based Textbook of Echocardiography*. 1st ed. Springer International Publishing AG, part of Springer Nature; 2018.

In the long axis view, the mitral valve (MV), leaflets and chordal apparatus, right ventricular outflow tract (RVOT), aortic valve (AV), left atrium (LA), long axis of the left ventricle (LV), and aorta may be assessed (Fig. 5.4).

Interestingly, the rightward and medial angulation of the probe permits a more complete study and imaging of the RV inflow and leftward angulation of the probe allows imaging of the anteriorly placed RVOT and PA (RV outflow view). The "RV inflow view" permits the evaluation of the right atrium (RA), proximal portion of the inferior vena cava (IVC), entrance of the coronary sinus (CS), tricuspid valve (TV), and base of the RV.

The parasternal short axis images are achieved as the transducer is rotated 90 degrees clockwise rotation from

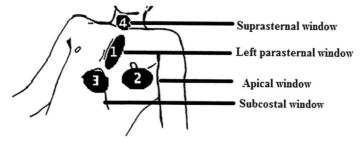

FIG. 5.2 Four standard windows in routine transthoracic echocardiography. *LA*, left atrium; *LV*, left ventricle; *MV*, mitral valve; *RVOT*, right ventricular outflow tract.

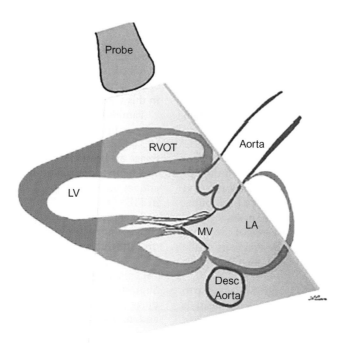

FIG. 5.3 Fan-shaped beam of ultrasound waves in left parasternal window showing parasternal long axis view.

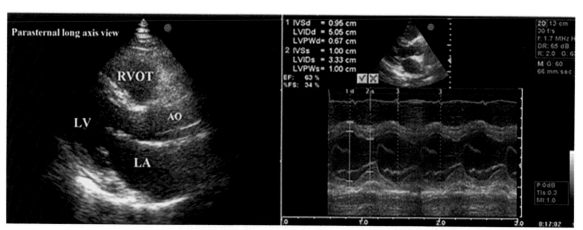

FIG. 5.4 (A) Standard 2D image of parasternal long axis view. (B) 2D guided M-mode study of parasternal long axis view for measurement of LV diameter.

the long axis view; also in this plane, the transducer may be swept from the cranial to the caudal position. Essentially, a series of cross-sectional images of the LV and RV are generated by moving the transducer caudally.

The RV resembles a crescentic structure alongside the right-anterior surface of the LV. At the basal level, the fish-mouthed shape of the MV is apparent. At midventricular level, both anterolateral and posteromedial papillary muscles are seen, and the most caudal angulation permits the imagining of LV apex[1-3] (Figs. 5.5–5.8).

The most cranial view provides the opportunity for the imagining of the AV, both atria, RVOT, and proximal portion of the pulmonary arteries. The three normal coronary cusps of the AV may be observed with the possible imaging of the proximal portion of the right coronary artery rising from the right coronary cusp at the 10 o'clock location and the left main coronary artery initiating from the left coronary cusp at the 3 o'clock location.

### Apical views

By placing the echocardiography transducer at the cardiac apex in a patient with left lateral decubitus and pointing the marker to the left shoulder and positioning the imaging sector toward the base of the heart, it is possible to obtain the essential apical views of the heart. This permits the imagining of all the chambers of the heart and the TV and the MV and their respective apparatus.

As the transducer is rotated 45 degrees, clockwise to this plane, the apical long axis view of the heart is acquired. A further clockwise rotation of the transducer to a complete 90 degrees yields the apical two-chamber view. The apical two-chamber view is vitally essential because it permits a direct imaging of the true inferior and anterior walls of the LV (Fig. 5.8A and B).

The superficial angulation of the apical four-chamber view brings the left ventricular outflow tract (LVOT) and AV into view and creates the five-chamber view (Figs. 5.9 and 5.10).

### Subcostal view

The subcostal window permits ultrasound access to the heart by placing the transducer on the abdomen below the xiphoid. The alignment of the heart relative to this approach permits a better imaging of both the interatrial and interventricular septa because the sound beam faces these structures in a perpendicular track. A series of essential long and short axis images are typically obtained from this chief window. The IVC and hepatic vein, liver, and abdominal aorta may also be assessed in this view (Fig. 5.11).

Familiarity with subcostal imaging is essential because in some circumstances, as in intensive care units (ICUs), it may be the only viewpoint from which to image the heart in a case with hyperinflated lungs, chest wall injury, or pneumothorax. Evaluation of the IVC size and respiratory collapse in the subcostal view is routine in TTE examination.[1-3]

Interestingly, in infants and small children, the subcostal window provides excellent images of all the cardiac structures.

### Suprasternal view

Suprasternal views are achieved by placing the transducer in the suprasternal notch. Both the longitudinal and transverse planes of the great vessels might be imaged in this view. The longitudinal plane is oriented through the long axis of the aorta and contains the origins of the innominate, left common carotid, and left subclavian arteries (Fig. 5.12).

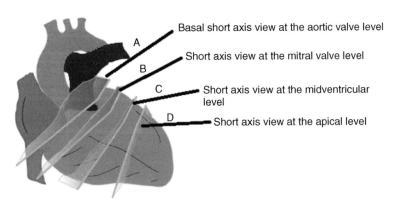

Basal short axis view at the aortic valve level

Short axis view at the mitral valve level

Short axis view at the midventricular level

Short axis view at the apical level

FIG. 5.5 Different imaging plane of parasternal short axis view from the left parasternal window.

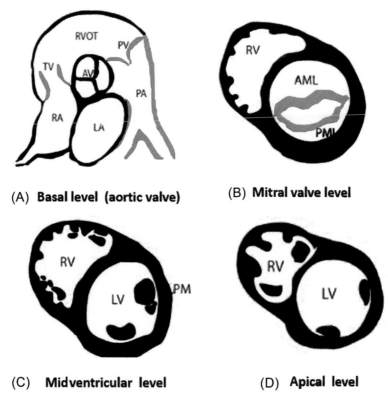

FIG. 5.6 Parasternal short axis view at the aortic valve (AV) level (A), mitral valve level (B), midventricular level (C), and apical level (D). *AML*, anterior mitral valve leaflet; *LA*, left atrium; *LV*, left ventricle; *PA*, pulmonary artery; *PM*, papillary muscle; *PML*, posterior mitral valve leaflet; *PV*, pulmonary valve; *RA*, right atrium; *RV*, right ventricle; *RVOT*, right ventricular outflow tract; *TV*, tricuspid valve.

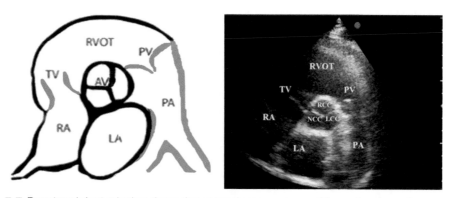

FIG. 5.7 Parasternal short axis view shows three normal coronary cusps of the aortic valve, pulmonary valve (PV), and pulmonary artery (PA) bifurcation. *AV*, aortic valve; *LA*, left atrium; *LCC*, left coronary cusp; *NCC*, noncoronary cusp; *RA*, right atrium; *RCC*, right coronary cusp; *RVOT*, right ventricular outflow tract; *TV*, tricuspid valve.

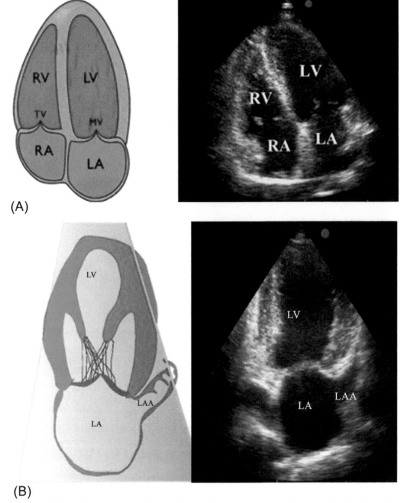

FIG. 5.8 (A) Apical four-chamber view in transthoracic echocardiography permits the imaging of all four chambers of the heart and the tricuspid valve (TV) and the mitral valve (MV). *LA*, left atrium; *LV*, left ventricle; *RA*, right atrium; *RV*, right ventricle. (B) Apical two-chamber view in transthoracic echocardiography permits the imaging of the left atrium (LA), left ventricle (LV), and left atrial appendage (LAA).

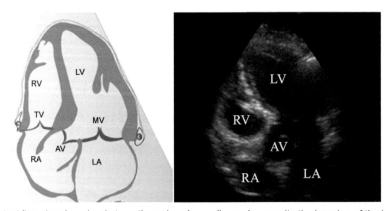

FIG. 5.9 Apical five-chamber view in transthoracic echocardiography permits the imaging of the left ventricular outflow tract and atrial valve (AV) in addition to the chambers, the mitral valve (MV), and the tricuspid valve (TV). *LA*, left atrium; *LV*, left ventricle; *RA*, right atrium; *RV*, right ventricle.

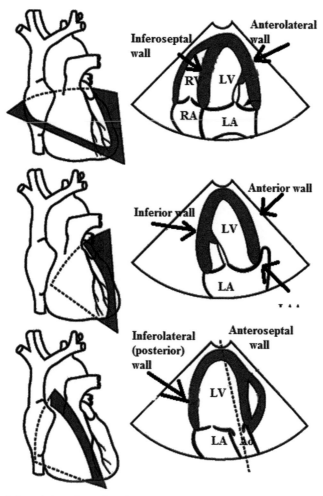

FIG. 5.10 Apical views in transthoracic echocardiography permit the imaging of all cardiac walls. *AO,* aorta; *LA,* left atrium; *LV,* left ventricle; *RA,* right atrium; *RV,* right ventricle.

The transverse plane contains a cross-section through the ascending aorta, with the right pulmonary artery (RPA) passage behind. Portions of the innominate vein and the superior vena cava (SVC) are observable anterior to the aorta. The LA and pulmonary veins are at the posterior site of the RPA.

### Right parasternal views

The right parasternal border may also be beneficial for viewing the heart in either longitudinal or transverse orientation. These views are principally helpful with medially positioned hearts, RV enlargement, and rightward orientation; with dilated ascending aorta; and for the measurement of the AV gradient (Fig. 5.13).[1-3]

## DOPPLER ECHOCARDIOGRAPHY

Doppler study is the bedrock of echocardiographic hemodynamic assessment in the cardiovascular system and is based on the Doppler effect found in 1842 by Christian Doppler.

The **Doppler effect** is the increase in sound frequency when the target [red blood cells (RBCs)] moves toward the transducer and vice versa (i.e., sound frequency decreases when RBCs move away) (Fig. 5.14). By using Doppler study, one can reliably calculate the intracardiac pressure gradients, stroke volume, and ventricular systolic and diastolic function and can conduct noninvasive assessment of the severities of shunts and valve regurgitation.

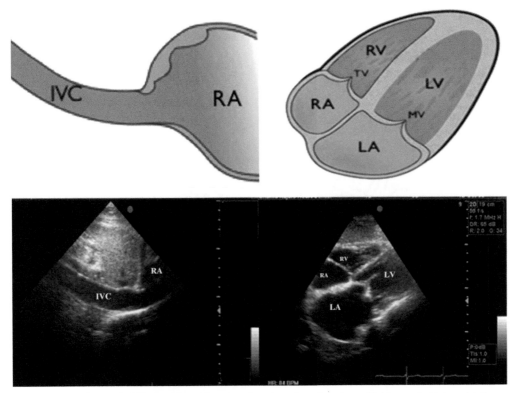

FIG. 5.11 *Left panel*: IVC to right atrium junction in subcostal view. *Right panel*: Subcostal four-chamber view.

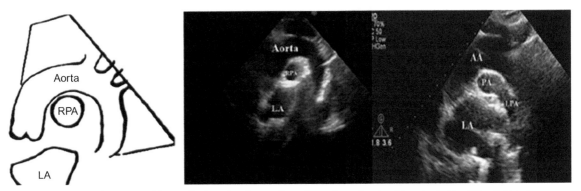

FIG. 5.12 Suprasternal long axis view showing aortic arch and branches besides short axis of the right pulmonary artery (RPA), *right panel* showing the main PA and LPA by anterior tilting of the probe.

By applying the Doppler source to ultrasound, the frequency shift of ultrasound waves reflected from moving RBCs essentially may be used to define the velocity and the direction of the blood flow. This may be done with either pulsed-wave (PW) or continuous-wave (CW) Doppler. PW Doppler permits the study of the velocity and direction of the blood flow at a particular site. However, the main shortcoming of PW Doppler is aliasing, which is an inability of the PW Doppler mode to measure high-velocity flows (Fig. 5.15).

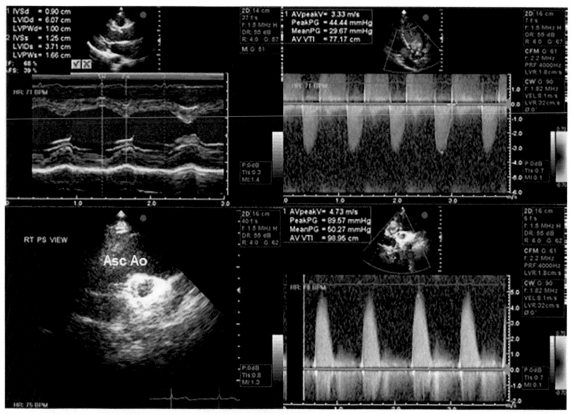

FIG. 5.13 Moderate aortic stenosis (AS) based on the apical view (*upper panels*) and severe AS when gradient obtained in right parasternal view (*lower panel*).

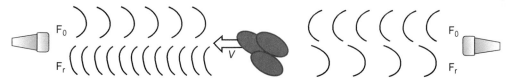

FIG. 5.14 Principle of Doppler effect, which means increase in sound frequency as the target moves toward the transducer and the decrease in sound frequency when it moves away from the transducer.

Continuous-wave Doppler permits the analysis of high-velocity flow alongside the whole length of the Doppler beam. The data may be revealed graphically and by agreement, the flow toward the transducer is represented as a deflection above, and the flow away from the transducer appears as a deflection below the baseline. The x-axis signifies "time," and the y-axis denotes "velocity" (Fig. 5.16).

Color-flow mapping also uses PW methodology; however, it maps flow velocity at multiple locations within an area and joins these data in color on a black-and-white two-dimensional (2D) image. By agreement, color coding for the flow velocity toward the transducer is red, and the flow velocity away from the transducer is blue. Higher velocities are mapped as brighter shades. A mosaic of color signifies turbulent flow. *Parallel alignment to the flow is crucial for precise Doppler quantitation, which is a vitally essential point to bear in mind.*

We should be aware of the artifacts and pitfalls that are Achilles' heels of echocardiography. They are unavoidable because they result from the physical principles of the ultrasound (Table 5.2).

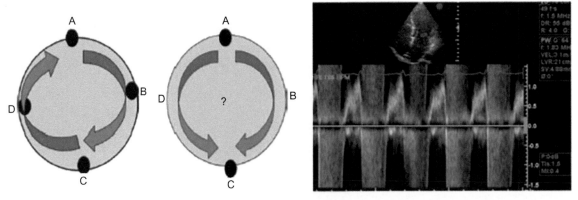

FIG. 5.15 In pulse wave Doppler study, sampling should be at least twice the wave frequency. *Left panel*: If the flow moves from place A to place C, the blood should be sampled at point B and D. *Middle panel*: Indeterminate blood flow direction. *Right panel*: Aliasing velocity of the pulse wave when detect high-velocity mitral regurgitation. Nyquist frequency limit is the maximum velocity, which is measured by PW without the occurrence of aliasing. Nyquist frequency limit = PRF/2 (one-half of the pulse repetition frequency).

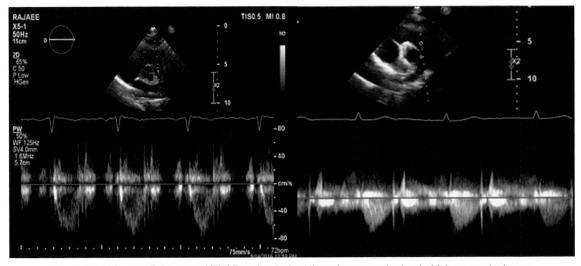

FIG. 5.16 *Left panel*: Pulse-waved (PW) Doppler study at the pulmonary valve level which uses a single crystal to send intermittent bursts of ultrasound waves and the same crystal waits to receive the returning signals. *Right panel*: Continuous-waved (CW) Doppler study along the pulmonary valve that can accurately estimate the maximum velocity without occurrence of aliasing.

It is important to know that Doppler study can measure the velocity of the flow, and pressure gradient is calculated by a simplified Bernoulli equation, which originally is a long and complicated formula and is simplified to four times the square of the velocity of the flow across the valve $(P = 4V^2)$. Indeed, direct measurement of the pressure gradient is best achieved by cardiac catheterization.[4–7]

## Doppler Study in Standard Views
### Parasternal long axis view
In this view, mitral regurgitation (MR) is seen as a distinct blue jet in the LA during systole. Small jets might be seen with normal valves. Aortic regurgitation (AR) is seen as a blue or red jet emanating from a closed AV. The jet is located in the LVOT and happens in diastole. The existence of this jet represents an abnormal AV.

**TABLE 5.2**
**Doppler Imaging Artifacts**

| Types of Doppler Artifacts | Origination | Elimination |
|---|---|---|
| *Signal aliasing*<br>Doppler signal wraps around the baseline, creates confusion to the flow direction, and precludes accurate measurement of maximal velocity | It happens when pulsed-wave Doppler is applied to flow velocities greater than the Nyquist limit in a nonlaminar disturbed flow or a high-velocity laminar flow | • By applying a lower-frequency transducer<br>• By decreasing the depth<br>• By using the continuous-wave Doppler mode |
| *Nonparallel intercept angle*<br>It leads to velocity underestimation | It happens with the malalignment of the interrogating beam and the blood flow direction | By placing the ultrasound beam parallel to the blood flow direction (0 degree to less than 20 degrees *intercept angle*) |
| *Beam width*<br>Superimposition of the 3D volume of the ultrasound beam on a single plane. Even the side lobe image merges with the main beam | It happens when there is simultaneous recording of different flows (e.g., simultaneous recording of the left ventricular inflow and outflow in the apical four-chamber view)<br>It is sometimes useful and permits measurement of the isovolumic relaxation time | By decreasing the power output or gain |
| *Mirror-image (or "cross-talk)*<br>Appearance of the symmetric Doppler signal, both above and below the baseline | It happens when there is interrogation of a flow (especially turbulent) at a perpendicular angle. Usually, the intensity is less than that of the actual signal | • By decreasing the power output<br>• By optimizing the alignment of the Doppler beam |
| *Electronic interference*<br>A band-like signal interfering with the Doppler flow | It is common during intraprocedural echocardiography and is a result of the inadequate shielding of electrical instruments | By shielding and avoiding electrical instruments (if possible) or strong magnetic fields nearby |

### Parasternal short axis view

IVC inflow has a continuous low-velocity red jet that enters through the RA floor next to the interatrial septum. A vigorous caval flow, like that seen in children, may be confused with a left-to-right interatrial shunt flow. Pulmonary outflow is a systolic blue jet in the pulmonary artery. The normal velocity through the pulmonary outflow tract is 0.6–0.9 m/s in adults and 0.7–1.2 m/s in children.[1–7]

### Apical views

Trans-MV and TV flow are best assessed in the four-chamber view as a result of the parallel position of the Doppler beam to the direction of the blood flow. Most likely, trans-AV flow can be evaluated in the apical long axis or five-chamber view.

The essential flows detected in this view are:

• MV inflow blood passing happens in diastole and may be quantified by PW with the sample volume placed at MV leaflet tips in the LV cavity (Fig. 5.17).

• The first positive deflection (E wave) signifies early passive LV filling, and the consequent deflection (A wave) imitates the late phase of LV filling, which is in consequence of LA contraction.

• Normal E wave velocity is less than 1.2 m/s and for A wave velocity is less than 0.8 m/s.

• AV and LVOT flow is seen as a blue flow detected in systole. The Doppler profile appears as a negative single uniform systolic contour.

• Pulmonary vein inflow from the right upper pulmonary vein is seen as a red jet arriving at the LA in the proximity of the interatrial septum. It might be quantified by PW, with the sample volume placed 1–2 cm into the pulmonary vein. There is a biphasic flow in systole and diastole.

Also, Doppler echocardiography makes it possible to estimate stroke volume (SV) and cardiac output (CO) by measuring the volumetric flow through the heart. SV is calculated by quantifying the cross-sectional area (CSA) of a vessel or valve and then integrating the flow

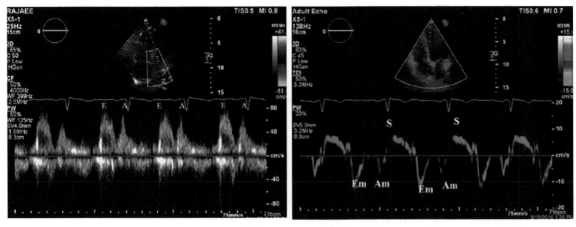

FIG. 5.17 *Left*, pulse wave Doppler study of MV inflow. *Right*, tissue Doppler myocardial velocity of the septal mitral annulus.

velocities across that particular region in the vessel or valve all over the period of flow (Fig. 5.18).

### Right ventricular inflow view

IVC inflow appears as a red jet at the inferior margin of the RA. It has both systolic and diastolic phases, and flow velocity is typically less than 1.0 m/s by PW. TV inflow is seen as a red jet passing the TV. It happens in diastole, with velocities less than 0.6 m/s.

Tricuspid regurgitation (TR) is a blue jet in the RA that happens in systole. Small jets are normal. The peak velocity of the regurgitant flow could be quantified by CW Doppler.

### Other views and doppler flow

Subcostal views are valuable for evaluating the flow within the IVC, hepatic veins, and abdominal aorta. The suprasternal window is used to record the flow in the ascending and descending aortas and in the SVC.

## MYOCARDIAL TISSUE DOPPLER IMAGING

TDI is an echocardiography mode, which detects low-velocity, high-amplitude myocardial velocity rather than high-velocity, low-amplitude signals of blood flow. TDI defines the velocity and direction of the myocardial motion. A sample volume (like to the PW) is

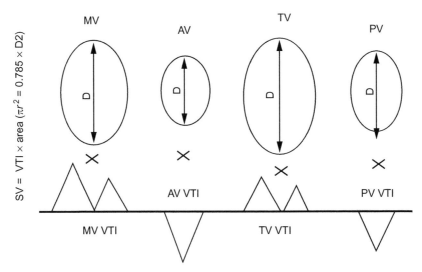

FIG. 5.18 Stroke volume across all heart valves in the absence of regurgitation and shunt is equal.

placed in the myocardium or valvular annulus to get a quantifiable spectral contour of myocardial motion. From the essential parameter of velocity, strain or strain rate imaging—which measures tissue deformation— might be derived. Doppler-derived tissue velocity, strain, and strain rate have been proven to improve the evaluation of myocardial mechanics compared with previous dealings such as wall thickening or motion.[8–12]

## TRANSESOPHAGEAL ECHOCARDIOGRAPHY

Transesophageal echocardiography (TEE) is a valuable modality in the imaging of the heart and great vessels in patients with suboptimal TTE windows. This may happen as a result of body physics and habitus as well as concomitant lung disease or in the operating room or the ICU, where appropriate access to the chest wall and optimal positioning are restrictive and prohibitive. TEE uses a particularly designed ultrasound probe combined within a standard gastroscope. This semi-invasive technique needs blind esophageal intubation (Fig. 5.19).

Because of the close proximity of the heart to the transducer, high-frequency transducers (5.0–7.5 MHz) are regularly used, allowing a better description of the small structures than the lower frequencies used in TTE (2.5–3.5 MHz). Accordingly, TEE is mainly valuable in the routine clinical setting for the detection of atrial

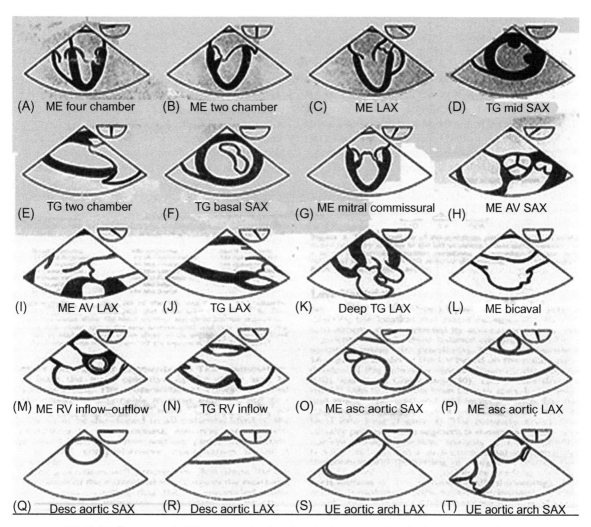

(A) ME four chamber  (B) ME two chamber  (C) ME LAX  (D) TG mid SAX

(E) TG two chamber  (F) TG basal SAX  (G) ME mitral commissural  (H) ME AV SAX

(I) ME AV LAX  (J) TG LAX  (K) Deep TG LAX  (L) ME bicaval

(M) ME RV inflow–outflow  (N) TG RV inflow  (O) ME asc aortic SAX  (P) ME asc aortic LAX

(Q) Desc aortic SAX  (R) Desc aortic LAX  (S) UE aortic arch LAX  (T) UE aortic arch SAX

FIG. 5.19 Recommended 20 cross-section imaging view in a comprehensive transesophageal exam.

septal defects (ASDs), patent foramen ovale (PFO), atrial and atrial auricle thrombi, small vegetations, abscesses, diseases of the aorta, and evaluation of the function of prosthetic valves. It is used in the operating room or in catheter or lead insertion to monitor and assess the repair of the cardiac valves and structures. Current instrumentation permits the imaging of multiple planes through the heart with multiplane TEE probes, in which the ultrasound plane is electronically steered over an arc of 180 degrees. In TEE, the anteroposterior (AP) orientation of the images from the esophagus is the reverse of the images from the TTE window because the ultrasound beam first meets the more posterior structures close to the esophagus.[1–4,13–15]

## CONTRAST ECHOCARDIOGRAPHY

Contrast echocardiography uses intravenous agents that result in augmented echogenicity of the myocardium or blood with ultrasound imaging.

Left-heart contrast agents form small microbubbles, which at low ultrasound power output disperse ultrasound at the gas and liquid interface, thereby increasing the signal detected by the transducer. Left-heart contrast agents with left ventricular opacification are useful in:

- Suboptimal images during stress echocardiography
- Apical hypertrophic cardiomyopathy
- LV noncompaction (LVNC)
- LV thrombosis or cardiac masses
- Differentiation between true LV aneurysm and pseudoaneurysm

Left-heart contrast agents contain air or fluorocarbon gas condensed with stabilizing materials such as denatured albumin or monosaccharides. The microbubbles

that are molded are small enough to pass through the pulmonary capillary bed, allowing opacification of the left heart after the intravenous injection. The opacification of the LV cavity improves the identification of the endocardial border and cardiac masses chiefly in cases of suboptimal acoustic windows.

Contrast echocardiography advances the analysis of regional wall motion abnormalities (RWMAs). Real-time myocardial contrast echocardiography is presently explored as an essential tool for the quantitative analysis of myocardial perfusion.

Right-heart contrast is done with the injection of agitated saline, and early appearance of bubbles in the left heart at the first three to five beats suggests intracardiac shunt.[1–4,16–20]

## STRESS ECHOCARDIOGRAPHY

Stress echocardiography (SE) is done with exercise, the administration of a pharmacologic agent, or transesophageal atrial pacing. The exercise protocol contains a treadmill exercise test, with speedy postexercise echocardiographic images or upright or supine bicycle echocardiographic images achieved at the peak of exercise. Because exercise-induced RWMAs caused by ischemia frequently last for a few minutes after the end of exercise, immediate post exercise images may be compared with the baseline preexercise images to detect exercise-induced RWMAs (Fig. 5.20). Thus, treadmill exercise with echocardiographic images achieved immediately after the end of exercise is the form of exercise echocardiography used most frequently to distinguish myocardial ischemia (coronary artery disease) (Tables 5.3 and 5.4).

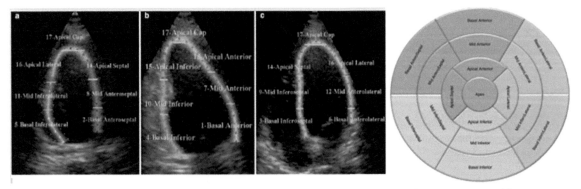

FIG. 5.20 Standard views during stress echocardiography: Apical long axis (A), two-chamber (B), and four-chamber (C) views showing 17-segment model in bull's eye map.

**TABLE 5.3**
**Interpretation by Regional Wall Motion (RWM) Analysis**

| Rest | Stress | Interpretation |
| --- | --- | --- |
| Normal RWM and contractility | Hyperdynamic | Normal |
| Normal RWM | New RWM abnormality or lack of hyperdynamic RWM | Ischemia |
| RWM abnormality | Worsening (hypokinesis → akinesis) | Ischemia |
| RWM abnormality | Unchanged | Infarcted tissue |
| Akinetic RWM | Improved to hypokinetic or to normal WM, biphasic response | Viable myocardium |

Modified from Oh JK, Seward JB, Tajik AJ. *The Echo Manual*. 3rd ed. Lippincott Williams and Wilkins; 2007.

**TABLE 5.4**
**Ischemic Features of Severe Ischemia**

| | Exercise | Dobutamine |
| --- | --- | --- |
| WMA | Multiple | Multiple |
| LV cavity | Dilate | Frequently not dilate |
| LVEF | Decrease | Might not decrease |
| ST-segment depression | Common | Uncommon |
| Hypotension | Specific | Nonspecific |

*LV*, left ventricular; *LVEF*, left ventricular ejection fraction; *WMA*, wall motion abnormality.
From Oh JK, Seward JB, Tajik AJ. *The Echo Manual*. 3rd ed. Lippincott Williams and Wilkins; 2007.

## STUDY OF MYOCARDIAL VIABILITY

Akinetic wall segments seen on echocardiography do not always indicate scarred or irreversibly dysfunctional myocardium. Because myocardial contractility ceases when 20% or more of the transmural thickness is involved by ischemia or infarction, a substantial amount of myocardium might still be alive or viable even when no mechanical contractility is imagined. Thus, it is important to define whether akinetic myocardium is irreversible or is a sign of stunned or hibernating myocardium with potential for functional recovery.

- **Stunned myocardium:** Reversible RWMA after reperfusion of transient coronary artery occlusion. Reperfusion may happen spontaneously or after thrombolytic therapy or percutaneous coronary angioplasty. Recovery of WMA might require days to weeks.
- **Hibernating myocardium:** Chronic depressed myocardial function subsequent to chronic myocardial ischemia; recovery of myocardial function afterward coronary revascularization is an example.[19–26]

## THREE-DIMENSIONAL ECHOCARDIOGRAPHY

Volumetric imaging, using a complex multiarray transducer to obtain three-dimensional (3D) pyramidal volume data, is used to acquire images of the heart structures in three spatial dimensions.

The structures might be viewed as a 3D image or shown simultaneously in multiple 2D tomographic image planes. Postacquisition processing involves cropping, which permits different views of the interior structures of the heart. The structure studied might be manipulated so that it is imaged from multiple angles similar to the surgical en face view of the interatrial septum and MV (Fig. 5.21).

Quantitative volumetric data, acquired by tracing the endocardial borders, enhance the accuracy of LV volume evaluation and allow the study of RV shape and volume. The usefulness of 3D echocardiography in quantification of LV volume and function is documented (3D TTE has better accuracy and reproducibility). The 3D echocardiography is a valuable method in imaging the enface view of the heart valves and showing the exact mechanism of valve pathology (Fig. 5.22).

Real-time 3D TEE is recommended in guiding the interventional valve procedure and assisting device implantation in cardiac catheterization laboratories. The current limitations of this method, which is frequently improving, include image quality, ultrasound artifact, and temporal resolution.[1–3,27,28]

## TWO-DIMENSIONAL (SPECKLED) STRAIN ECHOCARDIOGRAPHY

Speckle-tracking echocardiography or 2D strain is a relatively new method for segmental evaluation of myocardial function that analyzes motion by tracking speckles in the 2D ultrasound images. The geometric shift of each speckle signifies focal myocardial

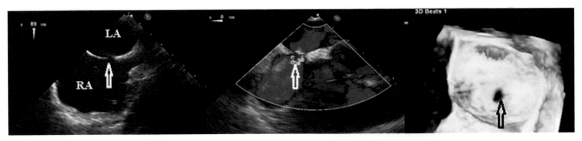

FIG. 5.21 Small defect in interatrial septum by 2D, color Doppler, and en face view in 3D TEE.

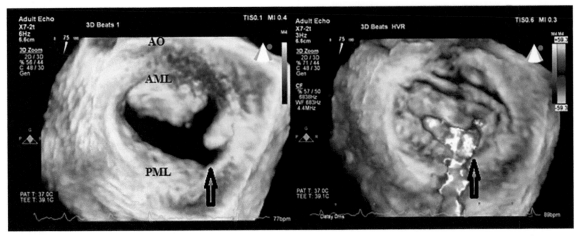

FIG. 5.22 Presence of a full cleft between P2 and P3 in 3D TEE MV (*arrow*), depth of cleft is more than 50% of the leaflet.

deformation. Software is available to process the temporal and spatial data, and by tracking the speckles, 2D tissue velocity, strain, and strain rate imaging may be calculated. This procedure, unlike Doppler measurement of strain, is not angle dependent. 2D strain can be applied to both ventricles and atria.

Global longitudinal strain is the average of the segmental strain in three apical views (apical four-, two-, and three-chamber views) (Fig. 5.23).

## STUDY OF THE CARDIAC CHAMBERS

By agreement, most research laboratories report the size of the LV, aortic root, and LA from the measurement of the linear dimensions of any structure in the parasternal long axis view. All linear dimensions have been revealed to bear a direct linear relation to body height. Normal chamber dimensions have also been defined for each of the standard 2D views to permit the quantitative evaluation of each chamber or great vessel from any view.

### Left Ventricular Volume

There are a number of modalities for calculating LV volume from 2D echocardiographic images that need the assumption of a geometric shape of the LV. The ellipsoid formula requires the measurement of the length of the LV and its diameter at the base. This volume approximation is valid in normal LVs (symmetric LVs); however, it is less reliable when there is an alteration of LV shape [e.g., after myocardial infarction (MI)]. The Simpson rule necessitates the measurement of the length of the LV from the apical views and then the definition of the volume of a predefined number of disks like cross-sectional segments from base to apex.

Three-dimensional volume measurement makes no geometric assumptions and may thus define the volume of both normal and distorted LVs[27–33] (Table 5.5).

### Left Ventricular Systolic Function

From 2D images, real-time echocardiographic evaluation of endocardial motion and the grade of wall thickening during systole permit an outstanding qualitative

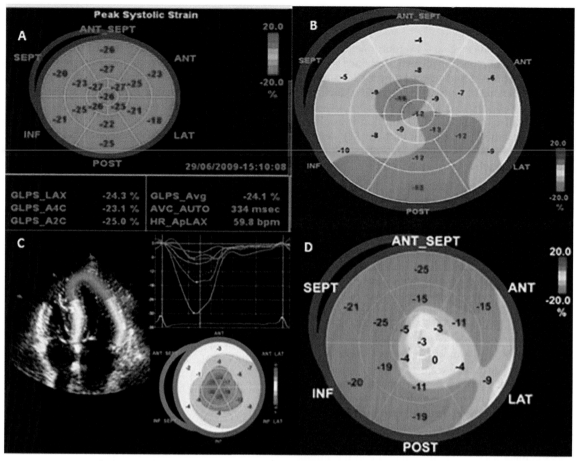

FIG. 5.23 Global longitudinal strain. (A) Normal individual with GLS −24%. (B) Hypertrophic cardiomyopathy with global 2D strain of −9.8%. (C) Amyloidosis with preserved red 2D color strain in apical segments. (D) Apical HCM with reduced 2D strain in apical segments and GLS −15.8%.

TABLE 5.5
Normal Values for Two-Dimensional Echocardiographic of Left Ventricular Size and Function

| Parameter | MALE | | FEMALE | |
|---|---|---|---|---|
| | Mean ± SD | 2-SD Range | Mean ± SD | 2-SD Range |
| **LV INTERNAL DIMENSION** | | | | |
| Diastolic dimension (mm) | 50.2 ± 4.1 | 42.0–58.4 | 45.0 ± 3.6 | 37.8–52.2 |
| Systolic dimension (mm) | 32.4 ± 3.7 | 25.0–39.8 | 28.2 ± 3.3 | 21.6–34.8 |
| **LV VOLUMES (BIPLANE)** | | | | |
| LV EDV (mL) | 106 ± 22 | 62–150 | 76 ± 15 | 46–106 |
| LV ESV (mL) | 41 ± 10 | 21–61 | 28 ± 7 | 14–42 |
| **LV VOLUME NORMALIZED BY BSA** | | | | |
| LV EDV (mL/m$^2$) | 54 ± 10 | 34–74 | 45 ± 8 | 29–61 |
| LV ESV (mL/m$^2$) | 21 ± 5 | 11–31 | 16 ± 4 | 8–24 |
| LV EF (biplane) | 62 ± 5 | 52–72 | 64 ± 5 | 54–74 |

BSA, body surface area; EDV, end-diastolic volume; EF, ejection fraction; ESV, end-systolic volume; LV, left ventricular; SD, standard deviation.
Modified from Lang RM, Badano LP, Mor-Avi V, et al. Recommendations for cardiac chamber quantification: a report from the American Society of Echocardiography and the European Association of Cardiovascular Imaging. J Am Soc Echocardiogr. 2015;28:1–39, with permission.

study of global and regional LV function. Using this technique, systolic function might be explained as either normal or depressed, and regional function for any segment is hyperkinetic, normal, hypokinetic, akinetic, or dyskinetic.

Quantitative evaluation of LV function is available by estimating the global ejection fraction (EF), defined by calculating the change in the volume of the LV among diastole and systole.

$$EF = \frac{(EDV - ESV)}{EDV}$$

The simplest way of estimating EF is to assume that the change in area at the base of the LV is demonstrative of global LV function. In this method, LVIDD is the internal diameter of the base of the LV in diastole, and LVISD is the internal diameter of the LV in systole.

Because this formula fails to describe apical function, 10% is empirically added if function at the apex is normal, 5% is added if the apex is hypokinetic, and 5%–10% is deducted if the apex is dyskinetic.

The Simpson rule mostly provides a more precise estimate of EF because it removes some of the assumptions about LV geometry. With present echocardiographic equipment, online and offline measurement skills provide an easy access to this quantitative method. To do the Simpson rule calculation, outline the full LV contour from the apical view in diastole. The automated measurement package will then draw a midline among the ventricular apex and the midpoint of the mitral annular plane and divide the LV into a series of small parallel disks of equal distances, which run perpendicular to the midline. Because the radius and the height of each disk are known, the volume of each disk may be calculated. Summing the volume of each disk permits the calculation of the diastolic LV volume. The same method is repeated for end-systolic LV volume, and EF is calculated as the difference in volume from diastole to systole, divided by the diastolic volume. The main limitation in this way is the inability to image the complete endocardial surface or the true length of the LV in some cases. The accuracy may be improved by using the biplane Simpson method, which averages the estimates of LV volume, acquired in orthogonal planes from apical four- and two-chamber views.

Two-dimensional echocardiographic estimates of EF make a number of expectations about LV shape; they are most useful in normal and symmetrically dilated LVs. The application of 3D technology may overcome the problems of estimating left ventricular ejection fraction (LVEF) in distorted and deformed ventricles. The product of SV and heart rate (HR) then gives an estimate of CO.

Although CO may be determined from the mitral, tricuspid, or pulmonary transvalvular flows, the AV diameter and flow velocities are the most precise. In clinical practice, mistakes in the measurement of the area of LVOT limit the use of the Doppler estimates of CO. This method is successful, however, in following relative changes in CO after pharmacologic intervention because the area of LVOT is presumed to remain constant.[1–4,28]

## Left Ventricular Diastolic Function

The impairment of LV diastolic filling has been progressively recognized as a clinical problem, either in connection with systolic dysfunction or as an isolated object. 2D echocardiography assesses LV size, volume, EF, and hypertrophy. The existence of an enlarged LA is found in more than 90% of cases with diastolic dysfunction. The echocardiographic Doppler valuation of LV filling properties includes trans-MV velocity and pulmonary vein flow characterization. The measurements of peak early (E) and late (A) diastolic flow velocities, isovolumic relaxation time, and deceleration time of early diastolic filling are all valuable measures of diastolic function. They are, however, limited by reduced accuracy in the detection of high LA pressure in cases with normal EF or left ventricular hypertrophy (LVH).

Essentially, flow propagation velocity by color M-mode and diastolic myocardial velocity by TDI (Ea) are the measurements of diastolic function that are independent of the effects of preload. Flow propagation velocity relates in reverse with the time constant of LV relaxation. Nevertheless, it may be difficult to measure and is thus less reproducible and might give erroneous results in patients with concentric LVH, small LV cavity, or high filling pressures.

Annular velocity by tissue Doppler is an index of myocardial relaxation, and multiple studies have revealed the ratio of trans-MV and E velocity to annular velocity. Em relates well with mean pulmonary capillary wedge pressure. Nonetheless, it is a regional index and may vary among sampling sites and in cases with abnormal regional wall motion (RWM). In addition, all diastology quantification measurements are not applicable for cases not in sinus rhythm or for patients who have inflow obstruction such as mitral stenosis (MS) and prosthetic valves.[1–4]

## Left Atrium

In subjects with normal EF, four parameters should be evaluated for diastolic dysfunction:

1. Annular e′ velocity (septal e′ <7 cm/s)
2. Average E/e′ >14 (lateral E/e′ >13 or septal E/e′ >15)
3. Peak TR jet velocity >2.8 m/s
4. Indexed LA volume >34 mL/m$^2$

If less than two parameters meet the cutoff values there is no diastolic dysfunction and if more than two of them meet the cut of values, diastolic dysfunction is present.

The left atrial appendage (LAA) is a "dog ear"-shaped extension of the LA located along the lateral aspect of the chamber near the MV annulus. Decisive imaging of the LAA is typically done with TEE for the most precise imaging of thrombi. It is essential to understand that the LAA is a trabeculated structure. These trabeculae may be confused with thrombi, which might form within the LAA.[1–5]

### Right Ventricle

The RV has been divided into inflow, apex, and outflow parts. The RV generally has a crescentic shape when imaged in the short axis, with its medial border made from the convexity of the interventricular septum (IVS). The lateral or free wall of the RV typically has a radius of curvature almost equal to the LV free wall. Because of the complex shape and anatomy of the RV, it is less agreeable to geometric modeling than the LV. Indeed, the accurate evaluation of RV volume and function is challenging by 2D echocardiography, and 3D echocardiography has been suggested to be more accurate and reproducible than 2D TTE.

Right ventricular enlargement may happen as a result of RV volume loading or RV infarction or as part of a general cardiomyopathic process. As dilatation progresses, the AP dimension of the RV increases, and IVS motion becomes progressively abnormal. Particularly in diastole, the IVS might appear to flatten—especially at the base—and in early systole, the IVS may move rightward rather than leftward (paradoxically) (Table 5.6).

Nevertheless, the pressure loading of the RV results in progressive hypertrophy. This might be problematic to distinguish with high confidence because of the degree of trabeculation of the RV chamber. An RV free wall thickness greater than 5 mm is a quantifiable criterion for RV hypertrophy. Marked pressure overload typically yields systolic flattening of the IVS.[1–4,28]

### Right Atrium

Study of RA size is typically made qualitatively by comparing it with the LA in the apical four-chamber view

**TABLE 5.6**
Normal Values for the Right Ventricle

| Parameter | Mean ± SD | Normal Range |
|---|---|---|
| RV basal diameter (mm) | 33 ± 4 | 25–41 |
| RV mid diameter (mm) | 27 ± 4 | 19–35 |
| RV longitudinal diameter (mm) | 71 ± 6 | 59–38 |
| RVOT PLAX diameter (mm) | 25 ± 2.5 | 20–30 |
| RVOT proximal diameter (mm) | 28 ± 3.5 | 21–35 |
| RVOT distal diameter (mm) | 22 ± 2.5 | 17–27 |
| RV wall thickness (mm) | 3 ± 1 | 1–5 |

*EDA*, end-diastolic area; *ESA*, end-systolic area; *PLAX*, parasternal, long axis view; *RVOT*, right ventricular outflow tract.
Modified from Lang RM, Badano LP, Mor-Avi V, et al. Recommendations for cardiac chamber quantification: a report from the American Society of Echocardiography and the European Association of Cardiovascular Imaging. *J Am Soc Echocardiogr.* 2015;28:1–39, with permission.

and quantitatively by measuring the maximal mediolateral and superoinferior dimensions in this window. The normal range of RA minor axis dimension is $1.9 ± 0.3$ cm/m$^2$ in male and female patients. There are some normal structures within the RA. These contain the eustachian valve, which crosses from the IVC to the region of the foramen ovale, and the crista terminalis. In the apical four-chamber view, the crista might be seen as a ridge of tissue that divides the smooth-walled part of the RA from its trabeculated anterior portion, frequently noted as a small mass located adjacent to the superior border of the RA. The RA appendage is a broad-based triangular structure that lies anterior to the atrial chamber close to the ascending aorta. It is most noticeable in the parasternal views of the RA and readily imaged by TEE.[1–4,29–34]

## STUDY OF VALVULAR HEART DISEASE
### Mitral Valve Disease
#### Mitral stenosis
TTE and TEE assist with the diagnosis and timing of intervention for MS by providing a precise valuation of valve morphology, valve area, and degree of pulmonary artery hypertension (PAH).

Acquired MS is unvaryingly caused by the scarring and inflammation of the MV and the chordal apparatus from past rheumatic fever. As a result of the disease, MV leaflets and chordal apparatus become diffusely thickened and jagged. Consequently, the valvular apparatus might shorten, fusing at the commissural margins, and finally harden and calcify. This results in a lessening in leaflet excursion so that MV leaflets appear dome shaped in diastole. As the degree of valvular obstruction progresses, the flow through the valve reduces, LA pressure begins to rise, LA size increases, and the potential for LA clot formation is increased. Characteristically, LV size is normal or even small. If there is severe MS, there may be paradoxic motion of the IVS as a result of slow ventricular filling. Furthermore, if there is PAH, the right cardiac chambers and the pulmonary arteries might dilate, and there may be severe TR. Almost all of these morphologic features are evident from the parasternal long axis view of the heart, but parasternal short axis images are crucial for the planimetry of MV stenotic orifice.

Echocardiographic classification of the MS is possible by evaluating the degree of leaflet thickening, calcification, anterior leaflet mobility, and degree of chordal shortening and thickening. When scientifically graded, a low value of 1 to a high value of 4 is given for each of these features. It is then possible to derive a numeric "score" that defines the extent of the MV disease. This system is useful in predicting the likelihood of the successful balloon dilatation of the valve, with scores greater than 8 predicting a poor outcome after percutaneous dilatation.

The direct planimetry of the valve orifice in the short axis plane of 2D echocardiography may provide a precise measurement of MV orifice area. 3D echocardiography may augment the accuracy of detecting the smallest MV orifice by providing perpendicular en face views in the multiple axis views of the MV orifice (Fig. 5.24).

Continuous-wave Doppler may help assess the severity of MS because it enables the calculation of peak and mean trans-MV pressure gradients in conjunction with MV area. For this purpose, the apical four-chamber view is desirable in that the Doppler beam may be directed through the MV plane, just parallel to the direction of LV inflow.

In contrast to the Doppler profile through a normal MV, the CW Doppler signal in cases with MS proves an increased velocity of the flow in early diastole, with a prolonged descent of the early filling wave (deceleration time). The degree of the prolongation of the phase of early filling associates directly to MV area and to the severity of MS. By the CW Doppler profile, it is possible to compute the trans-MV gradient by converting the velocity data into an estimate of pressure using the simplified Bernoulli equation. The Bernoulli formula states that the velocity (V) of the flow through a stenosis relates to the pressure gradient difference (P) across the stenosis. Precisely, the simplified Bernoulli equation forecasts that the pressure gradient across a valve approaches a value four times the square of the velocity of the flow across the valve ($P = 4V^2$). Knowing the peak velocity of the flow across the MV enables the calculation of the peak pressure gradient across the valve. Likewise, the average of the velocities throughout diastole yields the mean pressure gradient. Most echocardiographic equipment contains software that may spontaneously integrate the velocity profile contour after it is traced and determine the mean gradient using the Bernoulli equation. The Doppler estimates of MV area rely on the observation that the degree of the elongation of early filling relates directly to the grade of MS. The measurement of this is possible by calculating the time for the pressure gradient across the MV to decrease to half its max value, "pressure half-time" (PHT). PHT is achieved from the CW Doppler profile by defining velocity half-time, measuring the time interval among peak trans-MV velocity and the point where trans-MV velocity has dropped to half its peak value. In normal subjects, PHT is less than 60 ms. In contrast, in cases with MS, PHT is typically in excess of 200 ms, with higher values in cases with more severe disease. An empiric formula that relates PHT to MV orifice area is as follows: area = 220/PHT.[4,5,18,21,28]

### Mitral regurgitation

**Rheumatic mitral regurgitation.** Although the incidence of rheumatic MR is declining, the disease is still prevalent in older patients. Characteristically, the echocardiogram confirms MV leaflets and chordal thickening in relation with AV disease. As the rheumatic disease progresses and the leaflets become thicker and less mobile, MS might also be evident. In these cases, echocardiography is most beneficial in determining whether the valve is mainly stenotic or incompetent.

### Myxomatous mitral valve prolapse

Mitral valve prolapse (MVP) is a degenerative disease that principally affects the collagen of MV leaflets and chordae; still, it might also affect the AV and TV. Although it is frequently diagnosed clinically by the existence of a systolic murmur or click, echocardiography is often used to confirm the diagnosis. In

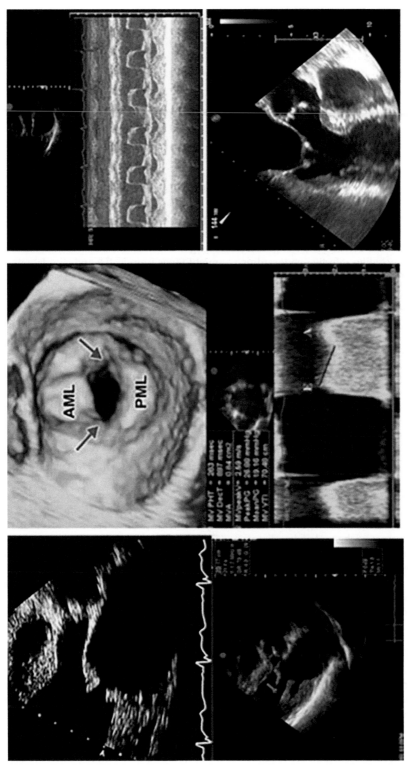

FIG. 5.24 *Left upper:* Thickened and dome-shaped mitral leaflets in 2D TTE, *middle upper:* bicommissural fusion in 3D TEE. *Right upper:* M-mode study showing thickened mitral leaflets with concomitant anterior and posterior motion in diastole. *Right lower:* Subvalve thickening in parasternal long axis view (*arrow*), *lower middle:* mitral valve area by pressure half-time method. *Right lower:* Rheumatic involvement of mitral and aortic valve in TEE.

echocardiography, MVP is suggested by the superior displacement of one or both MV leaflets into the LA during systole. Because of the complex saddle shape of the MV annulus, minor degrees of the superior movement of the anterior leaflet may normally be recorded from the apical four-chamber view. Consequently, the diagnosis of MVP must only be made when the long axis views (parasternal or apical long axis) display leaflet displacement. Color flow characteristically shows an eccentric regurgitation jet in the opposite direction to the leaflet that is prolapsed. In cases with more progressive disease, there is also evidence of leaflet thickening, which relates to the manifestation of the significant myxomatous infiltration of the valve. There might also be redundant or ruptured chordae. Definitely, patients with marked displacement, thickening, and irregularity of the leaflets are more likely to have severe MR and to be at greatest risk of complications, including infective endocarditis (IE). As in any patient with MR, LA size increases with the increasing severity of the regurgitant lesion, and LA size may act as an index of the severity and duration of MR. LV size may be normal or dilated. Systolic function is characteristically hyperdynamic in cases with primary compensated valvular MR. Although no single echocardiographic index yet precisely predicts the correct timing of MV surgery in cases with primary chronic valvular MR, those with an LV end-systolic diameter larger than 40 mm tend to have less recovery of LV function after surgery.

### Flail mitral leaflet
Complete or partial disruption of the support of one or both MV leaflets typically presents abruptly with the development of a new murmur or even acute pulmonary edema. In either setting, the echocardiogram in association with the clinical picture might provide a direct insight into the nature of the underlying disease process. Definitely, the echocardiogram may prove the systolic prolapse of the whole leaflet into the LA and significant MR by color Doppler flow. A flail leaflet is caused by IE, fundamental myxomatous MV disease (MVP), or papillary muscle rupture in relation with acute MI.

### Mitral annular calcification
Mitral annular calcification is common in older adults. It initiates as a focal process, affecting the posterior part of the annular ring, and then spreads laterally and anteriorly. As the process progresses, the base of MV leaflets and the chordal apparatus thicken and calcify. This impairs the normal mechanism of coaptation, leading to MR. It might also result in the restriction of MV inflow

with the development of a small trans-MV gradient. Although mitral annular calcification is visible in nearly any view, the parasternal short axis image at the base of the heart is the most valuable view for determining the circumferential extension of the disease.

### Functional mitral regurgitation
In some cases, the MV might appear morphologically normal when it is clearly incompetent, as evidenced by clinical or echocardiographic signs of moderate to severe MR. In these cases, the MR is caused by the abnormal and incomplete coaptation of MV leaflets caused by either annular dilatation or papillary muscle dysfunction. In both instances, the pattern of leaflet closure appears abnormal in the parasternal and apical views; MV leaflets appear to coapt only at their tips rather than along the distal third of the leaflet. The appearance might range from leaflet and chordal tethering to complete failure of coaptation. There is frequently associated LV dilatation and global or RWMA.

### Evaluation of mitral regurgitation
Color Doppler readily demonstrates MR. Regurgitant jets usually appear as a localized stream of flow emerging from the valve leaflets at valve closure and then expand into the distal chamber. From most sampling windows, the jets of MR are chiefly blue because they are directed away from the transducer. The introduction of yellow and green in the color-flow map specifies a high-velocity turbulent flow and results in a pattern referred to as "mosaic." Regurgitant flow typically initiates at the peak of the R wave on the electrocardiogram (ECG) and continues throughout systole. The peak velocity of these jets reflects the atrioventricular gradient, which may be calculated using the simplified PISA equation (explained earlier). Accordingly, the CW Doppler signal in cases with MR typically has a peak velocity of about 5 m/s, reflecting a peak atrioventricular gradient of 100 mmHg.

The semiquantitative evaluation of the severity of MR includes the integration of many 2D echocardiographic and Doppler-derived variables. First, it is helpful to consider the appearance of the valve leaflets, chordae, and pattern of leaflet coaptation. With this initial valuation, it is possible to gain a sense of whether the amount of regurgitation might be mild, moderate, or severe. In other words, it is not likely with a normal valvular structure, apparatus, and pattern of coaptation to have more than mild regurgitation. However, it is highly likely that with a flail or partially flail leaflet, there will be moderate to severe MR. After the valuation of valve morphology and the arrangement of coaptation, color

Doppler signals yield an additional insight into the amount and degree of regurgitation. Color-flow Doppler provides a color map of the net immediate velocity of the blood flow within the LA at varying time points during systole. From this map, it is possible to determine the size (area, length, and width at the orifice) and the direction (central or eccentric) of the MR regurgitant jet.

The descriptors of the jet size, mainly the size of the proximal jet at the vena contracta, relate to the angiographic amount of MR. Many factors affect the precise valuation of the degree of regurgitation. In other words, changes either in the gain or the pulse repetition frequency of the Doppler system may alter the relationship among the jet size and the degree of MR, resulting in either a false increase or decrease in the jet size (mostly jet length and area). In addition, the detection of the regurgitant jet might not be possible in all cases, such as in patients with prosthetic valves that block out or

reflect the Doppler signal and forbid its passage into the LA. Last, the association among the jet size and the severity of MR might be underestimated if the jet is directed eccentrically alongside the LA wall, as often happens with more significant regurgitation. In an effort to overcome some of the limitations related to the analysis of the distal jet, researchers have analyzed the size of the converging flow stream proximal to the valve (e.g., on the ventricular side of the MV). The analysis of the size of this proximal isovelocity surface area (PISA) provides a precise valuation of the regurgitant flow rate; however, it needs cautious technical manipulation and high-quality imaging to record a PISA that may be correctly measured (Fig. 5.25). Flow reversal in the pulmonary veins by PW Doppler offers further evidence that the degree of MR is likely to be severe. Because the LA bears the burden of chronic regurgitation, evaluation of LA size might also be valuable in defining its severity and chronicity. Nonetheless, because other parameters

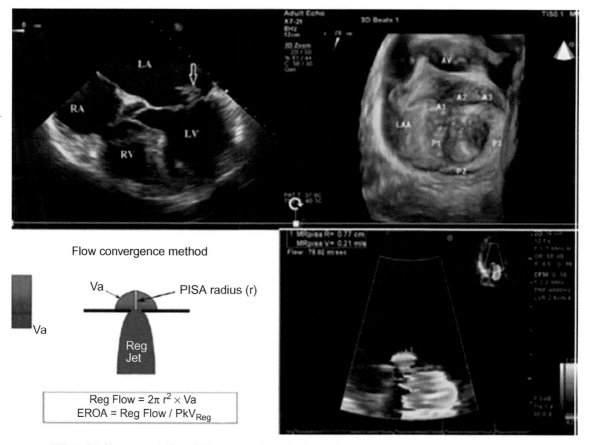

FIG. 5.25 *Upper panel*: 2D and 3D transesophageal echocardiography showing flail P2 scallop of the mitral valve. *Lower panel* shows proximal isovelocity surface area (PISA) formula.

such as AF and LV end-diastolic pressure might also influence LA size, the chamber size alone might be a deceptive marker of the severity of MR.[4–9,17,20,24,28]

## Aortic Valve Disease

### Aortic stenosis

The three fundamental features of AS are (1) leaflet deformity, thickening, and calcification; (2) reduced mobility; and (3) an absolute diminution in the size of the AV orifice resulting from decreased cusp separation. AS might be acquired or congenital. In congenital AS, the AV might be unicuspid; bicuspid; or infrequently, quadricuspid. Precise characterization is possible by imaging the AV in the short axis view to define the number of cusps and commissures. Although bicuspid valves are naturally stenotic, they might also dispose to significant AR. The identification of a bicuspid valve might be hard in older patients if the AV is significantly calcified.

Nothing like congenital AV disease, which often presents in the fourth decade of life, acquired calcific AS presents in the sixth or seventh decade. Classically, the AV is thickened and calcified and with decreased cusp separation. The finding of some residual leaflet motion commonly indicates that aortic valve area (AVA) is greater than $0.6 \text{ cm}^2$. None of the typical features of AS are essentially specific for the diagnosis of hemodynamically essential AS. Leaflet thickening is common in older adults, but it is seldom associated with significant stenosis. Although reduced cusp separation and the mobility of the leaflets are more specific and valuable for hemodynamically significant AS, this might also happen in cases with a low CO. The direct measurement of AV orifice is seldom precise by TTE; however, the direct planimetry of AVA from TEE may provide a precise and correct estimate in patients with a normal LV function and CO.

Essentially, in most patients with significant AS, LV size and function are usually normal; however, LVH is frequently apparent.

A precise valuation of the degree of AV stenosis is frequently possible using CW Doppler, which permits the estimation of the peak and mean AV gradients and AVA. To determine the peak and mean gradients across the valve, you must first obtain precise profiles of the flow originating from the valve, frequently from apical windows. It is also essential to interrogate the flow through the valve from the right parasternal window because the deformation of AV leaflets might eccentrically direct the jet of the blood flow toward the right sternal border as it enters the aorta. The typical CW Doppler profile of AS begins after the R wave on the ECG and is not holosystolic. Noting the time of the onset and the duration of the flow helps to discriminate the AS profile from the CW Doppler profile of the MR flow. The application of the Bernoulli equation to the CW Doppler interrogation of the transvalvular flow provides precise measures of the mean and peak instant gradients in AS. Classically, the simplified form of the formula ($\Delta P = 4V^2$) may be used. However, when LVOT velocity exceeds 1 m/s, the expanded version—$\Delta P = 4\,(V2^2 - V1^2)$, where $V^2$ is transaortic velocity and $V^1$ is LVOT velocity—must be used.

In recognition of the importance of recording Doppler signals parallel to the flow, AV gradients are best recorded from the apical five- or three-chamber, suprasternal notch, and right parasternal views. Generally, the highest velocities are found on the right parasternal window. The smaller footprint, provided by the nonimaging Pedoff probe, makes it crucial for the optimal valuation of cases with AS. When TEE is used, velocities are recorded from the deep transgastric views. It must be noted that although echocardiographically derived mean gradients are generally identical to those achieved invasively, the echocardiographically derivative peak instantaneous gradient is classically higher than the peak-to-peak gradient calculated in the catheterization laboratory.

Gradients alone might underestimate severity in the setting of low-flow states and overestimate severity when flow is higher (e.g., high-output states such as those caused by sepsis and anemia). For this reason, it is essential to define the AVA. Direct planimetry of TEE images might be used for this purpose, but TTE planimetry is not adequately precise. Therefore, the most common approach is by the application of the continuity equation. AVA is calculated as

$$AVA = \frac{(\text{CSA LVOT} \times \text{VTI LVOT})}{\text{VTI AV}}$$

Less desirable is the simplified version

$$AVA = \frac{(\text{CSA LVOT} \times \text{V LVOT})}{\text{“V” AV}}$$

where V predicates peak velocity. The CSA of LVOT is classically calculated by assuming a circular geometry with the equation $CSA = \pi\,(D/2)2$, where D is the systolic LVOT diameter measured on the parasternal long axis view of TTE or TEE-equivalent long axis view just proximal to AV annulus. It must be noted that because LVOT velocity incorporated into the calculation is the modal velocity, displayed as the densest part of the PW Doppler envelope, the velocity time integral (VTI) must not be traced by using the outer edge of the flow spectrum.

Ideal sample volume placement is in LVOT characteristically 1–2 mm proximal to the AV on the apical five- or three-chamber views (TTE) or in deep transgastric (TEE) views.[4–9,11,23,28]

### Low-gradient severe aortic stenosis

When there is a reduced stroke volume caused by significant LV systolic dysfunction, the measured effective orifice area (EOA) might be small despite low gradients, and it becomes essential to define whether the valve obstruction is really fixed (severe AS) or the valve is basically capable of opening more completely at higher flow rates (pseudo-severe AS). Also, dobutamine stress echocardiography is usually used in this setting to evaluate the true AVA and LV contractile reserve.

The ERO might also be severely reduced despite low gradients when LVEF is within the normal range. However, stroke volume is reduced, so-called paradoxic low-gradient preserved EF severe AS.

### Subvalvular aortic stenosis

The CW Doppler echocardiographic calculation of peak and mean pressure gradients is the cornerstone in assessing patients with LVOT obstruction below the AV. However, in regard to the site of flow acceleration, color Doppler might provide a clue that the obstruction is not at the level of the valve and more detailed imaging evaluation is essential to clarify the pathophysiology. In some patients, evaluation is complicated by the existence of obstruction at multiple levels. In such patients, it might be impossible to exactly delineate the gradients created at each level of obstruction.[4–9,11,23,26,28]

### Aortic regurgitation

Aortic regurgitation might result from abnormalities in the cusps of the valve, normal cusps whose coaptation is altered because of enlargement of the annulus or sinuses or, infrequently, prolapse of a dissection flap through the AV. TTE and TEE will establish a causative diagnosis and characteristically demonstrate LV end-diastolic enlargement if the AR is hemodynamically essential. The high-frequency fluttering of anterior MV leaflet, caused by the impact of the regurgitant jet on M-mode, and in cases of acute severe AR, the premature closure of the MV caused by a rise in LV pressure greater than the LA pressure are seen.

Color jet dimensions must be measured with the Nyquist settings in 50–60 cm/s. The best dimensional predictors of severity are jet area indexed to AV short axis area in the parasternal short axis view and jet diameter indexed to the LVOT diameter closely proximal to the valve in the parasternal long axis view. Jet length is not a good index of severity. PHT reflects the rate at which AV and LV pressures become equal and is most reliable in the setting of acute AR.

Vena contracta is the smallest diameter of the AI flow jet at the level of the valve measured in zoom mode in a parasternal long axis view or TEE-equivalent 120-degree view. Holodiastolic flow reversal in the proximal part of the descending thoracic aorta, as detected with the PW sample volume placed near the origin of the left subclavian artery, is a good marker of at least moderate aortic insufficiency (AI). The reversal flow of the abdominal aorta mostly reflects severe AI (Fig. 5.26). Although the PISA approach, which is broadly drawn on to evaluate the severity of MR and TR, has likely been used to calculate effective regurgitant orifice area and regurgitant volume for AR, it might be challenging to exactly measure the PISA radius when merely mild regurgitation is present (mainly with TTE). The quantitative Doppler approach, which determines regurgitant volume by matching the flow through LVOT with that across a competent nonstenotic valve, is strongest when the PV is used as the reference for normal flow (because

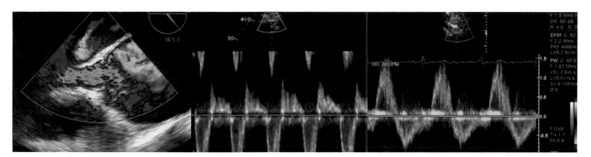

FIG. 5.26 *Left*: Severe aortic regurgitation associated with aortic root dilatation. *Middle*: Holodiastolic flow reversal in thoracic descending aorta. *Right*: Holodiastolic flow reversal in the abdominal aorta in severe aortic regurgitation.

of image quality). The MV may hypothetically be used as the reference; nonetheless, it is more geometrically complex and hence more susceptible to error.[4–9,23,28]

## Tricuspid Valve Disease

Tricuspid regurgitation might happen as a consequence of the abnormal development of the TV (Ebstein anomaly), disease affecting the valve leaflets or the chordal apparatus (myxomatous, degenerative, and endocarditis), or annulus dilatation (caused by RV dilatation). The evaluation of the degree of TR is very similar to that for MR. However, the peak velocity of the regurgitant flow through the TV is commonly 2.5 m/s, replicating a peak systolic gradient of 25 mmHg among the RV and RA. Ebstein anomaly is a congenital heart disease (CHD) characterized by the elongation and tethering of the anterior leaflet of the TV to RV endocardium. The septal and posterior leaflet origins are displaced apically, reducing the functional RV size, and the basal portion of the RV is atrialized. Ebstein anomaly may be diagnosed from the apical four-chamber view. In patients with Ebstein anomaly, the septal leaflet of the TV is more than 1 cm ($0.8 \text{ mm/m}^2$) apical to the MV. In most cases, TR is moderate to severe as evaluated by Doppler. Furthermore, color Doppler might detect some degree of right-to-left interatrial shunt flow through either a PFO or an ASD. TS most often occurs as a consequence of rheumatic fever, in which case it constantly occurs with MV or AV disease. More seldom, TS occurs with metastatic carcinoid tumors. In both instances, the leaflets and chordae appear thickened; the valve domes during diastole; and as a result of the stenosis, there is an increase in RA size.[4–9,28]

## Pulmonary Valve Disease

The PV is best imaged in the parasternal short axis view, although subcostal windows are also helpful in children. Cases with rheumatic heart disease might have thickening of the PV; however, significant PS is rare. By far the most common cause of PS is congenital deformity of the valve. This might occur in isolation or in relationship with other defects [e.g., tetralogy of Fallot (ToF)]. Characteristically, the valve appears mobile, but the leaflets dome during systole. In routine practice, CW Doppler is used to evaluate the peak velocity across the valve because this permits peak and mean transvalvular gradient calculation by the modified Bernoulli formula. This is often associated with the poststenotic dilatation of the proximal part of the main PA. In addition, the RV appears hypertrophied, and the IVS flattens in systole as a result of the increased pressure load. Color Doppler normally shows some degree of PR. More

marked degrees of PR occur with PAH, primary valve disease, congenital absence of the PV, or after pulmonary valvotomy. For clinical purposes, the degree of regurgitation is classified semiquantitatively based on the width and length of the regurgitant jet.[4–9,28]

## Prosthetic Heart Valves

Prosthetic heart valves might be either bioprosthetic or mechanical. Bioprosthetic valves might be heterografts from bovine or pig valves or the pericardium or homografts derived from human aorta or PA. Some bioprosthetic valves are supported by three struts that attach to a valve ring; others are strutless using the native valve leaflets and annulus.

The mechanical valve design is more diverse. Some older devices have a ball-in-cage design, and others have either a single or a double tilting disk. Owing to the variable and different nature of these prostheses, it is often possible to determine the particular type of prosthesis by echocardiography. Although surgical replacement of the heart valves has considerably improved outcome of patients with native valve disease, still there is a risk of life threatening malfunction in these patients. It is noteworthy to know that echocardiographic evaluation of prosthetic heart valves needs more knowledge and expertise comparing to the native valves assessment.

Not only correct diagnosis of the prosthetic valve malfunction is important, but also, mentioning the cause of PHV dysfunction has very important impact on proper treatment strategy.

Two-dimensional and Doppler echocardiography permit the valuation of the stability of the device, degree of the stenosis of the prosthesis, regurgitation through or around the valve, and vegetation or thrombus within or around the prosthesis. Poor seating of the prosthesis might occur as a result of paravalvular infection or wear of the sutures supporting the valve ring. As the valve seating becomes unstable, consistently there is some degree of paravalvular leakage. With this unsteadiness, the valve ring is seen to move independently during the cardiac cycle. Marked "rocking" of the prosthesis is a poor prognostic sign because it denotes that at least one third of the valve ring is unstable. CW Doppler may assess the gradient across the prosthesis in the same manner as for native valves.

- The Doppler pressure gradient might overestimate the catheter gradient through both the St. Jude tilting disk and Starr-Edwards valves up to 40%.
- Smaller prostheses will have higher gradients than larger prostheses of the same type.
- The gradient through an AV prosthesis is critically dependent on LV function.

So, to make a meaningful and precise statement about the importance of the Doppler gradient through a prosthesis, we need to consider the type, size, and location of the prosthetic valve as well as LV function. The detection of an essential increase in the gradient through a prosthesis is a critical clinical sign because it might indicate valve obstruction or partial occlusion. This might be the result of pannus ingrowth around the sewing ring or the existence of a large vegetation or thrombus within the prosthesis. To evaluate the importance of the degree of regurgitation through a prosthetic valve,

we must consider the type and the position of the prosthesis (Fig. 5.27). The type of prosthesis is of vital importance because bioprosthetic and Starr-Edwards valves do not usually leak. In contrast, the single-disk (Medtronic Hall) valve permits a small central leak, and the double-disk St. Jude Medical valve has small leakage, too (Fig. 5.28). Consequently, the detection of a small central jet of leakage is expected in cases with disk valves, is indicative of valve degeneration in a patient with a bioprosthetic valve, and might indicate either vegetation or pannus ingrowth around the valve

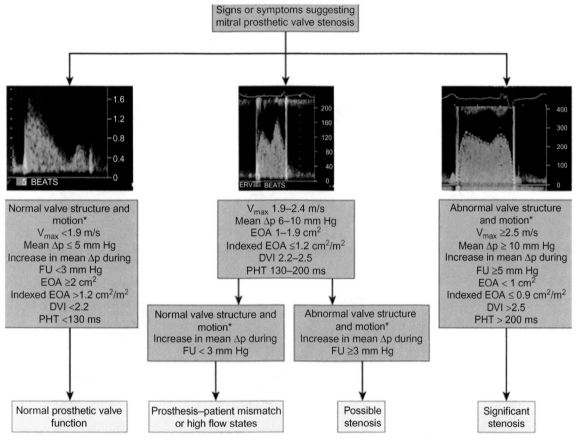

FIG. 5.27 Evaluation of mitral prosthetic valve stenosis starts with standard measures of stenosis severity, including maximal velocity ($V_{max}$; m/s, meters per second), mean pressure gradient (mean $\Delta p$), effective orifice area (EOA), and pressure half-time (PHT; ms, milliseconds); *FU*, follow-up. Doppler velocity index (DVI) is the ratio of mitral to left ventricular (LV) outflow tract velocity, and therefore a value greater than 2.2 is abnormal. Normal values for each valve type and size should be referenced, but the thresholds shown are a quick first step. In patients with intermediate measures of stenosis severity, the differential diagnosis includes significant stenosis, prosthesis–patient mismatch, and a high flow state. *Additional imaging, including transesophageal echocardiography, cinefluoroscopy, or computed tomography, may be needed to assess valve leaflet structure and motion. (Reproduced with permission from Zipes DP, Libby P, Bonow RO, Mann DL, Tomaselli GF. Braunwald's Heart Disease: A Textbook of Cardiovascular Medicine Internet. 11th ed. Elsevier Health Sciences; 2018, p. 1460 (chapter 71))

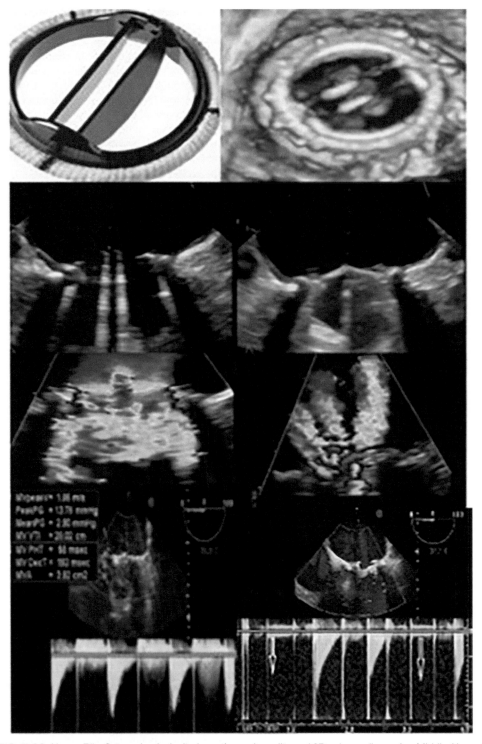

FIG. 5.28 *Upper*: Bileaflet mechanical mitral prostheses in reality and 3D echocardiography. *Middle*: Normal color Doppler flow in bileaflet mitral prostheses. *Lower*: *left*: Normal Doppler study of mitral prostheses. *Right*: Intermittent obstruction assessed by Doppler study.

ring in a Starr-Edwards valve. Irrespective of the valve type, a paravalvular leakage indicates the disruption of the valve ring as a result of the infection or wear of the valve sutures. Because regurgitant jets tend to be eccentric, they are easy to miss during a routine analysis. Although in some instances these problems may be overcome by imaging the heart in off-axis views, they may be totally overcome by using TEE because this permits a perfect view of both the valve and the LA[4-9,28,31] (Figs. 5.29 and 5.30).

Usually, 2D TTE is the first-line imaging modality when assessing PHV function.

2D TTE is useful method for diagnosis of the type of the heart valve prostheses and opening and closing motion of the occlude. Mechanical prostheses have their own specific echo patterns as in the monoleaflet prostheses: a single echo movement is seen going up and down and resulting in two major and minor orifices with a normal range of opening angle 60–80 degrees (which is the angle between the disk and the valve annulus). Besides the normal 2D and color-flow study of the prostheses, the normal function of prostheses should be confirmed by the normal Doppler parameters. Normal Doppler parameters for mitral prostheses are.

- MV peak E velocity <1.9 (m/s)
- MV mean gradient <6 mmHg
- PHT <100–130 ms
- VTI PrMV/VTI LVO ratio <2.2

In patients with suspected PHV dysfunction, 2D and 3D TOE are useful method. Distinguishing between thrombus and pannus as a cause of obstruction is important for proper management of these patients. Pannus is a highly echogenic immobile mass that happens late after valve implantation due to tissue ingrowth around the prostheses (Tables 5.7 and 5.8).

### Infective Endocarditis

Two-dimensional echocardiography is priceless in the valuation of patients with a clinical picture of IE.

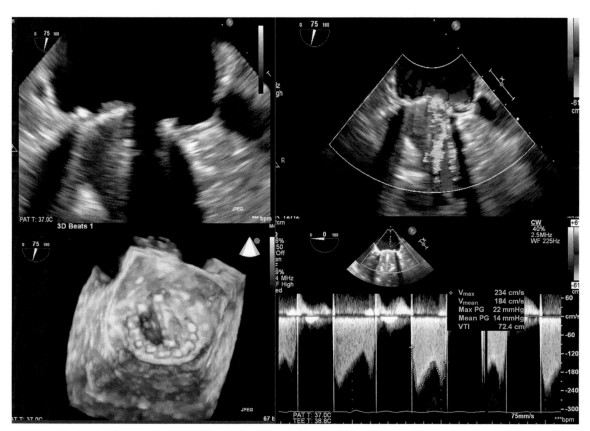

FIG. 5.29 Mitral prostheses malfunction by 2D, color Doppler, 3D, and Doppler study. Medial leaflet is stuck with no flow through it.

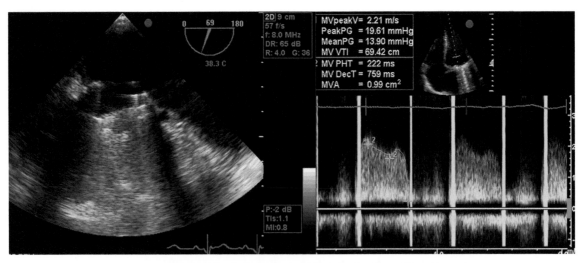

FIG. 5.30 Mono leaflet mitral prosthetic malfunction by 2D and Doppler study.

**TABLE 5.7**
**Doppler Parameters of Mitral Prostheses Function and Tricuspid Prostheses Function**

| Doppler parameters of mitral prostheses function | Normal[a] | Possible Stenosis[b] | Suggests Significant Stenosis[a,b] |
|---|---|---|---|
| Peak velocity (m/s)[c,d] | <1.9 | 1.9–2.5 | ≥2.5 |
| Mean gradient (mmHg)[c,d] | ≤5 | 6–10 | >10 |
| $VTI_{PrMv}/VTI_{LVO}$[c,d] | <2.2 | 2.2–2.5 | >2.5 |
| EOA (cm²) | ≥2.0 | 1–2 | <1 |
| PHT (ms) | <130 | 130–200 | >200 |

| Doppler parameters of tricuspid prostheses function | Consider Valve Stenosis[e] |
|---|---|
| Peak velocity[f] | >1.7 m/s |
| Mean gradient[f] | ≥6 mmHg |
| Pressure half-time | ≥230 ms |
| EOA and $VTI_{PrTV}/VTI_{LVO}$ | No data yet available for tricuspid prostheses |

*PHT*, pressure half-time; *PrMV*, prosthetic mitral valve; *PrTV*, prosthetic tricuspid valve.
[a]Best specificity for normality or abnormality is seen if the majority of the parameters listed are normal or abnormal, respectively.
[b]Values of the parameters should prompt a closer evaluation of valve function and/or other considerations such as increased flow, increased heart rate, or PPM.
[c]Slightly higher cutoff values may be seen in some bioprosthetic valves.
[d]These parameters are also abnormal in the presence of significant prosthetic MR.
[e]Because of respiratory variation, average ≥5 cycles.
[f]May be increased also with valvular regurgitation.
Modified from: Zoghbi WA, Chambers JB, Dumesnil JG, et al. Recommendations for evaluation of prosthetic valves with echocardiography and Doppler ultrasound. J Am Soc Echocardiogr. 2009;22(9):975–1014.

Whereas MV and TV vegetations are commonly on the atrial side of the valve, AV and PV vegetations tend to form on the ventricular surface. TEE also permits a precise valuation of vegetation morphology (size, mobility, and density), detection of the extravalvular extension of the infective course, and diagnosis of the degree of valvular dysfunction. Despite the clear value of TEE in the study of cases with suspected IE, the method may not

**TABLE 5.8**
Doppler Parameters of Prosthetic Aortic Valve Function in Mechanical and Stented Biologic Valves[a]

| Parameter | Normal | Possible Stenosis | Suggests Significant Stenosis |
|---|---|---|---|
| Peak velocity[b] (m/s) | <3 | 3–4 | >4 |
| Mean gradient[b] (mmHg) | <20 | 20–35 | >35 |
| DVI | ≥0.30 | 0.29–0.25 | <0.25 |
| EOA (cm²) | >1.2 | 1.2–0.8 | <0.8 |
| Contour of the jet velocity through the PrAV | Triangular, early peaking | Triangular to intermediate | Rounded, symmetrical contour |
| AT (ms) | <80 | 80–100 | >100 |

*PrAV*, prosthetic aortic valve.
[a]In conditions of normal or near normal stroke volume (50–70 mL) through the aortic valve.
[b]These parameters are more affected by flow, including concomitant AR.
Modified from: Zoghbi WA, Chambers JB, Dumesnil JG, et al. Recommendations for evaluation of prosthetic valves with echocardiography and Doppler ultrasound. J Am Soc Echocardiogr. 2009;22(9):975–1014.

exclude the diagnosis of IE with certainty for the following reasons. First, the vegetation might be too small to be revealed or may only be present as focal, nonspecific valvular thickening. Second, the differential diagnosis includes thrombi, tumors, fibrins, flail portions of the valve or chordae, old healed vegetations, or even aneurysm formations secondary to the IE process. Thus, it is crucial to correlate the echocardiographic findings with the clinical picture.[15,20,28,31]

## Ischemic Heart Disease

Because 2D echocardiography is noninvasive and has high spatial and temporal resolution, it is deemed the best tool for the valuation of serial changes in LV structure and function, which occur during LV myocardial ischemia and after MI. The hemodynamic situation, short- and long-term prognoses of the patient, and size of MI at autopsy also relate well with the echocardiographic site and the extent of MI. In addition, it is a valuable tool in the emergency setting to assist with the differential diagnosis of acute chest pain and in the early recognition of the acute mechanical complications of MI, including papillary muscle dysfunction and rupture, ventricular septal defect (VSD), and the late existence of apical aneurysms and thrombi.

## Regional Wall Motion Abnormalities

The echocardiographic valuation of RWMAs depends on the ability to consider both the grade of endocardial motion and the grade of myocardial thickening. The study of endocardial excursion is simple, but sometimes it might be misleading in the existence of noncardiac

motion (e.g., rotation and translation). Nevertheless, the valuation of myocardial thickening might be limited if the picturing of the epicardial and endocardial lines is inadequate. RWMA is most frequently defined qualitatively as being normal, hypokinetic (moving in the proper direction but at a slower than normal), akinetic (not moving), or dyskinetic (moving outward in systole). The Cardiac Imaging Committee of the American Heart Association has suggested a system with 17 segments to standardize echocardiographic segmental study with that of other cardiac imaging techniques.

## Acute Complications of Myocardial Infarction

The acute mechanical complications of MI, including papillary muscle rupture and VSD, are most common after large inferoposterior and inferoseptal MIs. Clinically, both situations present with a sudden deterioration in hemodynamic status and the creation of a new pansystolic murmur. In cases with papillary muscle rupture, one or the other MV leaflet becomes flail, and the head of the ruptured papillary muscle prolapses into the LA with each cardiac cycle. Furthermore, as a result of the acute onset of MR, the noninfarcted myocardium is hyperdynamic, and color flow confirms a large, frequently eccentric jet MR into a normal or slightly dilated LA. In cases with acute VSD, color Doppler may help exactly locate the VSD. CW Doppler may determine the peak velocity and gradient of the interventricular shunt flow. From these data, PA pressure may be estimated. The rupture of the free wall of the LV, which might occur even after small infarctions, is most often rapidly fatal as a result of acute tamponade. In some instances, however, pericardial adhesions may limit the extent of pericardial bleeding and lead to a localized pseudoaneurysm. In contrast, true aneurysms frequently form after large MIs affecting either the anterior or septal wall, or less frequently, the inferior base of the heart. Aneurysms are typically thinned and dyskinetic and predispose to thrombus formation. Apical thrombi are frequently evident in the region of abnormal wall motion. Thrombi might either embolize acutely or become organized, layering, or calcifying with time. LV remodeling may occur after MI, resulting in LV size and shape change with adverse effects on function.[1–3,19,28]

### Cardiomyopathies: Dilated Cardiomyopathy

Despite the large number of recognized causes of dilated cardiomyopathy (DCM), there is seldom a specific etiologic factor and most cases are presumed to be a result of viral infection. Classically, all the chambers are dilated, and both the RV and LV appear diffusely hypokinetic. The feature that most differentiates idiopathic DCM from ischemic cardiomyopathy is the existence of global, rather than regional, dysfunction. In some cases, though, regional dysfunction might be evident because of the preservation of systolic function at the base of the LV or because of the existence of left bundle branch block (LBBB), which causes paradoxic septal motion. Nonetheless, whereas RV function is regularly preserved in cases with ischemic cardiomyopathy, this is not typical of other causes. In most instances, both the MV and TV appear normal. Despite this, there might be significant central MR and TR resulting from the incomplete closure of MV and TV leaflets, giving rise to annular dilatation and leaflet tethering as a result of papillary muscle displacement with remodeling. The existence of LV thrombi raises the risk of systemic emboli.[1–3,21,28]

### Hypertrophic Cardiomyopathy

Hypertrophic cardiomyopathy (HCM) is familial in nature and is genetically determined. HCM is characterized by ventricular hypertrophy, which might be diffuse or local to the septum, apex, or ventricular free wall. HCM cases with septal hypertrophy are categorized with or without evidence of dynamic obstruction in LVOT. The most common and typical form of HCM is related with septal hypertrophy. Characteristically, the ratio of septal to posterior wall thickness is in excess of 1.3/1. The LV cavity often appears small, and the LV apex might be completely obliterated in systole. The MV might be morphologically normal; nonetheless, there are often subtle anomalies in the MV apparatus. These include the anterior displacement of the papillary muscles; redundancy of MV chordae or leaflets; and in some cases, prolapse of the MV. MR occurs frequently and relates to the anatomy of MV apparatus and to the grade of LVOT obstruction.

A symbolic sign of obstructive HCM (LVOT obstruction) is the systolic anterior motion (SAM) of the anterior leaflet of the MV. The interposition of this leaflet causes obstruction in mid-to-late systole (in LV emptying phase), so the CW Doppler profile typically has a late-peaking systolic pattern. LA enlargement is almost invariable in HCM. Of course, with AF, both atria are typically dilated. Asymmetric septal hypertrophy must be distinguished from discrete upper septal hypertrophy, which is common in old hypertensive cases and is not related to either midseptal hypertrophy or evidence of LVOT obstruction (Fig. 5.31).

### Restrictive Cardiomyopathy

The individual morphologic features of restrictive cardiomyopathy (RCM) are noticeable ventricular hypertrophy, small ventricular cavity, and enlargement of both atria. Classically, in the early stages, systolic function is normal or even hyperkinetic. Valvular leaflets might be thickened, and there is commonly significant MR and TR. The pericardium looks normal. The most prominent physiologic derangement is impaired diastolic relaxation. (Typically, the initial filling wave is large with rapid deceleration, resulting in increased early filling, and the late filling wave is either small or absent owing to a reduced late diastolic filling capability). Although a specific cause is seldom determined, attention must be given to the probability of an infiltrative course such as amyloidosis or hemochromatosis[1–3,21,26–28] (Figs. 5.32 and 5.33).

### Endomyocardial Fibrosis

Endomyocardial fibrosis is described by thickened endocardium, apical obliteration, global biventricular systolic and diastolic dysfunction, and MR. It is correlated with the hypereosinophilic syndrome and the changes resulting from endocardial inflammation and thrombus formation that dominantly affect the apex.

### Noncompaction Cardiomyopathy

The echocardiographic diagnosis is made by the detection of thickened LV walls with two distinct layers of noncompacted and compacted myocardium with deep intertrabecular recesses. The prominent trabecular network classically involves the apex or midventricular segments of the inferior and lateral walls with the hypokinesis of the affected segments. A ratio of noncompacted to compacted myocardial thickness greater than 2:1 measured at end systole is typical of LVNC. This form of cardiomyopathy is created by the intrauterine arrest of the compaction of the myocardial

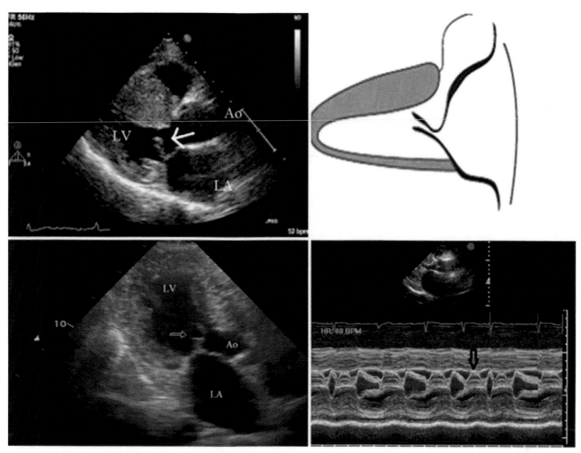

FIG. 5.31  (A, B) Systolic anterior motion (SAM) of the anterior mitral leaflet in parasternal long axis view (*white arrow*). (C) SAM in apical long axis view and (D) SAM of the anterior mitral leaflet in M-mode study in parasternal long axis view (*black arrow*) needs permission from Case Base text of Echocardiography by Springer.

fibers and network. Clinically, affected patients are at augmented risk of heart failure, embolic events, and arrhythmias.

### Arrhythmogenic Right Ventricular Dysplasia

Arrhythmogenic RV dysplasia predisposes to ventricular arrhythmias and sudden cardiac death. The RV myocardium is replaced by collagen and adipose tissue. This leads to the characteristic echocardiographic features of focal RV motion defects and aneurysm formation, RV dilatation and hypokinesis, and the existence of brightly echogenic areas in the RV myocardium revealing fatty-fibrous tissue replacement.[1–3,6,21,26–28]

### Pericardial Disease

The pericardium contains two separate layers: a visceral layer applied directly to the outer surface of the heart and proximal to the great vessels and a parietal layer that creates the free wall of the pericardial sac. Because the pericardial sac normally contains only 20–50 mL of fluid, it is frequently seen as a single extremely reflective border. In normal cases with an increased amount of fat overlying the visceral surface of the heart, division between the two layers might become obvious, predominantly anteriorly.

### Pericardial Effusion and Tamponade

Echocardiography is a sensitive method for the recognition and localization of pericardial effusion. Serous pericardial effusion appears as an echolucent area within the borders of the pericardial sac. The size of the pericardial effusion is frequently described semi-quantitatively as being small, moderate, or massive. The distinction among large fluid collections in the pleural space and pericardial effusion might be made on the parasternal long axis view. Pericardial effusion

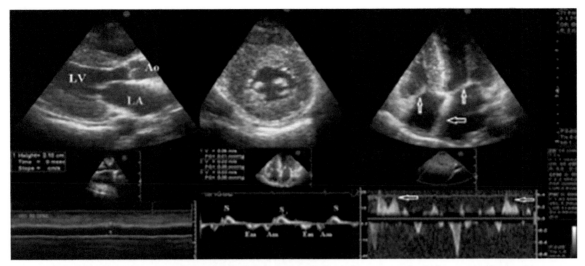

FIG. 5.32 Typical echocardiography finding in amyloidosis. *Left upper and middle panels*: Concentric increased myocardial thickness in parasternal long axis and short axis views, *upper right panel*: increase thickness of mitral and tricuspid valves and interatrial septum, biatrial enlargement (*arrows*). *Lower panel: left*: VC plethora, *middle*: Doppler tissue imaging of septum shows severely reduced septal velocities, *right*: inspiratory increased hepatic vein diastolic flow reversal, needs permission from Case Base text of Echocardiography by Springer.

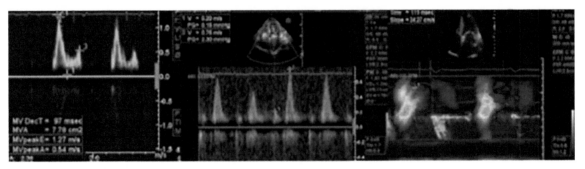

FIG. 5.33 *Left*: Increased peak E velocity and decreased A velocity with E/A ratio >2 and mitral deceleration time <150–160, *middle*: decreased systolic pulmonary venous flow velocity suggestive for high LA pressure. *Right*: Color M-mode velocity propagation in apical four-chamber view shows significantly reduced Vp (34 cm/s) needs permission from Case Base text of Echocardiography by Springer.

extends among the descending thoracic aorta and the LA. In contrast, the aorta remains closely apposed to the atrioventricular groove in the existence of pleural effusion. Also, the echocardiographic image might denote the existence of a particular pericardial abnormality such as tumor, fibrin, or organized hematoma. Echocardiography is also valuable in determining the hemodynamic significance of pericardial effusion collections. RV inversion is both sensitive and specific for cardiac tamponade. In contrast, RA inversion is a more sensitive but less specific marker of tamponade. Exaggerated respiratory phase variation in the cardiac valves is seen in tamponade, too, resulting in the inability of the heart both to fill normally and to eject a normal stroke volume in the existence of a tense fluid-filled pericardium.[1,2,22,28]

## Pericardial Constriction

The diagnosis of pericardial constriction by 2D echocardiography is difficult, but it might be proposed by abnormal pericardial thickening or calcification with impaired ventricular filling. Typically, pericardial thickening is noticeable as a thick, bright, echogenic layer surrounding all or a part (especially posterior) of the LV. In the existence of pericardial constriction, ventricular filling occurs early and stops abruptly at mid-diastole because of the restraining effect of the pericardium, which prevents the ventricular chambers from expanding as they fill. This configuration of rapid early diastolic filling and decreased late diastolic filling might also be inferred from the MV inflow Doppler flow, which typically displays a big early filling wave and a small or absent late filling wave. Other 2D echocardiographic features that might be visible include the lack of respiratory variation in the size of the IVC and a specific pattern of motion of the IVS. This "septal bounce" pattern is an initial diastolic leftward movement of the IVS, which is a result of the augmented RV inflow during peak inspiration followed by a rapid rightward shift as LV filling begins. Although none of these signs is either sensitive or specific for the diagnosis of pericardial constriction, with a harmonious picture, they provide support for the diagnosis. Moreover, some Doppler features might prove useful in the diagnosis of pericardial constriction and its distinction from RCM.

### Pericardial Cysts

Pericardial cysts are sporadic benign and developmental abnormalities that are frequently asymptomatic. They, however, might be detected on a routine chest radiography. Echocardiographically, they appear as a unilocular, fluid-filled, thin-walled structure placed adjacent to the RA or along the lateral border of the left or more in the right side of the heart.[1–3,22,24,28]

### Intracardiac Masses and Tumors

Intracardiac tumors might be either primary or secondary. Secondary tumors are meaningfully more frequent than primary ones and result from local thoracic malignancies that invade the heart directly or spread into the atria via the pulmonary vessels. Secondary hematologic spread might also occur from the abdomen, retroperitoneal space, skin, or breast. Secondary tumors grow within the myocardium, appearing as distinct, brightly echogenic masses. Rarely, secondary tumors might seed the endocardium and appear to grow into the ventricular cavity. Finally, the secondary invasion of the pericardium might be visible as the distinct regions of thickening of the visceral pericardium in relation with pericardial effusion. The primary tumors of the heart are definitely rare and most often benign. These include fibromas, fibroelastomas, rhabdomyomas, and myxomas.

The most frequent tumors are atrial myxomas. These commonly rise from the left side of the fossa ovalis, but they might arise anywhere in the atria and seldom involve the MV or the TV. They may be either single or multiple, sessile, or pedunculated. Myxomas have been associated with other signs, including lentiginosis and pituitary tumors (often familial). Echocardiographically, myxomas are discrete, multilobulated, and frequently homogeneous in appearance. They might contain focal areas of lucency caused by areas of hemorrhage, which occurs when the tumor outgrows its blood supply. Large and pedunculated myxomas might prolapse across the MV or the TV in diastole and impair ventricular filling.

From malignant primary tumors, rhabdomyosarcomas arise from striated muscles and infiltrate diffusely into the myocardium, dominantly the IVS. They might also grow into and obliterate the heart chambers. Angiosarcomas are the most common primary cardiac malignancy in adults and are more common in male patients. They most often arise in the RA in the region of the interatrial septum and might be polypoid. Fibrosarcomas arise from the endocardial parts and tend to be bulky fleshy tumors, which might infiltrate and involve more than one chamber.[1–5,10,27,28,31]

### Intracardiac Thrombi

Intracardiac thrombi form as a result of stasis and low flow within the heart or as a result of endocardial damage. Thrombi most commonly occur in AF, MS, DCM, and recent MI. Ventricular thrombi appear as focal echo adjacent to the normal endocardial contour with abnormal motion and might be laminar, sessile, or individually mobile. When organized, they might contain areas that are brighter than the myocardium. Thrombi must be differentiated from false tendons, apical scar, and artifacts. The risk of systemic embolism after MI is greater in patients with larger and hypermobile thrombi. LA clots most frequently arise in the LAA. TEE is often required to confirm the existence of thrombi with certainty. It is essential to distinguish thrombi from the normal trabeculae of the LAA and from the ridge among the LAA and the lower left pulmonary vein. A number of normal anatomic structures may mimic a mass lesion in the atria. Especially, the thickening of the tricuspid annulus, eminence of the trabeculae along the roof of the RA, and a noticeable eustachian valve might all be misdiagnosed as an RA tumor. Finally, the compression of the atrial wall by an intrathoracic mass or hiatal hernia might also yield the appearance of an LA tumor.[1,2,31]

## Aortic Disease

TTE permits the routine valuation of the ascending and abdominal portions of the aorta in adults and some imaging of the transverse arch and the descending thoracic aorta. It is often possible to obtain complete views of the entire aorta in the pediatric cases. TEE aids in a more complete study of the aorta in adults.

### Proximal Aorta Disease

An increase in aortic root dimension is common in proximal aortic root disease. In Marfan syndrome, dilatation classically occurs at the level of the aortic sinuses, and the aortic root appears relatively normal. In contrast, in patients with atherosclerotic aneurysms, the aorta looks diffusely thickened, and dilatation occurs beyond the level of the sinotubular junction. Aortic dissection is known by aortic root dilatation and a discrete dissection flap, which partitions the aortic lumen (Fig. 5.34). Classically, the true lumen is smaller than the false lumen, increases in size in systole, and has a high-velocity flow within it. When aortic dissection is definite, it is essential to define the involvement of the ostia of the coronary or arc vessels, AR, pericardial effusion, and tamponade. TEE permits the diagnosis of aortic dissection with much higher sensitivity and nearly complete specificity.

A rare disease of the proximal aorta is the development of an aneurysm of the sinus of Valsalva. The rupture of the aneurysm might occur spontaneously or as a result of infection and cases clinically with a continuous murmur. Color Doppler displays evidence of an abnormal aortoatrial or aortoventricular continuous shunt flow. The disease of the thoracic and abdominal aortic dissection might occur as a result of atheromatous disease or as a consequence of chest trauma. In cases of suspected aortic dissection, TEE is frequently necessary to confirm the diagnosis. The Doppler profile with a significant coarctation of the aorta (CoA) is a continuous systolic and diastolic flow in the abdominal aorta. Furthermore, CW Doppler directed through the descending thoracic aorta may define the gradient across the CoA, and the suprasternal window might allow a precise visualization and location of the CoA[1-3,20,27,28,35-37] (Fig. 5.35).

### Congenital Heart Disease

Approach to the patient with CHD needs a comprehensive evaluation of the central cyanosis, clubbing and looking for any history of surgery besides reading surgical notes before starting the echocardiography. Usually, TTE starts from subcostal view to determine the cardiac position, abdominal and atrial situs and IVC continuity to the right atrium (Fig. 5.36; Table 5.9).

### Atrial Septal Defects

ASDs are among the most common CHDs. Defects in the interatrial septum are categorized by their location. They include the ostium secundum ASD, placed in the midportion of the septum in the area of the fossa ovalis; ostium primum ASD, located inferiorly near the atrioventricular valves; sinus venosus type ASD, situated near the entry of the SVC or IVC; and CS septal defect at the mouth of the CS. 2D echocardiography may visualize the entire atrial septum and detect an ASD as a discrete absence of echoes in the appropriate area of the septal wall.

ASDs with low right-sided pressures predominantly have left-to-right shunting. When PAH develops, shunt flow is low in velocity and often bidirectional. Evidence of RA and RV chamber enlargement and paradoxic

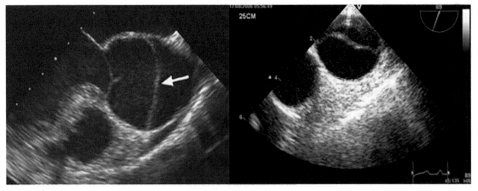

FIG. 5.34 Transesophageal echocardiography. *Left*: Midesophagus. Annuloaortic ectasia in Marfan syndrome with effacement of the sinotubular junction (STJ) and dissection flap in the ascending aorta. *Right*: Midesophagus. View, dissection flap in the descending thoracic aorta (*arrow*).

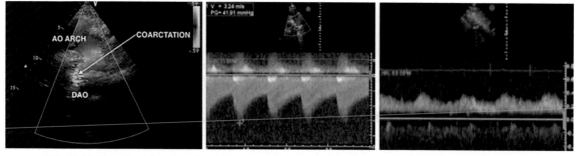

FIG. 5.35 The site of the stenosis may be seen properly in the suprasternal view. In significant coarctation, there is a turbulent flow in the proximal descending aorta and continuous-wave Doppler study will reveal increased velocity through the descending aorta, with a diastolic "tail" (high velocities maintained during diastole). Doppler flow study of the abdominal aorta demonstrating decreased pulsatility and absence of early diastolic flow reversal in the significant CoA.

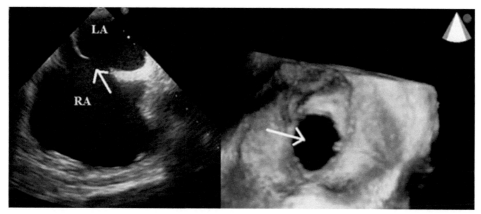

FIG. 5.36 Two- and three-dimensional (3D) transesophageal echocardiography (TEE) in a patient with secundum-type atrial septal defect (ASD) as indicated by *arrows*. 3D TEE has the advantage of demonstrating an en face view of the ASD. *LA*, left atrium; *RA*, right atrium.

motion of the IVS are indicative of RV volume overload and generally indicate a pulmonary-to-systemic shunt ratio greater than 1.5:1.

In addition to primary data from TTE, a different noninvasive method for distinguishing interatrial shunts is contrast echocardiography. By rapid intravenous injection of a small volume of agitated saline, the resulting turbulence and melted air creates multiple small ultrasound scatterers. This produces a "contrast effect" and permits the detection of right-to-left shunting by the passage of the contrast from the RA to the LA and the LV. Also, left-to-right shunting is visible as a "negative contrast effect" when unopacified LA blood enters the contrast-filled RA.

Essentially, with sinus venosus defects, and less commonly with secundum-type ASDs, the pulmonary veins, especially right ones, might drain to the RA. The diagnosis of partial anomalous pulmonary venous connection requires careful attention to the SVC, RA, and pulmonary veins by TEE.

Primum ASDs are frequently a part of the spectrum of endocardial cushion defects, which contain a deficiency in the atrioventricular septum and anomalies of the atrioventricular valves. Thus, a related cleft in the anterior MV leaflet and the existence of a VSD must be considered when a primum ASD is diagnosed.

The advent of the percutaneous closure of ASDs using a variety of devices has made decisive imaging of ASD size, location, and number a clinical imperative. Because of its proximity to the atrial septum from within the esophagus, TEE is frequently used to provide a clearer image of the ASD and to measure the size of

**TABLE 5.9**
**Basic Principles That Should Be Consider in the Imaging of Cases With Suspected Congenital Heart Disease (CHD)**

| | |
|---|---|
| A | In all probability, the presence of one congenital abnormality denotes the existence of more. Whether we seek to diagnose the most basic of communications amid the atria or we endeavor to identify the most complex of malformations, the objective of the sequential segmental modality is to prove normality. That is why we subject a patient with an isolated atrial septal defect (ASD) in the setting of a normally constructed heart to the same painstaking analysis as a patient with congenitally corrected transposition of the great arteries allied to multiple intracardiac defects |
| B | A patient's history and/or written surgical report are to be meticulously perused even prior to meeting the patient. The echocardiographer's thorough understanding of the particulars of the patient's earlier repairs affords a more clear-cut and efficient imaging examination |
| C | Inspection of the patient's color, fingers, and chest would be helpful. Is the patient cyanotic with clubbed fingers? After all, cyanotic patient is more likely to have complex malformations. The presence of the scars of sternotomy or lateral thoracotomy is proof of preceding surgical interventions |
| D | The so-called rules of cardiac development and congenital abnormalities arc not "gospel truth." The echocardiographer ought to, therefore, describe what is present, even if it does not chime in with the known conventional lesions |
| E | The philosophy of segmental analysis is based on the morphologic method. Therefore, the recognition of the cardiac chambers ought to be on the basis of their morphology rather than their position |
| F | Never hesitate to seek a second opinion if there is a complex anatomy |
| G | The consecutive segmental approach is a systematic and standard approach for echocardiography in CHD. In general, the sequential segmental approach consists of the following steps: cardiac position and orientation, viscera-atrial situs, ventricular position (ventricular looping), and the great arteries position (looping). Thereafter, the atrioventricular and ventriculoarterial connections are analyzed in terms of connections and relations |
| H | The key to the echocardiography of CHD is an appreciation of the sequential segmental approach for the diagnosis of both simple and complex lesions |
| I | In the valuation of eases with CHD, the echocardiographic study ought to be far more than a mere definition of the cardiac anatomy. Not only does a comprehensive echocardiographic valuation define the cardiovascular anatomy nevertheless also it seeks to provide a description of the function of the myocardium, abnormalities of the valves, and overall hemodynamic status |
| J | Atrioventricular and semilunar valves have common abnormalities, even with normal segmentation. Bicuspid aortic valves, Ebstein's anomaly of the tricuspid valve, and cleft MVs account for the most frequent findings. Echocardiography is deemed a frontline diagnostic modality inasmuch as it might provide information on the anatomy of the heart, morphology of the cardiac chambers, function and size of the ventricles, communications among the atria and the ventricles, origins of the great arteries, and venous return |
| K | There might be suboptimal echocardiography imaging in adult CHD cases due to the larger body habitus and chest deformity. Consequently, off-axis and nonstandard views are frequently used to evaluate complex anatomy |

Modified from Sadeghpour A, Alizadehasl A. *Case-Based Textbook of Echocardiography*. 1st ed. Springer International Publishing AG, part of Springer Nature; 2018.

the defect and its surrounding rims. The placement of ASD closure devices in the defects that are agreeable to percutaneous closure is accomplished in the cardiac catheterization laboratory under TEE guidance[5,37–42] (Fig. 5.37).

### Ventricular Septal Defects

The IVS is a complex arrangement composed of muscular and fibrous tissues. The defects in the septum are common and may occur at a single or multiple sites.

The echocardiographic recognition of a VSD depends on dropout in the IVS and the use of PW or color-flow Doppler to identify the turbulent shunt flow across the defect. Muscular VSDs occur frequently in children, and many of them close instinctively within the first 2 years of life. Nonetheless, muscular defects near the apex may be of considerable size. However, the fibrous part of the IVS (the membranous septum) lies adjacent to the AV annulus, and the TV septal leaflet, and its chordal apparatus lie along the RV aspect of the membranous

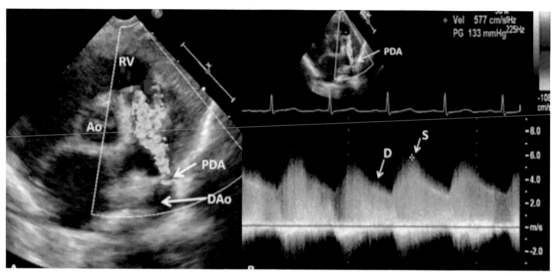

FIG. 5.37   Color (A) and Doppler (B) flow of patent ductus arteriosus.

septum. Consequently, the incorporation of this tissue into a septal aneurysm often causes the spontaneous closure of this type of VSD. The right coronary or non-coronary aortic cusps rarely prolapse into a high-membranous VSD, distorting AV coaptation and causing AR. Supracristal VSDs occur in that part of the IVS placed above the crista supraventricularis and beneath the pulmonary annulus. Echocardiographic views of RVOT are best for noticing this type of defect. Prolapse and distortion of the right coronary aortic leaflet also occur with supracristal VSDs.

Inlet VSDs occur in the region of the septum near the TV and MV annuli and are often correlated with the straddling of the TV or MV. Atrioventricular septal defects result from the absence of the atrioventricular septum, giving rise to large defects in the center of the heart that have an atrial as well as an inlet ventricular component. These are also known as "endocardial cushion" or "atrioventricular canal" defects. In patients with PAH, when pressures equalize among the LV and the RV, shunt flow is low in velocity and thus might be hard to detect by color-flow mapping. Echocardiography provides essential clinical data on shunt size and pulmonary artery pressure (PAP). Significant left-to-right shunting through a VSD enlarges the PA, LA, and LV. The estimates of Qp/Qs ratio may be made for shunts at ventricular level, as defined for atrial shunts. Using the simplified Bernoulli equation ($P = 4V^2$), the systolic pressure gradient among the LV and the RV may be derived from the peak flow velocity of the left-to-right jet across the VSD. Subtracting this gradient from the aortic systolic blood pressure gives an estimate of RV systolic pressure and PAP.[5,37–42]

## Patent Ductus Arteriosus

In fetal life, the patent ductus arteriosus (PDA) connects the PA and the aorta to permit passage of blood from the right heart to the systemic circulation without passing through the high-resistance pulmonary circuit. The persistence of this channel longer than the first few days or weeks of life is abnormal and is commonly an indication for noninvasive or surgical closure. 2D echocardiography may image the PDA in the left parasternal short axis view and suprasternal views, which display the PA bifurcation and the descending thoracic aorta. By TTE, it is often possible to image this channel through its length and measure its lumen size as well as the flow within the ductus and the main PA as a high-velocity jet coming into the PA (Fig. 5.38). Although the shunt flow is frequently continuous from the higher pressure aorta to the lower pressure PA, the normal systolic forward flow in the PA often obfuscates the systolic shunt flow, and the diastolic flow is the more readily detectable flow signal. With a significant volume of the shunt flow, the PA will be enlarged, as will the LA and LV. There might be a retrograde flow in the descending thoracic aorta by PW or color-flow Doppler, indicating substantial runoff from the aorta into the PDA.[5,37–42]

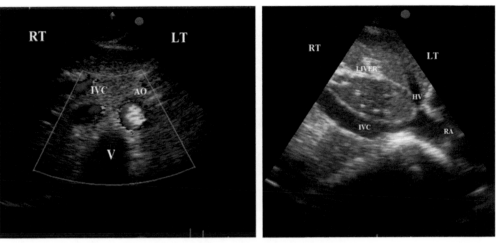

FIG. 5.38 In the subcostal short axis view, IVC is seen as an oval vessel located anterior and to the right of the abdominal aorta (AO). Normal abdominal situs and IVC continuity to RA.

### Tetralogy of Fallot

ToF is a well-recognized cyanotic CHD that results from the malalignment and anterior deviation of the conal septum. This creates obstruction to RVOT and a large subaortic VSD. The PA is often underdeveloped, and the RV develops hypertrophy in response to RVOT obstruction. Echocardiographically, the deviation of the conal septum is obviously visible as a muscular protrusion into the RVOT. The VSD is frequently large and simply imaged beneath the large overriding aortic root. PW and color-flow Doppler prove a low-velocity flow from the RV passing across the VSD and out the aorta and a high-velocity, turbulent flow in the RVOT. RVOT obstruction is frequently at multiple sites: the subvalvular muscular ridge, valvular and annular pulmonary levels, and rarely at the branch PAs.[35–38]

### Transposition of the Great Arteries

Another cyanotic CHD is the complete transposition of the great arteries (d-TGA). In this entity, the aorta arises from the RV, and the PA has its origin from the LV. Echocardiographically, the great arteries arise in parallel from the base of the heart instead of wrapping around one another. The semilunar valves are observable at roughly the same level relative to the long axis of the heart and thus may be imaged concurrently in the same plane. Following the course of the great arteries, whereas the anterior vessel arches and gives off brachiocephalic vessels, the posterior artery bifurcates into right and left pulmonary branches. Because the RV supplies the systemic circulation, it is characteristically enlarged and more globular in shape. d-TGA creates two circulations in parallel, with systemic venous return to the RA and RV being redirected to the systemic circulation and the pulmonary venous flow to the LA and LV returning to the lungs. So, some means of mixing these two circulations are essential. This most often occurs at atrial level via a PFO, but VSDs and a PDA are also means of intermixing and must be sought during echocardiographic Doppler study. The anatomy of the coronary arteries must also be defined because surgical correction needs the translocation of the coronary arteries from the anterior aorta to the posterior semilunar root.[5,37–41]

In the congenitally corrected TGA there is a discordant atrioventricular (AV) and ventriculoarterial (VA) connections (Fig. 5.39).

### Truncus Arteriosus

Persistent truncus arteriosus is an occasional malformation in which a single arterial trunk arising from the heart supplies the coronary, pulmonary, and systemic circulations. A large VSD is unvaryingly present, permitting both ventricles to eject blood into the single arterial vessel. Some patterns of truncus arteriosus are commonly documented. The most common patterns are those in which the PAs arise from the ascending part of the truncus arteriosus, either as a main PA—which then branches—or as separate branches from the posterior or lateral walls of the solitary arterial vessel. Echocardiographic diagnosis is based on signifying a large, single great vessel that overrides the IVS above a large VSD, nonexistence of an RVOT and pulmonary valve, and branching of the main PA or its independent branches from the large communal arterial trunk. The

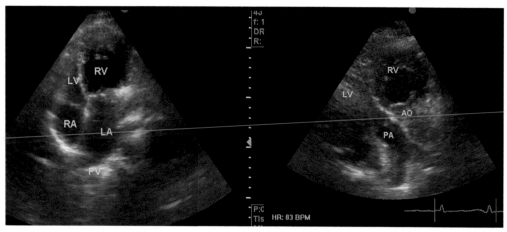

FIG. 5.39 Atrioventricular discordance, L loop ventricle with ventriculoarterial discordant: the morphologic right ventricle gives rise to the aorta and the morphologic LV drains into the PA suggestive for congenital corrected TGA.

truncal valve is regularly thickened, stenotic, or regurgitant and might have more than three cusps.

In type 1, there is a partially formed aorticopulmonary septum, and hence a main pulmonary artery segment is present. In type 2, there is absence of the aorticopulmonary septum, and thus no main pulmonary artery segment is present. The right and left branch pulmonary arteries arise from the truncus arteriosus, but their proximity to one another is not specified. In type 3, there is absence of one branch pulmonary artery from the truncus arteriosus. In type 4, the aortic arch is either hypoplastic or interrupted, and there is a large PDA.[36,37]

### Double-Outlet Right Ventricle

Double-outlet right ventricle (DORV) is an anomaly in which both great arteries rise completely or to a major extent from the RV. LV ejection must necessarily pass by a VSD to the right outflow vessels. There is widespread variability in the orientation of the great vessels relative to the position of the VSD. The clinical symptoms and signs might be simply those of a large VSD or might resemble the physiology of complete TGA. The existence of PS might create a physiology like ToF or TGA with RVOT obstruction.

The echocardiographic findings in DORV are of a large-outlet VSD and overriding of a great vessel. One main diagnostic feature is the absence of fibrous continuity among the anterior MV leaflet and the semilunar valve, which is close to the MV. The subarterial conal tissue is visible as muscle or fibrous tissue separating the MV from its adjacent semilunar valve. Because PS is frequent, echocardiographic study must define its

existence and severity. The size and location of the VSD in relation to the great arteries are other factors to be evaluated by echocardiography.[5,37–42]

### Cardiac Resynchronization Therapy

Cardiac resynchronization therapy (CRT) simultaneously paces the IVS and the lateral wall of the LV and leads to the concurrent contraction of LV walls in contrast to the dyssynchronous contraction seen in LBBB. Patients who respond to this therapy demonstrate improved LVEF; positive remodeling with reduced chamber size; and a decrease in MR, resulting in improvement in symptoms. The current criteria for CRT are based on electrical dyssynchrony and QRS duration. However, echocardiography may play an essential role in recognizing patients with significant mechanical dyssynchrony; therefore, it may improve the current method of patient selection for this expensive device therapy. The methods that have been used to date to evaluate the magnitude of dyssynchrony include measuring the delay among regional contraction using M-mode, TDI, and speckle tracking during 2D and 3D image acquisition. Myocardial contraction may be evaluated in terms of myocardial thickening, myocardial velocity, or myocardial strain and strain rate.[2,21,25,34,43–47]

### Ventricular Assist Devices

Mechanical devices may be used to manage patients with end-stage heart failure refractory to medical therapy. Echocardiography plays a crucial role in diagnosing patients with heart failure who would benefit from therapy and recognizing structural factors, which prohibit the use of these devices such as interatrial shunts, interventricular shunts, or significant AR. The ongoing monitoring of correct device function needs echocardiography to evaluate cardiac chamber size and function, valvular function, and device cannula flow profile. Finally, the finding of myocardial recovery and improved LV function may lead to defining the suitability for device insertion.

## Cardiac Interventional Procedures

TEE is frequently used to assist with interventional cardiac procedures, including balloon mitral valvuloplasty, percutaneous ASD and PFO closure, atrial appendage occluder device insertion for AF, percutaneous MV repair, and percutaneous AV replacement. TEE assists with defining the feasibility of procedures. For instance, an adequate tissue rim surrounding an ASD is necessary for successful device closure. It is critical for detecting contraindications to the procedures such as LA clots. During the intervention, TEE is used to screen the appropriate placement of the transseptal needles, guidewires, and devices. Finally, it may be used to evaluate the success of the procedure by recognizing residual shunts, valvular regurgitation, and some complications of the procedure such as pleural effusion and device impingement.[21,28,48–50]

## REFERENCES

1. Lang RM, Badano LP, Mor-Avi V, et al. Recommendations for cardiac chamber quantification by echocardiography in adults: an update from the American Society of Echocardiography and the European Association of Cardiovascular Imaging. *J Am Soc Echocardiogr.* 2015;28:1–39.
2. Nagueh SF, Smiseth OA, Appleton CP, et al. Recommendations for the evaluation of left ventricular diastolic function by echocardiography: an update from the American Society of Echocardiography and the European Association of Cardiovascular Imaging. *J Am Soc Echocardiogr.* 2016;29:277–314.
3. Rudski LG, Lai WW, Afilalo J, et al. Guidelines for the echocardiographic assessment of the right heart in adults: a report from the American Society of Echocardiography endorsed by the European Association of Echocardiography, a registered branch of the European Society of Cardiology, and the Canadian Society of Echocardiography. *J Am Soc Echocardiogr.* 2010;23:685–713.
4. Nishimura RA, Catherine M, Otto M, et al. 2014 AHA/ACC guideline for the management of patients with valvular heart disease: executive summary. *J Am Coll Cardiol.* 2014;63(22):2438–2488. https://doi.org/10.1016/j.jacc.2014.02.537.
5. Lancellotti P, Tribouilloy C, Hagendorff A, et al. Recommendations for the echocardiographic valuation of native valvular regurgitation: an executive summary from the European Association of Cardiovascular Imaging. *Eur Heart J Cardiovasc Imaging.* 2013;14:611–644.
6. Anavekar NS, Oh JK. Doppler echocardiography: a contemporary review. *J Cardiol.* 2009;54(3):347–358.
7. Zoghbi WA, Enriquez-Sarano M, Foster E, et al. Recommendations for evaluation of the severity of native valvular regurgitation with two-dimensional and Doppler echocardiography. *J Am Soc Echocardiogr.* 2003;16:777–802.
8. Lancellotti P, Tribouilloy C, Hagendorff A, et al. European Association of Echocardiography. European Association of Echocardiography recommendations for the valuation of valvular regurgitation. Part 1: aortic and pulmonary regurgitation (native valve disease). *Eur J Echocardiogr.* 2010;11:223–244.
9. Lancellotti P, Moura L, Pierard LA, et al. European Association of Echocardiography. European Association of Echocardiography recommendations for the valuation of valvular regurgitation. Part 2: mitral and tricuspid regurgitation (native valve disease). *Eur J Echocardiogr.* 2010;11:307–332.
10. Lang RM, Badano LP, Tsang W, et al. EAE/ASE recommendations for image acquisition and display using three-dimensional echocardiography. *Eur Heart J Cardiovasc Imaging.* 2012;13:1–46.
11. Aboulhosn J, Child JS. Left ventricular outflow obstruction: subaortic stenosis, bicuspid aortic valve, supravalvar aortic stenosis, and coarctation of the aorta. *Circulation.* 2006;114(22):2412–2422.
12. Abraham TP, Dimaano VL, Liang HY. Role of tissue Doppler and strain echocardiography in current clinical practice. *Circulation.* 2007;116(22):2597–2609.
13. Muralidhar K, Tempe D, Chakravarthy M, et al. Practice guidelines for perioperative transesophageal echocardiography: recommendations of the Indian association of cardiovascular thoracic anesthesiologists. *Ann Card Anesth.* 2013;16:268–278.
14. Acquatella H. Echocardiography in Chagas heart disease. *Circulation.* 2007;115(9):1124–1131.
15. Bayer AS, Bolger AF, Taubert KA, et al. Diagnosis and management of infective endocarditis and its complications. *Circulation.* 1998;98(25):2936–2948.
16. Bhatia VK, Senior R. Contrast echocardiography: evidence for clinical use. *J Am Soc Echocardiogr.* 2008;21(5):409–416.
17. Borer JS, Bonow RO. Contemporary approach to aortic and mitral regurgitation. *Circulation.* 2003;108(20):2432–2438.
18. Carabello BA. Modern management of mitral stenosis. *Circulation.* 2005;112(3):432–437.
19. Douglas PS, Khandheria B, Stainback RF, et al. ACCF/ASE/ACEP/AHA/ASNC/SCAI/SCCT/SCMR 2008 appropriateness criteria for stress echocardiography: a report of the American College of Cardiology Foundation Appropriateness Criteria Task Force, American Society of Echocardiography, American College of Emergency

Physicians, American Heart Association, American Society of Nuclear Cardiology, Society for Cardiovascular Angiography and Interventions, Society of Cardiovascular Computed Tomography, and Society for Cardiovascular Magnetic Resonance endorsed by the Heart Rhythm Society and the Society of Critical Care Medicine. *J Am Coll Cardiol.* 2008;51(11):1127–1147.

20. Douglas PS, Khandheria B, Stainback RF, et al. ACCF/ASE/ACEP/ASNC/SCAI/SCCT/SCMR 2007 appropriateness criteria for transthoracic and transesophageal echocardiography: a report of the American College of Cardiology Foundation Quality Strategic Directions Committee Appropriateness Criteria Working Group, American Society of Echocardiography, American College of Emergency Physicians, American Society of Nuclear Cardiology, Society for Cardiovascular Angiography and Interventions, Society of Cardiovascular Computed Tomography, and the Society for Cardiovascular Magnetic Resonance endorsed by the American College of Chest Physicians and the Society of Critical Care Medicine. *J Am Coll Cardiol.* 2007;50(2):187–204.

21. Elliott P, Andersson B, Arbustini E, et al. Classification of the cardiomyopathies: a position statement from the European Society of Cardiology Working Group on Myocardial and Pericardial Diseases. *Eur Heart J.* 2008;29(2):270–276.

22. Klein AL, Abbara S, Agler DA. American Society of Echocardiography clinical recommendations for multimodality cardiovascular imaging of patients with pericardial disease. *J Am Soc Echocardiogr.* 2013;26:965–1012.

23. Armstrong WF, Ryan T, eds. *Feigenbaum's Echocardiography.* 7th ed. Lippincott Williams & Wilkins; 2010.

24. Gardin JM, Adams DB, Douglas PS, et al. Recommendations for a standardized report for adult transthoracic echocardiography: a report from the American Society of Echocardiography's Nomenclature and Standards Committee and Task Force for a Standardized Echocardiography Report. *J Am Soc Echocardiogr.* 2002;15(3):275–290.

25. Gorcsan 3rd J, Abraham T, Agler DA, et al. Echocardiography for cardiac resynchronization therapy: recommendations for performance and reporting—a report from the American Society of Echocardiography Dyssynchrony Writing Group endorsed by the Heart Rhythm Society. *J Am Soc Echocardiogr.* 2008;21(3):191–213.

26. Ho CY, Seidman CE. A contemporary approach to hypertrophic cardiomyopathy. *Circulation.* 2006;113(24):e858–e862.

27. Hulot JS, Jouven X, Empana JP, et al. Natural history and risk stratification of arrhythmogenic right ventricular dysplasia/cardiomyopathy. *Circulation.* 2004;110(14):1879–1884.

28. Otto C. *The Practice of Clinical Echocardiography.* 3rd ed. Philadelphia: Saunders Elsevier; 2007.

29. Gaynor SL, Maniar HS, Prasad SM, Steendijk P, Moon MR. Reservoir and conduit function of right atrium: impact on right ventricular filling and cardiac output. *Am J Physiol Heart Circ Physiol.* 2005;288:H2140–H2145.

30. Muller H, Burri H, Lerch R. Evaluation of right atrial size in patients with atrial arrhythmias: comparison of 2D versus real time 3D echocardiography. *Echocardiography.* 2008;25:617–623.

31. Pibarot P, Dumesnil JG. Prosthetic heart valves. Selection of the optimal prosthesis and long-term management. *Circulation.* 2009;119:1034–1048.

32. Anita S, Azin A. The right ventricle: a comprehensive review from anatomy, physiology, and mechanics to hemodynamic, functional, and imaging evaluation. *Arch Cardiovasc Imaging.* 2015;3(4):e35717. https://doi.org/10.5812/acvi.35717.

33. Haghighi ZO, Alizadehasl A, Maleki M, et al. Echocardiographic valuation of right atrium deformation indices in healthy young subjects. *Am Heart J.* 2013;1(1):2–7.

34. Ojaghi-Haghighi Z, Alizadehasl A, Hashemi A. Reverse left ventricular apical rotation in dilated cardiomyopathy. *Arch Cardiovasc Imaging.* 2015;3(2).

35. Sadeghpour A, Kyavar M, Madadi S, Ebrahimi L, Khajali Z, Alizadeh SZ. Doppler-derived strain and strain rate imaging valuation of right ventricular systolic function in adults late after tetralogy of Fallot repair: an observational study. *Anatol J Cardiol.* 2013;13(6):536.

36. Naderi N, Haghighi ZO, Pezeshki S, Azin A. Quantitative valuation of right atrial function by strain imaging in adult patients with totally corrected tetralogy of Fallot. *Arch Cardiovasc Imaging.* 2013;1(1):8–12.

37. Sadeghpour A, Kyavar M, Alizadehasl A. *Comprehensive Approach to Adult Congenital Heart Disease.* 1st ed. London: Springer-Verlag; 2014.

38. Bossone E, D'Andrea A, D'Alto M, et al. Echocardiography in pulmonary arterial hypertension: from diagnosis to prognosis. *J Am Soc Echocardiogr.* 2013;26:1.

39. Klimezak C, Nihoyannopoulos P. *Challenges in Echocardiography.* Elsevier; 2008.

40. Forfia PR, Vachiéry JL. Echocardiography in pulmonary arterial hypertension. *Am J Cardiol.* 2012;110(suppl. 6):S16.

41. Mann D, Zipes D, Libby P, Bonow R. *Braunwald's Heart Disease, Textbook of Cardiovascular Medicine.* 10th ed. Philadelphia: Elsevier Saunders; 2015.

42. Quiñones MA, Otto CM, Stoddard M, Waggoner A, Zoghbi WA. Recommendations for quantification of Doppler echocardiography: a report from the Doppler quantification Task Force of the Nomenclature and Standards Committee of the American Society of Echocardiography. *J Am Soc Echocardiogr.* 2002;15:167–184.

43. Nagueh SF, Appleton CP, Gillebert TC, et al. Recommendations for the evaluation of left ventricular diastolic function by echocardiography. *J Am Soc Echocardiogr.* 2009;22(2):292–298.

44. Silbiger JJ. Mechanistic insights into ischemic mitral regurgitation: echocardiographic and surgical implications. *J Am Soc Echocardiogr.* 2011;24:707.

45. Solomon SD. *Essential Echocardiography. A Practical Handbook.* Totowa: Humana Press; 2007.

46. Williams LK, Frenneaux MP, Steeds RP. Echocardiography in hypertrophic cardiomyopathy diagnosis, prognosis, and role in management. *Eur J Echocardiogr.* 2009;10:iii9.

47. Sadeghpour A, Alizadehasl A. Stress echocardiography in prosthetic heart valves. *Arch Cardiovasc Imaging.* 2016;4(1):e39032.

48. Zahra OH, Azin A, Hassan M, et al. Left ventricular torsional parameters in patients with non-ischemic dilated cardiomyopathy. *Arch Cardiovasc Imaging.* 2015;3(1):e26751.

49. Alizadehasl A. Latent ventricular dysfunction in systemic lupus erythematosus. *Arch Cardiovasc Imaging.* 2015;3(2):e28299.

50. Sadeghpour A, Kyavar M, Madadi S, et al. Doppler-derived strain and strain rate imaging valuation of right ventricular systolic function in adults late after tetralogy of Fallot repair: an observational study. *Anadolu Kardiyol Derg.* 2013;13:536–542.

# CHAPTER 6

# Chest Radiography in Cardiovascular Disease

HAMIDREZA POURALIAKBAR
Rajaie Cardiovascular, Medical & Research Center, Iran University of Medical Sciences, Tehran, Iran

## KEY POINTS

- Chest radiography is the simple and useful imaging tool to evaluate the heart disease.
- The routine radiography study consists a frontal view and a lateral view.
- Chest radiography shows lungs, chest wall, and pleural space simultaneously.
- Cardiologist should be familiar to precisely interpret chest radiography in emergency heart disease, valvular heart disease, acquired heart disease congenital heart disease, and other incidental noncardiac findings.

The usual chest radiography study consists of a frontal view and a lateral view: a posteroanterior (PA) view of the patient while standing with the chest toward the recording medium and back to the X-ray tube and a lateral view of the patient while standing with the left side toward the film. For both views, the X-ray tube is positioned at a distance of 6 ft from the film, a 6-ft source-to-image distance (SID).[1]

Portable chest radiography has inherent practical limitations. Most of these radiographs are obtained with patients positioned supine or semisupine. Depth of inspiration is decreased in comparison with an erect film, so the heart appears relatively larger, with less optimal visualization of the lungs. The resolution is poorer with portable radiographs, thus making them less accurate and useful. In addition, the radiation dose to both patients and personnel is generally greater.[1]

Portable chest radiography is most useful for answering relatively simple mechanical questions, such as location of pacemaker or implantable cardioverter-defibrillator (ICD) or whether an endotracheal tube is in the correct location. These radiographs are not generally good at providing physiologic or complex anatomic information, and it is impossible to accurately evaluate heart size and contour or the status of the pulmonary vasculature. Although portable chest radiography may be convenient and provide some information, it should be performed only in limited situations when clearly needed to answer specific questions.[1]

The radiation exposure to the patient should always be kept in mind when any radiographic study is performed. The radiation necessary for PA and lateral chest radiographs is usually minimal, and the dose of a single study is generally less than 1 mSv.[1]

## NORMAL CHEST RADIOGRAPHS

There are multiple components in normal chest radiographs that we should know and evaluate; these components include the pulmonary parenchyma, heart, mediastinum, pleura, chest wall, aorta, pulmonary arteries, and soft tissues. It is imperative to take a systematic and standardized approach first based on assessment of the anatomy, then the physiology, and finally the pathology.[1]

In a standard PA chest radiograph, the heart size is normally less than half the transverse diameter of the thorax. The heart overlies the thoracic spine, roughly 75% to the left and 25% to the right of the spine. The pulmonary hila are seen below the aortic arch, slightly higher on the left than on the right. On a lateral chest radiograph, the left main pulmonary artery can be seen coursing superiorly and posteriorly relative to the right.

On a normal chest radiograph and on the PA view, the right contour of the mediastinum contains the right atrium (RA) and the ascending aorta and superior vena cava (SVC). The right ventricle (RV), as is clear from cross-sectional imaging, is located partially overlying the left ventricle (LV) on both frontal and lateral views. The left atrium (LA) is located just inferior to the left pulmonary hilum. Individuals with normal anatomy have a concavity at this level, the location of the LA appendage

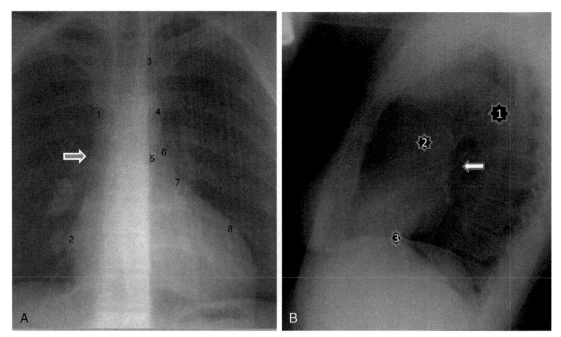

FIG. 6.1 Normal chest radiograph. (A) Posteroanterior view. *Arrow* indicates the ascending aorta. *1*, Superior vena cava; *2*, right atrium; *3*, subclavian artery; *4*, aortic knob; *5*, descending aorta; *6*, pulmonary trunk; *7*, left atrial auricle; *8*, left ventricle. (B) Lateral view. *1*, left hilum; *2*, right hilum; *3*, IVC.

(LAA). The LA makes the upper portion of the posterior contour of the heart on lateral radiographs (Fig. 6.1).

### Lungs and Pulmonary Vasculature

In normal subjects, the pulmonary arteries are easily visible centrally in the hila and become smaller peripherally. If the lung is divided in three zones, the major arteries are central; midsized pulmonary arteries (third- and fourth-order branches) are in the middle zone; and the small arteries and arterioles, which are normally below the limit of resolution, are in the outer zone. The visible small and midsized arteries (midzone) have sharp, clearly definable margin structures. On a standard, standing frontal (PA) chest radiography, the arteries in the lower zone are larger than those in the upper zone, at an equal distance from the hila, because of the effect of gravity on the normal, low-pressure lung circulation; gravity leads to slightly greater intravascular volume at the lung bases than in the upper zones.[1]

### THE CHEST RADIOGRAPH IN HEART DISEASE

#### Overview

A systematic approach to the evaluation of chest radiographs is imperative to distinguish normal from abnormal and to define the underlying pathology and pathophysiology. A systematic approach is directed toward discerning the findings from the radiograph and, for each finding, narrowing the differential diagnosis.

A five-step systematic approach allows the orderly examination of thoracic radiographs, and at each step, it is possible to narrow the diagnostic possibilities. A radiographic classification of acquired heart disease is used in association with this five-step examination.

The five steps in the examination of the chest radiography in patients with suspected cardiac disease are (1) thoracic musculoskeletal structures, (2) pulmonary vascularity, (3) overall heart size, (4) specific chamber enlargement, and (5) great arteries (ascending aorta, aortic knob, main pulmonary arterial segment).[2]

### Thoracic Musculoskeletal Structures

The thoracic should be examined for evidence of prior surgery, such as rib or sternal deformities or sternal wire sutures. Sternal deformities such as pectus excavatum may serve as a clue to cardiac lesions associated with it, such as Marfan syndrome and mitral valve prolapse. A narrow anteroposterior (AP) diameter of the thorax can be caused by pectus excavatum or a straight-back syndrome. A narrow AP diameter is defined as a distance between the sternum and the anterior border of the vertebral body that measures less than 8 cm and a ratio of the transverse diameter (determined by frontal view) to the AP diameter (determined by lateral view) exceeding 2.75. The AP diameter is the maximum diameter from the undersurface of the sternum to the anterior border of the vertebral body.[2]

## Pulmonary Vascularity

Evaluation of the pulmonary vascular pattern is difficult and imprecise but very important. As noted, the pattern varies with the patient's position (erect vs supine) and is altered substantially by underlying pulmonary disease. The information gained from analyzing the pulmonary vasculature, such as the shape of the heart, is very useful in arriving at a cardiac diagnosis.[3]

## Determining the Vascular Pattern
### Segmental analysis
Because the pulmonary arteries and veins have a complex branching pattern and are associated with many overlapping structures on a standard chest radiograph, there is moderate variability in interpreting which pulmonary pattern is present. Segmental analysis can help to classify pulmonary vasculature patterns. In a standard upright chest radiograph exposed at total lung capacity, the pulmonary vasculature can be divided into the following three areas:
1. The central pulmonary arteries
2. The hilar structures
3. The parenchymal arteries and veins

In a normal upright chest radiograph, the upper lung zone vessels are smaller in width than those in the lung bases because of gravitational effect. In a normal subject, the pulmonary artery in the hilum is roughly the same size as its adjacent bronchus. In the upper lung zones, the pulmonary artery diameter in an upright radiograph is 85% of the adjacent bronchial diameter. In the lower lung zones, the pulmonary arteries are one-third bigger than the nearby bronchus.[3]

### Pattern recognition
The first step in analyzing the pulmonary vasculature is to classify it into one of the following five patterns:
1. Normal
2. Diminished
3. Left-to-right shunt
4. Pulmonary arterial hypertension
5. Pulmonary venous hypertension (PVH)

**Diminished vasculature.** In the frontal view, a concave main pulmonary artery segment is the most reliable indicator of small main and central pulmonary arteries. There are diminished bronchovascular markings in the

hilum, and the diameters of the pulmonary arteries are smaller than their adjacent bronchi. The peripheral pulmonary arteries and veins are very small[2] (Fig. 6.2).

**Left-to-right shunt.** In patients with left-to-right shunt, the size of all pulmonary segments, including the central, hilar, and peripheral pulmonary arteries and veins, is enlarged. In a left-to-right shunt, the central pulmonary artery segment is convex, the hilum appears enlarged, and the peripheral vessels are large from the apex to the base. The chest film usually does not detect increased pulmonary flow until the flow ratio Qp/Qs is at least 2 (i.e., the pulmonary flow is twice than in the aorta,[2] Fig. 6.3).

**Pulmonary artery hypertension.** Pulmonary hypertension occurs when there is increased resistance in any part of the pulmonary circulation from the left heart to the pulmonary artery. The pattern of the pulmonary vasculature on the chest radiograph depends on the location of the increased resistance, the chronicity, and the severity. If the heart is structurally normal, the earliest sign of pulmonary artery hypertension is a convex main pulmonary artery segment. Severe, chronic pulmonary artery hypertension also enlarges the hilar branches but, unlike a left-to-right shunt, not the peripheral arteries within the

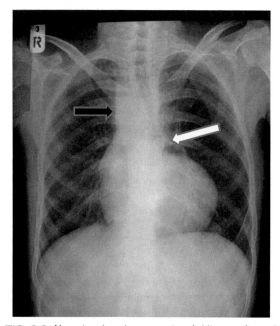

FIG. 6.2 Absent main pulmonary artery (*white arrow*), small hila, and severely decreased pulmonary blood vascularity in patient with diagnosis of tetralogy of Fallot. Right sided aortic arc (*black arrow*)

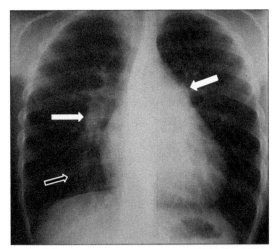

FIG. 6.3 Main pulmonary artery and main pulmonary artery branch enlargement (*white arrows*) and increased pulmonary blood vascularity (*black arrow*) in a patient with ventricular septal defect.

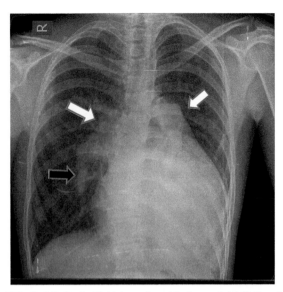

FIG. 6.4 Patient with history of ventricular septal defect and Eisenmenger syndrome. Cardiomegaly, enlargement of the main pulmonary artery and central pulmonary artery branches (*white arrows*), and tapering of peripheral branches (pruning) (*black arrow*) are seen.

lungs. The gradient of small vessels at the apex and large vessels at the base is preserved.

Note: In contrast, in patients with elevated pulmonary venous pressure, the vessel borders become hazy, the lower zone vessels constrict, and the upper zone vessels enlarge; vessels become visible farther toward the pleura, in the outer third of the lungs.

### Eisenmenger Syndrome

In adults with Eisenmenger syndrome, the pulmonary vasculature is unusually striking because of the central arterial enlargement. The arteries dilate longitudinally, forming a serpentine course. The rapid taper of the large aneurysmal hilar pulmonary arteries to the periphery looks like a "pruned tree." This phrase is correct angiographically and pathologically: there are fewer arterial side branches than in a normal arterial tree[3] (Fig. 6.4).

### Pulmonary Venous Hypertension

The major signs of PVH based on the severity of PVH are:
- Grade I (redistribution of pulmonary blood volume) (Fig. 6.5): equalization or larger diameter of the upper compared with the lower lobe vessels
- Grade II (interstitial pulmonary edema) (see Fig. 6.5): Kerley A or B lines, increased prominence of "interstitial markings," peribronchial cuffing, loss of the hilar angle, enlargement and indistinctness of hila, subpleural edema (increased thickness of pleura), and loss of visibility of much of the descending branch of the right pulmonary artery

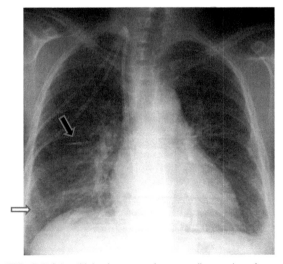

FIG. 6.5 Interstitial pulmonary edema, cardiomegaly, enlargement of the hila, haziness at the lower lungs, Kerley B line (*white arrow*), and subpleural effusion (*black arrow*).

- Grade III (alveolar pulmonary edema) (Fig. 6.6): confluent acinar shadows (pulmonary alveolar edema), perihilar alveolar filling, lower lobe, or more generalized alveolar filling

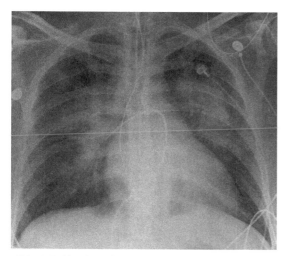

FIG. 6.6 Alveolar pulmonary edema with bat-wing sign.

There is usually a reasonably good correlation between the pulmonary vascular pattern and pulmonary capillary wedge pressure (PCWP). At a PCWP of less than 8 mmHg, the vascular pattern is normal. As PCWP increases to 10–12 mmHg, grade I changes appear. At pressures of 12–18 mmHg, grade II develops, and as PCWP increases above 18–20 mmHg, grade III occurs and shows the classic perihilar "bat-wing" appearance.[1]

The mentioned radiologic signs and PCWP are correlated to the acute phase, and in the chronic phase such as chronic mitral valve stenosis or chronic heart failure, the PCPW should be higher with the same radiologic appearance.

In patients with chronic pulmonary parenchymal disease, the radiologic findings of pulmonary edema may not be clearly visible. If the pulmonary edema is independent of LV dysfunction, such as at a high altitude or after cerebral trauma, the size of the heart may remain normal.

A more frequently encountered disparity is found in the setting of an acute, large transmural myocardial infarction; the heart is usually minimally or mildly enlarged despite a marked increase in LV end-diastolic pressure. Regardless of these limitations, it is important to evaluate the pulmonary vascular pattern routinely because it can provide a great deal of information.

## Cardiac Chambers and Great Vessels
Acquired heart disease can be divided into two groups, depending on the presence or the absence of substantial cardiomegaly.

The cardiothoracic (CT) ratio is calculated using the convention of measuring the thoracic diameter as the distance from the inner margin of the ribs at the level of the dome of the right hemidiaphragm and the cardiac diameter as the horizontal distance between the most rightward and most leftward margins of the cardiac shadow. We will set a CT ratio of less than 0.55 as normal in PA chest radiography.

"Small heart" disease is associated with a normal heart size or only mild cardiomegaly. The second group, called "big heart" disease, is characterized by substantial cardiomegaly (CT ratio >0.55). The pathophysiologic factors associated with "small heart" disease are pressure overload and reduced ventricular compliance. The pathophysiologic factors associated with "big heart" disease are volume overload and myocardial failure. Pericardial effusion also is included in this group[2] (Table 6.1 and Fig. 6.7).

The cardiac lesions included in the two groups are listed in Table 6.1.

### Specific Chamber Enlargement
After assessing the overall heart size, the individual chambers should be examined. The radiographic signs observed with enlargement of each of the cardiac chambers are given in the following sections.

#### Left atrial enlargement (Fig. 6.8)
1. Right retrocardiac double density: The distance from the middle of the double density (lateral border of the LA) to the middle of the left bronchus is smaller than 7 cm in more than 90% of normal subjects and larger than 7 cm in 90% of patients with LA enlargement proven by echocardiography. In cases of severe LA enlargement, the RA border may extend further to the right than the RA border.[2]

### TABLE 6.1
#### Cardiac Size and Acquired Cardiac Lesions

| Small Heart (CT Ratio <0.55) | Large Heart (CT Ratio >0.55) |
|---|---|
| Aortic stenosis | Aortic regurgitation |
| Arterial hypertension | Mitral regurgitation |
| Mitral stenosis | Tricuspid regurgitation |
| Acute myocardial infarction | High-output states |
| Hypertrophic cardiomyopathy | Congestive cardiomyopathy |
| Restrictive cardiomyopathy | Ischemic cardiomyopathy |
| Constrictive pericarditis | Pericardial effusion |
| | Paracardiac mass |

*CT*, cardiothoracic.

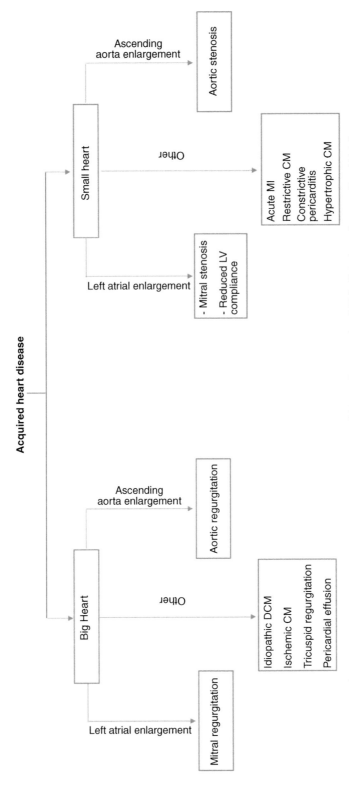

FIG. 6.7 Algorithm of acquired heart disease. *CM*, cardiomyopathy; *DCM*, dilated cardiomyopathy; *LV*, left ventricular.

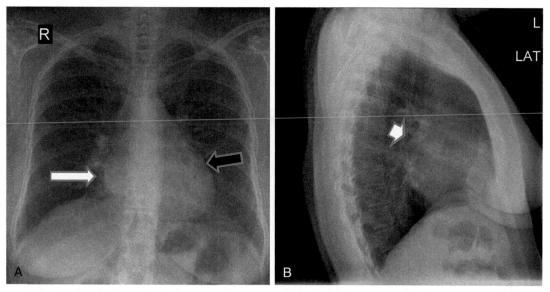

FIG. 6.8 (A) Dilatation of the left atrium, enlargement of the left atrial appendage (*black arrow*), and double-density sign (*white arrow*). (B) Displacement of the left bronchus (*white arrow*). *LAT*, lateral.

2. Enlargement of the LAA: This is seen as a bulge along the left cardiac border just beneath the main pulmonary artery segment. Using the left bronchus as an orientation point, the bulge above it is the main pulmonary artery segment, and the bulge at the level of or just below the left bronchus is the LAA.[2]
3. Widening of the carina or elevation of the left bronchus (or both)
4. Horizontal orientation of the distal portion of the left bronchus
5. Posterior displacement of the left upper lobe bronchus: On a normal lateral radiograph, the circular shadow of the right upper lobe and left bronchi is located within the tracheal air column. LA enlargement causes displacement of the left bronchus posterior to this level and beyond the plane of the trachea.[2]

### Right atrial enlargement (Fig. 6.9)
1. Lateral bulging of the right heart border more than 5 cm from midline spine on the PA radiograph
2. Elongation of the right heart border on the PA view: A rough rule is that an RA border exceeding 60% in length of the mediastinal cardiovascular shadow is a sign of substantial RA enlargement.

### Left ventricular enlargement (Fig. 6.10)
1. On the PA view, leftward and downward displacement of the cardiac apex is seen. The vector of

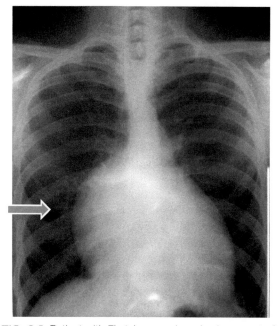

FIG. 6.9 Patient with Ebstein anomaly and enlargement of the right atrium (*arrow*).

enlargement of the LV is leftward and downward compared with the vector of RV enlargement, which is leftward only or perhaps leftward plus upward.

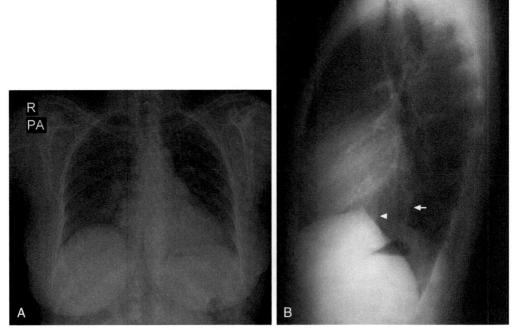

FIG. 6.10 (A) Patient with multivalvular disease and left ventricular (LV) enlargement in posteroanterior (PA) view. (B) Lateral view of the inferior vena cava (*arrowhead*) and LV (*arrow*).

2. On the lateral view, the posterior border of the heart is displaced posteriorly. The Hoffman-Rigler sign is measured 2.0 cm above the intersection of the diaphragm and the inferior vena cava. A positive measurement for LV enlargement is a posterior border of the heart extending more than 1.8 cm behind the inferior vena caval shadow at this level[2] (see Fig. 6.10B).

### Right ventricular enlargement (Fig. 6.11)

1. On the PA view, the left border of the heart is enlarged directly laterally or laterally and slightly superiorly. In some instances, this causes the apex to be displaced superiorly ("upward tipped apex"); in the extreme form, this causes a "boot shape."
2. On the lateral view, the retrosternal space is filled by the enlarged RV. RV enlargement is inferred by contact of the right heart border over more than one-third of the sternal length. A prominent convexity to the anterior border rather than the usual straight surface is an early sign of RV enlargement.[2]

## MITRAL VALVE DISEASE

### Mitral Valve Stenosis (Fig. 6.12)

Mitral valve stenosis usually is acquired and is caused by rheumatic fever. It is the salient lesion of rheumatic heart disease. Other rare causes are congenital valvular, subvalvular (parachute mitral valve), or supravalvular stenosis; LA myxoma; and severe mitral annular calcification. Mitral stenosis often is accompanied by a variable degree of mitral regurgitation (MR).

Mitral stenosis causes elevated LA pressure throughout diastole, and PVH produces pulmonary arterial hypertension. In long-standing mitral stenosis, pulmonary arterial hypertension may be severe, and pulmonary regurgitation eventually ensues across a dilated pulmonary annulus. The RV eventually dilates, causing tricuspid regurgitation from a dilated annulus.

### Chest radiography

Chest radiography provides good insight into the severity of mitral stenosis by showing the relative severity of PVH.

In mild disease, there may be only equalization or reversal of the diameter of upper and lower lobe

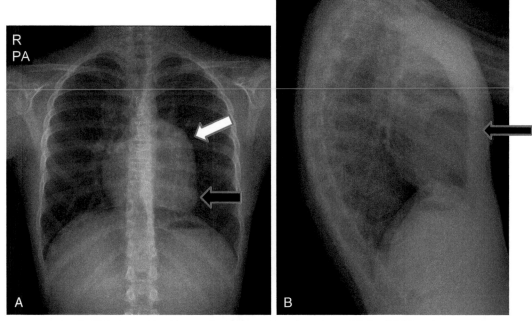

FIG. 6.11  (A, B) Patient with a history of total correction of tetralogy of Fallot (TFTC) and severe pulmonary valve insufficiency (PI), dilatation of the right ventricle (*black arrows*), and aneurysmal dilatation of the right ventricular outflow tract (*white arrow*). *PA*, posteroanterior.

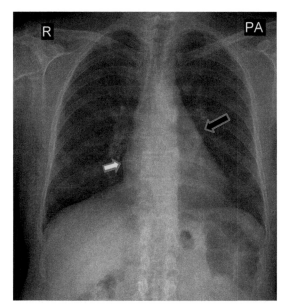

FIG. 6.12  Patient with severe mitral stenosis and increased pulmonary arterial pressure (PAP), a normal cardiothoracic ratio (small heart), double shadow (*yellow arrow*), dilatation of the left atrial appendage (*black arrow*), widening of carina, cephalization of the pulmonary blood pattern, and enlargement of the main pulmonary artery. *PA*, posteroanterior.

pulmonary vessels (cephalization). In more severe disease or with an imposed hypervolemic state, interstitial pulmonary edema or alveolar pulmonary edema becomes evident. In compensated mitral stenosis, only mild cardiomegaly or a normal heart size is seen. The LA and LAA invariably are enlarged.

Note: Enlargement of the pulmonary arterial segment and right heart indicates pulmonary arterial hypertension. Enlargement of the right heart in the absence of pulmonary arterial enlargement usually indicates concomitant tricuspid regurgitation.

The ascending aorta and aortic arch are characteristically small in isolated mitral valve disease. Even slight prominence of the thoracic aorta should raise suspicion of associated aortic valve disease[2] (Box 6.1).

---

**BOX 6.1**
**Main Radiographic Findings of Mitral Stenoses**

Enlargement of the left atrium is characteristic
Enlargement of the left atrial appendage
Mild cardiomegaly is seen in isolated mitral stenosis
Pulmonary venous hypertension or edema
Pulmonary edema may be observed intermittently

## Mitral Regurgitation

Mitral regurgitation may be caused by an abnormality of any portion of the mitral apparatus or by LV dilatation. The dysfunction may involve one or more of several components, including the leaflets, chordae, anterior and posterior papillary muscles, or annulus.

Myxomatous mitral valve disease is the most common cause of MR in the developed world followed by ischemic heart disease. In contrast, in the developing countries, the most common causes of MR appear to be rheumatic heart disease and ischemic heart disease.[2]

Chronic MR produces LA and LV enlargement. PVH or edema usually is less severe than with mitral stenosis. Pulmonary arterial hypertension is less common and less severe than with stenosis.[2]

### *Radiography* (Fig. 6.13)

The radiographic features of MR are regulated by the duration and severity of the lesion and associated lesions of the mitral and other valves. Isolated chronic MR is a volume overload lesion that causes LA and LV enlargement.

The right border of the LA may even extend beyond the border of the RA rather than causing a right retrocardiac double density[2] (Box 6.2).

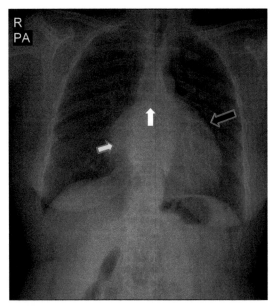

FIG. 6.13 Patient with severe mitral regurgitation, increased cardiothoracic ratio (big heart) double shadow (*yellow arrow*), widening of the carina (*white arrow*), and left atrial appendage enlargement (*black arrow*). *PA*, posteroanterior.

---

> **BOX 6.2**
> **Main Radiographic Features of Mitral Regurgitation**
>
> Moderate-to-severe cardiomegaly
> Left ventricular enlargement
> Left atrial enlargement
> Enlargement of left atrial appendage
> Variable degree of pulmonary venous hypertension or pulmonary edema (less severe than with mitral stenosis)

## AORTIC VALVE DISEASE

### Aortic Stenosis

Aortic valve stenosis of nonrheumatic or congenital origin is the most common valvular heart disease in the Western world and increases in prevalence with each decade of life. Conversely, rheumatic aortic stenosis (AS) is more prevalent worldwide. Stenosis in rheumatic aortic valve (AV) disease results from commissural fusion, aortic cusp thickening, and calcification. AS is a disease spectrum spanning from noncalcified to calcified etiologies.[4]

Aortic valve calcification is pathognomonic for significant AV disease, but it is usually difficult to see on a chest radiograph because of the overlying soft tissue densities and the minimal blurring caused by cardiac motion.[2]

**Radiography** (Fig. 6.14). Aortic stenosis is a pressure overload lesion that causes concentric LV hypertrophy. Consequently, AS, for much of its natural history, is a disease that is clearly "small heart" disease. There is little or no cardiac enlargement. The characteristic radiographic feature is enlargement of the ascending aorta. The pulmonary vascularity is also generally normal for much of the course of AS. However, in the decompensated phase of AS, there may be evidence of PVH caused by LV failure[2] (Box 6.3).

## AORTIC REGURGITATION

Aortic regurgitation is a volume overload lesion caused by retrograde flow across the aortic valve during diastole. Because of the excessive diastolic volume, the LV becomes dilated. Regurgitation may be caused by lack of coaptation of the valvular cusps, annular dilatation, or ascending aortic dilatation.

### Radiography (Fig. 6.15)

Aortic regurgitation is characterized by cardiomegaly on the chest radiographs, which are predominantly caused

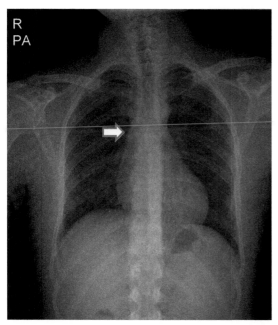

FIG. 6.14 Severe aortic stenosis, normal cardiothoracic ratio (small heart), normal cardiac chamber size, dilated ascending aorta (*arrow*), and normal pulmonary blood vascularity. *PA*, posteroanterior.

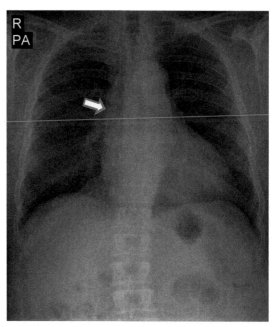

FIG. 6.15 Severe aortic valve insufficiency (AI), enlarged cardiothoracic ratio (big heart), left ventricular enlargement, dilatation of the ascending aorta (*arrow*) and aortic arc, normal size of other chambers, and normal pulmonary blood vascularity. *PA*, posteroanterior.

---

**BOX 6.3**
**Main Radiographic Features of Aortic Stenosis**

Enlargement of the ascending aorta caused by poststenotic dilatation
   Mild or no cardiomegaly in compensated stage
   Substantial cardiomegaly occurs only after myocardial failure has ensued
   No pulmonary venous hypertension or pulmonary edema is seen during most of the course of this disease
   Calcification of aortic valve may be seen on radiograph but is more readily shown on computed tomography

---

**BOX 6.4**
**Main Radiographic Features of Aortic Regurgitation**

Moderate-to-severe cardiomegaly
   Left ventricular enlargement
   Enlargement of ascending aorta and aortic arch
   The absence of pulmonary venous hypertension or pulmonary edema until late in the course of this lesion

---

by LV enlargement. Enlargement of the ascending aorta, aortic knob, and usually the descending thoracic aorta is seen. As opposed to AS, the enlargement of the thoracic aorta involves the aortic knob as well as the ascending aorta. Consequently, "big heart" disease with the aortic enlargement is indicative of aortic regurgitation.[2]

The severity of aortic regurgitation is depicted on chest radiographs. The extent of the increase in size of the heart is related to the severity and the duration of aortic regurgitation. For most of the course of aortic regurgitation, the pulmonary vascularity is normal. Consequently, the presence of pulmonary venous congestion in a patient with aortic regurgitation is suggestive of LV failure and is frequently associated with end-stage aortic valve disease (Box 6.4).

## PULMONARY STENOSIS

Pulmonary stenosis is an obstruction to RV outflow and can occur at the valvular, subvalvular, or supravalvular level. Most causes are congenital and occur in the valve.

### Valvular Pulmonary Stenosis

The most frequent cause of pulmonary valve stenosis is a congenital defect. The valve usually is a membrane with a central hole but can be bicuspid or tricuspid.

About 50% of patients with a carcinoid tumor that metastasized to the liver have pulmonary and tricuspid valve (TV) lesions.

## Radiography

The chest radiography findings in pulmonary valve stenosis are variable and depend on the age of the patient and on associated abnormalities. The classic chest radiograph of pulmonary valve stenosis shows mild enlargement of the RV and moderate enlargement of the main and left pulmonary artery (Fig. 6.16). The right pulmonary artery has normal size. Unless the pulmonary obstruction is so severe as to reduce cardiac output, the overall heart size is normal or mildly increased. The chest radiograph in supravalvular pulmonary stenosis shows a straight main pulmonary artery segment and small hilar structures.[3]

## PULMONARY REGURGITATION

Pulmonary valve regurgitation most often is caused by pulmonary arterial hypertension. It can occur in a congenitally absent pulmonary valve. It nearly always occurs after pulmonary valvuloplasty and surgical correction of tetralogy of Fallot. Many patients with pulmonary valve regurgitation also have tricuspid regurgitation caused by RV dilatation.[2]

## Radiography (Fig. 6.17)

The major feature of pulmonary regurgitation is enlargement of the main pulmonary arterial segment, central pulmonary arteries, and RV.

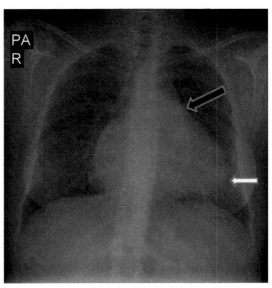

FIG. 6.17 Patient with severe pulmonary valve insufficiency (PI) and dilatation of the right ventricle (*white arrow*) and main pulmonary artery enlargement (*black arrow*). *PA*, posteroanterior.

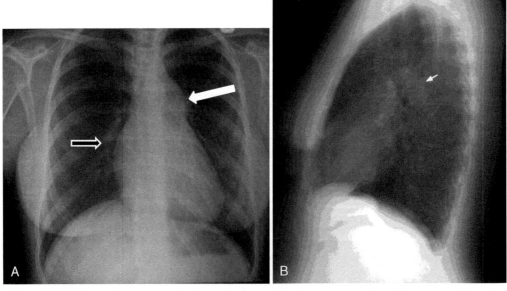

FIG. 6.16 Patient with severe valvular pulmonary stenosis, posteroanterior (PA) chest radiograph. (A) Dilatation of the main pulmonary artery (*white arrow*) and decreased pulmonary blood vascularity (*black arrow*), lateral (LAT) chest radiograph. (B) Dilatation of the left pulmonary artery (LPA) (*white arrow*).

## TRICUSPID VALVE DISEASE

The normal anatomy of the TV apparatus is complex. In a normal heart, the TV has three leaflets: anterior, posterior, and septal.[4] The valve is attached to the atrioventricular junction of the RV. The anterior leaflet is largest, the posterior is multiscalloped, and the septal leaflet is smallest. They are joined by papillary muscles; the medial papillary muscle has chordal attachments to septal and the posterior leaflets, and the anterior papillary muscle provides chordae to the posterior and the anterior leaflets. Comprehensive evaluation of this complex valvular apparatus still poses a challenge to all imaging modalities.[4]

### Tricuspid Stenosis

The chest radiograph in TV disease is quite variable. The abnormalities in tricuspid stenosis follow the principle that the chamber behind a severe stenosis is large. Although RA enlargement is always seen, because of association with rheumatic mitral valve stenosis, the RV and the left heart frequently are also enlarged. The SVC and azygos vein are also enlarged.[3]

### Tricuspid Valve Regurgitation

Tricuspid valve regurgitation occurs when there is an abnormality in one or several parts of the tricuspid apparatus: the annulus, leaflets, chordae, papillary muscles, or RV wall. Dilatation of the RV and the tricuspid annulus secondary to pulmonary artery hypertension is the most common cause of acquired regurgitation.[3]

### Radiography (Fig. 6.18)

The signs of tricuspid regurgitation may be difficult to see on a plain radiograph. Findings of RA enlargement are frequently not clearly detected from normal. In general, the best sign of RA enlargement is elongation of the RA border. The radiographic findings of tricuspid regurgitation are cardiomegaly or RA enlargement.

Cardiomegaly, with the signpost of RA enlargement, is suggestive of tricuspid regurgitation. The cardiac shape in patients with tricuspid regurgitation may be similar to that of congestive cardiomyopathy and pericardial effusion. Severe cardiomegaly is seen with longstanding severe tricuspid regurgitation; it can cause a "wall-to-wall" heart[2] (Box 6.5).

## CONGENITAL HEART DISEASE

### Radiography of Congenital Heart Disease

The radiographic diagnosis of congenital heart disease can be a confusing and difficult topic because of the myriad of congenital heart lesions that exist. Therefore,

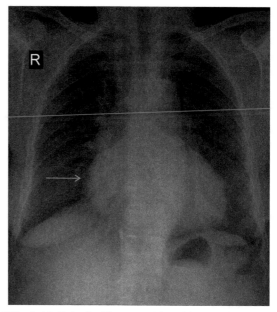

FIG. 6.18 Patient with severe tricuspid regurgitation and mitral stenosis, increased cardiothoracic ratio (big heart), and dilatation of the right atrium (*arrow*).

this part only reviews the main radiologic findings and prevalent and classic findings of them.

### Clinical-Radiographic Classification of Congenital Heart Disease

This classification depends on two pieces of clinical data: (1) whether it is cyanotic or noncyanotic and (2) symptoms of congestive heart failure, such as dyspnea, tachypnea, tachycardia, and frequent respiratory infections.

The main radiographic findings are (1) increased or decreased pulmonary arterial vascularity and (2) cardiomegaly or nearly normal heart size.

---

**BOX 6.5**
**Main Radiographic Features of Tricuspid Regurgitation**

Moderate-to-severe cardiomegaly
    Right atrial enlargement
    Right ventricular enlargement
    No pulmonary venous congestion or pulmonary edema
(isolated tricuspid regurgitation)
    Pulmonary venous congestion or edema suggestive of associated mitral valve disease

This classification system permits most major lesions involving right-to-left or left-to-right shunts to be classified into four categories. Therefore, when interpreting chest radiographs, the physician decides which category of congenital heart lesions exists.[2]

Based on the clinical and radiographic findings, there are four groups of congenital heart lesions. The groups and criteria as used in this classification system are as follows:

Group I: left-to-right shunts

Noncyanotic: sometimes symptoms of pulmonary congestion or congestive heart failure

Radiographic findings of pulmonary arterial overcirculation and cardiomegaly

Group II: right-to-left shunts with little or no cardiomegaly

Cyanosis

Decreased or normal pulmonary arterial vascularity and little or no cardiomegaly

Group III: right-to-left shunts with cardiomegaly

Cyanosis

Radiographic evidence of normal or decreased pulmonary blood flow and cardiomegaly

Group IV: admixture lesions (i.e., both right-to-left and left-to-right shunts)

It is frequently difficult to distinguish between normal and diminished pulmonary vascularity. This observation can be greatly simplified, however, when one remembers that normal pulmonary vascularity, in the radiographs of a patient with cyanosis, can be equated with decreased pulmonary vascularity. Consequently, the major observation on radiographs in terms of pulmonary vascularity in cyanotic patients is to determine whether the pulmonary vascularity is increased[2] (Box 6.6).

### Group I

Group I contains all of the left-to-right shunts; consequently, most of the patients with congenital heart disease are classified in this group. The criteria that place a patient within this category are the absence of cyanosis with increased pulmonary arterial vascularity in radiography. The degree of cardiomegaly is usually in proportion to the increase in pulmonary vascularity. The left-to-right shunts are volume overload lesions. So, there is usually cardiomegaly, and this is in general in proportion to the increased pulmonary blood vascularity.

---

**BOX 6.6**
**Classification of Shunt Lesions**

**GROUP I LESIONS: ACYANOTIC, PULMONARY ARTERIAL OVERCIRCULATION, CARDIOMEGALY**

Atrial septal defect

Partial anomalous pulmonary venous connection

Atrioventricular septal defect

Ventricular septal defect (VSD)

Patent ductus arteriosus

Other aortic level shunts (e.g., ruptured sinus of Valsalva aneurysm, aorticopulmonary window)

**GROUP II LESIONS: CYANOTIC, DECREASED PULMONARY VASCULARITY, NO CARDIOMEGALY**

Tetralogy of Fallot

Transposition with pulmonic stenosis and VSD

Double-outlet right ventricle with pulmonic stenosis and VSD

Double-outlet left ventricle with pulmonic stenosis and VSD

Single ventricle (univentricular atrioventricular connection) with pulmonic stenosis

Corrected transposition with pulmonic stenosis and VSD

Pulmonic atresia with intact ventricular septum, type I

Pulmonic stenosis with atrioventricular septal defect

Hypoplastic right ventricle syndrome

Some types of tricuspid atresias [large atrial septal defect (ASD) and pulmonary stenosis or atresia]

**GROUP III LESIONS: CYANOTIC, DECREASED PULMONARY VASCULARITY, CARDIOMEGALY**

Ebstein anomaly

Pulmonary stenosis (critical) with ASD or patent foramen ovale

Some types of tricuspid atresias (restrictive ASD)

Pulmonary atresia with intact ventricular septum, type II

Transient tricuspid regurgitation of the newborn

**GROUP IV LESIONS: CYANOTIC, PULMONARY ARTERIAL OVERCIRCULATION**

Transposition of great arteries

Truncus arteriosus

Total anomalous pulmonary venous connection

Tricuspid atresia

Single ventricle (univentricular atrioventricular connection)

Double-outlet right ventricle

Double-outlet left ventricle

Atrioventricular septal defect (complete form)

Hypoplastic left heart syndrome

Pulmonary arteriovenous fistulae

When cardiomegaly is out of proportion to the pulmonary arterial vascularity, then a decreased left-to-right shunt should be considered caused by a decreased size ventricular septal defect (VSD) or other cardiac lesions, such as primary myocardial disease or coarctation of the aorta.[2]

Two hallmarks can be used to help distinguish among the different types of left-to-right shunts (Table 6.2 and Fig. 6.19). The first of these is the LA. LA enlargement indicates that the main lesion is not at atrial level but rather a VSD or a patent ductus arteriosus (PDA) is present. The next hallmark is the aortic arch. A dilated aortic arch distinguishes between a PDA and a VSD. The aortic arch usually has a normal dimension or is small in VSD. PDA is associated with LA enlargement and a dilated aortic arch. Atrial septal defect and partial anomalous pulmonary venous connection lack both of these hallmarks.

The plain radiograph may be useful in determining the severity and progression of left-to-right shunts. The severe volume overload with large left-to-right shunts causes pulmonary venous congestion or pulmonary edema in addition to pulmonary arterial overcirculation.

Note: Disproportionate enlargement of central pulmonary arteries compared with the peripheral vasculature suggests the Eisenmenger complex but can also be observed with very large shunts. Pulmonary arterial calcification can occur in Eisenmenger complex (Boxes 6.7–6.9 and Figs. 6.20–6.22).

| TABLE 6.2 Distinguishing Features of Acyanotic Shunt Lesions | | |
|---|---|---|
| **Lesion** | **Chamber Enlargement** | **Dilated Aorta** |
| Atrial septal defect | Right atrium Right ventricle | No |
| Ventricular septal defect | Left atrium Left ventricle Right ventricle | No |
| Patent ductus arteriosus | Left atrium Left ventricle | Yes |

**BOX 6.7**
**Main Radiographic Features of Atrial Septal Defect (See Fig. 6.20)**

Enlargement of main and hilar pulmonary arterial segments
  Pulmonary arterial overcirculation: Generally a 2:1 shunt must exist before pulmonary overcirculation is present. About 50%–60% of patients with less than 2:1 shunts have only mild or no evident pulmonary overcirculation.
  Enlargement of the right atrium
  Enlargement of the right ventricle
  Small ascending aorta and aortic arch

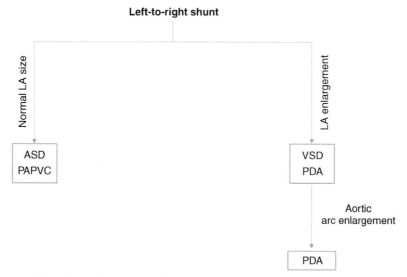

FIG. 6.19 Algorithm of left-to-right shunt. *ASD*, atrial septal defect; *LA*, left atrium; *LV*, left ventricle; *PAPVC*, partial anomaly of pulmonary venous connection; *PDA*, patent ductus arteriosus; *VSD*, ventricular septal defect.

### BOX 6.8
### Main Radiographic Features of Ventricular Septal Defect (See Fig. 6.21)

Pulmonary arterial overcirculation
    Enlargement of main and central pulmonary arterial segments
        Enlargement of the left atrium
        Enlargement of either or both ventricles
        Small thoracic aorta

### BOX 6.9
### Main Radiographic Features of Patent Ductus Arteriosus (See Fig. 6.22)

Pulmonary arterial overcirculation
    Enlargement of the main and central pulmonary arterial segments
        Enlargement of the left atrium
        Enlargement of the left ventricle
        Enlargement of the aortic arch
        **Abnormal contour of the posterior aortic arch** and proximal descending aorta: In many normal subjects, there is a localized dilatation of the aorta at the site of attachment of the ligamentum arteriosus, **the aortic spindle** (also called infundibulum). This aortic spindle is enlarged in patients with

*Continued*

### BOX 6.9—cont'd

patent ductus arteriosus. The combined shadows of the posterior arch and aortic spindle cause apparent elongation. The aorticopulmonary window may be obliterated or convex caused by the patent ductus arteriosus.
    Calcification of the walls of the ductus in older individuals

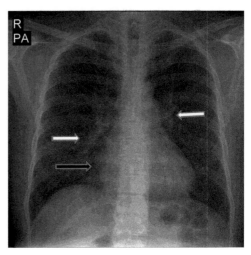

FIG. 6.20 Patient with left-to-right shunt (*white arrow*) and normal left atrial size and dilatation of the right atrium (*black arrow*) caused by atrial septal defect. *PA*, posteroanterior.

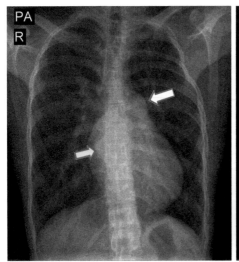
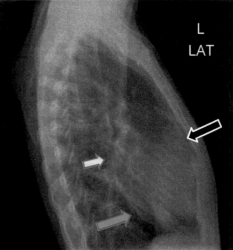

FIG. 6.21 Patient with left-to-right shunt pulmonary blood pattern, enlargement of the left atrium (*yellow arrow*), and enlargement of the left ventricle (*blue arrow*) and right ventricle (*black arrow*) caused by ventricular septal defect. *LAT*, lateral; *PA*, posteroanterior.

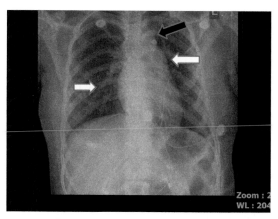

FIG. 6.22 Patient with patent ductus arteriosus, enlargement of the main pulmonary artery and left-to-right shunt (*white arrows*), dilatation of the left atrium, and dilatation of the aorta (*black arrow*).

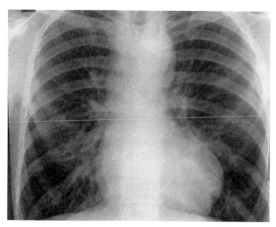

FIG. 6.23 Right ventricular enlargement (boot shape), decreased pulmonary vascularity, and absent MPA caused by tetralogy of Fallot.

## Group II

Group II lesions include cyanosis, and the plain radiograph demonstrates diminished or normal pulmonary vascularity and the absence of obvious cardiomegaly.

Statistically, the most frequent lesion in this group is tetralogy of Fallot. The remaining lesions are variants of tetralogy of Fallot [e.g., severe pulmonary stenosis and VSD with transposition of the great arteries (TGA) or double-outlet RV].

Normal vascularity in a cyanotic patient is equal to decreased vascularity because the distinction between normal and mildly decreased vascularity is frequently difficult. Asymmetric pulmonary vascularity is frequent because of associated branch pulmonary artery stenosis.[2]

Patients after total correction of tetralogy of Fallot (TFTC) show aneurysmal dilatation of the right ventricle (RV) outflow tract and enlargement of RV caused by pulmonary insufficiency (PI) (Figs. 6.23 and 6.24 and Box 6.10).

## Group III

Group III lesions differ from group II lesions by cardiomegaly seen on chest radiographs. These patients have cyanosis, normal or decreased pulmonary vascularity, and a substantial degree of cardiomegaly. The RA is frequently enlarged in this lesion. Many of the patients in this category have substantial tricuspid regurgitation, which is a major reason for the RA enlargement and cardiomegaly.[2]

In older children and adults, the most likely diagnosis is Ebstein anomaly. Uhl anomaly is a rare cause of a cardiac configuration similar to Ebstein anomaly[2] (Box 6.11 and Fig. 6.25).

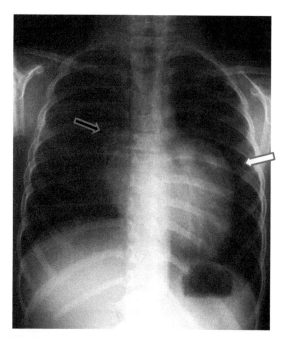

FIG. 6.24 Aneurysmal dilatation of the right ventricular outflow tract (*white arrow*) in a post-TFTC (total correction of tetralogy of Fallot) patient with severe pulmonary insufficiency (PI) and a stent in the right pulmonary artery (*black arrow*).

---

**BOX 6.10**
**Main Radiographic Features of Tetralogy of Fallot (Fig. 6.23)**

Decreased pulmonary vascularity
    Normal or nearly normal cardiac size
    Right ventricular enlargement or prominence: This may cause an uplifted cardiac apex (boot-shaped heart).
    Concave or absent main pulmonary arterial segment
    Small hilar pulmonary arteries
    Prominent ascending aorta and aortic arch
    Right aortic arc

---

**BOX 6.11**
**Main Radiographic Features of Ebstein Anomaly (See Fig. 6.25)**

Decreased pulmonary vascularity
    Main pulmonary arterial segment and hilar segments are small.
    Cardiomegaly
    Enlarged right atrium
    Enlargement of right ventricle. The right ventricle is less prominent than the atrium.
    Small thoracic aorta

---

### Group IV

Pulmonary arterial overcirculation in the presence of cyanosis is the main finding. The heart size is usually increased.

The most common diagnosis in this category is TGA, which is the most frequent cyanotic congenital heart lesion at birth. The lesion that is frequently forgotten in this group is multiple pulmonary arterial venous malformations.

### Coarctation of the Aorta

Coarctation of the aorta is a narrowing of the distal aortic arch or proximal descending aorta (or both) caused by a fibromuscular ring or a segmental tunnel narrowing of the aortic isthmus.

---

**BOX 6.12**
**Main Radiographic Findings in Coarctation (See Fig. 6.26)**

Rib notching
    Abnormal appearance of the aortic arch
    A notch on the proximal descending aorta followed by poststenotic dilatation causes a figure-3 sign on the aorta and a reverse figure-3 sign on the barium-filled esophagus.
    Left ventricular prominence
    Prominent ascending aorta

---

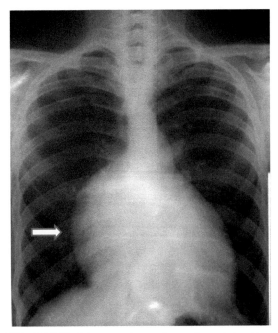

FIG. 6.25 Ebstein anomaly, cardiomegaly and decreased pulmonary blood vascularity, and dilatation of the right atrium (*white arrow*).

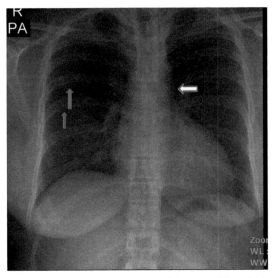

FIG. 6.26 Patient with coarctation of the aorta. Rib notching is indicated by the *blue arrow*, and 3 sign is indicated by the *white arrow*. *PA*, posteroanterior.

The coarctation usually occurs adjacent to the site of attachment of the ligamentum arteriosus and distal to the left subclavian artery. A bicuspid aortic valve occurs in a high percentage of patients.

Rib notching involves the fourth to eighth ribs. The notching includes scalloped regions on the undersurface of the posterior arc of the ribs. Coarctation proximal to the left subclavian arterial origin causes right-sided rib notching only, and an aberrant right subclavian artery from a site below the coarctation produces unilateral left-sided notching[2] (Box 6.12 and Fig. 6.26).

## REFERENCES

1. Mann DL, Zipes DP, Libby P, et al, eds. *Braunwald's Heart Disease: A Textbook of Cardiovascular Medicine.* 10th ed. Philadelphia: Elsevier; 2015.
2. Webb WR, Higgins CB. *Thoracic Imaging, Pulmonary and Cardiovascular Radiology.* Philadelphia: Lippincott Williams & Wilkins; 2005.
3. Miller SW. *Cardiac Imaging Tile Requisites.* 2nd ed. Philadelphia: Elsevier; 2005.
4. Kramer CM, ed. *Multimodality Imaging in Cardiovascular Medicine.* New York: Demos Medical Publishing; 2011.

# CHAPTER 7

# Cardiac Computed Tomography

HAMIDREZA POURALIAKBAR

Rajaie Cardiovascular, Medical & Research Center, Iran University of Medical Sciences, Tehran, Iran

---

**KEY POINTS**

- Cardiac computed tomography is a novel diagnostic imaging modality in cardiovascular disease.
- Cardiologists should know how to use and interpret the cardiac computed tomography.
- In this chapter, we learn the role of cardiac computed tomography in preventing medicine in cardiovascular disease, acute chest pain, stable chronic angina, ischemic heart disease, revascularization, and structural heart disease.

---

Progress in the clinical capabilities of cardiovascular computed tomography (CT) provides an array of applications for noninvasive cardiac and coronary artery assessment. Cardiac CT angiography now provides excellent image quality at low to extremely low effective radiation doses, which, coupled with ongoing progress in scanner technology and accumulating clinical trial evidence, establishes CT as a core technology for cardiovascular patient care. Beyond CT angiography, the technique now provides a detailed assessment of the arterial wall, left ventricular (LV) and right ventricular (RV) systolic function, and cardiac valve morphology. In addition, due to a decrease in the radiation dose, perfusion study is also available with cardiac CT.[1]

## MDCT TERMINOLOGY

The basic principle of CT technology harnesses ionizing radiation within a gantry rotating around the patient in which X-rays are detected on a detector array (Fig. 7.1) and converted through reconstruction algorithms to images. Physical limits to spatial and temporal resolution are recognized, based on minimum detector width for the detection of radiation signals and the speed at which the gantry can physically rotate. These physical limits are now being surmounted through software enhancements enabling preservation of or even improvements in diagnostic image quality at lower radiation exposures.[1]

In multidetector systems (MDCT), the gantry (X-ray tube and detector) rotates rapidly around the patient. Initial single-detector CT systems, introduced in 1972 for body imaging, were limited by very slow rotation

and long acquisition time. Fast gantry rotation, thin collimated detector rows, ECG-synchronized imaging, and acquisition of multiple slices per gantry rotation have since allowed the development of modern cardiovascular systems.[2–4] Multislice scanners with 8, 16, 64, 256, 320, 384, 512, and 640 slice acquisitions per rotation were introduced over the last decade.[5]

### Isotropic Data Acquisition

The most important advance in the newest systems is providing thinner slices, important for improving image quality as well as diminishing partial volume effects. The current systems allow for slice thicknesses between 0.5 and 0.75 mm (depending on manufacturer and scan model).[1,6]

### Spatial/Temporal Resolution

Spatial resolution compares the ability of the scanners to reproduce fine detail within an image, usually referred to as the high-contrast spatial resolution. Spatial resolution is important in all three dimensions when measuring coronary plaque.

Spatial resolution within the imaging plane (the $x$–$y$ axis) is broadly determined by the detector width, and the ability to create volumes of image data (voxels) of equal sides on all size, or *isotropism*. Currently, the narrow commercial detector width is 0.32 mm for "high-definition" CT.

The other major constraint with cardiac imaging is temporal resolution, a crucial factor in obtaining motion-free cardiac images. This requires fast gantry rotation (currently, maximum gantry rotation times are approximately 270–330 ms) and performing image

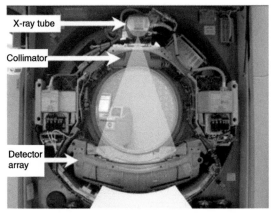

FIG. 7.1 View within the rotating multidetector computed tomography (CT) gantry. Key elements include the X-ray tube or source; a collimator to align the X-ray beam; and the detector array, consisting of narrow channels for detection of X-ray photons. The number of detector channels determines the nomenclature (e.g., 64-row multidetector CT). (From Taylor AJ. Cardiac computed tomography. In: Mann DL, Zipes DP, Libby P, et al., eds. *Braunwald's Heart Disease: A Textbook of Cardiovascular Medicine*. 10th ed. Philadelphia: Saunders; 2015, with permission.)

acquisition or reconstruction during periods of limited cardiac motion (end-systole to mid-late diastole). Currently, CT spatial resolution through the reconstruction of overlapping data sets is approximately 0.5 mm$^3$, and temporal resolution is approximately 63–165 ms, achieved with the use of half-scan reconstruction techniques. By coupling rapid image acquisition with ECG gating, images can be acquired in specific phases of the cardiac cycle. Although the temporal and spatial resolution of cardiac CT (approximately 0.23–0.4 mm) remains less than that of invasive coronary angiography (ICA <0.1 mm), it is sufficient for highly accurate, diagnostic coronary artery imaging.[1]

Software-based postprocessing techniques for selective reduction of coronary motion, also known as intracycle motion correction algorithms, are used to correct coronary motion artifacts by exploiting the trajectory data across time and "backtracking" to create motion-free images. Improvements in volume coverage by imaging greater lengths in the z-axis or craniocaudal direction have been achieved by increases in the number of detector rows. This has been termed *volumetric* CT imaging because, with enough detector elements to cover its entire length, the heart can be imaged in a single gantry rotation in less than 1 s.[7]

## SCAN MODES

There are two basic acquisition modes in cardiac CT, spiral (helical) and axial (sequence) scanning are now available (Table 7.1 and Fig. 7.2).

In the spiral mode, data are acquired during constant rotation of the gantry and continuous movement of the patient table through the gantry. For cardiac imaging, spiral data are retrospectively gated to the ECG. This scan mode relies on gathering of a redundant or overlapping data set so that complete image data can be reconstructed after CT data acquisition ("retrospective" reconstruction, Fig. 7.3A).

Data from specific periods of the cardiac cycle are then used for image reconstruction by retrospective referencing to the ECG signal (retrospective ECG gating). Because data are acquired throughout the cardiac cycle, spiral imaging allows reconstruction during multiple cardiac phases, which can be important for coronary imaging and is necessary for functional assessment (Fig. 7.3A).

A newer scan mode, high-pitch spiral CT, uses a very rapid rate of table feed (for movement of the patient through the X-ray beam) in a single cardiac cycle, enabling ultralow dose acquisitions by virtue of very short exposure times (approximate 250 ms). This scan mode must be performed only in optimally prepared patients with controlled heart rate and requires specific technology (dual-source CT).[7]

By contrast, *axial* imaging involves sequential scanner "step and shoot," in between which the X-ray tube is turned off and the table is moved to a different position for the next image to be acquired. For these cardiovascular sequential protocols, data acquisition is prospectively triggered by the ECG signal, typically in late diastole (Fig. 7.3B). The major relative advantage of spiral CT acquisition is the ability to reconstruct data throughout the cardiac cycle, enabling great flexibility for evaluation of ventricular function and data editing in the event of cardiac arrhythmias. The major relative advantage of sequential CT acquisition is the "on/off" X-ray exposure, with consequent marked (68%) reductions in radiation exposure but with limitations in data reconstruction, including the relative inability to evaluate ventricular function unless the study is performed using a widened acquisition window during systole. Both modes produce images of similar spatial and temporal resolution and thus provide the same diagnostic image quality, as demonstrated in the PROTECTION I clinical trial.[1]

### New Technologies

In addition to the CT hardware improvements previously described, other advances allow for enhanced

**TABLE 7.1**
**Scanning Modes for Cardiac Computed Tomography**

| Feature | Helical, Low Pitch | SCAN MODE Axial, Prospectively ECG Triggered With 64-Slice CT | Axial, Prospectively ECG Triggered With Wide-Area Detector | Helical, High Pitch, Prospectively ECG Triggered |
|---|---|---|---|---|
| Synonym(s) | Spiral, retrospectively gated | Triggered, step and shoot | Triggered | High-pitch helical |
| Bask principle | X-ray tube continuously "on," with patient moved through the beam | X-ray tube "on" and "off" triggered by the EGG, with no scanning between steps as the patient is moved through the scan range | Acquisition of CT data during a single heartbeat | X-ray tube "on" only for a single heartbeat during rapid helical acquisition without significant data overlap |
| CT data acquired | Systole and diastole | Set phase (diastole or systole) with some phase tolerance (temporal padding) | Set phase (diastole or systole) with some phase tolerance (temporal padding) | Can include systole and diastole for LVEF determination |
| Radiation-sparing maneuvers | ECG-based tube current modulation, limited scan length, use of 100 kVp in smaller patients | Limited scan length, use of 100 kVp in smaller patients | Single vs two- or three-beat scanning | Use of 100 kVp in smaller patients |
| Advantages | Enables flexible reconstruction in the event of arrhythmias or artifacts, evaluation of cine images for systolic and diastolic frames (ejection fraction) | Low radiation dose; no loss in image quality for purpose of coronary or structural diagnosis | Temporal uniformity of contract and absence of alignment artifacts | Extremely low radiation exposure |
| Disadvantage | Higher radiation dose | Loss of ventricular function evaluation | Less applicable to high heart rates or arrhythmias | Dual-source CT only in patients with low and stable heat rate |
| Uses | Patients who do not qualify for prospectively triggered CT | Standard methodology for patients with low, regular heart rates | Wide-area detectors only | Dual-source CT only |

*CT*, computed tomography; *ECG*, electrocardiography; *LVEF*, left ventricular ejection fraction.
From Taylor AJ. Cardiac computed tomography. In: Mann DL, Zipes DP, Libby P, et al., eds. *Braunwald's Heart Disease: A Textbook of Cardiovascular Medicine*. 10th ed. Philadelphia: Saunders; 2015, with permission.

CT image acquisition and reconstruction parameters. Iterative reconstruction (IR) has been introduced as an improvement over traditional filtered back projection (FBP) methods used in CT and employs system statistics to reconstruct high-quality, noise-reduced images.[8] IR improves image quality by accentuating signal-to-noise and contrast-to-noise ratios without increased radiation. An IR image can be acquired at a much lower radiation dose and can still achieve similar quality to images reconstructed by FBP.

Dual-energy computed tomography (DECT) techniques have also been recently introduced to improve material discrimination. This method acquires simultaneous or near-simultaneous, imaging at a low and high kVp.[9] The use of widely disparate energies allows for harnessing two polychromatic spectra (e.g., 80 and

- Axial (sequential)
- Helical

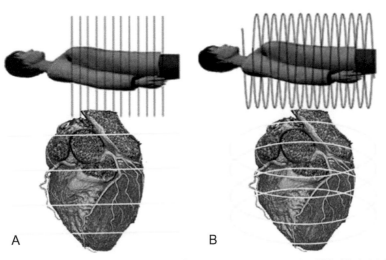

FIG. 7.2 The two basic acquisition modes in cardiac computed tomography (CT). (A) Axial (sequential). (B) Spiral (helical).

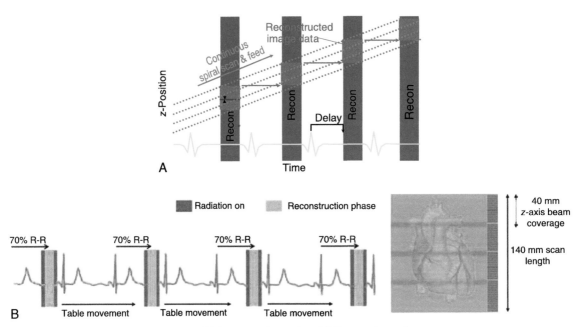

FIG. 7.3 (A) Retrospective gating. (B) Prospective gating.

140 kVp) to discriminate between the material densities of two basic materials by examining their attenuation characteristics at different X-ray energies. Methods of DECT acquisition have used DSCT (one detector array offering low-energy spectra and the other high-energy spectra), fast kVp switching (with microsecond changes in polychromatic spectra from low and high kVp), and energy-dependent dual detectors. From each of these methods, tissues can be reconstructed into single mono-chromatic energy (in kiloelectron volts, keV), which

may be used to improve current coronary and cardiac imaging interpretation, for example, the use of a monochromatic single energy, such as 40 keV, is closer to the k-edge of iodinated contrast, enabling a higher signal that cannot be achieved by traditional polychromatic spectral single-energy CT imaging, potentially allowing for more accurate assessment of contrast-enhanced structures (e.g., coronary arteries).[7]

## RADIATION EXPOSURE

Radiation protection of patients is based on the principles of justification and optimization. Justification implies that the benefit for the patient, for example, exclusion of pathology, diagnosis of disease, or follow-up of treatment, outweighs the risk of radiation exposure.

Optimization implies to choose the appropriate protocol and reduced the effective absorbed patient dose.

Radiation dosing is measured using the CT dose index and dose-length product (mGy cm). Determination of effective radiation dose [in sievert (Sv) units] entails the application of a constant determined by the relative radiation sensitivity of the tissue. The weighting factor for the chest is 0.14.[1]

To protect the patient we should minimize the radiation exposure with retains diagnostic image quality.

So briefly to reduce the radiation dose we should

1. Limit the number of scans
2. Decreased field of view
3. Decrease tube voltage
4. Decrease nominal tube current
5. Use ECG-based tube current modulation
6. Reduce exposure time
7. Use prospectively ECG-triggered scanning
8. Consider need coronary calcium scanning—omit if information obtained unlikely to add to the patient assessment
9. Use iterative reconstruction

Recent data on coronary CT angiographic imaging at 80 kVp using a high-pitch, prospectively ECG-triggered scan mode in patients with normal body mass index show mean radiation exposures of 0.4 mSv, or the equivalent of four chest X-ray examinations.[10] In the aggregate, this represents a 20- to 50-fold reduction in potential radiation exposure in less than a decade of technical progress in cardiac CT.

## PATIENT PREPARATION

Patient preparation steps include achieving intravenous access, typically in an antecubital vein suitable for contrast administration at a flow rate of 4–6 mL/s, and administering preprocedure beta blockade when needed to achieve the desired heart rate and rhythm. Administration of sublingual nitroglycerin can be used to increase coronary vasodilatation at the time of imaging. Cooperate with breathing instructions and hold their breath for the duration of the scan.

Relative contraindications include severe sensitivity or anaphylaxia to contrast media, inability to hold the breath, unstable patient such as acute infarction or hypotension, and pregnancy. In addition to mentioned above, some factors can influence on the image quality and should be considered and include high or irregular heart rates (particularly atrial fibrillation), morbid obesity, or severe coronary artery calcium (CAC), defined as CAC scores above 400–1000. Each of these conditions can degrade scan quality or interpretability.[1]

These relative contraindications continue to be partially relieved by technical advances in the field. High heart rates (addressed using dual-source scanners or multisegment reconstruction techniques), irregular heart rates (arrhythmia rejection software), atrial fibrillation (prospective ECG-triggered acquisitions), morbid obesity, and CAC (iterative reconstruction techniques) each can be partially overcome through recent advances in CT technology.[1]

Practical note: Generally, acceptable heart rate is less than 65 beats/min and usually using beta-blockers administered either orally (e.g., metoprolol 25–100 mg 1 h before the scan) or intravenously (e.g., metoprolol 5 mg in repeated doses). In a patient with a history of bronchospasm, the beta-blocker should not be used.

In a patient with sick sinus syndrome, presyncope and severely reduced LV and RV dysfunction, beta-blocker should be prescribed cautiously.

Some scanners with faster gantry rotations or dual-source configurations can obtain diagnostic image quality at higher heart rates, but in general, scan quality is lower at higher heart rates.

Nitroglycerin (400–800 μg sublingually) typically is administered just before CT angiography, to increase coronary artery diameter and improve the image quality. Screening patients for contraindications to nitrates such as sildenafil should be routine.

Preprocedure for cardiac CT angiography included:
- No food for 3–4 h before examination
- Drink water
- Take all regular medication by patient
- No caffeine 12 h before examination
- Take premedications for contrast allergy as needed
- Take premedications for renal protection as needed

- Serum creatinine by institutional protocol (diabetics, age >60 years, known chronic kidney disease)
  During procedure:
- Intravenous line 18 or 20 gauge, antecubital site
- Pulse/blood pressure/ECG monitor
- Beta-blocker (IV or PO) (metoprolol)
  - 25–100 mg metoprolol PO 1 h before scan
  - 5 mg metoprolol intravenous bolus; repeat as needed
- Positioning
- Breath-hold training—observe heart rate response
- Nitroglycerin—400–800 µg sublingual
  Post procedure:
- Drink oral fluids
- Hold metformin 48 h after contrast administration

## Image Acquisition

A typical sequence of scan acquisition and a postprocessing algorithm are included:

1. Scout the film; determine cardiac location
2. Set the scan range; limit scan range to cardiac and other relevant structures of interest
3. Perform the calcium scan
   If indicated: use a calcium scan to refine CT angiography scan range
4. Nitroglycerin administration: 400–800 µg sublingual
5. Contrast test bolus or bolus tracking
6. Breath-hold initiated
7. CT angiogram; check vital signs after procedure
8. Image reconstruction and postprocessing/analysis

Use of interpretation and reporting standards is recommended. Novel applications, such as evaluation of late myocardial enhancement or myocardial perfusion during vasodilator stress, require specific alterations to the imaging protocol.

## CARDIAC COMPUTED TOMOGRAPHY ANATOMY[11–13]

Evaluation of the coronary arteries begins with an axial review of their origin and proximal course.

The right and left coronary arteries arise from the right and left sinuses of Valsalva, respectively. The locations of the sinuses are anatomic misnomers: the left sinus is posterior in location and the right sinus is anterior (Figs. 7.4 and 7.5).

The left main coronary artery normally arises from the left sinus of Valsalva and normally gives rise to the LAD artery and the LCX artery. In approximately 15% of patients, a third branch, the ramus intermedius branch, arises at the division of the LM, resulting in a trifurcation (see Figs. 7.4 and 7.5).

The LAD courses anteriorly and inferiorly in the anterior interventricular groove to the cardiac apex, giving rise to septal and diagonal branches.

LCX courses in the left AV groove, giving rise to obtuse marginal branches. The LCX and branches supply the lateral aspect of the LV (see Figs. 7.4 and 7.5).

The RCA normally courses in the right AV groove toward the crux of the heart. The first branch of RCA is conus branch in 50%–60% of patient. In approximately 60% of patients, the sinoatrial node artery arises from the RCA. This artery gives off branches that supply the RV myocardium and called "RV marginals" or "acute marginals." The other branches of the RCA include atrioventricular nodal branch (see Figs. 7.4 and 7.5).

The coronary artery that gives rise to posterior descending artery (PDA) and posterolateral branch is referred to as the "dominant" artery. Variable dominance rates are reported; right dominance occurs in 70%–85% of the population, left dominance in 8%–10%, and codominance in the remainder (see Figs. 7.4–7.6).

## Cardiac Chambers

The left and right cardiac chambers are typically visualized in two-chamber, three-chamber, four-chamber, and short-axis views (Fig. 7.7).

- The two-chamber view of the left ventricle (LV) is comparable to the right anterior oblique ventriculogram performed during angiography (see Fig. 7.7).
- The three-chamber view includes the left atrium (LA), left ventricle, and aortic root. It visualizes the relationship between the LV, mitral valve, and left ventricular outflow tract (LVOT). It is also the basis to reconstruct additional images of the aortic root (see Fig. 7.7).
- The four-chamber view allows simultaneous assessment of the left and right ventricles (LV and RV), the atria (LA and RA), and the atrioventricular valves (mitral and tricuspid valves) (see Fig. 7.7).

## Image Reconstruction

Thin-slice cardiac CT reconstructions allow the acquisition of isotropic voxels. A variety of postprocessing techniques, including maximum intensity projection, multiplanar reformation (MPR), curved reformation (CR), and volume rendering (VR), allow noninvasive assessment of every view of the cardiovascular system.

Multiplanar reformation is the basic tool for interpreting cardiac CTA studies. This technique allows optimal evaluation of the heart and coronary arteries (Fig. 7.8).

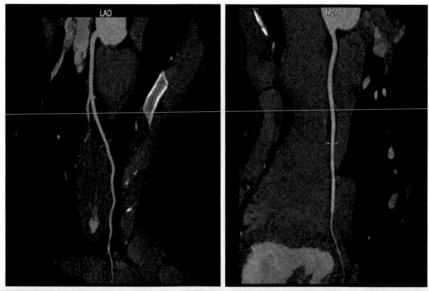

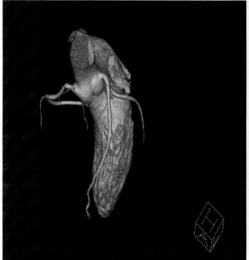

| | Scan | kV | mAs / ref. | CTDIvol˙ | DLP | TI | cSL |
|---|---|---|---|---|---|---|---|
| | | | | mGy | mGycm | s | mm |
| Physician: | | | | | | | |
| Patient position H-SP | | | | | | | |
| Topogram | 1 | 120 | 19  mA | 0.07 L | 1.9 | 2.9 | 0.6 |
| Fl_CaSc | 2D | 120 | 68 /  80 | 1.15 L | 19.4 | 0.25 | 0.6 |
| contrast | | | | | | | |
| Premonitoring | 3 | 80 | 23 | 0.30 L | 0.3 | 0.25 | 10.0 |
| contrast | | | | | | | |
| Monitoring | 4 | 80 | 23 | 3.89 L | 3.9 | 0.25 | 10.0 |
| Fl_CorCTA | 17D | 80 | 382 / 430 | 1.76 L | 30.5 | 0.25 | 0.6 |
| Operator: | | | | | | | |

22-Sep-2016  13:59

Ward:

Total mAs 941   Total DLP 56 mGycm

| Medium | Type | Iodine Conc. | Volume | Flow | CM Ratio |
|---|---|---|---|---|---|
| | | mg/mL | mL | mL/s | |

**FIG. 7.4** Patient with atypical chest pain referred from the emergency department to rule out coronary artery disease. The heart rate of the patient is appropriate for a high-pitch spiral study. The coronary arteries show normal total patient radiation dose measured at 0.78 mSv. *LAD*, left anterior descending coronary artery; *RCA*, right coronary artery; *R/O*, ruled out.

Maximum intensity projection is a postprocessing technique that takes the highest attenuation voxels in the slab volume. They can allow quick assessment for significant coronary artery stenosis but can obscure details, particularly when highly attenuating structures (such as a stent or calcified plaques) are present (see Fig. 7.8).

Curved MPR provides a planar image from the entire tortuous coronary arteries along its center line (see Fig. 7.8).

Volume rendering is useful for revealing general structural relationships and especially for evaluating coronary artery anomalies, bypass grafts, and fistulas (see Fig. 7.8). Volume rendering can facilitate

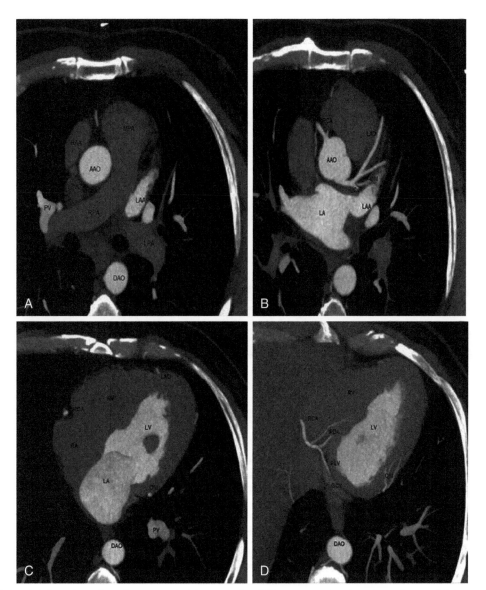

FIG. 7.5 Overview of cardiac computed tomography (CT) cross-sectional anatomy from axial images. (A) Thick-slice axial projection at the level of the superior vena cava (SVC) and main pulmonary artery (MPA). (B) Thick-slice axial maximum intensity projection showing the origin of the left main coronary artery (LMCA) and the left anterior descending coronary artery (LAD) (arrow). (C) Midlevel four-chamber ventricular view showing the right atrium (RA), right ventricle (RV), left atrium (LA), and left ventricle (LV). (D) Thick-slice maximum intensity projection showing the distal right coronary artery (RCA). AAo, ascending aorta; DAO, descending aorta; LAA, left atrial appendage; LCx, left circumflex; LPA, left pulmonary artery; OM, obtuse margin; PV, pulmonary vein; RAA, right atrial appendage.

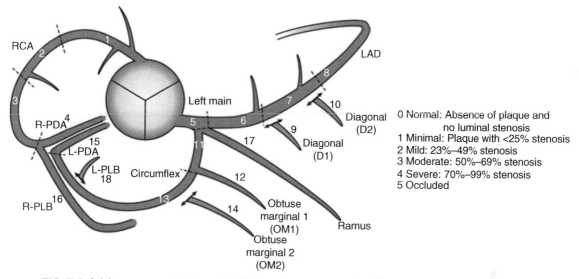

FIG. 7.6 Axial coronary anatomic model of the coronary segments described in cardiac computed tomography. *LAD*, left posterior descending artery; *L-PLB*, left posterolateral branch; *RCA*, right main coronary artery; *R-PDA*, right posterior descending artery; *R-PLB*, right posterolateral branch. (From Taylor AJ. Cardiac computed tomography. In: Mann DL, Zipes DP, Libby P, et al., eds. *Braunwald's Heart Disease: A Textbook of Cardiovascular Medicine*. 10th ed. Philadelphia: Saunders; 2015, with permission.)

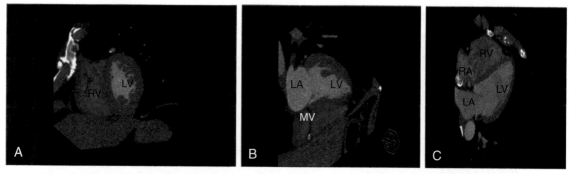

FIG. 7.7 Standard cardiac chamber view in cardiac computed tomography, including short-axis (A), long axis (B), and four-chamber (C) views. *LA*, left atrium; *LV*, left ventricle; *MV*, mitral valve; *RA*, right atrium; *RV*, right ventricle.

significantly the relation between complicated 3D structures to the interpreter and also surgeons. However, it is not appropriate for the detection and quantification of coronary stenosis. The most useful application of this reconstruction is understanding the spatial relationship of the great vessels, chest wall, and coronary arteries.

## CALCIUM SCORING

Around 650,000 asymptomatic patients with no known coronary artery disease (CAD) present with acute coronary events annually. These patients represent a failure of the current risk assessment system for CAD, which consists primarily of conventional cardiac risk factor assessment. Substantial evidence indicates that CAC scoring is underused clinically and is the most powerful predictor of subclinical atherosclerosis today. CAC scoring may be the key to preventing asymptomatic patients with subclinical CAD from experiencing coronary events.

CAC scanning is a noncontrast-enhanced image acquisition technique that is performed during a single

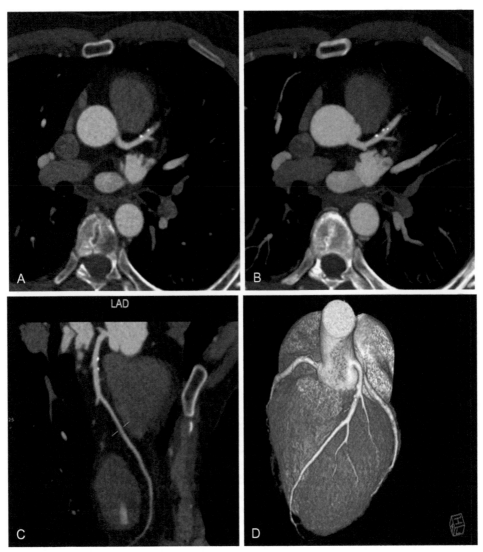

FIG. 7.8 (A) Thin-slice multiplanar reconstruction. (B) Thick-slice maximum intensity projection. (C) Curved multiplanar reformation. (D) Vendor three-dimensional reconstruction. *LAD*, left anterior descending coronary artery.

breath-hold. Current guidelines recommend prospective ECG-triggered scanning from the bifurcation of the main pulmonary artery to the apex of the heart, with a 2.5- to 3-mm slice thickness and a tube voltage 120 kVp. No beta blockade is required, and the scan time is 3–5 s.[7,14]

Agatston et al. originally determined a calcium score by the summation of the product of the calcified plaque area and a factor for maximum calcium density (1 for lesions with a maximal density of 130–199 Hounsfield units (HU), 2 for 200–299 HU, 3 for 300–399 HU, 4 for >400 HU) in each lesion. Calcium scores are generally classified in as follows: 1–10, minimal; 11–100, mild; 101–400, moderate; and greater than 400, severe (Fig. 7.9).

## Prognostic Implications of CACS

The prognostic value of CAC has been demonstrated consistently across many cohorts worldwide, most notably in the Multi-Ethnic Study of Atherosclerosis (MESA),

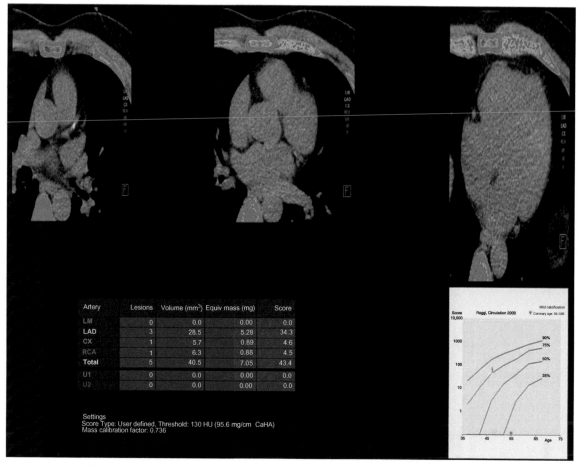

| Artery | Lesions | Volume (mm³) | Equiv mass (mg) | Score |
|--------|---------|--------------|-----------------|-------|
| LM | 0 | 0.0 | 0.00 | 0.0 |
| LAD | 3 | 28.5 | 5.28 | 34.3 |
| CX | 1 | 5.7 | 0.89 | 4.6 |
| RCA | 1 | 6.3 | 0.88 | 4.5 |
| Total | 5 | 40.5 | 7.05 | 43.4 |
| U1 | 0 | 0.0 | 0.00 | 0.0 |
| U2 | 0 | 0.0 | 0.00 | 0.0 |

Settings
Score Type: User defined, Threshold: 130 HU (95.6 mg/cm CaHA)
Mass calibration factor: 0.736

**FIG. 7.9** Example of coronary artery calcium scoring from a noncontrast computed tomography scan in which calcified foci are identified within the left anterior descending (*yellow*), right coronary artery (*red*), and left circumflex (*blue*) coronary arteries. The number of lesions, volume, and equivalent mass and scores are in the table along with the curves.

a population-based prospective cohort study of asymptomatic US adults. Risk of incident adverse events for individuals with a CAC score of 0 was very low, with a major adverse cardiovascular event (MACE) rate of 0.5% over 4 years (Fig. 7.10). However, higher levels of CAC showed a correspondingly higher risk of MACE; patients with a CAC score of 400 or higher experienced events more than 10% of the time, a rate exceeding the traditional definitions of a "coronary heart disease equivalent."[15] This prognostic value of CAC is incremental to clinical CAD risk factors, increasing the discrimination of future adverse clinical events [area under the receiver operating characteristic (ROC) curve 0.77 vs 0.82; $P < 0.001$].[16] The MESA study demonstrated higher CAC in Caucasians and Hispanics, male

sex, and advancing age and also importantly provided population-based reference standards by which individual scores may be compared.[17] A CAC score greater than the 75th percentile for age, sex, and ethnicity may be considered "high risk," irrespective of the absolute score; however, the prognostic value of the absolute CAC score demonstrates uniformity across ethnic groups and by sex, and thus it has been suggested that absolute CAC rather than CAC percentiles be used for prediction of events.[15–18] The Heinz Nixdorf Recall Study similarly showed in an older population-based cohort that the upper quartile of CAC had an event rate 11.1 times that of the lowest quartile in men and 3.2 times that of the lowest quartile in women ($P < 0.01$ for both).[7,19]

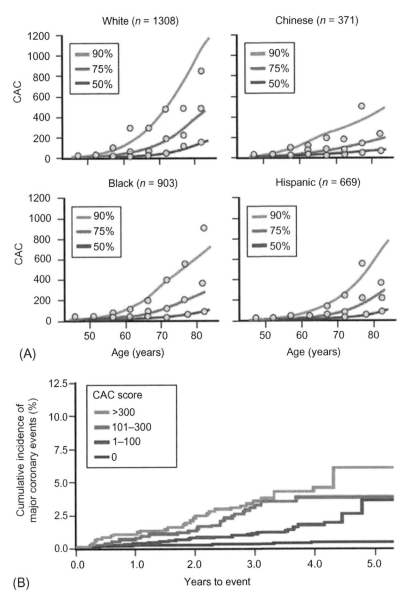

FIG. 7.10 (A) Data from the Multi-Ethnic Study of Atherosclerosis (MESA) for the distribution of coronary artery calcium (CAC) scores among men relative to age and ethnicity. (B) Major cardiovascular outcomes observed in MESA in association with higher thresholds of coronary calcium scores. (From Taylor AJ. Cardiac computed tomography. In: Mann DL, Zipes DP, Libby P, et al., eds. *Braunwald's Heart Disease: A Textbook of Cardiovascular Medicine.* 10th ed. Philadelphia: Saunders; 2015, with permission.)

CACS has been repeatedly demonstrated to be a robust predictor of atherosclerotic cardiovascular disease (ASCVD) events, including CHD, stroke, and fatal ASCVD and is associated with a significantly better *c*-statistic (improved discrimination) as compared to traditional risk factors, particularly in patients who are deemed to be in the intermediate-risk category.[15,20–33]

CACS has emerged as the most powerful predictor of risk in asymptomatic individuals as demonstrated in every cohort in which it has been studied. One stunningly consistent observation is the approximate ten-fold increased hazard of hard events associated with high CACS compared to CACS = 0.[20,34] In a head-to-head comparison of novel risk markers (CACS, ABI, hs-CRP, and family history) for improvement in ASCVD risk assessment in intermediate-risk individuals, all were independent risk markers, but CACS provided markedly superior discrimination and risk reclassification compared to other markers.[35] In MESA, findings suggested that CACS was associated more strongly than carotid intima-media thickness (cIMT) with the risk of incident ASCVD with a $c$-statistic of 0.81 (95% CI 0.78–0.83) for CACS vs 0.78 for cIMT (95% CI 0.75–0.81).[36]

The data from five large prospective randomized studies provide approximate 10-year event rates associated with increasing levels of CACS (ASCVD events defined in three studies as CHD death, MI, and revascularization and in two studies as CHD death and MI) (Table 7.2).[19,23,28,32,33,37,38] Asymptomatic patients with CACS 101–400 Agatston had a 10-year event rate of 12.8%–16.4%, and patients with CACS 1–100 Agatston had an approximate 10-year event rate between 2.3% and 5.9%. According to the 2018 ACC/AHA Guideline on the Management of Blood Cholesterol, patients with 10-year ASCVD risk of $\geq$7.5% to <20% are identified as one of the four statin benefit groups in primary prevention. Patients with risk from 5% to <7.5% may also be considered for statin therapy in the setting of shared decision-making.[39,40] Thus, the 10-year risk of ASCVD events as estimated by CACS may help to inform the patient–clinician discussion regarding preventive therapies.

Historically, the duration of follow-up after baseline CACS was only approximately 4–5 years. This is a significant shortcoming given the fact that contemporary risk assessment algorithms, such as the ACC/AHA Pooled Cohort Equations, predict 10-year and lifetime risk of ASCVD events.[41] However, two recent studies have demonstrated that CACS accurately predicts 15-year mortality and support effective long-term risk prediction and reclassification.[42,43]

The net reclassification index is used for calibration of risk markers to measure the improvement in risk prediction or risk reclassification when comparing new biomarkers or measures of subclinical atherosclerosis to traditional risk prediction strategies.[44] Several large prospective, population-based studies have demonstrated that CACS improves not only risk stratification and discrimination but also improves accurate reclassification of ASCVD risk beyond traditional risk factors and risk assessment algorithms.[16,35,38,45–47] Though CACS has primarily been recommended for use in patients at intermediate ASCVD risk as determined by conventional risk assessment algorithms, there has also been considerable interest in defining its potential role in individuals at low risk. An early analysis of the MESA study included 2684 women followed for a mean of 3.75 years who were classified as low risk based on the FRS.[31] The prevalence of any CAC in these low-risk women was 32%. There was a sixfold greater risk for a CHD event in women with CACS >0 compared to women with no evidence of CAC (HR 6.5; 95% CI 2/6–16.4, $P < 0.001$).[48]

Among another cohort of 9715 patients referred for CACS, a total of 2363 asymptomatic men and women were classified as low–intermediate risk using the FRS.[46] After a mean follow-up of 14.6 years, the total mortality ranged from 5.0% for women with a CACS = 0%–23.5% for those with CACS >400 ($P < 0.001$). For men, the 15-year mortality ranged from 3.5% among those with CACS = 0%–18% for those with CACS >400 ($P < 0.001$). Thus, even among men and women with low–intermediate risk factor burden, the presence of CAC effectively identifies those who are at significantly higher risk than predicted by the FRS alone. Women with CACS >10 were noted to have higher mortality risk compared to men with similar CACS. The fact that risk assessment based on the traditional risk factor-based algorithm performed poorly in women suggests that CACS may play an important role to improve risk prediction in women.[48]

A recent meta-analysis assessed the utility of CACS for ASCVD risk estimation among 6739 women with 10-year risk <7.5% by the Pooled Cohort Equations in five large population-based cohorts (the

**TABLE 7.2**

Summary of Absolute Event Rates by Coronary Artery Calcium Score (CACS) From 14,856 Patients in Live Prospective Studies

| CACS | FRS Equivalent[a] | 2013 ACC/AHA Statin Benefit Group[b] | 10-Year Event Rate (%) |
|---|---|---|---|
| 0 | Very low | No | 1.1–1.7 |
| 1–100 | Low | May consider | 2.3–5.9 |
| 101–400 | Intermediate | Yes | 12.8–16.4 |
| >400 | High | Yes | 22.5–28.6 |
| >1000 | Very high | Yes | 37.0 |

[a]FRS indicates Framingham Risk Score.[6]
[b]2013 ACC/AHA statin benefit group indicates eligibility for statin therapy based on 10-year ASCVD risk as calculated by the Pooled Cohort Equations.
Adapted from Hecht,[35] with permission. Joseph Schoepf U, ed. *CT of the Heart*. 2nd ed. © Humana Press 2005, 2019:321.

Dallas Heart Study, the Framingham Heart Study, the Heinz Nixdorf Recall Study, MESA, and the Rotterdam Study).[49] The median follow-up period ranged from 7.0 to 11.6 years. CAC was present in 36.1% of these low-risk women. Compared to women with CACS = 0, the presence of any CAC (CACS >0) was associated with increased risk of ASCVD event [multivariable-adjusted hazard ratio, 2.04 (95% CI, 1.44–2.90)] and modest improvement in prognostic accuracy compared to traditional risk factor-based algorithm [$c$-statistic 0.77 (95% CI, 0.74–0.81) vs 0.73 (95% CI, 0.69–0.77)].[48]

In evaluating individuals without evident CAC, a long-term "warranty period" appears to be present. In a single-center study, 422 individuals with a baseline CAC score of 0 underwent annual CAC for 5 consecutive years and were compared to a matched cohort of 621 individuals with a baseline CAC greater than 0. In those without CAC, conversion to CAC greater than 0 occurred in 25% at an average of 4 years, suggesting no need for repeat imaging until at least this point. Evaluation of the matched cohort with CAC at baseline demonstrated CAC greater than 0 to be the strongest predictor of CAC progression [hazard ratio (HR) >12].[50] The slow conversion of 0 score to a CAC greater than 0 appears to translate to the predictability of clinical outcomes. In a large study of 4864 participants with a baseline CAC of 0, the warranty period, defined by less than 1% mortality per year, extended to 15 years for individuals at low and intermediate risk for CAD events, as defined by the National Cholesterol Education Program and Adult Treatment Panel III (NCEP/ATP III) risk categories, regardless of age or sex. For individuals considered at high clinical risk, the warranty period extended only to 5 years and was 14 years for individuals older than 60.[7,16]

Notably, CAC is a measure of not only coronary atherosclerotic burden but also overall vascular atherosclerotic burden. In this regard, CAC is useful to predict cerebrovascular disease events. In the MESA study, among participants followed for almost 10 years, CAC was an independent predictor of cerebrovascular risk, even after accounting for traditional cerebrovascular disease events, and improved discrimination as well.[19] CAC is also associated with other adverse future clinical events, including atrial fibrillation, cancer, stroke, and congestive heart failure (CHF).[51–55]

Although the negative predictive value (NPV) of a CAC score of 0 has been consistently demonstrated with an event rate in asymptomatic patients, with an annualized event rate of 0.5% over 5 years in recent meta-analyses, it should not be considered similarly in symptomatic patients.[56] Recent data from the multinational CONFIRM registry showed that 4% of symptomatic patients with CAC of 0 had obstructive CAD of 50% stenosis or more, and CAC offered no incremental discriminatory utility above CCTA. Similarly, in the ROMICAT study, a CAC of 0 in acute chest pain patients did not adequately exclude acute coronary syndrome (ACS).[57,58]

In a study of 10,377 asymptomatic patients (903 diabetics), there are 4800 patients without diabetes and 267 patients with diabetes who had CACS = 0. Over a mean follow-up period of 5.0 years, participants with diabetes and CACS = 0 demonstrated a survival similar to that of individuals without diabetes and CACS = 0.[48]

Progression of CAC is clearly associated with an increased risk of future ASCVD events. Despite significant event reduction in patients treated with statin therapy and evidence of reduction in atheroma volume by IVUS, CAC progression is not retarded and may even be accelerated on treatment. Greater progression of CAC on statin therapy has been interpreted by many as a benign conversion of preexisting noncalcified to calcified plaque. However, the greater progression of CAC on statin therapy has been associated with higher MACE rates and does not support this prevailing view. Instead, the progression of CAC, irrespective of statin therapy, supports the predominant formation of new atherosclerotic plaque that then becomes calcified. At the current time, there are no medical therapies which have been demonstrated to achieve reductions.[48,59]

2018 AHA/ACC/AACVPR/AAPA/ABC/ACPM/ADA/AGS/APhA/ASPC/NLA/PCNA Guideline on the Management of Blood Cholesterol increased the number of people recommended to receive statins.[48]

CAC evaluation is a class IIa recommendation for performance that is reserved for **adults 40–75 years of age without diabetes mellitus and with LDL-C levels ≥70–189 mg/dL (≥1.8–4.9 mmol/L), at a 10-year ASCVD risk of ≥7.5%–19.9%, if a decision about statin therapy is uncertain, consider measuring CAC.** If CAC is zero, treatment with statin therapy may be withheld or delayed, except in cigarette smokers, those with diabetes mellitus, and those with a strong family history of premature ASCVD. A CAC score of 1–99 favors statin therapy, especially in those ≥55 years of age. For any patient, if the CAC score is ≥100 Agatston units or ≥75th percentile, statin therapy is indicated unless otherwise deferred by the outcome of clinician–patient risk discussion.

## CORONARY COMPUTED TOMOGRAPHIC ANGIOGRAPHY

### Diagnostic Accuracy

Since its introduction, the primary interest in the clinical use of coronary CT angiography (CCTA) has been as a noninvasive alternative to coronary angiography. An array of single-center studies and three prospective multicenter studies evaluated the diagnostic performance of CCTA, primarily compared to an ICA reference standard (Table 7.3, Fig. 7.11). Of the three multicenter studies, with a CAD prevalence of 25%–68%, the Assessment by Coronary Computed Tomographic Angiography of Individuals Undergoing Invasive Coronary Angiography (ACCURACY) trial[60] and the study by Meijboom and colleagues[39] enrolled only patients without known CAD, observing a sensitivity of 95% and 99% and specificity of 83% and 64%, respectively. In contrast, the Coronary Artery Evaluation Using 64-Row Multidetector Computed Tomography Angiography (CORE-64) study enrolled a heterogeneous group of patients with and without known CAD with a CAC score less than 600, noting the sensitivity and specificity to be 85% and 90%, respectively.[61] Based on these results, it is usually noted that CCTA is an excellent imaging modality for the exclusion of CAD. Further, its specificity for detection of coronary artery stenosis is similar or superior to more traditional stress testing methods, with or without imaging. With each improvement of CT technology, diagnostic performance of CCTA has been evaluated in smaller single-center studies of 30–160 patients. The sensitivity and specificity of CCTA vs ICA—both a per-patient and a per-vessel basis—have generally been observed to be higher than those using conventional 64-detector row CCTA with both values generally above 90% (Table 7.4).[7]

Studies directly comparing CCTA to traditional stress testing methods are less common but have been evaluated in a single, large-scale multicenter trial. Contemporary evidence to date suggests a value to CCTA over other imaging methods for the diagnosis of high-grade coronary stenoses. In the prospective multicenter Evaluation of Integrated Cardiac Imaging in Ischemic Heart Disease (EVINCI) study of 475 patients across several European centers, patients underwent CCTA, MPI by single-photon emission computed tomography (SPECT), or positron emission tomography (PET) and left ventricular wall motion analysis by stress echocardiography (SE) or cardiac magnetic resonance (CMR) imaging.[62] Significant CAD, as defined by greater than 70% luminal stenosis, was observed in 29% of patients. Among all the imaging modalities CCTA demonstrated the highest diagnostic accuracy, with a sensitivity and specificity of 91% and 92%, respectively, and an area under ROC curve of 0.91. In contrast, MPI was observed to have a sensitivity and specificity of 74% and 73%, respectively, and area under ROC curve of 0.74. Wall motion analysis by SE or CMR demonstrated a higher specificity but lower sensitivity at 92% and 49%, respectively.[7]

### Prognostic Implications

Numerous potential coronary artery and cardiac characteristics observable by CCTA beyond luminal stenosis severity offer prognostic utility for risk stratification of patients with suspected CAD. These features include extent, severity, and location of CAD, as well as atherosclerosis measures of plaque composition, plaque burden, high-risk plaque (HRP) features, and arterial remodeling.[7]

To date, the largest study evaluating the prognostic value of these CAD findings is the Coronary CT Angiography Evaluation For Clinical Outcomes: an International Multicenter Registry (CONFIRM) study[63] (Fig. 7.12). At its inception, this dynamic observational cohort study comprised 27,125 stable patients with suspected CAD who underwent CCTA and were followed for all-cause mortality, nonfatal myocardial infarction (MI), and other MACE events. The first published study from CONFIRM examined differences in all-cause mortality rates based on CCTA CAD findings, as stratified by single-, double-, and triple-vessel CAD.[64] In a 2.3-year follow-up, a 2.6-fold increased risk of death was observed for patients with any stenosis greater than 70%, as well as a 1.6-fold increased risk of death for those with milder stenosis (<50%). Increasing risk of mortality was observed for patients with greater numbers of coronary artery distribution involved for one-vessel (HR 2.00), two-vessel (HR 2.92), and three-vessel or left main CAD (HR 3.7) (P < 0.01 for all). A gender–CAD relationship was observed, with women experiencing greater risk of mortality than men for three-vessel CAD (HR 4.21 vs 3.27). Importantly, incident rates of all-cause death were very low in the absence of CAD by CCTA, with an annualized rate of 0.28%. Subsequent studies have validated this very low rate of events and suggest a warranty period of CCTA to extend beyond 5 years for patients with no evident stenosis or atherosclerosis by CCTA.[7]

One potential benefit of CCTA imaging is its ability to discern nonobstructive CAD stenosis that can be present even in the setting of high overall atherosclerotic plaque burden. Prior studies have demonstrated that the majority of individuals experiencing their first

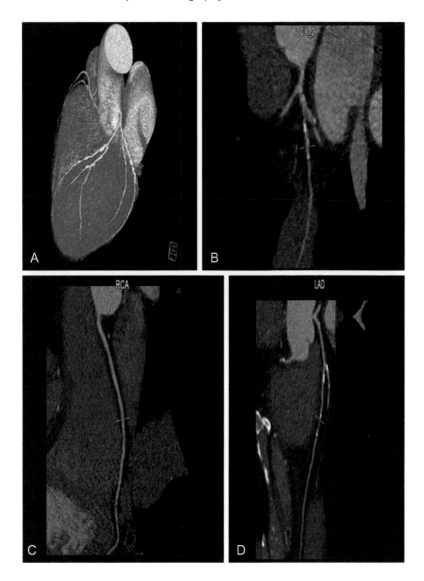

FIG. 7.11 Coronary computed tomography angiography scan from a patient with a history of hypertension and diabetes and exertional dyspnea. (A–F) Multiple calcified plaques three-vessel disease are seen. (G–K) Coronary angiography shows three-vessel disease, making the patient a candidate for coronary artery bypass graft. *LAD*, left anterior descending coronary artery; *RCA*, right coronary artery.

unheralded MI do not possess obstructive CAD stenosis. This was demonstrated first in a two-center prospective CCTA study of 2583 patients with suspected CAD.[65] At a 3.1-year follow-up, this population, limited only to those with maximum per-patient stenosis less than 50%, demonstrated differential outcomes based on the number of epicardial coronary artery distributions with any nonobstructive atherosclerosis, which were associated with a nearly twofold increased risk of mortality. A nearly fivefold increased risk of mortality was observed for individuals with nonobstructive CAD in all three epicardial vessel distributions.

The one potentially important clinical question arising from a normal CCTA without evidence of stenosis or atherosclerosis is its relatively benign nature. Prior studies have observed a very low risk of future mortality or MACE in individuals with normal CCTA. Annualized event rates have been reported at 0.01%–0.24%.[66] These

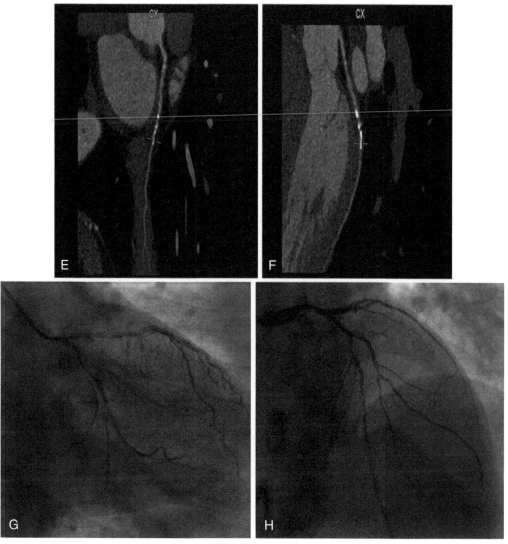

FIG. 7.11, CONT'D

data emphasize the importance of the NPV of CCTA not only to exclude the presence of AD but also to effectively rule out the risk of future events. Currently, a normal CCTA appears to confer at least a 5-year warranty period. Given these propitious findings, prior studies have evaluated whether CCTA as a screening test offers incremental prognostic role over CAC in asymptomatic individuals. In a study of 7590 patients without chest pain syndrome who were followed for 24 months, CCTA added no prognostic value for future death or MACE (c-statistic, 0.75 vs 0.77), with no significant net reclassification of patients to higher or lower risk groups.[67] As

such, routine performance of CCTA in asymptomatic individuals appears to have no tangible clinical benefit and, as per contemporary ACC multimodality imaging appropriate use criteria, should be avoided.[68]

### Imaging of Coronary Stents

CCTA has been studied extensively for this purpose and has been incorporated into the currently accepted guidelines for the evaluation of larger coronary stents ($\geq 3$ mm)[10] (Fig. 7.13).

It is commonly believed that stent size is the only factor that influences the visualization of stents by CCTA,

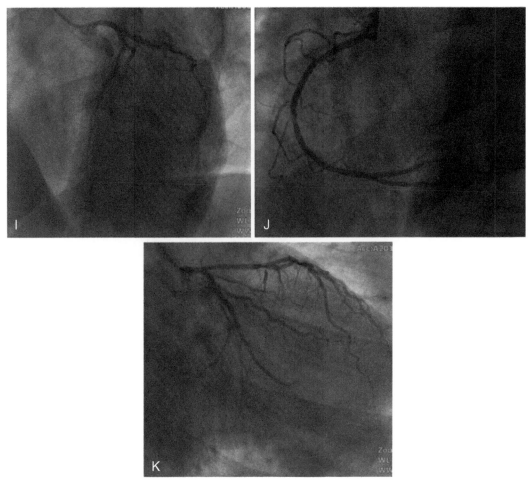

FIG. 7.11, CONT'D

but CT scan parameters and stent alloy type also play a significant role. Comparatively, current generation drug-eluting stents are better visualized than older stents with different metallic makeup. Several meta-analyses have reported high diagnostic performance for stent imaging by CCTA, with sensitivity and specificity of 82%–91% and 91%–93%, respectively.[69–72]

However, blooming and beam-hardening artifacts caused by stent struts and stents with diameters <3 mm are the existing challenges that limit the diagnostic accuracy of CCTA in the evaluation of stent patency.[73,74] Improvements in image acquisition and postprocessing, including several new approaches to enhance the evaluation of stent patency, ISR, and stent structure, have been developed. Iterative reconstruction techniques, use of high convolution kernels, and DECT acquisitions have shown promising results[75–78].

Notably, improvements in coronary stent technology may enhance the evolution of CCTA. Bioabsorbable drug-eluting vascular scaffolds comprised of poly-L-lactide and poly-D,L-lactide particularly accommodate CCTA visualization with little to no blooming artifacts. These revascularization methods, if proven effective, may allow for more routine assessment of patency by CCTA.

Stent fracture is a well-established cause of ISR typically observed after drug-eluting stent implantation due to the reduced stent strut thickness and fewer stent cell connections. These characteristics have led to weaker longitudinal strength in the new-generation DES.[79]

**TABLE 7.3**

Multicenter Trials Assessing the Diagnostic Accuracy of Cardiac Computed Tomography Angiography for Detection of Coronary Artery Stenosis

| Study | Patients (n) | Prevalence of CAD (%) | Sensitivity (%) | Specificity (%) | Positive Predictive Value (%) | Negative Predictive Value (%) |
|---|---|---|---|---|---|---|
| Budoff et al.,[60] ACCURACY | 230 | 25 | 95 | 83 | 64 | 99 |
| Meijboom et al.,[30] prospective multivendor study | 360 | 68 | 94 | 83 | 48 | 99 |
| Miller et al.,[28] CORE-64 | 291 | 56 | 85 | 90 | 91 | 83 |

*ACCURACY,* Assessment by Coronary Computed Tomographic Angiography of Individuals Undergoing Invasive Coronary Angiography; *CAD,* coronary artery disease; *CORE-64,* Coronary Artery Evaluation Using 64-Row Multidetector Computed Tomography Angiography.
From Taylor AJ. Cardiac computed tomography. In: Mann DL, Zipes DP, Libby P, et al., eds. *Braunwald's Heart Disease: A Textbook of Cardiovascular Medicine.* 10th ed. Philadelphia: Saunders; 2015, with permission.

## Coronary CT Angiography in Patient With Prior CABG

Contemporary studies evaluating CCTA have reported very high diagnostic accuracy for both stenosis and occlusion in CABGs (Fig. 7.14). A recent meta-analysis comparing 64-slice CCTA to ICA in the evaluation of graft occlusion and stenosis also yielded excellent results for CCTA.[41] This meta-analysis by Chan et al. comprised 31 studies with 1975 total patients and demonstrated a sensitivity of 96.3% for identifying stenosis or occlusion compared to ICA. They did note, however, that CCTA was significantly better ($P = 0.004$) for identifying abnormalities of saphenous vein grafts compared to arterial grafts, indicating once again spatial resolution as a potential limiting factor. Data from 64-slice CT showed a sensitivity, specificity, and accuracy of 100% for evaluating venous graft occlusion vs 83.3%, 100%, and 98.9% for evaluating arterial graft occlusion, respectively.[44] This study also evaluated the severity of stenosis in patent grafts and found sensitivity, specificity, and accuracy of 94.4%, 98.4%, and 96.9% in evaluating significant stenoses in venous grafts vs 100%, 97.7%, and 98% in arterial grafts, respectively.[48]

Despite its high performance to identify and exclude CABG disease, such patients often have extensive native CAD. No study to date has evaluated the accuracy of CCTA for those undergoing CABG on a per-patient basis in which the accuracy is evaluated for both CABG and native coronary arteries.

## Atherosclerotic Plaques

Early reports of atherosclerosis findings were limited to classifications of noncalcified, calcified, and "mixed" plaques. In general, a cutoff point of 130 HU has been historically defined as a calcified plaque with values below this threshold interpreted as noncalcified. Given the fact that the vast majority of cardiac events are caused by plaque rupture, the detection and characterization not only of calcified but also of noncalcified plaque components is a promising tool for improved risk stratification. In comparison to IVUS, accuracy for detecting noncalcified plaque has been found to be approximately 80%–90% but these studies were performed in selected patients.[6]

## High-Risk Plaque Features

Multiple coronary artery plaque features have been identified that are independently linked with adverse outcomes. These have been termed high-risk plaque (HRP) features and are important to recognize clinically. The four most commonly referenced are low-attenuation plaque, spotty calcium, positive remodeling, and the "napkin-ring" sign (Fig. 7.15). Low-attenuation plaque has been defined as attenuation less than 30 HU in three regions of interest within the noncalcified portion of a plaque.[67,68] Low-attenuation plaque is thought to reflect lipid-rich plaque which is histologically vulnerable to rupture (Fig. 7.16). Spotty calcium has been defined as the presence of calcified plaque with a diameter of less than 3 mm in direction,

**TABLE 7.4**

Diagnostic Accuracy of Coronary CT Angiography With Prospective ECG Gating Based on Step-and-Shoot, Flash, and Volume Modes for Patient- and Vessel-Based Detection of Significant Coronary Stenosis Exceeding 50%

| | | | | | | | DIAGNOSTIC ACCURACY, % | | | | | | | | |
| | | | | | | | PER-PATIENT BASIS | | | | PER-VESSEL BASIS | | | |
| Author | Year | Patients | Vessels | Scanner | ECG Gating | No. of Slices | Sens | Spec | PPV | NPV | Sens | Spec | PPV | NPV |
|---|---|---|---|---|---|---|---|---|---|---|---|---|---|---|
| Pelliccia[139] | 2013 | 118 | 375 | Toshiba | Volume | 320 | 98 | 91 | 93 | 98 | 93 | 95 | 92 | 96 |
| Maffei[140] | 2012 | 160 | 637 | Siemens | Flash | 128 | 100 | 83 | 72 | 100 | 98 | 91 | 61 | 100 |
| Van Veben[141] | 2011 | 106 | 255 | Toshiba | Volume | 320 | 100[a] | 87[a] | 93[a] | 100[a] | 99[a] | 95[a] | 92[a] | 99[a] |
| Stolzmann[42] | 2011 | 100 | — | Siemens | SAS | 64 | 100 | 93 | 95 | 100 | 99 | 97 | 95 | 99 |
| Bamberg[143] | 2011 | 33 | 96 | Siemens | Flash | 128 | 100[b] | 18[b] | 71[b] | 100[b] | 91 | 69 | 79 | 85 |
| Achenbach[144] | 2011 | 50 | 200 | Siemens | Flash | 128 | 100 | 82 | 72 | 100 | 100 | 94 | 74 | 100 |
| Scheffel[145] | 2010 | 43 | 129 | Siemens | SAS | 64 | 100 | 93 | 97 | 100 | 96 | 89 | 90 | 95 |
| Nasis[146] | 2010 | 63 | 260 | Toshiba | Volume | 320 | 94 | 87 | 88 | 93 | 89 | 95 | 82 | 97 |
| Husmann[147] | 2010 | 61 | 244 | GE | SAS | 64 | 100 | 86 | 89 | 100 | 93 | 86 | 73 | 97 |
| De Graaf[148] | 2010 | 64 | 177 | Toshiba | Volume | 320 | 100 | 88 | 92 | 100 | 94 | 92 | 83 | 97 |
| Carrascosa[149] | 2010 | 50 | 210 | Philips | SAS | 64 | 100 | 75 | 81 | 100 | 96 | 94 | 83 | 99 |
| Alkadhi[150] | 2010 | 50 | 199 | Siemens | SAS | 128 | 94 | 91 | 85 | 99 | 97 | 98 | 88 | 99 |
| Alkadhi[150] | 2010 | 50 | 245 | Siemens | Flash | 128 | 94 | 94 | 89 | 97 | 96 | 97 | 83 | 99 |

[a]Excluding nondiagnostic segments vessels and patients.
[b]Hemodynamically significant coronary artery stenosis ≤0.75.

*ECG*, electrocardiogram; *Sens*, sensitivity; *Spec*, specificity; *PPV*, positive predictive value; *NPV*, negative predictive value; *SAS*, step and shoot.
Zipes DP, Libby P, Bonow RO, Mann DL, Tomaselli GF, eds. *Braunwald's Heart Disease: A Textbook of Cardiovascular Medicine.* 11th ed. Copyright © 2019 by Elsevier Inc., 2018:328.

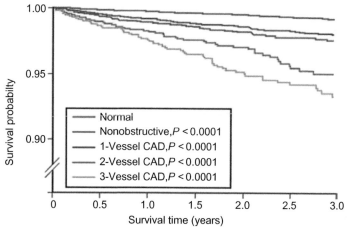

FIG. 7.12 Data from the Coronary CT Angiography Evaluation For Clinical Outcomes: An International Multicenter Registry (CONFIRM) registry showing worse cardiovascular prognosis based on increasing severity of coronary artery disease (CAD), as defined by cardiac computed tomography angiography. An adverse prognosis was noted for nonobstructive CAD in addition to one-, two-, or three-vessel CAD. (From Taylor AJ. Cardiac computed tomography. In: Mann DL, Zipes DP, Libby P, et al., eds. *Braunwald's Heart Disease: A Textbook of Cardiovascular Medicine.* 10th ed. Philadelphia: Saunders; 2015, with permission.)

length less than 1.5 times the vessel diameter, and width less than two-thirds of the vessel diameter.[80–82] Positive remodeling is generally defined as a ratio of outer vessel diameter in the region of plaque to the uninvolved vessel of 1.1 or greater.[83,84] The "napkin-ring" sign is defined as a noncalcified portion of coronary artery plaque with a higher attenuation peripheral ring and a lower attenuation core.[85–87] The "napkin-ring" sign is thought to correspond by histology to a thin-cap fibroatheroma which may be vulnerable to rupture. HRP features increase the rate of plaque rupture, which can be responsible for the ACS secondary to atherothrombosis, which is the development of coronary thrombosis superimposed on a ruptured plaque. Atherothrombosis is the main cause of unstable angina and acute myocardial infarction.[88]

In the initial large-scale study evaluating the prognostic utility of atherosclerotic plaque characteristics, low-attenuation plaques with HU less than 30 and positive arterial remodeling were assessed for their ability to risk-stratify 1059 stable patients who underwent CCTA and were followed for ACS occurrence to 27-month follow-up.[68] Atherosclerotic plaques were categorized as having no high-risk features, one-feature positive or two-feature positive plaques Compared to patients with no high-risk features, significantly higher rates of ACS occurred in patients with one- and two-feature positive plaques (0.49% vs 3.7% vs 22.2%,

respectively; $P < 0.001$). In a follow-up study of 3158 patients, CCTA-defined HRP was an independent predictor of future ACS incremental to high-grade stenosis.[89] In this study, for the 449 patients who underwent serial CCTA imaging, atherosclerotic plaque progression was also strongly associated with future ACS. These findings supporting the additive value of atherosclerotic plaque burden and plaque composition are also seen in patients presenting with non-ST-segment elevation MI (NSTEMI). In an evaluation of 312 patients presenting with NSTEMI or stable angina, lesions responsible for events demonstrated lower attenuation patterns by CCTA in those with NSTEMI.[7]

### Relationship of Findings to Ischemia

Coronary CTA, like invasive angiography, is a purely morphologic imaging modality and cannot demonstrate the functional relevance of stenosis (ischemia). The correlation of CT results with the presence of ischemia is poor. Especially in the case of lesions with a borderline degree of stenosis, this may be a limitation for the clinical application of CT angiography. Not surprisingly, CCTA is a better predictor of angiographic findings than testing for ischemia. A "negative" CCTA result is a reliable predictor to rule out the presence of coronary artery stenosis and the need for revascularization, and it may therefore be used as a "gatekeeper" to avoid invasive angiograms.[6]

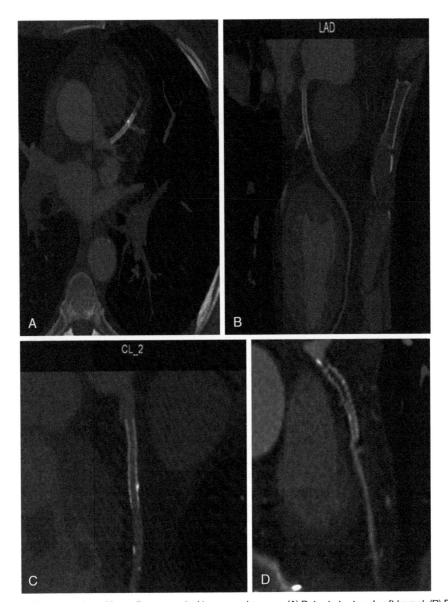

FIG. 7.13 Stent imaging with cardiac computed tomography scan. (A) Patent stent and soft kernel. (B) Patent stent with sharp kernel. (C) Sharp kernel and wide window. (D) Occluded stent. *LAD*, left anterior descending coronary artery.

CCTA has been compared to a host of physiologic stress tests, including SPECT, PET, and fractional flow reserve (FFR) for the correlation of anatomic stenosis to myocardial perfusion deficits. These studies have been generally small in sample size, 42–110 patients.[90–92] In the largest study comparing CCTA findings to rubidium-82 PET, CCTA was associated with myocardial perfusion defects, but only to a moderate

degree. With worsening coronary stenosis on CCTA, as defined by less than 50%, 50%–70%, and more than 70% stenosis, the positive predictive value (PPV) was only 29%, 44%, and 77%, respectively, at the per-patient level. Conversely, the NPV to exclude myocardial ischemia was remarkably high, at 92%, 91%, and 88%, respectively. Similarly, using FFR in 79 patients with stable symptomatic CAD, CCTA showing 50% or

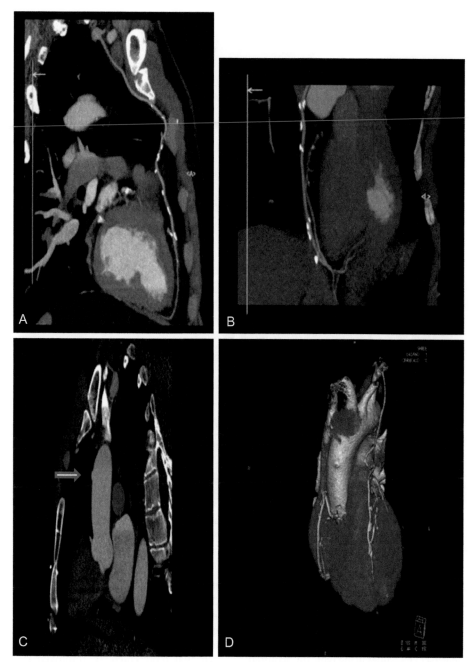

FIG. 7.14 Coronary artery bypass graft (CABG) imaging by cardiac computed tomography. (A) Patent left internal mammary artery (LIMA) graft on the distal left anterior descending coronary artery with good distal flow on oblique multiplanar reformat. (B) Patent saphenous vein graft (SVG) on the posterior descending artery on oblique multiplanar reformation. (C) Occluded SVG on lateral maximum intensity projection (*arrow*). (D) Volume render technique (VRT) from a patient with CABG.

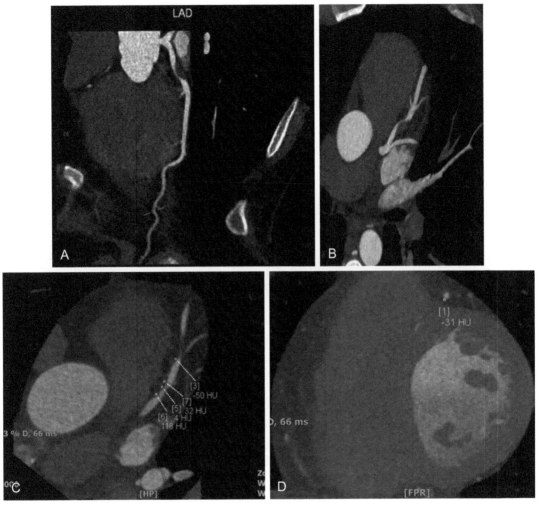

FIG. 7.15 (A, B) Noncalcified plaque and positive remodeling in thin-slice curve multiplanar reconstruction. (C, D) Vulnerable lipid-rich (<30 HU) plaque without significant stenosis. *LAD*, left anterior descending coronary artery.

more stenosis identified less than half of lesions that demonstrated coronary pressure differences.[93] The findings are generally consistent across studies and have raised.

FFR derived from CCTA (FFRCT) is a method for deriving three-vessel FFR values using typically acquired CCTA (Fig. 7.17). In this regard, FFRCT requires no additional testing or radiation and no medications but can be performed on any acquired CCTA. As with invasive FFR, FFRCT enables precise localization of ischemia-causing coronary stenosis. The diagnostic performance of FFRCT has been evaluated in three prospective multicenter trials: Diagnosis of Ischemia-Causing Stenosis Obtained Via Noninvasive Fractional Flow Reserve (DISCOVER-FLOW), Determination of Fractional Flow Reserve by Anatomic Computed Tomographic Angiography (DeFACTO), and Analysis of Coronary Blood Flow Using CT Angiography: Next Steps (NXT).[94–96] Each trial represented an improved generation over the last, with the NXT trial most recently reported. In this study of 254 patients referred for clinically indicated ICA, CCTA and FFRCT were performed, with 484 vessels directly interrogated by invasive FFR. The primary endpoint of this study was the area under ROC curve for FFRCT, 0.90 and 0.93 on a per-patient and per-vessel basis, respectively, which corresponded to an overall

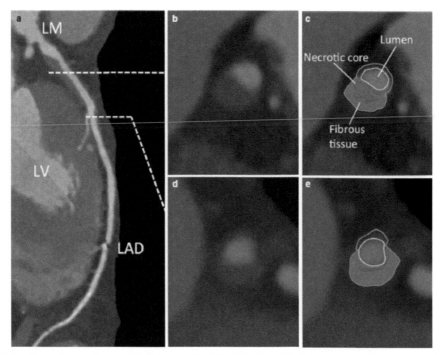

FIG. 7.16 Curved multiplanar reconstruction (A) of the LM-LAD with the presence of noncalcified plaques. Horizontal lines represent two different plaque types. Cross-sectional images of the first plaque without (B) and with color overlay (C) represent an unstable plaque, with positive remodeling, large necrotic core (*red*), and smaller amount of fibrous tissue (*green*). Cross-sectional images of the second plaque without (D) and with (E) color overlay show a stable plaque with a smaller necrotic core and more pronounced fibrous tissue. (Joseph Schoepf U, ed. *CT of the Heart*. 2nd ed. © Humana Press 2005, 2019:321.)

per-vessel diagnostic accuracy of 86%. These performance characteristics compared favorably to anatomic evaluation alone by ICA or CCTA, which revealed modest accuracies for diagnosis of invasive FFR-determined ischemia (77% vs 53%). A recent meta-analysis of diagnostic imaging modalities evaluated the comparative diagnostic performance of FFRCT to SPECT SE, CMR, and ICA. For invasive FFR-verified ischemia, highest sensitivities of testing modalities were observed for CCTA (90%), CMR (90%), and FFRCT (90%), with more moderate specificities observed for FFRCT (71%).

FFRCT has been assessed for its ability to alter the clinical management of patients undergoing noninvasive and invasive testing. In the crossover-design Prospective Longitudinal Trial of FFRCT Outcome and Resource Impacts (PLATFORM), 584 symptomatic patients with suspected CAD were assigned to either usual care or a CCTA-FFRCT-based evaluation, to determine the rates of no obstructive CAD of 50% or greater stenosis at ICA.[48] Two separate cohorts were studied, referred for invasive assessment and for noninvasive stress testing. Compared with a CCTA-FFRCT-based approach, usual care resulted in a significantly lower rate of obstructive CAD at ICA (12% vs 73%) and also resulted in 61% of ICAs being canceled after CCTA-FFRCT findings were known.

Given the ascendancy of ischemia-guided intervention over anatomic-guided intervention, the ability of computerized tomography fractional flow reserve (FFRCT) to detect lesion-specific ischemia opens a door for FFRCT-guided PCI. In the RIPCORD study, 200 consecutive patients from the NXT trial underwent sequential decision-making for the most optimal treatment strategy (optimal medical therapy alone, PCI, coronary artery bypass grafting, or more information required) based on coronary CTA alone or the hybrid anatomic-physiological approach of coronary CTA plus FFRCT. The decision was made by consensus of three experienced interventional cardiologists reporting on the changes in their management plan after disclosure of FFRCT. Overall, there was a change in management in 36% of patients, with a 23% increase in the use of

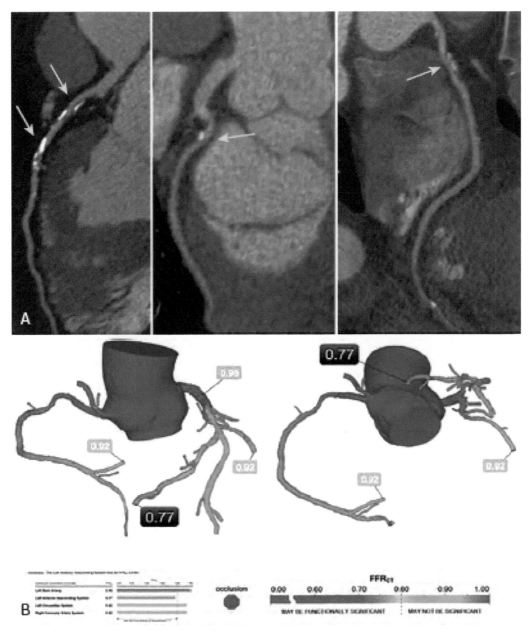

FIG. 7.17 Fractional flow reserve derived from CCTA (FFR<sub>CT</sub>). (A) CCTA demonstrates moderate stenosis in proximal portion of the left anterior descending artery (LAD). Midportion of LAD cannot be adequately visualized due to severely calcified plaque. Mild nonstenotic plaque is noted in the left circumflex artery and moderate stenosis in the midportion of the right coronary artery. (B) FFR<sub>CT</sub> demonstrates significant ischemia in LAD (FFR<sub>CT</sub> 0.77) the spares the diagonal branch (FFR<sub>CT</sub> 0.92). Note that FFR<sub>CT</sub> allows for interrogation of ischemia at all points in the coronary artery tree. (Zipes DP, Libby P, Bonow RO, Mann DL, Tomaselli GF, eds. *Braun-wald's Heart Disease: A Textbook of Cardiovascular Medicine.* 11th ed. Copyright © 2019 by Elsevier Inc., 2018:326.)

optimal medical therapy alone, a 5% decrease in PCI, and a 0.5% increase in CABG. Among patients assigned to PCI, in 18% the target vessel for PCI was changed, whereas 30% were reallocated to optimal medical therapy.[48]

## Use in Patients With Acute Chest Pain

There is nearly one death from heart disease every 38 s in the United States.[97] Acute chest pain is the single most common complaint of patients older than 15 years of age presenting to the emergency department (ED)[98] and accounts for about 4% of ED visits in the United States.[99] Origins of chest pain include diseases of the heart, aorta, pulmonary system, esophagus, upper abdomen, and chest wall and even psychiatric disorders. Determination of the etiology of the chest pain is often difficult although different types of chest pain are classically ascribed to different corresponding diseases. ACS is estimated to be responsible for 20% of all clinical encounters for acute chest pain.[100] Patients with ACS present with unstable angina, acute myocardial infarction, or sudden cardiac death (SCD)[101]; therefore, timely triage of ACS is important as it affects treatment and prognosis. Also, timely triage may save significant costs. Using coronary CTA to evaluate patients instead of admitting patients for a rule-out approach with serial troponin has the potential to save significant costs to the health-care system.

CCTA has shown its safety and efficiency in excluding CAD or relevant stenosis for advanced risk stratification over the past decade in the setting of ambiguous acute chest pain of a low-to-intermediate risk of ACS with 86%–100% sensitivity, 92%–98% specificity, 93%–100% NPV, and 50%–90% PPV.[48]

A recent meta-analysis examined the relative diagnostic performance of CCTA vs other diagnostic methods, including stress echocardiography and SPECT, when using ICA or ACS as a reference standard. In this analysis, CCTA demonstrated favorable diagnostic performance that was superior to stress echocardiography and SPECT (CT sensitivity/specificity, 95%/99%; stress echocardiography, 84%/94%; SPECT, 85%/86%).[102] Based on these favorable diagnostic findings several observational cohort studies—both from research initiatives as well as site-specific clinical care have attempted to determine the natural clinical outcomes of patients with low-to-intermediate acute chest pain [as defined primarily by the Thrombolysis in Myocardial Ischemia (TIMI) risk score] who present with suspected ACS.[103] In the largest observational study to date, the Rule-Out Myocardial Infarction Using Computed Assisted Tomography (ROMICAT), 368 patients

with negative initial myocardial necrosis biomarkers and a nondynamic ECG underwent CCTA for diagnosis and exclusion of ACS.[104] In this population of individuals undergoing evaluation, 31 patients (8.4%) were diagnosed with ACS. CCTA identified approximately half these individuals as having no stenosis or atherosclerosis and 20% who had high-grade coronary stenosis. On discharge, none of those individuals without stenosis or atherosclerosis experienced ACS. Similarly, patients with nonobstructive CAD enjoyed a 98% NPV for ACS. In contrast, the PPV of CCTA for those with CCTA identified obstructive coronary stenosis was only 35%, suggesting an overdiagnosis phenomenon in which CCTA may identify stenosis that is ultimately not the cause of the acute chest pain syndrome. In a low-risk population of 600 patients presenting with acute chest pain, more than four of five patients could be effectively discharged with a 30-day ACS rate of 0%.

To assess this, several prospective randomized trials sought to determine the differential clinical and economic outcomes of a CCTA-based ACS evaluation vs the standard of care (SOC) (Table 7.5). These trials differed in their inclusion criteria as well as the mode of evaluation in the standard-of-care arms. In the ROMI-CAT II and CT Coronary Angiography Compared to Exercise ECG (CT-COMPARE) studies low-to-intermediate risk patients were enrolled, whereas the American College of Radiology Imaging Network (ACRIN-PA) and Coronary Computed Tomographic Angiography for Systematic Triage of Acute Chest Pain Patients to Treatment (CT-STAT) studies enrolled low-risk patients.[105–108] Uniform to these trials was a high NPV for ACS that was safe (i.e., with few reported adverse cardiovascular outcomes in a follow-up of 30 days to 6 months). Other important clinical, workflow, and resource utilization parameters were evaluated, including the time to diagnosis, length of stay, rates of ED discharge, total and ED costs, and rates of downstream ICA. In both ACRIN-PA and ROMICAT II trials, a CCTA-based strategy resulted in immediate discharge of approximately half of patients, which was approximately two to four times the rate of the standard-of-care practice. Among these large-scale trials, only ROMICAT II observed no ED cost-savings, whereas the other studies observed a 15%–38% reduction. These cost-savings were in part the result of shorter lengths of stay but were offset by higher rates of ICA and coronary revascularization. Consistently, the latter is observed and evokes unease about the potential for CCTA findings to provoke unnecessary procedures in these low-risk or low-to-intermediate risk individuals.

**TABLE 7.5**
Primary and Secondary Diagnostic Findings of CT-STAT, ROMICAT II, ACRIN/PA, and PROSPECT Trials

| Study | CT-STAT[96] (2011) | | ROMICAT II[95] (2012) | | ACRIN/PA[94] (2012) | | PROSPECT[100] (2015) | |
|---|---|---|---|---|---|---|---|---|
| Design | Multicenter randomized | | Multicenter randomized | | Multicenter randomized | | Single-center randomized | |
| No. of patients | 699 | | 1000 | | 1370 | | 400 | |
| Patient presentation | Troponin (−), normal ECG | | Troponin (−), normal ECG | | Troponin (−), normal ECG | | Troponin (−), normal ECG | |
| Controls | MPI | | Standard evaluation | | Standard evaluation | | MPI | |
| **INDEX VISIT** | CCTA | Control | CCTA | Control | CCTA | Control | CCTA | Control |
| Length of stay (h), median (IQR) | — | — | 8.6 (6.4–27.6) | 26.7 (21.4–30.4) | 18 (7.6–27.2) | 24.8 (19.2–30.5) | 28.9 (11.0–48.4) | 30.4 (23.9–51.3) |
| Time to diagnosis (h), median (IQR) | 2.9 (2.1–4.0) | 6.2 (4.2–19.0) | 5.8 (4.0–90) | 21.0 (8.5–23.8) | — | — | — | — |
| Direct ED discharge (%) | — | — | 47 | 12 | 50 | 23 | — | — |
| Total ED costs (USD), median (IQR) | 2137 (1660–3077) | 3458 (2900–4297) | 1937 (1504–4057) | 2742 (1755–3832) | — | — | — | — |
| Radiation dose (mSv) | 11.5[a] (6.8–16.8) | 12.8 (11.6–13.9) | 14.3 ± 10.9[b] | 5.3 ± 9.6[b] | — | — | 96[a] (6.2–23.0) | 27[a] (19.0–27.0) |
| **INDEX VISIT + FOLLOW-UP** | | | | | | | | |
| Follow-up duration | 6 months | | 28 days | | 30 days | | 1 year | |
| ACS diagnosis (%) | 1 | 3 | 9 | 6 | 1 | 1 | — | — |
| ICA (%) | 8 | 7 | 12 | 8 | 5 | 4 | 15 | 16 |
| Revascularization (%) | 4 | 3 | 6 | 4 | 3 | 1 | 8 | 6 |
| MACE (%) | 0.8 | 0.4 | 0.4 | 1 | 1 | 1 | 5 | 8 |

[a]Median value reported.
[b]Mean value reported.

ACS, acute coronary syndrome; CCTA, coronary computed tomographic angiography; ECG, electrocardiogram; ED, emergency department; ICA, invasive coronary angiography; IQR, interquartile range; MACE, major adverse cardiac events; MPI, stress myocardial perfusion imaging; USD, United States Dollar.

MACE definitions:

CT-STAT ACS: cardiac death or revascularization 6 months in patients who had normal or near-normal index testing.

ROMICAT II: death, myocardial infarction unstable angina, or urgent coronary revascularization within 28 days.

ACRIN/PA: cardiac death or myocardial infarction within 30 days.

PROSPECT: all-cause death, myocardial infarction, cardiac arrest and cerebrovascular accident.

Zipes DP, Libby P, Bonow RO, Mann DL, Tomaselli GF, eds. *Braunwald's Heart Disease: A Textbook of Cardiovascular Medicine.* 11th ed. Copyright © 2019 by Elsevier Inc., 2018:328.

The Cardiac CT in the Treatment of Acute Chest Pain (CATCH) trial aimed to determine the prognostic utility of CCTA compared to the SOC in 299 patients presenting with acute chest pain and normal ECG and blood biomarkers.[109] In the CCTA-guided group referral for ICA required coronary stenosis >70% or >50% in the left main, and for intermediate stenosis (50%–70%), a stress test was used. Significant stenosis on ICA was defined as a stenosis ≥70% or reduced FFR ≤0.75 in intermediate stenoses (50%–70%). Referral rate for ICA was 17% with CCTA vs 12% with standard care ($P = 0.1$). ICA confirmed significant coronary artery stenoses in 12% vs 4% ($P = 0.001$), and 10% vs 4% were subsequently revascularized ($P = 0.005$). PPV for the detection of significant stenoses was 71% with CCTA vs 36% with standard care ($P = 0.001$). Clinical events (cardiac death, myocardial infarction, unstable angina pectoris, revascularization, and readmission for chest pain), during 120 days of follow-up, were recorded in 8 patients (3%) in the CCTA-guided group vs 15 patients (5%) in the standard care group ($P = 0.1$).[109] These results are consistent with a recent meta-analysis of four randomized trials and three case–control studies totaling more than 3300 patients. CCTA-based care resulted in a 74% reduction in downstream events and a 42% reduction in repeat ED visits.[110]

The most contemporary RCT, the Better Evaluation of Acute Chest Pain with Computed Tomography Angiography (BEACON), evaluated the use of a CCTA-based strategy vs the SOC at seven sites where high-sensitivity troponins were used for early diagnosis of ACS.[111] The 500 patients were evaluated for a primary endpoint of coronary revascularization within 30 days following the index ED visits for which there was no difference between strategies. Although a CCTA-based strategy did not increase ED discharge rates or change lengths of stay, CCTA patients did incur lower medical costs and less outpatient testing after ED discharge.

CCTA vs MPI stress testing was evaluated in the Study Comparing CT Scan and Stress Test in Diagnosing Coronary Artery Disease in Patients Hospitalized for Chest Pain (PROSPECT) trial.[112] The 400 patients represented an ethnically diverse population of more than 50% Hispanic and 37% African American patients of low socioeconomic status and were stratified to either CCTA or MPI testing at the index ED visit. The primary outcome—the rate of ICA without revascularization within 1 year—was no different between testing groups. At a median average follow-up of 40 months, no differences were observed for MACE in this underpowered

study, although radiation exposure was lower for patients undergoing CCTA over MPI, and CCTA was regarded with higher patient satisfaction.

## Use in Patients With Stable Suspected Coronary Artery Disease

Chronic chest pain is a multifactorial clinical problem, and the diagnosis is based on patients' history. It is characterized by recurrent episodes of chest pain occurring in a relatively stable pattern. About 4 million cardiac stress tests (in 87% of cases combined with imaging) are performed annually in the United States for chest pain evaluation. There is concern regarding the rising health-care costs, inappropriate utilization, and patient safety of diagnostic testing, with approximately one-third of cardiac stress tests being likely inappropriately requested. In addition, around 25% of ICA is performed among asymptomatic patients.[48] Currently, almost 10 million CAD imaging tests are performed each year in the United States, which annually represents 25% of the total number of individuals diagnosed with CVD. The vast majority of these tests are stress tests with imaging, typically by SPECT MPI.

Given the relatively recent introduction of CCTA, there is intense interest to determine whether anatomic imaging by CCTA vs physiologic imaging by stress MPI offers any relative advantage in the care of stable patients with CAD. To this end, numerous large-scale observational cohort registries and randomized trials have been performed to determine the efficacy of each of these modes of workup (Table 7.6).

In the large-scale Prospective Multicenter Imaging Study for Evaluation of Chest Pain (PROMISE) randomized trial, 10,003 patients underwent either CCTA or "functional" testing, which included not only SPECT MPI but also stress echocardiography and stress ECG testing without imaging.[113] At a median-follow-up of 25 months, the primary endpoint—defined as all-cause mortality, nonfatal MI, unstable angina hospitalization, or procedural complication—was no different for the CCTA group than for the functional testing group (HR 1.04). Median average radiation exposure was lower for CCTA patients than those in the functional assessment arm (10.0 mSv vs 11.3 mSv). CCTA was associated with a higher rate of ICA within the 90 days following the index test (12.2% vs 8.1%), although those undergoing ICA in the CCTA arm were observed to have a higher rate of high-grade coronary stenosis. Despite higher rates of ICA, 3-year costs for CCTA were similar to functional testing, at 1 and 3 years of follow-up.[114] Similarly, quality-of-life measures, as

**TABLE 7.6**
Primary and Secondary Diagnostic Outcome Findings From PROMISE and SCOT-HEART Trials

| | PROMISE[103] (2015) | | | | SCOT-HEART[107] (2015) | | | |
|---|---|---|---|---|---|---|---|---|
| Study design | Prospective multicenter | | | | Prospective multicarrier | | | |
| Population | Symptomatic patients without diagnosed CAD | | | | Recent-onset chest pain, suspected CAD | | | |
| Patients (n) | 10,0003 | | | | 4146 | | | |
| Disease prevalence (%, >50% stenosis) | 11 | | | | 42 | | | |
| Modalities (population, n) | CCTA (4996) | Functional testing[a] (5007) | HR[b] (95% CI) | P value | Standard care plus CCTA (2073) | Standard care (2073) | HR[c] (95% CI) | P value |
| Primary composite endpoint | 164 | 151 | 1.04 (0.83–1.29) | 0.75 | — | — | — | — |
| Death force any cause | 74 | 75 | — | — | 17 | 20 | 0.86 (0.45–1.64) | 0.65 |
| Nonfatal MI | 30 | 40 | — | — | 22 | 35 | 0.63 (0.37–1.07) | 0.09 |
| Hospitalization for unstable angina | 61 | 41 | — | — | 76 | 69 | 1.12 (0.81–1.55) | 0.51 |
| Major procedural complication | 4 | 5 | — | — | — | — | — | — |
| Primary endpoint plus catheterization showing no obstructive CAD | 332 | 353 | 0.91 (0.78–1.06) | 0.22 | — | — | — | — |
| Death or nonfatal MI | 104 | 112 | 0.88 (0.67–1.15) | 0.35 | — | — | — | — |
| Death, nonfatal MI, or hospitalization for unstable angina | 162 | 148 | 1.04 (0.84–1.31) | 0.70 | — | — | — | — |

| | | | | | | | |
|---|---|---|---|---|---|---|---|
| CAD death[d] | — | — | — | 4 | 7 | 0.57 (0.17–1.97) | 0.38 |
| CAD death[d] and MI | — | — | — | 26 | 42 | 0.62 (0.38–1.01) | 0.05 |
| CAD death,[d] MI, and stroke | — | — | — | 31 | 48 | 0.64 (0.41–1.01) | 0.06 |
| Nonfatal stroke | — | — | — | 5 | 7 | 0.73 (0.23–2.32) | 0.59 |
| Noncardiovascular death | — | — | — | 13 | 13 | 1.01 (0.47–2.17) | 0.99 |
| Invasive catheterization showing no obstructive CAD | 170 | 213 | 0.02 | — | — | — | — |
| Coronary revascularization | — | — | — | 233 | 201 | 1.20 (0.99–1.45) | 0.06 |
| PCI | — | — | — | 184 | 160 | 1.19 (0.96–1.47) | 0.11 |
| CABG | — | — | — | 54 | 45 | 1.22 (0.82–1.81) | 0.33 |
| Hospitalization for noncardiac chest pain | — | — | — | 183 | 208 | 0.86 (0.71–1.05) | 0.15 |

[a]Functional testing included exercise electrocardiograms, nuclear steam testing, or stress echocardiography.

[b]Hazard ratios were adjusted for age, sex, CAD risk equivalent (i.e., history of diabetes, peripheral arterial disease, or cerebrovascular diseases), and the prespecification of the intended functional test if patients were randomly assigned to the functional testing group.

[c]Hazard ratios were adjusted for study center and minimization variables, excluding baseline diagnosis.

[d]CAD death was defined as death due to myocardial infarction in all cases.

CABG, coronary artery bypass graft surgery; CAD, coronary artery disease; CCTA, coronary computed tomography angiography; CI, confidence interval; HR, hazard ratios; MI, myocardial infarction; PCI, percutaneous coronary intervention; PROMISE, Prospective Multicenter Imaging Study for Evaluation of Chest Pain; SCOT-HEART, Scottish Computed Tomography of the HEART.

Zipes DP, Libby P, Bonow RO, Mann DL, Tomaselli GF, eds. Braunwald's Heart Disease: A Textbook of Cardiovascular Medicine. 11th ed. Copyright © 2019 by Elsevier Inc., 2018:335.

determined by the Duke Activity Status Index and Seattle Angina Questionnaire, were consistently similar during the entire follow-up period.[115] These nonsignificant differences in quality-of-life and clinical outcomes occurred despite significantly higher rates of prescribed primary prevention medical therapies for patients undergoing CCTA over functional testing for aspirin (11.8% vs 7.8%) and statins (12.7% vs 6.2%).[116] Compared with patients undergoing functional testing, CCTA patients were more likely to adopt a heart-healthy diet and achieve weight loss. Prognostically, compared with functional testing, CCTA was associated with greater predictive abilities for future adverse clinical outcomes when an abnormal test was reported (HR 5.86 vs 2.27).

In contrast to the clinical outcomes-based endpoint of the PROMISE trial, the Scottish Computed Tomography of the Heart (SCOT-HEART) trial examined an endpoint of diagnostic certainty of angina caused by CAD at a 6-week endpoint.[117] "Diagnostic certainty" was defined by the caring physician and categorized by presence vs absence, as well as unlikely vs probable angina. Importantly, this study was not a direct comparison of anatomic vs functional testing, but rather a test of the SOC plus CCTA vs SOC alone, which included clinical evaluation plus symptom-limited exercise testing if considered clinically necessary. For the primary endpoint, there was a significant increase in the diagnostic certainty [relative risk (RR) 3.76] among imaging physicians, associated with a lower frequency of angina diagnosis (RR 0.78). A similar pattern emerged for the attending clinician, whose certainty rose by 1.75-fold with negligible effects on the frequency of diagnosis. Increases in diagnostic certainty resulted in significant changes in downstream planned diagnostic evaluations in the SOC plus CCTA group vs SOC alone (15% vs 1%). Contrary to the PROMISE trial, average median radiation doses of CCTA were significantly lower (4.1 mSv). In the 6-week follow-up of patients in the SCOT-HEART study, marginal differences were observed for near-term death or MI (1.3% vs 2.0%; $P = 0.053$). At 20 months' follow-up, however, when prognostic evaluations began at the initiation of preventive therapy, those undergoing CCTA experienced a 50% reduction in fatal and nonfatal MI compared to SOC alone.[118] These findings were associated with similar rates of ICA between CCTA and SOC groups, but higher rates of confirmation of obstructive CAD in CCTA patients as well as higher rates of preventive medical therapies (HR 4.03).

The precise reasons for the improvement in clinical outcomes after CCTA have yet to be proved in an RCT. Large-scale observational evidence suggests the clinical outcomes benefit following CCTA may result from the efficacy of primary preventive medical therapies. In 10,418 patients from the CONFIRM registry followed for 27 months with no or nonobstructive CAD, defined by a maximal per-patient coronary stenosis between 1% and 50%, those with evident mild coronary stenosis experienced a 56% reduction in mortality.[7] Independent of NCEP/ATP III guidelines, statins conferred a clinical benefit only for patients with evident CAD on CCTA. A subsequent study from CONFIRM evaluated the effects of primary vs secondary medical therapy on outcomes in patients with obstructive CAD of 50% or greater stenosis on CCTA. In this cohort, statins were similarly associated with a 43% reduction in the risk of MACE, with no decrement in this risk for patients prescribed aspirin, beta-blockers, and ACE inhibitors.

## Anomalous Coronary Arteries

Angelini et al. defined a coronary anomaly as any coronary artery pattern seen only rarely in the general population (i.e., <1% of cases). Defining features of an anomalous artery may relate to the number of ostia or proximal course, as well as a host of other deviations from patterns commonly encountered in the physiologically normal population. Although the incidence of coronary anomalies encountered during conventional coronary angiography ranges from 0.6% to 1.6%, data indicate that they may account for almost 12% of deaths in high school and college athletes in the United States. Similar data from the American Heart Association suggest that coronary anomalies may be responsible for up to 19% of cases of SCD in athletes. The exact pathophysiologic mechanism for the anomaly-induced SCD remains unclear, although certain abnormal anatomic features have been associated with myocardial ischemia resulting from possible compression, torsion, or vasospasm of the anomalous coronary artery. Investigators have postulated that this situation, in turn, may precipitate syncope or malignant arrhythmias. Approximately 80% of adults with coronary anomalies are asymptomatic.

The incidental finding of a morphologically abnormal coronary artery on cardiac computed tomography may present a dilemma resulting from the continued uncertainty of the clinical significance of coronary anomalies with regard to morbidity and risk of SCD[16,42–45] (Figs. 7.18 and 7.19).

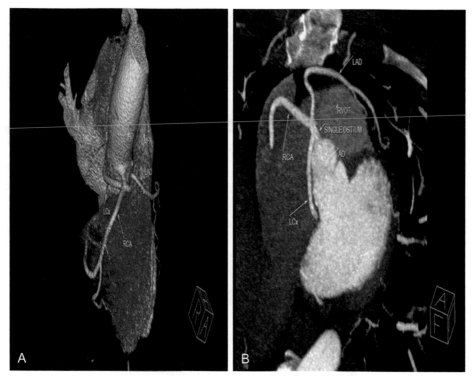

FIG. 7.18   (A, B) Single coronary artery from right sinus Valsalva. *AO*, aorta; *LAD*, left anterior descending coronary artery; *LCx*, left circumflex; *RCA*, right coronary artery; *RVOT*, right ventricular outflow tract.

## ASSESSMENT OF CARDIOVASCULAR STRUCTURE AND FUNCTION

Beyond coronary artery stenosis and atherosclerosis, ECG-gated CT allows for a comprehensive assessment of cardiac structure and function. Because cardiac function evaluation requires retrospective ECG helical gating, with significantly greater amounts of radiation exposure, cardiac CT functional evaluation is less frequently performed. In specific cases, however, it may be useful, and techniques to acquire optimal image acquisition and measurements should be known.[7]

Left ventricular (LV) assessment can be determined by continuous image acquisition throughout the cardiac cycle in an array of patient subsets.[119] In most cases, image reconstruction is performed at every 5% or 10% increment of the R-R interval, which enables cardiac motion assessment. Current software algorithms allow for semiautomated segmentation with manual correction of LV cavities, which offers ease of volumetric measurement. Despite current CT temporal resolution being significantly poorer than other imaging modalities, CT has generally demonstrated a high correlation

with other methods. Using a CMR gold standard, cardiac CT quantification demonstrated $r$ values for comparison of LV ejection fraction (EF), end-systolic volume, and end-diastolic volume and mass: 0.93, 0.95, 0.93, and 0.86, respectively.[7] Partly because of these findings, cardiac CT is considered appropriate for use by recent multimodality AUC to be useful to differentiate etiologies of CHF.

In order to employ CT to define the cardiac chambers and separate them from the surrounding myocardium, it is necessary to use intravenous contrast. In general, this can be accomplished with <100 mL of nonionic contrast, and it is possible to perform complete imaging of the heart chambers, the coronary arteries, and the proximal great vessels (aorta and pulmonary artery) in a single setting with a single injection of contrast.[6]

Cardiac CT can be used to quantitate left and right ventricular volumes, left and right atrial volumes, left and right ventricular muscle mass, regional left ventricular function, wall thickening and contractility, rates of diastolic filling of the right and left ventricles, postinfarction left and right ventricular remodeling,

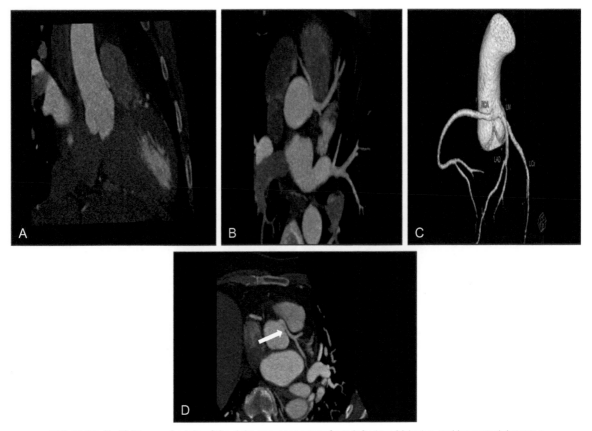

FIG. 7.19 (A, B) Abnormal origin of the right coronary artery from left sinus Valsalva and interarterial course (malignant course) and compression on the ostioproximal portion of it. (C) Volume rendering image. (D) Abnormal origin of the left main coronary artery from right sinus Valsalva and interarterial course (*white arrow*). *LCx*, left circumflex; *RCA*, right coronary artery.

cardiac remodeling following cardiac and lung transplantation, and ejection fraction in patients with no contraindication to the use of iodinated contrast medium.[6]

All available postprocessing workstations can provide quantitative and often noninteractive (i.e., automatic) measurements of the LV in particular. Reproducibility of CT in performing right and left ventricular volume and function measurements has also been established. Cardiac CT imaging using thin sections allows postprocessing of images into end-diastolic and end-systolic short and "long" axis images at multiple ECG phases to facilitate identification of structures and salient features of the ventricular anatomy.[6]

Using short and long axis imaging also allows identification of infarct locations. Demonstrated in this latter example is a common CT finding in contrast-enhanced images from patients with remote myocardial infarction. The "negative" contrast is actually due to lack of contrast opacification in the infarcted region causing "contrast rarefaction."[6]

Other important pathologies, such as LV apical thrombus, ventricular aneurysms, and pseudoaneurysms, are diagnosed and serve as an added diagnostic benefit of cardiac CT.[7]

## Valvular Heart Disease

The Society for Computed Cardiac Tomography recently released consensus guidelines for the appropriate use of cardiac CT to evaluate noncoronary structures including cardiac valves. It is appropriate to use cardiac CT to evaluate native and prosthetic valves with suspected clinically significant valvular dysfunction if the images from other noninvasive methods are inadequate. It is not recommended as the initial imaging modality to assess valvular anatomy and function.[120]

Given current contrast protocols that aim to selectively opacify the LV cavity over the right, the general focus for valvular evaluation by cardiac CT has been on left-sided valves. Aortic stenosis is generally accurately diagnosed by cardiac CT. Double-oblique localization of the aortic valve at the level of the leaflet insertions can be easily performed by initial start planes in the left sagittal oblique and left coronary oblique axes, which allows visualization of the phasic motion of the valve throughout the cardiac cycle. Meta-analytic data from 14 studies suggest an overestimation of AVA by cardiac CT compared to transthoracic echocardiography (TTE), with better correlation to transesophageal echocardiography (TEE). Numerous other aortic valvular conditions are easily visualized by cardiac CT, including congenital bicuspid or quadricuspid aortic stenosis and extent and severity of aortic valve calcium.

Aortic valve calcification can be accurately quantified using CT, and interscan reproducibility is >90%. The amount of calcification is directly correlated with the severity of AS although the relationship is curvilinear with stenosis severity increasing more rapidly at lower than higher calcium loads. The incremental value of the information derived from the aortic valve calcium score may be particularly useful in patients with low cardiac output and reduced transvalvular gradients.

CT may be useful in evaluating the mechanism leading to aortic regurgitation (AR). AR caused by degenerative valve disease is characterized by thickened and/or calcified leaflets, and the area of lack of coaptation may be visualized in diastolic phase reconstructions centrally or at the commissures. Regurgitant orifice areas (ROAs) measured by planimetry using MDCT correlate well with echocardiographic parameters of AR severity, such as the vena contracta width and the ratio of the regurgitant jet to LVOT height, and allow for the detection of moderate and severe AR with high accuracy.[6]

Among 53 patients with AR, compared to 29 patients without AR, undergoing cardiac CT and TTE, cardiac CT demonstrated a sensitivity and specificity of 98% and 98% to grade AR severity.[121] The utility of cardiac CT for AR evaluation is for moderate-to-severe cases since cardiac CT misses more than one-fourth of mildly regurgitant valves. Aortic regurgitant volume can be quantified when cardiac CT is performed by retrospective helical gating methods. Calculation of LV and right ventricular (RV) end-systolic and end-diastolic volumes enables calculation of their respective stroke volumes. RV stroke volumes subtracted from LV stroke volumes represent the aortic regurgitant volume.

Mitral valve (MV) evaluation can be more challenging than for the aortic valve because of its complex anatomic structure and highly mobile valvular apparatus.[122] As in the case of aortic valve calcification, the presence of calcium in the mitral annulus is associated with systemic atherosclerosis and carries negative prognostic implications. MS is often accompanied by marked atrial enlargement involving the appendage. The presence or absence of thrombus in the left atrial appendage can be determined after contrast administration with very high sensitivity although lower specificity since slow flow may impair opacification, which may be increased by adding delayed imaging.[6] Planimetry of mitral valve opening by CT provides an accurate assessment of MS severity.

At its greatest area, short-axis planimetry will offer measurements of the anatomic regurgitant orifice in a manner highly correlative to TTE for the diagnosis of moderate or severe mitral stenosis. Comparisons to TEE reveal a general overestimation of the MV area by cardiac CT.

Mitral regurgitation on cardiac CT can be quantified by two methods: calculation of the regurgitant volume and measurement of the anatomic ROA. Measurement of mitral regurgitant volume by differences in LV and RV stroke volumes shows high correlation to TTE ($r = 0.95$) with no significant biases.[123] Importantly, planimetry of the MV by cardiac CT provides only the *anatomic* ROA, which may differ from the hemodynamically dependent *effective* ROA. Numerous other MV pathologies can be readily interpreted on cardiac CT scans and may offer assistance in diagnosis of mitral regurgitation, including prolapse, flail leaflet, paravalvular abscess, endocarditis, or in the case of prosthetic valves, thrombus formation, or dehiscence.

## Structural Heart Disease Interventions

Given the anatomic and physiologic data afforded by cardiac CT, coupled with recent advances in complex percutaneous therapies for structural heart disease, CT has evolved to become an important imaging modality for preprocedural guidance and postprocedural follow-up for many of these interventions. These include imaging for transcatheter heart valve replacement, left atrial appendage occlusion, and arrhythmia ablation.

Since its demonstrated superiority over conservative therapy and similar outcomes to surgical therapy in high-risk patients with severe aortic stenosis, transcatheter aortic valve replacement (TAVR) is finding expanding clinical utility in patients with less severe aortic valvular disease.[124–126] Almost coincident with this has been the examination of the potential of cardiac CT findings to provide information that may improve procedural TAVR outcomes or prevent unnecessary complications.[126] Specific to TAVR, cardiac and vascular CT scans are routinely performed and provide information related to (1) aortic annular size and calcifications, (2) prediction of TAVR deployment angles, (3) coronary ostial heights, (4) aortoiliac size and atherosclerotic burden, and (5) postprocedural evaluation of TAVR devices for evidence of leaflet thickening suggestive of thrombosis.

Cardiac CT scanning for TAVR is largely performed with retrospective helical gating. Patients undergoing TAVR are generally elderly, and the need for dynamic assessment of the aortic annulus often outweighs the risk of radiation from a cardiac CT.

The aortic annulus is a complex three-dimensional virtual ring at the base of the aortic cusps. The annulus is oval in nature, and hence 3D imaging modalities including 3D TEE and MDCT are, by far, superior to 2D modalities such as 2D TTE or angiography. Thus, MDCT is considered the gold standard for device sizing.[48] The anatomical structures at the aortic root change throughout the cardiac cycle. These annular cyclic changes need to be taken into consideration when choosing the device that needs to withstand them. Recently, some authors have advocated the utilization of systolic phases in order to refrain from prosthesis undersizing.[48] Accurate annular sizing should be performed using two orthogonal planes along the aortic root. The perpendicular plane immediately below the nadir of the aortic cusps represents the annulus. At this location, measurements should include diameters (shortest and longest), annular perimeter and area, and the calculated derived virtual diameters from both perimeter and area.[127–132] MDCT perimeter- and area-derived virtual diameters have been shown to change the least during the cardiac cycle and are considered to be the most reliable diameter measurement.[127–132] Prosthesis sizing is undertaken using dedicated tables for each device. When sizing a device, one should consult with the most updated manufacturer instructions (Fig. 7.20).

Other components of the aortic root should be addressed, including the distance of the coronary ostia location, aortic cusp length and calcification, aortic sinuses width and degree of calcification, and sinotubular junction and ascending aorta size. These data are essential in fitting the appropriate device to the specific anatomy.[128] Prosthesis inappropriate sizing is associated with coronary occlusion, annular rupture, paravalvular regurgitation, and device embolization.

The presence, quantity, and distribution of aortic root calcification are related to procedure outcome.[48] TAVR prosthesis anchoring requires some degree of calcification; however, high calcification burdens in the aortic valve and LVOT are strong predictors for paravalvular aortic regurgitation.[48] Greater calcium burden in the left coronary cusp has been implicated as an independent predictor for the need for permanent pacemaker following the procedure []. LVOT calcification adjacent to the noncoronary cusp was demonstrated as a predictor for aortic root injury.[48]

The specific aortic root orientation is different for every patient with a general anterior right-sided angulation in most cases. The accurate position for each patient is easily depicted using MDCT data. Thus, providing a correct fluoroscopic (C-arm) angle in which all three coronary cusps are aligned in the same plane allows ease of utilization with the physical constraints of a catheterization suite. Further, in candidates of TAVR, aortoiliac angiography is often simultaneously performed to assess the dimensions of the vasculature for planned transfemoral approaches. Several important imaging features can predict periprocedural complications, including minimum aortoiliac artery diameter less than the diameter of external sheath, severe calcifications in femoral and superficial femoral arteries, "horseshoe" calcifications, and severe aortic atheromatous plaque.

Patients undergoing TAVR who have underlying renal insufficiency may undergo low-dose iodinated contrast protocols, which have included the use of monochromatic DECT imaging and selective aortoiliac angiography.

Percutaneous repair or replacement of the mitral valve presents as a viable option for patients deemed too high a surgical risk. Current American College of Cardiology/American Heart Association (ACC/AHA) guidelines list criteria for patients with mitral regurgitation that are potentially suitable for minimally invasive approach and include:

- Severely symptomatic heart failure (NYHA class III/IV) despite medical therapy.
- Chronic mitral regurgitation caused by leaflet degeneration (primary MR) as opposed to MR resulting from left ventricular remodeling (secondary MR).
- MR graded as moderate/severe to severe on echocardiography.
- The anatomy permits to repair or replacement.
- The patient otherwise has a reasonable life expectancy.
- Comorbidities place the patient as an unacceptable surgical risk.

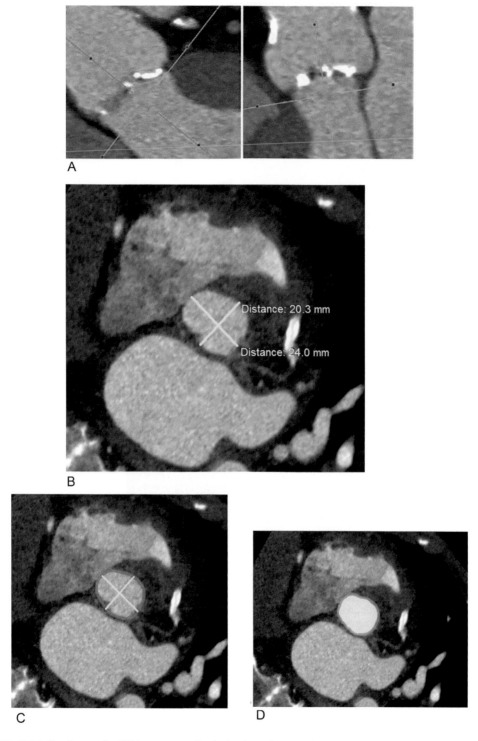

FIG. 7.20 Cardiovascular CT for preprocedural planning of transcatheter aortic valve replacement (TAVR). Aortic annulus. (A) The aortic annulus obtained using two perpendicular pales through the nadir of the aortic cusps. (B) Annulus diameters longest and shortest.(C) Aortic annulus perimeter and derived diameters. (D) Aortic annulus area.

*Continued*

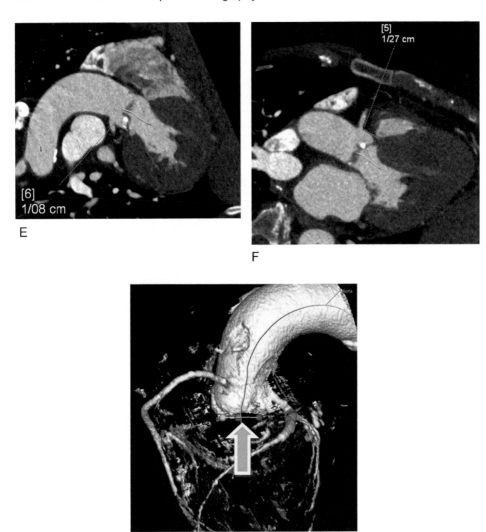

FIG. 7.20, CONT'D   (E, F) Measurement of the right coronary ostial height (E), and left coronary ostial height (F). (G) Fluoroscopic projection angle predicted by MDCT. Volume rendering of the aortic root aligning all three cusps in the same plane: volume-rendered imaging of the aorta, aortic annulus, and aortic valve. *Arrow* indicates the plane of the aortic annulus. When all points in the aortic annular plane are aligned, these CT projection angles can be helpful during the procedure as a guide to which angles may be useful at the time of the TAVR procedure.

Transcutaneous mitral valve procedures have predominantly involved mitral repair rather than replacement. The MitraClip device (Abbott Vascular) has a widespread use, is the only FDA-approved device, and has ongoing registry-based evidence to its utility.[133] The concept of the MitraClip is derived from the Alfieri surgical repair of the mitral valve, where a double stitch between the anterior and posterior leaflets fixes the cusps where regurgitation is maximal. A double orifice is thereby created with two smaller inflow orifices. Access is gained by the femoral vein and transseptal puncture. Experience with the MitraClip device has been presented in several registries and trials. The EVEREST I trial assessed feasibility and followed 24 patients with clips. Of these 13 had reduced MR sustained at 6 months.[134] The subsequent EVEREST II trial randomly assigned 279 patients to either surgical repair or percutaneous repair in a 2:1 ratio.[135] Outcomes were assessed at 30 days and 12 months with primary endpoints being survival, 30-day adverse outcomes, requirement for additional surgery, and continued grade 3/4 MR. The overall findings were of greater efficacy in the surgical cohort (73% vs 55%), though with less adverse outcomes within the percutaneous repair group (15% vs 48%). The safety of percutaneous repair was confirmed in an analysis of high-risk candidates from the EVEREST II cohort. Current guidelines recommend percutaneous mitral repair in patients with chronic primary MR, who are severely symptomatic despite optimal medical therapy and at prohibitive risk for surgery.[6] Devices specific for TMVR are currently undergoing feasibility trials. These include Tiara (Neovasc Inc., Richmond, BC, Canada), CardiAQ (CardiAQ Valve Technologies, Irvine, CA, USA), Tendyne (Tendyne Holdings, Roseville, MN, USA), and Twelve (Twelve Inc., Redwood City, CA, USA). The devices incorporate distinct features to aid positioning. These include atrial skirts to aid apposition against the left atrial wall, tabs to engage the myocardium, anchors to engage the annulus and leaflets, and paddles to engage the leaflets or apical tether. Transseptal implantation has not been successful, and the devices are designed for transapical delivery.[136]

Radiofrequency ablation to isolate arrhythmogenic foci surrounding the pulmonary veins is an interventional procedure to treat atrial fibrillation. CT has a role in defining the pulmonary vein anatomy, presence of thrombus and proximity to the esophagus. Additionally, CT imaging can be merged with electrical mapping systems to define the atrial border and vein location for the proceduralist. The number, position, and presence of accessory veins can be determined in preprocedural CT. Most commonly there are four, two on each side. Occasionally there can be a single ostium with the merger of the veins. Knowledge of vein anatomy is required to prevent injury and ensure all veins draining into the left atrium are isolated. Ostial size can also be determined, with smaller ostia more susceptible to stenosis. The presence of thrombus in the left atrium or left atrial appendage can be shown on CT. Delayed phase imaging can discriminate filling defects due to thrombus from defects due to slow contrast filling as thrombus will persist in delayed phases. The presence of thrombus contraindicates proceeding with ablation.[48]

Proximity to the esophagus can be determined, with the left pulmonary veins commonly lying anterior. There is the potential risk of atrial-esophageal fistula formation with ablation of ostia in close proximity to the esophagus.[48]

## REFERENCES

1. Maleki M, Alizadehasl A, Haghjoo M, eds. *Practical Cardiology*. 1st ed. Elsevier; 2018.
2. Kronmal RA, McClelland RL, Detrano R, et al. Risk factors for the progression of coronary artery calcification in asymptomatic subjects: results from the Multi-Ethnic Study of Atherosclerosis (MESA). *Circulation*. 2007; 115:2722.
3. Raggi P, Callister TQ, Shaw LJ. Progression of coronary artery calcium and risk of first myocardial infarction in patients receiving cholesterol-lowering therapy. *Arterioscler Thromb Vasc Biol*. 2004;24:1272.
4. Raggi P, Cooil B, Ratti C, et al. Progression of coronary artery calcium and occurrence of myocardial infarction in patients with and without diabetes mellitus. *Hypertension*. 2005;46:238.
5. Schultz CJ, Halliburton SS, Schoenhagen P, eds. *Cardiac CT Made Easy: An Introduction to Cardiovascular Multidetector Computed Tomography*. Taylor & Francis Group; 2014.
6. Budoff MJ, Shinbane JS, eds. *Cardiac CT Imaging Diagnosis of Cardiovascular Disease*. 3rd ed. Springer International Publishing; 2016.
7. Zipes DP, Libby P, Bonow RO, Mann DL, Tomaselli, GF, eds. 2018 Braunwald's Heart Disease: A Textbook of Cardiovascular Medicine, 11th ed., Copyright © 2019 by Elsevier Inc.
8. Naoum C, Blanke P, Leipsic J. Iterative reconstruction in cardiac CT. *J Cardiovasc Comput Tomogr*. 2015;9:255–263.
9. Danad I, Fayad ZA, Willemink MJ, et al. New applications of cardiac computed tomography: dual-energy, spectral, and molecular CT imaging. *JACC Cardiovasc Imaging*. 2015;8:710–723.
10. Raff GL, Abidov A, Achenbach S, et al. SCCT guidelines for the interpretation and reporting of coronary computed tomographic angiography. *J Cardiovasc Comput Tomogr*. 2009;3:122.
11. Higgins CB, de Roos A, eds. *MRI and CT of the Cardiovascular System I*. 3rd ed. Lippincott Williams & Wilkins; 2013 ISBN 978-1-4511-3731-6.
12. O'Brien JP, Srichai MB, Hecht EM, Kim DC, Jacobs JE. Anatomy of the heart at multidetector CT: what the radiologist needs to know. *Radiographics*. 2007; 27:1569–1582.
13. Sundaram B, Patel S, Bogot N, Kazerooni EA. Anatomy and terminology for the interpretation and reporting of cardiac MDCT: part 1, structured report, coronary calcium screening, and coronary artery anatomy. *AJR Am J Roentgenol*. 2009;192:574–583.
14. Voros S, Rivera JJ, Berman DS, et al. Guideline for minimizing radiation exposure during acquisition of coronary artery calcium scans with the use of multidetector computed tomography: a report by the Society for Atherosclerosis Imaging and Prevention Tomographic Imaging and Prevention Councils in collaboration with the Society of Cardiovascular

Computed Tomography. *J Cardiovasc Comput Tomogr.* 2011;5:75–83.

15. Detrano R, Guerci AD, Carr JJ, et al. Coronary calcium as a predictor of coronary events in four racial or ethnic groups. *N Engl J Med.* 2008;358:1336–1345.

16. Polonsky TS, McClelland RL, Jorgensen NW, et al. Coronary artery calcium score and risk classification for coronary heart disease prediction. *JAMA.* 2010;303: 1610–1616.

17. McClelland RL, Chung H, Detrano R, et al. Distribution of coronary artery calcium by race, gender, and age: results from the Multi-Ethnic Study of Atherosclerosis (MESA). *Circulation.* 2006;113:30–37.

18. Budoff MJ, Nasir K, McClelland RL, et al. Coronary calcium predicts events better with absolute calcium scores than age-sex-race/ethnicity percentiles: MESA (Multi-Ethnic Study of Atherosclerosis). *J Am Coll Cardiol.* 2009;53:345–352.

19. Erbel R, Mohlenkamp S, Moebus S, et al. Coronary risk stratification, discrimination, and reclassification improvement based on quantification of subclinical coronary atherosclerosis: the Heinz Nixdorf Recall Study. *J Am Coll Cardiol.* 2010;56:1397–1406.

20. Weber LA, Cheezum MK, Reese JM, et al. Cardiovascular imaging for the primary prevention of atherosclerotic cardiovascular disease events. *Curr Cardiovasc Imaging Rep.* 2015;8:36.

21. Arad Y, Spadaro LA, Goodman K, et al. Prediction of coronary events with electron beam computed tomography. *J Am Coll Cardiol.* 2000;36:1253–1260.

22. Raggi P, Callister TQ, Cooil B, et al. Identification of patients at increased risk of first unheralded acute myocardial infarction by electron-beam computed tomography. *Circulation.* 2000;101:850–855.

23. Wong ND, Hsu JC, Detrano RC, et al. Coronary artery calcium evaluation by electron beam tomography and its relation to new cardiovascular events. *Am J Cardiol.* 2000;86:495–498.

24. Vliegenthart R, Oudkerk M, Song B, et al. Coronary calcification detected by electron-beam computed tomography and myocardial infraction: the Rotterdam Coronary Calcification Study. *Eur Heart J.* 2002;23:1596–1603 Park R, Detrano RC, Xiang M, et al. Combined use of computed tomography coronary calcium scores and C-reactive protein levels in predicting cardiovascular events in nondiabetic individuals. *Circulation.* 2002;106:2073–2077.

25. Kondos GT, Hoff JA, Sevrukov A, et al. Electron-beam tomography coronary artery calcium and cardiac events. *Circulation.* 2003;107:2571–2576.

26. Shaw LJ, Raggi P, Schisterman E, et al. Prognostic value of cardiac risk factors and coronary artery calcium screening for all-cause mortality. *Radiology.* 2003;228: 826–833.

27. Greenland P, LaBree L, Azen SP, et al. Coronary artery calcium score combined with Framingham score for risk prediction in asymptomatic individuals. *JAMA.* 2004;291:210–215.

28. Arad Y, Goodman KJ, Roth M, et al. Coronary calcification, coronary disease risk factors, C-reactive protein, and atherosclerotic cardiovascular disease events. *J Am Coll Cardiol.* 2005;46:158–165.

29. Taylor AJ, Bindeman J, Feuerstein I, et al. Coronary calcium independently predicts incident premature coronary heart disease over measure cardiovascular disease risk factors. *J Am Coll Cardiol.* 2005;46:807–814.

30. Budoff MJ, Shaw LJ, Liu ST, et al. Long-term prognosis associated with coronary calcification. *J Am Coll Cardiol.* 2007;49:1860–1870.

31. Lakoski SG, Greenland P, Wong ND, et al. Coronary artery calcium scores and risk for cardiovascular events in women classified as "low risk" based on Framingham risk score. *Arch Intern Med.* 2007;167:2437–2442.

32. Becker A, Leber A, Becker C, Knez A. Predictive value of coronary calcifications for future cardiac events in asymptomatic individuals. *Am Heart J.* 2008;155:154–160.

33. Erbel R, Mohlenkamp S, Moebus S, et al. Coronary risk stratification, discrimination, and reclassification improvement based on quantification of subclinical coronary atherosclerosis. *J Am Coll Cardiol.* 2010;56: 1397–1406.

34. Hecht HS, Narula J. Coronary artery calcium scanning in asymptomatic patients with diabetes. *J Diabetes.* 2012;4:342–350.

35. Yeboah J, McClelland RL, Polonsky TS, et al. Comparison of novel risk markers for improvement in cardiovascular risk assessment in intermediate-risk individuals. *JAMA.* 2012;308:788–795.

36. Folsom AR, Kronmal RA, Detrano RC, et al. Coronary artery calcification compared with carotid intima-media thickness in the prediction of cardiovascular disease incidence: the Multi-Ethnic Study of Atherosclerosis. *Arch Intern Med.* 2008;168:1333–1339.

37. Hecht HS. Coronary artery calcium scanning: past, present, and future. *JACC Cardiovasc Imaging.* 2015;8:580–596.

38. Elias-Smale SE, Vliegenthart R, Koller MT, et al. Coronary calcium score improves classification of coronary heart disease in the elderly. *J Am Coll Cardiol.* 2010;56:1407–1414.

39. Stone NJ, Robinson JG, Lichtenstein AH, et al. The 2013 ACC/AHA guideline on the treatment of blood cholesterol to reduce atherosclerotic cardiovascular risk in adults. *J Am Coll Cardiol.* 2014;63:2889–2934.

40. Grundy SM, Stone NJ, Bailey AL, et al. 2018 ACC/AHA/AACVPR/AAPA/ABC/ACPM/ADA/AGS/APhA/ASPC/NLA/PCNA guideline on the management of blood cholesterol: a report of the American College of Cardiology Foundation and the American Heart Association Task Force on Clinical Practice Guidelines. *J Am Coll Cardiol.* 2018;https://doi.org/10.1016/j.jacc.2018.11.003.

41. Goff DF, Lloyd-Jones DM, Bennett G, et al. 2013 ACC/AHA guideline on the assessment of cardiovascular risk. *J Am Coll Cardiol.* 2014;63:2935–2957.

42. Shaw LJ, Giambrone AE, Blaha MJ, et al. Long-term prognosis after coronary artery calcification testing in asymptomatic patients: a cohort study. *Ann Intern Med.* 2015;163:14–21.

43. Valenti V, Hartaigh BÓ, Heo R, et al. A 15-year warranty period for asymptomatic individuals without coronary artery calcium: a prospective follow-up of 9,715 individuals. *JACC Cardiovasc Imaging.* 2015;8:900–909.

44. Cook NR. Statistical evaluation of prognostic versus diagnostic models: beyond the ROC curve. *Clin Chem.* 2008;54:17–23.

45. Sarwar A, Shaw LJ, Shapiro MD, et al. Diagnostic and prognostic value of absence of coronary artery calcification. *JACC Cardiovasc Imaging.* 2009;2:678–688.

46. Kelkar AA, Schultz WM, Khosa F, et al. Long-term prognosis after coronary artery calcium scoring among low-intermediate risk men and women. *Circ Cardiovasc Imaging.* 2016;9:e003742(2016). https://doi.org/10.1161/circimaging.115.003742.

47. Blaha MJ, Cainzos-Achirica M, Greenland P, et al. Role of coronary artery calcium score of zero and other negative risk markers for cardiovascular disease: the Multi-Ethnic Study of Atherosclerosis (MESA). *Circulation.* 2016;133:849–858.

48. Schoepf UJ, ed. *CT of the Heart.* 2nd ed. Humana Press; 2019.

49. Kavousi M, Desai CS, Ayers C, et al. Prevalence and prognostic significance of coronary artery calcification in low-risk women: a meta-analysis. *JAMA.* 2016;316:2126–2134.

50. Min JK, Lin FY, Gidseg DS, et al. Determinants of coronary calcium conversion among patients with a normal coronary calcium scan: what is the "warranty period" for remaining normal? *J Am Coll Cardiol.* 2010;55:1110–1117.

51. Gibson AO, Blaha MJ, Arnan MK, et al. Coronary artery calcium and incident cerebrovascular events in an asymptomatic cohort: the MESA study. *JACC Cardiovasc Imaging.* 2014;7:1108–1115.

52. Gepner AD, Young R, Delaney JA, et al. Comparison of coronary artery calcium presence, carotid plaque presence, and carotid intima-media thickness for cardiovascular disease prediction in the Multi-Ethnic Study of Atherosclerosis. *Circ Cardiovasc Imaging.* 2015;8.

53. O'Neal WT, Efird JT, Qureshi WT, et al. Coronary artery calcium progression and atrial fibrillation: the Multi-Ethnic Study of Atherosclerosis. *Circ Cardiovasc Imaging.* 2015;8.

54. Whitlock MC, Yeboah J, Burke GL, et al. Cancer and its association with the development of coronary artery calcification: an assessment from the Multi-Ethnic Study of Atherosclerosis. *J Am Heart Assoc.* 2015;4.

55. Leening MJ, Elias-Smale SE, Kavousi M, et al. Coronary calcification and the risk of heart failure in the elderly: the Rotterdam Study. *JACC Cardiovasc Imaging.* 2012;5:874–880.

56. Nasir K, Clouse M. Role of nonenhanced multidetector CT coronary artery calcium testing in asymptomatic and symptomatic individuals. *Radiology.* 2012;264:637–649.

57. Pursnani A, Chou ET, Zakroysky P, et al. Use of coronary artery calcium scanning beyond coronary computed tomographic angiography in the emergency department evaluation for acute chest pain: the ROMICAT II trial. *Circ Cardiovasc Imaging.* 2015;8.

58. Villines TC, Hulten EA, Shaw LJ, et al. Prevalence and severity of coronary artery disease and adverse events among symptomatic patients with coronary artery calcification scores of zero undergoing coronary computed tomography angiography: results from the CONFIRM (Coronary CT Angiography Evaluation For Clinical Outcomes: An International Multicenter) Registry. *J Am Coll Cardiol.* 2011;58:2533–2540.

59. Nicholls SJ, Ballantyne CM, Barter PJ, et al. Effect of two intensive statin regimens on progression of coronary disease. *N Engl J Med.* 2001;365:2078–2087.

60. Budoff MJ, Dowe D, Jollis JG, et al. Diagnostic performance of 64-multidetector row coronary computed tomographic angiography for evaluation of coronary artery stenosis in individuals without known coronary artery disease: results from the prospective multicenter accuracy (Assessment by Coronary Computed Tomographic Angiography of Individuals Undergoing Invasive Coronary Angiography) trial. *J Am Coll Cardiol.* 2008;52:1724–1732.

61. Miller JM, Rochitte CE, Dewey M, et al. Diagnostic performance of coronary angiography by 64-row CT. *N Engl J Med.* 2008;359:2324–2336.

62. Neglia D, Rovai D, Caselli C, et al. Detection of significant coronary artery disease by noninvasive anatomical and functional imaging. *Circ Cardiovasc Imaging.* 2015;8.

63. Min JK, Dunning A, Lin FY, et al. Rationale and design of the CONFIRM (Coronary CT Angiography Evaluation For Clinical Outcomes: An International Multicenter) Registry. *J Cardiovasc Comput Tomogr.* 2011;5:84–92.

64. Min JK, Dunning A, Lin FY, et al. Age- and sex related differences in all-cause mortality risk based on coronary computed tomography angiography findings results from the international multicenter CONFIRM (Coronary CT Angiography Evaluation For Clinical Outcomes: An International Multicenter) Registry of 23,854 patients without known coronary artery disease. *J Am Coll Cardiol.* 2011;58:849–860.

65. Lin FY, Shaw LJ, Dunning AM, et al. Mortality risk in symptomatic patients with nonobstructive coronary artery disease: a prospective 2-center study of 2,583 patients undergoing 64-detector row coronary computed tomographic angiography. *J Am Coll Cardiol.* 2011;58:510–519.

66. Marwick TH, Cho I, Ó Hartaigh B, et al. Finding the gatekeeper to the cardiac catheterization laboratory:

coronary CT angiography or stress testing? *J Am Coll Cardiol.* 2015;65:2747–2756.

67. Motoyama S, Sarai M, Harigaya H, et al. Computed tomographic angiography characteristics of atherosclerotic plaques subsequently resulting in acute coronary syndrome. *J Am Coll Cardiol.* 2009;54(1):49–57.

68. Motoyama S, Kondo T, Sarai M, et al. Multislice computed tomographic characteristics of coronary lesions in acute coronary syndromes. *J Am Coll Cardiol.* 2007;50(4):319–326.

69. Vanhoenacker PK, Decramer I, Bladt O, et al. Multidetector computed tomography angiography for assessment of in-stent restenosis: meta-analysis of diagnostic performance. *BMC Med Imaging.* 2008;8:14.

70. Sun Z, Almutairi AM. Diagnostic accuracy of 64 multislice CT angiography in the assessment of coronary in stent restenosis: a meta-analysis. *Eur J Radiol.* 2010;73:266–273.

71. Carrabba N, Schuijf JD, de Graaf FR, et al. Diagnostic accuracy of 64-slice computed tomography coronary angiography for the detection of in-stent restenosis: a meta-analysis. *J Nucl Cardiol.* 2010;17:470–478.

72. Kumbhani DJ, Ingelmo CP, Schoenhagen P, et al. Meta-analysis of diagnostic efficacy of 64-slice computed tomography in the evaluation of coronary in stent restenosis. *Am J Cardiol.* 2009;103:1675–1681.

73. Sheth T, Dodd JD, Hoffmann U, et al. Coronary stent assessability by 64 slice multi-detector computed tomography. *Catheter Cardiovasc Interv.* 2007;69:933–938.

74. Chung SH, Kim YJ, Hur J, et al. Evaluation of coronary artery in-stent restenosis by 64-section computed tomography: factors affecting assessment and accurate diagnosis. *J Thorac Imaging.* 2010;25:57–63.

75. Eisentopf J, Achenbach S, Ulzheimer S, et al. Low-dose dual-source CT angiography with iterative reconstruction for coronary artery stent evaluation. *JACC Cardiovasc Imaging.* 2013;6:458–465.

76. Bamberg F, Dierks A, Nikolaou K, Reiser MF, Becker CR, Johnson TR. Metal artifact reduction by dual energy computed tomography using monoenergetic extrapolation. *Eur Radiol.* 2011;21:1424–1429.

77. Meinel FG, Bischoff B, Zhang Q, Bamberg F, Reiser MF, Johnson TR. Metal artifact reduction by dual-energy computed tomography using energetic extrapolation: a systematically optimized protocol. *Invest Radiol.* 2012;47:406–414.

78. Mangold S, Cannao PM, Schoepf UJ, et al. Impact of an advanced image-based monoenergetic reconstruction algorithm on coronary stent visualization using third generation dual-source dual-energy CT: a phantom study. *Eur Radiol.* 2016;26:1871–1878.

79. Park KW, Park JJ, Chae IH, et al. Clinical characteristics of coronary drug-eluting stent fracture: insights from a two-center des registry. *J Korean Med Sci.* 2011;26:53–58.

80. van Velzen JE, de Graaf FR, de Graaf MA, et al. Comprehensive assessment of spotty calcifications on computed tomography angiography: comparison to plaque characteristics on intravascular ultrasound with radiofrequency backscatter analysis. *J Nucl Cardiol.* 2011;18(5):893–903.

81. Kitagawa T, Yamamoto H, Horiguchi J, et al. Characterization of noncalcified coronary plaques and identification of culprit lesions in patients with acute coronary syndrome by 64-slice computed tomography. *JACC Cardiovasc Imaging.* 2009;2(2):153–160.

82. Kashiwagi M, Tanaka A, Kitabata H, et al. Feasibility of noninvasive assessment of thin-cap fibroatheroma by multidetector computed tomography. *JACC Cardiovasc Imaging.* 2009;2(12):1412–1419.

83. Gauss S, Achenbach S, Pflederer T, Schuhback A, Daniel WG, Marwan M. Assessment of coronary artery remodelling by dual-source CT: a head-to-head comparison with intravascular ultrasound. *Heart.* 2011;97(12):991–997.

84. Hoffmann U, Moselewski F, Nieman K, et al. Noninvasive assessment of plaque morphology and composition in culprit and stable lesions in acute coronary syndrome and stable lesions in stable angina by multidetector computed tomography. *J Am Coll Cardiol.* 2006;47(8):1655–1662.

85. Ito T, Terashima M, Kaneda H, et al. Comparison of in vivo assessment of vulnerable plaque by 64-slice multislice computed tomography versus optical coherence tomography. *Am J Cardiol.* 2011;107(9):1270–1277.

86. Otsuka K, Fukuda S, Tanaka A, et al. Napkin-ring sign on coronary CT angiography for the prediction of acute coronary syndrome. *JACC Cardiovasc Imaging.* 2013;6(4):448–457.

87. Maurovich-Horvat P, Hoffmann U, Vorpahl M, Nakano M, Virmani R, Alkadhi H. The napkin-ring sign: CT signature of high-risk coronary plaques? *JACC Cardiovasc Imaging.* 2010;3(4):440–444.

88. Fuster V, Moreno PR, Fayad ZA, Corti R, Badimon JJ. Atherothrombosis and high-risk plaque: part I: evolving concepts. *J Am Coll Cardiol.* 2005;46(6):937–954.

89. Motoyama S, Ito H, Sarai M, et al. Plaque characterization by coronary computed tomography angiography and the likelihood of acute coronary events in mid-term follow-up. *J Am Coll Cardiol.* 2015;66:337–346.

90. Di Carli MF, Dorbala S, Curillova Z, et al. Relationship between CT coronary angiography and stress perfusion imaging in patients with suspected ischemic heart disease assessed by integrated PET-CT imaging. *J Nucl Cardiol.* 2007;14:799–809.

91. Gaemperli O, Schepis T, Valenta I, et al. Functionally relevant coronary artery disease: comparison of 64-section CT angiography with myocardial perfusion SPECT. *Radiology.* 2008;248:414–423.

92. Schuijf JD, Wijns W, Jukema JW, et al. Relationship between noninvasive coronary angiography with multi-slice computed tomography and myocardial perfusion imaging. *J Am Coll Cardiol.* 2006;48:2508–2514.

93. Meijboom WB, Van Mieghem CA, van Pelt N, et al. Comprehensive assessment of coronary artery stenoses: computed tomography coronary angiography versus conventional coronary angiography and correlation with fractional flow reserve in patients with stable angina. *J Am Coll Cardiol.* 2008;52:636–643.

94. Koo BK, Erglis A, Doh JH, et al. Diagnosis of ischemia-causing coronary stenoses by noninvasive fractional flow reserve computed from coronary computed tomographic angiograms. results from the prospective multicenter DISCOVE-FLOW (Diagnosis of Ischemia-Causing Stenoses Obtained Via Noninvasive Fractional Flow Reserve) study. *J Am Coll Cardiol.* 2011;58: 1989–1997.

95. Min JK, Leipsic J, Pencina MJ, et al. Diagnostic accuracy of fractional flow reserve from anatomic CT angiography. *JAMA.* 2012;308:1237–1245.

96. Norgaard BL, Leipsic J, Gaur S, et al. Diagnostic performance of noninvasive fractional flow reserve derived from coronary computed tomography angiography in suspected coronary artery disease: the NXT Trial (Analysis of Coronary Blood Flow Using CT Angiography: Next Steps). *J Am Coll Cardiol.* 2014;63:1145–1155.

97. Lloyd-Jones D, Adams RJ, Brown TM, et al. Heart disease and stroke statistics—2010 update: a report from the American Heart Association. *Circulation.* 2010;121(7): e46–e215. (2010). https://doi.org/10.1161/CIRCULATIONAHA.109.192667.

98. Pitts SR, Niska RW, Xu J, Burt CW. National Hospital Ambulatory Medical Care Survey: 2006 emergency department summary. *Natl Health Stat Report.* 2008;7:1–38.

99. McCaig LF, Burt CW. National Hospital Ambulatory Medical Care Survey: 2002 emergency department summary. *Adv Data.* 2004;340:1–34.

100. Pozen MW, D'Agostino RB, Selker HP, Sytkowski PA, Hood Jr. WB. A predictive instrument to improve coronary-care-unit admission practices in acute ischemic heart disease. A prospective multicenter clinical trial. *N Engl J Med.* 1984;310(20):1273–1278.

101. Virmani R, Burke AP, Farb A, Kolodgie FD. Pathology of the vulnerable plaque. *J Am Coll Cardiol.* 2006;47(suppl 8):C13–C18.

102. Romero J, Husain SA, Holmes AA, et al. Non-invasive assessment of low risk acute chest pain in the emergency department a comparative meta-analysis of prospective studies. *Int J Cardiol.* 2015;187:565–580.

103. Maffei E, Seitun S, Guaricci AI, et al. Chest pain: coronary CT in the ER. *Br J Radiol.* 2016;89:20150954.

104. Hoffmann U, Bamberg F, Chae CU, et al. Coronary computed tomography angiography for early triage of patients with acute chest pain: the ROMICAT (Rule Out Myocardial Infarction Using Computer Assist d Tomography) trial. *J Am Coll Cardiol.* 2009;53:1642–1650.

105. Hamilton-Craig C, Fifoot A, Hansen M, et al. Diagnostic performance and cost of CT angiography versus stress ECG: a randomized prospective study of suspected acute coronary syndrome chest pain in the emergency department (CT-COMPARE). *Int J Cardiol.* 2014;177: 867–873.

106. Litt HI, Gatsonis C, Snyder B, et al. CT angiography for safe discharge of patients with possible acute coronary syndromes. *N Engl J Med.* 2012;366:1393–1403.

107. Hoffmann U, Truong QA, Schoenfeld DA, et al. Coronary CT angiography versus standard evaluation in acute chest pain. *N Engl J Med.* 2012;367:299–308.

108. Goldstein JA, Chinnaiyan KM, Abidov A, et al. The CT-STAT (Coronary Computed Tomographic Angiography For Systematic Triage of Acute Chest Pain Patients To Treatment) trial. *J Am Coll Cardiol.* 2011;58:1414–1422.

109. Linde JJ, Kofoed KF, Sorgaard M, et al. Cardiac computed tomography guided treatment strategy in patients with recent acute-onset chest pain: results from the randomised, controlled trial: cardiac CT in the Treatment of Acute Chest Pain (CATCH). *Int J Cardiol.* 2013;168:5257–5262.

110. El-Hayek G, Benjo A, Uretsky S, et al. Meta-analysis of coronary computed tomography angiography versus standard of care strategy for the evaluation of low risk chest pain: are randomized controlled trials and cohort studies showing the same evidence? *Int J Cardiol.* 2014;177:238–245.

111. Dedic A, Lubbers MM, Schaap J, et al. Coronary CT angiography for suspected ACS in the era of high-sensitivity troponins: randomized multicenter study. *J Am Coll Cardiol.* 2016;67:16–26.

112. Levsky JM, Spevack DM, Travin MI, et al. Coronary computed tomography angiography versus radionuclide myocardial perfusion imaging in patients with chest pain admitted to telemetry: a randomized trial. *Ann Intern Med.* 2015;163:174–183.

113. Douglas PS, Hoffmann U, Patel MR, et al. Outcomes of anatomical versus functional testing for coronary artery disease. *N Engl J Med.* 2015;372:1291–1300.

114. Mark DB, Federspiel JJ, Cowper PA, et al. Economic outcomes with anatomical versus functional diagnostic testing for coronary artery disease. *Ann Intern Med.* 2016;165:94–102.

115. Mark DB, Anstrom KJ, Sheng S, et al. Quality-of-life outcomes with anatomic versus functional diagnostic testing strategies in symptomatic patients with suspected coronary artery disease: results from the PROMISE randomized trial. *Circulation.* 2016;133:1995–2007.

116. Ladapo JA, Hoffmann U, Lee KL, et al. Changes in medical therapy and lifestyle after anatomical or functional testing for coronary artery disease. *J Am Heart Assoc.* 2016;5.

117. Newby D, Williams M, Hunter A, et al. CT coronary angiography in patients with suspected angina due to coronary heart disease (SCOT-HEART): an open-label, parallel-group, multicentre trial. *Lancet.* 2015;385:2383–2391.

118. Williams MC, Hunter A, Shah AS, et al. Use of coronary computed tomographic angiography to guide

management of patients with coronary disease. *J Am Coll Cardiol.* 2016;67:1759–1768.

119. Levine A, Hecht HS. Cardiac CT angiography in congestive heart failure. *J Nucl Med.* 2015;56(suppl 4): 46s–51s.

120. Taylor AJ, Cerqueira M, Hodgson JM, et al. ACCF/SCCT/ ACR/AHA/ASE/ASNC/NASCI/SCAI/SCMR 2010 appropriate use criteria for cardiac computed tomography. A report of the American College of Cardiology Foundation Appropriate Use Criteria Task Force, the Society of Cardiovascular Computed Tomography, the American College of Radiology, the American Heart Association, the American Society of Echocardiography, the American Society of Nuclear Cardiology, the North American Society for Cardiovascular Imaging, the Society for Cardiovascular Angiography and Interventions, and the Society for Cardiovascular Magnetic Resonance. *J Am Coll Cardiol.* 2010;56:1864–1894.

121. Feuchtner GM, Spoeck A, Lessick J, et al. Quantification of aortic regurgitant fraction and volume with multidetector computed tomography comparison with echocardiography. *Acad Radiol.* 2011;18:334–342.

122. Blanke P, Naoum C, Webb J, et al. Multimodality imaging in the context of transcatheter mitral valve replacement: establishing consensus among modalities and disciplines. *JACC Cardiovasc Imaging.* 2015;8:1191–1208 56(22):1864–1894.

123. Guo YK, Yang ZG, Ning G, et al. Isolated mitral regurgitation: quantitative assessment with 64-section multidetector CT: comparison with MR imaging and echocardiography. *Radiology.* 2009;252:369–376.

124. Leon MB, Smith CR, Mack MJ, et al. Transcatheter or surgical aortic-valve replacement in intermediate-risk patients. *N Engl J Med.* 2016;374:1609–1620.

125. Smith CR, Leon MB, Mack MJ, et al. Transcatheter versus surgical aortic-valve replacement in high-risk patients. *N Engl J Med.* 2011;364:2187–2198.

126. Makkar RR, Fontana GP, Jilaihawi H, et al. Transcatheter aortic-valve replacement for inoperable severe aortic stenosis. *N Engl J Med.* 2012;366:1696–1704.

127. Leipsic J, Gurvitch R, Labounty TM, et al. Multidetector computed tomography in transcatheter aortic valve implantation. *JACC Cardiovasc Imaging.* 2011;4(4):416–429.

128. Achenbach S, Delgado V, Hausleiter J, Schoenhagen P, Min JK, Leipsic JA. SCCT expert consensus document on computed tomography imaging before transcatheter aortic valve implantation (TAVI)/transcatheter aortic valve replacement (TAVR). *J Cardiovasc Comput Tomogr.* 2012;6(6):366–380.

129. Apfaltrer P, Henzler T, Blanke P, Krazinski AW, Silverman JR, Schoepf UJ. Computed tomography for planning transcatheter aortic valve replacement. *J Thorac Imaging.* 2013;28(4):231–239.

130. Blanke P, Schoepf UJ, Leipsic JA. CT in transcatheter aortic valve replacement. *Radiology.* 2013;269(3):650–669.

131. Gurvitch R, Webb JG, Yuan R, et al. Aortic annulus diameter determination by multidetector computed tomography: reproducibility, applicability, and implications for transcatheter aortic valve implantation. *JACC Cardiovasc Interv.* 2011;4(11):1235–1245.

132. Korosoglou G, Gitsioudis G, Waechter-Stehle I, et al. Objective quantification of aortic valvular structures by cardiac computed tomography angiography in patients considered for transcatheter aortic valve implantation. *Catheter Cardiovasc Interv.* 2013;81(1):148–159.

133. Nishimura RA, Vahanian A, Eleid MF, Mack MJ. Mitral valve disease—current management and future challenges. *Lancet.* 2016;387:1324–1334.

134. Feldman T, Wasserman HS, Herrmann HC, et al. Percutaneous mitral valve repair using the edge-to-edge technique: six-month results of the EVEREST Phase I Clinical Trial. *J Am Coll Cardiol.* 2005;46:2134–2140.

135. Feldman T, Foster E, Glower DD, et al. Percutaneous repair or surgery for mitral regurgitation. *N Engl J Med.* 2011;364:1395–1406.

136. Gilard M, Cornily JC, Pennec PY, et al. Accuracy of multislice computed tomography in the preoperative assessment of coronary disease in patients with aortic valve stenosis. *J Am Coll Cardiol.* 2006;47(10):2020–2024.

## Further reading

137. American College of Cardiology Foundation Task Force on Expert Consensus Documents, Mark DB, Berman DS, et al. ACCF/ACR/AHA/NASCI/SAIP/SCAI/SCCT 2010 expert consensus document on coronary computed tomographic angiography, a report of the American College of Cardiology Foundation Task Force on Expert Consensus Documents. *J Am Coll Cardiol.* 2010;55 (23):2663–2699.

# CHAPTER 8

# Cardiac Magnetic Resonance Imaging

HAMID MOJIBIAN[a] • HAMIDREZA POURALIAKBAR[b]
[a]Department of Radiology and Biomedical Imaging, Yale University School of Medicine, New Haven, CT, United States, [b]Rajaie Cardiovascular, Medical & Research Center, Iran University of Medical Sciences, Tehran, Iran

---

**KEY POINTS**

- Magnetic resonance imaging (MRI) is a robust technology in cardiovascular imaging.
- MRI is the gold standard technique to measure ejection fraction of ventricles and their volumes.
- In this chapter, we learn about tissue characterization which is one of the unique features of this modality to show edema, fibrosis, iron, etc.
- In addition, how to use T1 mapping, T2 mapping, and measurement of ECV in cardiomyopathy and myocarditis.

---

Magnetic resonance imaging (MRI) has probably changed medicine in a way that no other technology has in the past few years. Although MRI generates high-resolution still images of internal organs, it traditionally had significant limitations in imaging moving organs such as beating hearts, which limited its role in cardiology. Recent technological advances in MR technology have made cardiac MRI (cMR) practical and an essential part of the practice of cardiology in many places. However, both technical demands and unfamiliarity of practicing cardiologists with cMR have been significant barriers to making the technology more widely used in the care of patients with cardiovascular conditions.

Discussion of the technical aspects of cMR is beyond this chapter, and no one should expect to master performing and interpreting MRI studies without going through proper training as outlined in professional society guidelines.[1] This chapter discusses very basic principles of MRI physics that are important in understanding how MRI can be used in the evaluation of cardiovascular conditions as well as knowing its limitations and pitfalls. Having a basic knowledge of MRI terminology will help practitioners to better understand examination reports.

## BASIC PHYSICS, TECHNICAL CONSIDERATIONS, AND IMAGING TOOLS

In a nutshell, MRI images are the result of digitally converting signals generated from excitation of the protons inside the body by radiofrequency (RF) waves into pictures. Each organ in the human body consists of millions of protons. Each proton molecule consistently spins around an axis that generates a small magnetic field around that molecule very similar to the Earth's magnetic field spinning around its axis. After placing the patient in an MRI magnet with the magnetic strength that is usually 1.5 or 3.0 T, all protons in the patient's body align themselves in parallel or antiparallel to the MRI magnetic field. However, protons align slightly more parallel than antiparallel to the magnetic field because that requires lower energy. At the same time, the spinning protons rotate around an external axis very similar to a spinning top. This rotation is called *precession*, and the speed of it is called *precession frequency*, which directly depends on the strength of the external magnetic field of the MRI scanner.[2]

By sending RF waves at the same speed as precession frequency, the protons pick up the energy and get excited as part of the process called *resonance*. Protons start to rotate in the same phase, knocking out protons from their stable status, changing the magnetic vector of rotating protons, and forming transverse magnetization. The moving vector of spinning protons creates a current that can be picked up by coils surrounding the patient.

When RF waves stop, protons simultaneously start to recover to their original longitudinal state and get out of the spinning phase, respectively, called *longitudinal relaxation* and *transverse relaxation*. The time it takes for protons to recover to the longitudinal state is called the *longitudinal relaxation* time or *T1 time*. The time it takes for protons to completely get out of phase is called the *transverse relaxation time* or *T2 time*. T1 is several times longer than T2 time, and both relaxations happen

**TABLE 8.1**
**Magnetic Resonance Imaging Signal Intensities**

|  | T1-Weighted Image | T2-Weighted Image |
|---|---|---|
| Liquid (edema) | Dark | Bright |
| Fat | Bright | Dark |
| Acute blood | Dark | Intermediate |
| Subacute blood | Bright | Bright |
| Cyst | Dark | Bright |
| Calcium | Dark | Dark |

separately from each other. This means that if we wait long enough to read signals, longitudinal relaxation will contribute more to the contrast of the image, while signals from transverse relaxation are mostly dispersed, known as a T1-weighted image. Organs containing material with higher T1 value have higher signals than materials with lower T1 value. For example, fat has a high T1 value, and water has a low T1 value. Therefore, it is expected that in a T1-weighted image, fat is bright (higher signal), and liquids such as cerebrospinal fluid are dark (low signal) (Table 8.1 and Fig. 8.1). T1 mostly is inherent to the material structure.

Gadolinium-based contrast agents shorten the longitudinal relaxation (T1) time that allows for performing magnetic resonance angiography (MRA) with highest signal in the blood vessels, allowing creating images closely similar to the real angiogram. In addition, if an organ shows increased uptake of gadolinium or delayed washout, it will be bright on T1-weighted imaging, allowing diagnosis of a broad spectrum of pathologies. For example, after myocardial infarction, fibrous tissue entraps gadolinium with delayed washout compared with normal myocardium, allowing visualizing of a post-myocardial infarction (MI) scar as areas of increased T1 signal intensity (Fig. 8.2).

However, the transverse relaxation time (T2) is related to inhomogeneity in the magnetic fields, both at the external and molecular levels. For example, fast movement of water molecules diminishes aggravating factors of the external magnetic field, but for larger particles with slower movement, the external magnetic field has a more pronounced effect. In other words, liquids have longer transverse relaxation times (T2), and more complex liquid molecules may have shorter T2 times. In a T2-weighted image, liquids show higher signal and are bright (Fig. 8.3).

The signals that are picked up by antennas in the form of coils surrounding the patient (image) are digitally processed and through very complex mathematical calculation converted to images. However, this process

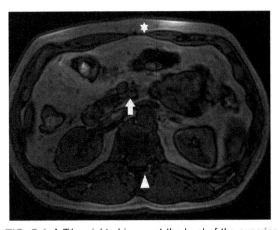

FIG. 8.1 A T1-weighted image at the level of the superior mesenteric artery (SMA) in a patient with suspected SMA dissection. Low signal intensity of cerebrospinal fluid (*arrowhead*) and high signal intensity of abdominal wall fat (*star*) are typical of a T1-weighted image. The increased signal intensity along the posterior aspect of SMA (*arrow*) is suggestive of blood in the vessel wall, confirming the suspected diagnosis of SMA dissection.

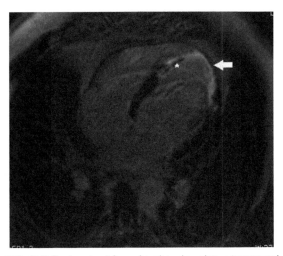

FIG. 8.2 Postcontrast four-chamber view shows transmural increased signal intensity or myocardial delayed enhancement of the apex and septum (*arrow*). This is caused by delayed washout of gadolinium from the scarred infarcted myocardium in distribution of the left anterior descending coronary artery. A higher concentration of gadolinium shortens T1, increasing the signal and allowing the distinction of normal viable myocardium from abnormal infarcted myocardium. The image also shows an area of microvascular obstruction (*star*).

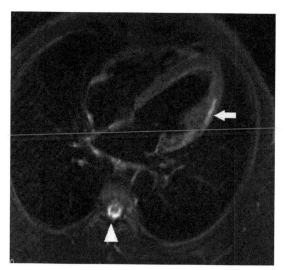

FIG. 8.3 A T2-weighted four-chamber image in a patient with suspected myocarditis. Increased signal intensity of cerebrospinal fluid (*arrowhead*) is seen on the T2-weighted image. The epicardial increased signal intensity along the left ventricular lateral wall (*arrow*) indicates edema that can be seen in the setting of acute myocarditis.

needs to be repeated several times to fill a mathematical space called the *K-space*. This repetition is one of the reasons MRI studies take a long time to complete because each slice of an image may take up to several minutes to be completely acquired and processed. In addition, this has been one of the reasons that until recently, MRI was not able to image a moving organ such as a beating heart. Any displacement of the imaging organ causes

disruption of the K-space calculation; so, it distorts the images. The introduction of electrocardiography (ECG)-gated imaging revolutionized cardiac MRI by allowing filling the K-space during the cardiac cycle with minimal artifact from cardiac motion.

In computed tomography (CT), images can be manipulated after acquisition to different contrast levels or reformatted to different planes from the original axial images. Unlike CT, in MRI, everything, including the plane of imaging, needs to be planned and executed while the patient is in the scanner. Many parameters affect the type of image, including if it would be T1 or T2 weighted or it is a still image or cine image. MRI sequences are small pieces of software, allowing programming of the MRI scanner to generate a picture based on the desired clinical need. There are many MRI sequences, and each vendor also has specific names unique to its system. Table 8.2 shows the MRI sequences commonly used in cardiovascular imaging and their applications.

## HARDWARE AND TECHNICAL REQUIREMENTS

There are special requirements to allow a center to perform and interpret cardiovascular MRI examinations. Both 1.5- and 3.0-T scanners are appropriate for performing cMR studies. Scanners with lower strength are not suitable, and scans with 1.5-T scanners have fewer technical challenges than 3.0-T scanners. Special cardiac software with specific sequences and hardware packages including ECG- or vector cardiogram (VCG)-based gating capabilities are required. In addition, a postprocessing software to allow volumetric and flow calculations is essential (Fig. 8.4).

**TABLE 8.2**
**Commonly Used Magnetic Resonance Imaging Sequences and Their Applications**

| Generic Sequence | Siemens | GE | Philips | Application |
|---|---|---|---|---|
| SE | SE | SE | SE | AI, TC |
| Fast SE | Turbo SE | Fast SE | Turbo SE | AI, TC (faster than SE) |
| STIR | STIR | STIR | STIR | TC, edema |
| GRE | GRE | GRE | FFE | CI, TC, AI |
| Ultra-fast GE | Turbo flash | FGRE | TFE | CI, TC, AI |
| Balanced GE | True FISP | FIESTA | Balanced FFE | CI |
| Phase contrast | PC | PC | PC | FL, VL |
| MRA | MRA | MRA | MRA | AI |

*AI*, anatomic imaging; *CI*, cine imaging; *FFE*, fast field echo; *FGRE*, fast gradient echo; *FIESTA*, fast imaging employing steady-state acquisition; *FISP*, fast imaging with steady-state precession; *FL*, flow; *GRE*, gradient echo; *MRA*, magnetic resonance angiography; *PC*, phase contrast; *STIR*, short-TI inversion recovery; *TC*, tissue characterization; *VL*, velocity.

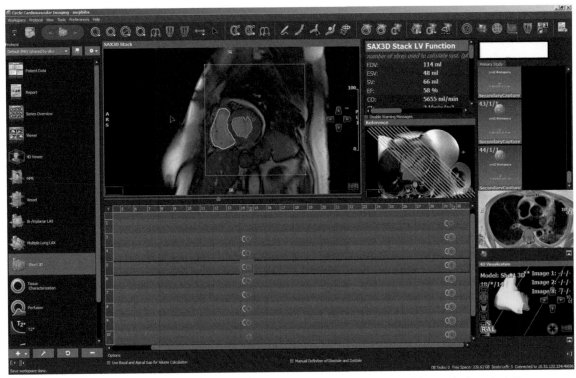

FIG. 8.4 A screenshot from postprocessing software shows volumetric left and right ventricular calculations.

However, the most important element for a successful cardiac MRI program is the human factor, including both well-trained cardiac imagers and technologists.

## CLINICAL APPLICATIONS

Many features make MRI an ideal tool for the evaluation of cardiovascular conditions. Among these functions are the capability of creating high-resolution images without limitation of the acquisition window, high reproducibility, the unique ability of tissue characterization, simultaneous anatomic and hemodynamic imaging without exposing patients to any harmful radiation, and being completely noninvasive.[3]

New indications for cMR are being introduced at a very fast pace. Rather than discussing specific indications and uses of cMR, we will review MRI technologies and tools to guide clinicians in picking the appropriate tests for their patients in a clinical practice setting.

### Anatomic Visualization

MRI is an excellent tool for anatomic visualization of cardiac, vascular, and extracardiac structures in different planes that does not suffer from the limitations of other

imaging modalities such as echocardiography (Fig. 8.5). Most studies do not need contrast, including when visualizing the vasculature, except when dynamic images are required, such as in evaluation of fistulas, leaks, or shunts (Fig. 8.6).

Clinical examples include:
- Congenital heart disease
- Hypertrophic cardiomyopathy
- Cardiac and extracardiac tumors
- Vascular anomalies such as vascular aneurysms, dissection, venous anomalies, and vascular shunts
- Interventional planning such as in ablation therapy or structural heart disease

### Functional Evaluation

Cine-cMR images allow both visualization and quantification of cardiac functions. cMR is now the gold standard for cardiac function evaluation.[4] Calculation and not just estimation of left and right ventricular function, end-diastolic volume, end-systolic volume, and many other parameters (including atrial volumetric measurements) are possible with cMR. Table 8.3 shows the most common volumetric measurements provided on a regular cMR report. Phase-contrast images allow flow

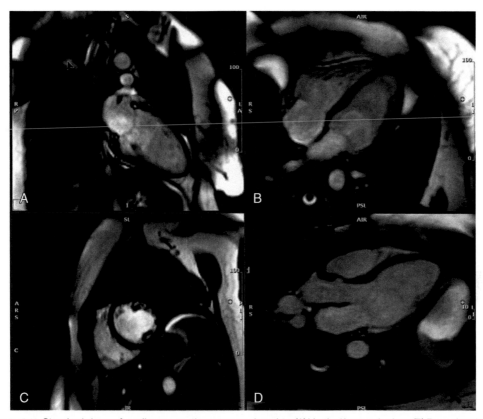

FIG. 8.5 Standard views of cardiac magnetic resonance imaging. (A) Vertical long-axis view. (B) Four-chamber view. (C) Short-axis view. (D) Left ventricular outflow view, also called the three-chamber view.

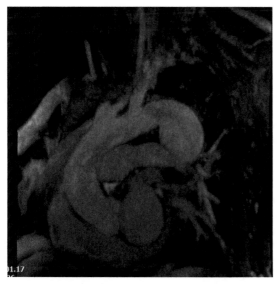

FIG. 8.6 An example of noncontrast magnetic resonance angiography of the thoracic aorta showing aneurysm of the proximal descending aorta.

**TABLE 8.3**
**Most Commonly Used Quantitative Measurements**

| Ventricles | Valves | Vessels |
| --- | --- | --- |
| End-diastolic volume | Diameter | Diameter |
| End-systolic volume | Surface area | Flow |
| Stroke volume | Regurgitation volume | Velocity |
| Ejection fraction | Regurgitation fraction | |
| Cardiac output | Valve gradient | |
| Ventricular diameter | | |
| Wall thickness | | |

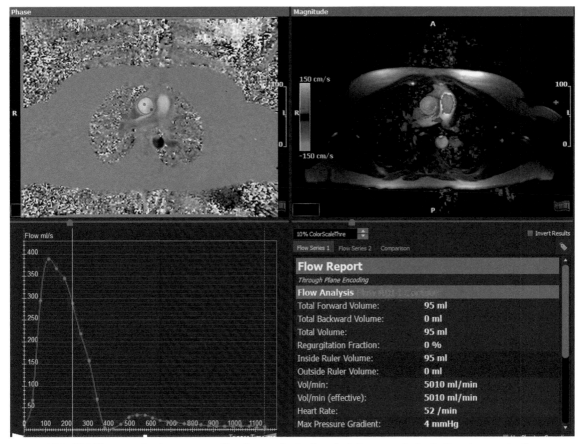

FIG. 8.7 Phase-contrast sequences allow flow and velocity calculation very similar to Doppler examination studies.

measurements and velocity measurements very similar to Doppler examinations (Fig. 8.7).

Clinical examples include:

- Accurate calculation of left ventricular ejection fraction in decision making for automatic implantable cardioverter defibrillator (AICD) placement after myocardial infarction
- Calculation of right ventricular end-diastolic volume and aneurysm detection in diagnosis of arrhythmogenic right ventricular cardiomyopathy as part of new diagnostic criteria
- Accurate calculation of mitral and aortic regurgitation fraction. cMR is potentially more precise than echocardiography in the computation of regurgitation fraction.
- Gradient calculation through a stenotic area in aortic stenosis or across aortic coarctation
- Dynamic visualization of intracardiac shunts
- Serial follow-up of ventricular functions such as in patients with congenital heart disease or myocardial insult
- Right ventricular function calculation in patients with congenital heart disease
- Dynamic evaluation of aortic dissection flap
- First-pass perfusion imaging in ischemic heart disease

## Tissue Characterization

Cardiac MRI has the unique capability for tissue characterization. cMR allows noninvasive evaluation of myocardial edema by T2 imaging, scar and myocardial fibrosis by the acquisition of postcontrast delayed myocardial images (myocardial delayed enhancement [MDE]), quantification of iron by T2*-weighted imaging, and identification of amyloid deposition using newer technique such as T1 mapping.

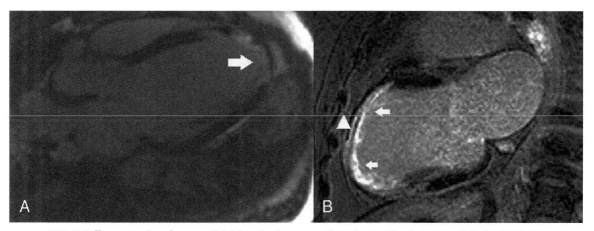

FIG. 8.8 Two examples of myocardial delayed enhancement in patients with prior myocardial infarction in the left anterior descending coronary artery distribution (*arrow*). (A) A subendocardial myocardial delayed enhancement pattern with a better chance of functional recovery after possible revascularization compared with (B) which shows transmural delayed enhancement (*arrows*) with areas of no perfusion (*arrowhead*).

Clinical examples include:
- Calculation of extent and thickness of myocardial scar after a myocardial infarction that may correlate with patient's outcome and response to revascularization[5] (Fig. 8.8)
- Identification of myocardial scar in the diagnosis of infiltrative processes such as sarcoidosis, cardiac amyloid, and myocarditis (Fig. 8.9)
- Iron quantification in patients with hemosiderosis directly related to prognosis

- Myocardial scar and mapping of arrhythmias focus
- Myocardial fibrosis and scar burden calculation for risk stratification in patients with hypertrophic cardiomyopathy

## PATIENT SELECTION AND PREPARATION

Cardiac MRI is usually not the first imaging modality in the evaluation of patients with cardiovascular conditions because of a lack of widespread availability,

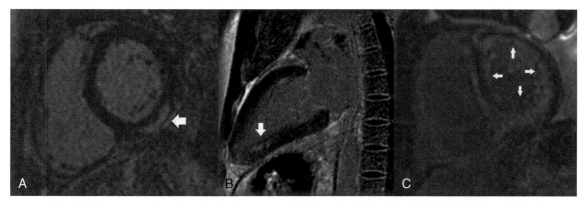

FIG. 8.9 Three examples of nonischemic myocardial delayed enhancement. (A) Epicardial linear delayed enhancement of the inferolateral wall in a patient with viral myocarditis (*arrow*). (B) Midmyocardial foci of myocardial delayed enhancement in the inferior wall in a patient with sarcoidosis (*arrow*). (C) Circumferential subendocardial delayed enhancement (*arrows*) with poor blood pool contrast in a patient with amyloidosis.

expense, lack of expertise to perform and interpret the studies, and the unfamiliarity of clinicians. CMR's roles still mostly remain in confirming or excluding a suspected diagnosis or shining the light on cases that otherwise are unresolved.

In many instances, patients need to travel to a center equipped with the proper scanner. The scan usually takes between 30 and 90 min and involves multiple breath holds. The newer scanners, called *wide-bore scanners*, have wider openings. However, these scanners are not widely popular, and patients still need to stay in a closed space for the period of the scan. Patients who have claustrophobia either are not able to tolerate the examination or need medication to calm them down for the duration of the scan. Pediatric patients require anesthesia in many cases to provide the best motion-free images.

Having arrhythmias during the examination is the primary reason for a suboptimal study or even incomplete examination. Arrhythmias mainly affect cine images, resulting in inaccurate functional evaluation and calculation. MRA sequences are less affected than cine images.

Patients with many medical devices such as older pacemakers, brain aneurysm clips, stimulators, and different types of pumps cannot get into scanners. However, cardiac prosthetic valves, most of the nondrug-eluting coronary and peripheral stents, inferior vena cava filters, and aortic stent grafts are not contraindications for cMR. Patients with abandoned venous pacemaker and AICD leads cannot be placed in MRI scanners. Epicardial pacer wires are safe. MRISafety.com is an excellent source to check the MRI compatibility of many devices.[6] It should be noted that if a device is considered safe for a 3-T scan, it is not necessarily also safe for a 1.5-T scan.

Many newer pacemakers are MRI compatible. However, this does not mean that patients with these pacemakers can be placed in a magnet without proper preparation, which is usually done in coordination with the electrophysiology team to disable and reprogram the device after completion of the examination. MRI-compatible pacemakers still may cause artifacts over the chest, limiting scans of the heart and thoracic structures. Review of the instructions for use of each device is necessary before clearing a patient for any types of cardiac scans.

Patients with glomerular filtration rates of less than $30 \text{ mL/min}/1.73 \text{ m}^2$ should not receive gadolinium because of the increased risk of nephrogenic systemic fibrosis.[7] However, gadolinium does not affect kidney function, unlike iodinated contrast agents.

## SPECIFIC INDICATIONS AND MAGNETIC RESONANCE TECHNIQUES

- Myocardial disease:
  - Acute edema (black blood T2 images)
  - Amyloid infiltration (T1 map, early postcontrast images)
  - Myocardial scar (MDE postcontrast image) pattern of enhancement helps to distinguish between ischemic and nonischemic cardiomyopathies.
  - Iron quantification (T2 imaging)
  - Ventricular clot (early postcontrast images with high T1)
  - MR stress perfusion in patients with suspected coronary artery disease
- Cardiac masses and tumors
  - Confirming the mass (black blood images, cine images)
  - Thrombus versus tumor (early postcontrast images with high T1 in thrombus, perfusion imaging, delayed enhancement in tumors)
  - Associated findings such as tumors outside the heart (magnetic resonance angiography [MRA], black blood, or steady-state free precession (SSFP) noncine image)
- Congenital heart disease
  - Anatomic imaging (black blood, magnetic resonance angiography [MRA])
  - Function (cine balanced steady-state free precession [bSSFP])
  - Shunt calculation (phase-contrast [PC] imaging)
  - Gradient calculation (PC)
- Valvular and pericardial heart disease
  - Regurgitation fraction (PC and cine imaging)
  - Gradient calculation (PC)
  - Anatomic visualization (cine bSSFP, MRA)
  - Ventricular decoupling imaging (real-time cine imaging)
- Electrophysiology
  - Scar imaging
  - MRA for interventional planning
- Pericardial disease
  - Hemodynamic evaluation (cine image and phase-contrast imaging)
  - Pericardial characterization (black blood images and postcontrast MDE for pericardial enhancement)
- Vascular disease
  - Vascular sizing (black blood, bSSFP, and MRA images)
  - Aortitis (black blood T2 images)
  - Shunt, fistula (time-resolved MRA)

## Tissue Characterization and Parametric Mapping

Cardiac MRI has the unique capability for tissue characterization. cMR images allow noninvasive evaluation of myocardial edema by T2 imaging, scar and myocardial fibrosis by the acquisition of postcontrast delayed myocardial images (myocardial delayed enhancement [MDE]), and characterization of masses and thrombi. Parametric cMR allows quantification of myocardial process giving more objective insight into disease processes. Examples of parametric cMR such as quantification of iron by T2*-weighted imaging, quantification of amyloid protein using T1 mapping, or quantification of fluid content and edema imaging using T2 mapping. Clinical examples include:

- Calculation of extent and thickness of myocardial scar after a myocardial infarction that may correlate with patient's outcome and response to revascularization[5] (Fig. 8.8)
- Identification of myocardial scar in the diagnosis of infiltrative processes such as sarcoidosis, cardiac amyloid, and myocarditis (Fig. 8.9)
- Iron quantification in patients with hemosiderosis directly related to prognosis (T2*)
- Myocardial scar and mapping of arrhythmias focus
- Myocardial fibrosis and scar burden calculation for risk stratification in patients with hypertrophic cardiomyopathy
- Calculation of T1 map and extracellular volume (ECV) in conditions like amyloidosis

## REFERENCES

1. Pohost GM, Kim RJ, Kramer CM, Manning WJ. Resonance SfCM. Task Force 12: training in advanced cardiovascular imaging (cardiovascular magnetic resonance [CMR]) endorsed by the Society for Cardiovascular Magnetic Resonance. *J Am Coll Cardiol.* 2008;51(3):404–408.
2. Ridgway JP. Cardiovascular magnetic resonance physics for clinicians: part I. *J Cardiovasc Magn Reson.* 2010;12:71.
3. Constantine G, Shan K, Flamm SD, Sivananthan MU. Role of MRI in clinical cardiology. *Lancet.* 2004;363(9427): 2162–2171.
4. Collins JD. Global and regional functional assessment of ischemic heart disease with cardiac MR imaging. *Radiol Clin North Am.* 2015;53(2):369–395.
5. Sawlani RN, Collins JD. Cardiac MRI and ischemic heart disease: role in diagnosis and risk stratification. *Curr Atheroscler Rep.* 2016;18(5):23.
6. MRIsafety.com. Information Resource for MRI Safety. (2017). http://www.mrisafety.com/; 2017. Accessed 2 January 2017.
7. Fraum TJ, Ludwig DR, Bashir MR, Fowler KJ. Gadolinium-based contrast agents: a comprehensive risk assessment. *J Magn Reson Imaging.* 2017;46(2):338–353.

# CHAPTER 9

# Nuclear Cardiology

HADI MALEK

Rajaie Cardiovascular Medical & Research Center, Iran University of Medical Sciences, Tehran, Iran

---

**KEY POINTS**

- There are several nuclear medicine procedures in the field of nuclear cardiology, among which myocardial perfusion imaging (MPI) is a widely available and sensitive method for evaluation of ischemic heart disease, left ventricular function, and myocardial viability.
- MPI can be interpreted visually and quantitatively; however, the interpreting physician should be aware of pitfalls and potential sources of artifacts.

---

## INTRODUCTION

Myocardial perfusion imaging (MPI) using single-photon emission computed tomography (SPECT) is the most frequently performed nuclear cardiology procedure and provides a sensitive means for detection, localization, and risk stratification of ischemic heart disease, assessment of left ventricular (LV) function, and myocardial viability.[1]

In MPI, a radiotracer is injected intravenously, and the distribution pattern, which is proportional to regional myocardial perfusion, is detected by a gamma camera. A series of multiple planar projection images are collected by rotation of the gamma camera head around the patient at regular angular intervals in a 180-degree arc for SPECT acquisition. The two-dimensional projections are then reconstructed mathematically into three-dimensional images and are oriented manually or automatically to be displayed in a series of slices in short axis, vertical long axis, and horizontal long axis orientations.

## RADIOPHARMACEUTICALS

The common characteristic of all the radiotracers that are used in MPI is that they are accumulated in viable myocytes in proportion to the regional blood flow.

Thallium-201 ($^{201}$Tl) is a cyclotron-produced radionuclide with a half-life of 73.1 h and emitted X-rays of primarily 68–80 keV and γ-rays of 137 and 167 keV, respectively.[2] $^{201}$Tl needs no in-house preparation and a single injection suffices for both stress and rest imaging.[3] Initial uptake of $^{201}$Tl in the myocardium is

according to myocardial perfusion and viability; however, as it redistributes over time, prolonged uptake depends on viability. Although $^{201}$Tl has a higher first-pass extraction as compared to the $^{99m}$Tc compounds, it suffers from higher radiation burden for the patient and lower image quality, limiting its use in obese patients and high-quality electrocardiography (ECG)-gated SPECT studies.[4]

$^{99m}$Tc-sestamibi and $^{99m}$Tc-tetrofosmin are lipid-soluble, cationic radiotracers with a half-life of 6 h and emitted photons of 140 keV. The first-pass extraction of both is less than $^{201}$Tl and after mitochondrial uptake, their myocardial washout and redistribution is negligible. Therefore, two separate injections are needed for stress and rest imaging.[5] However, high-energy photons of these $^{99m}$Tc compounds decrease the problems related to attenuation artifacts, providing images of higher quality.[3]

## DETECTION OF CORONARY ARTERY DISEASE AND STRESS TESTS

The basis of MPI is the visualization of heterogeneity of myocardial radiotracer uptake as a result of difference of myocardial blood flow secondary to coronary flow reserve impairment. In the resting state, the regional blood flow of normal and stenosed arteries may be equal, resulting in homogeneous distribution of radiotracers. However, the regional blood flow of the regions supplied by normal coronary arteries increases significantly during exercise or pharmacologic stress by vasodilators, but no such increase occurs in regions supplied by significantly stenosed coronary arteries, resulting in heterogeneous radiotracer uptake.[6] To demonstrate this heterogeneity, a linear relationship must exist between myocardial blood flow and radio-tracer uptake. Even though the relationship between these two is more linear in low flow, the radiotracer uptake demonstrates a plateau at higher rates, known as the *roll-off phenomenon*.[7] Fortunately, the identification of patients with high-degree (>70%) coronary stenosis is not significantly affected, whereas normal MPI might be seen in patients with a less severe degree of stenosis as a result of the roll-off phenomenon.[8]

Various methods of stress tests have been introduced for MPI. The appropriate stress test depends mostly on the clinical condition and physical ability of the patients.[5] However, dynamic exercise is the first test of choice.[4, 9] In patients with left bundle branch block (LBBB) or paced rhythm, pharmacologic stress with vasodilators (dipyridamole or adenosine) is the accepted modality of stress because reversible perfusion defects may appear in the anteroseptal wall in higher heart rates even in the absence of stenosis of left anterior descending artery (LAD).[1, 10]

In patients who are not able to perform exercise or an appropriate heart rate target or complain is not achieved, vasodilators with low-level ergometer exercise is preferred. If there is any contraindication, dobutamine (with atropine in patients with submaximal heart rate response) can be substituted. Medications, food, and beverages that may interfere with stress should be interrupted for a certain period of time.[4, 5] Selective adenosine A2A receptor agonists have also been developed, providing selective coronary vasodilation along with reduction of incidence and severity of side effects.[11]

## ELECTROCARDIOGRAPHY-GATED SPECT

By ECG gating, a cardiac cycle is created representing the average of cardiac beats acquired during the acquisition. In this method, the QRS complex of the patient's ECG triggers the count accumulation and each R-R interval is divided into 8 or 16 frames; therefore, each frame demonstrates a particular phase of the cardiac cycle.[12] Then, the collected data can be analyzed quantitatively, providing global systolic function (LV ejection fraction and end-systolic and end-diastolic volumes), regional systolic parameters (wall motion and wall thickening), and global diastolic function.[13] The synchrony of LV, both regionally and globally, can also be assessed by phase analysis.[14, 15] Gated study is recommended as a part of the MPI study to assess both LV functional parameters and distinguish true perfusion abnormalities from artifacts.[16, 17]

## IMAGE INTERPRETATION

A systematic approach should be observed in clinical interpretation of the MPI images. Assessment of cine display of rotating planar projection images, reviewing stress and acquisition work sheets, and evaluation of reconstructed image as well as ECG-gating quality and possible artifacts and quantification of SPECT MPI should all be incorporated in interpretation.[8, 18]

To have a common nomenclature with other imaging modalities and standardizing interpretation, the cardiac slices are divided into 20 or, more optimally, 17 segments.[19] The name of each myocardial segment defines its location relative to the LV long axis as basal, midventricular, and apical, and 360 degree circumferential locations (Fig. 9.1).[20]

Different patterns of SPECT MPI and high-risk nonperfusion findings are summarized in Table 9.1.

## SEMIQUANTITATIVE VISUAL ANALYSIS

In semiquantitative visual analysis, a score is applied to each segment of the LV 17-segments model. Each score characterizes the amount of perfusion or functional abnormality. A summed score can then be derived by adding the scores of all segments of poststress perfusion as summed stress score (SSS), resting state perfusion as summed resting score (SRS), wall motion as summed motion score (SMS), or wall thickening as summed thickening score (STS). The sum of the difference between stress and resting scores of each segment is defined as summed difference score (SDS), representing the amount of myocardial ischemia.[19] The amount of perfusion abnormality in terms of extent and severity is incorporated into the perfusion semiquantitative variables, providing more prognostic information.[29]

## NORMAL VARIATIONS, ARTIFACTS, AND PITFALLS

Normal variations and artifacts in MPI can be falsely interpreted as perfusion abnormality, leading to deterioration of the SPECT specificity. The most common normal variations and artifacts are listed in Table 9.2. The interpreting physician should be aware of the potential sources of artifacts and the means to avoid them in order to improve the specificity of the SPECT MPI studies.[32, 33] Quality control procedures, repeating acquisitions, applying attenuation correction techniques, and incorporating ECG gating with SPECT can improve diagnostic accuracy by minimizing some of the artifacts (Fig. 9.2).[34, 35]

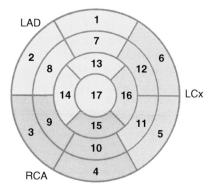

1. Basal anterior
2. Basal anteroseptal
3. Basal inferoseptal
4. Basal inferior
5. Basal inferolateral
6. Basal anterolateral

7. Mid anterior
8. Mid anteroseptal
9. Mid inferoseptal
10. Mid inferior
11. Mid inferolateral
12. Mid anterolateral

13. Apical anterior
14. Apical septal
15. Apical inferior
16. Apical lateral
17. Apex

FIG. 9.1 Standardized left ventricular (LV) segmentation and nomenclature on bull's eye plot. *LAD*, left anterior descending coronary artery; *LCx*, left circumflex coronary artery; *RCA*, right coronary artery. (Reproduced with permission from Cerqueira MD, Weissman NJ, Dilsizian V, et al. Standardized myocardial segmentation and nomenclature for tomographic imaging of the heart. A statement for healthcare professionals from the Cardiac Imaging Committee of the Council on Clinical Cardiology of the American Heart Association. *J Nucl Cardiol.* 2002;9(2):240–245.)

**TABLE 9.1**
**Interpretation Patterns in Myocardial Perfusion Imaging**

| Pattern | Finding | Interpretation |
| --- | --- | --- |
| **PERFUSION FINDINGS** | | |
| Normal | Rather homogeneous radiotracer uptake throughout the LV myocardium with higher activity in areas closer to the camera and lower activity in the attenuated areas with quantitative uptake which is above lower limits of normal distribution | Normal (On condition that balanced ischemia does not exist as SPECT MPI shows relative and not absolute flow)[21, 22] |
| Defect | A localized area of decreased relative radiotracer uptake with quantitative uptake, which is below lower limits of normal distribution | |
| Reversible defect | A defect presented on stress images that is normalized partially or completely on the rest or redistribution images | Ischemia |
| Fixed defect | A defect presented on both stress and rest (or redistribution) images with no significant change | Infarction |
| Paradoxical or reverse defect | A defect on the rest (or redistribution) images which does not exist or exists with less severe degree on stress images | Controversial (artifact, prior revascularization, prior MI, cardiomyopathy, etc.)[23] |

*Continued*

TABLE 9.1

| Pattern | Finding | Interpretation |
|---|---|---|
| **NONPERFUSION FINDINGS** | | |
| Lung uptake | Increased lung uptake associated with an elevated LV end-diastolic pressure and can be quantified as LHR | Stress-induced LV dysfunction or severely decreased resting LVEF[8, 24, 25] |
| Transient LV dilation | Increased LV size after stress as compared with the rest images (even in an otherwise normal MPI)[26] | Most likely indicates subendocardial ischemia and systolic LV dysfunction[27] |
| Transient RV visualization | More prominent visualization of RV on postexercise images compared with the rest images | Stress-induced LV dysfunction associated with severe CAD[28] |

CAD, coronary artery disease; LHR, lung-to-heart uptake ratio; LV, left ventricular; LVEF, left ventricular ejection fraction; MI, myocardial infarction; MPI, myocardial perfusion imaging; RV, right ventricular; SPECT, single-photon emission computed tomography.

TABLE 9.2
Common Normal Variations and Artifacts in Myocardial Perfusion Imaging With Single-Photon Emission Computed Tomography

| | Mechanisms | Findings |
|---|---|---|
| **NORMAL VARIATIONS** | | |
| Shortening of septum | Membranous septum | Decreased count density of the basal septum |
| Apical thinning | Partial volume effect | Decreased count density of the apex |
| Higher lateral-to-septal wall activity | Closer location of lateral wall to gamma camera | Relatively lower count density of the septum compared with the lateral wall |
| **ARTIFACTS** | | |
| Breast attenuation | Attenuation of photons by overlapping breast | Variable (depending on the breast size, position and density of breast) |
| Diaphragmatic attenuation | Attenuation of photons by left hemidiaphragm and right ventricle | Decreased count density of inferior wall |
| Patient's motion | Image misregistration in the process of SPECT reconstruction | Variable (depending on the extent, plane, and time of motion) |
| Subdiaphragmatic activity | Prominent activity in the liver, stomach, or intestine | Decreased or increased count density of the adjacent wall (usually inferior wall) |
| Technical artifacts | Flood field nonuniformity, incorrect center of rotation, inconsistent orientation and alignment of stress and rest studies | Variable |
| Quantification artifacts | LV localization failure, inappropriate determination of the LV boundaries, etc. | Inaccurate quantitative results[30] |
| **HEART-RELATED ISSUES** | | |
| Regional myocardial hypertrophy | Increased count density | Hot spot formation with relatively decreased count density in the other regions[31] |
| Left bundle branch block | Probably due to diastolic blood flow impairment secondary to delayed septal contraction | Decreased count density of septum (more prominent in higher heart rates) |
| Balanced ischemia | Relative measurement of uptake in MPI with SPECT | Absence of perfusion abnormality |

LV, left ventricular; MPI, myocardial perfusion imaging; SPECT, single-photon emission computed tomography.

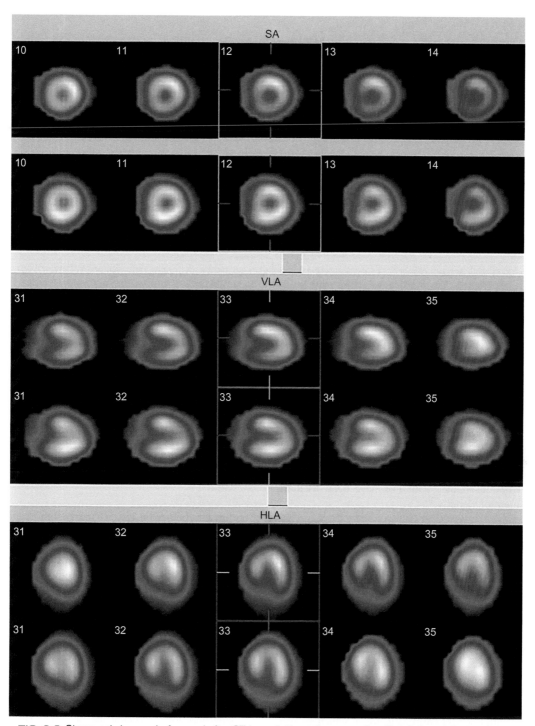

FIG. 9.2 Stress-only images before and after CT-based attenuation correction. Resolution of diaphragmatic attenuation artifact, with mild perfusion defect of the inferior and inferolateral walls in noncorrected images.

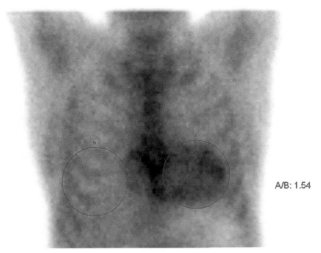

A/B: 1.54

FIG. 9.3 Anterior planar $^{99m}$Tc-pyrophosphate imaging in a patient with transthyretin-related (ATTR) amyloidosis. There is diffuse myocardial uptake with a heart (A) to contralateral chest (B) uptake ratio of greater than 1.5.

## ASSESSMENT OF VIABILITY

Nuclear cardiology plays an important role in identifying viable dysfunctional myocardium with the potential of improving regional or global function of LV after revascularization. As cellular viability depends on sufficient blood flow, membrane integrity, and preserved metabolic activity, resting tracer uptake ($^{201}$Tl, $^{99m}$Tc-sestamibi, or $^{99m}$Tc-tetrofosmin) with SPECT or evidence of metabolic activity ($^{18}$F-2-fluorodeoxyglucose [FDG] or $^{11}$C-acetate) with PET have been used for assessment of viability.[1]

## RADIONUCLIDE ANGIOGRAPHY

Radionuclide angiography (RNA), also known as radionuclide ventriculography (RVG), is performed by either first-pass or equilibrium methods for assessment of right ventricular and LV function and volume. The latter can be performed in the SPECT method and provides a highly producible and accurate method for the determination of LVEF.[36]

## POSITRON EMISSION TOMOGRAPHY

Positron emission tomography (PET) radiotracers are labeled with positron-emitting isotopes, which are usually elements that can be incorporated into compounds that are comparable to naturally occurring substances in the human body. Absolute quantification of myocardial blood flow is one of the advantages of PET, which can provide diagnostic and prognostic information before SPECT findings. The ability to assess coronary artery disease, myocardial perfusion, and viability as well as ventricular function makes PET an imperative modality in the field of clinical cardiology.[37] PET/CT has been shown to be encouraging in the imaging of cardiac device and prosthetic heart infections.[38, 39]

## RADIONUCLIDE IMAGING OF CARDIAC AMYLOIDOSIS

Cardiac amyloidosis is characterized by the deposition of extracellular amyloid fibrils in myocardium, resulting in restrictive cardiomyopathy, heart failure, and arrhythmias. Radionuclide imaging modalities are noninvasive methods that may facilitate early diagnosis and distinguish various forms of cardiac amyloidosis. $^{99m}$Tc-pyrophosphate has been found to have both high sensitivity and specificity for differentiating between transthyretin-related (ATTR) and light chain (AL) amyloidosis (Fig. 9.3).[40, 41]

## REFERENCES

1. Klocke FJ, Baird MG, Lorell BH, et al. ACC/AHA/ASNC guidelines for the clinical use of cardiac radionuclide imaging—executive summary: a report of the American College of Cardiology/American Heart Association Task Force on Practice Guidelines (ACC/AHA/ASNC

Committee to Revise the 1995 Guidelines for the Clinical Use of Cardiac Radionuclide Imaging). *J Am Coll Cardiol.* 2003; 42(7):1318–1333.

2. Pagnanelli RA, Basso DA. Myocardial perfusion imaging with 201Tl. *J Nucl Med Technol.* 2010; 38(1):1–3.

3. Gnanasegaran G, Ahmed A, Croasdale J, Buscombe JR. Planar and SPECT radiopharmaceuticals in nuclear cardiology: current status and limitations. In: Movahed A, Gnanasegaran G, Buscombe J, Hall M, eds. *Integrating Cardiology for Nuclear Medicine Physicians.* Berlin Heidelberg: Springer-Verlag; 2009:221–229.

4. Verberne HJ, Acampa W, Anagnostopoulos C, et al. EANM procedural guidelines for radionuclide myocardial perfusion imaging with SPECT and SPECT/CT: 2015 revision. *Eur J Nucl Med Mol Imaging.* 2015; 42(12):1929–1940.

5. Henzlova MJ, Duvall WL, Einstein AJ, Travin MI, Verberne HJ. ASNC imaging guidelines for SPECT nuclear cardiology procedures: stress, protocols, and tracers. *J Nucl Cardiol.* 2016; 23(3):606–639.

6. Wackers F. Exercise myocardial perfusion imaging. *J Nucl Med.* 1994; 35(4):726–729.

7. Kailasnath P, Sinusas AJ. Comparison of Tl-201 with Tc-99m-labeled myocardial perfusion agents: technical, physiologic, and clinical issues. *J Nucl Cardiol.* 2001; 8(4):482–498.

8. Russell RR, Wackers FJT. Coronary artery disease detection: exercise stress SPECT. In: Zaret BL, Beller GA, eds. *Clinical Nuclear Cardiology: State of the Art and Future Directions.* Mosby Elsevier; 2010:225–243.

9. Levine MG, Ahlberg AW, Mann A, et al. Comparison of exercise, dipyridamole, adenosine, and dobutamine stress with the use of Tc-99m tetrofosmin tomographic imaging. *J Nucl Cardiol.* 1999; 6(4):389–396.

10. Iskandrian AE. Detecting coronary artery disease in left bundle branch block. *J Am Coll Cardiol.* 2006; 48(10):1935–1937.

11. Udelson JE, Heller GV, Frans JT, et al. Randomized, controlled dose-ranging study of the selective adenosine A2A receptor agonist binodenoson for pharmacological stress as an adjunct to myocardial perfusion imaging. *Circulation.* 2004; 109(4):457–464.

12. Udelson JE, Dilsizian V, Bonow RO. Nuclear cardiology. In: Zipes DP, Libby P, Bonow RO, Mann DL, Braunwald E, Tomaselli GF, eds. *Braunwald's Heart Disease: A Textbook of Cardiovascular Medicine.* 11 ed. Elsevier Health Sciences; 2019:261–300.

13. Germano G, Van Kriekinge SD, Berman DS, Beller GA. Regional and global ventricular function and volumes from SPECT perfusion imaging A2. In: Zaret BL, ed. *Clinical Nuclear Cardiology.* 4th ed. Philadelphia: Mosby; 2010:194–222.

14. Rastgou F, Shojaeifard M, Amin A, et al. Assessment of left ventricular mechanical dyssynchrony by phase analysis of gated-SPECT myocardial perfusion imaging and tissue Doppler imaging: comparison between QGS and ECTb software packages. *J Nucl Cardiol.* 2014; 21(6):1062–1071.

15. Malek H, Rayegan F, Firoozabadi H, et al. Determination of normal ranges of regional and global phase parameters using gated myocardial perfusion imaging with Cedars-Sinai's QGS software. *Iran J Nucl Med.* 2018; 26(1):16–21.

16. Brindis RG, Douglas PS, Hendel RC, et al. ACCF/ASNC appropriateness criteria for single-photon emission computed tomography myocardial perfusion imaging (SPECT MPI): a report of the American College of Cardiology Foundation Quality Strategic Directions Committee Appropriateness Criteria Working Group and the American Society of Nuclear Cardiology endorsed by the American Heart Association. *J Am Coll Cardiol.* 2005; 46(8):1587–1605.

17. Hansen CL, Goldstein RA, Akinboboye OO, et al. Myocardial perfusion and function: single photon emission computed tomography. *J Nucl Cardiol.* 2007; 14(6):e39–e60.

18. Malek H, Ghaedian T, Yaghoobi N, Rastgou F, Bitarafan-Rajabi A, Firoozabadi H. Focal breast uptake of 99mTc-sestamibi in a man with spindle cell lipoma. *J Nucl Cardiol.* 2012; 19(3):618–620.

19. Berman DS, Abidov A, Kang X, et al. Prognostic validation of a 17-segment score derived from a 20-segment score for myocardial perfusion SPECT interpretation. *J Nucl Cardiol.* 2004; 11(4):414–423.

20. Heller GV, Cerqueira MD, Weissman NJ, et al. Standardized myocardial segmentation and nomenclature for tomographic imaging of the heart. A statement for healthcare professionals from the Cardiac Imaging Committee of the Council on Clinical Cardiology of the American Heart Association. *J Nucl Cardiol.* 2002; 9(2):240–245.

21. Lima RS, Watson DD, Goode AR, et al. Incremental value of combined perfusion and function over perfusion alone by gated SPECT myocardial perfusion imaging for detection of severe three-vessel coronary artery disease. *J Am Coll Cardiol.* 2003; 42(1):64–70.

22. Parkash R, deKemp RA, Ruddy TD, et al. Potential utility of rubidium 82 PET quantification in patients with 3-vessel coronary artery disease. *J Nucl Cardiol.* 2004; 11(4):440–449.

23. Pizzi MN, Sabaté-Fernández M, Aguadé-Bruix S, et al. Paradoxical scintigraphic pattern in regions with myocardial necrosis on myocardial perfusion gated SPECT with 99mTc-tetrofosmin. *J Nucl Cardiol.* 2012; 19(3):515–523.

24. Aksut SV, Mallavarapu C, Russell J, Heo J, Iskandrian AS. Implications of increased lung thallium uptake during exercise single photon emission computed tomography imaging. *Am Heart J.* 1995; 130(2):367–373.

25. Iskandrian AS, Heo J, Nguyen T, Lyons E, Paugh E. Left ventricular dilatation and pulmonary thallium uptake after single-photon emission computer tomography using thallium-201 during adenosine-induced coronary hyperemia. *Am J Cardiol.* 1990; 66(10):807–811.

26. Abidov A, Bax JJ, Hayes SW, et al. Transient ischemic dilation ratio of the left ventricle is a significant predictor

of future cardiac events in patients with otherwise normal myocardial perfusion SPECT. *J Am Coll Cardiol.* 2003; 42(10):1818–1825.

27. McLaughlin MG, Danias PG. Transient ischemic dilation: a powerful diagnostic and prognostic finding of stress myocardial perfusion imaging. *J Nucl Cardiol.* 2002; 9(6): 663–667.

28. Williams KA, Schneider CM. Increased stress right ventricular activity on dual isotope perfusion SPECT: a sign of multivessel and/or left main coronary artery disease. *J Am Coll Cardiol.* 1999; 34(2):420–427.

29. Hachamovitch R, Berman DS, Shaw LJ, et al. Incremental prognostic value of myocardial perfusion single photon emission computed tomography for the prediction of cardiac death differential stratification for risk of cardiac death and myocardial infarction. *Circulation.* 1998; 97(6):535–543.

30. Malek H, Yaghoobi N, Hedayati R. Artifacts in Quantitative analysis of myocardial perfusion SPECT, using Cedars-Sinai QPS Software. *J Nucl Cardiol.* 2017; 24(2):534–542.

31. Hambye A-S, Vervaet A, Dobbeleir A. Variability of left ventricular ejection fraction and volumes with quantitative gated SPECT: influence of algorithm, pixel size and reconstruction parameters in small and normal-sized hearts. *Eur J Nucl Med Mol Imaging.* 2004; 31(12): 1606–1613.

32. Depuey EG. Coronary artery disease detection: exercise stress SPECT. In: Zaret BL, Beller GA, eds. *Clinical Nuclear Cardiology: State of the Art and Future Directions.* Mosby Elsevier; 2010:72–95.

33. Burrell S, MacDonald A. Artifacts and pitfalls in myocardial perfusion imaging. *J Nucl Med Technol.* 2006; 34(4): 193–211.

34. Hendel RC, Corbett JR, Cullom SJ, DePuey EG, Garcia EV, Bateman TM. The value and practice of attenuation correction for myocardial perfusion SPECT imaging: a joint position statement from the American Society of Nuclear Cardiology and the Society of Nuclear Medicine. *J Nucl Med.* 2002; 43(2):273–280.

35. Johansen A, Lomsky M, Gerke O, et al. When is reacquisition necessary due to high extra-cardiac uptake in myocardial perfusion scintigraphy? *EJNMMI Res.* 2013; 3(1):1.

36. Wright GA, Thackray S, Howey S, Cleland JG. Left ventricular ejection fraction and volumes from gated blood-pool SPECT: comparison with planar gated blood-pool imaging and assessment of repeatability in patients with heart failure. *J Nucl Med.* 2003; 44(4):494–498.

37. Dilsizian V, Bacharach SL, Beanlands RS, et al. ASNC imaging guidelines/SNMMI procedure standard for positron emission tomography (PET) nuclear cardiology procedures. *J Nucl Cardiol.* 2016; 1–40.

38. Bensimhon L, Lavergne T, Hugonnet F, et al. Whole body [18F] fluorodeoxyglucose positron emission tomography imaging for the diagnosis of pacemaker or implantable cardioverter defibrillator infection: a preliminary prospective study. *Clin Microbiol Infect.* 2011; 17(6): 836–844.

39. Tanis W, Scholtens A, Habets J, et al. Fusion of cardiac computed tomography angiography and 18F-fluorodesoxyglucose positron emission tomography for the detection of complicated prosthetic heart valve endocarditis. *Eur Heart J.* 2013; 34(suppl. 1):4545.

40. Brown A, Btokin C, Frye S, Muzaffar R, Osman M. 99mTc Pyrophosphate (PYP) imaging Transthyretin Cardiac Amyloidosis Imaging: a new an application for an old tracer. *J Nucl Med.* 2019; 60(suppl. 1):2068.

41. Minamimoto R, Hotta M. Radionuclide imaging for diagnosis of cardiac amyloidosis. *J Nucl Med.* 2017; 58 (suppl. 1):983.

# CHAPTER 10

# Catheterization and Angiography

ALI ZAHED MEHR
Cardiovascular Intervention Research Center, Rajaie Cardiovascular, Medical & Research Center, Iran University of Medical Sciences, Tehran, Iran

---

**KEY POINTS**

- Cardiologists need to be familiar with cath lab equipment, tools, and devices.
- It is important to learn how to prepare patients for catheterization and manage a step-by-step approach to routine procedures in the cath lab.
- Interpreting catheterization findings is of paramount value.
- Catheterization is an almost safe procedure, but the operator should be ready to confront and manage possible catheterization complications.

---

## INTRODUCTION

The information derived from catheterization laboratory (cath lab) diagnostic procedures is very valuable in the evaluation of cardiac structural and functional diseases. In addition, coronary angiography is the gold standard for precise diagnosis of coronary artery disease.

*Interventional cardiology* refers to many therapeutic procedures being done in a cath lab. This subspecialty has made cardiac surgery unnecessary in a wide spectrum of cardiac diseases.

## RADIATION SAFETY

Consider the ALARA principle,[1] "as low as reasonably achievable":

1. Reduce fluoroscopy time.
2. Reduce the frame rate per second.
3. Avoid unnecessary cineangiographies.
4. Use beam collimation (limit the field).
5. Approximate the detector (camera) to the patient.
6. Avoid unnecessary magnifications.
7. Change projection views during long procedures to reduce the patient's skin exposure.
8. The personnel should keep the maximal distance from the x-ray source.
9. Use lead aprons, collars, eyeglasses, and movable shields.
10. Avoid deep left anterior oblique (LAO) or left lateral projections if possible.

## PRECATHETERIZATION PREPARATIONS[1]

1. Full explanation of the procedure to the patient.
2. Taking a complete history, including functional class; coronary risk factors; history of any allergy, gastrointestinal bleeding, cerebrovascular accident, or kidney disease; and previous procedures such as cardiac catheterization, percutaneous coronary intervention (PCI), or cardiac surgery.
3. Complete physical examinations with emphasis on vital signs, cardiopulmonary examinations, and distal pulses.
4. Electrocardiography.
5. Chest radiography.
6. Routine laboratory data: complete blood count, platelets, erythrocyte sedimentation rate, hemoglobin A1C, fasting blood glucose, lipid profile, blood urea nitrogen, creatine, Na, K, prothrombin time, partial thromboplastin time, international normalized ratio (INR), and urinalysis.
7. Intravenous (IV) line and hydration ($\approx 1$ L).
8. Sedation with benzodiazepines and antihistamines.
9. Hold warfarin for 2–3 days and switch to heparin (INR needs to be less than 1.8).
10. Discontinue metformin until 48 h after the procedure.
11. Use oral or IV corticosteroids possibly with antihistamines 12 h and immediately before the procedure for patients with a history of asthma or allergy to contrast agents.

## ACCESS

The usual access sites are femoral, radial, and brachial.

In the femoral region, the acronym NAVEL can describe the position of different structures: The **n**erve is the most lateral element; then there are **a**rtery, **v**ein, **e**mpty space, and **l**ymphatics.

After passing beneath the inguinal ligament, the external iliac artery becomes the common femoral artery, which is over the femoral head. Then it bifurcates to the superficial femoral artery (SFA) and deep femoral artery.

To puncture the common femoral artery, the femur head can be found using fluoroscopy. Another way is to palpate the anterior superior iliac spine and symphysis pubis. The line that connects these two anatomic landmarks suggests the location of the inguinal ligament. The common femoral artery is then punctured 2–3 cm caudal to this line[2] (Fig. 10.1).

Before puncturing the artery, the location must be anesthetized with 10 mL of 1% or 2% lidocaine. Try to do a front-wall puncture with a needle. The angle between the needle and the skin should be 30–45 degrees, and the needle must be beveled up.

The strong pulsatile blood jet shows that the needle is in a good position, and the 0.035-in. guidewire is introduced through the needle. This step is very important to avoid complications: If the wire encounters any difficulty, it should not be pushed forcefully; it might be in the vessel wall or outside the vessel! Fluoroscopy is useful, but usually the whole procedure must be repeated.

If the wire moves easily, fluoroscopy is needed to show the proper position of the wire on the left-hand side of the spine. Then the needle is removed, and the skin is slightly opened with a scalpel and the sheath and dilator, which are fixed together, go over the wire into the artery. Then the wire and dilator are removed; the sheath remains in the artery as the access. The side lumen is connected to the pressure transducer. There should not be any leak from the sheath valve or around the sheath shaft.

To have venous access, the femoral vein is punctured 1–2 cm medial and inferior to the arterial access site. A 10-mL syringe is used to make suction through the needle because the vein does not have a jet similar to the artery. After introducing the wire, fluoroscopy is used to see the wire on the right-hand side of the spine. Then the sheath and dilator are inserted over the wire similar to arterial access.

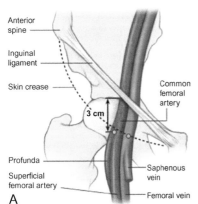
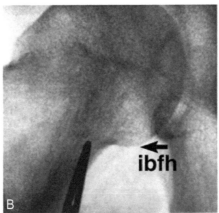
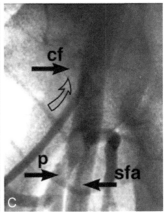

FIG. 10.1 Regional anatomy relevant to percutaneous femoral arterial and venous catheterization. (A) Schematic diagram showing the right femoral artery and vein coursing underneath the inguinal ligament, which runs from the anterior superior iliac spine to the pubic tubercle. The arterial skin nick should be placed approximately 3 cm below the ligament and directly over the femoral arterial pulsation; the venous skin nick should be placed at the same level but approximately 1 fingerbreadth more medially. Although this level corresponds roughly to the skin crease in most patients, anatomic localization relative to the inguinal ligament provides a more constant landmark. (B) Fluoroscopic localization of the skin nick (marked by the tip of the clamp) to the inferior border of the femoral head (ibfh). (C) A catheter (*open arrow*) inserted through this skin nick has entered the common femoral artery (cf) above its bifurcation into the superficial femoral artery (SFA) and profunda (p) branches. (From Davidson CJ, Bonow RO. Cardiac catheterization. In: Mann DL, Zipes DP, Libby P, et al., eds. *Braunwald's Heart Disease: A Textbook of Cardiovascular Medicine.* 10th ed. Philadelphia: Saunders; 2015; with permission.)

## Radial Access

The Allen test is used to make sure that the palmar arc is intact. Then the whole upper limb is prepped and draped. A gauze roll is placed under the wrist. The hand becomes hyperextended. Then the site is anesthetized 2–3 cm above the styloid process with 1 mL of 1%–2% lidocaine through an insulin syringe.

Then a small radial access needle is used to puncture the radial artery. The angle between the needle and the skin must be about 30 degrees. After a small blood jet is observed, the 0.018- or 0.025-in. guidewire is introduced through the needle. Then the needle is removed; the skin is opened slightly with a scalpel; and the hydrophilic sheath, which has been made wet, is inserted.

A cocktail containing 100–200 µg of nitroglycerine with or without calcium blocker and lidocaine is injected. Heparin can be injected intravenously or through the sheath (5000 units). It is better to inject the cocktail slowly and mixed with blood to avoid arterial spasm.[3]

## SHEATHS AND CATHETERS

Sheaths can have different lengths and diameters. The size of a sheath is specified by the largest catheter that can move easily through it. The size of a catheter is its outer diameter in French units. Every French unit is about 0.33 mm.

The catheter lengths most commonly used in the left cardiac cath and angiography are 100 cm. The longer catheters (125 cm) can be used for tortuous aortas.

The 6-Fr sheaths and catheters are standard for cardiac cath and diagnostic angiography. Smaller catheters and sheaths can lower the risk of vascular complications. Larger catheters such as 7 and 8 Fr are used in some complex interventional procedures (e.g., bifurcation stenting, rotablation).

### Coronary Angiography Catheters

These catheters can be 4–8 French catheter scale (Fr) in size. The 5- or 6-Fr Judkins catheters are the most popular.[4]

The left Judkins catheter can be 3.5, 4, 4.5, 5, or 6. These numbers show the distance between the primary and secondary curves in centimeters. The right Judkins catheter can be 3.5, 4, 5, or 6 (Fig. 10.2). Larger catheters are used for dilated aortas.

Other popular coronary catheters are the left and right Amplatz catheters (Fig. 10.3). The size of these catheters can be I, II, or III. The left Amplatz II is usually appropriate for left coronary injection, and the right

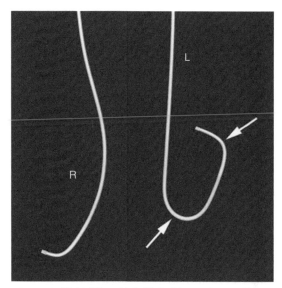

FIG. 10.2 Right (R) and left (L) Judkins catheters. The primary (*upper arrow*) and secondary (*lower arrow*) curves of the Judkins left catheter are shown. (From Popma JJ, Kinlay S, Bhatt DL. Coronary arteriography and intracoronary imaging. In: Mann DL, Zipes DP, Libby P, et al., eds. *Braunwald's Heart Disease: A Textbook of Cardiovascular Medicine*. 10th ed. Philadelphia: Saunders; 2015; with permission.)

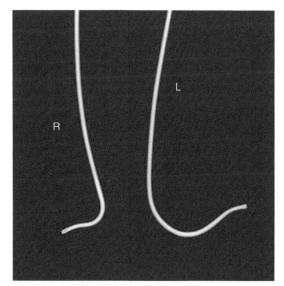

FIG. 10.3 Amplatz right (R) and left (L) catheters. (From Popma JJ, Kinlay S, Bhatt DL. Coronary arteriography and intracoronary imaging. In: Mann DL, Zipes DP, Libby P, et al., eds. *Braunwald's Heart Disease: A Textbook of Cardiovascular Medicine*. 10th ed. Philadelphia: Saunders; 2015; with permission.)

Amplatz I is a good option for the right coronary artery (RCA).

Multipurpose catheters were frequently used for diagnostic angiography in the past.

There are different kinds of catheters for coronary angiography via radial access. A single catheter can be used for engagement of both left and right coronaries.

## GUIDEWIRES

The guidewires used for diagnostic catheterization and coronary angiography are usually 0.035 in in diameter and 150 cm in length. The shorter wires (30 cm) are used just for introducing short access sheaths.

Some of the diagnostic wires are hydrophilic; these are suitable for tortuous or atherosclerotic aortas.

Smaller guidewires are available that are used for interventional purposes. For example, the 0.014 in guidewires are routinely used for coronary interventions.

## LEFT HEART CATHETERIZATION

The standard catheter for this procedure is the pigtail catheter. It is traumatic with multiple side holes, which makes it the safest catheter for movement through the aorta and aortic valve (AV) and for injection into cardiac chambers. It is also very reliable for measuring cardiac and vascular pressures.

It is usually needed to manipulate the catheter to cross the AV. By pushing the wire back and forth through the pigtail catheter, we can try different ways to cross the AV:

1. The pigtail head is toward the patient's left-hand side. The wire is pushed through the AV.
2. The pigtail is pushed farther and crosses the AV without the upfront wire.
3. The pigtail bends in the root over the wire; then the wire is retracted a little to lessen the catheter's support. The catheter may drop into the left ventricle (LV).

When the pigtail is in the LV, it is connected to a pressure transducer to see the LV pressure curves and find out the left ventricular end-diastolic pressure (LVEDP). Then contrast agent is injected into the LV by an injector in the right anterior oblique (RAO) projection providing that the LVEDP is less than 30 mmHg.

The injection volume is about 30–40 mL.

Left ventriculography data:

- LV size and ejection fraction
- Regional wall motion abnormalities and aneurysms
- Filling defects (clots)
- Mitral regurgitation (MR) severity:

- 1+ trivial or mild: scant opacification of the left atrium (LA)
- 2+ mild to moderate: LA opacification less than LV
- 3+ moderate to severe: LA opacification similar to LV
- 4+ severe: LA opacification more than LV[1]

After injection, the postangiographic LVEDP, which shows the amount of rising after stress, is evaluated. Then the pigtail catheter is pulled back through the AV to investigate any difference in peak systolic pressures of the LV and aorta (transvalvular aortic gradient), which shows the severity of aortic stenosis.

Aortic root injection can show the size of the ascending aorta, the number of AV cusps, any possible saphenous vein grafts (SVGs), and the severity of aortic insufficiency (AI). Estimation of AI severity is done similar to that for MR (see earlier).

## RIGHT HEART CATHETERIZATION

This section describes the simple right cardiac catheterization, which is used to measure pulmonary artery (PA) pressure. For detailed right heart catheterization, see Chapter 11.

The access is often femoral. The multipurpose catheter is widely used. The catheter is pushed with or without a wire through venous access toward the right atrium (RA). Then it may enter the right ventricle (RV) without any maneuver, but usually, it needs a little rotation to form a loop in the RA. The guidewire can be used to enter the RV before the catheter. In some situations, making a loop in the RA is difficult. If so, the catheter can be pushed toward a hepatic vein, and then with more force, the bent catheter can enter the RA.

When the catheter is in the RV, clockwise rotation and a pullback maneuver place the tip of the catheter in the RV outflow tract. This maneuver is easier with the wire inside the catheter. Then the catheter is pushed into the PA, the wire is removed, and the catheter is connected to the pressure transducer.

In some difficult cases, the "reverse catheter loop" technique can be used. In this method, the loop in the RA is laterally and then inferiorly directed. Then by pushing the wire, it enters the RV and goes straight toward the PA.

If all of these techniques fail, a pigtail or a floating catheter can be used.

## CORONARY ANGIOGRAPHY INDICATIONS

Indications for coronary angiography in patients with stable angina include[4,5] history of aborted sudden cardiac death, symptoms of heart failure, moderate- to high-risk noninvasive tests, and low ejection fraction with evidence of ischemia in a noninvasive test. Another indication is when noninvasive tests cannot be done or are equivocal.

Almost all patients with unstable angina need angiography, which can be done as an early invasive or a delayed approach. The exceptions are (1) severe comorbidity when revascularization risks are more than its benefits and (2) relieved chest pain with a low probability of acute coronary syndrome (ACS). In severe persistent chest pain and a low probability of ACS, a good option is coronary computed tomography angiography (CTA).

All patients with ST-segment elevation myocardial infarction (STEMI) also need coronary angiography as an intention to do primary PCI or as a delayed approach. The exceptions are those who are not revascularization candidates or refuse to have it done.

For valvular or congenital cardiac surgeries, coronary angiography is indicated if the information derived from noninvasive tests or imaging is not enough or the patient is older than 35 years of age.

Indications for angiography before a noncardiac surgery are a high-risk noninvasive test, refractory angina, and an equivocal test before a high-risk surgery.

In heart transplant donors, the indications are determined from the person's age and risk factors. In heart transplant recipients, coronary angiography is done every year.

## CORONARY CATHETER MANIPULATION

### Left Judkins Catheter

When the catheter and guidewire enter the ascending aorta, the wire is removed, and with a little push-and-pull movement, the catheter tip will align with the left main (LM) artery. Sometimes it needs some rotations. In such a situation, the most successful method is a forward movement with counterclockwise rotation and then pullback with a little clockwise rotation.[6]

If these maneuvers fail and the catheter bends over, a bigger catheter can be used. If the catheter tip position is inferior to the LM artery, a smaller catheter may help. In very difficult cases, other kinds of left coronary catheters such as the left Amplatz catheter can be used.

In radial approach, deep breath helps to navigate the wire from the right subclavian artery to the ascending aorta, then it is better to push the wire and the catheter with clockwise rotation until entering into the left aortic cusp; then the wire is removed slowly and with slow pullback and a little counterclockwise rotation, the tip of the catheter would engage in the LM ostium.

### Right Judkins Catheter

When the catheter tip reaches the aortic cusps, the wire is removed, and clockwise rotation accompanied with slow pullback will engage the catheter tip in the RCA.

This catheter is also used for SVGs in postcoronary artery bypass graft patients. For this purpose, first, the aortic root is injected with a pigtail catheter in LAO projection to determine the origin of the SVGs. Then with a somewhat similar technique for RCA engagement, we try to select every SVG.

The right Judkins catheter is also used for left internal mammary artery (LIMA) injection. In LAO projection with some counterclockwise rotation at the distal aortic arc, we can enter the left subclavian artery. The wire and then the catheter is pushed distal to the origin of the LIMA. Then the wire is removed, and in anteroposterior (AP) projection, a little counterclockwise rotation with pulling back will engage the tip of the catheter in the ostium of the LIMA. The engagement is not a necessity; usually, injection near the origin can opacify the artery acceptably. Inflating a left-arm pressure cuff makes the image even better.

## CORONARY ANATOMY

The LM coronary artery originates from the left aortic cusp. Its length is usually shorter than 20 mm. Then it bifurcates into the left anterior descending coronary artery (LAD) and left circumflex artery (LCx).

The LAD travels down the anterior interventricular groove toward the apex. In some situations, it does not reach the apex; in others, it finishes at the apex. A wraparound LAD continues toward posterior interventricular groove and gives some posterior septal branches.

The LAD main branches are diagonal and septal arteries. The first branches are called S1 and D1; then there may be S2, D2, and so on.

The LAD length is arbitrarily divided into three segments: (1) proximal LAD (before S1), (2) midpart LAD, and (3) distal LAD (the distal one third). The LCx travels in the left atrioventricular groove. Obtuse marginals (OMs) are its main branches; they provide flow to the inferolateral parts of LV.

The LCx has also one or two LA branches. The LCx artery is often nondominant and becomes very narrow after OM branches. In about 15% of people, it is dominant and reaches the crux (the spot where atrioventricular and interventricular grooves meet at the back of the heart). Before reaching the crux, it has some posterior LV (PLV) branches. After the crux, it continues as the left posterior descending artery (PDA). In some people, the LCx is codominant. This means that all PLVs have left origin, and only the PDA is from the right side or there are two PDAs (one from the left and another from right).

In about 25% of cases, there is another vessel originating from the LM located between the LAD and LCx. This artery is called the *ramus intermedius*. It can have the role of a high diagonal or a high OM branch.

The RCA originates from the right coronary cusp. The first branch is the conus artery. This artery may have a separate ostium in some cases. The second branch is the sinus node artery (SNA); however, the SNA sometimes originates from the LA branches of the LCx. The next RCA branches are the right ventricular arteries (RV branches). In about 80% of cases, the RCA reaches the crux and then bifurcates into the PDA and PLV.

Similar to the LAD, the RCA is divided into three segments: proximal, midpart, and distal.

Apart from the LAD and RCA, lesions in all other coronary vessels are described as proximal or distal (i.e., LCx, diagonals, OMs, PDA, PLV, and ramus).[4]

## ANGIOGRAPHIC PROJECTIONS

Coronary injections must be done in different views to be able to see coronary arteries separately. This strategy is also useful to detect eccentric stenosis. Such lesions may be hidden in some views and prominent in others.

For describing the position of the C-arm around a patient, the location of the detector is used: LAO means the detector is on the left-hand side of the patient; RAO means the detector is on the right-hand side of the patient; and *cranial* and *caudal* are terms to show the inclination of the detector toward the head or leg of the patient, respectively.

There are four routine projections for the left coronary artery and two for the RCA. Other views may be used for better evaluation in some patients.

Suitable coronary views for evaluation of different coronary segments can be summarized as follows: Left coronary views:

- RAO caudal: LM, proximal LAD, distal LAD, and OMs
- AP cranial: midpart LAD, diagonals, and septals
- LAO cranial: ostium of LM and diagonals, midpart LAD, and distal of dominant LCx
- LAO caudal (spider view): LM, proximal LAD, proximal LCx
- AP caudal: LM, ostioproximal LAD, proximal LCx
- RAO cranial: the whole length of the LAD
- Left lateral: midpart LAD, distal LADRCA views

- LAO: proximal RCA, midpart RCA, and distal RCA
- AP cranial: PDA, PLV, and distal RCA
- LAO cranial: ostioproximal RCA and distal RCA
- Left lateral: midpart RCASVG views
- LAO: the whole length of the SVG
- AP cranial: RCA or diagonal after anastomosis
- RAO caudal: ramus or LCx after anastomosis LIMA views
- AP cranial: the whole length of the LIMA and midpart LAD
- Left lateral: anastomosis site, midpart LAD, and distal LAD

## CORONARY FINDINGS AND INTERPRETATION

### Calcification

Before dye injections, possible coronary and valvular calcifications can be seen by fluoroscopy. AV calcification is seen in aortic stenosis. Mitral annular calcification is seen like a crescent. Mitral leaflet calcification is a specific finding for mitral stenosis. Coronary calcifications show the burden of plaques and the difficulty of intervention.

### Thrombus

Thrombotic lesions are usually hazy. Typically, a filling defect can be detected in the lumen. We expect to see such lesions in ACSs.

### Stenosis

To determine the percentage of a stenotic lesion, we consider the normal vessel diameter distal to the plaque as a reference. Lesions less than 50% stenosis is regarded as mild or nonsignificant. Lesions with 50%–70% diameter reduction are considered moderate. Lesions with more than 70% reduction in lumen diameter are severe and can induce ischemia on exertion. Some lesions with critical stenosis (>90%) may be symptomatic at rest.

### Lesion Complexity for Intervention

Type A lesions are the simplest ones for PCI, and type C lesions are the most difficult ones (Table 10.1).

### Ectasia

Irregular luminal dilation and aneurysmal formation may predispose patients to clot formation in the lumen. The result may be acute luminal stenosis or distal embolization.

Coronary flow speed is reduced in some patients with or without ectasia. This slow-flow pattern (Thrombolysis In Myocardial Infarction [TIMI] 2 instead of

| Characteristic | Description |
|---|---|
| **TABLE 10.1** **Characteristics of Type A, B, and C Coronary Lesions** | |
| **TYPE A LESIONS (HIGH SUCCESS, >85%; LOW RISK)** | |
| Discrete (<10 mm) | Little or no calcium |
| Concentric | Less than totally occlusive |
| Readily accessible | Not ostial in locations |
| Nonangulated segment, <45 degrees | No major side branch involvement |
| Smooth contour | Absence of thrombus |
| **TYPE B LESIONS (MODERATE SUCCESS, 60%–85%; MODERATE RISK)** | |
| Tubular (10–20 mm in length) | Moderate to heavy calcification |
| Eccentric | Total occlusions <3 months old |
| Moderate tortuosity of proximal segment | Ostial in location |
| Moderately angulated segment, ≥45 degrees, <90 degrees | Bifurcation lesion requiring double guidewire |
| Irregular contour | Some thrombus present |
| **TYPE C LESIONS (LOW SUCCESS, <60%; HIGH RISK)** | |
| Diffuse (>2 cm in length) | Total occlusion >3 months old |
| Excessive tortuosity of proximal segment | Inability to protect major side branches |
| Extremely angulated segments, ≥90 degrees | Degenerated vein grafts with friable lesions |

From Popma JJ, Kinlay S, Bhatt DL. Coronary arteriography and intracoronary imaging. In: Mann DL, Zipes DP, Libby P, et al., eds. *Braunwald's Heart Disease: A Textbook of Cardiovascular Medicine.* 10th ed. Philadelphia: Saunders; 2015; with permission.

normal TIMI 3)[4] can be restricted to just one coronary artery, but it is usually diffuse. Patients with slow-flow coronaries often have typical refractory angina even without stenosis. Microvascular disease and endothelial dysfunction have some role in such situations.

### Coronary Spasm

Transient arterial wall constrictions can occur spontaneously or be precipitated by catheter engagement. Intracoronary nitroglycerine dissipates them.

## CORONARY ANOMALIES AND VARIATIONS

### Absent Left Main Artery

In patients with separate ostia of LAD and LCx from the aorta, two catheters with different sizes may be needed to be able to cannulate them.

### Anomalous Origin of the Left Circumflex Artery From the Right Coronary Artery

In such patients, the LCx origin can be from the proximal RCA or from the right coronary cusp near the RCA ostium. The course of the LCx is usually retroaortic.

### Anomalous Origin of the Left Main or Left Anterior Descending Coronary Artery From the Right Coronary Artery

The LAD or LM can travel in four different courses: (1) anterior to the aorta, (2) retroaortic, (3) septal course, or (4) interarterial or malignant type in which it locates between the aorta and pulmonary trunk. This situation may be associated with ischemia, arrhythmias, and sudden death. The best way to determine the course of the LM or LAD is CTA. Malignant types may need surgery. Other courses rarely cause ischemia; slit-like coronary ostia and ostial bending are two conditions that can induce ischemia and deserve appropriate treatment.

### Anomalous Origin of the Right Coronary Artery From the Left Cusp

The RCA course can be malignant or benign.

### Coronary Fistula

These fistulas can drain to the coronary veins, pulmonary artery, or cardiac chambers (arteriocameral fistulas). Large fistulas can produce significant left-to-right shunts with prominent $O_2$ step-up. One therapeutic option is interventional closure of fistulas.

### Muscle Bridge

Major coronary arteries are epicardial, but according to the findings from CTA and autopsies, in about one third of people, some segments pass beneath the myocardium. These coronary segments are compressed during systole. Because coronary arteries flow essentially in diastole, these compressions are not often harmful. Some patients complain of chest pain or dyspnea. Treatment approaches are administering beta-blockers or calcium blockers, avoiding nitrates, and surgery in a minority of patients.

## CATHETERIZATION COMPLICATIONS

Cardiac catheterization and coronary angiography are low-risk procedures. The major complications occur in fewer than 1% of patients and include myocardial infarction, heart failure, tamponade, arrhythmias, stroke, renal failure, major bleeding, vascular damages, anaphylactic reactions, and death. More frequent events are vasovagal reactions and contrast allergies such as nausea and vomiting, rashes, bronchospasm, edema, and hives.

Contrast-induced nephropathy is a major concern in procedures done with contrast agents. Newer low osmolar or isosmolar agents have reduced the incidence of this event. Prehydration and avoiding large amounts of contrast during the procedure are very important in prevention.

Vascular access complications, including bleedings, occlusions, and infections, are the most common catheterization complications. Among these, bleeding is the more frequent:

Local hematomas are very common. They produce pain and discomfort. Large ones may need packed cell (PC) transfusions.

### Pseudoaneurysm

Sometimes the connection between the hematoma site and vessel lumen hinders thrombosis of the blood in the hematoma region. A to-and-fro flow can be seen in duplex sonography. Femoral puncture below the femoral head is a predisposing factor for this condition and for AV fistula caused by difficult hemostasis. Treatment includes manual compression of the pseudoaneurysm neck and then complete bed rest for some hours. Discontinuation of anticoagulants and antiplatelets (if possible) is very important. Another option is thrombin injection into the pseudoaneurysm sac under ultrasound guidance. The last option is vascular surgery. Some lesions close spontaneously in follow-up (usually those that are <2 cm).

### Arteriovenous Fistula

Iatrogenic connection between femoral vein and artery is more resistant to manual compression than pseudoaneurysm. If manual compression fails, vascular surgery is suggested after some months of follow-up. Deploying a covered stent is another option.

### Retroperitoneal Hematoma

When manual compression of the femoral access site is not effective, bleeding into the retroperitoneal space accumulates as a large hematoma. This massive bleeding may be fatal. Puncturing the artery proximal to the inguinal ligament is a risk factor. Initially, the patient has only mild abdominal or back pain. Any hypotension or significant rate change should be considered suspicious. Abdominal CT (or ultrasonography) can be diagnostic. Distorted bladder shadow in fluoroscopy is other evidence supporting the diagnosis. Serial hemoglobin check and fluid resuscitation with PC transfusion plus anticoagulation reversal are the cornerstones of a conservative approach. A more successful strategy is doing digital subtraction angiography from contralateral femoral access. Finding the site of bleeding can be helpful for both the vascular surgeon (to explore and close it) and the interventionist (to deploy a coil or a covered stent).

## REFERENCES

1. Davidson CJ, Bonow RO. Cardiac catheterization. In: Mann DL, Zipes DP, Libby P, Bonow RO, Braunwald E, eds. *Braunwald's Heart Disease: A Textbook of Cardiovascular Medicine.* 10th ed. Philadelphia: WB Saunders; 2015:364–391. International Textbook of Medicine; vol. 1.
2. B aim DS, Grossman W. Percutaneous approach, including transseptal and apical puncture. In: Baim DS, Grossman W, eds. *Cardiac Catheterization, Angiography, and Intervention.* 7th ed. Philadelphia: Lea & Febiger; 2006.
3. Archbold RA, Robinson NM, Schilling R. Radial artery access for coronary angiography and percutaneous coronary intervention. *BMJ.* 2004; 329:443.
4. Popma JJ, Kinlay S, Bhatt DL. Coronary arteriography and intracoronary imaging. In: Mann DL, Zipes DP, Libby P, Bonow RO, Braunwald E, eds. *Braunwald's Heart Disease: A Textbook of Cardiovascular Medicine.* 10th ed. Philadelphia: WB Saunders; 2015:392–428. International Textbook of Medicine; vol. 1.
5. Fihn SD, Gardin JM, Abrams J, et al. ACCF/AHA/ACP/AATS/PCNA/SCAI/STS guideline for the diagnosis and management of patients with stable ischemic heart disease: a report of the American College of Cardiology Foundation/American Heart Association Task Force on Practice Guidelines, and the American College of Physicians, American Association for Thoracic Surgery, Preventive Cardiovascular Nurses Association, Society for Cardiovascular Angiography and Interventions, and Society of Thoracic Surgeons. *J Am Coll Cardiol.* 2012; 60:e44.
6. Rassi AN. Left heart catheterization. In: Griffin BP, Callahan TD, Menon V, et al., eds. *Manual of Cardiovascular Medicine.* 4th ed. New York: Lippincott Williams & Wilkins; 2013.

# CHAPTER 11

# Hemodynamic Study

NASIM NADERI

Rajaie Cardiovascular, Medical & Research Center, Iran University of Medical Sciences, Tehran, Iran

## INTRODUCTION

When the diagnostic challenges in patients with structural heart disease cannot be answered through clinical evaluation and noninvasive testing, the problem should be solved by cardiac catheterization.

Hence, in the current era, a hemodynamically directed cardiac catheterization should be a goal-directed procedure, specifically individualized for each patient, based on the problem and the results of the noninvasive testing. To fully understand hemodynamics, one must learn how to make proper measurements, calculate derived values, and interpret the results in relation to specific disease conditions.

In hemodynamic studies, Ohm's law is used to calculate and interpret the measurement results. According to Ohm's law, pressure difference and resistance are the main determinants of flow. Flow or cardiac output (CO) is calculated by the following formula: $Q = \Delta P / R$, where $Q$ is the flow or CO, $\Delta P$ is the pressure difference across the vascular bed, and $R$ is the systemic or pulmonary vascular resistance (PVR).[1-5]

## PRESSURE MEASUREMENT

A fluid-filled catheter connected to the pressure transducer of a specific monitor is commonly used for measuring pressure in cardiac catheterization laboratories. The monitor can be set up to show both the pressure curve and the measured pressure through a vessel or chamber.

Before starting the pressure measurement, it is necessary to set the zero point on the monitor. All pressures should be measured at end expiration. In patients with spontaneous breathing, the top curve should be considered for measurement, and in patients on mechanical ventilation, the bottom curve should be considered for measurement.

It is better to consider the average of three beats, particularly in patients with irregular rhythms such as atrial fibrillation rhythm.[1-7]

## OXIMETRY MEASUREMENTS

Oximetry measurements are necessary for the calculation of CO by the Fick method and to assess the presence of shunts. The oxygen saturation of blood is measured, and the $O_2$ content of blood is calculated with the following formula:

$$O_2\,\text{content}\,(\text{mL}/100\,\text{mL}) = Hb \times 1.36 \times (O_2\text{sat}/100)$$

where Hb is the hemoglobin in grams per deciliter, 1.36 is the oxygen-carrying capacity of blood in milliliters of oxygen per gram of hemoglobin, and $O_2$sat is the oxygen saturation of the blood.

The dissolved oxygen in blood is generally negligible in these calculations and is usually ignored.[1-7]

## TEMPERATURE MEASUREMENTS

A thermistor is mounted at the tip of the Swan-Ganz catheter or pulmonary artery catheter (PAC) to measure the temperature of the blood as it passes through the pulmonary artery (see the discussion of Thermodilution Cardiac Output for more detail).

## CARDIAC PERFORMANCE

The cardiac performance is the volume ejected by each heartbeat [stroke volume (SV)].

The physiologic determinants of cardiac performance are contractility, preload (filling pressures), afterload (resistances), and heart rate (HR).

Cardiac output is calculated with the following formula:

$$CO = SV \times HR$$

Cardiac output is the blood flow out of the heart in liters per minute and is the measurement of how much blood is ejected by the left ventricle each minute, which is affected by several factors, including the patient's age, body size, and metabolic demands. Normal CO is about 5 L/min.

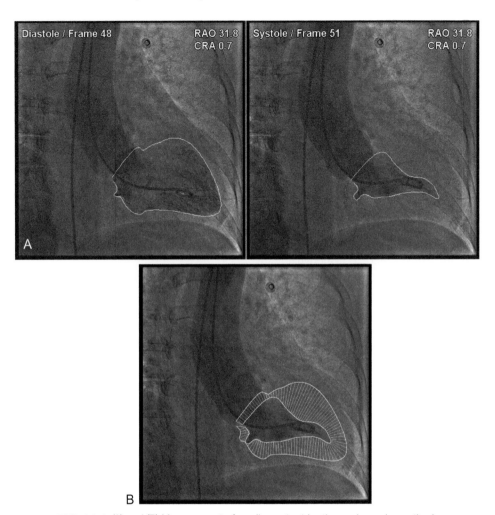

FIG. 11.1 (A) and (B) Measurement of cardiac output by the angiography method.

Cardiac output is commonly measured clinically by two thermodilution or Fick techniques. Left ventriculography is a method in which CO can be indirectly estimated (Fig. 11.1).

## Cardiac Index

The CO should be normalized among different body sizes.

Normal cardiac index (CI) = 2.5–4.0 L/min/m$^2$

$$CI(L/min/m^2) = CI(L/min)/body\ surface\ area\ (BSA)(m^2)$$

$$BSA = \sqrt{[Height\ (cm) \times weight\ (kg)/3600]}$$

## Thermodilution Cardiac Output

A Swan-Ganz catheter or PAC is used for the measurement of CO by this technique. The blood temperature is used as an indicator for measuring the CO with the thermodilution technique. The change in pulmonary artery blood temperature vs time is graphed and inversely proportionate to the blood flow. The CO is computed considering the graphed curves automatically by dedicated software in vigilance monitors and shown quickly. If the area under the curve is small, there is a high CO state and vice versa.[1–7]

## Limitations of the Thermodilution Technique

1. Severe tricuspid or pulmonary valve regurgitation
2. Very low CO (<2.5 L/min); in this situation, the CO may be overestimated

## Fick Cardiac Output

The Fick CO calculation is considered the "gold standard" for determining CO. The oxygen consumption ($VO_2$) and the blood oxygen content in arterial ($CaO_2$) and venous ($CvO_2$) blood are required to calculate the Fick CO.

The arteriovenous oxygen difference is calculated by subtracting the oxygen content of mixed venous blood, usually pulmonary arterial blood in most clinical settings, from pulmonary venous blood, which is estimated by systemic arterial blood.

The calculation of oxygen content was described earlier in this chapter.

$$\text{Arteriovenous } O_2 \text{ difference} = (\text{Aortic oxygen saturation} - \text{Pulmonary artery oxygen saturation})/100$$

$$\text{Fick CO(L/min)} = \frac{\text{Oxygen consumption(mL/min)}}{[(\text{Ao\%Sat} - \text{PA\%sat})/100]} \times 1.36 \times \text{Hgb (mg/dL)} \times 10$$

## Oxygen Consumption

$O_2$ consumption or resting $O_2$ uptake is proportional to the basal metabolic rate. It can be measured using a Douglas bag or estimated as 3 mL $O_2$/kg or 125 mL/min/m$^2$.

$$\text{Estimated } O_2 \text{ consumption (mL/min)} = 125 \times \text{BSA}$$

## Cardiac Output by Left Ventriculography

$$\text{Angiographic SV} = \text{End-diastolic volume} - \text{End-systolic volume}$$

End-diastolic volume and end-systolic volume are calculated using quantitative measurements of the left ventricular angiography (see Fig. 11.1). Average SV for adults is 70 mL.

## Filling Pressures (Preload)

Filling pressures show the preload condition of the subject. The atrial pressures and end-diastolic pressures of the ventricles are considered as the filling pressure.

## Right and left heart Catheterization

Measurement and interpretation of right atrial, right ventricular, and pulmonary capillary wedge pressure (PCWP) as well as the determination of CO and screening of intracardiac shunts are performed by right heart catheterization (RHC). RHC is performed using a PAC, Swan-Ganz catheter, or ordinary end-hole catheters. The procedure is carried out via venous access (jugular, subclavian, cephalic/basilic, or femoral veins).

Left heart catheterization is performed via arterial approaches (usually femoral), and systemic arterial and left ventricular pressure waveforms can be obtained.[1-7]

Table 11.1 depicts the normal values of hemodynamic parameters.

### TABLE 11.1
### Normal Hemodynamic Parameters

| Parameter | Equation | Normal Range |
|---|---|---|
| Arterial oxygen saturation (SaO$_2$) | | 95%–100% |
| Mixed venous saturation (SvO$_2$) | | 60%–80% |
| Arterial blood pressure (BP) | Systolic (SBP) | 100–140 mmHg |
| | Diastolic (DBP) | 60–90 mmHg |
| Mean arterial pressure (MAP) | SBP + (2DBP)/3 | 70–105 mmHg |
| Right atrial pressure (RAP)/central venous pressure (CVP) | | 2–6 mmHg |
| Right ventricular pressure (RVP) | Systolic (RVSP) | 15–30 mmHg |
| | Diastolic (RVDP) | 2–8 mmHg |
| Pulmonary artery pressure (PAP) | Systolic (SPAP) | 15–30 mmHg |
| | Diastolic (DPAP) | 8–15 mmHg |
| Mean pulmonary artery pressure (MPAP) | SPAP + (2DPAP)/3 | 9–18 mmHg |
| Pulmonary capillary wedge pressure (PCWP) | | 6–12 mmHg |
| Left atrial pressure (LAP) | | 4–12 mmHg |

*Continued*

**TABLE 11.1**
Normal Hemodynamic Parameters—cont'd

| Parameter | Equation | Normal Range |
|---|---|---|
| Stroke volume (SV) | CO/HR × 1000 | 60–100 mL/beat |
| Cardiac output (CO) | | 4–8 L/min |
| Cardiac index (CI) | | 2.5–4 L/min/m² |
| Systemic vascular resistance (SVR) | 80 × (MAP − RAP)/CO | 800–1200 dyn s/cm⁻⁵ |
| Pulmonary vascular resistance (PVR) | 80 × (MPAP − PCWP)/CO | <250 dyn s/cm⁻⁵ |

BSA, body surface area; HR, heart rate.

## Pulmonary Artery Catheter and Swan-Ganz Catheter

The pulmonary artery or Swan-Ganz catheters are flexible balloon-tipped, flow-directed catheters (Fig. 11.2) that are widely used for RHC. The Swan-Ganz catheter is a PAC that has a thermistor and is used when thermodilution CO is measured.

The PAC passes through the right-side cardiac chambers to the pulmonary artery and provides the measurement of right heart chamber pressures and oxygen saturation. It is ultimately placed in the pulmonary capillary wedge position to obtain PCWP. PCWP reflects left atrial pressure (LAP) (see Fig. 11.3).

## Central Venous Pressure Measurement and Interpretation

Knowing the status of the central venous pressure (CVP) is very important in taking care of critically ill patients. CVP is measured from the superior or inferior vena cava and reflects right atrial pressure.

Right atrial and right ventricular end-diastolic pressures reflect right ventricular filling pressures (right ventricular preload).

$$CVP \sim \text{right atrial pressure} \sim \text{right ventricular end-diastolic volume (preload)}$$

Remember that right atrial pressure (and thus CVP) is a reflection of venous return, an important component of cardiac performance (preload).

The preload and cardiac functions are interrelated, so it can be difficult to interpret the influence of each one on the other. If the right atrial pressure (preload) remains constant, CO can still be influenced by changes in the other three determinants of cardiac performance.

Although the cardiac performance status cannot be determined by CVP alone, a good approximation of the hemodynamic status and right-sided cardiac function can be obtained by measuring the right-sided filling pressures of the patient.[1-7]

## Central Venous Pressure Waveforms

Central venous pressure (right atrial) and PCW (left atrial) pressure tracings have similar morphologies, but the right-sided pressures are slightly lower than the left.

The atrial waveform has two or three distinctive low-amplitude waves for each cardiac cycle in a normal sinus rhythm. This means that between each RR interval of the electrocardiogram (ECG), there are three positive waves (a, c, and v) and two negative waves (x and y), and they correlate with different phases of the cardiac cycle and ECG (Fig. 11.4).

a wave = atrial contraction

c wave (not always visible) = bulging of the tricuspid valve into the atrium at the beginning of ventricular contraction

x descent = the atrium relaxes, and the tricuspid valve is pulled downward

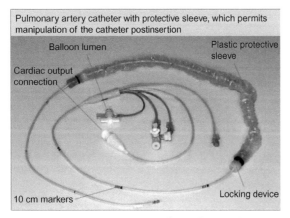

Pulmonary artery catheter with protective sleeve, which permits manipulation of the catheter postinsertion

Balloon lumen

Plastic protective sleeve

Cardiac output connection

10 cm markers

Locking device

FIG. 11.2 Swan-Ganz catheter. (From Scales K. How to remove a pulmonary artery catheter. *Nurs Stand.* 2016;30 (26):36–39; with permission.)

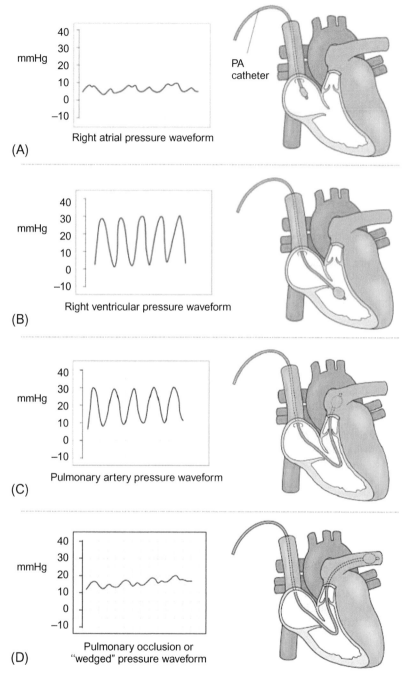

FIG. 11.3 Pressure waveforms seen as the pulmonary artery catheter (PA) is advanced through the heart: (A) right atrial pressure waveform, (B) right ventricular pressure waveform, (C) pulmonary artery pressure waveform, and (D) pulmonary capillary wedge pressure waveform. (From Scales K. How to remove a pulmonary artery catheter. *Nurs Stand*. 2016;30(26):36–39; with permission.)

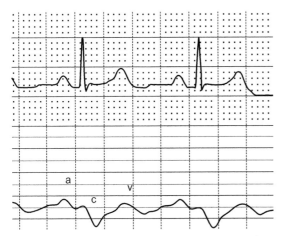

FIG. 11.4 A central venous pressure waveform. (From Morgan BL. Hemodynamic waveforms interpretation. *Critical Care Concepts*. 2005. http://www.caccn.ca/en/pdfs/4A%20Hemodyn_waves%20(B%20Morgan).pdf; with permission.)

v wave = passive filling of the right atrium and vena cavae when the tricuspid valve closes. In a CVP tracing, the v is generally located immediately after the peak of the T wave on the ECG

y descent = the tricuspid valve opens and blood flows into the right ventricle

The easiest way to evaluate a CVP tracing is to locate the v wave at first, immediately after T wave on ECG. After the v wave is identified, a and c can be identified. An a wave should be present if the patient has a sinus rhythm. The a is seen during the PR interval.

If present, the c wave is generally within the QRS.[1-7]

### Abnormal Central Venous Pressure Waveforms

Abnormal CVP waveforms are described in detail earlier.

### Left Heart Filling Pressures

Pulmonary capillary wedge pressure reflects left atrial and left ventricular end-diastolic pressure (LVEDP). PCWP can be easily measured by RHC, and left heart catheterization allows direct measurement of LVEDP.

The morphologies of PCWP or LAP waveforms are similar to CVP.

### Ventricular Pressure

Systole is during the QT interval in the ECG and consists of three phases (Fig. 11.5)—the isovolumic contraction, rapid ejection, and reduced ejection phases.

Diastole is coincident with the TQ period on the ECG and consists of four phases—the isovolumic relaxation, early rapid filling, atrial systole, and end-diastolic phases.

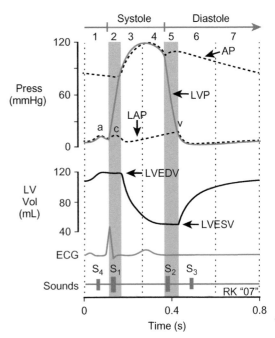

FIG. 11.5 A ventricular pressure tracing. *AP*, aortic pressure; *ECG*, electrocardiogram; *LAP*, left atrial pressure; *LVEDV*, left ventricular end-diastolic volume; *LVP*, left ventricular pressure; *LVSEV*, left ventricular end-systolic volume. (From Klabunde RE. *Cardiovascular Physiology Concepts*. 2nd ed. Philadelphia: Lippincott Williams & Wilkins; 2011; with permission.)

### Vascular Resistances

As explained earlier in this chapter, according to Ohm's law, vascular resistance is defined as the pressure difference across a vascular bed divided by the blood flow through that bed. The two clinically calculated resistances are systemic vascular resistance (SVR) and PVR.

### *Systemic Vascular Resistance*

SVR is the quantitative value for left ventricular afterload. In most patients, changes in vascular resistance reflect changes in arteriolar tone or changes in the viscosity of blood (often secondary to anemia or polycythemia). In patients who are in shock or hypotensive, SVR calculation helps to differentiate among etiologies and can guide therapy. For example, whereas a hypotensive patient with a low SVR may have sepsis, a patient in cardiogenic shock often has hypotension with an elevated SVR. Normal SVR is between 900 and 1440 $dyn/s/cm^{-5}$.

SVR (in Wood units or mmHg/L/min) =
  Mean arterial pressure (MAP) – Right atrial pressure/CO

SVR (in Wood units) × 80 = SVR in $dyn/s/cm^{-5}$

MAP = (Systolic blood pressure [BP] + [2 diastolic BP])/3

## Pulmonary Vascular Resistance

Pulmonary vascular resistance is the quantitative value for right ventricular afterload. The pulmonary vascular bed is very low resistance. The normal PVR is usually less than 2 Wood units (between 30 and 180 dyn/s/cm$^{-5}$). PVR is increased by anything that causes increased resistance in the pulmonary vascular system, including pulmonary emboli, hypoxia, and so on.

$$PVR \text{ (Wood units or mmHg/L/min)} =$$
$$MPAP - LAP(PCWP)/CO$$

$$PVR \text{ (in Wood units)} \times 80 = PVR \text{ in dyn/s/cm}^{-5}$$

$$\text{Mean pulmonary arterial pressure (MPAP)} =$$
$$[\text{Systolic PAP} + (2 \text{ diastolic PAP})]/3$$

## CLINICAL IMPLICATIONS OF RIGHT HEART CATHETERIZATION

Routine insertion of a PAC has no benefit in all critically ill patients. However, in selected cases, valuable information can be obtained from RHC.

### Heart Failure Hemodynamics

The most common indications for RHC in the setting of heart failure include:

1. Shock: RHC is indicated in patients with low BP or shock with unknown volume status to discriminate volume depletion from severe cardiac failure.
2. Cardiorenal syndrome: Right heart catheterization is indicated in patients with acute heart failure who have worsening renal function (WRF).
3. Pretransplant evaluation: Right heart catheterization is mandatory in patients who might be candidates for heart transplantation. In these patients, a full assessment of PVR and its reversibility (if elevated) should be undertaken. The right ventricle of the donor heart may not tolerate the irreversible elevated PVR, and the recipient will develop acute right-sided heart failure, which could be lethal. However, there is no absolute cutoff value for PVR in this setting.[8,9]

The RHC should be performed in optimally treated patients, and a vasodilator challenge test should be carried out when the pulmonary artery systolic pressure is 50 mmHg or greater and either the PVR is greater than 3 Wood units (>240 dyn/s/cm$^{-5}$) or the transpulmonary gradient (TPG = mean PAP − PCWP) is 15 mmHg or greater.

The drugs usually used for the vasodilator challenge test are inotropes such as milrinone or dobutamine, pulmonary vasodilators such as prostacyclin or nitric oxide, and systemic vasodilators such as nitroglycerin or nitroprusside. If the PVR can be reduced to less than 2.5 with a vasodilator in the absence of systemic hypotension (systemic BP <85 mmHg), the high PVR is reversible.

In patients who have a fixed pulmonary artery systolic pressure greater than 60 mmHg in conjunction with PVR greater than 5 Wood units (>400 dyn/s/cm$^{-5}$) or when the TPG exceeds 16–20 mmHg, the risk of right-sided heart failure and mortality after heart transplantation is severely increased.[9]

4. Unexplained dyspnea: In some circumstances, determining the cause of dyspnea by noninvasive methods is difficult, particularly in patients with normal left ventricular systolic function and the absence of significant valvular dysfunction. In these instances, performing RHC and direct measurement of filling pressures are required to determine the cause of shortness of breath[5,10] (Fig. 11.6).

In these situations, some maneuvers may be required in the catheterization laboratory if the results of resting hemodynamic measures are inconclusive.

1. Fluid challenge or exercise is very useful in the evaluation of patients with dyspnea and normal resting filling pressures.
2. Vasodilator challenge: In patients with unexplained dyspnea and high diastolic pressures, afterload reduction with vasodilators is extremely useful to determine whether the elevation of filling pressures is reversible with lowering the systemic BP. This maneuver can be a guide for outpatient medical management.

### Pulmonary Hypertension Hemodynamics

Right heart catheterization in the setting of pulmonary hypertension (PH)[11–14] is for the following:

1. To confirm the diagnosis of PH: If the mean of PAP is 20 mmHg or greater in RHC, the diagnosis is confirmed.
   - To determine whether the PH is postcapillary (secondary to left-sided heart diseases), precapillary (intrinsic pulmonary vascular disease), or a combination of both.
   - Precapillary: Mean PAP ≥20 mmHg and PCWP ≤ 15 mmHg, PVR ≥3 Wood Unit.
   - Isolated postcapillary PH: Mean PAP ≥20 mmHg and PCWP >15 mmHg, PVR <3 Wood unit.
   - Combined precapillary and postcapillary PH: Mean PAP ≥20 mmHg and PCWP >15 mmHg, PVR ≥3 Wood unit.
   - Diastolic pressure gradient = Diastolic PAP– PCWP.

Fig. 11.7 shows pulmonary hypertension hemodynamics.

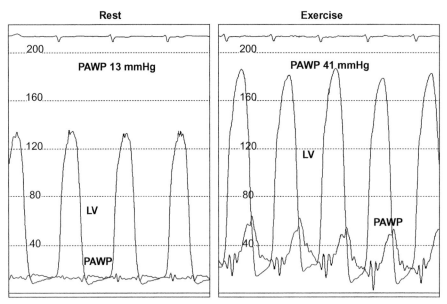

FIG. 11.6 Elevation of pulmonary capillary wedge pressure after exercise in a patient with dyspnea and no significant abnormality on echocardiography. (From Nishimura RA, Carabello BA. Hemodynamics in the cardiac catheterization laboratory of the 21st century. *Circulation.* 2012;125(17):2138–2150; with permission.)

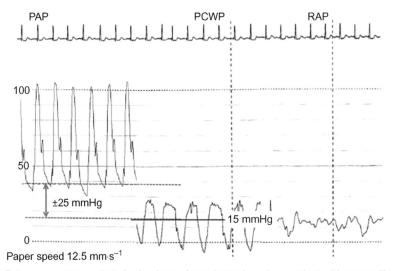

FIG. 11.7 Pulmonary artery catheterization hemodynamic tracings in a patient with precapillary PH. The increase in pulmonary arterial pressure (PAP) is associated with an increase in the gradient between pulmonary artery diastolic pressure and PCWP known as diastolic pressure gradient (DPG) to 25 mmHg. (From Mehta S, Vachiéry JL. Pulmonary hypertension: the importance of correctly diagnosing the cause. *Eur Respir Rev.* 2016;25(142s):372–380 (Fig. 1).)

2. To evaluate the severity of hemodynamic impairment
   - Low risk: Right atrial pressure (RAP) <8 mmHg, cardiac index ≤2.5 L/min/m$^2$, mixed venous oxygen saturation >65%.
   - Moderate risk: RAP 8–14 mmHg, cardiac index 2–2.4 L/min/m$^2$, mixed venous oxygen saturation 60%–65%.
   - High risk: RAP >10 mmHg, cardiac index <2 L/min/m$^2$, mixed venous oxygen saturation < 60%.
3. To perform vasoreactivity testing in selected patients
   - In patients with diagnosis of idiopathic pulmonary arterial hypertension (IPAH), hereditary pulmonary arterial hypertension (HPAH), and PAH associated with drugs.
   - To find patients who can be treated with high doses of calcium channel blockers.
4. Together with pulmonary angiography (digital subtraction angiography or high-quality multidetector computed tomography pulmonary angiography) to support management decisions in patients with chronic thromboembolic pulmonary hypertension.

## The Hemodynamics of Valvular Heart Disease[15]

In the setting of valvular heart disease, hemodynamic study is used to more precisely define the physiologic determinants of cardiac performance (preload, afterload, and contractility) and their relationship in order to better decision-making about the different therapeutic strategies.

Although the echocardiography has recently become the technique of choice for the evaluation and follow-up of valvular heart disease, the invasive hemodynamic study remains a crucial tool in the following cases:
1. When the patient's symptoms are out of proportion to the hemodynamics assessed by echocardiography.
2. When echocardiography shows a pulmonary hypertension out of proportion to the severity of left-sided valvular disorders or detected in those with right-sided valvular disorder (particularly in patients with severe tricuspid regurgitation).

Hemodynamic study in this setting is necessary to clarify; whether the patient has pulmonary hypertension or not. If the patient has PH in which hemodynamic category it is placed (precapillary, isolated postcapillary, or combined postcapillary) and which therapeutic strategy should be chosen for controlling pulmonary hypertension before, during, and after the specific management for the valvular heart disease (see earlier and Chapter 12).
3. The right heart performance which is an important predictor of left-sided valvular surgeries can be better assessed in cases with the equivocal right ventricular echocardiographic assessment.
4. Invasive hemodynamic monitoring is crucial before and during percutaneous valvular interventions such as transcatheter balloon mitral valvuloplasty, edge-to-edge mitral repair, transcatheter aortic valve replacement, and valve-in-valve procedures.

## Assessment of Valvular Stenosis

The assessment of valve stenosis requires the measurement of the valve gradient and calculation of left-sided valve area. The Gorlin equation is used for calculation of the valve area. The cardiac output, heart rate, systolic ejection period (for aortic valve stenosis) or diastolic filling period (for mitral valve stenosis), the pressure difference across the stenotic valve, acceleration of gravity factor, and an empirical constant to calculate valve area.

Gorlin equation:

$$\text{Aortic valve area} = (\text{Cardiac output}/\text{heart rate} \times \text{systolic ejection period})/44.5 \times \sqrt{\Delta P}$$

$$\text{Mitral valve area} = (\text{Cardiac output}/\text{heart rate} \times \text{diastolic ejection period})/44.5 \times \sqrt{\Delta P}$$

$$\sqrt{\Delta P} = \text{mean pressure gradient}$$

Hakki equation:

$$\text{Valve area} = \text{Cardiac output}/\sqrt{\Delta P}$$

$$\sqrt{\Delta P} = \text{peak pressure gradient}$$

Practical points in the estimation of valve area:
1. Hakki equation is a simplified form of Gorlin formula which can be used to calculate aortic valve area.
2. Fick method is the gold standard for estimating the cardiac output.
3. The limitations of Gorlin equation are as follows:
   a. The calculated valve area is more significantly influenced by the cardiac output than the pressure gradient because the square root of the pressure gradient is used, so any error in measuring the cardiac output can strongly influence the calculation of valve area particularly in patients with low cardiac outputs (less than 3 L/min).
   b. In patients with concomitant regurgitation and stenosis of a valve, it is needed to use total cardiac output determined by the angiographic method in Gorlin formula. Because cardiac output measured by Fick or thermodilution methods shows the sum of regurgitant flow and total CO, the valve area may be overestimated.

Practical points in hemodynamic study of aortic valve stenosis (AS):

1. To measure the mean aortic transvalvular pressure gradient, a simultaneous assessment of left ventricular and ascending aorta is required with a dual lumen pigtail catheter or the use of one catheter in left ventricle and a second in the ascending aorta just above the aortic valve (Fig. 11.8).
2. The location of aortic pressure measurement is important because a true central aortic pressure is different from the peripheral artery pressure. The peak arterial pressure in the periphery is often higher than ascending aorta due to peripheral amplification.
3. Carabello sign: The presence of a catheter across the stenotic aortic valve leads to reducing the effective orifice area and an increase in transvalvular gradient during the pullback technique, so it is possible to observe an increase in arterial blood pressure during catheter pullback in a patient with severe AS. This sign is called Carabello sign.
4. Low pressure-low-gradient AS:

The severity of AS is defined by the mean transvalvular pressure gradient (a mean pressure gradient of 40 mmHg or greater in severe AS); so, a small decrease in flow may result in significant reductions in the valve gradient. This entity is called low-flow low-gradient AS which is seen in patients with severe left ventricular dysfunction. So, in patients with severe left ventricular dysfunction who may have reduced cardiac output, a pharmacological stimulation of cardiac output using dobutamine and recalculation of aortic valve area is recommended.

Practical points in hemodynamic study of mitral valve stenosis (MS):

1. The mitral valve gradient is estimated as the difference between mean left atrial pressure (or mean PCWP) and mean LV diastolic pressure. For better estimation of pressure gradient, the PCWP and LV pressure should be traced simultaneously (Fig. 11.9).
2. The precise measurement of PCWP in MS may be difficult because the right-side chambers and pulmonary artery may be dilated secondary to pulmonary hypertension.
3. In those with atrial fibrillation rhythm, the average of valve gradients over at least 10 cardiac cycles should be measured.
4. A high v wave in LAP or PCWP tracing shows concomitant mitral regurgitation.

### Practical Points In Hemodynamic Study of Valvular Regurgitation

1. The degree of pulmonary hypertension can show the severity of mitral regurgitation (MR).
2. The severity of MR can also be estimated by the height of v wave in left atrial or PCWP tracing. However, the height of V wave is a sensitive, not a specific marker and it depends on left atrial volume and compliance. A large v wave can be seen in the setting of acute severe MR in which left atrium has low compliance (Fig. 11.10).
3. The severity of aortic regurgitation can be assessed by angiography using a side-hole catheter (such as pigtail catheter). The left ventricular end-diastolic pressure should be measured before and after injection.

### The Hemodynamics of Pericardial Disease[16]

Among the three entities of pericardial disease including constrictive pericarditis (CP), acute pericarditis, and cardiac tamponade, hemodynamic impairment occurs most frequently in CP and cardiac tamponade than acute pericarditis.

The practical points regarding the hemodynamic evaluation of CP and for differentiating restrictive cardiomyopathy (RCM) and CP have been discussed in detail in Chapter 29.

The hard and scarred pericardium limits the ventricular filling and a characteristic square root or dip-and-plateau pattern is seen in pressure tracing of left and right ventricle in CP. This pattern of hemodynamic tracing is due to the rapid early ventricular filling and an abrupt cessation of ventricular filling in mid-to-late diastole.

Fig. 11.11 shows a clinical scenario of CP.

A 40-year-old gentleman who had been managed as arrhythmogenic right ventricular cardiomyopathy (ARVC) in other center since 3 years ago, referred to heart failure clinic due to aggravation of right-sided heart failure symptoms in terms of peripheral edema and abdominal distension. Transthoracic echocardiography was in favor of constrictive pericarditis and his right heart catheterization showed the following tracings (Fig. 11.11). The patient was successfully undergone the pericardiectomy surgery.

### Cardiac Tamponade

In cardiac tamponade, the cardiac chambers are compressed and ventricular filling throughout the diastolic period is impaired. The reason is that the intrapericardial pressure exceeds intracardiac pressure secondary to fluid accumulation in the pericardial space. Cardiac catheterization is usually not necessary to make the diagnosis of cardiac tamponade. In these patients, the atrial pressure is typically elevated with a prominent x descent and blunted or absent y descent (Fig. 11.12).

The x descent is preserved because during the systolic ejection, the intracardiac volume decreases and leads to a temporary reduction in intrapericardial pressures. The

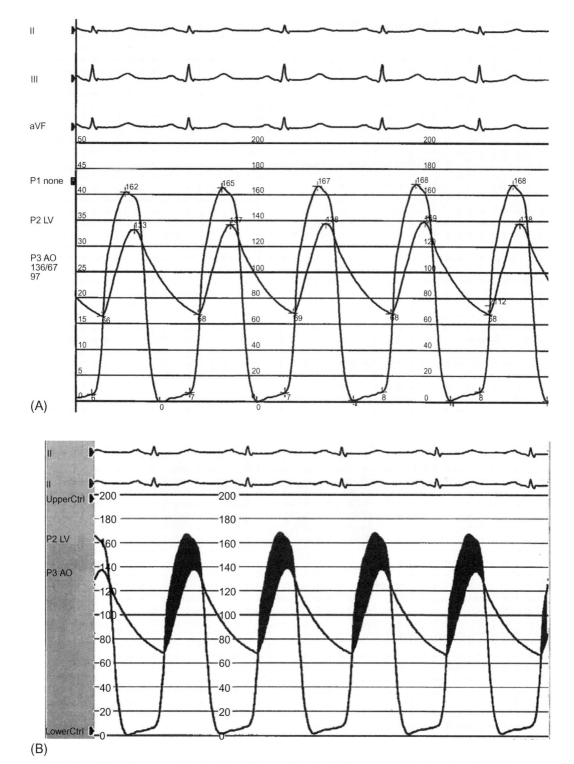

FIG. 11.8 (A) Aortic pressure tracings in an 82-year-old patient with severe aortic valve stenosis. Aortic pressure tracing demonstrating delayed upstroke in the setting of severe obstruction. (B) Simultaneous LV and aortic pressure measurements in aortic stenosis. A slight delay can be seen in the upstroke of both the aortic and left ventricular pressure tracing with the presence of a mean transvalvular gradient of 32 mmHg for a calculated valve area of 0.86 cm$^2$ in the setting of cardiac output of 4.0 L/min. (From Pighi M, Asgar AW. Invasive hemodynamics of valvular heart disease. *Interv Cardiol Clin*. 2017;6(3):319–327 (Fig. 1).)

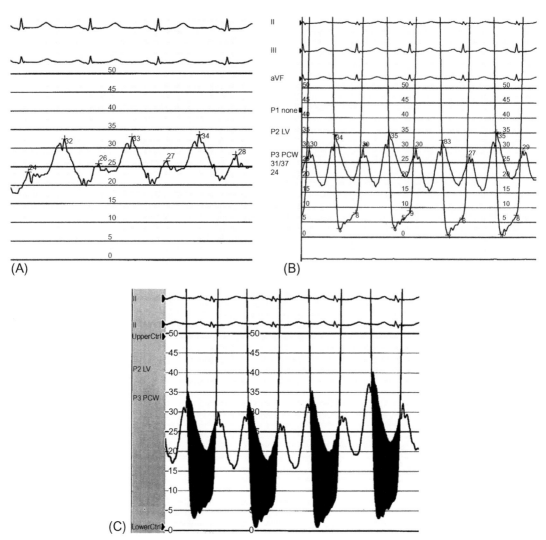

**FIG. 11.9** Simultaneous left ventricular and pulmonary capillary wedge pressure tracings in mitral stenosis. (A) The "a" wave is prominent and measures approximately 28–30 mmHg with an increased "v" wave as well. (B, C) The mean mitral valve gradient is 17 mmHg for a calculated valve area of 0.92 cm$^2$ in the setting of a cardiac output of 4.0 L/min. (From Pighi M, Asgar AW. Invasive Hemodynamics of valvular heart disease. *Interv Cardiol Clin.* 2017;6(3):319–327 (Fig. 2).)

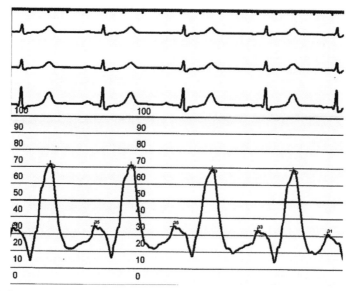

FIG. 11.10 Left atrial pressure tracing in a patient with severe mitral regurgitation referred for a MitraClip procedure. The patient is in sinus rhythm, there is an elevation of the mean left atrial pressure with a prominent "v" wave measuring 70 mmHg. (From Pighi M, Asgar AW. Invasive hemodynamics of valvular heart disease. *Interv Cardiol Clin*. 2017;6(3):319–327 (Fig. 3).)

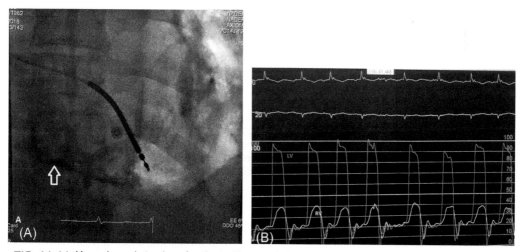

FIG. 11.11 Hemodynamic tracing of patient with constrictive pericarditis. (A) The fluoroscopy image shows calcifications around the heart (*arrow*). (B) Simultaneous pressure recording of right and left ventricles shows elevated and equalized diastolic pressure in RV and LV. Dip-and-plateau pattern (*arrow*).

*Continued*

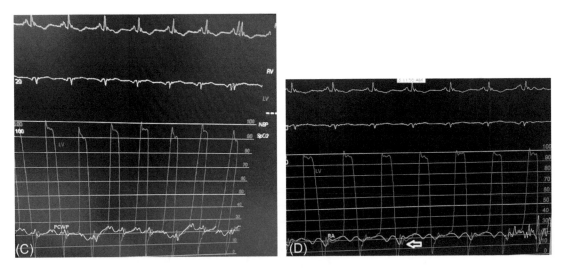

FIG. 11.11, cont'd (C) Simultaneous pressure recording of PCWP and left ventricle shows elevated and equalized diastolic pressure of LV and PCWP. (D) Simultaneous pressure recording of right atrium and left ventricles shows elevated and equalized diastolic pressure in RA and LV. In the RA pressure tracing, the rapid x and y descents can be seen. The y descent of the RA pressure corresponds to the early rapid filling phase of the ventricular pressure tracing, which shows the typical dip-and-plateau pattern (arrow).

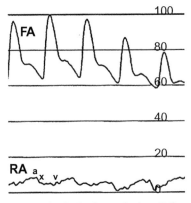

FIG. 11.12 Cardiac tamponade. Hypotension in the femoral artery (FA) pressure with loss of the y descent in the RA pressure tracing is evident. With inspiration, there is a decrease in the aortic pulse pressure. (From Athappan G, Sorajja P. Invasive hemodynamics of pericardial disease. *Interv Cardiol Clin.* 2017;6(3): 309–317 (Fig. 8).)

elevated intrapericardial pressure during the rest of the cardiac cycle leads to impairment of ventricular filling and a blunted y descent (Fig. 11.12).

The equalization of end-diastolic ventricular pressures, reduced stroke volume and cardiac output, and alterations in the pulse pressure or systolic ejection period which is secondary to a reduced stroke volume are the other hemodynamic findings of tamponade.

## INTRA-AORTIC BALLOON PUMP[17]

**Normal intra-aortic balloon pump (IABP) waveform:** When the balloon inflation and deflation are correctly timed, it results in optimal hemodynamic effects (Fig. 11.13).

The balloon inflates about 40 ms before the dicrotic notch. This is timed by the end of the T wave on the ECG. The deflation of the balloon is with the R wave of the ECG.

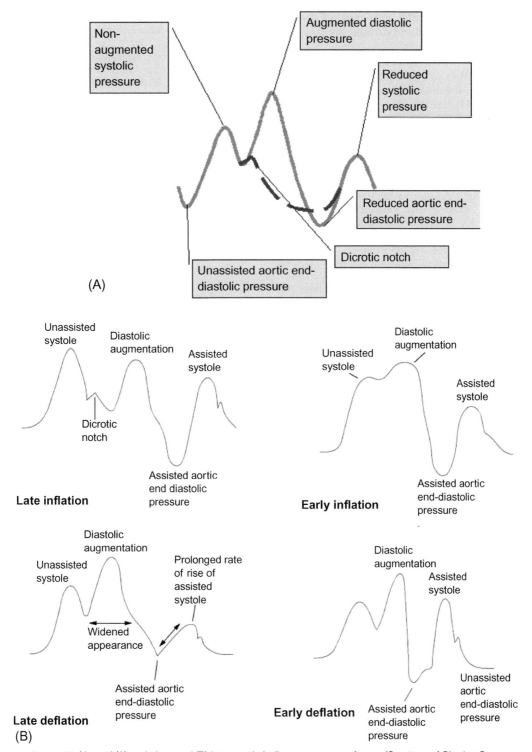

FIG. 11.13 Normal (A) and abnormal (B) intra-aortic balloon pump waveforms. (Courtesy of Charles Gomersall. https://www.aic.cuhk.edu.hk/web8/IABP pressure waveforms.htm.)

The pulse waveform after augmentation shows a reduced aortic systolic and end-diastolic pressure.

## REFERENCES

1. Wiggers CJ. Determinants of cardiac performance. *Circulation*. 1951;4(4):485–495.
2. Bangalore S, Bhatt DL. Right heart catheterization, coronary angiography, and percutaneous coronary intervention. *Circulation*. 2011;124(17):e428–e433.
3. Al Ajmi AM. *Invasive Hemodynamics Manual for Adult Cardiac Catheterization*. Cath. Lab; 2013.
4. Davis MJ, Gore RW. Determinants of cardiac function: simulation of a dynamic cardiac pump for physiology instruction. *Adv Physiol Educ*. 2001;25(1):13–35.
5. Nishimura RA, Carabello BA. Hemodynamics in the cardiac catheterization laboratory of the 21st century. *Circulation*. 2012;125(17):2138–2150.
6. Daily EK. Hemodynamic waveform analysis. *J Cardiovasc Nurs*. 2001;15(2):6–22.
7. Scales K. How to remove a pulmonary artery catheter. *Nurs Stand*. 2016;30(26):36–39.
8. Costanzo MR, Dipchand A, Starling R, et al. The International Society of Heart and Lung Transplantation Guidelines for the care of heart transplant recipients. *J Heart Lung Transplant*. 2010;29(8):914–956.
9. Mehra MR, Kobashigawa J, Starling R, et al. Listing criteria for heart transplantation: International Society for Heart and Lung Transplantation guidelines for the care of cardiac transplant candidates—2006. *J Heart Lung Transplant*. 2006;25(9):1024–1042.
10. Keusch S, Bucher A, Müller-Mottet S, et al. Experience with exercise right heart catheterization in the diagnosis of pulmonary hypertension: a retrospective study. *Multidiscip Respir Med*. 2014;9(1):1.
11. Galiè N, Humbert M, Vachiery J-L, et al. ESC/ERS guidelines for the diagnosis and treatment of pulmonary hypertension. *Eur Heart J*. 2015;2015, ehv317.
12. Galiè N, McLaughlin VV, Rubin LJ, Simonneau G. An overview of the 6th World Symposium on Pulmonary Hypertension. *Eur Respir Soc*. 2019;53(1), 1802148.
13. Simonneau G, Montani D, Celermajer DS, et al. Haemodynamic definitions and updated clinical classification of pulmonary hypertension. *Eur Respir J*. 2019;53(1), 1801913.
14. Mehta S, Vachiéry J-L. Pulmonary hypertension: the importance of correctly diagnosing the cause. *Eur Respir Rev*. 2016;25(142):372–380.
15. Pighi M, Asgar AW. Invasive hemodynamics of valvular heart disease. *Interv Cardiol Clin*. 2017;6(3):319–327.
16. Athappan G, Sorajja P. Invasive hemodynamics of pericardial disease. *Interv Cardiol Clin*. 2017;6(3):309–317.
17. Myat A, McConkey H, Chick L, Baker J, Redwood S. The intra-aortic balloon pump in high-risk percutaneous coronary intervention: is counterpulsation counterproductive? *Interv Cardiol*. 2012;4(2):211–234.

# CHAPTER 12

# Heart Failure and Pulmonary Hypertension

NASIM NADERI

Rajaie Cardiovascular, Medical & Research Center, Iran University of Medical Sciences, Tehran, Iran

## HEART FAILURE DEFINITION

Heart failure (HF) is a syndrome in which the heart is unable to act as a pump because of abnormalities in loading conditions, myocardial contractility, or relaxation performance. The impaired cardiac performance leads to HF-related symptoms, including dyspnea, leg or abdomen swelling, fatigue, excessive tiredness, nocturia, and signs such as elevated jugular venous pressure, increase in liver size and hepatojugular reflux, lung crackles, ascites, and lower limb edema.[1–3]

The presence of signs and symptoms of HF should force the physician to refer the patient for diagnostic workup regarding cardiac dysfunction. Although the clinical response to HF-specific therapies such as diuretic therapy may be helpful in decision-making, a thorough cardiovascular workup is necessary in these patients.

Heart failure syndrome has four stages based on structural changes and symptoms. The clinical approach and management strategies are different in each stage (Fig. 12.1).[2]

However, the description of HF is based on left ventricular ejection fraction (LVEF) throughout the word. Demographics, underlying etiology, comorbidities, and therapeutic approaches are different in patients with different types of HF in terms of LVEF.

Three types of HF have been defined based on LVEF[1]:
1. HFpEF: HF with preserved LVEF—patients who have normal LVEF ($\leq 50\%$)
2. HFrEF: HF with reduced EF ($<40\%$)
3. HFmrEF: HF with midrange ejection fraction (40%–49%)

### Key Points

For the diagnosis of HF, specific symptoms and signs of HF should be present.

Patients who have structural heart disease and are asymptomatic are at stage B of HF.

Signs of HF may not be present in the early stages of HF—in particular in patients with HFpEF.

Patients who have received diuretics may not present with signs of HF.

In the setting of HFmrEF and HFpEF, the presence of elevated B-type natriuretic peptide (BNP) or N-terminal pro-B-type natriuretic peptide (NT-proBNP) levels accompanied by evidence of structural heart disease or diastolic dysfunction is necessary to diagnose HF.

## DIAGNOSTIC WORKUP FOR HEART FAILURE

Natriuretic peptides (NPs), electrocardiography, and echocardiography are essential initial investigations.[1,2,4]

### Key Points About Natriuretic Peptides

The elevated plasma levels of NPs help identify those who need further cardiology workup. If the plasma concentration of NPs is normal, a diagnosis of HF will be unlikely.

In nonacute settings, BNP less than 35 pg/mL and NT-proBNP less than 125 pg/mL are the upper limits of normal.

In acute settings, a BNP less than 100 pg/mL and NT-proBNP less than 300 pg/mL should be considered as the upper limits of normal.

Remember that the negative predictive values of these cut points are higher; therefore, it is recommended to use NPs for ruling out HF, not for making the diagnosis.

There are many cardiac and noncardiac conditions in which NPs are elevated.

Cardiac causes include acute coronary syndrome (ACS), pulmonary emboli, pulmonary hypertension, myocarditis, different types of cardiomyopathies, contusion of heart after trauma, valvular and congenital heart diseases, and cardioversion with direct current (DC) shock.

Noncardiac causes include advanced age, cerebrovascular events, renal failure, liver failure, chronic

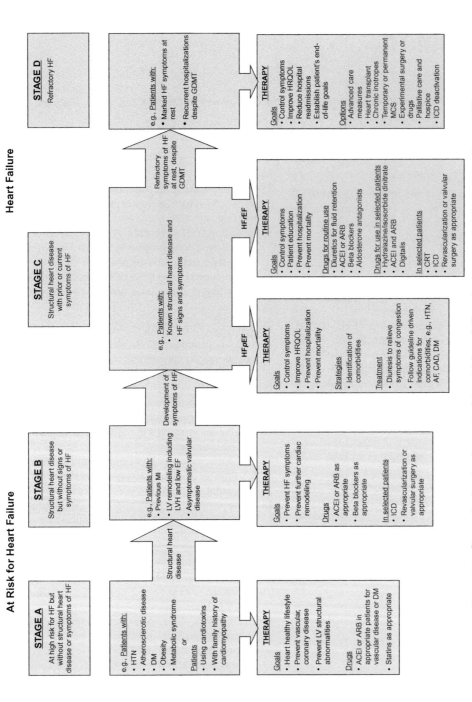

FIG. 12.1 Stages in the development of heart failure (HF) and recommended therapy by stage. *ACE,* angiotensin-converting enzyme; *AF,* atrial fibrillation; *ARB,* angiotensin receptor blocker; *CAD,* coronary artery disease; *CRT,* cardiac resynchronization therapy; *DM,* diabetes mellitus; *EF,* ejection fraction; *GDMT,* guideline-directed medical therapy; *HFpEF,* heart failure with preserved left ventricular ejection fraction; *HFref,* heart failure with reduced ejection fraction; *HRQOL,* health-related quality of life; *HTN,* hypertension; *ICD,* implantable cardioverter defibrillator; *LV,* left ventricular; *LVH,* left ventricular hypertrophy; *MCS,* mechanical circulatory support; *MI,* myocardial infarction. (From Yancy CW, Jessup M, Bozkurt B, et al. 2013 ACCF/AHA guideline for the management of heart failure: a report of the American College of Cardiology Foundation/American Heart Association Task Force on Practice Guidelines. *J Am Coll Cardiol.* 2013;62(16):e147–239; with permission.)

obstructive pulmonary disease (COPD), severe infection and sepsis, anemia, thyrotoxicosis, diabetic ketoacidosis, and paraneoplastic syndromes. NPs may be low in obese patients.

## Electrocardiography

The presence of any abnormality on the electrocardiogram (ECG) increases the likelihood of HF. ECG might also provide some information about the cause of HF (e.g., ischemic heart disease), and the findings of ECG are helpful in implementing of some of the specific therapies [e.g., anticoagulation in atrial fibrillation rhythm or cardiac resynchronization therapy in the setting of HF with left bundle branch block (LBBB) pattern].[1,2,4]

## Echocardiography

The assessment of cardiac structure and function in patients suspected to each type of HF is by transthoracic echocardiography. Transesophageal echocardiography is not routinely recommended in patients with HF (see also Chapter 5 for more details about echocardiography in HF).

## Other Diagnostic Tests
### Chest radiography

Chest radiography is more helpful in acute settings than in nonacute HF. Recently, computed tomography (CT) has become the standard diagnostic test for diagnosis of pulmonary pathologies (see also Chapter 6 for more details).

### Cardiac magnetic resonance imaging

In subjects with poor echocardiography window, cardiac magnetic resonance imaging (MRI) is the method of choice for assessment of cardiac structure and function, particularly in patients with right HF and complex congenital heart diseases.

Cardiac MRI is also recommended in cases in which myocarditis, amyloidosis, sarcoidosis, noncompaction cardiomyopathy, hypertrophic cardiomyopathy, and other infiltrative cardiomyopathies for myocardial tissue characterization are suspected (see also Chapter 8 for more details).

### Coronary angiography

Selective coronary angiography is recommended in patients with HF who have angina pectoris and has a high pretest probability for coronary artery disease (CAD).

An algorithmic approach for the diagnosis of HF in nonacute settings is shown in Fig. 12.2.

## ACUTE HEART FAILURE

Acute heart failure (AHF) is a sudden onset or worsening of symptoms and signs of HF caused by fluid overload and severe congestion in multiple organs or inadequate cardiac output that requires immediate evaluation and treatment.

Acute HF has three stages of management, and the goals of treatment are different in each stage:
1. Immediate stage: The patient is in the emergency department (ED), intensive care unit (ICU), or critical care unit (CCU)
2. Intermediate stage: The hospital course in the step-down ward
3. Predischarge stage

In the ED, the diagnosis of AHF should be established quickly, and appropriate management should be initiated as soon as possible.

In the first step, the clinical conditions and the precipitating factors that need urgent treatment should be identified. These include hypertension crisis, acute coronary syndrome (ACS), acute pulmonary emboli, tachyarrhythmias, bradyarrhythmias or conduction disturbances, and acute mechanical causes [aortic dissection or thrombosis, myocardial rupture complicating ACS (acute mitral regurgitation, free wall rupture, and ventricular septal defect), acute native or prosthetic valve incompetence secondary to endocarditis, chest trauma, or cardiac intervention].

The second step is amelioration of the congestive symptoms, improvement of cardiac output and oxygenation, and optimization of volume status.

The next measures during hospital course and predischarge stage are:
- Identification of other precipitating factors (Box 12.1)
- Starting diagnostic workups to identify the cause of HF if it remains unclear
- Starting and optimization of guideline-directed medical therapies for HF
- Selecting the patients who need revascularization or device therapy
- Selecting the patients who are at risk of thromboembolic events and starting appropriate anticoagulation therapies
- Implementing the educational and self-care programs for patients and their families and starting cardiac rehabilitation programs[1]

## Acute Heart Failure in the Emergency Department
### Indications for admission

Evidence of severe decompensated HF, hypoperfusion, and end-organ damage, including loss of consciousness, hypotension, pulmonary edema, and kidney or liver dysfunction

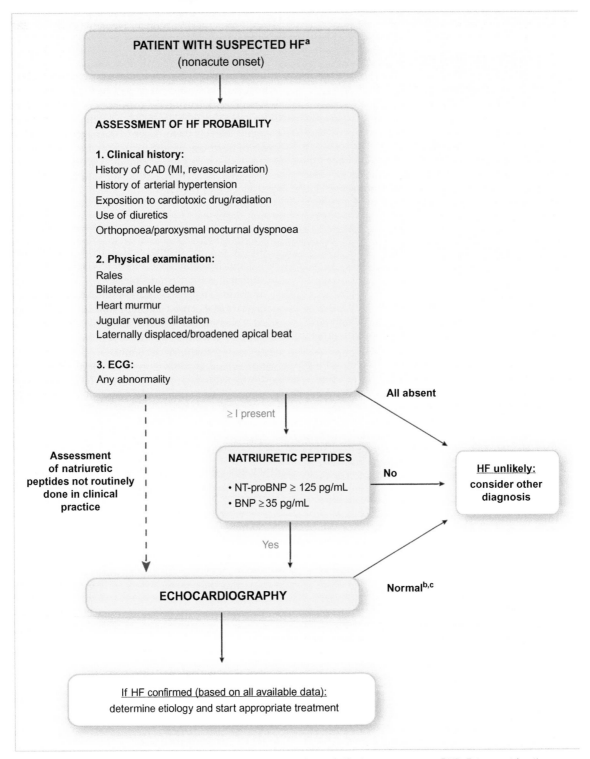

FIG. 12.2 Diagnostic algorithm for a diagnosis of heart failure (HF) of nonacute onset. *BNP*, B-type natriuretic peptide; *CAD*, coronary artery disease; *ECG*, electrocardiogram; *MI*, myocardial infarction; *NT-proBNP*, N-terminal pro-B-type natriuretic peptide. (From Ponikowski P, Voors AA, Anker SD, et al. 2016 ESC guidelines for the diagnosis and treatment of acute and chronic heart failure: the task force for the diagnosis and treatment of acute and chronic heart failure of the European Society of Cardiology (ESC) developed with the special contribution of the Heart Failure Association (HFA) of the ESC. *Eur Heart J.* 2016;37(27):2129–200; with permission.)

The presence of dyspnea at rest accompanied with rapid breathing or arterial oxygen saturation less than 90% at room air

Arrhythmias with hemodynamic impairment, including atrial fibrillation with rapid ventricular response and ventricular tachycardia

ACS

Aggravated edema or the presence of severe peripheral congestion even in the absence of dyspnea

Significant electrolyte imbalance

The presence of other critical conditions such as pneumonia, pulmonary emboli, cerebrovascular accidents, prosthetic valve malfunction, or diabetic ketoacidosis

Frequent implantable cardioverter defibrillator (ICD) firing

Acute de novo HF (first occurrence of HF)

## Diagnosis and Prognosis

The diagnostic approach and management measures should be in parallel in patients with AHF. The other differential diagnoses (i.e., acute renal failure, pulmonary infections, and severe anemia) should also be considered and ruled out in the initial assessment. In the initial assessment of patients suspected of having AHF, it is essential to take a thorough history of the present illness, past medical and cardiovascular history, and potential cardiac and noncardiac precipitant factors and to look for signs and symptoms of fluid overload and hypoperfusion by physical examination.[1,2,4]

### Diagnostic Investigations

A careful clinical evaluation of patients with AHF should be followed by appropriate diagnostic investigations.

#### *Key points about diagnostic investigations*

ECG findings are usually abnormal and can be useful in the diagnosis of myocardial ischemia and arrhythmias.

Chest radiography: Cardiomegaly, pulmonary congestion, edema, and pleural effusion are specific findings of AHF. Chest radiography results are normal in 20% of patients with AHF. Chest radiography is also a useful test in the diagnosis of concomitant problems such as pneumonias. Portable chest radiography in a supine position has limited value in the evaluation of patients with AHF.[1,5]

Lung ultrasound: Lung ultrasound is better than chest radiography in ruling out pleural effusions and interstitial edema. B-lines originating from extravasated fluid into the interstitium and alveoli can be detected by lung ultrasound. The diagnostic findings for interstitial and alveolar edema in acute heart failure are more than three B-lines in more than two intercostal spaces bilaterally.[5]

Echocardiography: Limited bedside echocardiography in the ED can be very useful in patients who are critically ill (i.e., cardiogenic shock) or suspected to have acute structural complications (i.e., acute valvular regurgitations, acute prosthetic dysfunction, and aortic dissection). Echocardiography can also be used to estimate right- and left-sided filling pressure, however, the measured data have less certainty in the setting of acute heart failure. Estimation of left-sided filling pressures can be performed by Doppler imaging and tissue Doppler right atrial pressures. The collapsibility and width of the inferior vena cava can be used to assess right-sided filling pressures. Early echocardiography should be considered for patients who present with AHF for the first time (acute de novo HF).[1,3,5]

Table 12.1 presents different echocardiographic parameters for detecting the congestion in AHF.

**TABLE 12.1**
**Echocardiographic Parameters for Detecting Congestion in Acute Heart Failure**

| Echocardiographic Parameter | Comparator | Comment |
|---|---|---|
| IVC collapse <50% | RAP >7 mmHg | Using in positive pressure ventilated patients is difficult |
| Inspiratory diameter IVC <12 mm | RAP >7 mmHg | In positive pressure ventilated patients cannot be used |
| Mitral inflow E-wave velocity >50 cm/s | PCWP >18 mmHg | Difficult when E and A wave are fused, low specificity |
| Lateral E/Em >12 | PCWP >18 mmHg | Less accurate in CRT and advanced heart failure |
| Mitral inflow E wave Deceleration time <130 ms | PCWP >18 mmHg | Difficult when of E and A wave are fused |
| Pulmonary vein S/D <1 | PCWP >18 mmHg | Intra-observer variability in Doppler measurements of the vein |

Abbreviations: *CRT*, cardiac resynchronization therapy; *IVC*, inferior vena cava; *PCWP*, pulmonary capillary wedge pressure; *RAP*, right atrial pressure.

Laboratory tests: The following laboratory assessments should be performed in all patients with AHF at admission: complete blood count with white blood cell differentiation (CBC/diff), blood urea nitrogen (BUN), creatinine, serum electrolytes (sodium, potassium, and magnesium), serum lactate level, liver function tests [alanine aminotransferase (ALT), aspartate aminotransferase (AST), total and direct bilirubin, and lactate dehydrogenase (LDH)], blood sugar, cardiac troponins and NT-proBNP or BNP, thyroid function test, and iron profile (serum iron, total iron-binding capacity, and ferritin).[1,3]

### Key points about laboratory tests in acute heart failure[1,3,6–8]

The *D-dimer* should be checked if the patient is suspected of having acute pulmonary emboli.

Routine *arterial blood gas (ABG)* measurement is not mandatory unless the precise measurement of $pO_2$ and $pCO_2$ is needed.

The *$O_2$ saturation* can be easily assessed by pulse oximetry, and for the assessment of pH and $pCO_2$, a venous sample is usually enough.

*CBC/diff* is helpful in patients with suspected infection as a precipitating factor of AHF.

The assessment of *procalcitonin level* is recommended in some patients to differentiate pneumonia and guide antibiotic therapy.

*BUN, creatinine, and electrolytes* should be measured at admission and on a daily basis or every 1 or 2 days during hospital stays and on the discharge day.

More frequent sampling is recommended in critical patients according to the severity of the case, particularly in patients with electrolyte imbalance.

*Liver function test (LFT)* results may be abnormal in patients with AHF. This condition is called acute cardiogenic liver injury. It may be secondary to severe congestion or a low output state and is a poor prognostic factor. Patients having portal hypertension or chronic congestion may exhibit acute cardiogenic liver injury even after mild hemodynamic disturbances.

The ratio of first measured ALT to LDH is usually helpful for differentiating the liver causes of abnormal LFT results. A ratio less than 1.5 is more probably related to AHF than hepatic dysfunction secondary to, for example, hepatitis.[5,6]

*Cardiac troponins* are useful for diagnosis of ACS and myocardial infarction. Cardiac troponins are often elevated in the majority of patients with AHF in the absence of an acute coronary event, which shows ongoing myocardial damage and is a poor prognostic factor. They can also be elevated in the setting of acute myocarditis.

A *plasma level of natriuretic peptide (BNP or proBNP)* should be measured in all patients with acute dyspnea and suspected AHF. It helps to differentiate AHF from noncardiac causes of acute dyspnea.

NP levels can be detected low in patients with end-stage HF, flash pulmonary edema, and right-sided HF.

The plasma level of NPs should be measured before discharge for prognostic evaluation.

*Thyroid function test* should be assessed in all patients with AHF, particularly in those with newly diagnosed AHF, because both hypothyroidism and hyperthyroidism may precipitate AHF.

Many patients with chronic HF are receiving amiodarone, and it is needed to evaluate regarding the thyroid side effects of this drug.

It should be kept in mind that amiodarone-induced hyperthyroidism is an important cause of frequent ICD firing.

Hypothyroidism is one of the most important causes of diuretic resistance, particularly in patients with advanced end-stage HF.

*Iron profile*: Considering the high prevalence of iron deficiency (ID) in chronic HF and its prognostic importance in these patients, the iron profile needs to be assessed in all patients diagnosed with HF.

It should be kept in mind that the ferritin level may be increased in the setting of AHF as an acute-phase reactant, and if the ferritin level is within normal limits in patients with AHF, the iron profile study should be repeated after discharge.

Although hemodynamic study by right heart catheterization (RHC) is gold standard method in diagnosing the congestion and, may be helpful in the diagnosis of AHF, the invasive nature of this procedure limits its routine use in clinical practice. The utility of right heart catheterization (RHC) in patients with HF is discussed in Chapter 11.

## Management of AHF[1,3]

As mentioned earlier, the first step in the management of patients with AHF is identifying the critical clinical conditions such as cardiogenic shock or respiratory failure that needs urgent treatment (Fig. 12.3). The diagnostic workups and appropriate nonpharmacologic and pharmacologic treatments should be started promptly and in parallel. These patients should be transferred immediately to a place with resuscitation facilities.

High-risk patients include all of the following:
* Patients with ACS
* Patients with hypertensive crisis
* Patients with rapid arrhythmias or severe bradycardia or conduction disturbances
* Patients with acute mechanical causes such as mechanical complications of ACS, intervention complications, native or prosthetic valve dysfunction, aortic dissection, or cardiac tumors
* Patients with acute pulmonary emboli

The management protocol of these patients is explained in detail elsewhere in this book.

Patients with any of the following criteria should be admitted to an ICU or CCU:

Hemodynamic instability: patients with a systolic blood pressure (BP) less than 90 mmHg or signs or symptoms of hypoperfusion

Respiratory failure: severe respiratory distress, tachypnea with a respiratory rate greater than 25 breaths/min or use of accessory breathing muscles, oxygen saturation less than 90% despite supplemental oxygen, and intubated patients and those who need intubation

Rhythm disturbances: the presence of bradyarrhythmia (heart rate <40 beats/min) or tachyarrhythmia (heart rate >130 beats/min)

The remaining patients with AHF usually can be hospitalized in a step-down unit or an ordinary ward. A few patients who have subtle signs of congestion can be managed with small doses of diuretics and some adjustments of oral medications in the ED and discharged with instructions to make an appointment in the outpatient clinic. The patients who are admitted to the ICU or CCU should be transferred to the step-down unit after resolution of morbid conditions and clinical stabilization.

## Management of the early phase[1,3]

The clinical profile should be assessed in the early phase, and management should begin based on the identified hemodynamic profile (Table 12.2). The hemodynamic profile is identified clinically after answering two questions:
1. Is the patient congested?
2. Is the peripheral perfusion adequate?

Patients with AHF are divided into two groups based on the presence or the absence of congestion:
1. Wet patients (95% of AHF patients)
2. Dry patients (5% of AHF patients)

After assessment of patients regarding the degree of congestion, they should be assessed for the adequacy of peripheral perfusion. With this approach, each patient with AHF may be placed into one of the four groups presented in Table 12.2.

### Key points about oxygen therapy

Oxygen therapy is not indicated in all patients with AHF.

It is reserved for patients who have a decreased systemic $O_2$ saturation ($O_2$ saturation <90% or $PO_2$ <60 mmHg).

Patients should be monitored with transcutaneous arterial oxygen saturation ($SpO_2$) during oxygen therapy.

Intensive $O_2$ therapy may be dangerous in patients with COPD because hyperoxygenation may suppress ventilation and lead to hypercapnia.

Measurement of PH and $PCO_2$ is advised during oxygen therapy, particularly in patients with COPD or pulmonary edema.

Venous sample would be enough, but in patients with cardiogenic shock, ABG analysis and serum lactate level are preferred.

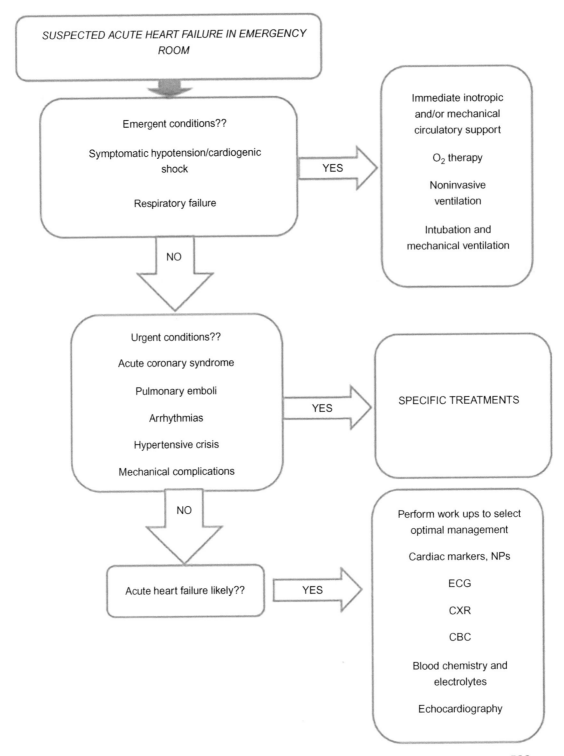

FIG. 12.3 Initial management algorithm for acute heart failure (AHF). *CBC,* complete blood count; *ECG,* electrocardiogram; *ED,* emergency department; *NP,* natriuretic peptide.

**TABLE 12.2**
**Management of Acute Heart Failure Based on Hemodynamic Profile**

| Hemodynamic Profile | Description | Treatment |
|---|---|---|
| Dry and warm | Compensated | Adjust oral medications |
| Dry and cold | Hypoperfused and hypovolemic | IV fluid challenge If failed, start inotrope |
| Wet and warm | Hypertensive (elevated BP) Vascular-type fluid redistribution | Vasodilators Diuretics |
| | Congestive (normal BP) Cardiac-type fluid retention | Diuretic Vasodilators If failed, approach to diuretic resistance |
| Wet and cold | Cardiogenic shock (systolic BP <85 mmHg) | Pharmacologic and/or mechanical circulatory support Address causes |
| | Peripheral hypoperfusion syndrome Systolic BP: 85–110 mmHg and imminent end-organ failure anticipated | Inotrope therapy |

*BP*, blood pressure; *IV*, intravenous.

### Key points about noninvasive positive-pressure ventilation and intubation

To prevent endotracheal intubation, noninvasive positive-pressure ventilation (NIPPV) should be considered as soon as possible in patients with hypoxemia and respiratory distress ($SpO_2$ <90% and respiratory rate >25 breaths/min).

NIPPV should be used with caution in patients with hypotension because it may reduce BP.

If the patient has a respiratory failure refractory to non-invasive management [hypoxemia ($PaO_2$ <60 mmHg), hypercapnia ($PaCO_2$ >50 mmHg),

and acidosis (pH <7.35)], then the patient should be intubated.

For sedation in patients with AHF and cardiogenic shock, midazolam is the preferred drug because of its less cardiac side effects, and it is better to avoid propofol because of its cardiodepressive side effects and hypotension.[1,2,4,7–9]

The routine use of opiates in AHF is not recommended. There are some concerns regarding the increasing mortality risk in patients receiving morphine.

Opiates should be used cautiously in patients with pulmonary edema.[1,2,4]

### Practical points in management of congestion and diuretic therapy[1,3,5,9–15]

1. Intravenous (IV) a loop diuretic is usually the first-line diuretic.
2. The initial dose of loop diuretics in patients who are not receiving oral diuretic (loop diuretic naïve) should be low (20–40 mg of furosemide equivalent intravenously).
3. The initial IV dose of loop diuretic in patients who are chronically receiving oral loop diuretic should be one to two times of 24 h oral home dose intravenously.
4. Patients with renal failure and those with severe congestive symptoms may require higher IV loop diuretic doses.
5. The treatment of congestion in first 24 h of admission can be categorized into the three phases (Fig. 12.4A):
   - Acute treatment phase in which the patient receives intravenous bolus loop diuretic within 1 h of admission
   - Early evaluation phase which is first 6 h after loop diuretic administration
   - Early response phase which is the remaining time of first 24 h
6. Spot urine sodium analysis is a useful tool for evaluating the diuretic response.
7. During IV diuretic therapy, symptoms and signs of congestion, urinary output, body weight, renal function, and serum electrolyte levels (Na, K, Mg) should be regularly and closely monitored.
8. For the second day of admission until discharge the diuretic dose should be adjusted considering the urinary output (Fig. 12.4B).
9. In patients who are presented with severe edema or have refractory symptom despite IV diuretic therapy, combination diuretic therapy is recommended an oral thiazide-type diuretic (metolazone is preferred) is the first line of choice. Acetazolamide or amiloride

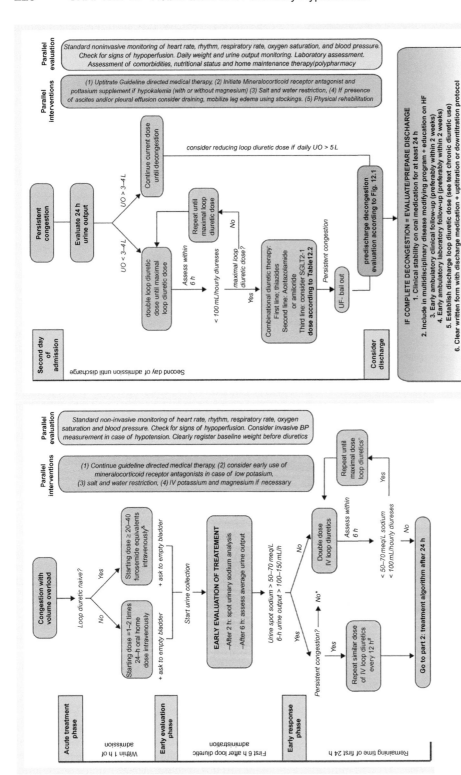

FIG. 12.4 Algorithmic approach to diuretic use in acute heart failure. (A) Congestion with volume overload. (B) Treatment algorithm after 24 h. Total loop diuretic dose can be administered as either bolus infusion or continuous infusion. *BP*, blood pressure; *HF*, heart failure; *IV*, intravenous; *SGLT2-I*, sodium-glucose linked transporter 2 inhibitor; *UF*, ultrafiltration; *UO*, urine output. ^Higher dose should be considered in patients with reduced glomerular filtration rate. *Consider other reasons for dyspnoea given the quick resolution of congestion. °The maximal dose for IV loop diuretics is generally considered furosemide 400–600 or 10–15 mg bumetanide. #In patients with good diuresis following a single loop diuretic administration, once a day dosing can be considered. (From Mullens W, Damman K, Harjola VP, et al. The use of diuretics in heart failure with congestion—a position statement from the Heart Failure Association of the European Society of Cardiology. *Eur J Heart Fail.* 2019;21(2):137–155.)

can be considered as the second choice and sodium-glucose cotransporter-2 (SGLT2) inhibitors as the third choice (Table 12.7).[1,2,4]

**Combination diuretic therapy.** The potential risks and benefits of combination diuretic therapy are presented in Table 12.3. The most commonly used diuretic for combination diuretic therapy (CDT) is metolazone, which is a thiazide-type diuretic. Acetazolamide, which is a carbon anhydrase inhibitor that acts in the proximal tubule, can also be used. Amiloride inhibits the sodium channels of distal nephron and increases urinary output. Sodium-glucose cotransporter-2 (SGLT2) inhibitors are new diabetic drug classes, which inhibit the proximal sodium absorption. The recent studies have shown the beneficial effects of these drugs in patients with heart failure with or without diabetes mellitus.[1,5,10,12,15]

**Key points about combination diuretic therapy**
CDT should be used only in patients with severe fluid overload refractory to adequate doses of IV loop diuretics, particularly patients with decompensated advanced HF and those who have chronic renal failure.

## TABLE 12.3
## Potential Risks and Benefits of Combined Diuretic Therapy

| Adverse Effects | Benefits |
|---|---|
| Electrolyte imbalance<br>• Hypokalemia<br>• Hyponatremia<br>• Hypomagnesemia | Earlier symptomatic improvement<br>• Relief of edema and systemic congestion<br>• Weight loss |
| Hypotension | Overcoming diuretic resistance |
| Hypovolemia or dehydration | Earlier hospital discharge |
| Worsening renal function | Diuresis in chronic renal failure |
| Hypochloremic metabolic alkalosis | Decrease readmission |
| Hyperuricemia | |
| Arrhythmias (secondary to electrolyte imbalance) | |
| Worsening of hepatic encephalopathy | |

There is no general agreement about the adequate dose of loop diuretic, and it should be defined individually. A dose of 160–320 mg/day of IV furosemide or its equivalent is the dose range used in several studies.

Close monitoring of serum electrolytes is very important. Severe hypokalemia and hypomagnesemia may be developed with CDT.

Some increase in serum creatinine level may be seen with CDT, which usually is reversible.

In patients who are severely congested, reduction in creatinine can occur.

Acetazolamide should be used with caution in low glomerular filtration rates (GFRs).

Short-term acetazolamide (1–2 days) in combination with other diuretics may be useful, particularly in patients who have metabolic alkalosis.

**Practical points in intravenous vasodilator therapy**[1,16–18]
1. IV vasodilators are used to reduce congestion and improve symptoms in warm and wet patients.
2. IV vasodilators are the initial therapy in patients with hypertensive AHF (vascular type of fluid redistribution).
3. For symptomatic relief in patients with AHF with congestion (cardiac type of fluid accumulation), IV vasodilators should be considered if the systolic BP (SBP) is greater than 90 mmHg. In patients with low SBP, renal perfusion may be severely diminished, leading to increased risk of renal failure.
4. BP and symptoms should be monitored frequently during administration of IV vasodilators.
5. In patients with significant aortic or mitral stenosis, IV vasodilators should be used with caution.

*Choice of vasodilator in acute heart failure*
Currently available drugs for this purpose are presented in Table 12.4.

**Key points about vasodilator therapy**
For patients with lower SBPs (patients who are not hypertensive), IV nitroglycerin can be started with smaller doses.

Continuous infusion of IV nitrates for more than a few hours is associated with reduced efficacy because of tolerance.

Sodium nitroprusside should be administered almost exclusively in CCUs and sometimes with invasive hemodynamic monitoring. Careful noninvasive BP monitoring is also reasonable.

**TABLE 12.4**
**Currently Available Intravenous Vasodilators**

| Drug Name | Typical Dosage Range | Adjustment Dose | Adverse Effects |
|---|---|---|---|
| Nitroglycerin | 5–200 µg/min | 10–20 µg/min each 5–15 min | Headache, hypotension, flushing |
| Sodium nitroprusside | 0.2–0.5 µg/kg/min | 0.25–0.5 µg/kg/min each 5–15 min | Hypotension, palpitation, arrhythmias, cyanide poisoning |
| Nesiritide | 0.01–0.03 µg/kg/min | No available data Use for more than 48 h is not recommended | Hypotension, rise in creatinine |

Prolonged use of nitroprusside can be rarely associated with thiocyanate toxicity.

Rebound vasoconstriction has been reported after abrupt withdrawal of nitroprusside.

Nesiritide is BNP, a vasodilator that helps sodium and water excretion. Nesiritide has favorable hemodynamic effects; it reduces preload and afterload and increases cardiac output.

**Practical recommendations for the use Inotropes in acute heart failure[1,17–20].** Inotrope therapy in AHF should be reserved for patients with severely reduced cardiac output who are prone to compromised vital organ perfusion. In these patients, an inotrope should be immediately started to restore end-organ perfusion and stabilize the patient's hemodynamics until a definite treatment is planned according to the underlying cause of the shock.

There are two categories of AHF patients who require inotropic therapy:

1. Patients with cardiogenic shock (SBP <85 mmHg)
2. Patients without evidences of cardiogenic shock but with marginal BP (SBP 85–110 mmHg) and signs of peripheral hypoperfusion and deterioration of vital organs (kidney, liver, and brain) function

Currently available inotropes and their dosages are presented in Table 12.5.

Three steps can be considered for the inotrope therapy in a patient with decompensated HF:

1. Step 1: Is there a real need for starting inotrope therapy?
   1. Inotropes should not be used in patients who are hypovolemic. Hypovolemia should always be excluded based on clinical signs and tests of adequate intravascular volume such as lack of IVC collapse, the presence of normal or elevated central venous pressure, negative fluid challenge test (no improvement in blood pressure or cardiac

**TABLE 12.5**
**Currently Available Inotropes**

| Drug Name | Dosage (µg/kg/min) | Pulmonary Vasodilatory Effects |
|---|---|---|
| **INODILATORS** | | |
| Dobutamine | 2–10 | 0–↑ |
| Milrinone | 0.25–0.75 | ↑↑ |
| Levosimendan | 0.05–0.2 | ↑↑ |
| Low-dose dopamine[a] | <3 | 0 |
| **VASOPRESSORS** | | |
| Epinephrine | 0.05–0.5 | 0 |
| Norepinephrine | 0.05–0.4 | 0 |
| High-dose dopamine[a] | >5 | 0 |

[a]Opamine in doses of 3–5 µg/kg/min has inotropic effects.

index accompanied with increasing in filling pressures following a bolus fluid administration), negative passive leg rising test.

2. Inotropes could be used in combination with management of the treatable causes of AHF or as a bridge to casual managements.

2. Step 2: What is the most appropriate inotrope?
   3. The inotropes can be divided into two groups: inodilators and vasopressors (Table 12.5).
   4. Inotropes should be started and continued with the lowest possible doses because of their deleterious effects on survival.
   5. Inodilators are not suitable for patients with an SBP less than 85 mmHg unless in combination with a vasopressor.

6. The combination of a vasopressor plus an inodilator at moderate doses is preferred over any single agent at maximal dosages.

7. Among vasopressor inotropes, norepinephrine has lower mortality rate and fewer side effects than dopamine.

8. Norepinephrine plus levosimendan or dobutamine is the best inotrope choice for cardiogenic shock and septic cardiomyopathy.

9. Epinephrine should be reserved for the last choice if there is persistent hypotension despite the use of other vasopressors and adequate filling pressures.

10. Hypoperfused patients with AHF may not always have an SBP less than 85 mmHg. Some patients with AHF have marginal SBPs (85–110 mmHg) because of significant peripheral vasoconstriction after neurohormonal activation. These patients may have signs of hypoperfusion such as cool extremities, reduced pulse pressure, impaired mentation, decrease in urinary output and worsening renal function (increasing BUN and creatinine), hepatic failure (hepatic enzymes and bilirubin elevation), and hyponatremia. Inodilators (milrinone and levosimendan) are preferred in these patients.

11. Milrinone and levosimendan are also preferred inotropes for reversing the effect of beta blockade.

12. In HF patients with pulmonary hypertension who are candidates for heart transplantation (HTx) and have a high pulmonary vascular resistance (PVR), inodilators (milrinone and levosimendan) are suitable inotropes because these agents have vasodilatory effects in the pulmonary arterial system and help in reducing PVR.

13. Milrinone is not a good choice in ischemic cardiomyopathy because this agent can increase medium-term mortality. Levosimendan and dobutamine are preferred in this setting.

14. In severe takotsubo syndrome, levosimendan is preferred inotrope.

15. Milrinone and levosimendan are not good choices in patients with primary renal insufficiency, and dobutamine is the preferred agent in this setting.

16. In patients with acute cardiorenal syndrome, levosimendan is a good choice because it improves renal blood flow and has renoprotective effects.

17. In patients with AHF and cardiohepatic dysfunction, levosimendan seems to be beneficial.

However, it should not be used in patients who have primary hepatic dysfunction because it has hepatic excretion.

18. Levosimendan and milrinone can be considered for repetitive use for advanced heart failure (see later).

3. Step 3: The proper time to wean the inotrope

19. Alleviation of congestion and improvement of vital signs ($SpO_2$, systolic blood pressure, heart rate, and respiratory rate) and invasive parameters [PCWP, CI, and mixed venous $O_2$ saturation ($SvO_2$)]

20. Improvement of echocardiographic indices

21. Improvement of renal function shown by increasing in urinary output and decreasing BUN, creatinine levels

22. Reduction of serum lactate level

23. During the time of inotrope weaning, standard guideline-directed oral HF treatment should be started, and maximal tolerable doses should be reached after complete weaning from the inotropic support.

24. Some patients are inotropic dependent and are unable to maintain adequate hemodynamics and perfusion without inotropic support despite multiple attempts to withdraw them. These patients are usually supported with inotropes for prolonged periods of time either as a part of palliative strategies for symptomatic relief or as a bridge to transplant or a left ventricular assist device.

### Indications for Invasive and Swan-Ganz Monitoring

The indications for invasive hemodynamic monitoring are discussed in detail in Chapter 11. Some clinical scenarios are presented next.

### First scenario

A 68-year-old man is admitted to the CCU with a diagnosis of severe systolic HF. A pulmonary artery catheter is placed because of developing hypotension. He also has cold extremities and is a little confused. His urinary output has decreased compared with 3 h ago. The initial readings are: BP = 83/56 mmHg, heart rate = 112 beats/min, pulmonary capillary wedge pressure (PCWP) = 18 mmHg, pulmonary artery pressure (PAP) = 34/21 mmHg, right atrial pressure (RAP) = 13 mmHg, cardiac output (CO) = 3.6 L/min, cardiac index (CI) = 2 L/min/m$^2$, stroke volume (SV) = 32 mL.

Based on these measures, milrinone is started at 0.1 μg/kg/min, and the following values are acquired after 1 h: BP = 87/58 mmHg, heart rate = 110 beats/min, PCWP = 20 mmHg, PAP = 36/22 mmHg, RAP = 14 mmHg,    CO = 4.4 L/min,    CI = 2.4 L/min/m$^2$, SV = 40 mL.

The milrinone action as an inotrope was effective in improving the stroke volume. Although there is no change in filling pressures, the improved contractility after the treatment with an inotrope caused an improvement in cardiac output. This example demonstrates that the physician should be careful about both filling pressures (preload) and contractility. The low cardiac output is responsible for hypotension and oliguria (low output state) in this scenario, so it is rational to start an inotrope.

### Second scenario

A 71-year-old woman with a history of acute extensive anterior myocardial infarction becomes hypotensive, and a pulmonary artery catheter is placed for her. The following hemodynamic values are measured: BP = 85/52 mmHg,    HR = 115    beats/min,    RAP = 8 mmHg, PCWP = 14 mmHg,    PAP = 30/17 mmHg,    CO = 3.1 L/min, CI = 1.6 L/min/m$^2$, SV = 27 mL.

About 100 mL of IV fluid (normal saline) is infused over 10 min, and the following values are obtained after 10 min:  BP = 98/60 mmHg,   HR = 104   beats/min, RAP = 12 mmHg,   PCWP = 22 mmHg,   PAP = 40/25 mmHg,        CO = 4.3 L/min,        CI = 2.4 L/min/m$^2$, SV = 41 mL.

This example demonstrates that the increase in preload in a patient who is hypovolemic can increase the stroke volume and cardiac output.

### Key points about renal replacement therapy in acute heart failure[1,5,14,17]

Ultrafiltration (UF) is recommended for renal replacement therapy (RRT) in AHF patients.

UF has no advantage over loop diuretics as first-line therapy in AHF.

UF should be considered for patients with acute renal failure and refractory fluid overload.

Other indications of UF in patients with refractory volume overload include:
- Oliguria unresponsive to fluid replacement
- Severe hyperkalemia (potassium >6.5 mmol/L)
- Severe acidosis (pH <7.2)
- Urea  >150 mg/dL  and  serum  creatinine >3.4 mg/dL[1,2,13,15]

### Some Practical Recommendations About Patients With Acute Heart Failure[1,3,9,11,17,21]

Prophylaxis for thromboembolic events with heparin or other anticoagulants is recommended unless contraindicated.

Thromboembolism prophylaxis is not necessary for patients who are already taking oral anticoagulants.

IV digoxin can be used in patients with AF rhythm who have rapid ventricular response (>110 beats/min) if not used previously.

The IV doses of digoxin are 0.25–0.5 mg and 0.0625–0.125 mg in patients with normal kidney function and moderate to severe renal dysfunction, respectively.

It is better to adjust the maintenance dose of digoxin based on the blood levels of digoxin, particularly in older adults and patients who have other factors affecting  digoxin  metabolism  (e.g.,  other medications).

Patients with fluid overload and resistant hyponatremia can be treated with aquaretics such as tolvaptan.

Sedative and antianxiety medications may be needed in agitated patients. Benzodiazepines should be used with caution in AHF, particularly in those with hepatic impairment.

Pleurocentesis is only recommended for patients who have severe dyspnea caused by massive pleural effusion or if an infectious process or malignancy is needed to be ruled out.

Ascites paracentesis in AHF is indicated in patients with increased intra-abdominal pressure to improve renal function.

### Monitoring the patient's status when admitted for AHF[1,3,11,13,17]

- Routine monitoring of BP, heart rate and pulses, respiratory rate, and temperature should be continued during the hospital stay.
- The patient's daily fluid balance (urinary intake and output) and weight chart should be maintained.
- Routine use of a Foley catheter is not recommended.
- Routine invasive monitoring is not recommended for all patients with AHF except for those with cardiogenic shock.
- BUN, creatinine, and electrolytes should be measured on a daily basis.
- Measurement of NPs at baseline and during the hospital course is helpful for discharge planning. Patients with decrease in their NP levels have a greater than 6 months' prognosis after discharge.[1,2]

### Discharge Plan[1,3–5,11,13,17]

The plan of discharge is made if:
- The patient has stable hemodynamic and is euvolemic for at least 48 h on oral diuretics. Fig. 12.5 shows integrative euvolemia/congestion evaluation at discharge.
- Standard guideline-directed medical treatment has been established.

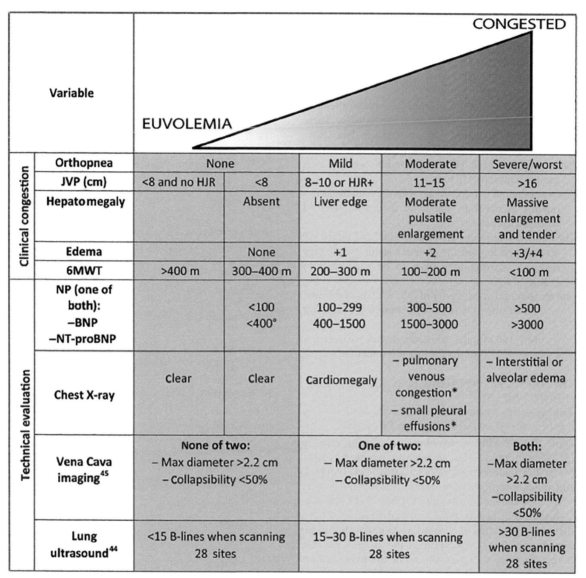

| | Variable | EUVOLEMIA → CONGESTED | | | | |
|---|---|---|---|---|---|---|
| **Clinical congestion** | Orthopnea | None | | Mild | Moderate | Severe/worst |
| | JVP (cm) | <8 and no HJR | <8 | 8–10 or HJR+ | 11–15 | >16 |
| | Hepatomegaly | | Absent | Liver edge | Moderate pulsatile enlargement | Massive enlargement and tender |
| | Edema | | None | +1 | +2 | +3/+4 |
| | 6MWT | >400 m | 300–400 m | 200–300 m | 100–200 m | <100 m |
| **Technical evaluation** | NP (one of both): −BNP −NT-proBNP | | <100 <400° | 100–299 400–1500 | 300–500 1500–3000 | >500 >3000 |
| | Chest X-ray | Clear | Clear | Cardiomegaly | − pulmonary venous congestion* − small pleural effusions* | − Interstitial or alveolar edema |
| | Vena Cava imaging[45] | None of two: − Max diameter >2.2 cm − Collapsibility <50% | | One of two: − Max diameter >2.2 cm − Collapsibility <50% | | Both: −Max diameter >2.2 cm −collapsibility <50% |
| | Lung ultrasound[44] | <15 B-lines when scanning 28 sites | | 15–30 B-lines when scanning 28 sites | | >30 B-lines when scanning 28 sites |

FIG. 12.5 Integrative euvolemia/congestion evaluation at discharge. *6MWT*, 6-min walk test; *BNP*, B-type natriuretic peptide; *HJR*, hepatojugular reflux; *HR*, heart rate; *JVP*, jugular venous pulsation; *NP*, natriuretic peptide; *NT-proBNP*, N-terminal pro-B-type natriuretic peptide; *SBP*, systolic blood pressure. °The cutoff for NT-proBNP to exclude congestion as endorsed by the Heart Failure Association position paper on grading congestion is higher than the cutoff endorsed by the European Society of Cardiology guidelines to exclude acute heart failure. *Chest X-ray can be clear but the presence of abnormalities suggests higher degree of congestion. Partially adapted from the Heart Failure Association position paper on assessing and grading congestion in acute heart failure. (From Mullens W, Damman K, Harjola VP, et al. The use of diuretics in heart failure with congestion—a position statement from the Heart Failure Association of the European Society of Cardiology. *Eur J Heart Fail.* 2019;21(2):137–55.)

- Renal function and serum electrolytes are stable for at least 24 h.
- Essential education and advice about self-care have been provided.

### Key points about discharge plans

Patients should be visited within 1–2 weeks after discharge by a family physician or cardiologist. These patients should have an ambulatory laboratory follow-up at the first after discharge visit.

Patients with chronic HF should be followed up by a multidisciplinary HF team.

It is recommended to follow-up with the patients as frequently as necessary based on their risk to avoid rehospitalization.

The frequency of visits may be individualized by the HF team depending on the patient's status (some very high-risk patients may need to be seen weekly) (Table 12.6).

The recommended frequency of follow-up is as follows:
- At least one or two visits per month for high-risk patients
- Every 1–6 months for moderate-risk patients
- Every 6–12 months for low-risk patients

## THERAPEUTIC APPROACH TO CHRONIC HEART FAILURE[1–5,12,15,17,22]

### Therapeutic Approach to Patients With Heart Failure and Reduced Ejection Fraction

Triple therapy with an angiotensin-converting enzyme (ACE) inhibitor [or an angiotensin receptor blocker (ARB) if ACE inhibitors are not tolerated], beta blockers, and mineralocorticoid receptor antagonists (MRAs) is the base of the standard treatment of HFrEF (LVEF <40%).

It should be kept in mind that in patients who have signs and symptoms of congestion, diuretics should be started as the first step to optimize the patient's volume status. The dose of diuretic should be titrated based on the patient's signs and symptoms.

The treatment is started with an ACE inhibitor (or ARB) and beta blocker, and if the patient remains symptomatic despite uptitration of the beta blocker and ACE (or ARB) to the maximally tolerated dose, an MRA is introduced. Because both drugs exert effects on serum creatinine and potassium, it is recommended that an MRA is added when the ACE inhibitor titration is completed. It is advised that the titration of the recommended drugs to their maximally tolerated dose be completed within 4–6 months.

### Novel therapies

According to the latest guidelines, ivabradine and angiotensin receptor antagonists plus neprilysin inhibitors (ARNIs) are recommended for eligible patients.

**TABLE 12.6**
**Risk Groups of Heart Failure Patients for Follow-up Programs**

| High Risk | Intermediate Risk | Low Risk |
|---|---|---|
| Stage D of heart failure who are highly symptomatic (NYHA class of IIIb–IV, frequent symptomatic hypotension) | Patients have no clear features of low or high risk | Asymptomatic patients (NYHA class of I–II) with are optimal guideline-directed medical therapies with no history of hospitalization in past year |
| History of frequent hospitalization or recent admission in past month | | |
| Patients who have nonadherence to their therapies and diet | | |
| New-onset HF | | |
| During up- and downtitration of HF medications | | |
| Patients with complications of treatment such as electrolyte imbalance and worsening renal function | | |
| Patients with comorbidities such as renal failure or chronic lung diseases | | |
| History of frequent ICD firing | | |

*HF,* heart failure; *ICD,* implantable cardioverter defibrillator; *NYHA,* New York Heart Association.

The algorithmic approach for evidence-based therapy in HFrEF is shown in Fig. 12.6.

### Diuretics

The initial doses and maximal doses of loop diuretics in patients with normal GFRs and renal insufficiency are depicted in Table 12.7.

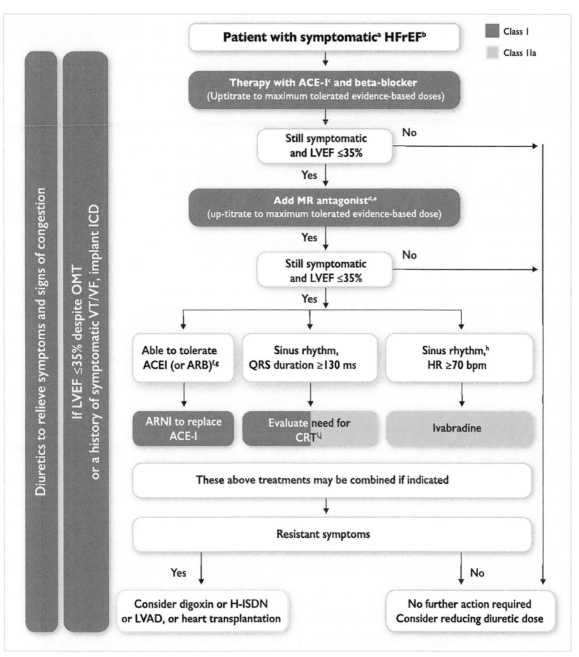

FIG. 12.6 Therapeutic algorithm for a patient with symptomatic heart failure with reduced ejection fraction. *Green* indicates a class I recommendation and *yellow* indicates a class IIa recommendation. *ACEI*, angiotensin-converting enzyme inhibitor; *ARB*, angiotensin receptor blocker; *ARNI*, angiotensin receptor neprilysin inhibitor; *BNP*, B-type natriuretic peptide; *CRT*, cardiac resynchronization therapy; *HF*, heart failure; *HFrEF*, heart failure with reduced ejection fraction; *H-ISDN*, hydralazine and isosorbide dinitrate; *HR*, heart rate; *ICD*, implantable cardioverter defibrillator; *LBBB*, left bundle branch block; *LVAD*, left ventricular assist device; *LVEF*, left ventricular ejection fraction; *MR*, mineralocorticoid receptor; *NT-proBNP*, N-terminal pro-B-type natriuretic peptide; *NYHA*, New York Heart Association; *OMT*, optimal medical therapy; *VF*, ventricular fibrillation; *VT*, ventricular tachycardia. [a]Symptomatic, NYHA class II-IV. [b]HFrEF, LVEF, 40%. [c]If ACE inhibitor not

**TABLE 12.7**
Currently Available Diuretics Recommended in Heart Failure

| Drug Class | Potency FENa%[a] | Starting Dose/Usual Chronic Dose | Maximum Total Recommended Daily Dose |
|---|---|---|---|
| **LOOP DIURETICS** | | | |
| Dose of intravenous and oral loop diuretics are similar | | | |
| Furosemide | | 20–40 mg/40–240 mg | 400–600 mg |
| Bumetanide | | 0.5–1 mg/1–5 mg | 10–15 mg |
| Torsemide | | 5–10 mg/10–20 mg | 200–300 mg |
| **THIAZIDE-LIKE DIURETICS** | | | |
| Only PO use in acute HF | | | |
| Hydrochlorothiazide | | 25 mg/12.5–100 mg | 200 mg |
| Chlorthalidone | | 12.5–25 mg/25–200 mg | 100 mg |
| Chlorothiazide (IV formulation available) | | 250–500 mg | 1000 mg |
| Indapamide | | 2.5 mg | 5 mg |
| Metolazone | | 2.5 mg/2.5–10 mg | 20 mg |
| **CARBONIC ANHYDRASE INHIBITOR** | | | |
| Acetazolamide | | Oral: 250–375 mg Intravenous: 500 mg | Oral: 500 mg 3×/day Intravenous: 500 mg 3×/day |
| **MINERALOCORTICOID RECEPTOR ANTAGONISTS (MRA)** | | | |
| Spironolactone | | 12.5–25 mg | |
| Eplerenone | | 12.5–25 mg | |
| Potassium canrenoate Intravenous form of MRA not for chronic use | | 25–200 mg | 50–100 mg Up to 400 mg can be used in hepatic patients |
| **POTASSIUM-SPARING DIURETICS** | | | |
| Amiloride | | 5 mg | 20 mg |
| Triamterene | | 50–75 mg | 200 mg |

[a]Defined in non-HF patients. FENa = 100 × (urine sodium × serum creatinine)/(serum sodium × urine creatinine). FENa is the percentage of the sodium filtered by the kidney and excreted in the urine. In clinical use, FENa can be a surrogate of diuretic effectiveness. The normal value depends on the glomerular filtration rate of the patient. It is commonly <2% in patients with relatively intact renal function. Diuretic agents increase FENa.

tolerated/contraindicated, use ARB. [d]If MR antagonist not tolerated/contraindicated, use ARB. [e]With a hospital admission for HF within the last 6 months or with elevated natriuretic peptides (BNP 250 pg/mL or NT-proBNP 500 pg/mL in men and 750 pg/mL in women). [f]With an elevated plasma natriuretic peptide level (BNP ≤ 150 pg/mL or plasma NT-proBNP ≤ 600 pg/mL), or if HF hospitalization within recent 12 months plasma (BNP ≤ 100 pg/mL or plasma NT-proBNP ≥ 400 pg/mL). [g]In doses equivalent to enalapril 10 mg bid. [h]With a hospital admission for HF within the previous year. [i]CRT is recommended if QRS ≤ 130 ms and LBBB (in sinus rhythm). [j]CRT should/may be considered if QRS ≥ 130 ms with non-LBBB (in a sinus rhythm) or for patients in AF provided a strategy to ensure biventricular capture in place (individualized decision). For further details, see Sections 7 and 8 and corresponding web pages. (From Ponikowski P, Voors AA, Anker SD, et al. 2016 ESC guidelines for the diagnosis and treatment of acute and chronic heart failure: the task force for the diagnosis and treatment of acute and chronic heart failure of the European Society of Cardiology (ESC) developed with the special contribution of the Heart Failure Association (HFA) of the ESC. *Eur Heart J.* 2016;37(27):2129–200; with permission.)

## Practical points about diuretics

Diuretics are an essential component of treatment in HF patients who are overloaded.

The goal of diuretic therapy is to decrease and eliminate signs and symptoms of fluid overload, while adverse effects are monitored.

Diuretics cannot exert their full effects without sodium restriction.

The optimum sodium intake in the setting of HF is unknown, but experts suggest less than 3 g/day of sodium restriction in patients with symptomatic HF.

Patients with refractory HF should have fluid restriction, particularly those who have worsening or severe hyponatremia (Na <125 mg/dL).

Using an oral loop diuretic accompanied by a low-sodium diet is the initial step in the treatment of congestion in patients with HF.

The diuretic response in patients with HF is less than in normal individuals for several reasons:

1. The renal blood flow is reduced in HF, so diuretic delivery to the kidney is decreased.
2. The sodium reabsorption at other sites of renal tubules is increased because of activation of renin–angiotensin–aldosterone and sympathetic nervous systems because of renal hypoperfusion.
3. In HF patients who have significant edema, intestinal absorption of oral loop diuretics may be delayed, and there is a lower serum peak concentration of drug leading to reduced diuretic effect.

Furosemide is the most commonly used diuretic in HF and is usually the first step. The starting dose of furosemide for patients without prior loop diuretic therapy is 20–40 mg once or twice a day. Further dosing is adjusted after considering the diuretic response, and the initial dose can be increased. If the patient achieves dry body weight, the diuretic dose should be adjusted to the minimum dose required to maintain dry body weight.

Dosing in patients with prior IV loop diuretic therapy is based on the response to the IV therapy. The oral dose of furosemide is almost twice the IV dose.

The bioavailability of oral furosemide has a range from 10% to 100% (average ≈50%), so the response to furosemide may be inadequate. If the diuretic response is suboptimal, diuretic therapy can be switched to torsemide or bumetanide, which have better absorption and bioavailability. Torsemide has longer half-life than bumetanide and furosemide.

If a patient does not respond to the maximum oral doses of loop diuretic, then IV doses may be prescribed. In carefully selected patients with refractory edema, combination diuretic therapy may be started to prevent hospitalization.

Careful monitoring of kidney function (BUN and creatinine) and serum electrolytes is recommended in patients receiving diuretics, particularly in those who are taking high doses. Serum BUN and creatinine often increase during diuretic therapy. Nonsteroidal antiinflammatory drugs (NSAIDs) should be avoided in patients with HF because they interfere with the response to their medication, particularly diuretics.

## *Angiotensin-converting enzyme inhibitors and angiotensin receptor antagonists*

The types and doses of ACE inhibitors and ARBs are presented in Table 12.8.

## Key points about angiotensin-converting enzyme inhibitors and angiotensin receptor antagonists

ACE inhibitors and ARBs should be given to all HFrEF patients to reduce the risk of death and HF hospitalization unless there is a remarkable intolerance or contraindication.

ACE inhibitors and ARBs should begin at a low dose and slowly increase to the target dose as tolerated. Doubling the dose should not be done sooner than 2 weeks in outpatient settings. If the patient is hospitalized or is under close observation, uptitration can be faster. The maximum tolerated dose should be continued in patients with HF.

Serum potassium and BUN and creatinine levels should be checked 1–2 weeks after each dose adjustment.

The diuretic dose should be optimally adjusted to maintain the proper fluid balance. Overdiuresis compromises renal function and leads to electrolyte imbalance and hypotension, so uptitration of ACE inhibitors and ARBs will not be possible.

In patients who have severe volume overload, particularly if renal failure or hypotension is present, it is recommended to reduce or temporarily discontinue the ACE inhibitors or ARBs until the patient's condition becomes stable.

In the setting of volume depletion (e.g., diarrhea, dehydration, and blood loss), it may be necessary to discontinue ACE inhibitors or ARBs because an acute decrease in angiotensin II in this setting may lead to severe hypotension.

NSAIDs should not be prescribed for HF patients because they may interfere with the effects of ACE inhibitors or ARBs.

**TABLE 12.8**
**Currently Available Disease-Modifying Drugs for Heart Failure With Reduced Ejection Fraction**

| Drug Class | Starting Dose | Maximum Dose |
|---|---|---|
| **BETA BLOCKERS** | | |
| Bisoprolol | 1.25 mg OD | 10 mg OD |
| Metoprolol succinate | 12.5–25 mg OD | 200 mg OD |
| Carvedilol | 3.125 mg bid | 25 mg bid |
| Nebivolol | 1.25 mg OD | 10 mg OD |
| **ACE INHIBITORS** | | |
| Captopril | 6.25 mg tid | 50 mg TDS |
| Enalapril | 2.5 mg bid | 10–20 mg bid |
| Lisinopril | 2.5–5 mg OD | 20–40 mg OD |
| Ramipril | 1.25–2.5 mg OD | 10 mg OD |
| Trandolapril | 0.5 mg OD | 4 mg OD |
| **ARBS** | | |
| Losartan | 50 mg OD | 150 mg OD |
| Valsartan | 40 mg bid | 160 mg bid |
| Candesartan | 4–8 mg OD | 32 mg OD |
| **MRAS** | | |
| Spironolactone | 25 mg OD | 50 mg OD |
| Eplerenone | 25 mg OD | 50 mg OD |
| **ARNIS** | | |
| Sacubitril/valsartan | 49/51 mg bid | 97/103 mg bid |
| **IF CHANNEL BLOCKER** | | |
| Ivabradine | 5 mg bid | 7.5 mg bid |

ACE, angiotensin-converting enzyme; ARNI, angiotensin receptor antagonists plus neprilysin inhibitor; bid, twice a day; MRA, mineralocorticoid receptor antagonist; OD, daily.

Adverse effects of ACE inhibitors include hypotension, cough, angioedema, rash, hyperkalemia, renal insufficiency, neutropenia, taste disturbances, and fetal abnormalities.

Hypotension may be present at the initiation of therapy, and it is not necessary to abandon the drug. Patients should be reassured that dizziness and lightheadedness improve with time. To control hypotensive symptoms, as a first step, other vasodilators such as nitrates or calcium channel blockers (CCBs) should be withheld. The patient should be assessed regarding volume status, and downtitration of diuretics can be considered. If the patient has symptomatic postural hypotension, decreasing or discontinuing the drug is recommended. In patients who are prone to develop hyperkalemia, the potassium level should be carefully monitored.

The risk factors for hyperkalemia are diabetes mellitus, renal insufficiency, the use of MRAs or potassium-sparing diuretics, high potassium diets, and using low-sodium salts with high K content. Mild fluctuations in serum potassium levels (<5.5 mmol/L is acceptable) are often self-limited and can be carefully followed without any change in ACE inhibitor or ARB doses.

Azotemia may be seen with ACE inhibitor or ARB therapy and does not mean therapy must be discontinued. Mild azotemia can be well tolerated by many HF patients, and stopping other nephrotoxic drugs (NSAIDs) and reducing diuretic dose (if the patient is not congested) help recovery of kidney function. Up to a 50% increase in serum creatinine, above baseline is acceptable.

Renal insufficiency with ACE inhibitor or ARB therapy is more common in patients with more severe symptoms and higher New York Heart Association (NYHA) class. Development of renal insufficiency after the initiation of ACE inhibitors or ARB therapy warrants further evaluation for bilateral renal artery stenosis. It is recommended to consider dose adjustment of ACE inhibitors or ARBs if the serum creatinine increases by more than 50% and discontinuing the drug if serum creatinine increases by more than 100%. In patients who cannot be given ACE inhibitors or ARBs because of renal insufficiency, the combination of isosorbide dinitrate and hydralazine may be considered to reduce the risk of death.

Up to 40%–50% of patients on ACE inhibitor therapy may develop chronic dry cough. It is more common in women and Asian people. There is no need to withdraw the drug in the presence of mild cough. It should be kept in mind that cough may be caused by congestion of the lung, which warrants intensification of therapy rather than withdrawal of therapy. If it is proved that the cough is due to an ACE inhibitor (recurred after ACE inhibitor withdrawal and rechallenge) and cannot be tolerated, then the ACE inhibitor can be replaced with an ARB.

Angioedema is very rare (0.1%–0.2% of patients), but if it occurs the drug should be permanently discontinued and avoided. The safety of ARBs in patients who experience angioedema with ACE inhibitors is uncertain.

Contraindications of ACE inhibitors and ARB include bilateral renal artery stenosis, history of angioedema and known drug allergy, and pregnancy.

ARBs are recommended in HF patients who cannot tolerate ACE inhibitors accompanied by beta blockers and MRAs.[1–3] ARBs may be considered in combination with ACE inhibitors in symptomatic HF patients receiving beta blockers who cannot tolerate MRAs. This combination should be used under strict supervision.

### Beta blockers

The types and doses of approved beta blockers for HFrEF are presented in Table 12.8.

### Key points on beta blockers

Beta blockers are recommended for all HFrEF patients (symptomatic and asymptomatic) who are on standard therapy with ACE inhibitors and optimal doses of diuretics to reduce risk of death and HF hospitalization. Beta blockers and ACE inhibitors should be started together. Beta blockers should be started in patients who are clinically stable and their fluid overload is controlled (euvolemic and compensated state).

It is recommended to start beta blockers at low doses and uptitrate slowly to the maximum tolerated dose. There should be at least 2-week intervals between each dose adjustment, and patients should be reevaluated at each titration for worsening HF symptoms (increasing edema and dyspnea, fatigue, and weight gain). Uptitration of beta blockers may be slower in some patients.

The first step in the setting of increasing congestive signs and symptoms is increasing the diuretic dose. If the increased diuretic dose does not work, the beta-blocker dose should be halved.

If a patient taking a beta blocker develops severe fatigue, the beta-blocker dose should be halved, and the patient should be reevaluated 1–2 weeks later.

In the setting of severe decompensation, the beta-blocker dose should be halved, or the treatment should be stopped.

Asymptomatic hypotension does not require beta-blocker dose adjustment. To control hypotensive symptoms, as a first step, other vasodilators such as nitrates or CCBs should be held. The patient should be assessed regarding volume status, and downtitration of diuretics may be considered if the patient is euvolemic. The reduction of ACE inhibitor dose may allow continuing beta blockers in patients with orthostatic hypotension. Low doses of both drugs are preferred to one of them.

In the setting of bradycardia (heart rate <50 beats/min) and worsening symptoms, the beta-blocker dose should be halved. In severely symptomatic patients with bradycardia, beta blockers should be stopped. In patients taking beta blockers who have bradycardia, it is better to reduce or hold the other rate-lowering drugs such as digoxin and amiodarone.

Contraindications of beta blockers
1. High-degree atrioventricular (AV) blocks (second- and third-degree AV block) in the absence of a pacemaker
2. Asthma: In patients with asthma, beta$_1$-selective blockers may be used with careful and closed monitoring
3. Critical limb ischemia
4. Known allergy to the drug

### Mineralocorticoid antagonists

Mineralocorticoid antagonists should be given to all HFrEF patients (LVEF <35%) who are persistently symptomatic despite treatment with beta blockers and ACE inhibitors to reduce mortality and HF hospitalization.[1–3] Currently available MRAs are spironolactone and eplerenone (see Table 12.8).

### Key points on mineralocorticoid antagonists

The drug should be initiated at low doses and uptitrated to the target dose over 4–8 weeks. BUN, creatinine, and electrolytes (potassium) should be checked at 1 and 4 weeks after starting or dose adjustment and at 2, 3, 6, 9, and 12 months and each 4 months thereafter.

The main concern about MRAs is hyperkalemia, which is more common in patients with renal insufficiency. If the potassium rises above 5.5 mmol/L or creatinine is more than 2.5 mg/dL (GFR <30 mL/min/1.73 m$^2$), the prescribed dose should be halved, with careful and close follow-up for creatinine and potassium.

MRAs should be immediately stopped if potassium rises to more than 6 mmol/L or creatinine is more than 3.5 mg/dL (GFR <20 mL/min/1.73 m$^2$).

If a patient has vomiting, diarrhea, or excessive sweating caused by infection and fever, electrolyte imbalance should be carefully monitored.

Triple therapy with an ACE inhibitor, ARB, and MRAs is not recommended.

The initial diuretic dose of MRAs in combination with ACE inhibitors or ARBs is 12.5–25 mg/day and can be uptitrated to a maximum of 50 mg/day.

If a patient is not already taking an ACE inhibitor or ARB, the MRAs can be uptitrated to 100–200 mg/day as a diuretic.

Drug allergy is a contraindication of MRAs.

Interactions with the following drugs should be kept in mind when a patient is given an MRA: NSAIDs, cotrimoxazole, ACE inhibitors, ARBs, renin inhibitors, K$^+$ supplements, K$^+$-sparing diuretics, high K salts, and CYP3A4 inhibitors, including ketoconazole, itraconazole, nefazodone, clarithromycin, telithromycin, and HIV protease inhibitors (ritonavir and nelfinavir).

Spironolactone should be switched to eplerenone if a male patient develops breast discomfort or gynecomastia.

### Key points about ivabradine

Ivabradine is recommended in stable symptomatic HFrEF patients (LVEF <35%) who have sinus rhythm and a heart rate greater than 70 beats/min when an ACE inhibitor, ARB, beta blocker, or MRA is given to the maximal tolerated dose.[1-3]

The starting dose is 5 mg twice a day; the target dose is 7.5 mg twice a day.

Drug should be started with a low dose and up- or downtitrated depending on the patient's resting heart rate (from 2.5 mg twice a day to 7.5 mg twice a day).

In patients older than 75 years, ivabradine should be started with 2.5 mg twice a day.

Ivabradine is well tolerated, particularly in those with lower BPs, and can be titrated over 2–4 weeks. The drug should be stopped if the resting heart rate is less than 50 beats/min or there is symptomatic bradycardia.

In the setting of bradycardia:
- Rhythm disturbances other than sinus bradycardia should be excluded.
- Secondary causes of bradyarrhythmias such as hypothyroidism should be excluded.
- Other rhythm-lowering drugs (CCBs, digoxin, and amiodarone) should be adjusted.
- Drugs with liver metabolism interfering with ivabradine should be reviewed and adjusted. These drugs include antifungal azoles (e.g., ketoconazole and itraconazole), macrolide antibiotics (e.g., clarithromycin and erythromycin), nefazodone, and HIV protease inhibitors (ritonavir and nelfinavir).

Contraindications for ivabradine:
- ACS
- Cardiogenic shock and severe hypotension
- Cerebrovascular events and transient ischemic attack
- Severe renal and liver dysfunction
- Pregnancy and breastfeeding
- Allergy to the drug

### Key points about angiotensin receptor antagonist/neprilysin inhibitors

Sacubitril/valsartan is a replacement for ACE inhibitors and ARBs in patients with HFrEF who remain symptomatic despite optimal medical treatment with beta blockers, ACE inhibitors, ARBs, and MRA to reduce the risk of hospitalization and death.

The starting dose is 49/51 mg twice a day and the target dose is 97/103 mg twice a day.

ARNIs should not been used in the setting of symptomatic hypotension, history of angioedema, or severe hepatic and renal impairment. This drug should not be used concomitantly with an ACE inhibitor. It should not be administered within 36 h of switching from or to an ACE inhibitor. A 24-h washout period is needed before switching from an ARB to an ARNI.

It should not be used concomitantly with aliskiren in patients with diabetes.

It should be stopped when pregnancy is detected.

Adverse effects include hyperkalemia, hypotension, and renal failure.

It can increase lithium levels and predispose patients to lithium toxicity, so careful monitoring of serum lithium level is needed.

### Some practical points on other treatments in HFrEF

Isosorbide/hydralazine should not be used in all patients with HFrEF. It can be added to the treatment with beta blockers, ACE inhibitors, ARBs, and MRAs in African blacks if they remain symptomatic to reduce hospitalization and death. Isosorbide/hydralazine can be used in patients who have contraindication of ACE inhibitors or ARBs or cannot tolerate them.

Digoxin is recommended for patients with symptomatic HFrEF and sinus rhythm to reduce hospitalization. In HFrEF patients with AF rhythm, digoxin is recommended if there is a rapid ventricular response. It should not be used if the ventricular response is appropriate. Digoxin should be prescribed with an adjusted dose and under careful supervision, in particular in older adults, women, and patients with renal impairment.

Aliskiren (a direct renin inhibitor) is not recommended in HFrEF patients.

Anticoagulant therapy with warfarin in HFrEF patients is only recommended in patients with AF rhythm.

There is not enough evidence for using nonvitamin K antagonist oral anticoagulants (NOACs) in patients with advanced HFrEF who may have marginal liver and kidney function.

ASA is only recommended in patients with concomitant coronary artery disease.

There is not enough evidence for using vitamins and dietary supplements in patients with HF.

The only guideline-recommended supplement is omega-3.

There is some evidence about the usefulness of Co Q10 in patients with ischemic cardiomyopathy.[23]

HF patients should be vaccinated against influenza every year and against pneumococcal infections every 5 years.

**Practical points about the frequency of performing laboratory tests in heart failure patients[1,3,4]**

BUN, creatinine, and serum electrolytes should be measured every 1–3 months in stable patients (in some high-risk patients during each follow-up visit).

BUN, creatinine, and serum electrolytes should be measured within 5–7 days of intensification of diuretic dose and within 7–10 days of ACE inhibitor, ARB, or MRA initiation or dose adjustment.

Potassium should be measured within 3–5 days after a high potassium measurement (>5–5.5 mmol/L).

*Heart failure comorbidities*[1,3,4,24–26]

The iron deficiency and muscle wasting (cachexia and sarcopenia) have currently considered as important comorbidities, which need to be considered in follow-up and management of patients with heart failure.

**Iron deficiency and heart failure.** Iron deficiency is seen in up to 60% of patients with HF and, regardless of the presence of anemia or severity of HF, is associated with significant mortality and morbidity.

**Definitions.** Absolute ID is a ferritin level equal to or less than 100 µg/L. Functional ID is a ferritin level between 100 and 299 µg/L with transferrin saturation less than 20%.[2,21]

**Key points about iron therapy in heart failure**

IV or oral iron supplements should be initiated for patients with documented ID with a goal of improving symptoms, functional capacity, and quality of life.

Ferric carboxymaltose is the drug of choice in IV iron therapy, but other IV iron agents can be used.

Serious side effects, including anaphylactic reactions, may be seen with use of iron dextran.

Oral iron supplements are usually intolerable because of gastrointestinal side effects. There is some evidence that shows polysaccharide iron complexes can be well tolerated in patients with HF and are effective in increasing ferritin level.

The erythropoiesis-stimulating agents should not be routinely used to treat anemia in HF because of the increased risk of thromboembolic events with use of these drugs.

Patients with end-stage kidney disease and anemia should be referred to a nephrologist for optimal therapy of anemia.

**Cachexia and sarcopenia.** The muscle mass declines by 1%–2% annually and the muscle strength decreases by 1.5% after 50 years. There are four main reasons for loss of muscle mass; sarcopenia, cachexia, anorexia, and dehydration.

Cachexia is a generalized wasting process affecting all body compartments [lean tissue (skeletal muscle), fat tissue (energy reserves), and bone tissue (osteoporosis)]. It may occur in 5%–15% of patients with HF, especially those with HFrEF, and more advanced disease status. Cachexia in HF can be defined as involuntary non-edematous weight loss 6% or greater of body weight within the previous 6–12 months.

Skeletal muscle wasting or sarcopenia occurs in 30%–50% of patients with HF particularly in those with reduced LVEF. Sarcopenia can be seen in patients with HF even before age 50 and in its most severe form it is associated with frailty and poor morbidity and mortality.

The sarcopenia is diagnosed when a patient has both low muscle mass and low gait speed.

Dual-energy X-ray absorptiometry (DXA) is currently considered the gold standard. Other diagnostic methods for measurement of skeletal muscle mass are bioelectrical impedance, computed tomography, magnetic resonance imaging, urinary excretion of creatinine, anthropometric assessments, and neutron activation assessments.

**Treatment approaches to sarcopenia.** Exercise and physical activity accompanied with nutritional interventions are important considerations for both sarcopenia prophylaxis and sarcopenia management. Other therapeutic approaches include the use of growth hormones, testosterone, estrogens, and vitamin D.

**Advanced heart failure[27].** All the following criteria should be present despite optimal guideline-directed therapies for the identification of patients with advanced heart failure are:

1. Persistent and severe symptoms of HF (NYHA functional class of III or IV).
2. Severe cardiac dysfunction defined by an LVEF ≤30% or isolated severe RV failure by any cause or nonoperable severe valvular or congenital abnormalities or persistently high (or increasing) NT-proBNP or BNP values and data of severe diastolic dysfunction or left ventricular structural abnormalities according to the definition of HFpEF and HFmrEF.
3. Episodes of systemic or pulmonary congestion requiring high-dose intravenous diuretics (or combination diuretic therapy) or episodes of low output state requiring inotropes or vasoactive drugs or malignant arrhythmias causing more than one unplanned visit or hospital admission in the last 12 months.
4. Severe impairment of functional capacity with inability to exercise or a 6 min' walk distance (6MWD) less than 300 m or peak $VO_2$ (<12–14 mL/kg/min), estimated to be of cardiac origin.

In addition to the above, extra-cardiac organ dysfunction due to heart failure (e.g., cardiac cachexia, liver, or renal dysfunction) or type 2 pulmonary hypertension (see later) may be present, but are not required.

Criteria 1 and 4 can be met in patients who have cardiac dysfunction (as described in criterion #2), but who also have substantial limitation due to other diseases (most commonly by kidney disease or severe pulmonary disease, chronic liver disease, or noncardiac cirrhosis). These patients have also limited quality of life and survival due to advanced disease and can be considered as advanced heart failure, however, the therapeutic options for these patients are usually more limited.

It is recommended that clinical cardiologists refer these patients for advanced heart failure therapies to specialized advanced heart failure centers before their clinical conditions worsen greatly because the surgical risk increases dramatically in patients with advanced conditions.

The Interagency Registry for Mechanically Assisted Circulatory Support (INTERMACS) profiles (Table 12.9) are also useful to further describe clinical parameters and characteristics consistent with a need for advanced therapies.

Advanced heart failure therapies refer to long-term mechanical circulatory support (MCS) or heart transplantation (HTx). However, short-term therapies may be needed in situations where the patient's clinical condition deteriorates, or end-organ dysfunction develops,

**TABLE 12.9**

**Interagency Registry for Mechanically Assisted Circulatory Support (INTERMACS) Classification for Patients With Advanced Heart Failure**

| INTERMACS Level | Description |
|---|---|
| 1. Critical cardiogenic shock: crash and burn | Patient has unstable hemodynamics, life-threatening hypotension, and vital organ hypoperfusion |
| 2. Progressive decline | Patient is dependent on inotropic support but shows signs of continuing renal dysfunction, refractory fluid retention, and deterioration of nutrition |
| 3. Stable but inotrope dependent | Patient is stable on mild to moderate doses of inotropes or temporary mechanical circulatory support but is dependent on support |
| 4. Resting symptoms | Patient is on oral medications and has weaned from inotropic support but frequently has symptoms of congestion at rest or with daily living activities |
| 5. Exertion intolerant | Patient is stable at rest but unable to perform any activity and may have chronic volume overload frequently with renal dysfunction |
| 6. Exertion limited | Patient is stable at rest with no evidence of congestion and can do minor activities |
| 7. Advanced NYHA class 3 | Patient is at NYHA class III with no recent (during previous month) decompensation history |

*NYHA*, New York Heart Association.

while the patient is waiting for HTx or until MCS can be implanted.

The short-term therapies include temporary MCS or repetitive inotrope ±IV diuretic therapy.

Inotropes can be used as short-term therapy in patients with low cardiac output and evidence of end-organ dysfunction, accompanied with the strategies used for decongestion (see earlier).

The repetitive inotrope ±IV diuretic therapy can be used as palliative therapy where MCS is not available and the patient cannot be a candidate for HTx.

Temporary MCSs include intra-aortic balloon pump (IABP), extracorporeal membrane oxygenation (ECMO), TandemHeart percutaneous ventricular assist device, Impella ventricular support systems, and Centri-Mag acute circulatory support system.

The muscle wasting or sarcopenia, defined as aging-related muscle mass loss, is generally considered a problem in people aged 60 years and above.

### Indications for Heart Transplantation and Mechanical Circulatory Support[1–3,27–29]

#### Current indications for heart transplantation

The decision for HTx in acute settings should be made by a multidisciplinary team. The INTERMACS profile (Table 12.9) and the heart failure prognostic models can be used to support clinical decision-making and estimate the risk of transplantation in urgent situation.

Listing should be based on both cardiopulmonary exercise test and HF prognostic score calculator results.

HF prognostic score calculators include the Seattle Heart Failure Model (SHFM; http://depts.washington.edu/shfm), Heart Failure Survival Score (HFSS; http://www.mortalityscore.org/heart_failure), Meta-Analysis Global Group in Chronic Heart Failure (MAGGIC; https://www.mdcalc.com/maggic-risk-calculator-heart-failure), and metabolic exercise test data combined with cardiac and kidney indexes (MECKI).

Right heart catheterization should be performed for all HTX candidates before listing.

Obese candidates [body mass index (BMI) $>35$ kg/m$^2$] should lose weight to achieve a BMI of 35 kg/m$^2$ or less.

HTx should be considered for the following unstable patients unless there are contraindications:

Severe refractory cardiogenic shock requiring high-dose inotropic support or short-term MCS and when a long-term assist device cannot be considered for a patient.

Patients with long-term MCS who have developed MCS-related complications that cannot be resolved or MCS replacement is impossible.

In ambulatory chronic heart failure setting, HTx should be considered for the following patients unless there are contraindications:

The presence of a peak VO$_2$ 12 mL/kg/min or less in HF patients receiving beta blockers and 14 mL/kg/min or less in HF patients intolerant to beta blockers.

In women and young patients ($<50$ years), the percent of predicted peak VO$_2$ ($\leq50\%$) should also be considered in conjunction with peak VO$_2$.

The presence of a ventilation equivalent of carbon dioxide (VE/Vco$_2$) slope of greater than 35 in the presence of a submaximal cardiopulmonary exercise test (CPX) test [respiratory exchange ratio (RER) $<1.05$].

Patients with an estimated 1-year survival of less than 80% calculated by the SHFM or medium or high risk for mortality in HFSS should be listed.

Severe or intractable angina chest pain in patients with CAD who cannot be revascularized.

Intractable life-threatening arrhythmias unresponsive to medical therapy, catheter ablation, or implantation of an ICD.

Hypertrophic cardiomyopathy, restrictive cardiomyopathy, or right-sided cardiomyopathies refractory or unresponsive to medical management.

#### Contraindications for heart transplantation

Fixed pulmonary hypertension; PVR greater than six Wood units

Active or recent solid organ or blood malignancy within 5 years

AIDS

Sepsis

Systemic lupus erythematosus, sarcoidosis, or amyloidosis

Irreversible renal (GFR $<30$ mL/min/1.73 m$^2$) or hepatic dysfunction unless concomitant kidney or liver transplantation is considered

Significant obstructive pulmonary disease (forced expiratory volume in 1 s $<1$ L/min)

Severe diabetes mellitus with end-organ damage

Clinical severe peripheral vascular or cerebrovascular disease

Substance abuse

Psychosocial problems

#### Current indications for mechanical circulatory support in acute and chronic heart failure[1,3,28]

Bridge to decision (BTD)/bridge to bridge (BTB): Short-term MCS (e.g., ECMO) for patients with cardiogenic shock until stabilization of hemodynamics and vital organ perfusion. The management team will have enough time to evaluate the patient for HTx or long-term MCSs and exclude contraindications for HTx or long-term assist device.

Bridge to candidacy (BTC): MCS [usually left ventricular assist device (LVAD)] in an end-stage HF patient who has a relative contraindication for HTx to make him or her eligible for HTx.

Bridge to transplantation (BTT): LVAD or biventricular assist device (BiVAD) for an advanced HF patient who is at high risk for death to keep him or her alive until a donor organ becomes available.

Bridge to recovery (BTR): MCS (usually LVAD) in patient with reversible HF (e.g., acute myocarditis) to keep him or her alive until cardiac function recovery.

Destination therapy (DT): Use of long-term MCS (LVAD) in end-stage HF patients who are ineligible for HTx as an alternative for HTx.

### Interagency Registry for Mechanically Assisted Circulatory Support (INTERMACS) classification[28]

INTERMACS classification (Table 12.9) is used to describe the clinical condition of advanced HF patients. This classification puts HF patients into seven levels based on their hemodynamic profile and level of end-organ damage. It helps better prediction of perioperative risk and selection of alternative treatments.[2,23]

**Practical points in acute and chronic right ventricular failure.** The definitions of RV dysfunction and RV failure are different. RV dysfunction is a state in which the RV stroke volume increases despite elevated RV end-diastolic volume (preserved contractility), but RV stroke volume cannot be increased in RV failure (failed contractility).

The most important hemodynamic findings of RV failure include elevated right atrial (RA) pressure and reduced cardiac index. Both have prognostic significance.

The diagnostic pathway for RV failure is shown in Fig. 12.7.

### Management of Right Ventricular Failure[30]

Unfortunately, there is no specific guideline for the treatment of right HF in acute or chronic settings.

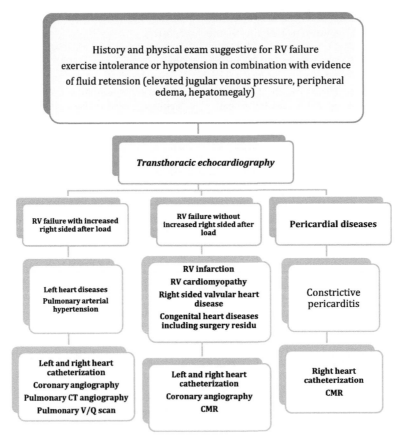

FIG. 12.7 Diagnostic pathway for right ventricular (RV) failure. *CMR*, cardiac magnetic resonance; *CT*, computed tomography; *V/Q*, ventilation/perfusion.

Tailoring therapy to right HF's specific cause is the most important part of management. The main aim of the RV is to keep RA pressure and RV end-diastolic pressure as low as possible to optimize the venous return. Acute RV failure is a clinical diagnosis, but biomarker tests and echocardiography are also necessary for accurate assessment and management.

### Key points on acute right ventricular failure

Many cases of acute RV failure are acute-on-chronic RV failure such as decompensated chronic pulmonary hypertension and acute-on-chronic pulmonary emboli.

The most important causes of acute RV failure are:
- Acute pulmonary thromboemboli
- Acute decompensation of chronic pulmonary hypertension
- Right ventricular infarction
- Cardiac tamponade
- Decompensation of cardiomyopathies [dilated cardiomyopathy, arrhythmogenic right ventricular cardiomyopathy (ARVC), and restricted cardiomyopathy]
- RV failure after cardiac surgery
- RV failure after LVAD

In management of acute RV failure, both general supportive measures and cause-specific treatment should be considered. With successful treatment of the underlying cause, the RV can recover substantially.

### Steps in management of acute right ventricular failure

1. Assessment the severity of RV failure (Is there any sign or risk for low output state?)
   Clinical evaluation: BP, mental status, urinary output
   Laboratory tests: NPs, troponins, renal function test, liver function test, ABG, and lactate level
   Imaging: transthoracic echocardiography (severity of RV dysfunction and concomitant cardiac pathologies), chest CT scan (lung and chest pathologies), and pulmonary CT angiography (the presence of acute or chronic pulmonary thromboemboli and burden of clot)
   Invasive monitoring: Swan-Ganz monitoring [central venous pressure (CVP) and cardiac index]
2. General supportive measures
   Adequate oxygenation
   Lung-protective mechanical ventilation
   Infection prevention measures
   Thromboembolism and peptic ulcer prophylaxis
   Early nutritional support

Glucose control
Control of anemia
For lung-protective mechanical ventilation, the following points should be considered:
   ○ P-plato ≤30 mmHg
   ○ Tidal volume: 4–6 mL/kg/predicted body weight
   ○ Minimize positive end-expiratory pressure (PEEP)
   ○ Avoid acidosis, hypercarbia, hypoxemia, and auto-PEEP
It is recommended that patients with RV failure who are on mechanical ventilation to have daily episodes of spontaneous breathing.
3. Identifying and addressing the trigger factors
   Treatment of infections, sepsis, and arrhythmias
   Cause-specific treatments: revascularization and percutaneous coronary intervention for RV infarction, thrombolysis or embolectomy for acute massive PTE, and thromboendarterectomy for chronic thromboembolic pulmonary hypertension (CTEPH)
4. Optimize volume status (Fig. 12.8)
5. Strategies for improvement of RV contractility: increase RV perfusion pressure and minimize RV afterload

The ideal agent should augment RV contractility through positive inotropic effects and improve RV perfusion by lowering filling pressure and restoring coronary perfusion gradient without increasing pulmonary vascular resistance.
- Norepinephrine (0.2–10 μg/kg/min) is an ideal agent in hypotensive patients.
- Levosimendan, dobutamine, and phosphodiesterase (PDE)-3 inhibitors (milrinone) are inodilators and can reduce right-sided filling pressures and dilated pulmonary artery and reduce PVR.

### Key points about management of acute right ventricular failure

If a patient is in cardiogenic shock, norepinephrine should be initiated as the first step for maintaining arterial pressure. Then, after initial stabilization of SBP, an inodilator can be added to reduce filling pressures and PVR.

A further measure for reducing the RV afterload is using the selective pulmonary vasodilators including prostaglandins (IV or inhaled) and inhaled nitric oxide (iNO).

These agents are most commonly used in patients with pulmonary arterial hypertension.

IV prostaglandins may cause ventilation/perfusion (V/Q) mismatch by vasodilating the poorly ventilated areas of the lung.

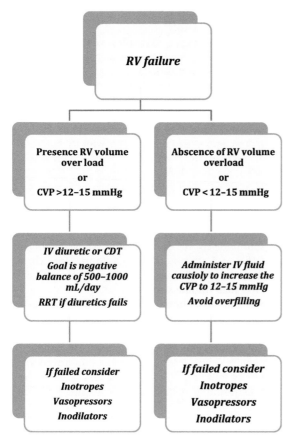

FIG. 12.8 Optimization of volume status in right ventricular (RV) failure. *CDT*, combination diuretic therapy; *CVP*, central venous pressure; *IV*, intravenous; *RRT*, renal replacement therapy.

Prostaglandins should not be used in patients with concurrent severe LV dysfunction because it increases pulmonary capillary wedge pressure (PCWP).

iNO improves V/Q mismatch by vasodilating well-ventilated areas of the lung.

iNO reduces right-side afterload and enhances the efficacy of inotropic therapy, which leads to greater right-sided stroke volume and cardiac output.

Some patients with severe RV failure who not respond to pharmacologic therapies should be referred for mechanical circulatory supports such as ECMO or right ventricular assist device (RVAD).

### Key points for chronic right ventricular failure
The main aim is to treat the underlying cause—for example, treatment of LV failure, pulmonary arterial hypertension, thromboendarterectomy in CTEPH (see also pulmonary hypertension), and corrective surgery for right-sided valvular heart diseases.

Diuretics are recommended for right-sided congestion and fluid overload (peripheral edema and ascites). In the cases of refractory edema, combined diuretic therapy is recommended. Overdiuresis should be avoided because the left atrial pressure is not high in these patients, so they are very sensitive to reduction of preload and may develop hypotension and renal failure.

MRAs are recommended in patients with RV failure with other diuretics to reduce the risk of hypokalemia. MRAs may also have antifibrosis effects on the RV.

Digoxin is recommended in symptomatic patients with RV failure who have more than moderate RV dysfunction.

**Practical points in heart failure with preserved ejection fraction**[1,3,31–33]. There is no specific treatment for HEpEF yet, and clinical trials failed to show any reduction in mortality and morbidity after commonly recommended treatments. HFpEF is usually seen in older adults (75 years of age or older) who are highly symptomatic and have a poor quality of life; therefore, the treatment is mainly directed toward symptoms and concomitant conditions and comorbidities.

### Key points
Treatment of comorbidities and associated conditions has considerable impact on the clinical course of HFpEF. The most common associated conditions include hypertension, CAD, diabetes mellitus, anemia, chronic lung disease, chronic kidney disease, obesity, and sleep disorders.

The general principles of HFpEF include:
- Control of peripheral edema and pulmonary congestion with diuretics
- Optimal treatment of systemic hypertension
- Revascularization for CAD in the presence of ischemia as a cause of HF symptoms
- Restoration of sinus rhythm or heart rate control in patients with AF rhythm

Diuretic and venodilators such as nitrates should be used with caution in patients with LV diastolic dysfunction who have small and stiff LV cavities. Because cardiac performance in these patients is largely dependent on the preload and excessive preload reduction may lead to underfilling of the ventricle, reduction of cardiac output, and hypotension.

MRAs are suggested for patients with definite diagnosis of HFpEF because of MRAs' preventive effects on the development of myocardial fibrosis.

Cardiac rehabilitation programs are strongly recommended in patients with HFpEF. Clinical trials showed that dynamic exercise training can improve functional capacity and quality of life in these patients.

## PULMONARY HYPERTENSION[34–46]

Pulmonary hypertension is a chronic disease with multiple causes and a grave prognosis. Although pulmonary hypertension is a devastating and life-threatening condition, with prompt diagnosis and appropriate management, patients with pulmonary hypertension have fewer symptoms and live longer.

Pulmonary hypertension is defined as a mean of pulmonary arterial pressure of 20 mmHg or greater in RHC. The hemodynamic classification and risk stratification of pulmonary hypertension by RHC is discussed in detail in Chapter 11.

Pulmonary hypertension is classified into five groups according to the clinical presentation, hemodynamic characteristics, pathologic findings, and management strategy[29] (Table 12.10).

An algorithmic approach to the diagnosis of pulmonary hypertension is shown in Fig. 12.9.

The signs and symptoms of pulmonary hypertension are nonspecific. Patients with pulmonary hypertension usually present with HF symptoms such as dyspnea, fatigue, abdominal swelling, and lower limb edema. Patients may have signs of RV failure during physical examination.

### Approach to the pulmonary hypertension

The first step in the approach of pulmonary hypertension is to evaluate its probability by echocardiography.

The echocardiographic findings showing a high probability of pulmonary hypertension include:

1. A tricuspid regurgitation (TR) velocity greater than 3.4 m/s
2. TR velocity between 2.9 and 3.4 m/s accompanied by other signs of pulmonary hypertension in echocardiography

Other signs of pulmonary hypertension in echocardiography include:

1. RV enlargement [RV/left ventricle (LV) basal diameter >1] or flattening of the interventricular septum (LV eccentricity index >1.1 in diastole and systole)

---

**TABLE 12.10**
**Updated Pulmonary Hypertension Classification**

1. Pulmonary arterial hypertension
   1.1. Idiopathic PAH
   1.2. Heritable PAH
   1.3. Drugs and toxins induced PAH
   1.4. PAH Associated with:
        1.4.1. Connective tissue disease
        1.4.2. Human immunodeficiency virus (HIV) infection
        1.4.3. Portal hypertension
        1.4.4. Congenital heart disease
        1.4.5. Schistosomiasis
   1.5. Long-term responder to calcium channel blockers
   1.6. PAH with overt features of venous/capillaries (PVOD/PCH) involvement
   1.7. Persistent pulmonary hypertension of the newborn
2. Pulmonary hypertension due to left heart disease
   2.1. PH due to heart failure with preserved LVEF
   2.2. PH due to heart failure with reduced LVEF
   2.3. Valvular heart disease
   2.4. Congenital/acquired cardiovascular conditions leading to postcapillary PH
3. Pulmonary hypertension due to lung diseases and/or hypoxia
   3.1. Obstructive lung disease
   3.2. Restrictive lung disease
   3.3. Other lung disease with mixed restrictive/obstructive pattern
   3.4. Hypoxia without lung disease
   3.5. Developmental lung disorders
4. Pulmonary hypertension due to pulmonary artery obstructions
   4.1. Chronic thromboembolic PH
   4.2. Other pulmonary artery obstructions
5. Pulmonary hypertension with unclear and/or multifactorial mechanisms
   5.1. Hematological disorders
   5.2. Systemic and metabolic disorders
   5.3. Others
   5.4. Complex congenital heart disease

*LVEF*, left ventricular ejection fraction; *PAH*, pulmonary arterial hypertension; *PCH*, pulmonary capillary hemangiomatosis; *PVOD*, pulmonary veno-occlusive disease. From Simonneau G, Montani D, Celermajer DS, et al. Haemodynamic definitions and updated clinical classification of pulmonary hypertension. Eur Res J. 2019;53 (1):1801913. © ERS 2020: European Respiratory Journal; https://doi.org/10.1183/13993003.01913-2018.

---

2. Pulmonary artery dilatation (PA diameter >25 mm)
3. Early diastolic pulmonary regurgitation velocity >2.2 m/s
4. RV outflow Doppler acceleration time <105 ms or midsystolic notching

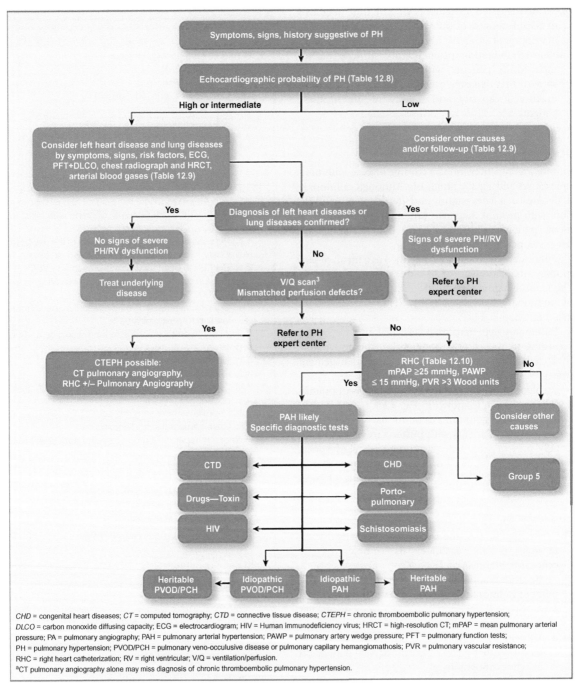

FIG. 12.9 Diagnostic algorithm of pulmonary hypertension (PH). Note that computed tomography (CT) pulmonary angiography alone may miss the diagnosis of chronic thromboembolic PH. (From Galie N, Humbert M, Vachiery JL, et al. 2015 ESC/ERS guidelines for the diagnosis and treatment of pulmonary hypertension: the Joint Task Force for the Diagnosis and Treatment of Pulmonary Hypertension of the European Society of Cardiology (ESC) and the European Respiratory Society (ERS): endorsed by: Association for European Paediatric and Congenital Cardiology (AEPC), International Society for Heart and Lung Transplantation (ISHLT). *Eur Heart J.* 2016;37(1):67–119; with permission.)

5. RA enlargement (RA area $>18$ cm$^2$)
6. Increased inferior cava diameter with decreased inspiratory collapse ($>21$ mm with $<50\%$ collapse with a sniff or $<20\%$ with quiet inspiration)

The probability of pulmonary hypertension is moderate if:

There is a TR velocity between 2.9 and 3.4 m/s without other signs of pulmonary hypertension on echocardiography or

There is a TR velocity 2.8 m/s or less accompanied with other signs of pulmonary hypertension in echocardiography.

A TR velocity of 2.8 m/s or less without other signs of pulmonary hypertension on echocardiography shows a low probability for pulmonary hypertension.

Other diagnostic tools in evaluation of pulmonary hypertension are summarized in Table 12.11.

**Key points about diagnostic tools in pulmonary hypertension**

A normal ECG and chest radiograph do not exclude pulmonary hypertension.

The differential diagnosis of a low diffusion capacity for carbon monoxide (DLCO) in pulmonary artery hypertension (PAH) includes PAH associated with scleroderma, parenchymal lung disease, and pulmonary veno-occlusive disease (PVOD).

A DLCO less than 45% of predicted is associated with a poor outcome.

The spirometry results may be falsely normal in combined emphysema and pulmonary fibrosis, although the DLCO result is almost always abnormal.

The interpretation of pulmonary function test should always be alongside lung imaging.

Overnight oximetry or polysomnography should be performed if the patient is suspected of having obstructive sleep apnea or hypoventilation syndromes.

Anticardiolipin antibody may be positive in patients with systemic lupus erythematosus.

Thrombophilia screening is essential in patients with CTEPH, including antiphospholipid antibodies, anticardiolipin antibodies, and lupus anticoagulant.

**Practical points in pulmonary artery hypertension (Group 1), general measures, and supportive care**

In patients with PAH, the severity of disease should be assessed with data derived from clinical assessment, exercise tests, biomarkers, and echocardiographic and hemodynamic findings (Table 12.12).

Regular follow-up assessments every 3–6 months in stable patients are recommended.

Achieving a low-risk status (good exercise capacity, good quality of life, good RV function, and low mortality risk) is the treatment goal in patients with PAH.

Age, sex, underlying disease, and comorbidities also have a significant impact on disease manifestation and prognosis and cannot be affected by PAH therapy.

Patients with PAH should avoid pregnancy.

Influenza and pneumococcal infection vaccinations are recommended for patients with PAH.

Excessive physical exertion is not recommended in patients with PAH; however, deconditioned patients with PAH should participate in supervised cardiac rehabilitation programs.

In patients with NYHA class III or IV and those with persistent hypoxemia (PO$_2$ $<60$ mmHg), O$_2$ should be administered during flight.

Epidural anesthesia is preferred in elective surgeries.

**Key points in the treatment of pulmonary artery hypertension**

In patients with PAH with signs and symptoms of right HF, diuretic therapy is recommended.

Patients with persistent hypoxemia (PO$_2$ $<60$ mmHg) should get continuous long-term O$_2$ therapy.

Oral anticoagulant therapy is considered in patients with idiopathic pulmonary arterial hypertension (IPAH), hereditary pulmonary arterial hypertension (HPAH), and PAH because of the use of anorexigens.

Correction of anemia and ID is recommended in patients with PAH.

Patients with IPAH, HPAH, and drug-induced pulmonary arterial hypertension (DPAH) who are responders to vasoreactivity testing should be treated with high doses of CCBs.

For vasoreactivity testing, inhaled nitric oxide (NO) at 10–20 ppm is the preferred agent, but IV adenosine and/or inhaled or IV prostaglandins can be used as alternatives.

The criteria for vasoreactivity are:
1. Reduction of mean PAP, 10 mmHg or greater to reach an absolute value of 40 mmHg or less
2. Unchanged or increased cardiac output

Recommended CCBs are nifedipine and amlodipine in patients with severe RV dysfunction and bradycardia and diltiazem for patients with tachycardia.

The recommended daily doses of CCBs are:

Nifedipine: 120–240 mg

Diltiazem: 240–720 mg

Amlodipine: up to 20 mg

Long-term response to CCBs is defined by clinical improvement (NYHA functional class I or II) and sustained hemodynamic improvement after at least 1 year on CCBs only (same or better than achieved in the acute test and usually to obtain mean PAP less than 30 mmHg with a normal or increased CO).

**TABLE 12.11**
**Diagnostic Tools in Pulmonary Hypertension**

| Diagnostic Tool | Comments |
|---|---|
| Electrocardiogram | P pulmonale, right axis deviation, RV hypertrophy, RV strain, right bundle branch block, and QTc prolongation |
| Chest radiography | Central pulmonary arterial dilatation, "pruning" (loss) of the peripheral blood vessels, RA and RV enlargement<br>Findings depending on the etiology of PH: signs suggesting lung disease, pulmonary venous congestion caused by left heart diseases |
| Pulmonary function test | Mild to moderate reduction of lung volumes, decreased lung DLCO<br>Findings of obstructive or restrictive lung disease in patients with chronic lung diseases (COPD or interstitial lung disease) |
| Arterial blood gas | Decreased systemic arterial oxygen saturation with or without hypercarbia depending on etiology of PH |
| Ventilation/perfusion lung scan | Screening method of choice for CTEPH<br>Small peripheral unmatched and nonsegmental defects in perfusion in PAH and PVOD |
| High-resolution computed tomography | Increased PA diameter $\geq$29 mm<br>Pulmonary to ascending aorta diameter ratio $\geq$1.0<br>A segmental artery to bronchus ratio >1:1 in three or four lobes<br>Ground-glass abnormalities<br>Characteristic changes of interstitial lung disease and emphysema<br>Characteristic changes of PVOD: interstitial edema, diffuse central ground-glass opacification, thickening of interlobular septa, parahilar lymphadenopathy, pleural effusion<br>HRCT findings in pulmonary capillary hemangiomatosis: diffuse bilateral thickening of the interlobular septa; small, centrilobular, poorly circumscribed nodular opacities |
| Pulmonary computed tomography angiography | Evidence of surgically accessible CTEPH<br>Typical angiographic findings in CTEPH: complete obstruction; bands, webs, and intimal irregularities |
| Cardiac magnetic resonance imaging | Findings that are highly predictive for pulmonary hypertension: late gadolinium enhancement, reduced pulmonary arterial distensibility, retrograde flow<br>Very useful in accurate assessment of RV function and defining cardiac structure precisely in patients with congenital heart disease<br>Magnetic resonance angiography is useful in patients suspected with CTEPH who have contraindication for computed tomography angiography such as pregnant women |
| Blood tests and immunology | Routine biochemistry, hematology, thyroid function, and liver function tests<br>ProBNP has prognostic significance<br>Serologic testing for detecting connective tissue diseases, hepatitis, and HIV infection<br>Looking for evidence of scleroderma is very important, including anticentromere, dsDNA, anti-Ro, U3-RNP, B23, Th/To, and U1-RNP |
| Abdominal ultrasound scan and Doppler study | Useful for identification of some of the etiologies of PAH, including portal hypertension |
| Right heart catheterization and vasoreactivity | RHC is recommended in all patients suspected with PAH (group 1) and CTEPH for assessment of the severity of hemodynamic impairment<br>Vasoreactivity is recommended in selected patients with PAH, including IPAH, HPAH, and FPAH, to detect patients who can be treated with CCBs<br>RHC is recommended in patients with CHD to support decision for correction<br>RHC is recommended in groups 2 and 3 to help in the differential diagnosis and support treatment decisions or if organ transplantation is considered |

*CCB,* Calcium channel blocker; *CHD,* congenital heart disease; *COPD,* chronic obstructive pulmonary disease; *CTEPH,* chronic thromboembolic pulmonary hypertension; *DLCO,* diffusion capacity for carbon monoxide; *FPAH,* familial pulmonary arterial hypertension; *HRCT,* high-resolution computed tomography; *HPAH,* hereditary pulmonary arterial hypertension; *PAH,* pulmonary artery hypertension; *PH,* pulmonary hypertension; *proBNP,* pro B-type natriuretic peptide; *PVOD,* pulmonary veno-occlusive disease; *RA,* right atrium; *RHC,* right heart catheterization; *RV,* right ventricular.

**TABLE 12.12**
**Risk Assessment in Pulmonary Hypertension**

| Determination of Prognosis[a] (Estimated 1-Year Mortality Risk) | Low Risk (<5%) | Intermediate Risk (5%–10%) | High Risk (>10%) |
|---|---|---|---|
| Clinical signs of right heart failure | Absent | Absent | Present |
| Progression of symptoms | No | Slow | Rapid |
| Syncope | No | Occasional syncope[b] | Repeated syncope[c] |
| WHO functional class | I, II | III | IV |
| 6MWD | >440 m | 165–440 m | <165 m |
| Cardiopulmonary exercise testing | Peak $VO_2$ >15 mL/min/kg (>65% predicted) VE/$VCO_2$ slope <36 | Peak $VO_2$ 11–15 mL/min/kg (35%–65% predicted) VE/$VCO_2$ slope 36–44.9 | Peak $VO_2$ <11 mL/min/kg (<35% predicted) VE/$VCO_2$ slope $\geq$45 |
| NT-proBNP plasma levels | BNP <50 ng/L NT-proBNP <300 ng/L | BNP 50–300 ng/L NT-proBNP 300–1400 ng/L | BNP >300 ng/L NT-proBNP >1400 ng/L |
| Imaging (echocardiography, CMR imaging) | RA area <18 cm$^2$ No pericardial effusion | RA area 18–26 cm$^2$ No or minimal pericardial effusion | RA area >26 cm$^2$ Pericardial effusion |
| Hemodynamics | RAP <8 mmHg CI $\geq$2.5 L/min/m$^2$ $SvO_2$ > 65% | RAP 8–14 mmHg CI 2.0–2.4 L/min/m$^2$ $SvO_2$ 60%–65% | RAP >14 mmHg CI <2.0 L/min/m$^2$ $SvO_2$ <60% |

*6MWD*, 6-min walking distance; *BNP*, Brain natriuretic peptide; *CI*, cardiac index; *CMR*, cardiac magnetic resonance; *NT-proBNP*, N-terminal pro B-type natriuretic peptide; *RA*, right atrium; *RAP*, right atrial pressure; *SvO₂*, mixed venous oxygen saturation; *VE/VCO₂*, ventilator equivalents for carbon dioxide; *VO₂*, oxygen consumption; *WHO*, World Health Organization.

[a]Most of the proposed variables and cutoff values are based on expert opinion. They may provide prognostic information and may be used to guide therapeutic decisions, but application to individual patients must be done carefully. One must also note that most of these variables have been validated mostly for IPAH, and the cut-off levels used above may not necessarily apply to other forms of PAH. Furthermore, the use of approved therapies and their influence on the variables should be considered in the evaluation of the risk.

[b]Occasional syncope during brisk or heavy exercise, occasional orthostatic syncope in an otherwise stable patient.

[c]Repeated episodes of syncope, even with little or regular physical activity.

From Galie N, Humbert M, Vachiery JL, et al. 2015 ESC/ERS guidelines for the diagnosis and treatment of pulmonary hypertension: the Joint Task Force for the Diagnosis and Treatment of Pulmonary Hypertension of the European Society of Cardiology (ESC) and the European Respiratory Society (ERS): endorsed by: Association for European Paediatric and Congenital Cardiology (AEPC), International Society for Heart and Lung Transplantation (ISHLT). *Eur Heart J.* 2016;37(1):67–119; with permission.

In patients without marked hemodynamic improvement after high doses of CCBs, specific PAH therapies should be initiated.

PAH treatment pathways are shown in Fig. 12.10.

PAH-specific therapies (pulmonary vasodilators) should be started in patients who are not candidates for CCBs (nonreactive).

Patients with PVOD may develop pulmonary edema in response to PAH-specific therapies.

The NYHA functional class should be considered to guide the choice of PAH-specific therapies (Fig. 12.11).

NYHA FC II: Monotherapy may be initiated with a currently approved phosphodiesterase-5 (PDE5) inhibitor, endothelin receptor antagonist (ERA), or the soluble guanylate cyclase stimulator riociguat.

NYHA FC III (treatment naïve): Monotherapy can be initiated with a currently approved a PDE5 inhibitor, ERA, or riociguat.

NYHA FC III (treatment naïve with markers of poor prognosis or rapid progression): Parenteral prostacyclin analogs.

NYHA FC III (nontreatment naïve with markers of poor prognosis or rapid progression): Parenteral or inhaled prostacyclin analogs.

NYHA FC IV (treatment naïve): Parenteral prostacyclin analogs or inhaled prostacyclin analogs in

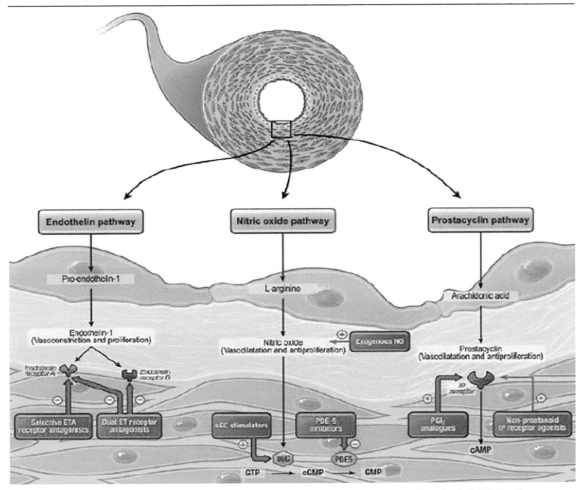

FIG. 12.10 Established vasomotor pathways targeted by current and emerging therapies in PAH. The three major pathways (endothelin-1, nitric oxide, and prostacyclin) involved in the regulation of pulmonary vasomotor tone are shown. These pathways represent the targets of all currently approved PAH therapies. Endothelial dysfunction results in decreased production of endogenous vasodilatory mediators (nitric oxide and prostacyclin) and the upregulation of endothelin-1, which promotes vasoconstriction and smooth muscle cell proliferation. The endothelin-1 pathway can be blocked by either selective or nonselective endothelin-1 receptor antagonists; the nitric oxide pathway can be manipulated by direct administration of exogenous nitric oxide, inhibition of phosphodiesterase type-5, or stimulation of soluble guanylate cyclase; and the prostacyclin pathway can be enhanced by the administration of prostanoid analogs or nonprostanoid IP receptor agonists. *ET*, endothelin; *ETA*, endothelin type A; *IP*, prostaglandin I2; *NO*, nitric oxide; *PAH*, pulmonary arterial hypertension; *PDE-5*, phosphodiesterase type 5; *sGC*, soluble guanylate cyclase. (From Humbert M, Lau EM, Montani D, et al. Advances in therapeutic interventions for patients with pulmonary arterial hypertension. *Circulation.* 2014;130(24):2189–208; with permission.)

combination with an ERA if unable to manage IV prostaglandin therapy.

For NYHA FC III or IV PAH patients with poor clinical status despite PAH-specific monotherapy, a second class of PAH therapy should be added to improve exercise capacity. These patients should also be referred to a pulmonary hypertension expert center for further evaluations.

PAH-specific drugs are presented in Table 12.13. An algorithmic treatment approach for PAH patients is shown in Fig. 12.11.

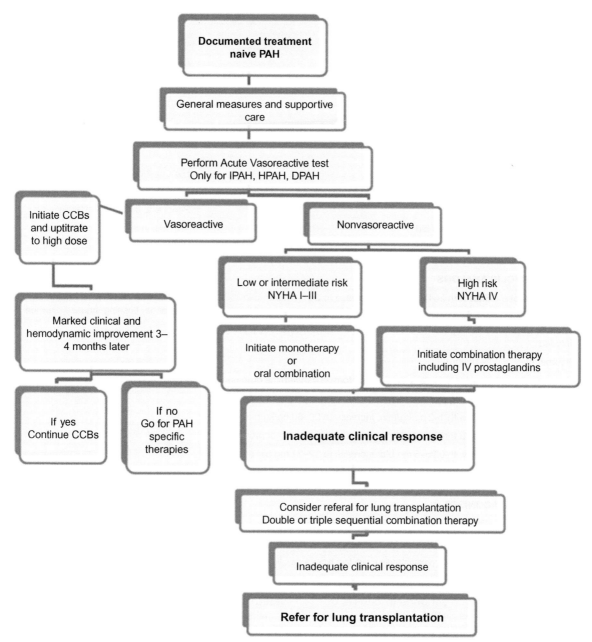

FIG. 12.11 Algorithmic treatment approach for patients with pulmonary artery hypertension. *CCB*, calcium channel blocker; *DPAH*, drug-induced pulmonary arterial hypertension; *HPAH*, hereditary pulmonary arterial hypertension; *IPAH*, idiopathic pulmonary arterial hypertension; *IV*, intravenous; *NYHA*, New York Heart Association; *PAH*, pulmonary artery hypertension.

**TABLE 12.13**
**PAH-Specific Drugs**

| Drug Classes | Recommended Dose Ranges | Adverse Effects |
|---|---|---|
| **PHOSPHODIESTERASE TYPE 5 INHIBITORS** | | |
| Sildenafil | 20 mg tid | Headache, flushing, epistaxis |
| Tadalafil | 2.5–40 mg/day | |
| Vardenafil | 5 mg bid | |
| **GUANYLATE CYCLASE STIMULATORS** | | |
| Riociguat | 1–2.5 mg tid | Hypotension, syncope |
| **ENDOTHELIN RECEPTOR ANTAGONISTS** | | |
| Ambrisentan | 5–10 mg | Peripheral edema, headache |
| Bosentan | 62.5–125 mg bid | Anemia, increased transaminases, headache |
| Macitentan | 10 mg/day | Nasopharyngitis, headache, anemia |
| **PROSTACYCLIN ANALOGS** | | |
| Epoprostenol IV | Start with 2–4 ng/kg/min; increase to 20–40 ng/kg/min | Infusion site reaction and pain, headache, flushing, nausea diarrhea jaw pain, rash |
| Iloprost inhaled | 2.5–5 µg inhaled six to nine times daily; median, 30 µg/day | |
| Iloprost IV | 2–12 µg/h | |
| Treprostinil | The doses for treprotinil in four form is beneath the drug name | |
| Inhaled | 18–54 µg per treatment qid | |
| Subcutaneous | Start with 1–2 ng/kg/min; increase to 20–80 ng/kg/min | |
| IV | Two to three times higher than the dose of IV epoprostenol | |
| Oral | Start with 0.25–5 mg bid; increase to 12–21 mg bid over 12 weeks | |
| Beraprost | 120 µg qid | |
| **IP RECEPTOR AGONISTS** | | |
| Selexipag (oral) | 200–1600 µg bid | Headache, diarrhea, jaw pain |

*bid*, twice a day; *IV*, intravenous; *PI*, prostaglandin I; *qid*, four times a day; *tid*, three times a day.

**Key points about treatment of other causes of pulmonary hypertension (PH)**

Patients with PAH associated with connective tissue diseases should be treated as patients with IPAH.

Patients with PAH associated with portal hypertension should be treated as patients with IPAH. The severity of liver disease should be taken into account.

Anticoagulation is not recommended for PAH patients with liver disease.

Patients with PAH associated with HIV should be treated as patients with IPAH. Comorbidities and drug–drug interactions should be considered.

Anticoagulation is not recommended for PAH patients with HIV disease.

The association of PAH with amphetamines/methamphetamines and dasatinib is now considered definite.

Occupational exposure to organic solvent trichloroethylene can be the cause of PVOD.

In patients with pulmonary hypertension secondary to left heart disease, medical treatment should be optimized, structural heart disease should be corrected, and other causes of pulmonary hypertension (i.e., pulmonary emboli, CTEPH, sleep apnea, and COPD) should be identified.

The definition for PH in the context of chronic lung disease (CLD):

(1) CLD without PH: mean PAP <21 mmHg or mean PAP 21–24 mmHg with pulmonary PVR <3 Wood unit

(2) CLD with PH: mean PAP 21–24 mmHg with PVR 3 Wood unit or greater, or mean PAP 25–34 mmHg

(3) CLD with severe PH: mean PAP 35 mmHg or greater, or mean PAP 25 mmHg or greater accompanied with low cardiac index (CI <2 L/min/m$^2$)

Long-term oxygen therapy is recommended in patients with lung disease who are hypoxemic.

Some studies suggest that currently available pulmonary vasoactive medications such as sildenafil may have a benefit in COPD patients with mean PAP 35 mmHg or greater.

RHC is not recommended for patients with lung disease and pulmonary hypertension unless an alternative diagnosis such as PAH or CTEPH is suspected or another therapeutic option (lung transplantation) is considered.

**Practical points about chronic thromboembolic pulmonary hypertension.** Chronic thromboembolic pulmonary hypertension is precapillary pulmonary hypertension in the presence of occlusive thromboemboli within the pulmonary arteries. Screening for CTEPH in patients with pulmonary emboli who are symptomatic after 3 months of effective anticoagulation is necessary.

The diagnostic findings of CTPEH are:
- The presence of precapillary pulmonary hypertension after at least 3 months of anticoagulation therapy for acute pulmonary emboli
- Mismatched perfusion defects on V/Q lung scan
- Chronic total occlusions (pouch lesions or tapered lesions), ring-like stenoses, or webs or slits in pulmonary conventional, CT, or MR angiography

Pulmonary thromboendarterectomy is the best treatment option for CTEPH.

Surgery should be considered for all patients with CTEPH, and these patients should be referred to an experienced center for determination of operability.

For determining operability, three questions should be answered:

1. Does the severity of hemodynamic impairment observed in RHC correlate with the clot burden observed on pulmonary artery imaging?

2. Are the diseased arteries surgically accessible?

3. Does the patient have comorbidities that may prohibit surgery?

**Key points**

Lifelong anticoagulation should be prescribed for patients with CTEPH.

There is no PVR threshold for CTEPH surgery.

The surgical risk is higher in patients with PVR greater than 1000 dyne/s/cm$^{-5}$ in RHC.

The aim of surgery is to decrease PVR to less than 300 dyn/s/cm$^{-5}$.

Surgery should be performed in an ECMO facility.

Nonoperable patients and patients who have recurrent CTEPH after surgery should be medically treated with riociguat.

Other PAH-specific therapies can be used in inoperable patients who are symptomatic.

Balloon pulmonary angioplasty may be a therapeutic option in inoperable patients.

## REFERENCES

1. Ponikowski P, Voors AA, Anker SD, et al. 2016 ESC Guidelines for the diagnosis and treatment of acute and chronic heart failure. *Eur Heart J*. 2015;ehw128.

2. Yancy CW, Jessup M, Bozkurt B, et al. 2013 ACCF/AHA guideline for the management of heart failure: a report of the American College of Cardiology Foundation/American Heart Association Task Force on Practice Guidelines. *J Am Coll Cardiol*. 2013;62(16):e147–e239.

3. Yancy CW, Jessup M, Bozkurt B, et al. 2016 ACC/AHA/HFSA focused update on New Pharmacological Therapy for Heart Failure: an update of the 2013 ACCF/AHA Guideline for the Management of Heart Failure: a report of the American College of Cardiology/American Heart Association Task Force on Clinical Practice Guidelines and the Heart Failure Society of America. *J Am Coll Cardiol*. 2016;68(13):1476–1488.

4. Howlett JG, Chan M, Ezekowitz JA, et al. The Canadian Cardiovascular Society heart failure companion: bridging guidelines to your practice. *Can J Cardiol*. 2016;32(3):296–310.

5. Mullens W, Damman K, Harjola VP, et al. The use of diuretics in heart failure with congestion—a position statement from the Heart Failure Association of the European Society of Cardiology. *Eur J Heart Fail*. 2019;21(2):137–155.

6. Xanthopoulos A, Starling RC, Kitai T, Triposkiadis F. Heart failure and liver disease: cardiohepatic interactions. *JACC: Heart Fail*. 2019;7(2):87–97.

7. Samsky MD, Patel CB, DeWald TA, et al. Cardiohepatic interactions in heart failure: an overview and clinical implications. *J Am Coll Cardiol*. 2013;61(24):2397–2405.

8. Nikolaou M, Parissis J, Yilmaz MB, et al. Liver function abnormalities, clinical profile, and outcome in acute decompensated heart failure. *Eur Heart J*. 2012;ehs332.

9. Ter Maaten JM, Valente MA, Damman K, Hillege HL, Navis G, Voors AA. Diuretic response in acute heart

failure—pathophysiology, evaluation, and therapy. *Nat Rev Cardiol.* 2015;12(3):184–192.

10. Valente MAE, Voors AA, Damman K, et al. Diuretic response in acute heart failure: clinical characteristics and prognostic significance. *Eur Heart J.* 2014;35(19):1284–1293.

11. Gheorghiade M, Braunwald E. A proposed model for initial assessment and management of acute heart failure syndromes. *JAMA.* 2011;305(16):1702–1703.

12. Jentzer JC, DeWald TA, Hernandez AF. Combination of loop diuretics with thiazide-type diuretics in heart failure. *J Am Coll Cardiol.* 2010;56(19):1527–1534.

13. Gheorghiade M, Follath F, Ponikowski P, et al. Assessing and grading congestion in acute heart failure: a scientific statement from the Acute Heart Failure Committee of the Heart Failure Association of the European Society of Cardiology and endorsed by the European Society of Intensive Care Medicine. *Eur J Heart Fail.* 2010;12(5):423–433.

14. London GM, Pannier B. Renal replacement therapy for heart failure patients: in whom, when and which therapy to use? *Nephrol Dial Transplant.* 2009;24(8):2314–2315.

15. Sica DA. Metolazone and its role in edema management. *Congest Heart Fail.* 2003;9(2):100–105.

16. Metra M, Teerlink JR, Voors AA, et al. Vasodilators in the treatment of acute heart failure: what we know, what we don't. *Heart Fail Rev.* 2009;14(4):299–307.

17. Howlett JG, McKelvie RS, Arnold JMO, et al. Canadian Cardiovascular Society Consensus Conference guidelines on heart failure, update 2009: diagnosis and management of right-sided heart failure, myocarditis, device therapy and recent important clinical trials. *Can J Cardiol.* 2009;25(2):85–105.

18. Elkayam U, Tasissa G, Binanay C, et al. Use and impact of inotropes and vasodilator therapy in hospitalized patients with severe heart failure. *Am Heart J.* 2007;153(1):98–104.

19. Farmakis D, Agostoni P, Baholli L, et al. A pragmatic approach to the use of inotropes for the management of acute and advanced heart failure: an expert panel consensus. *Int J Cardiol.* 2019;297:83–90.

20. Felker GM, Benza RL, Chandler AB, et al. Heart failure etiology and response tomilrinone in decompensated heart failure: results from the OPTIME-CHF study. *J Am Coll Cardiol.* 2003;41(6):997–1003.

21. Verbrugge FH, Grieten L, Mullens W. Management of the cardiorenal syndrome in decompensated heart failure. *Cardiorenal Med.* 2014;4(3–4):176–188.

22. McMurray JJ, Packer M, Desai AS, et al. Angiotensin–neprilysin inhibition versus enalapril in heart failure. *N Engl J Med.* 2014;371(11):993–1004.

23. Mortensen SA, Rosenfeldt F, Kumar A, et al. The effect of coenzyme Q10 on morbidity and mortality in chronic heart failure: results from Q-SYMBIO: a randomized double-blind trial. *JACC: Heart Fail.* 2014;2(6):641–649.

24. Taghavi S, Amiri A, Amin A, Ehsani A, Maleki M, Naderi N. Oral iron therapy with polysaccharide-iron complex may be useful in increasing the ferritin level for a short time

in patients with dilated cardiomyopathy. *Res Cardiovas Med.* 2017;6(1):e39816.

25. Hajahmadi M, Shemshadi S, Khalilipur E, et al. Muscle wasting in young patients with dilated cardiomyopathy. *J Cachexia Sarcopenia Muscle.* 2017;8(4):542–548.

26. von Haehling S. Muscle wasting and sarcopenia in heart failure: a brief overview of the current literature. *ESC Heart Fail.* 2018;5(6):1074–1082.

27. Crespo-Leiro MG, Metra M, Lund LH, et al. Advanced heart failure: a position statement of the Heart Failure Association of the European Society of Cardiology. *Eur J Heart Fail.* 2018;20(11):1505–1535.

28. Holman WL. Interagency registry for mechanically assisted circulatory support (INTERMACS) what have we learned and what will we learn? *Circulation.* 2012;126(11):1401–1406.

29. De Jonge N, Kirkels J, Klöpping C, et al. Guidelines for heart transplantation. *Neth Heart J.* 2008;16(3):79–87.

30. Harjola VP, Mebazaa A, Čelutkienė J, et al. Contemporary management of acute right ventricular failure: a statement from the Heart Failure Association and the Working Group on Pulmonary Circulation and Right Ventricular Function of the European Society of Cardiology. *Eur J Heart Fail.* 2016;18(3):226–241.

31. Sharma K, Kass DA. Heart failure with preserved ejection fraction mechanisms, clinical features, and therapies. *Circ Res.* 2014;115(1):79–96.

32. Pitt B, Pfeffer MA, Assmann SF, et al. Spironolactone for heart failure with preserved ejection fraction. *N Engl J Med.* 2014;370(15):1383–1392.

33. Edelmann F, Wachter R, Schmidt AG, et al. Effect of spironolactone on diastolic function and exercise capacity in patients with heart failure with preserved ejection fraction: the Aldo-DHF randomized controlled trial. *JAMA.* 2013;309(8):781–791.

34. Simonneau G, Montani D, Celermajer DS, et al. Haemodynamic definitions and updated clinical classification of pulmonary hypertension. *Eur Respir J.* 2019;53(1):1801913.

35. Nathan SD, Barbera JA, Gaine SP, et al. Pulmonary hypertension in chronic lung disease and hypoxia. *Eur Respir J.* 2019;53(1):1801914.

36. Galiè N, Humbert M, Vachiery J-L, et al. 2015 ESC/ERS Guidelines for the diagnosis and treatment of pulmonary hypertension. *Eur Heart J.* 2015;ehv317.

37. Taichman DB, Ornelas J, Chung L, et al. Pharmacologic therapy for pulmonary arterial hypertension in adults: CHEST guideline and expert panel report. *Chest J.* 2014;146(2):449–475.

38. Tapson VF, Jing Z-C, Xu K-F, et al. Oral treprostinil for the treatment of pulmonary arterial hypertension in patients receiving background endothelin receptor antagonist and phosphodiesterase type 5 inhibitor therapy (the FREEDOM-C2 study): a randomized controlled trial. *Chest J.* 2013;144(3):952–958.

39. Kim NH, Delcroix M, Jenkins DP, et al. Chronic thromboembolic pulmonary hypertension. *J Am Coll Cardiol.* 2013;62:25_S.

40. Galiè N, Corris PA, Frost A, et al. Updated treatment algorithm of pulmonary arterial hypertension. *J Am Coll Cardiol.* 2013;62:25_S.

41. Tapson VF, Torres F, Kermeen F, et al. Oral treprostinil for the treatment of pulmonary arterial hypertension in patients on background endothelin receptor antagonist and/or phosphodiesterase type 5 inhibitor therapy (the FREEDOM-C study): a randomized controlled trial. *Chest J.* 2012;142(6):1383–1390.

42. Madani MM, Auger WR, Pretorius V, et al. Pulmonary endarterectomy: recent changes in a single institution's experience of more than 2,700 patients. *Ann Thorac Surg.* 2012;94(1):97–103.

43. Mayer E, Jenkins D, Lindner J, et al. Surgical management and outcome of patients with chronic thromboembolic pulmonary hypertension: results from an international prospective registry. *J Thorac Cardiovasc Surg.* 2011;141 (3):702–710.

44. Naderi N, Ojaghi Haghighi Z, Amin A, et al. Utility of right ventricular strain imaging in predicting pulmonary vascular resistance in patients with pulmonary hypertension. *Congest Heart Fail.* 2013;19(3):116–122.

45. Amin A, Navid H, Chitsazan M, Ghaleshi B, Taghavi S, Naderi N. Safety of adenosine for acute pulmonary vasoreactivity testing in pulmonary hypertension. *Multidiscip Cardiovas Ann.* 2016;7:1.

46. Shafie D, Dohaei A, Amin A, Taghavi S, Naderi N. Pulmonary vascular capacitance as a predictor of vasoreactivity in idiopathic pulmonary arterial hypertension tested by adenosine. *Res Cardiovas Med.* 2015;4(4):1–5.

# CHAPTER 13

# Tachyarrhythmias

MAJID HAGHJOO
Department of Cardiac Electrophysiology, Rajaie Cardiovascular, Medical & Research Center, Iran, University of Medical Sciences, Tehran, Iran

## KEY POINTS

- Tachyarrhythmias are broadly categorized as narrow complex tachycardia (NCT, <120 ms) or wide complex tachycardia (WCT, ≥120 ms).
- Tachyarrhythmias are frequently symptomatic and present with palpitations, diaphoresis, dyspnea, chest pain, dizziness, syncope, and heart failure.
- NCTs include sinus tachycardia, atrioventricular nodal reentrant tachycardia, orthodromic atrioventricular reciprocating tachycardia, focal atrial tachycardia, atrial flutter, atrial fibrillation (AF), multifocal atrial tachycardia, inappropriate sinus tachycardia, and sinoatrial nodal reentrant tachycardia.
- WCTs include monomorphic ventricular tachycardia, aberrant supraventricular tachycardia, antidromic atrioventricular reciprocating tachycardia, and pacemaker-mediated tachycardia, AF with aberrant conduction, preexcited AF, artifactual tachycardia, and polymorphic ventricular tachycardia.
- The first step in evaluation of all tachycardias is the determination of hemodynamic stability. The second step is to determine whether the rhythm is regular or irregular. The third step is identification of P wave during regular NCT.
- In NCT, treatment options depend on the hemodynamic status of the patient and regularity of the tachycardia. If a patient has hemodynamic instability, synchronized direct current cardioversion is recommended if the rhythm is not sinus tachycardia. The Valsalva maneuver and carotid sinus massage can be tried if it does not delay cardioversion.
- Pulseless patients with WCT should be treated according to advanced cardiac life support recommendations. In hemodynamically unstable but conscious patients, immediate synchronized cardioversion is recommended. Stable patients should be treated similarly to NCT patients.

## INTRODUCTION

Tachyarrhythmia is defined as a heart rhythm with a ventricular rate of 100 beats/min or greater. Tachyarrhythmias are broadly categorized as narrow complex tachycardia (NCT; <120 ms) or wide complex tachycardia (≥120 ms). NCT reflects rapid activation via the normal His–Purkinje system and therefore tachycardia origin above or within the His bundle [i.e., supraventricular tachycardia (SVT)].[1,2] However, wide complex tachycardia (WCT) indicates abnormally slow ventricular activation.[3] Tachycardia origin can be below the His bundle within bundle branches, Purkinje system, or ventricular myocardium [i.e., ventricular tachycardia (VT)]. Otherwise, it may reflect SVT with preexisting bundle branch block (BBB), rate-dependent aberrancy, or conduction over an accessory pathway.

## CLINICAL PRESENTATION

Tachyarrhythmias are frequently symptomatic; patients present with palpitations, diaphoresis, dyspnea, chest pain, dizziness, syncope, and heart failure.

Patients with NCT usually present with palpitations. Although dyspnea or chest pain can occur in any patient, those with underlying heart diseases (e.g., coronary heart disease) are more likely to present in this way, particularly at heart rates of greater than 150 beats/min. Syncope is a rare manifestation of NCT because heart rate is not so fast as to impair cardiac output. However, atrial flutter (AFL) and atrial fibrillation (AF) may present with syncope caused by a very rapid ventricular rate (>250 beats/min).

Patients with WCT may present with syncope, dizziness, chest pain, sudden cardiac arrest, or heart failure.

However, stable patients complain of palpitations or rarely may be asymptomatic.

### Narrow Complex Tachycardia

#### Etiology

Narrow complex tachycardia occurs in normal hearts in most cases. An abnormal connection between the atria and ventricles (accessory pathway) may be responsible for some episodes of these tachycardias. Other causes include digitalis toxicity, coronary artery disease, heart failure, thyrotoxicosis, myocarditis, pericarditis, cardiomyopathy, and hypertensive heart disease.

#### Classification

Narrow complex tachycardias are generally classified according to the regularity of ventricular response. Regular tachycardias include sinus tachycardia, atrioventricular nodal reentrant tachycardia (AVNRT), orthodromic atrioventricular reciprocating tachycardia (AVRT), focal atrial tachycardia (FAT), AFL, inappropriate sinus tachycardia, and sinoatrial nodal reentrant tachycardia.[2] Irregular tachycardias consist of AF, AFL with variable conduction, and multifocal atrial tachycardia (MAT).

**Atrioventricular nodal reentrant tachycardia.** Atrioventricular nodal reentrant tachycardia is the most common (60%) paroxysmal supraventricular tachycardia (PSVT) in adults. The term *PSVT* is applied to SVTs with abrupt onset and offset other than AF, AFL, and MAT. It is more common in women and, in most cases, symptoms begin after the age of 20 years.[4]

*Pathophysiology.* The electrical substrate for AVNRT consists of dual atrioventricular (AV) nodal pathways.[1] Whereas *fast pathway* has rapid conduction and a relatively long refractory period, the *slow pathway* is characterized by slow conduction and a shorter refractory period.[5] Slow and fast AV nodal pathways originate from perinodal atrial tissues and then enter a common pathway within the AV node.[5] The rest of the atria, His–Purkinje system, and the ventricles are not necessary parts of the reentry circuit. Based on the contribution of fast and slow pathways in the antegrade or retrograde limbs of the tachycardia circuit, AVNRT is divided into typical and atypical forms.[6]

*Typical AVNRT* (also called common form) accounts for 80%–90% of the patients with AVNRT.[6] In this form of the arrhythmia, tachycardia is initiated by a critically timed premature atrial beat. This beat arrives at the AV node when the fast pathway is in a refractory state; therefore, the impulse conducts antegradely via the slow pathway with a shorter refractory period. When the impulse reaches the end of the slow pathway, the fast

pathway is ready for retrograde conduction. Therefore, typical AVNRT is also called "slow–fast" AVNRT.

*Atypical AVNRT* (uncommon form) comprises 10%–20% of the total AVNRT population.[6] In "fast–slow" AVNRT, antegrade conduction occurs down the fast pathway with retrograde conduction up the slow pathway. Some patients have "slow–slow" AVNRT in which both the antegrade and retrograde limbs of the circuit use slow AV nodal pathways.

*Electrocardiographic characteristics.* Atrioventricular nodal reentrant tachycardia is characterized by a ventricular rate of 150–250 beats/min. In typical AVNRT (Fig. 13.1), the RP interval is very short, and the P wave is usually hidden within the QRS (no visible P wave) or appears at the end of QRS and present as pseudo-r in leads V1 or aVR, pseudo-s in inferior leads, or notching at the end of aVL.[7] In atypical AVNRT (Fig. 13.2), the RP interval is longer, and P waves are manifested as negative deflections within the ST segment or shortly before the next QRS complex in the inferior leads.[8]

Although it is more common with orthodromic AVRT, ST-segment depression has been reported in 25%–50% of patients with AVNRT.[9] ST-segment depression is related to the repolarization abnormality and does not indicate myocardial ischemia. Memory T wave (T-wave inversion) has been observed in 40% of patients after acute tachycardia termination. Similar to ST-segment depression, these changes represent repolarization abnormalities, and they are not the result of coronary artery disease.

*Electrophysiologic characteristics.* In typical AVNRT (slow–fast), earliest retrograde atrial activation is recorded near the His bundle.[6] The atrial–His bundle (AH) interval is relatively long (>180 ms), and the His–atrial (HA) interval is relatively short (<70 ms), resulting in a short RP tachycardia (Fig. 13.3).

Atypical fast–slow AVNRT uses the same circuit as typical AVNRT but in the reverse direction. Therefore, the earliest retrograde atrial activation is recorded near the coronary sinus (CS) ostium or proximal part of CS.[6] The AH interval (<180 ms) is shorter than the HA interval, resulting in a long RP tachycardia (Fig. 13.4).

Atypical slow–slow AVNRT has a long AH interval (>180 ms), with early retrograde atrial activation recorded near the CS ostium[6] (Fig. 13.5).

**Orthodromic atrioventricular reciprocating tachycardia.** Orthodromic AVRT is the second most common (30%) PSVT in adults.[10] Orthodromic AVRT accounts for about 95% of all AVRTs. Patients with this arrhythmia typically present at a younger age than those with AVNRT.[11]

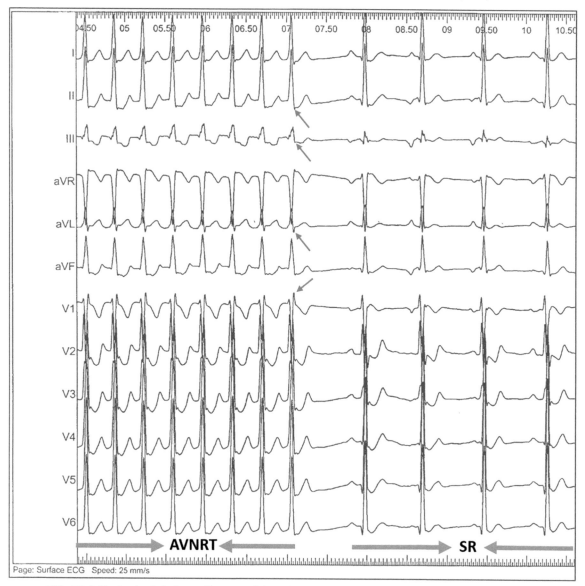

FIG. 13.1 Twelve-lead electrocardiograms of sinus rhythm and tachycardia in a patient with typical atrioventricular nodal reentrant tachycardia (AVNRT). There is characteristic pseudo-s in inferior leads and pseudo-r′ in V1.

*Pathophysiology.* In orthodromic AVRT, the normal AV conduction system serves as the antegrade limb, and an AV accessory pathway serves as the retrograde limb. Common proximal atrial and distal ventricular tissues are essential parts of the tachycardia circuit. About half of the participating accessory pathway is manifest (with delta wave in sinus rhythm), and the other half is concealed (only conduct retrogradely). Orthodromic AVRT may be initiated by atrial or ventricular ectopies.[11]

To initiate orthodromic AVRT, properly timed premature atrial complexes (PACs) are blocked in the accessory pathway but conduct antegradely to the ventricles via the normal AV conduction system. The impulse then returns to the atria in a retrograde fashion via the AV accessory pathway. Regarding the premature ventricular beats (PVCs), these beats are blocked in the normal AV conduction system but conduct retrogradely to the atria via the accessory pathway. The impulse then comes back to the

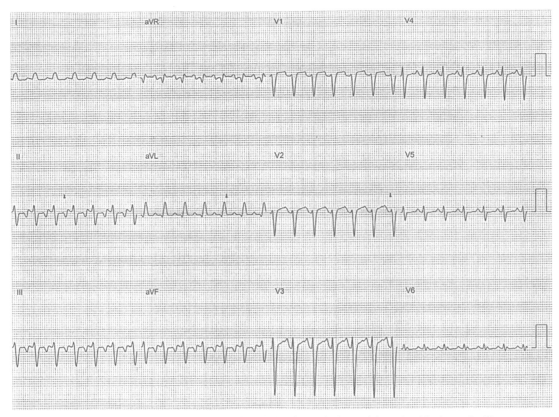

FIG. 13.2 Twelve-lead electrocardiogram of atypical atrioventricular nodal reentrant tachycardia. There are clear P waves in the ST segment with long RP and short PR intervals.

ventricles in an antegrade fashion via the normal AV conduction system to complete the reentrant circuit.

*Electrocardiographic characteristics.* Orthodromic AVRT is characterized by a regular ventricular rate of 150–250 beats/min and clear P waves in the ST segment (Fig. 13.6). Other characteristic electrocardiographic (ECG) findings (see Fig. 13.6) are ST-segment depression of 2.0 mm or greater (horizontal or downsloping ST segment) at the J point and lasting for 80 ms in inferior (II, III, aVF) and precordial leads (V2–V6), RP interval of 100 ms or greater, and ST-segment elevation of 1.0 mm, or greater at the J point (horizontal or upsloping ST segment), or 1.5 mm or greater at the J point (downsloping ST segment) lasting 80 ms in lead aVR.[12–14]

*Electrophysiologic characteristics.* In the presence of the manifest accessory pathway, incremental atrial pacing progressively increases the degree of preexcitation or even can unmask preexcitation if it is not manifested during sinus rhythm.

Ventricular pacing in all retrogradely conducting accessory pathways (manifest or concealed) is associated with conduction over the accessory pathway at short pacing cycle length (CL). Contrary to the normal AV conduction system, retrograde conduction over the accessory pathways is nondecremental (constant over a wide range of pacing CLs), and earliest retrograde atrial activity can show the atrial origin of the accessory pathway.

Initiation of orthodromic AVRT with an atrial extra stimulation requires anterograde block in the accessory pathway, anterograde conduction over the normal AV conduction system, and subsequent retrograde conduction over the accessory pathway. Delivery of ventricular ectopy when the His bundle is refractory results in atrial advancement in the presence of a retrogradely conducting accessory pathway (Fig. 13.7). In free-wall accessory pathways, ipsilateral BBB during orthodromic AVRT results in prolongation of the surface VA interval (≥35 ms) and tachycardia CL (≥35 ms) because more time is needed for the impulse to travel from the AV

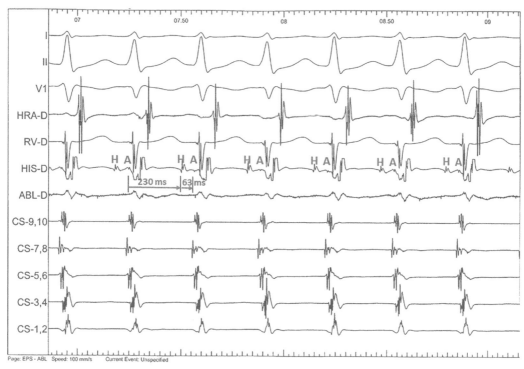

FIG. 13.3 Intracardiac recording during typical slow–fast atrioventricular nodal reentrant tachycardia. Note that there are characteristic short His–atrial (HA) (63 ms) and ventriculoatrial (VA) intervals and a long atrial–His bundle (AH) interval (230 ms). Retrograde atrial activation is concentric, and the earliest activity is recorded in the His catheter.

node and His bundle and contralateral bundle branch and transseptally to the ipsilateral ventricle to reach the accessory pathway and then activate the atrium.[15] Smaller prolongation (≥25 ms) indicates septal AVRT. However, contralateral BBB has no influence on surface VA interval or tachycardia CL.

**Focal atrial tachycardia.** FAT is the third most common SVT (≈10%).[16] Men and women seem to be equally affected.
*Pathophysiology.* FAT arises from a single atrial focus. FATs have a characteristic distribution within the right and left atria.[17,18] Right atrial FATs originate in most cases from the crista terminalis and tricuspid annulus. Other less common origins are the coronary sinus ostium, perinodal tissues, and right atrial appendage. Left atrial FATs predominantly arise from pulmonary veins. Mitral annulus, coronary sinus body, left interatrial septum, and left atrial appendage are less common sites of origin.
*Electrocardiographic characteristics.* The atrial rate during FAT is generally between 110 and 250 beats/min. AV conduction is usually 1:1 (Fig. 13.8); however, second-degree AV block may occur depending on the

atrial rate and conduction properties of the AV node. The PR interval is usually within the normal range and leads to a long RP tachycardia.
P-wave morphology is helpful in determining tachycardia origin.[18] Negative or biphasic (positive–negative) P wave in V1 indicates a right atrial origin; however, positive or biphasic (negative–positive) points to a left atrial origin. A negative P wave in leads I and aVL are highly suggestive of a left atrial location for FAT. Negative P waves in the right precordial leads suggest an anterior right atrium (RA) (RA appendage or tricuspid annulus). Negative P waves in the inferior leads suggest a low atrial origin (coronary sinus ostium, inferior part of tricuspid, or mitral annulus).
*Electrophysiologic characteristics.* Microreentrant and triggered-activity AT can be initiated by atrial extra stimulation or atrial pacing; however, automatic AT cannot be reproducibly induced by atrial extra stimulation or atrial pacing and usually requires isoproterenol infusion.
The AH interval during AT is usually longer than those during sinus rhythm. AV block may occur during tachycardia because neither the AV node nor ventricle is

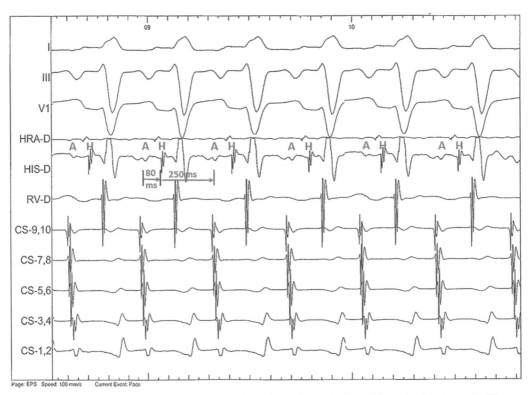

FIG. 13.4 Intracardiac recording during atypical fast–slow atrioventricular nodal reentrant tachycardia. There are characteristic short atrial–His bundle (AH) (80 ms) interval and long His–atrial (HA) interval (250 ms). Retrograde atrial activation is concentric, and the earliest activity is recorded in the proximal electrodes of the coronary sinus catheter.

part of the tachycardia circuit. BBB has no effect on tachycardia CL because ventricles are not part of the tachycardia circuit. Variability in CL is not characteristic of FAT, but changes in the atrial CL preceding changes in the ventricular CL are pathognomonic for AT.

**Atrial flutter.** AFL is uncommon in normal hearts (1.7%).[19,20] AFL is 2.5 times more common in men.[19] *Pathophysiology.* Typical AFL uses the isthmus between the tricuspid annulus and inferior vena cava as necessary components of the reentry circuit. Therefore, typical AFL is also called cavotricuspid isthmus (CTI)-dependent AFL.[21]

Atypical AFL is a macroreentrant AT that is not dependent on CTI.[21] The tachycardia circuit may be in the right or left atrium and usually occurs around a prior incisional scar, postablation lesion, congenital heart disease lesion, or idiopathic fibrosis. This kind of flutter is also known as non-CTI dependent AFL.[21]

*Electrocardiographic characteristics.* Characteristic ECG features of the typical AFL include an atrial rate of 250–350 beats/min, "sawtooth" (counterclockwise)

or "sine wave" (clockwise, reverse typical) flutter waves, absence of isoelectric interval between flutter waves, and usually a regular ventricular response of 150 beats/min. In counterclockwise typical AFL, there is negative flutter wave in inferior leads, a positive wave in V1, and a negative wave in V6 (Fig. 13.9). However, clockwise typical AFL has reverse morphology with positive waves in inferior leads, broad negative wave in V1, and positive wave in V6 (Fig. 13.10).

Atypical AFL is characterized by an atrial rate of 350–450 beats/min, regular but low-amplitude flutter waves, and sometimes the presence of an isoelectric interval between flutter waves. A negative flutter wave in V1 is in favor of right-sided AFL, but a positive or isoelectric flutter wave in V1 indicates a left atrial origin. Counterclockwise perimitral AFL has positive flutter waves in V1–V6 and inferior leads with negative waves in a VL. Clockwise perimitral AFL is positive in V1–V3, negative and then positive in V4–V6, negative in inferior leads, and positive in I and aVL.

*Electrophysiologic characteristics.* In counterclockwise typical AFL, the impulse travels through the low

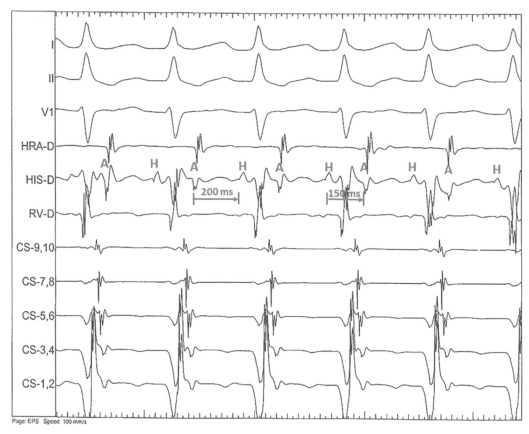

FIG. 13.5 Intracardiac recording during atypical slow–slow atrioventricular nodal reentrant tachycardia. There are characteristic long atrial–His bundle (AH) (200 ms) and His–atrial (HA) intervals (150 ms). Retrograde atrial activation is concentric, and the earliest activity is recorded in the proximal electrodes of coronary sinus catheter.

septum, ascends superiorly and anteriorly up the septal and posterior walls of the right atrium, and descends over the anterior and lateral free wall.[21] Finally, the circuit is completed across the region between the tricuspid valve and the inferior vena cava, cavotricuspid isthmus. A reverse direction of rotation is seen in reverse typical AFL.[21]

Atypical left AFLs are most commonly caused by incomplete ablation lines related to the Maze procedure or catheter ablation. They are usually seen in the anterior wall, through the roof, or on the septum. Mapping can often be difficult because of low voltages.

Atypical right AFLs are most frequently caused by atriotomy scar, where the scar is vertical along the lateral right atrium. The anterior right atrial wall may have ascending or descending activation depending on whether the circuit is clockwise or counterclockwise, but the septum may have more variable conduction.

The flutter circuit can be recognized in all types of AFLs by concealed entrainment. First postpacing interval 30 ms or less longer than tachycardia CL confirms that pacing sites are within the tachycardia circuit (Fig. 13.11).

**Atrial fibrillation.** AF is the most common cardiac arrhythmia in humankind. The prevalence of AF is higher in men than in women. The overall prevalence of AF is 1%, and 70% of the patients are at least 65 years old.[22] *Pathophysiology.* The majority of AF episodes are initiated by ectopies from pulmonary veins. However, a minority of AF attacks are triggered by AFL, FAT, AVNRT, and AVRT. Sustained AF requires abnormal substrate such as atrial enlargement, increase in atrial pressure, atrial inflammation, or fibrosis. These abnormal substrates are related to underlying heart diseases. The most common underlying diseases are systemic hypertension and coronary artery disease.[22,23] Other important but

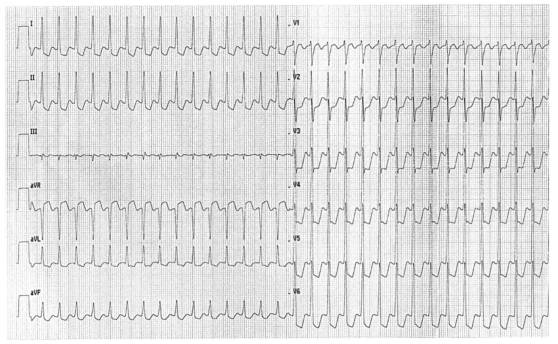

FIG. 13.6 Twelve-lead electrocardiogram of orthodromic atrioventricular reciprocating tachycardia. There is downsloping ST-segment depression 2.0 mm or greater in inferior (II, aVF) and precordial leads (V2–V6) and upsloping ST-segment elevation 1.0 mm or greater in aVR.

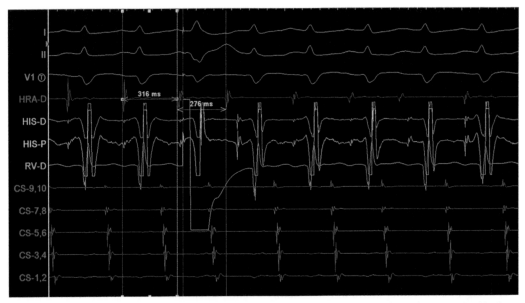

FIG. 13.7 Delivery of a programmed ventricular stimulation during His bundle refractoriness resulted in the atrial activity advancement (from 316 to 276 ms). This finding is in favor of orthodromic atrioventricular reciprocating tachycardia.

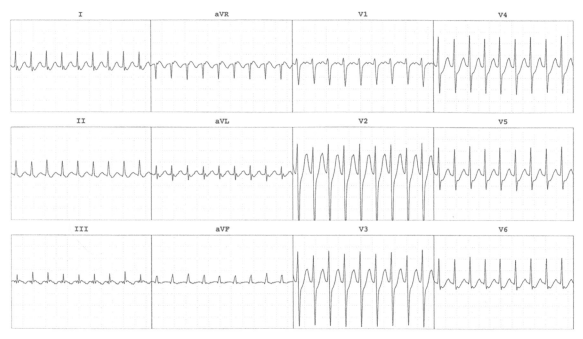

FIG. 13.8 Twelve-lead electrocardiogram during focal atrial tachycardia. Atrioventricular conduction of 1:1 is normal, and the P wave is clearly seen with a normal PR interval.

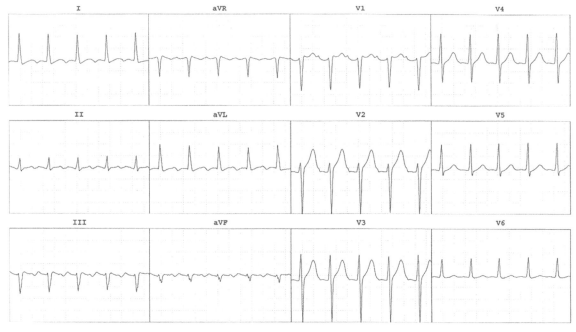

FIG. 13.9 Twelve-lead electrocardiogram during typical counterclockwise atrial flutter. There are "sawtooth" flutter waves, the absence of an isoelectric interval between flutter waves, and usually a regular ventricular response. In addition, flutter waves are negative in inferior leads, positive in V1, and negative in V6.

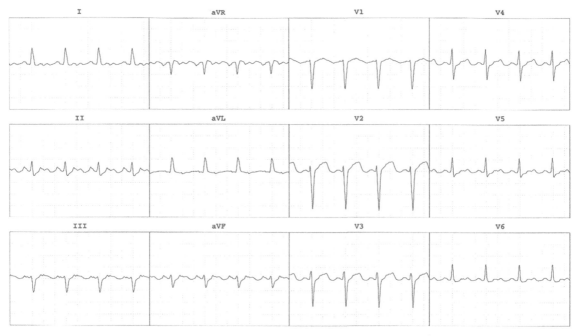

FIG. 13.10 Twelve-lead electrocardiogram during typical clockwise atrial flutter (AFL). There are "sine wave" flutter waves, absence of isoelectric interval between flutter waves, and usually a regular ventricular response. In clockwise typical AFL, flutter waves are positive in inferior leads, negative in V1, and positive in V6.

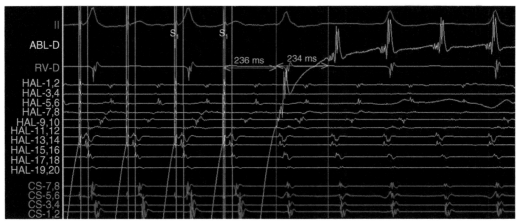

FIG. 13.11 Entrainment in typical atrial flutter. First postpacing interval 30 ms or less longer than tachycardia cycle length confirms that pacing sites are within the tachycardia circuit.

less common predisposing disorders are rheumatic heart disease, congenital heart disease, cardiomyopathies, and heart failure.

*Electrocardiographic characteristics.* In AF, there is no organized atrial activity; therefore, no discrete P waves are seen. Fibrillatory waves (with varying amplitude and morphology) are present at a rate of 350–600 beats/min (Fig. 13.12). Ventricular response varies between 90 and 170 beats/min and follows no regular pattern (i.e., irregularly irregular). However, AF may

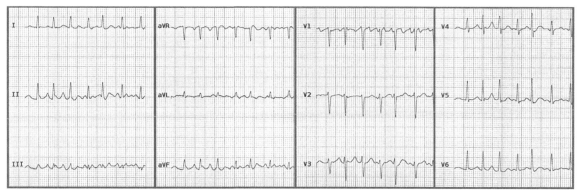

FIG. 13.12 Twelve-lead electrocardiogram during atrial fibrillation. There is baseline chaotic atrial activity with irregular ventricular response.

be associated with faster ventricular response in younger patients, those with thyrotoxicosis, and patients with preexcitation.

*Electrophysiologic characteristics.* Intracardiac recordings clearly show beat-to-beat variability in the atrial electrogram (EGM) amplitude, morphology, and CL. The different patterns of conduction during AF may be reflected in the morphology of atrial EGMs. Single potentials usually specify rapid uniform conduction, short double potentials may indicate collision, long double potentials are usually suggestive of conduction block, and fragmented potentials and complex fractionated atrial EGMs are markers for slow conduction.

**Sinus tachycardia (including inappropriate sinus tachycardia and sinoatrial nodal reentrant tachycardia).** Sinus tachycardia is one of the most common rhythm disturbances in humans.[24] It is a normal heart response to exercise and physical stress. Inappropriate sinus tachycardia is an uncommon arrhythmia that occurs in the absence of identifiable causes of sinus tachycardia, such as hyperthyroidism or fever, and is generally considered a diagnosis of exclusion. Sinoatrial nodal reentrant tachycardia (SANRT) is also an infrequent condition that rarely causes symptoms and occurs most commonly in adults with structural heart disease.[25–27]

*Pathophysiology.* Sinus tachycardia is a normal physiologic response to conditions in which there is enhanced catecholamine release.[24] Parasympathetic withdrawal is a less common cause of sinus tachycardia. A long list of identifiable causes has been reported for sinus tachycardia, including fever, dehydration, sepsis, anemia, heart failure, pulmonary emboli, myocardial infarction, hypoxia, pain, anxiety, thyrotoxicosis,

beta-blocker withdrawal, and cardiac stimulants. The pathophysiologic mechanism behind inappropriate sinus tachycardia is poorly understood; however, it may be related to sinus node hyperactivity in association with autonomic perturbations.[26]

*Electrocardiographic characteristics.* In sinus tachycardia, P-wave axis and morphology are similar or identical to sinus rhythm. The only difference is the heart rate of 100 beats/min or greater. An upright P wave in leads I and II indicates a sinus node origin. However, P waves may be difficult to identify at a heart rate of greater than 140 beats/min because they are superimposed on the preceding T wave. Inappropriate sinus tachycardia is identical electrocardiographically to other kinds of sinus tachycardias.[25] From the ECG point of view, SANRT is indistinguishable from sinus tachycardia.[23] The sudden onset and termination can help to distinguish SANRT from sinus tachycardia.

*Electrophysiologic characteristics.* Sinus tachycardia can be initiated by sympathomimetic agents in the electrophysiology laboratory. Warm-up and cool-down are characteristic features. Inappropriate sinus tachycardia is an incessant arrhythmia that cannot be terminated by overdrive atrial pacing or extra stimulation. SANRT can be induced and terminated by atrial or ventricular extra stimulation and overdrive pacing.

### Evaluation

After an NCT has been identified, further scrutiny of the ECG is required to identify the specific arrhythmia in a particular patient because diagnostic evaluation and therapy will differ depending on the underlying arrhythmia. The first step in the evaluation of NCT is the determination of hemodynamic stability. The second step is to determine whether the rhythm is regular or irregular.

Regular rhythms include sinus tachycardia, SANRT, AVNRT, orthodromic AVRT, FAT, and AFL with fixed AV conduction. Irregular rhythms consist of AF, AFL with variable AV conduction, and multifocal AT. The third step is identification of the P wave during regular narrow complex tachycardia. If P waves are superimposed on the preceding T waves, there are several methods to help in identification of the P wave during tachycardia. The Valsalva maneuver, carotid sinus massage (CSM), and intravenous (IV) adenosine are the well-known methods used to reveal hidden P waves. After the Valsalva maneuver, CSM, or the IV administration of adenosine to patients with NCT, four possible results may be observed:

1. Transient slowing of tachycardia CL (sinus tachycardia).
2. Termination of tachycardia (AVNRT, AVRT, and some forms of AT): Termination with a QRS complex may be observed with AVNRT, AVRT, or AT. However, termination with a P wave rules out AT and can be seen with AVNRT or AVRT.
3. Transient AV block with tachycardia persistence (AFL, AT).
4. No change is usually due to inadequate CSM or inadequate dose of adenosine.

### Treatment

Treatment options depend on the hemodynamic status of the patient and the regularity of the tachycardia. If a patient has hemodynamic instability, an attempt should be made as quickly as possible to determine whether the rhythm is sinus tachycardia. If the rhythm is not sinus tachycardia, direct current (DC) cardioversion is recommended. The Valsalva maneuver and CSM can be tried if those do not delay cardioversion.

**Regular narrow complex tachycardia.** In hemodynamically stable tachycardia, vagal maneuvers, IV adenosine, IV calcium antagonists, or IV beta-blockers are recommended.

Vagal maneuvers are safe and highly effective for acute termination of NCT. Although there are several types of vagal maneuvers, only a small number of these maneuvers are used clinically for therapeutic purposes (e.g., the Valsalva maneuver and CSM). There are several techniques for performing the Valsalva maneuver; in the most common approach, the patient is placed in a supine or semi-sitting position and instructed to exhale forcefully against a closed glottis after a normal inspiratory effort. Adequate maneuver is defined as neck vein distention, increased tone in the abdominal wall muscles, and a flushed face. The patient should maintain the strain for 10–15 s and then release it and resume normal breathing.

Carotid sinus massage is performed after auscultating for carotid bruit. The maneuver is done in the supine position with the neck hyperextended. The pressure is applied for 5–10 s inferior to the angle of the mandible at the level of the thyroid cartilage near the carotid arterial impulse. If no response is observed, the maneuver is repeated on the opposite side. If CSM in the supine position is ineffective, it can be repeated in the semi-sitting position. CSM is contraindicated in patients with carotid bruit (unless significant stenosis has been excluded by Doppler ultrasonography) and history of transient ischemic attack or stroke within the past 3 months.

After vagal maneuvers, the first-line drug is IV adenosine. The initial dose is 6 mg over 1–2 s via the brachial vein. If no response is detected within 1–2 min, 12 mg may be given; a 12-mg bolus may be repeated if needed (maximum single dose, 12 mg). After each dose, 20 mL of normal saline flush is recommended. Use 12 mg of the initial dose in patients receiving theophylline or caffeine. However, the initial dose should be reduced to 3 mg in patients receiving carbamazepine or dipyridamole, those with transplanted hearts, or if adenosine is administered via a central line.

If IV adenosine is ineffective or contraindicated (in patients with bronchial asthma and ischemic heart disease), IV verapamil is recommended as the second-line agent. The initial recommended dose is 5 mg over 2 min. If the patient does not respond to the initial dose, the second dose of 5–10 mg ($\approx 0.15$ mg/kg) may be given 15–30 min after the initial dose; the maximum total dose of verapamil is 20–30 mg.

If tachycardia persists after IV verapamil, IV betablockers (esmolol, propranolol, or metoprolol) are recommended. The IV loading dose of esmolol is 500 µg/kg over 1 min followed by a 50-µg/kg/min infusion for 4 min. If the response is inadequate, the infusion can be increased by 50 µg/kg/min every 4 min to a maximum of 200 µg/kg/min. In refractory tachycardia, procainamide or amiodarone may be considered.

**Irregular narrow complex tachycardia.** In stable tachycardia, rate control and antithrombotic are recommended to improve symptoms and prevent systemic thromboembolism. Beta-blockers and nondihydropyridine calcium channel blockers are preferred as first-line agents in most patients. For patients with AF or AFL less than 48 h in duration in whom cardioversion is planned, the use of antithrombotic therapy is not necessary before cardioversion. However, for patients with AF or AFL for longer than 48 h in duration (or unknown duration) 4 weeks of therapeutic oral anticoagulation before cardioversion is essential. Transesophageal echocardiography (TEE) screening for the presence of atrial thrombi is recommended if cardioversion is desired before 4 weeks. Anticoagulation must be continued for a minimum of 4 weeks after cardioversion. In MAT, correction of associated electrolyte abnormalities and management of underlying cardiac or pulmonary diseases are necessary before initiation of additional medical therapy.

## Wide Complex Tachycardia
### Etiology
Wide complex tachycardia usually occurs in patients with underlying heart disease. VT is the most prevalent cause of WCT,[28,29] especially in patients with a history of heart disease ($\leq$80%). SVT may also present with WCT because of aberrant conduction or conduction over an accessory pathway.[28,29] Among patients with WCT caused by SVT, aberrant conduction is the most common reason for a widened QRS.[30] Antidromic AVRT is a relatively uncommon cause of WCT (6%).[30] Regular WCT in patients with a cardiac pacemaker may be caused by tracking one of the SVTs or may be caused by endless loop tachycardia (ELT). Congenital or acquired QT prolongation may be responsible for some cases of irregular WCT. ECG artifact, particularly when observed on a single-lead rhythm strip, may be misdiagnosed as VT.[31]

### Classification
Similar to NCT, WCT is divided into those with a regular or irregular ventricular rate. Regular WCTs include monomorphic VT, aberrant SVT, antidromic AVRT, and pacemaker-mediated tachycardia (PMT). Irregular rhythms consist of AF with aberrant conduction, preexcited AF, artifactual tachycardia, and polymorphic VT.

**Aberrant supraventricular tachycardia.** All previously mentioned NCTs may present with WCT caused by baseline or rate-dependent aberrancy.
*Pathophysiology.* The supraventricular impulse can be delayed or blocked in the His–Purkinje system, giving rise to a wide QRS. This phenomenon is known as aberrancy. In the presence of baseline left BBB (LBBB), right BBB (RBBB), or a nonspecific intraventricular conduction delay, any SVT will have a wide QRS. In some patients, conduction is normal during sinus rhythm but aberrant during the tachycardia caused by rate-related aberration. Such a delay in recovery may also be caused by underlying His–Purkinje system disease;

hyperkalemia; or the effects of antiarrhythmic drugs, particularly the class IC agents.
*Electrocardiographic characteristics.* If available, a previous ECG when the patient was in normal sinus rhythm may be helpful. The presence of a BBB on the baseline ECG does not prove that the tachycardia is SVT with aberrancy; however, the similarity of the QRS during the tachycardia to the QRS during sinus rhythm points to an SVT with aberrancy (Fig. 13.13).
*Electrophysiologic characteristics.* Electrophysiologic characteristics of the aberrant SVT are similar to the SVT with narrow complex tachycardia.

**Antidromic atrioventricular reciprocating tachycardia.** Antidromic AVRT is the least common arrhythmia associated with Wolff–Parkinson–White (WPW) syndrome, occurring in fewer than 10% of patients.[11]
*Pathophysiology.* In antidromic AVRT, antegrade conduction occurs over an accessory pathway, and retrograde conduction occurs over the AV node or a second accessory pathway. Therefore, the QRS complex will be wide with characteristic morphology. To initiate antidromic AVRT, *atrial ectopies* should be blocked in the AV node–His–Purkinje system but able to conduct antegradely to the ventricles over the accessory pathway.[11] Then the impulse returns to the atria via the AV node–His–Purkinje system to complete the reentrant circuit. *Ventricular ectopies* initiating antidromic AVRT are blocked in the accessory pathway but conduct retrogradely to the atria over the AV node–His–Purkinje system.[11] The impulse then travels back to the ventricles via the accessory pathway to complete the reentrant circuit.
*Electrocardiographic characteristics.* Electrocardiography during antidromic AVRT typically shows a regular ventricular rate of 150–250 beats/min, wide QRS complexes, and inverted P waves with an RP interval that is usually more than half the tachycardia CL (Fig. 13.14). Antidromic AVRT is difficult to differentiate from VT because ventricular activation starts outside the normal intraventricular conduction system in both types of tachycardias.
*Electrophysiologic characteristics.* The initial site of atrial activation in classic antidromic AVRT is consistent with retrograde conduction over the AV node. If the antidromic AVRT is using a second accessory pathway for retrograde conduction, then the atrial activation sequence will depend on the location of that accessory pathway. In addition, ventricular activation precedes His bundle activation (negative HV interval) during antidromic AVRT (Fig. 13.15).

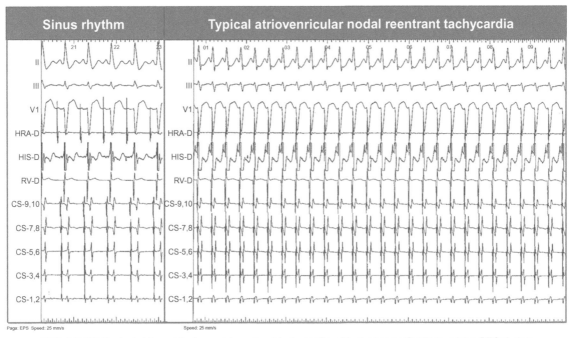

FIG. 13.13 Typical atrioventricular nodal reentrant tachycardia with aberrancy. Similarity of the QRS during the tachycardia to the QRS during sinus rhythm points to a supraventricular tachycardia with aberrancy. Intracardiac recording is in favor of typical atrioventricular nodal reentrant tachycardia.

**Monomorphic ventricular tachycardia.** Monomorphic VT is the most frequent cause of WCT (≤80%), especially in patients with structural heart disease (>90%).[28,29]

*Pathophysiology.* Monomorphic VT may be idiopathic, but most of the patients have underlying cardiac disease. VT usually originates from the ventricular myocardium; therefore, ventricular activation results in wide QRS. Rare cases of VT arise from bundle branches and the Purkinje system. Abnormal myocardium or scar tissue provides the necessary environment for the initiation and maintenance of VT.

*Electrocardiographic characteristics.* Monomorphic VT is characterized by three or more consecutive uniform ventricular ectopies at a ventricular rate of 100 beats/min or greater (Fig. 13.16). Definitive ECG diagnosis requires AV dissociation, capture or fusion beat, and ventriculoatrial association of 2:1 or more. Other suggestive features for VT are as follows:

- **Negative or positive concordance:** Negative concordance is strongly suggestive of VT. However, SVT with LBBB aberrancy may rarely yield a similar picture. The positive concordance also suggests VT but not as strong as a negative concordance. Antidromic

AVRT using the left posterior accessory pathway typically produces positive concordance.[32]

- **Axis:** Right superior axis is extremely rare in sinus rhythm and strongly suggests VT. In the presence of RBBB pattern VT, a QRS axis to the left of −−30 degrees favors VT. In LBBB pattern VT, a QRS axis more positive than +90 degrees suggests VT.[33]

- **QRS morphology:** Monophasic R or qR complex in V1 and rS in V6 favors VT in WCT with RBBB morphology[32,33]; RSR′ or RsR′ in V1 and Rs in V6 suggests SVT. Broad (≥40 ms) initial R wave in V1 or V2, a notch in downslope of V1 or V2, onset of the QRS complex to the nadir of the S wave of 60 ms or greater in V1 or V2, and Q or QS wave in V6 favor VT with LBBB morphology. By contrast, absence of initial R wave or narrow initial R wave in V1 or V2, downslope of S wave less than 60 ms and absence of Q wave in V6 favor SVT.

- **QRS duration:** In an LBBB pattern WCT, a QRS duration greater than 160 ms suggests VT.[32,33] However, a QRS duration greater than 140 ms favors VT in RBBB pattern WCT.[32,33]

*Electrophysiologic characteristics.* Ventricular tachycardia is characterized by AV dissociation and a negative

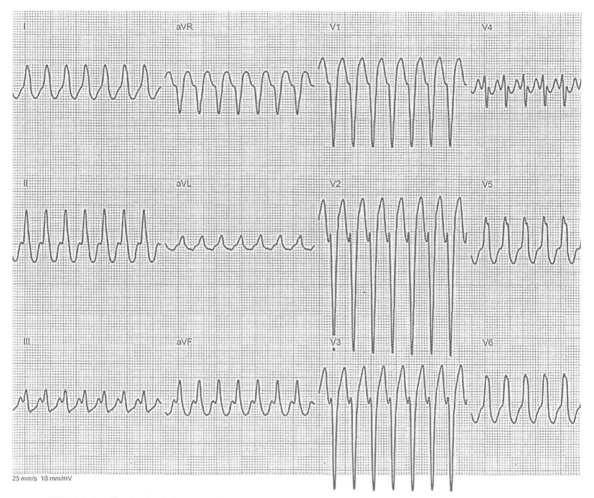

25 mm/s  10 mm/mV

FIG. 13.14  Twelve-lead electrocardiogram during antidromic atrioventricular reentrant tachycardia. This figure typically shows a regular ventricular rate of 190 beats/min, wide QRS complexes, and an RP interval that is usually more than half the tachycardia cycle length.

HV interval or HV interval shorter than that in sinus rhythm (Fig. 13.17). Sometimes no His potential is visible during VT. A negative HV interval or HV during tachycardia shorter than the HV interval in sinus rhythm may also be observed in antidromic AVRT.

**Pacemaker-mediated tachycardia.** A variety of tachycardias may be encountered in which the pacing system is functioning normally. PMT is not as rare as initially thought.

*Pathophysiology.* Regular WCT in patients with a pacemaker may be due to tracking of a native atrial tachyarrhythmia,[34] ELT,[35] or repetitive nonreentrant ventriculoatrial synchronous rhythm (RNRVAS).[36] In

the presence of sinus tachycardia, AT, AFL, and AF, the pacemaker tracks the atrial impulse and increases the ventricular rate, resulting in WCT. ELT can result if ventricular ectopies conduct retrogradely to the atrium, resulting in atrial activation and then ventricular tracking. This cycle repeats indefinitely. A third mechanism for PMT, RNRVAS, also creates a wide complex rhythm but usually at the lower rate limit or sensor-mediated rate rather than at the upper rate limit.

*Electrocardiographic characteristics.* Most transvenous ventricular pacemakers pace the right ventricle, causing an LBBB pattern in V1 and a broad R wave in lead I (Fig. 13.18). However, a biventricular pacemaker paces both ventricles. The QRS complex is usually

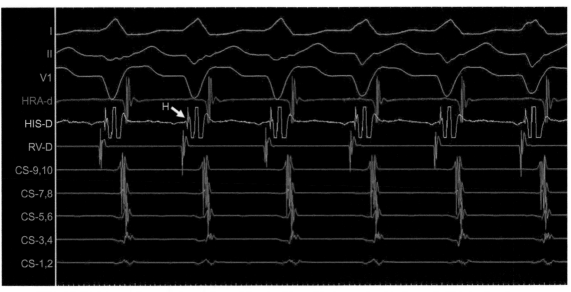

FIG. 13.15 Intracardiac recording during antidromic atrioventricular reentrant tachycardia. This tracing shows a negative HV interval (the *arrow* shows His potential) with 1:1 atrioventricular association.

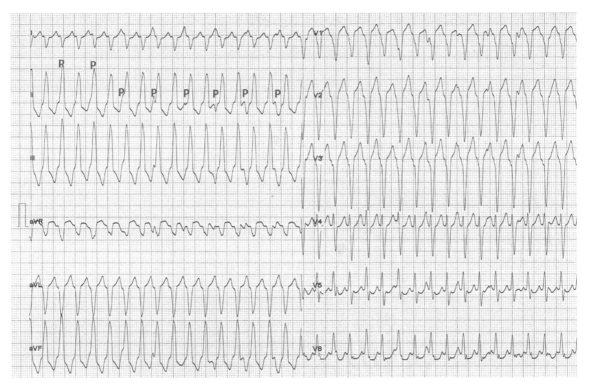

FIG. 13.16 Twelve-lead electrocardiogram during monomorphic ventricular tachycardia. Atrioventricular dissociation definitely proves the ventricular origin of the tachycardia.

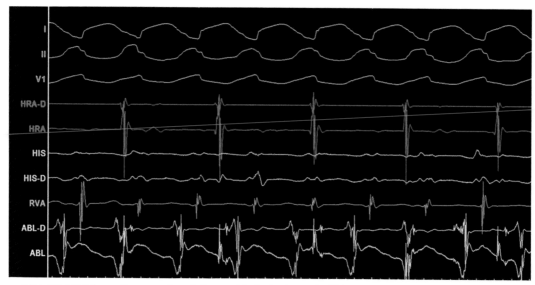

FIG. 13.17 Intracardiac recording during ventricular tachycardia. This tracing clearly shows a lack of association between atrial and ventricular electrograms.

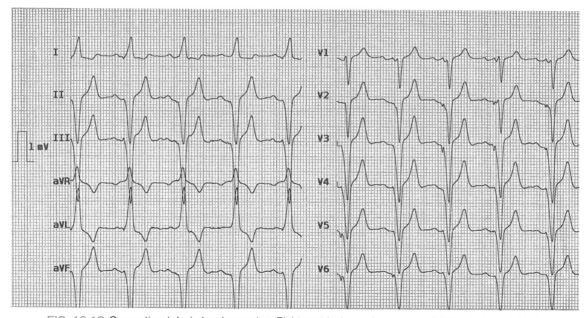

FIG. 13.18 Conventional dual-chamber pacing. Right ventricular pacing causes a left bundle branch block pattern in V1 and a broad R wave in lead I.

narrower than baseline in patients with biventricular pacemakers, and the surface ECG typically shows dominant positive QRS complex in V1 and QS or qR in leads I and aVL (Fig. 13.19). The presence of pacing spike before QRS complex is helpful in relating WCT to

PMT; however, bipolar pacing artifact may not be easily detected in some patients.

*Electrophysiologic characteristics.* Pacemaker-mediated tachycardia caused by sinus tachycardia or atrial tachyarrhythmias is easily detected by reviewing intracardiac

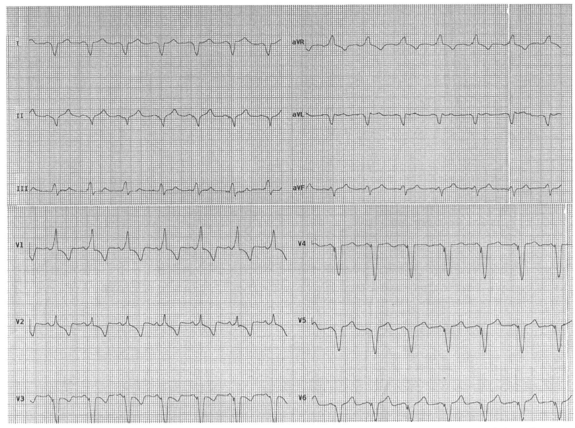

FIG. 13.19 Biventricular pacing. This figure shows a typical electrocardiogram pattern of right bundle branch block pattern in V1, QS in I, and aVL.

EGMs recorded by pacemakers or defibrillators. ELT is diagnosed by initiation of tachycardia by ventricular ectopies and termination by placing a magnet on the device or prolonging the postventricular atrial refractory period (PVARP). Excessive extension of PVARP for prevention of ELT predisposes the patient to RNRVAS. At the onset of RNRVAS, the retrograde P wave coincides with the PVARP and is not being sensed. As a result, there may be failure to capture with the next atrial stimulus, which occurs at the end of a relatively short atrial escape interval. The cycle will repeat and result in sustained retrograde conduction followed by ineffective atrial impulse. Therefore, the AR (atrium in refractory) marker is seen before all AP (atrial pacing) markers.

**Preexcited atrial fibrillation.** Preexcited AF is one of the major causes of irregular WCT. AF with aberrant conduction is the most common cause of irregular WCT.
*Pathophysiology.* The risk of AF or AFL is increased in patients with WPW.[37,38] There is usually variable QRS morphology, depending on how much conduction is through the AV node and how much is through the accessory pathway. There is a possibility that the ventricular rate will be very rapid (>300 beats/min) caused by 1:1 conduction from the atrium to the ventricles and can degenerate into VF.[39]
*Electrocardiographic characteristics.* Preexcited AF is characterized by irregular tachycardia with variable QRS morphology. There may be both narrow and wide QRS complexes. A closer look at the ECG will reveal

initial slurring of the QRS complex (delta wave). Those with the shortest R-R interval of 240 ms or less are more susceptible for AF degeneration to VF.

*Electrophysiologic characteristics.* The risk of AF is higher in the patients with a short antegrade effective refractory period of the accessory pathway, inducible orthodromic AVRT, and multiple accessory pathways.

**Artifactual tachycardia.** Sometimes ECG artifact may mimic WCT such as VT or VF. The presence of narrow-complex beats marching within the wide complex rhythm, absence of hemodynamic deterioration, an unstable baseline before and/or after wide QRS rhythm, and association with body movements strongly support the diagnosis of artifact.

**Polymorphic ventricular tachycardia.** Polymorphic VT is a rare cause of irregular WCT.

*Pathophysiology.* Polymorphic VT may occur in the setting of a normal or prolonged QT interval. For patients with polymorphic VT and a normal baseline QT interval, the most likely cause is myocardial ischemia. However, cardiomyopathies (hypertrophic cardiomyopathy and dilated cardiomyopathy) and other channelopathies (Brugada syndrome, short QT syndrome, and catecholaminergic polymorphic VT) may present with polymorphic VT.

*Electrocardiographic characteristics.* Polymorphic VT is defined as an unstable rhythm with a continuously varying QRS complex morphology in any recorded ECG lead. Polymorphic VT that occurs in the setting of QT prolongation is considered as a distinct arrhythmia, known as torsades de pointes. Baseline sinus rhythm may show ECG hallmarks of the underlying heart disease such as ischemic ST-T changes, prolonged QT interval, Brugada type ECG pattern, and short QT.

*Electrophysiologic characteristics.* Polymorphic VT is characterized by irregular WCT and AV dissociation. This type of VT can be induced in an electrophysiology laboratory during programmed ventricular stimulation or rapid ventricular pacing.

*Evaluation*

After a WCT has been identified, prompt diagnosis and management are important. The first step in evaluation of a patient with a WCT is an immediate assessment of hemodynamic status. Signs of hemodynamic instability include hypotension, altered mental status, chest pain, or heart failure. In stable WCT or unstable WCT after cardioversion, the second step is to determine the regularity

of WCT. An irregular WCT usually represents AF with aberrant conduction or preexcitation, although polymorphic VT and artifact mimicking tachycardia should also be considered. Regular WCTs include monomorphic VT, SVT with aberrant conduction, antidromic AVRT, and PMT. A brief history with special emphasis on structural heart disease (particularly prior myocardial infarction), known arrhythmias, pacemaker or implantable cardioverter-defibrillator implantation, and patient medications can aid in identifying the most likely cause of WCT. Reviewing the previous ECGs is highly useful in the diagnosis of SVT with aberrancy and antidromic AVRT. Differentiation between monomorphic VT and antidromic AVRT is particularly difficult because there is direct myocardial activation in both types of tachycardias. To differentiate between monomorphic VT and SVT with aberrant conduction, the AV relationship and morphologic criteria would be highly helpful in determining the tachycardia mechanism (see "ECG Characteristics of Monomorphic VT" earlier).

*Treatment*

Unresponsive or pulseless patients should be treated according to advanced cardiac life support (ACLS) recommendations. In a patient who is hemodynamically unstable but conscious, immediate synchronized cardioversion is recommended. Recommended energy levels for cardioversion in different settings are listed in Table 13.1. In a stable patient with WCT, treatment depends on the specific tachycardia mechanism. Patients with SVT with aberrant conduction should be treated

**TABLE 13.1**
**Recommended Energy Level for Electrical Cardioversion**

| Tachycardia | Biphasic Device (J) | Monophasic Device (J) |
|---|---|---|
| SVT other than AF | 50–100 | 100 |
| AF | 120–200 | 200 |
| Monomorphic VT with pulse | 100 | 200 |
| VF or pulseless VT | 120–200 | 360 |

*AF*, atrial fibrillation; *SVT*, supraventricular tachycardia; *VT*, ventricular tachycardia.

## TABLE 13.2
Recommended Dosing of Different Antiarrhythmic Drugs

| Antiarrhythmic Drug | Dose | Indications |
|---|---|---|
| Flecainide | 2 mg/kg IV over 10 min or 200–300 mg PO | AF, AFL |
| Propafenone | 2 mg/kg IV over 10 min or 450–600 mg PO | AF, AFL |
| Ibutilide | 1 mg IV over 10 min; if necessary can be repeated once after 20 min | AF, AFL |
| Amiodarone | 150 mg IV over 10 min followed by 1 mg/min for 6 h; then 0.5 mg/min for 18 h; a loading 300 mg over 20–30 min is recommended for VT | AF, AFL, VT |
| Lidocaine | 1–1.5 mg/kg IV; if refractory VF or pulseless VT, repeat 0.5–0.75 mg/kg bolus every 5–10 min (maximum cumulative dose, 3 mg/kg) | VT |
| Procainamide | 15–18 mg/kg IV over 25–30 min or 100 mg every 5 min as needed to a total dose of 1 g | AF, AFL, VT |

*AF*, atrial fibrillation; *AFL*, atrial flutter; *IV*, intravenous; *PO*, oral; *VF*, ventricular fibrillation; *VT*, ventricular tachycardia.

similarly to the narrow-complex counterpart. Patients with stable regular monomorphic VT and antidromic AVRT should be treated similarly. Procainamide is the drug of choice. IV amiodarone is the next choice. As a last choice, lidocaine is less effective than either procainamide or amiodarone. Recommended dosing of different antiarrhythmic drugs is summarized in Table 13.2.

## REFERENCES

1. Ganz LI, Friedman PL. Supraventricular tachycardia. *N Engl J Med.* 1995;332(3):162–173.
2. Katritsis DG, Josephson ME. Differential diagnosis of regular, narrow-QRS tachycardias. *Heart Rhythm.* 2015;12(7):1667–1676.
3. Garmel GM. Wide complex tachycardias: understanding this complex condition: part 1-epidemiology and electrophysiology. *West J Emerg Med.* 2008;9(1):28–39.
4. Akhtar M, Jazayeri MR, Sra J, Blanck Z, Deshpande S, Dhala A. Atrioventricular nodal reentry. Clinical, electrophysiological, and therapeutic considerations. *Circulation.* 1993;88(1):282–295.
5. Katritsis DG, Becker A. The atrioventricular nodal reentrant tachycardia circuit: a proposal. *Heart Rhythm.* 2007;4:1354–1360.
6. Heidbüchel H, Jackman WM. Characterization of subforms of AV nodal reentrant tachycardia. *Europace.* 2004;6(4):316–329.
7. Haghjoo M, Bahramali E, Sharifkazemi M, Shahrzad S, Peighambari M. Value of the aVR lead in differential diagnosis of atrioventricular nodal reentrant tachycardia. *Europace.* 2012;14(11):1624–1628.
8. Ng KS, Lauer MR, Young C, Liem LB, Sung RJ. Correlation of P-wave polarity with underlying electrophysiologic mechanisms of long RP′ tachycardia. *Am J Cardiol.* 1996;77(12):1129–1132.
9. Imrie JR, Yee R, Klein GJ, Sharma AD. Incidence and clinical significance of ST segment depression in supraventricular tachycardia. *Can J Cardiol.* 1990;6(8):323–326.
10. Colucci RA, Silver MJ, Shubrook J. Common types of supraventricular tachycardia: diagnosis and management. *Am Fam Physician.* 2010;82(8):942–952.
11. Josephson ME. Preexcitation syndromes. In: Josephson ME, ed. *Clinical Cardiac Electrophysiology.* Philadelphia: Lippincott Williams & Wilkins; 2008:339.
12. Cain ME, Luke RA, Lindsay BD. Diagnosis and localization of accessory pathways. *Pacing Clin Electrophysiol.* 1992;15(5):801–824.
13. Green M, Heddle B, Dassen W, et al. Value of QRS alteration in determining the site of origin of narrow QRS supraventricular tachycardia. *Circulation.* 1983;68(2):368–373.
14. Kay GN, Pressley JC, Packer DL, Pritchett EL, German LD, Gilbert MR. Value of the 12-lead electrocardiogram in discriminating atrioventricular nodal reciprocating tachycardia from circus movement atrioventricular tachycardia utilizing a retrograde accessory pathway. *Am J Cardiol.* 1987;59(4):296–300.
15. Yang Y, Cheng J, Glatter K, Dorostkar P, Modin GW, Scheinman MM. Quantitative effects of functional bundle branch block in patients with atrioventricular reentrant tachycardia. *Am J Cardiol.* 2000;85:826–831.
16. Wellens HJ, Brugada P. Mechanisms of supraventricular tachycardia. *Am J Cardiol.* 1988;62(6):10D–15D.
17. Roberts-Thomson KC, Kistler PM, Kalman JM. Focal atrial tachycardia II: management. *Pacing Clin Electrophysiol.* 2006;29(7):769–778.
18. Kistler PM, Roberts-Thomson KC, Haqqani HM, et al. P-wave morphology in focal atrial tachycardia: development of an algorithm to predict the anatomic site of origin. *J Am Coll Cardiol.* 2006;48(5):1010–1017.
19. Granada J, Uribe W, Chyou PH, et al. Incidence and predictors of atrial flutter in the general population. *J Am Coll Cardiol.* 2000;36(7):2242–2246.

20. Garson Jr. A, Bink-Boelkens M, Hesslein PS, et al. Atrial flutter in the young: a collaborative study of 380 cases. *J Am Coll Cardiol.* 1985;6(4):871–878.

21. Saoudi N, Cosío F, Waldo A, et al. Working Group of Arrhythmias of the European of Cardiology and the North American Society of Pacing and Electrophysiology. A classification of atrial flutter and regular atrial tachycardia according to electrophysiological mechanisms and anatomical bases; a statement from a Joint Expert Group from the Working Group of Arrhythmias of the European Society of Cardiology and the North American Society of Pacing and Electrophysiology. *Eur Heart J.* 2001;22:1162–1182.

22. Go AS, Hylek EM, Phillips KA, et al. Prevalence of diagnosed atrial fibrillation in adults: national implications for rhythm management and stroke prevention: the AnTicoagulation and Risk Factors in Atrial Fibrillation (ATRIA) Study. *JAMA.* 2001;285(18): 2370–2375.

23. Krahn AD, Manfreda J, Tate RB, Mathewson FA, Cuddy TE. The natural history of atrial fibrillation: incidence, risk factors, and prognosis in the Manitoba Follow-Up Study. *Am J Med.* 1995;98(5):476–484.

24. Yusuf S, Camm AJ. The sinus tachycardias. *Nat Clin Pract Cardiovasc Med.* 2005;2(1):44–52.

25. Pahlajani DB, Miller RA, Serratto M. Sinus node re-entry and sinus node tachycardia. *Am Heart J.* 1975;90(3): 305–311.

26. Gomes JA, Mehta D, Langan MN. Sinus node reentrant tachycardia. *Pacing Clin Electrophysiol.* 1995;18(5 pt. 1): 1045–1057.

27. Blaufox AD, Numan M, Knick BJ, Saul JP. Sinoatrial node reentrant tachycardia in infants with congenital heart disease. *Am J Cardiol.* 2001;88(9):1050–1054.

28. Akhtar M, Shenasa M, Jazayeri M, Caceres J, Tchou PJ. Wide QRS complex tachycardia. Reappraisal of a common clinical problem. *Ann Intern Med.* 1988;109(11):905–912.

29. Antunes E, Brugada J, Steurer G, Andries E, Brugada P. The differential diagnosis of a regular tachycardia with a wide QRS complex on the 12-lead ECG: ventricular tachycardia, supraventricular tachycardia with aberrant intraventricular conduction, and supraventricular tachycardia with anterograde conduction over an accessory pathway. *Pacing Clin Electrophysiol.* 1994;17(9): 1515–1524.

30. Miller JM, Hsia HH, Rothman SA, Buxton AE. Ventricular tachycardia versus supraventricular tachycardia with aberration: electrocardiographic distinctions. In: Zipes DP, Jose J, eds. *Cardiac Electrophysiology From Cell to Bedside.* Philadelphia: W.B. Saunders; 2000:696.

31. Knight BP, Pelosi F, Michaud GF, Strickberger SA, Morady F. Physician interpretation of electrocardiographic artifact that mimics ventricular tachycardia. *Am J Med.* 2001;110(5):335–338.

32. Gupta AK, Thakur RK. Wide QRS complex tachycardias. *Med Clin North Am.* 2001;85(2):245–266.

33. Wellens HJ. Electrophysiology: ventricular tachycardia: diagnosis of broad QRS complex tachycardia. *Heart.* 2001;86(5):579–585.

34. Greenspon AJ, Greenberg RM, Frankl WS. Tracking of atrial flutter during DDD pacing: another form of pacemaker-mediated tachycardia. *Pacing Clin Electrophysiol.* 1984;7(6 pt. 1):955–960.

35. Frumin H, Furman S. Endless loop tachycardia started by an atrial premature complex in a patient with a dual chamber pacemaker. *J Am Coll Cardiol.* 1985;5(3): 707–710.

36. Barold SS, Levine PA. Pacemaker repetitive nonreentrant ventriculoatrial synchronous rhythm. A review. *J Interv Card Electrophysiol.* 2001;5(1):45–58.

37. Campbell RW, Smith RA, Gallagher JJ, Pritchett EL, Wallace AG. Atrial fibrillation in the preexcitation syndrome. *Am J Cardiol.* 1977;40(4):514–520.

38. Sharma AD, Klein GJ, Guiraudon GM, Milstein S. Atrial fibrillation in patients with Wolff-Parkinson-White syndrome: incidence after surgical ablation of the accessory pathway. *Circulation.* 1985;72(1):161–169.

39. Timmermans C, Smeets JL, Rodriguez LM, Vrouchos G, van den Dool A, Wellens HJ. Aborted sudden death in the Wolff-Parkinson-White syndrome. *Am J Cardiol.* 1995; 76(7):492–494.

# CHAPTER 14

# Cardiac Implantable Electronic Devices

MAJID HAGHJOO

Department of Cardiac Electrophysiology, Rajaie Cardiovascular, Medical & Research Center, Iran
University of Medical Sciences, Tehran, Iran

## KEY POINTS

- A five-letter NBG (North American Society of Pacing and Electrophysiology [NASPE]/British Pacing and Electrophysiology Group [BPEG]) and four-letter NBD (NASPE/BPEG Defibrillator) codes have been developed to describe basic functions of various implantable pacemakers and defibrillators, respectively.
- Most of the temporary cardiac implantable electronic devices (CIEDs) are implanted percutaneously; however, epicardial systems are now implanted in a small number of patients. Novel leadless pacemaker and subcutaneous implantable cardioverter defibrillators (ICDs) are now available to decrease the long-term complications of transvenous systems.
- All CIEDs consist of a pulse generator and one or more electrodes transmitting electrical impulses to the heart and receiving cardiac signals. There are two types of pulse generators: pacemaker and defibrillator.
- All pacemakers operate according to the programmed pacing modes and timing cycles.
- The ICD should be programmed based on the patient's disease state and indications for which the ICD was considered. Together with programming the device in terms of arrhythmia protection and termination, clinicians should also consider a multitude of other parameters that focus on reduction of shock therapy and right ventricular pacing.
- The three most common factors affecting cardiac resynchronization therapy (CRT) response are suboptimal atrioventricular (AV) timing, arrhythmias, and anemia. There are several strategies to improve CRT response: appropriate patient selection, optimizing left ventricular lead location, biventricular capture optimization, and optimal atrioventricular/interventricular (AV/VV) interval programming.
- Troubleshooting must be approached in a systematic manner. Identifying the cause(s) of pacemaker malfunction is essential to implement an effective solution. Solutions must be verified to ensure that they have effectively resolved the original problem.

## INTRODUCTION

Cardiac implantable electronic devices (CIEDs) are established treatments for a variety of cardiac arrhythmias. Permanent pacemakers reestablish effective circulation and near normal hemodynamics by providing an appropriate heart rate and heart rate response. Implantable cardioverter defibrillators (ICDs) provide antitachycardia pacing (ATP) for termination of ventricular tachycardia (VT) and high-voltage shock, which are used to defibrillate ventricular fibrillation (VF) or to cardiovert ATP-refractory VT. Cardiac resynchronization therapy (CRT) or biventricular devices contain all capabilities of standard pacemakers and ICDs in addition to correcting inter- and intraventricular dyssynchrony. Since the first pacemaker implantation in a human in 1958 by Dr. Senning, there have been major new developments in CIED technology, including reduced size, increased battery longevity, and remote monitoring capability, as well as the addition of magnetic resonance imaging (MRI)-compatible CIEDs. This chapter presents an overview of important topics related to cardiac pacing, defibrillation, and resynchronization.

## NBG CODES FOR PACEMAKERS

A three-letter code describing the basic function of the various pacing systems was first proposed in 1974 by a combined task force from the American Heart Association and the American College of Cardiology and subsequently revised by a committee from the North American Society of Pacing and Electrophysiology (NASPE) and the British Pacing and Electrophysiology Group (BPEG). The code (Table 14.1), which has five letters or positions, is called the NBG (NASPE/BPEG Generic) code.[1]

**TABLE 14.1**
**NBG Pacemaker Codes**

| First Position:<br>Chamber Paced | Second Position:<br>Chamber Sensed | Third Position:<br>Response to Sensing | Fourth Position:<br>Rate Modulation | Fifth Position:<br>Multisite Pacing |
|---|---|---|---|---|
| O = None | O = None | O = None | O = None | O = None |
| A = Atrium | A = Atrium | T = Triggered | R = Rate modulation | A = Atrium |
| V = Ventricle | V = Ventricle | I = Inhibited | | V = Ventricle |
| D = Dual<br>(A + V) | D = Dual<br>(A + V) | D = Dual<br>(T + I) | | D = Dual<br>(A + V) |

*NBG*, North American Society of Pacing and Electrophysiology (NASPE)/British Pacing and Electrophysiology Group (BPEG) Generic.

*First position* refers to the pacing chamber. "A" indicates atrium, "V" indicates ventricle, and "D" indicates both atrium and ventricle. "O" means absence of pacing.

*Second position* refers to the sensing chamber. "A" indicates atrium, "V" indicates ventricle, and "D" indicates both atrium and ventricle. "O" means the absence of sensing.

*Third position* refers to the response to sensing. "I" indicates pacemaker inhibition in response to sensing. "T" indicates that the pacemaker is triggered in response to sensing. "D" indicates dual modes of response. This designation is unique for dual-chamber systems. An event sensed in the atrium inhibits the atrial output but triggers a ventricular output. "O" indicates no response to sensing.

*Fourth position* refers to rate modulation. "R" indicates that the pacemaker has rate-adaptive capability to increase heart rate in response to patient physical activity. "O" indicates the absence of rate responsiveness.

*Fifth position* refers to multisite pacing. "A" indicates multisite pacing in one atrium or both atria. "V" indicates multisite pacing in one ventricle or both ventricles. "D" indicates multisite pacing both in the atrium and ventricle. "O" indicates the absence of multisite pacing.

Most commonly, a code containing only the first three or four letters is used. Then it can be assumed that the positions not mentioned are "O" or absent.

## NBD CODES FOR DEFIBRILLATORS

After the NBG code, the mode code committee of the NASPE and BPEG developed another nomenclature system for defibrillator, known as the NBD (NASPE/BPEG Defibrillator Code), in January 1993.[2] Similar to the NBG code, the NBD code is a generic code, but it gives more information regarding the cardioversion and shocking capabilities without providing more information regarding the antibradycardia-pacing capabilities. The code has four letters with the following descriptions (Table 14.2).

*First position* refers to the shock chamber. "A" indicates atrium, "V" indicates ventricle, and "D" indicates both atrium and ventricle. "O" indicates no shocking capability.

*Second position* refers to the ATP chamber. "A" indicates atrium, "V" indicates ventricle, and "D" indicates both atrium and ventricle. "O" indicates no ATP capability.

*Third position* refers to the way that the device detects a tachycardia. "E" indicates that the device detects a

**TABLE 14.2**
**NBD Defibrillator Codes**

| First Position:<br>Shock Chamber | Second Position:<br>Antitachycardia Pacing | Third Position:<br>Tachycardia Detection | Fourth Position: Antibradycardia-<br>Pacing Chamber |
|---|---|---|---|
| O = None | O = None | E = Electrogram | O = None |
| A = Atrium | A = Atrium | H = Hemodynamic | A = Atrium |
| V = Ventricle | V = Ventricle | | V = Ventricle |
| D = Dual<br>(A + V) | D = Dual<br>(A + V) | | D = Dual<br>(A + V) |

*NBD*, North American Society of Pacing and Electrophysiology (NASPE)/British Pacing and Electrophysiology Group (BPEG) Defibrillator.

tachycardia by electrogram signal processing alone. "H" indicates that the device senses one or more hemodynamic-related variables as well, such as blood pressure or transthoracic impedance.

The fourth letter refers to the antibradycardia-pacing chamber. "A" indicates atrium, "V" indicates ventricle, and "D" indicates both atrium and ventricle. "O" indicates no pacing capability.

## CLASSIFICATION OF CARDIAC IMPLANTABLE ELECTRONIC DEVICES

### Transvenous Systems

Most of the temporary CIEDs are implanted percutaneously in the infraclavicular region of the anterior chest wall. CIEDs are usually implanted prepectorally; however, submuscular implantation has advantages in some patients (e.g., those without subcutaneous fat). Electrical impulses were conducted from the pulse generator to the cardiac chambers using one or more electrodes (leads). Devices with one atrial or ventricular electrode are called single-chamber pacemakers or ICDs; devices with atrial and ventricular electrodes are known as dual-chamber pacemakers or ICDs; and devices with atrial, right ventricular (RV), and left ventricular (LV) leads are called triple-chamber pacemakers or ICDs. Triple-chamber devices are also referred to as biventricular pacemaker/ICDs or CRT-P/CRT-D.

### Epicardial Systems

Epicardial systems are now implanted in a small number of the patients. In this system, the pulse generator is usually placed in the upper portion of the abdominal free wall, and leads are surgically attached directly to the epicardial surface of the heart. Although epicardial systems have mainly been replaced by transvenous systems, there are a few indications, including the absence of venous access, congenital cardiac anomalies, intracardiac shunts, tricuspid prosthesis, and small children. Similar to transvenous counterpart, epicardial systems may have one, two, or three electrodes.

### Novel Systems

In response to the limitations of both transvenous and epicardial systems, efforts have been made to develop new CIEDs. Leadless pacemakers (generator and electrode in a single unit) are implanted into the RV via a femoral approach. One leadless pacemaker, the Micra Transcatheter Pacing System (TPS) (Medtronic), are now available for implantation in patients who require single-chamber ventricular pacing.[3–5] Similarly a novel defibrillator, subcutaneous ICD (S-ICD), was developed over the past decade.[6] All components of the S-ICD—the pulse generator and leads—are implanted subcutaneously. The need in some patients for a system that avoids the use of transvenous leads has been long recognized. Indications of S-ICD implantation includes all indications of epicardial systems plus individuals with inherited channelopathies (rarely need pacing), history of previous endocarditis or device infections, patients anticipating cardiac transplantation, hypertrophic cardiomyopathy, young patients, women (cosmetic reasons), prosthetic heart valve (higher risk for infection), and primary prevention of ischemic and dilated cardiomyopathies.

## COMPONENTS OF CARDIAC IMPLANTABLE ELECTRONIC DEVICES

All CIEDs consist of a pulse generator and one or more electrodes transmitting electrical impulses to the heart and receiving cardiac signals. There are two types of pulse generators: pacemaker and defibrillator.

### Pulse Generator

Pulse generators consist of a battery, circuitry, can, antenna, reed switch, and connectors. Lithium-iodine is the most commonly used power source for today's pacemakers. Circuitry contains microprocessors to control sensing, output, telemetry, and diagnostic circuits. Connectors are used to attach the pacing or the high-voltage leads to the pulse generators. An antenna is used for communication with the programmer. The can contains all components, keeps out body fluids, and acts as a conductor. There are additional components in defibrillators: high-voltage capacitors for storing energy, a high-voltage transformer for changing the small battery voltage to high voltage, activity sensors, and audible alarms.

### Pacing or High-Voltage Leads (Electrodes)

Also, there are dedicated leads for the pacing and high-voltage leads for the cardioversion/defibrillation. Transvenous leads have different fixation mechanisms: passive fixation and active fixation. Passive fixation leads are typically entrapped within the trabecula of the right heart chambers. Current active fixation leads rely on a screw helix to attach to cardiac chambers. High-voltage leads have multilumen design with sense/pace conductors in the center and shocking conductors in the periphery. Single-coil leads have only a distal coil, but dual-coil leads have additional proximal coils. Epicardial leads are applied directly to the surface of the heart, and fixation mechanisms include stab-in, screw-in, and suture-on mechanisms. S-ICD leads are specifically designed; each lead has an 8-cm shock coil flanked by two sensing electrodes.

## PACING MODES

### VOO/AOO Mode

VOO/AOO mode paces in the ventricle or the atrium but will not sense and therefore has no response to cardiac events. Pacemakers programmed to the VVI, VVIR, and VDD modes revert to VOO mode upon magnet application. Pacemakers programmed to the AAI and AAIR modes revert to AOO mode upon magnet application. In these asynchronous modes, intrinsic beats have no effect on the timing cycle.

### VVI/AAI Mode

In inhibited modes (VVI/AAI), intrinsic events that occur before the lower rate interval expires reset the lower rate interval. As with paced events, sensed events also initiate blanking and refractory periods.

### VVIR/AAIR

Single-chamber rate-responsive pacing (VVIR/AAIR) is identical to non-rate-responsive pacing operation, with the exception that the pacing rate is driven by a sensor. The sensor determines whether or not a rate increase is indicated and adjusts the rate accordingly. The highest rate that the pacemaker is allowed to pace is the upper rate limit or interval.

### Hysteresis

Hysteresis allows the sensed intrinsic rate to decrease to a value below the programmed lower rate. Hysteresis provides the ability to maintain the patient's own intrinsic rhythm as long as possible while pacing at a faster rate if the intrinsic rhythm falls below the hysteresis rate. The hysteresis rate is always programmed to a value less than the lower rate. The lower rate limit is initiated by a paced event, and the hysteresis rate is initiated by a nonrefractory-sensed event.

### Noise Reversion

The portion of the refractory period after the blanking period ends is commonly called the "noise sampling period." This is because a sensed event in the noise sampling period will initiate a new refractory period and blanking period. If events continue to be sensed within the noise sampling period, causing a new refractory period each time, the pacemaker will asynchronously pace at the lower rate because the lower rate timer is not reset by events sensed during the refractory period. This behavior is known as "noise reversion."

### VDD Mode

In the VDD mode, the pacemaker will pace only in the ventricle and will sense in both chambers. In response to sensing in the ventricle, the pacemaker will inhibit. If a P wave is sensed, a sensed atrioventricular (AV) interval (SAV) will be triggered. There is no paced AV interval (PAV) in the VDD mode because the pacemaker will not pace in the atrium. Because the VDD mode does not have the ability to pace in the atrium, the pacemaker will operate as if in the VVI mode in the absence of atrial activity faster than the programmed lower rate.

### DOO Mode

DDI and DDD modes revert to DOO mode upon magnet application.

### DDI/DDIR Mode

In the DDI/DDIR mode, the pacemaker will pace in both chambers and sense in both chambers. In response to sensing, the pacemaker will inhibit, but a sensed P wave will not trigger an AV interval (therefore, there is no SAV interval in the DDI/DDIR mode). DDI/DDIR pacing can be thought of as AAI/R with VVI/R backup.

### DDD/DDDR Mode

In these modes, the pacemaker will pace and sense in both chambers. In response to sensing in the ventricle, the pacemaker will inhibit. If a P wave is sensed, an SAV will be triggered. If there is no intrinsic atrial beat at the end of the ventriculoatrial (VA) interval, the pacemaker will deliver an impulse in the atrium that initiates PAV.

## TIMING CYCLE OF PACING

The timing cycle of the pacemaker differs depending on the type of pacemaker:

*Single-chamber timing* has three components: the lower rate, refractory period, and blanking period (Fig. 14.1). There is a fourth component, the upper rate, in the rate-responsive mode.

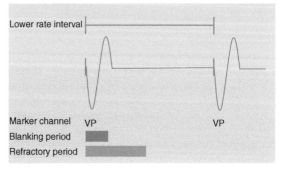

FIG. 14.1 Timing cycle of a single-chamber ventricular pacemaker. Timing cycle consists of lower rate interval, blanking period, and refractory period.

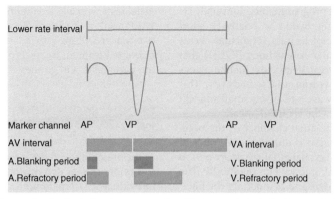

FIG. 14.2 Timing cycle of a dual-chamber pacemaker. Timing cycle includes lower rate interval, AV interval, VA interval, upper tracking rate, and dedicated blanking and refractory periods for each channel.

*Dual-chamber timing* has basic components of each chamber and additional components to permit chamber interaction: lower rate, refractory period, blanking period, AV and VA intervals, upper tracking rate, and upper sensor rate in the rate-responsive mode (Fig. 14.2).

### Single-Chamber Timing

The *lower rate* defines the lowest rate that the pacemaker will pace. For example, if the lower rate is programmed to 70 ppm in the VVI mode, the pacemaker is required to pace at a rate of 70 ppm if the patient's intrinsic ventricular rate is less than 70 beats/min. A paced or nonrefractory-sensed event restarts the rate timer at the programmed rate. The upper sensor rate in single-chamber pacing is available only in rate-responsive modes. The *upper rate* defines the limit at which sensor-driven pacing can occur.

Events that fall into the *refractory period* are sensed by the pacemaker, but the timing interval will remain unaffected by the sensed event. A refractory period is started by a paced, nonrefractory, or refractory-sensed event.

During the *blanking period*, the pacemaker is "blind" to any electrical activity. A paced or sensed event will initiate a blanking period. Blanking is a method to prevent multiple detection of a single-paced or sensed event by the sense amplifier.

### Dual-Chamber Timing

In dual-chamber pacemakers, the *lower rate* is the rate at which the pacemaker will pace the atrium in the absence of intrinsic atrial activity. The *upper tracking rate* limits the rate at which the ventricle can pace in the presence of high atrial rates. In rate-responsive modes, the *upper activity (sensor) rate* provides the limit for sensor-indicated pacing.

The *refractory period* after a ventricular event (paced or sensed) is designed to avoid restarting of the VA interval because of a T wave. Ventricular sensed events occurring in the noise sampling portion of the ventricular refractory period are "seen" (and marked "VR" on the marker channel) but will not restart the VA interval. The atrial channel is refractory after a paced or sensed event during the AV interval. This allows atrial senses occurring in the AV interval to be "seen" but not restart another AV interval. The postventricular atrial refractory period (PVARP) is the period of time after a ventricular pace or sense when the atrial channel is in refractory mode. In other words, atrial senses outside of blanking that occur during this period are "seen" (and marked "AR" on the marker channel) but do not initiate an AV interval. The purpose of PVARP is to avoid allowing retrograde P waves, far-field R waves, or atrial ectopies to start an AV interval, which would cause the pacemaker to pace in the ventricle at a high rate.

DDD/DDDR modes have four types of *blanking periods*: A nonprogrammable atrial blanking period (varies from 50 to 100 ms) is initiated each time the atrium paces or senses. This is to avoid the atrial lead sensing its own pacing pulse or P wave (intrinsic or captured). The postventricular atrial blanking period is initiated by a ventricular pace or sensed event (nominally set at 220 ms) to avoid the atrial lead sensing the far-field ventricular output pulse or R wave. In dual-chamber timing, a nonprogrammable ventricular blanking period occurs after a ventricular paced or sensed event to avoid sensing the ventricular pacing pulse or the R wave (intrinsic or captured). This period is 50–100 ms in duration and is dynamic, based on signal strength. There also is a ventricular blanking period after an atrial pacing pulse in order to avoid sensing the far-field atrial stimulus (crosstalk). This period is programmable (nominally set at 28 ms). This blanking period is relatively short because it is important not to miss ventricular events (e.g., premature ventricular contractions [PVCs]) that occur early in the AV interval. Ventricular blanking does not occur coincidentally with an atrial sensed event. This is because the intrinsic P wave is relatively small and will not be far-field sensed by the ventricular lead.

The total time that the atrial chamber of the pacemaker is in refractory period is during the AV interval and during the PVARP. The total atrial refractory period (TARP) is equal to the SAV interval plus the PVARP. The TARP is important to understand as it defines the highest rate that the pacemaker will track atrial events before 2:1 block occurs.

### Upper Rate Behavior

When the intrinsic atrial rate approaches (and exceeds) the programmed upper rate (assuming the TARP is less than the upper rate interval), pacemaker operations will change from 1:1 tracking operations to blocking operations (Wenckebach vs 2:1 AV block), which are designed to prevent tracking atrial arrhythmias that are too fast and that will likely cause patients to become symptomatic.[7]

#### Wenckebach pattern

The pattern of sensing a P wave, starting an SAV, waiting for the upper rate interval to time out, and pacing in the ventricle repeats until a P wave falls into the PVARP and does not start an SAV. The amount of delay created by the time from the sensed P wave until the upper rate interval expires is a little longer each time, producing the gradually lengthening of the P wave to ventricular pace intervals. When a P wave falls into the PVARP and does not initiate an SAV, the pacemaker looks for the next sensed P wave, and the pattern starts all over again. The rate at which the pacemaker will exhibit Wenckebach behavior is at the upper tracking rate (or upper rate if the pacemaker does not have a separate upper tracking rate and upper activity rate).

#### 2:1 AV block

The sequence begins with a sensed P wave. This P wave initiates an SAV followed by a paced ventricular event. The next P wave falls into the PVARP, started by the ventricular pace, so no SAV is initiated. The following P wave is sensed outside of the PVARP, so an SAV is started. Again, no ventricular event occurs during the SAV, so the pacemaker paces in the ventricle. The rate at which the pacemaker will exhibit a 2:1 block pattern is determined by the SAV and the PVARP (or the TARP).

Atrial rates with a P–P coupling interval shorter than the TARP result in 2:1 block. To determine at what rate the pacemaker will go into 2:1 block, the TARP is simply converted from an interval to a rate. Therefore, the rate the pacemaker will go into 2:1 block is 60,000/TARP.

## PROGRAMMING CONSIDERATIONS FOR IMPLANTABLE CARDIOVERTER DEFIBRILLATORS

At the present time, there is a significant amount of clinical evidence that demonstrates the significance of the individual ICD programming for the *reduction of shock therapy* and for the benefits that painless ATP pacing may provide to a patient for termination of ventricular arrhythmias.

The ICD should be programmed based on the patient's disease state and indications for which the ICD was considered. Together with programming the device in terms of arrhythmia protection and termination, clinicians should also consider a multitude of other parameters that focus on *reduction of RV pacing*.

### Minimizing Right Ventricular Pacing

Right ventricular pacing may induce significant dyssynchrony, and this induced dyssynchrony is associated with increased risk of heart failure (HF), atrial fibrillation (AF), and death. The Dual Chamber and VVI Implantable Defibrillator (DAVID) Trial[8] showed that RV pacing greater than 40% results in an increase in death and HF hospitalization. The Syncope and Falls in the Elderly—Pacing and Carotid Sinus Evaluation (PACE SAFE) Trial[9] clearly revealed an increased risk for AF in the DDD pacing group vs the minimized ventricular pacing (MVP) group. The Danish II Trial[10] demonstrated that long-term DDDR pacing induces left atrial dilation and, in the case of a high proportion of RV pacing, also reduces LV function. The Mode Selection Trial (MOST) Substudy[11] showed that for every 1% of incremental unnecessary ventricular pacing (VP), the risk of AF increases by 1%. Therefore, clinical evidence showed that unnecessary pacing should be reduced wherever possible. There are several ways to achieve this goal:

1. In single-chamber pacing, a lower rate should be programmed to a level below the patient's intrinsic rate.
2. In dual-chamber pacing, there are three main strategies by which RV pacing can be reduced: DDD pacing with a fixed long AV delay, AV hysteresis, and AAI(R)-DDD(R) mode switch algorithms. Among these three algorithms, the newer AAI(R)-DDD(R) mode switch algorithms are the most effective algorithms

to minimize RV pacing. These algorithms use a functional AAI(R) pacing mode; however, the device continually monitors AV conduction on a beat-to-beat basis (therefore, in reality, they function in ADI(R) mode as both chambers are sensed). In the event of persistent loss of AV conduction, the algorithm can switch to DDD(R) mode but can revert to AAI(R) when conduction returns to minimize RV pacing. MVP algorithm by Medtronic, Boston Scientific RYTHMIQ algorithm, SafeR algorithm by Sorin, and VP Suppression algorithm by Biotronik are well-known AAI(R)-DDD(R) mode switch algorithms.

### Shock Reduction

Implantable cardioverter defibrillators are lifesaving devices; however, inappropriate shocks occur in up to 20% of patients over the lifetime of these devices.[12–14] Clinical studies showed that avoiding ICD shocks reduces patients' anxiety, improves the quality of life, reduces HF risk, and improves survival.[15–17] There are several methods to avoid ICD shocks:

1. Programming ATP in VF zone: In the Pacing Fast Ventricular Tachycardia Reduces Shock Therapies (PainFREE RxII) trial,[15] 76% of detected episodes in the programmed VF zone were fast VTs that have a high success rate in being terminated with ATP therapy as opposed to shock.
2. Reducing inappropriate shocks caused by oversensing: Oversensing of physiologic and nonphysiologic signals accounts for a small but significant proportion of inappropriate shock.[18] There are several algorithms in ICDs to reduce T-wave oversensing and detect lead problems in the early stage before resulting in ICD shocks.[19,20]
3. Reducing shocks caused by nonsustained VT: These shocks are avoided by programming longer detection intervals or durations.

### OPTIMIZING CARDIAC RESYNCHRONIZATION THERAPY BY DEVICE PROGRAMMING

Although CRT is a highly effective therapy, a significant percentage of the patients get no benefit from CRT. The three most common factors affecting CRT response are suboptimal AV timing, arrhythmias, and anemia. There are several strategies to improve CRT response:

1. Select the appropriate candidate for CRT: Patients with sinus rhythm, left bundle branch block and QRS duration of 150 ms or greater are most likely to benefit from CRT.

2. Optimal LV lead location: Lateral branches of the coronary venous system are the most appropriate locations for LV lead placement. The middle cardiac vein and anterior interventricular vein are not appropriate targets for LV lead implantation.
3. Optimize the percentage of biventricular pacing: AF, frequent ventricular ectopies, and elevated LV lead threshold may decrease the percentage of biventricular capture. Medical or interventional treatment of these causes improves CRT response.
4. Optimize the AV and interventricular (VV) intervals: There are both echocardiographic methods and device-based algorithms to improve CRT response. AdaptivCRT is a dynamic and physiologic pacing algorithm that enhances cardiac resynchronization by adjusting CRT parameters automatically with changes in patient activity levels and conduction status.

### TROUBLESHOOTING

Troubleshooting must be approached in a systematic manner. Identifying the cause(s) of pacemaker malfunction is essential to implement an effective solution. Solutions must be verified to ensure that they have effectively resolved the original problem without introducing new concerns. There are pseudomalfunctions caused by normally functioning pacemaker algorithms that mimic true malfunctions. Therefore, these conditions should be ruled out before the diagnosis of true malfunction. True malfunctions are divided into pacing and sensing problems.

### Undersensing

*Undersensing* refers to underdetection of intrinsic cardiac activity in each chamber (Fig. 14.3). Therefore, the pacemaker sends an inappropriate pacing impulse to that

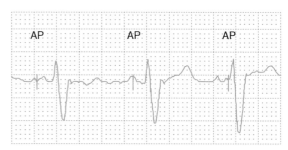

FIG. 14.3 Undersensing in a single-chamber atrial pacemaker. The pacemaker fails to detect the native P wave and sends an inappropriate stimulation to the atrium with functional noncapture.

chamber. Undersensing may be caused by inappropriately programmed sensitivity, lead dislodgment, insulation break, conductor fracture, lead maturation, or a change in native signal.

*Lead dislodgment* usually occurs early in the life of the pacemaker before the lead has attached to the endocardial tissue. The primary causes of lead dislodgment are inadequate initial positioning and patient movement (e.g., bringing arms overhead).

*Lead failure,* including insulation break and conductor fracture, is related to chronic stress imposed on the lead as a result of its placement in the subclavian region.

*Lead maturation* arises because of the trauma to cells surrounding the electrode, which causes edema and subsequent development of a fibrotic capsule. The inexcitable capsule reduces the current at the electrode interface, requiring more energy to capture the heart.

*Change in native signal* may occur because of myocardial infarction, electrode abnormalities, and changes in medications.

### Oversensing

*Oversensing* refers to sensing of inappropriate signal (Fig. 14.4). The sensed signal can be physiologic or nonphysiologic. Oversensing may be caused by lead failure,

a loose connection, or exposure to interference. The source of interference may be electromagnetic interference (EMI) signals or myopotentials. Sources of EMI are often found in hospitals and include surgical equipment such as electrocautery, transthoracic defibrillation, lithotripsy, radiofrequency ablation, and transelectrical nerve stimulation units. Myopotentials are more problematic with unipolar devices than bipolar devices. Oversensing is the most common cause of pause in pacing function.

### Loss of Capture

*Loss of capture* refers to the absence of myocardial capture despite the presence of a pacing spike (Fig. 14.5). Loss of capture may be related to lead dislodgment, lead failure, loose connection, lead maturation, inappropriately programmed low amplitude, Twiddler syndrome, electrolyte abnormalities, drug therapy, battery depletion, exit block, and myocardial infarction.

*Loose connection* at the connector block usually occurs because the lead has been inadequately secured at implant. Therefore, it is an early complication of pacemaker implantation or generator change. The poor connection may be viewed radiographically.

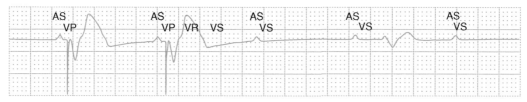

FIG. 14.4 Oversensing in the ventricular channel of a dual-chamber pacemaker. There is inappropriate sensing in the ventricular channel in the absence of native ventricular activity.

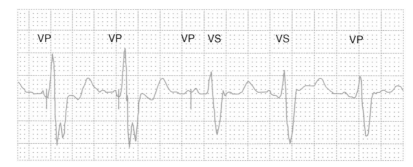

FIG. 14.5 Intermittent ventricular loss of capture. After appropriate ventricular capture in the first two beats, there is an intermittent loss of capture in third and fifth beats (pacing spike with no capture).

*Twiddler syndrome* usually occurs in older patients who manipulate the device pocket. This complication is more common after replacement of a large-sized device with a smaller new one. Twiddler syndrome can be identified radiographically.

*Electrolyte abnormalities*, especially hyperkalemia, may adversely affect the pacing threshold. Hyperkalemia increases the pacing threshold and may result in loss of capture.

*Drug therapy* may affect capture thresholds and result in significant changes from the patient's baseline. The most common drugs with this effect are class IC antiarrhythmic medications, such as flecainide and propafenone.

## No Output

In this situation, there is no pacing spike, and the heart rate is lower than the programmed lower rate (Fig. 14.6). No output may be caused by a loose connection, conductor fracture, battery depletion, or circuit failure.

## Pseudomalfunctions

*Pseudomalfunctions* refer to electrocardiogram (ECG) findings that appear to result from pacemaker malfunction but that represent normal pacemaker function. Pseudomalfunctions should be ruled out as the cause(s) of an anomalous ECG strip before corrective measures are taken. Pseudomalfunctions may be caused by changes in rate, AV interval or refractory periods, or mode.

*Rate changes* may be related to magnet operation, upper rate behavior, electrical reset, battery depletion, pacemaker-mediated tachycardia (PMT) intervention, rate response, hysteresis, sleep function, mode switching, and rate drop response. Magnet operation varies within different product lines and from manufacturer to manufacturer but usually involves asynchronous pacing when the magnet is applied. Upper rate behavior has been described in detail before. Electrical reset is usually characterized by a rate change and often a mode change.

Electrical reset may occur because of exposure to EMI such as electrocautery, defibrillation, and causing reversion to a "backup mode." Battery depletion indicators, including EOS (end of service) and RRT (relative replacement time), are often similar to backup mode. Dual-chamber mode will downgrade to single-chamber mode upon reaching to EOS. PMT intervention is designed to interrupt a kind of PMT known as endless-loop tachycardia. PMT intervention will extend the PVARP to 400 ms after eight consecutive events. Rate response can result in rate acceleration or deceleration. This finding is quite typical when the patient is active. However, sensors may cause a false-positive increase in the pacing rate. For example, a piezoelectric crystal may increase the pacing rate when the patient is either lying on the side in which pacemaker is implanted or experiencing a bumpy car ride.

*Abnormalities of AV interval/refractory periods* may be caused by safety pacing, blanking, rate-adaptive AV delay, sensor-varied PVARP, PVC response, and noncompetitive atrial pace (NCAP). *Ventricular safety pacing* is designed to prevent inhibition caused by "cross talk." In this situation, the pacemaker delivers a ventricular pace 110 ms after an atrial pacing. *Rate-adaptive AV delay* is designed to mimic the intrinsic response to increasing heart rate. In a normal heart, PR intervals decrease as the heart rate increases. Conversely, as the heart rate decreases, PR intervals increase. When *sensor-varied PVARP* is enabled, the duration of the PVARP will shorten as the heart rate increases. When a PVC is detected and the *PVC response* is programmed on, the PVARP is extended in order to avoid sensing the retrograde P wave that could occur as a result of the PVC. NCAP prevents atrial pacing from occurring too close to the relative refractory period, which may trigger atrial arrhythmias. If NCAP is activated, the scheduled atrial pace will be delayed until at least 300 ms have elapsed since the refractory-sensed P wave occurred. To keep the ventricular rate from experiencing the same delay, the ensuing PAV can be shortened.

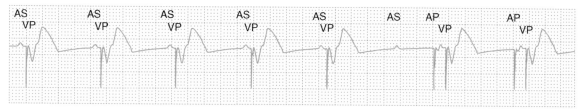

FIG. 14.6 No output in the ventricular channel of a dual-chamber pacemaker. After appropriate atrial sensing and ventricular capture in the first five beats, atrial sensing is not followed by a pacing spike and capture in the ventricle.

*Mode changes* may be caused by battery depletion indicators, electrical reset, mode switching, and noise reversion. The *RRT*, previously known as the elective replacement indicator, is designed to alert the clinician at least 3 months before the battery voltage drops to a level at which noncapture or inconsistent pacing would result. The *EOS*, previously known as the end-of-life (EOL) indicator, is designed to give the patient and physician adequate time to replace the device. Patients with EOS should be admitted immediately. Sensing occurring during atrial or ventricular refractory periods will restart the refractory period. Continuous refractory sensing is called *noise reversion* and causes pacing to occur at the sensor-indicated rate for rate-responsive modes and at the lower rate for non-rate-responsive modes.

## REFERENCES

1. Bernstein AD, Daubert JC, Fletcher RD, et al. The revised NASPE/BPEG generic code for antibradycardia, adaptive-rate, and multisite pacing. North American Society of Pacing and Electrophysiology/British Pacing and Electrophysiology Group. *Pacing Clin Electrophysiol.* 2002; 25(2):260–264.
2. Bernstein AD, Camm AJ, Fisher JD, et al. North American Society of Pacing and Electrophysiology policy statement. The NASPE/BPEG defibrillator code. *Pacing Clin Electrophysiol.* 1993;16(9):1776–1780.
3. Ritter P, Duray GZ, Steinwender C, et al. Early performance of a miniaturized leadless cardiac pacemaker: the Micra Transcatheter Pacing Study. *Eur Heart J..* 2015;36 (37):2510–2519.
4. Reynolds D, Duray GZ, Omar R, et al. A leadless intracardiac transcatheter pacing system. *N Engl J Med.* 2016;374(6):533–541.
5. Knops RE, Tjong FV, Neuzil P, et al. Chronic performance of a leadless cardiac pacemaker: 1-year follow-up of the LEADLESS trial. *J Am Coll Cardiol.* 2015;65(15): 1497–1504.
6. Weiss R, Knight BP, Gold MR, et al. Safety and efficacy of a totally subcutaneous implantable-cardioverter defibrillator. *Circulation.* 2013;128(9):944–953.
7. Furman S. Dual chamber pacemakers: upper rate behavior. *Pacing Clin Electrophysiol.* 1985;8(2):197–214.
8. Wilkoff BL, Cook JR, Epstein AE, et al. Dual-chamber pacing or ventricular backup pacing in patients with an implantable defibrillator: the Dual Chamber and VVI Implantable Defibrillator (DAVID) Trial. *JAMA.* 2002; 288(24):3115–3123.
9. Sweeney MO, Bank AJ, Nsah E, et al. Minimizing ventricular pacing to reduce atrial fibrillation in sinus-node disease. *N Engl J Med.* 2007;357(10):1000–1008.
10. Nielsen JC, Kristensen L, Andersen HR, Mortensen PT, Pedersen OL, Pedersen AK. A randomized comparison of atrial and dual-chamber pacing in 177 consecutive patients with sick sinus syndrome: echocardiographic and clinical outcome. *J Am Coll Cardiol.* 2003;42(4): 614–623.
11. Sweeney MO, Hellkamp AS, Ellenbogen KA, et al. Adverse effect of ventricular pacing on heart failure and atrial fibrillation among patients with normal baseline QRS duration in a clinical trial of pacemaker therapy for sinus node dysfunction. *Circulation.* 2003; 107(23):2932–2937.
12. Kadish A, Dyer A, Daubert JP, et al. Prophylactic defibrillator implantation in patients with nonischemic dilated cardiomyopathy. *N Engl J Med.* 2004;350: 2151–2158.
13. Daubert JP, Zareba W, Cannom DS, et al. Inappropriate implantable cardioverter-defibrillator shocks in MADIT-II: frequency, mechanisms, predictors, and survival impact. *J Am Coll Cardiol.* 2008;5:1357–1365.
14. Poole JE, Johnson GW, Hellkamp AS, et al. Prognostic importance of defibrillator shocks in patients with heart failure. *N Engl J Med.* 2008;359:1009–1017.
15. Wathen MS, DeGroot PJ, Sweeney MO, et al. Prospective randomized multicenter trial of empirical antitachycardia pacing versus shocks for spontaneous rapid ventricular tachycardia in patients with implantable cardioverter-defibrillators. *Circulation.* 2004;110:2591–2596.
16. Ahmad M, Bloomstein L, Roelke M, Bernstein AD, Parsonnet V. Patients' attitudes toward implantable defibrillator shocks. *Pacing Clin Electrophysiol.* 2000;23(6): 934–938.
17. Sweeney MOL, Sherfesee L, DeGroot PJ, Wathen MS, Wilkoff BL. Differences in effects of electrical therapy type for ventricular arrhythmias on mortality in implantable cardioverter-defibrillator patients. *Heart Rhythm.* 2100;7(3):353–360.
18. Swerdlow CD, Gunderson BD, Ousdigian KT, et al. Downloadable algorithm to reduce inappropriate shocks caused by fractures of implantable cardioverter-defibrillator leads. *Circulation.* 2008;118:2122–2129.
19. Kallinen LM, Hauser RG, Tang C, et al. Lead integrity alert algorithm decreases inappropriate shocks in patients who have Sprint Fidelis pace-sense conductor fractures. *Heart Rhythm.* 2010;7:1048–1055.
20. Sweeney MO, Ruetz LL, Belk P, Mullen TJ, Johnson JW, Sheldon T. Bradycardia pacing-induced short-long-short sequences at the onset of ventricular tachyarrhythmias: a possible mechanism of proarrhythmia? *J Am Coll Cardiol.* 2007;50:614–622.

# CHAPTER 15

# Bradyarrhythmias

MAJID HAGHJOO

Department of Cardiac Electrophysiology, Rajaie Cardiovascular, Medical & Research Center, Iran University of Medical Sciences, Tehran, Iran

## KEY POINTS

- Bradyarrhythmias encompass a number of rhythm disturbances, including sinus node dysfunction (SND) and atrioventricular (AV) block.
- Bradyarrhythmias may be asymptomatic and detected during routine electrocardiographic (ECG) examination or presented with dizziness, fatigue, syncope, presyncope, exercise intolerance, and poor concentration. Symptomatic SND is called sick sinus syndrome (SSS).
- ECG presentations of SND are sinus bradycardia, sinus pause or arrest, sinoatrial exit block, chronotropic incompetence, and tachy-brady syndrome.
- Symptom–rhythm correlation is highly important in SSS diagnosis. The initial clues to the diagnosis of SSS are most often gleaned from the patient's history, and the diagnosis is confirmed by a 12-lead surface ECG, ambulatory ECG recording, or exercise stress testing.
- In SND, treatment should be limited to patients with a good symptom–rhythm correlation. Asymptomatic patients do not need any treatment.
- AV block is traditionally classified as first-, second-, or third-degree (complete) AV block. On the basis of intracardiac recordings, supra-, intra-, or infra-Hisian block can be differentiated.
- Diagnosis of AV block can be established in most cases noninvasively by the 12-lead ECG. In intermittent AV block, ambulatory ECG monitoring and exercise testing are important to establish a symptom–rhythm correlation.
- Except for asymptomatic first-degree, type 1 second-degree AV block, and reversible types, other types of AV blocks need a pacemaker, irrespective of associated symptoms.

## INTRODUCTION

Bradyarrhythmias are a common clinical problem and encompass a number of rhythm disturbances, including sinus node dysfunction (SND) and atrioventricular (AV) blocks. The normal adult heart rate has been considered historically to range from 60 to 100 beats/min, with bradyarrhythmias being defined as a heart rhythm with a rate below 60 beats/min.[1] In this chapter, clinical presentation, etiology, diagnosis, treatment options, and prognosis are reviewed.

## CLINICAL PRESENTATION

Bradyarrhythmia may be asymptomatic and detected during routine electrocardiographic (ECG) examination or presented with a broad variety of symptoms, including dizziness, fatigue, syncope, presyncope, exercise intolerance, and poor concentration.[2] A patient with comorbid conditions that might be exacerbated by reduced cardiac output (e.g., angina and heart failure) may present with worsening symptoms related to the comorbidity. Presenting symptoms can be intermittent or permanent.

## SINUS NODE DYSFUNCTION

### Etiology

SND consists of a variety of conditions affecting sinus node impulse generation and transmission and may be responsible for bradyarrhythmias.[3] SND can occur as a physiologic response in well-trained athletes[4] or during sleep; however, it may also occur as a pathologic response in a variety of disorders.[5] Symptomatic SND is called *sick sinus syndrome* (SSS).

Sinus bradycardia with a heart rate as low as 30 beats/min or sinus pauses up to 2 s are common, especially in athletes, children, and young adults.[6] SND may also occur secondary to numerous pathologic causes (Table 15.1).

## TABLE 15.1
### Etiology of Sinus Node Dysfunction

| Extrinsic Causes | Intrinsic Causes |
|---|---|
| Pharmacologic agents | Idiopathic degeneration |
| Beta blockers | Ischemic heart disease |
| Calcium antagonists | Endocarditis |
| Cardiac glycosides | Myocarditis |
| Class I and III antiarrhythmics | Infiltrative diseases |
| Sympatholytic antihypertensives | Collagen vascular diseases |
| Parasympathomimetic agents | Muscular dystrophies |
| Opioids and sedatives | Congenital heart disease |
| Chemotherapy agents | Cardiac surgery |
| Organophosphate compounds | |
| Others: lithium, cimetidine | |
| Electrolyte disturbances | |
| Hypothyroidism | |
| Obstructive sleep apnea | |
| Hypoxia | |
| Hypothermia | |
| Increased vagal tone (coughing, vomiting, defecation, micturition) | |

## Classification

Electrocardiographic presentations of SND are sinus bradycardia, sinus pause or arrest, sinoatrial (SA) exit block, chronotropic incompetence, and tachycardia-bradycardia (tachy-brady) syndrome.

**Sinus bradycardia** is defined as sinus rhythm with heart rate less than 60 beats/min. Except for the rate, other features, including P-wave morphology, PR interval, and 1:1 AV conduction, are similar to the normal sinus rhythm. Sinus bradycardia is a common transient clinical finding with no hemodynamic consequence, especially in children and young adults. However, it can be persistent and produce symptoms in older adult patients with heart rates less than 40 beats/min.

**Sinus pause or arrest** is characterized by temporary cessation of sinus node discharges. Electrocardiographically, there are no P waves and associated QRS-T during sinus pause. This pause is sometimes followed by junctional rhythm or idioventricular rhythm. The absence of

escape rhythm results in asystole. Sinus pause less than 3 s usually needs no investigation and may be seen in normal people; however, longer pauses ($\geq$3 s) require further investigation and treatment.[7,8]

**Sinoatrial exit block:** This type of SND has similar ECG presentation to sinus pause. In SA exit block, sinus node depolarization is normal, but it fails to conduct to surrounding atrial tissues.

In *first-degree SA exit block*, the conduction time between sinus node impulse and atrial tissue depolarization increases. Sinus node depolarization produces no wave on surface ECG; therefore, first-degree SA exit block cannot be recognized on surface ECG. Thus, first-degree SA exit block cannot be diagnosed without electrophysiologic study (EPS).

In *type 1 second-degree SA exit block*, there is progressive shortening of the P-P interval before a P-QRS-T complex is dropped (Fig. 15.1). This P-P interval shortening may be helpful in discriminating this condition from sinus pause.

In *type 2 second-degree SA exit block*, the P-P interval surrounding the dropped complexes is two times (or a multiple) of the baseline P-P interval. This point can distinguish this type of SA exit block from sinus pause.

*Third-degree SA exit block* is characterized by asystole or junctional rhythm in ECG, and diagnosis on surface ECG is often difficult or impossible, and it often requires invasive EPS.

In SA exit block, diagnostic approach and treatment of SA exit block are similar to the sinus pause.

**Chronotropic incompetence** is defined as an inappropriate increase in heart rate in response to changing metabolic needs during activity.[9] It is often missed in clinical practice, which may be partly because of an absence of universally accepted diagnostic criteria. A generally accepted criterion for chronotropic incompetence is inability to achieve at least 80% of maximum predicted heart rate (220 − age) at peak exercise.[9]

**Tachy-brady syndrome:** Alternative episodes of paroxysmal brady- and supraventricular tachyarrhythmias (Fig. 15.2) have been defined as tachy-brady syndrome.[10,11] Rapid heart rate is mainly caused by atrial fibrillation (AF) or atrial flutter (AFL). Hence, the ventricular rate may abruptly increase with the onset of AF or AFL, especially in patients with an intact AV conduction system. With their abrupt cessation of tachycardia, prolonged bradycardia or asystole occurs because of exaggerated overdrive suppression of abnormal pacemakers.[2]

## Diagnostic Modalities

To diagnose SSS, it is essential to find a correlation between the patient's symptoms and the ECG

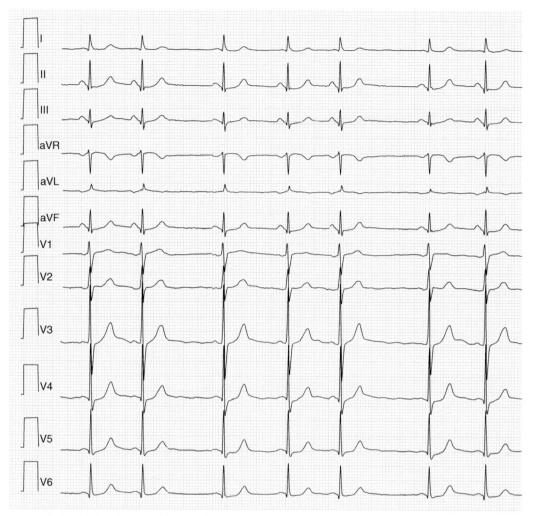

FIG. 15.1 Type 1 second-degree sinoatrial exit block. There is progressive shortening of the P-P interval before a P-QRS-T complex is dropped.

abnormalities. There are no standardized criteria for establishing a diagnosis of SSS, and the initial clues to the diagnosis of SSS are most often gleaned from the patient's history. Apart from a thorough medical history, a 12-lead surface ECG and ambulatory ECG recording may confirm the diagnosis if typical ECG findings (e.g., sinus bradycardia, sinus pauses, alternating bradycardia, and atrial tachyarrhythmias) can be correlated with symptoms. Exercise stress testing can help in identifying SND and excluding myocardial ischemia. Although there is no uniform definition, most clinicians diagnose chronotropic incompetence as the inability to achieve at least 80% of the maximum predicted heart rate with exercise testing. Whenever surface ECG and repetitive ambulatory recordings 1–14 days are incapable of documenting the cause of a patient's symptoms, an external event recorder (symptoms occurring more than once a month) or an implantable loop recorder (patients with less frequent symptom) should be considered.[12] In patients with suspected SSS but without a confirmed diagnosis after ambulatory ECG monitoring, invasive EPS may also be considered.[13]

Treatment should be limited to patients with a good symptom–rhythm correlation.[14] Asymptomatic patients do not need any treatment.[14]

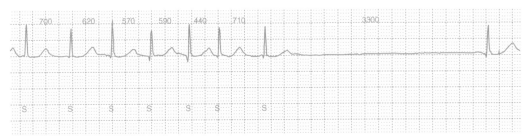

FIG. 15.2 Tachy-brady syndrome. Sudden termination of atrial fibrillation is followed by a long asystole (3.3 s).

## ATRIOVENTRICULAR BLOCK

### Etiology

AV block is divided to acquired or congenital subtypes. Congenital AV block may be caused by intrauterine exposure to maternal antibodies[15] or may be associated with congenital heart disease.[16] The most common cause of acquired AV block is idiopathic degeneration of the conduction system disease (referred to as Lenègre or Lev disease).[17] Increased vagal tone caused by sleep, athletic training, pain, carotid sinus massage, or hypersensitive carotid sinus syndrome can result in slowing of the sinus rate or the development of AV block. Major causes of pathologic AV block are listed in Box 15.1.

### Classification

Electrocardiographically, AV block is traditionally classified as first-, second-, or third-degree (complete) AV block. On the basis of intracardiac electrophysiologic recordings, supra-, intra-, or infra-Hisian blocks can be differentiated.

**First-degree AV block** is characterized by abnormal prolongation of the PR interval to more than 0.2 s. Every P wave is followed by one QRS complex but with a constantly prolonged PR interval. The location of delayed conduction may be within the AV node or His-Purkinje conduction.

**Second-degree AV block** is defined as intermittent failure of AV conduction. Based on ECG patterns, second-degree AV block can be divided into four subtypes: Mobitz type I (Wenckebach), Mobitz type II, 2:1 AV block, and advanced second-degree AV block.

*Mobitz type I* is characterized by a progressive PR interval prolongation before the nonconducted P wave (Fig. 15.3). The first conducted P wave after the nonconducted P wave has the shortest PR interval of such a cycle; so the pauses between the QRS complexes encompassing the nonconducted P wave are less than twice the P-P interval. Mobitz type I is usually indicative of AV node disease.

*Mobitz type II* is defined as the occurrence of a single nonconducted P wave without prior PR interval prolongation (Fig. 15.4). The pause encompassing the blocked P wave equals two P-P intervals. This kind of AV block is usually caused by infranodal disease within the bundle of His or both bundle branches.

*2:1 AV block* is a specific form of second-degree AV block. In this condition, every other P wave is nonconducted (Fig. 15.5), and it is not possible to categorize AV block as Mobitz type I or type II. The anatomic site of the block can be in the AV node or in the His-Purkinje system.

Advanced second-degree AV block (high-degree AV block) is characterized by at least two consecutive

---

**BOX 15.1**
**Major Causes of Acquired Atrioventricular Block**

Pathologic
  Idiopathic degeneration of the conduction system
  Ischemic heart disease
  Cardiomyopathy and myocarditis
  Congenital heart disease
  Metabolic: hyperkalemia, severe hypo- or
    hyperthyroidism
  Autoimmune disease, e.g., systemic lupus
    erythematosus
  Neuromuscular disorders
  Infiltrative malignancies
  Trauma
  Familial AV block
Iatrogenic
  Drugs: digitalis, calcium channel blockers, beta
    blockers, amiodarone, adenosine
  Cardiac surgery
  Catheter ablation of arrhythmias
  Transcatheter VSD closure
  Alcohol septal ablation for HCM
  Transcatheter aortic valve implantation

*ASD*, atrioventricular; *HCM*, hypertrophic cardiomyopathy; *VSD*, ventricular septal defect.

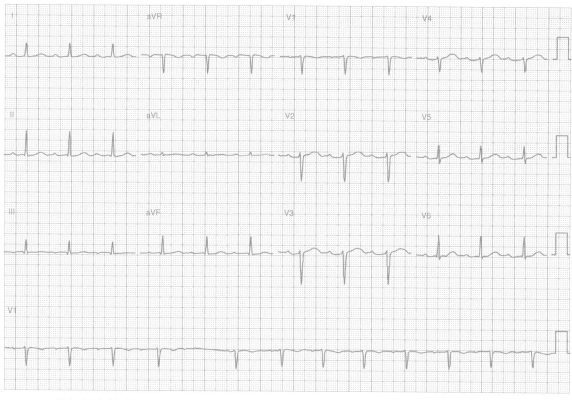

FIG. 15.3 Mobitz type I second-degree atrioventricular block. Note that there is progressive PR interval prolongation before a P-wave fails to conduct to the ventricle.

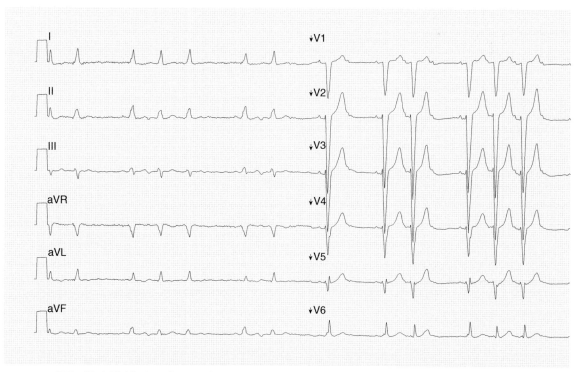

FIG. 15.4 Mobitz type II second-degree atrioventricular block. There is no PR interval prolongation before a nonconducted P-wave.

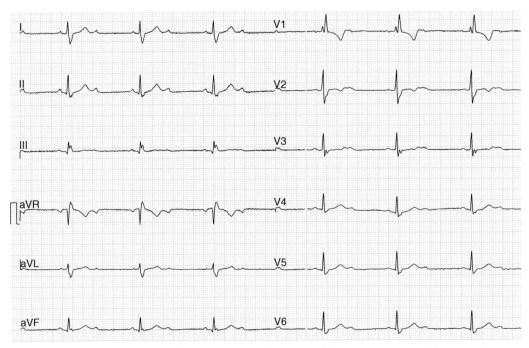

FIG. 15.5 Two-to-one atrioventricular (AV) block. Every other P wave is nonconducted, and it is not possible to categorize the AV block as Mobitz type I or type II.

nonconducted P waves. AV conduction ratio may be regular or not.

**Third-degree AV block:** Complete or third-degree AV block is defined as complete failure of AV conduction so that no atrial impulses can reach ventricles (Fig. 15.6). The site of the block can be localized to the AV node, the His bundle, or the bundle branches. A complete AV block within the AV node is characterized by a regular narrow QRS escape rhythm of 40–60 beats/min. However, more distal block with the His-Purkinje system gives rise to a wide QRS escape rhythm with a rate of 20–40 beats/min.

### Diagnostic Modalities

The diagnosis of AV block can be established noninvasively in most cases. The 12-lead ECG usually provides the information to characterize the type and localize

the level of the block. In patients with intermittent AV block, ambulatory ECG monitoring and exercise testing are important to establish a correlation between symptoms and rhythm. Except for the 2:1 AV block, invasive EPS has no significant role in decision-making.

### Treatment

Treatment of AV block should start with looking for potentially reversible causes such as Lyme disease, obstructive sleep apnea, or myocardial ischemia. Drugs hindering AV node conduction (e.g., beta blockers, digitalis, and calcium channel antagonists) should be discontinued, if possible. Except for patients with asymptomatic first-degree and type 1 second-degree AV block, other types need permanent pacemaker implantation irrespective of associated symptoms.[17]

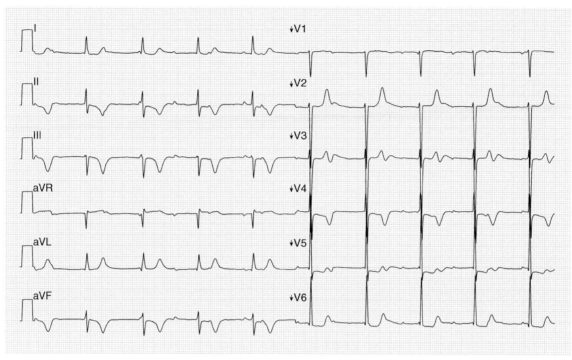

FIG. 15.6 Complete atrioventricular block. There is no relation between P waves and QRS complexes.

## REFERENCES

1. Spodick DH. Normal sinus heart rate: sinus tachycardia and sinus bradycardia redefined. *Am Heart J.* 1992; 124:1119–1121.
2. Dreifus LS, Michelson EL, Kaplinsky E. Bradyarrhythmias: clinical significance and management. *J Am Coll Cardiol.* 1983;1:327–338.
3. Sneddon JF, Camm AJ. Sinus node disease. Current concepts in diagnosis and therapy. *Drugs.* 1992; 44:728–737.
4. Talan DA, Bauernfeind RA, Ashley WW, Kanakis Jr. C, Rosen KM. Twenty-four hour continuous ECG recordings in long-distance runners. *Chest.* 1982;82:19–24.
5. Vogler J, Breithardt G, Eckardt L. Bradyarrhythmias and conduction blocks. *Rev Esp Cardiol.* 0122;65(7):656–667.
6. Brodsky M, Wu D, Denes P, Kanakis C, Rosen KM. Arrhythmias documented by 24 hour continuous electrocardiographic monitoring in 50 male medical students without apparent heart disease. *Am J Cardiol.* 1977;39(3):390–395.
7. Ector H, Rolies L, De Geest H. Dynamic electrocardiography and ventricular pauses of 3 seconds and more: etiology and therapeutic implications. *Pacing Clin Electrophysiol.* 1983; 6:548–551.
8. Hilgard J, Ezri MD, Denes P. Significance of ventricular pauses of three seconds or more detected on twenty-four-hour Holter recordings. *Am J Cardiol.* 1985;55: 1005–1008.
9. Brubaker PH, Kitzman DW. Chronotropic incompetence: causes, consequences, and management. *Circulation.* 2011;123:1010–1020.
10. Short DS. Syndrome of alternating bradycardia and tachycardia. *Br Heart J.* 1954;16:208–214.
11. Moss AJ, Davis RJ. Brady-tachy syndrome. *Prog Cardiovasc Dis.* 1974;14:439–454.
12. Paruchuri V, Adhaduk M, Garikipati NV, Steinberg JS, Mittal S. Clinical utility of a novel wireless implantable loop recorder in the evaluation of patients with unexplained syncope. *Heart Rhythm.* 2011;8(6): 858–863.
13. Strauss HC, Bigger JT, Saroff AL, Giardina EG. Electrophysiologic evaluation of sinus node function in patients with sinus node dysfunction. *Circulation.* 1976; 53(5):763–776.

14. Epstein AE, DiMarco JP, Ellenbogen KA, et al. ACC/AHA/ HRS 2008 Guidelines for Device-Based Therapy of Cardiac Rhythm Abnormalities: a report of the American College of Cardiology/American Heart Association Task Force on Practice Guidelines (Writing Committee to Revise the ACC/AHA/NASPE 2002 Guideline Update for Implantation of Cardiac Pacemakers and Antiarrhythmia Devices): developed in collaboration with the American Association for Thoracic Surgery and Society of Thoracic Surgeons. *Circulation.* 2008;117(21):e350–e408.

15. Silverman E, Mamula M, Hardin JA, Laxer R. Importance of the immune response to the Ro/La particle in the development of congenital heart block and neonatal lupus erythematosus. *J Rheumatol.* 1991; 18(1):120–124.

16. Clark BC, Berul CI. Arrhythmia diagnosis and management throughout life in congenital heart disease. *Expert Rev Cardiovasc Ther.* 2016;14(3):301–320.

17. Zoob M, Smith KS. The aetiology of complete heart block. *Br Med J.* 1963;2(5366):1149–1153.

# CHAPTER 16

# Electrophysiology Tracing Interpretation

AMIR FARJAM FAZELIFAR
Department of Cardiac Electrophysiology, Rajaie Cardiovascular, Medical & Research Center, Iran University of Medical Sciences, Tehran, Iran; Cardiac Electrophysiology Research Center, Rajaie Cardiovascular, Medical & Research Center, Iran University of Medical Sciences, Tehran, Iran

---

**KEY POINTS**

- An electrophysiology study could diagnose and treat many types of cardiac rhythm disturbances.
- Cardiac surgery prolonged life in many patients with ischemic and congenital heart disease. Arrhythmia ablation, besides antiarrhythmic drugs and cardiac electronic devices, could improve the quality of life in symptomatic patients. Arrhythmology and interpretation of intracardiac electrophysiology tracing are important steps to understand the mechanism of many effective curative procedures in cardiology.

---

## INTRODUCTION

Cardiac mechanical performance depends on electrical activity. Heart auscultation, jugular vein observation, and pulse wave pattern were instruments for tachy- or bradyarrhythmia detection for many years before the electrocardiogram was innovated by Einthoven more than 100 years ago.[1] By using different maneuvers such as the carotid sinus massage, Valsalva maneuver, diving reflex, exercise test and drug injection such as atropine, adenosine, and verapamil, arrhythmia management progressed significantly.[2] However, there were patients with arrhythmic symptoms without abnormal ECG. Some of these patients did not respond to drug therapy. In the middle of the 20th century, invasive electrophysiology diagnostic and therapeutic procedures were innovated by physicians such as Dr. Forssmann, Dr. Scherlag, Dr. Henrick, JJ Wellens, and Dr. Durrer.[1]

## WHAT IS ELECTROPHYSIOLOGY (EP) PROCEDURE?

During EP procedure, via peripheral veins and arteries, different electrophysiology catheters with signal recording and pacing ability are deployed in heart chambers and well-known electrical structures. All spontaneous or paced depolarization signals are transferred to the EP equipment. We can analyze cardiac electrical map by comparing intracardiac signals and surface ECG. The physician analyzes arrhythmia mechanism and can destroy abnormal structures with a catheter and preferred energy source such as radiofrequency or cryoablation.[3]

## EP CATHETER IMPLANTATION

For cardiac electrical map creation, electrical data should be retrieved from all heart chambers and conductive structures (AV node and His bundle). For this reason, catheters are implanted in the right atrium and ventricle. A multipolar catheter, which is established parallel to the mitral valve in coronary sinus, simultaneously collects left atrium and ventricle signals. The proximal part is beside the coronary sinus ostium in the right posteroseptal area and the distal part is in the lateral part of the mitral ring (Fig. 16.1). The His catheter is the most important catheter that sits on the septal side of the tricuspid valve. It can record the atrial, ventricular, and His-bundle potentials simultaneously. The His potential is a sharp potential with less than 30 ms duration. The normal HV interval means normal conduction from the atrium to the ventricle via the AVN–His–Purkinje system.

Sino-atrial activity after conduction through atrial chambers reaches the AVN. The A–H interval on the His catheter is the time interval between atrial activity at the entrance site of AVN and the His-bundle potential recording. The PR interval in surface ECG is the summation of intra-atrial conduction time, A–H and H–V intervals (Fig. 16.2).

There are several multipolar mapping catheters in different shapes for more accurate arrhythmia evaluation in specific chambers, such as the Halo catheter in the right atrium or the Lasso catheter in pulmonary veins (Fig. 16.3). The conventional ablation catheter is not only able to map and pace the specific areas, but also

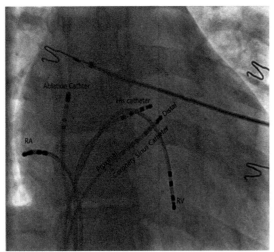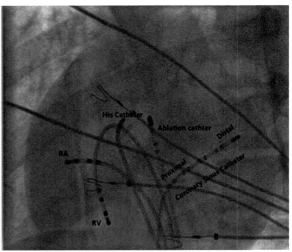

FIG. 16.1 Electrophysiology catheters in RAO (*left*) and LAO (*right*) views.

with energy delivery can destroy the target tissue. This process is named arrhythmia ablation.

## ELECTROPHYSIOLOGY TRACING STRUCTURE

The normal ECG recording speed is 25 mm/s. We usually use higher speeds, 100–200 mm/s, in electrophysiology work for better observation and evaluation (Fig. 16.4). A standard diagram is available in each tracing to measure intervals in milliseconds. We should always remember that each tracing is a static feature of signals, but arrhythmia mechanism detection is a dynamic process. Therefore, we describe them in differential diagnosis.

## SIGNAL RECORDING AND SEQUENCES IN NORMAL HEART

Electrical activity initiates from the sinoatrial node (SAN). It spreads from the right atrium (RA) to the left atrium (LA) via several specific ways and lasts for less than 70 ms.[2] The next important station of the conduction system is AVN. In more than 80% of people, there are two fast and slow pathways in atrioventricular node (AVN), which are considered to be functionally and anatomically distinct. The fast pathway with a faster conduction velocity and longer refractory period emanates from the interatrial septum and is usually recorded on the His catheter on the top of the triangle of Koch. A slow pathway with longer conduction time but shorter

effective refractory period crosses the isthmus between the coronary sinus ostium and the septal leaflet of the tricuspid annulus. The AVN structure is very complex, and in the normal atrium the A–H interval on His catheter shows its conduction time. The electrical impulse, after leaving the AVN, depolarizes the His bundle and spreads to the left and right bundles and continues depolarization through the purkinje system to provide rapid ventricular activation. The conduction time between the His-bundle activation and beginning of the QRS complex in surface ECG is named the H–V interval and is usually between 35 and 55 ms (Fig. 16.2). The His bundle, unlike AVN, does not have a decremental conduction pattern. The surface PR interval is a combination of intra-atrial, AVN, and H–V interval conduction times (Fig. 16.5).[4]

The His-bundle security is very high and any slow conduction (for example, HV interval more than 100 ms) or spontaneous or paced block feature in a physiologic range in the intra- or infra-His-bundle heralds catastrophic fate (Fig. 16.6).[5] During tachyarrhythmias, the normal HV interval usually explains that the AVN–His bundle with or without dependency on the infra-His structure is the main passage for impulse propagation.

The coronary sinus catheter can record both left atrial and ventricle signals from proximal (left posteroseptal area) to distal (lateral aspect of the mitral valve). Atrial signals are sharp, but ventricular signals are wide and show low amplitude on this catheter (Fig. 16.2).

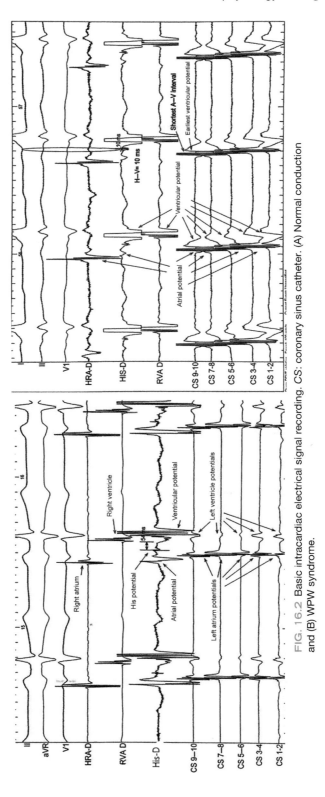

FIG. 16.2 Basic intracardiac electrical signal recording. CS: coronary sinus catheter. (A) Normal conduction and (B) WPW syndrome.

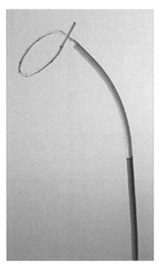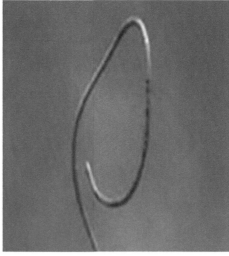

FIG. 16.3 Multipolar diagnostic catheters for specific arrhythmia mapping.

## PACING MANEUVERS IN AN ELECTROPHYSIOLOGY STUDY

Pacing maneuvers are used for evaluation of conduction system refractoriness, arrhythmia induction or termination, and detection of arrhythmia mechanism.

Pacing maneuvers are usually divided into two subgroups:

1. Overdrive pacing with or without decrement in cycle length.
2. Programmed extra stimuli.

During pacing maneuvers, capture should always be confirmed. Extra stimuli are usually delivered after a sequence of pacing beats to reduce the autonomic effect on the conduction system.

## OVERDRIVE PACING EFFECT ON CONDUCTION SYSTEM

### Atrium

Overdrive pacing usually starts in the right atrium for evaluation of SAN performance in patients suspected to have sick sinus syndrome. In different pacing cycle lengths, for 15–60 s, SAN recovery time (SANRT) shows normal or indolent function. It is measured from the last paced beat to the first spontaneous sinus beat (Fig. 16.7). If we subtract it from the basic sinus rhythm, corrected SNRT (CSNRT) is calculated. Normal CSNRT is less than 525 ms. Atrial tachycardia or flutter, reentrant arrhythmias such as AVNRT or AVRT and even ventricular arrhythmias such as left septal VT or arrhythmias with triggered activity mechanism can be induced by atrial overdrive pacing from RA or CS catheter pacing.

### AVN and His Bundle

AVN has decremental conduction against His-bundle conduction behavior. During atrial incremental pacing, the A–H interval gradually increases up to a level where one-to-one conduction fails and the A–H interval after a blocked paced beat is shorter than the last conducted paced beat (Fig. 16.8). This cycle length pacing is called the atrioventricular wenckebach point (AVWP). The H–V interval is normal during pacing and the QRS shape is constant. Sometimes aberrant conduction (functional left or right bundle branch block) appears and the H–V interval is normal or minimally increased. If the H–V interval decreases or surges to negative values and the QRS morphology changes, antegrade accessory conduction dominates and the delta wave will be more noticeable in surface ECG. The obvious delta wave does not see in slowly decremental conducting accessory pathways. This type of accessory pathway has been named the Mahaim preexcitation syndrome and it appears usually in an LBBB pattern (Fig. 16.9).

Any intra- or infra-His block in symptomatic patients (syncope or presyncope) and/or pacing cycle length more than 400 ms is pathologic (Fig. 16.10).

Overdrive His pacing is a maneuver for the detection of a concealed accessory pathway. Different pacing amplitude is used to capture the His bundle and/or ventricle. In the absolute His-bundle pacing, the captured QRS is identical to the native ECG and spike to QRS is equal to the H–V interval. Atrial activation pattern and H–A interval reveal the presence or absence of an accessory pathway (Fig. 16.11).

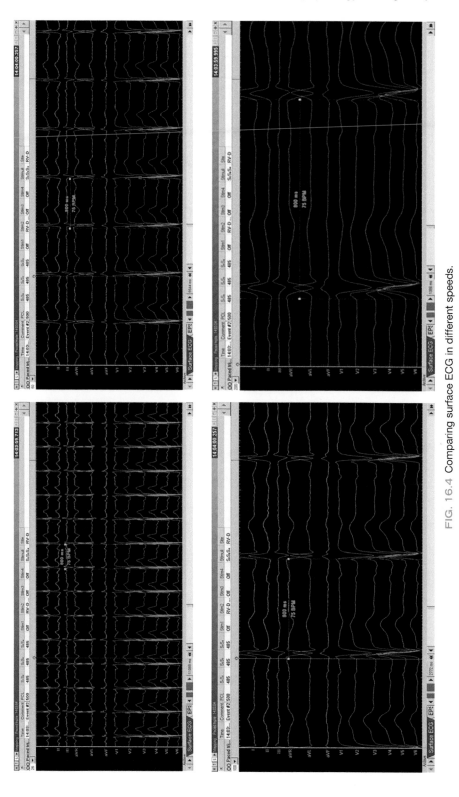

FIG. 16.4 Comparing surface ECG in different speeds.

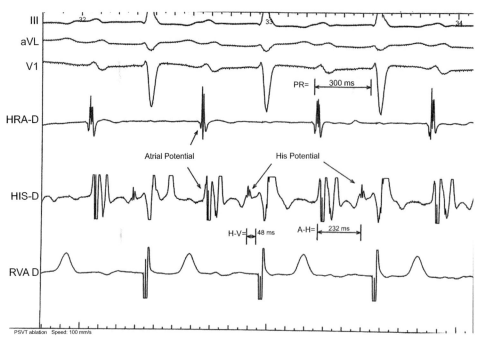

FIG. 16.5 Surface PR is a combination of intra-atrial conduction time with A–H and H–V intervals.

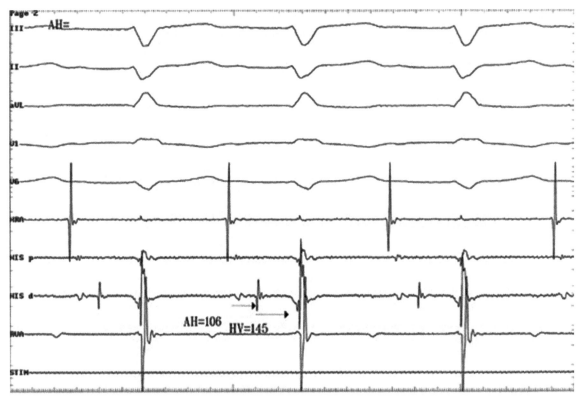

FIG. 16.6 Abnormal H–V interval recording in a patient with a history of traumatic syncope and wide QRS pattern. An H–V interval of more than 100 ms increases the risk of sudden cardiac death.

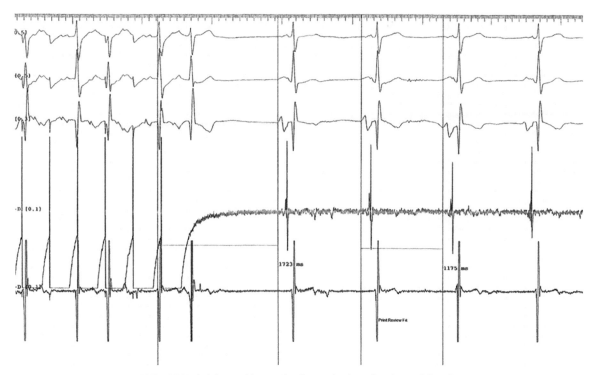

FIG. 16.7 Atrial overdrive pacing for evaluation of a sino-atrial node.

## Ventricle

Overdrive ventricular pacing has several indications. It is usually used for ventricular or supraventricular arrhythmia induction or termination, dissociation atrial activity from ventricle for arrhythmia mechanism diagnosis, and pace mapping for detection of the best ablation target. If the atrium and ventricle are not dissociated after ventricular pacing in drives minimally less than the basic cycle length, the atrial activation pattern is important. In the normal conduction system, the earliest retrograde atrial activation should appear on the His catheter (concentric pattern) and ventricular incremental pacing reveals retrograde decremental conduction. The ventriculoatrial wenckebach point (VAWP) means no one-to-one conduction from the ventricle to the atrium during ventricular incremental pacing and V–A (or His-A) in ventricular paced beat after block is shorter than V–A (or His-A) in captured beat before block (Fig. 16.12). Concentric pattern without decremental conduction pattern unmasks a concealed septal accessory pathway. The earliest atrial signal on other mapping catheters is usually named the eccentric pattern and is related to the presence of an accessory pathway (Fig. 16.13). The ablation catheter is used for finding the earliest atrial activation during ventricular pacing.

## PROGRAMMED ELECTRICAL STIMULATION MANEUVER

Programmed electrical stimulation will provide information regarding the behavior of impulse propagation from the antegrade perspective. The interval between the last basic paced complex and the premature stimulus is a coupling interval and is usually used for determination of refractoriness. Myocardial cells during the period of repolarization response to electrical stimulation and refractoriness refer to a state of absent or reduced cell excitability. Refractoriness is "cycle length dependent," and therefore 8–10 constant beats are used before the premature beat to allow the tissue to accommodate to a steady-state condition. This period of pacing is named the basic pacing cycle length (BCL). During prematurity decline, electrical conduction slows before impulse block. This delay can induce arrhythmia in susceptible tissues.

## Atrium

The sinus node recovery time was described before. Sino-atrial conduction time (SACT) is another maneuver to evaluate sick sinus syndrome (SSS). In the Strauss method, progressively premature atrial extra stimuli are

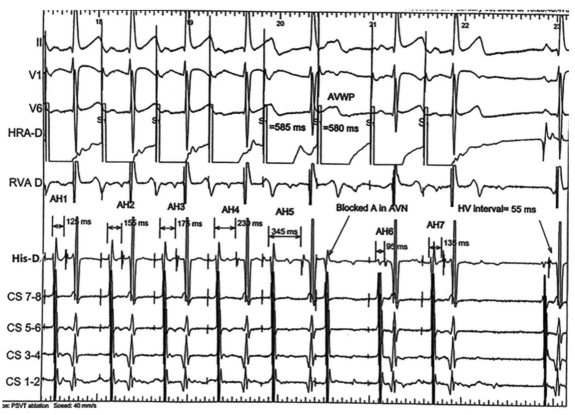

FIG. 16.8 Atrioventricular wenckebach point during atrial decremental pacing. Notice the A–H interval prolongation before block. AVWP = 580 ms.

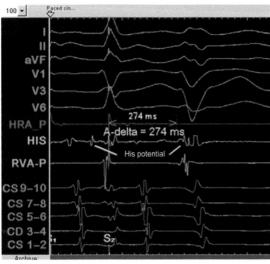

FIG. 16.9 Atrial pacing reveals Mahaim fiber conduction. A–H interval prolongation with H–V interval shortening.

introduced after every 8–10th beat of the stable sinus rhythm. The time interval between premature stimulus and spontaneous sinus beat minus stable sinus rhythm equals conduction of the impulse into and out of sinus node tissue and SACT is half of the measured time. Normal SACT times generally range from 40 to 150 ms.

### AVN and His Bundle

The atrial signal on the His catheter is the entrance area of the AVN and the His potential is the node's exit site. During progressively atrial extra-stimulation, the A–H interval increases. An A–H interval of less than 150 ms conducts through the fast pathway and more than 200 ms uses the slow pathway. Programmed atrial extra-stimulation determines fast and slow refractoriness. Prematurity interval decreases by either 10 or 20 ms and the AH interval gradually increases, but sudden A–H prolongation (more than 50 ms) means the extra-stimulus reaches the fast pathway's refractory period and jumps to the slow pathway (Fig. 16.14).

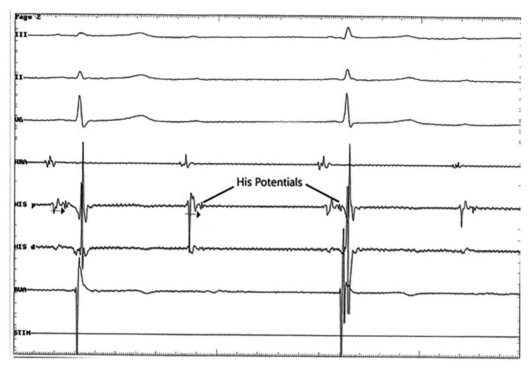

FIG. 16.10 Spontaneous infra-His block in a patient with a narrow QRS pattern.

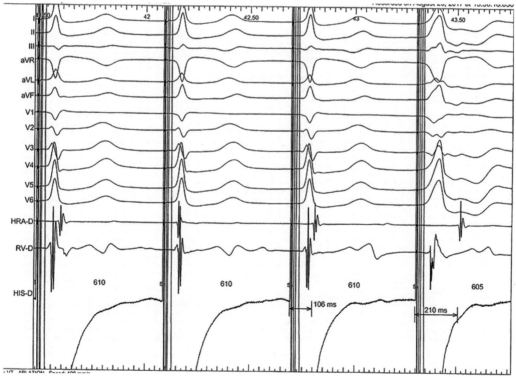

FIG. 16.11 His-bundle pacing. This maneuver helps to detect the presence of an accessory pathway conduction. In this picture, atrial conduction is over the AV node.

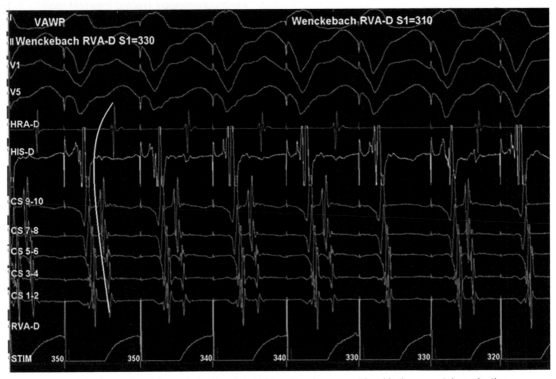

FIG. 16.12 Ventriculoatrial wenckebach point. Atrial pattern is concentric with decremental conduction.

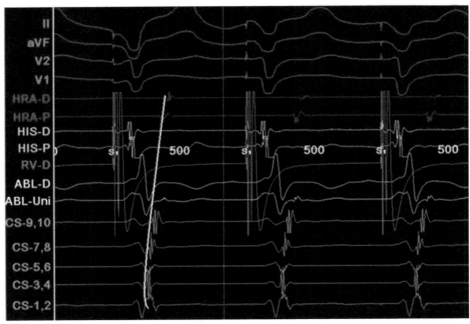

FIG. 16.13 Eccentric atrial pattern during ventricular pacing. Earliest atrial activation is recorded on CS-3,4. Accessory pathway is located on the posterolateral area of the mitral ring.

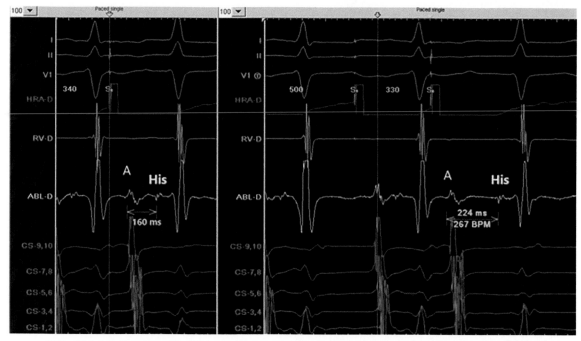

FIG. 16.14 A–H prolongation during programmed atrial stimulation. A 10 ms decrease in prematurity suddenly increased the A–H interval by more than 50 ms (antegrade jump or antegrade effective refractory period of fast pathway is 330 ms).

Continuing a further decrease in prematurity leads to the input limit of the AVN (Antegrade Effective Refractory Period of AVN)[6,7] (Fig. 16.15). A decrease in prematurity can reveal the atrial refractory period. It means atrial pacing cannot depolarize the atrial muscle (Fig.16.16). Sometimes the propagating impulse not only penetrates the His bundle and ventricles but also come backs to the atrium via the fast pathway (Echo beat) (Fig. 16.17). The HV interval is normal during assessment of the AVN function. In prematurity intervals of more than 350–400 ms, any intra or infra-His potential is pathologic (Fig. 16.18).[8]

Fast or decremental conducting accessory pathways are determined by progressive H–V interval shortening and QRS morphology change.[9,10] Any sudden H–V interval normalization and disappearance of delta wave means an antegrade accessory pathway conduction block (Fig. 16.19). Atrial tachycardia, AVN reentrant tachycardia (AVNRT), and atrioventricular reentrant tachycardia (AVRT) can be induced by atrial programmed stimulation (Fig. 16.20).

### Ventricle

Sometimes programmed electrical stimulation in a ventricle shows retrograde AVN conduction. In this situation, atrial activation on the His catheter is the earliest recorded signal (concentric pattern) and with a decrease in interval prematurity, the ventriculoatrial time increases. Retrograde jump (retrograde fast pathway block) can be seen (Fig. 16.21). Any eccentric atrial activation pattern or concentric pattern without decremental conduction is a sign of the presence of an accessory pathway. A sudden change in retrograde atrial activation and transition from an eccentric pattern to a concentric atrial sequence means a retrograde accessory pathway block. This is named the retrograde refractory period of the accessory pathway (Fig. 16.22).

Ventricular extra stimuli can be delivered concomitant with the His-bundle potential during supraventricular tachyarrhythmias. Any advancement in atrial activation timing means the presence of accessory pathway conduction[11] (Fig. 16.23).

Ventricular programmed stimulation is frequently used for ventricular arrhythmia induction.

### ROLE OF EPS IN BRADYARRHYTHMIA DETECTION

In patients with syncope or presyncope symptoms, EPS has a fundamental role for bradyarrhythmia detection. SNRT, CSNRT, and SACT are used to reveal SSS in suspected patients. In patients without sinus node activity,

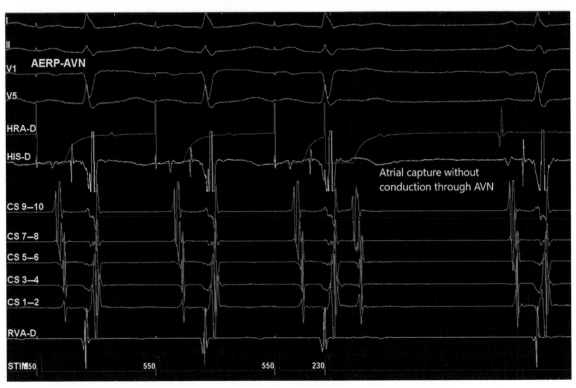

FIG. 16.15 Antegrade effective refractory period of AVN = 230 ms.

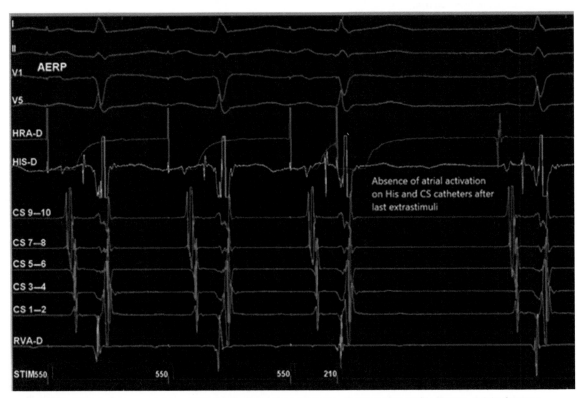

FIG. 16.16 Absence of atrial capture during programmed electrical stimulation. In this picture, atrial refractory period is 210 ms.

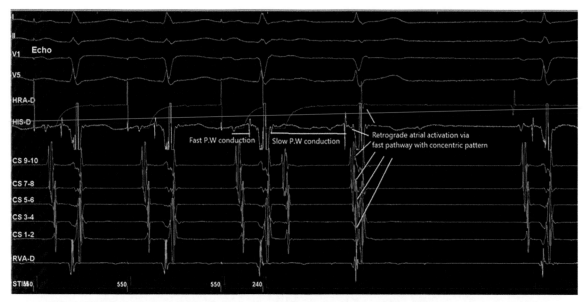

FIG. 16.17 During antegrade slow pathway conduction, fast pathway gain its ability to conduct retrogradely electrical impulse to the atrium. This atrial concentric activation is named echo beat.

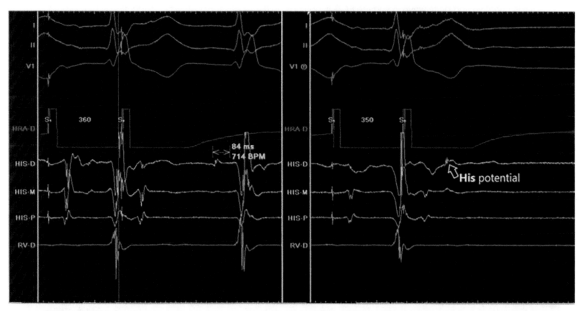

FIG. 16.18 Infra-His block during programmed stimulation, in a patient with a history of syncope and abnormal QRS pattern.

A–V node or subnodal structures escape to save the patients. The H–V interval defines the trigger point (Fig. 16.24).

In patients without atrial activity, even retrograde atrial depolarization, pacing maneuvers help to differentiate SSS from an atrial standstill. In an atrial standstill, atrial pacing from right and left in high outputs does not capture the atrium and surface P waves are absent in ECG with and without atrial pacing.

AV node and the His-bundle conduction patterns can be evaluated during EPS maneuvers. Level of block, AV

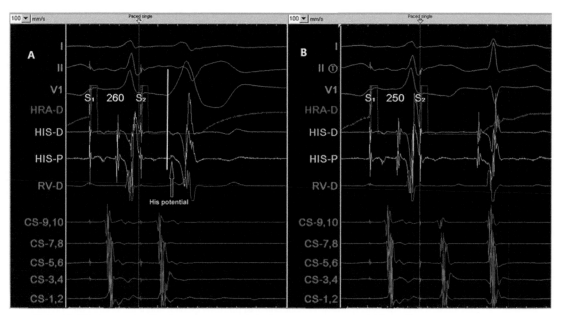

FIG. 16.19 Antegrade effective refractory period of accessory pathway (AERP-AP) can be evaluated during PES. Usually AERP-AP of less than 250 ms has more sudden cardiac death risk for patient. In (A), the H–V interval is negative and delta wave in surface ECG is obvious. In (B), accessory pathway conduction is blocked and atrial activation reaches ventricle through normal AVN–His purkinje system.

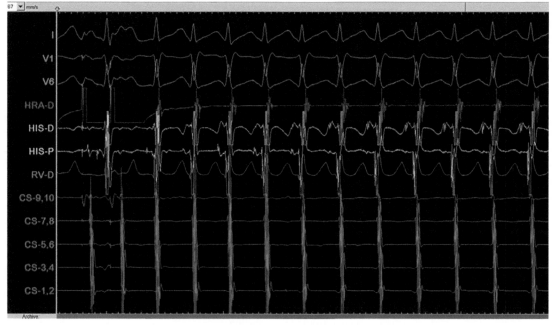

FIG. 16.20 AVNRT induction with atrial programmed stimulation. Atrial and ventricular signals are superimposed on each other and H–V interval is normal.

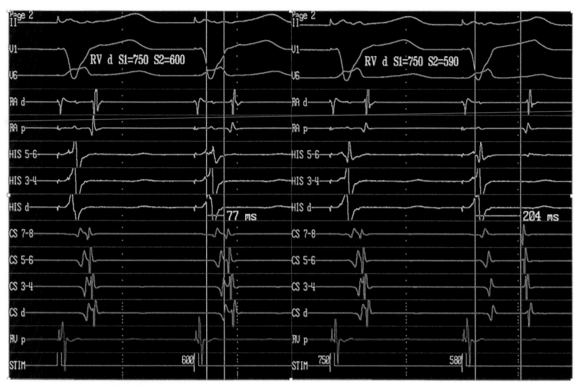

FIG. 16.21 Retrograde jump. With a 10 ms decrease in prematurity, V–A conduction increases more than 50 ms. Retrograde conduction pattern is concentric.

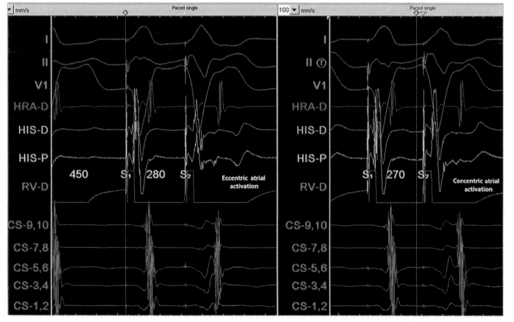

FIG. 16.22 During ventricular programmed stimulation, eccentric retrograde atrial activation suddenly changes to a concentric pattern. It means retrograde accessory pathway conduction is blocked in 270 ms. Retrograde effective refractory period of accessory pathway (RERP-AP) is 270 ms.

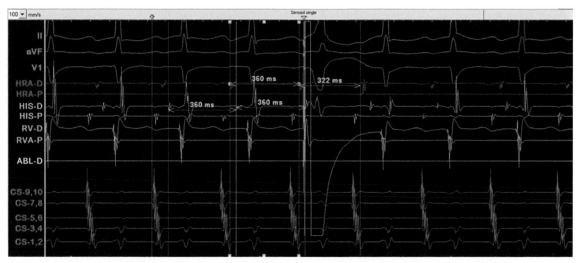

**FIG. 16.23** Right ventricular premature pacing during His-bundle refractoriness advances atrial activation by more than 10 ms (here: 38 ms). This arrhythmia shows concentric atrial activation. This maneuver confirms the presence of an accessory pathway with slow conduction characteristic in this tracing.

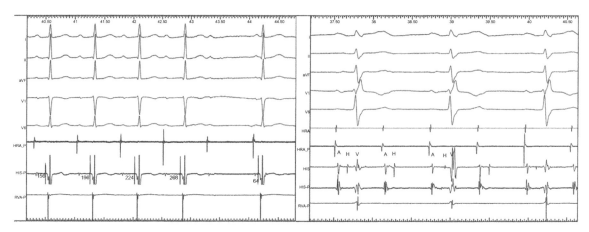

**FIG. 16.24** Spontaneous block in AVN (A) and His–Purkinje (B) systems.

node intra-His, or infra-His helps to decide about pacemaker implantation in symptomatic patients (Fig. 16.25). In highly suspected patients, procainamide infusion is used for stress on the His–Purkinje system to reveal subtle abnormalities (Fig. 16.25).

## HOW TO INTERPRET TACHYARRHYTHMIA TRACING?

1. In the first step, we should note the surface ECG. P and QRS morphology, rate, relationship, and regularity are helpful for interpretation.

2. The H–V interval in arrhythmia and comparison with basic H–V, all through the tracing, is a fundamental step. A normal H–V interval means ventricular depolarization is via the AVN–His-bundle system (except for the bundle branch reentrant VT). The new bundle branch block pattern with a normal H–V interval or minimal prolongation is aberrant conduction. A decline in the H–V interval or negative values means QRS is formed in the ventricle out of the normal conduction system and the routine pattern is bypassed.

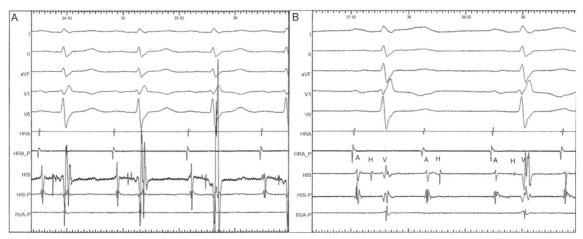

FIG. 16.25 Procainamide His–Purkinje stress in a patient suspicious for conduction system disorder. Plane A, before drug stress test. Plane B, after procainamide infusion with infra-His block. H-H′ pattern reveals intra-His conduction disorder.

3. Atrial and ventricular signal correlation. If atrial signals are more than ventricular signals, the arrhythmia is atrial tachycardia (Fig. 16.26), but AVNRT with block might be seen in this situation (Fig. 16.27). In a one-to-one atrium and ventricle correlation and normal H–V interval, atrial tachycardia, AVNRT, AVRT, and junctional tachycardia are differential diagnoses. In the presence of a short or negative H–V interval, antidromic AVRT or ventricular tachycardia can be recognized (Fig. 16.28). If ventricular signals are more than atrial signals and a normal H–V interval, AVNRT and junctional tachycardia with block can be seen and in a negative H–V interval, ventricular tachycardia is at the top of the differential diagnosis list.

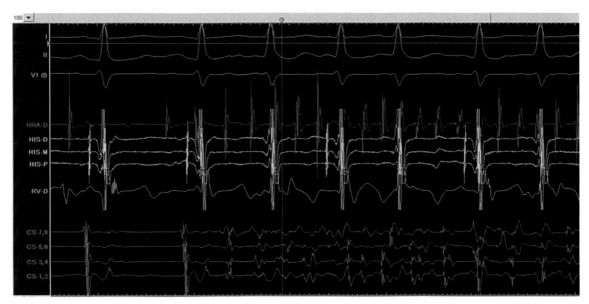

FIG. 16.26 Atrial fibrillation initiation with irregular conduction to ventricle via normal AVN–His–Purkinje system.

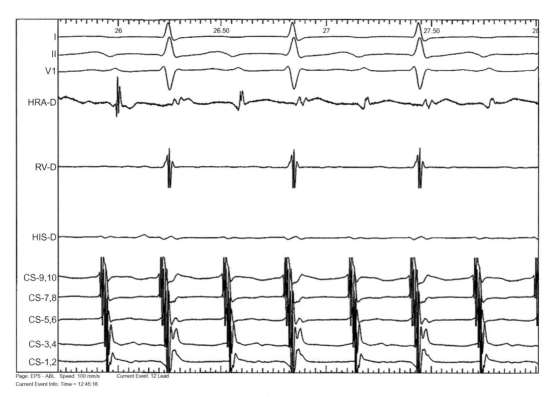

FIG. 16.27 AVNRT with AV block.

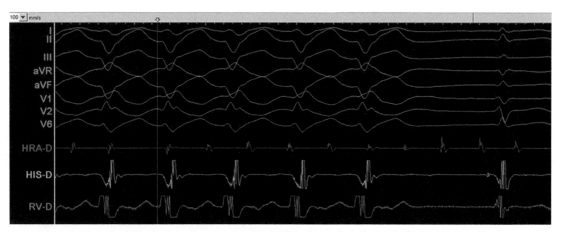

FIG. 16.28 In the *left side* of tracing, regular wide QRS tachycardia with a negative H–V interval is shown. Atrial signals are more than ventricular signals, but they are dissociated. After arrhythmia termination, a narrow QRS with a normal H–V interval appears. In this tracing, double arrhythmia is detected: atrial and ventricular tachycardia.

4. Type of arrhythmia initiation and termination can help to diagnose arrhythmia. AVNRT and AVRT usually initiate with A–H prolongation. Arrhythmia termination with P cannot usually be seen in atrial tachycardia, but termination with P wave after carotid sinus massage is in favor of AVRT. Ventricular depolarization near the His potential can terminate tachycardia in patients with a concealed accessory pathway conduction (Fig. 16.29).

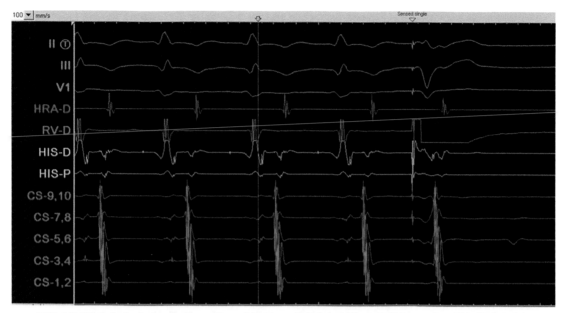

FIG. 16.29 Arrhythmia termination with ventricular pacing during His potential recording. This finding is in favor of AVRT.

## USUAL ARRHYTHMIA CHARACTERISTICS

### Atrial Tachycardia

Atrial pacing helps atrial tachycardia induction with or without A–H prolongation. Change in arrhythmia cycle length is frequently seen and ventricular cycle length variation is after atrial cycle length variation. Transient conduction block in the AV node or His–Purkinje system is not able to terminate arrhythmia. Atrioventricular dissociation during ventricular pacing helps to diagnose atrial tachycardia and is usually seen with a V–A–A–V pattern.[12] Atrial tachycardia terminates with QRS, and warm-up and cooldown patterns might be seen.

### AVN Reentrant Tachycardia

All arrhythmia mechanism is in the AVN and there is no dependency on the atrium or ventricle for arrhythmia continuation. AVNRT with a normal H–V interval and one-to-one atrium and ventricle signals, atrial signals more than ventricular signals or ventricular signals more than atrial signals are reported.[11] Arrhythmia initiates after atrial or ventricular pacing with A–H prolongation. Aberrant conduction with LBBB or RBBB patterns does not change arrhythmia cycle length or patterns of intracardiac signals (Fig. 16.30). Advancement maneuver or PVC resetting is negative in AVNRT (Fig. 16.31).

### Junctional Tachycardia

This arrhythmia is usually irregular with a normal H–V interval and one-to-one conduction between atrial and ventricular signals. Junctional tachycardia with atrial block can be seen.

### Orthodromic AVRT

An atrial activation pattern is usually eccentric. Any block in atrial or ventricular level terminates this arrhythmia. Aberrant conduction might change the arrhythmia cycle length or atrial and ventricular time intervals (accessory pathway and bundle branch block are ipsilateral).[12] Advancement maneuver frequently detects this arrhythmia (Fig. 16.23). Arrhythmia cycle length change is dependent on the A–H interval (AV node conduction) and V–A conduction is constant.

### Antidromic AVRT

The H–V interval is negative in this arrhythmia. An atrium is part of arrhythmia and premature pacing maneuvers in the atrium can impact on arrhythmia cycle length.

### Ventricular Tachycardia

The H–V interval is negative (bundle branch VT is an exception with a normal or prolonged H–V interval). There is no correlation between atrial and ventricular signals, but one-to-one or wenckebach conduction patterns can be seen. Arrhythmia irregularity does not rule

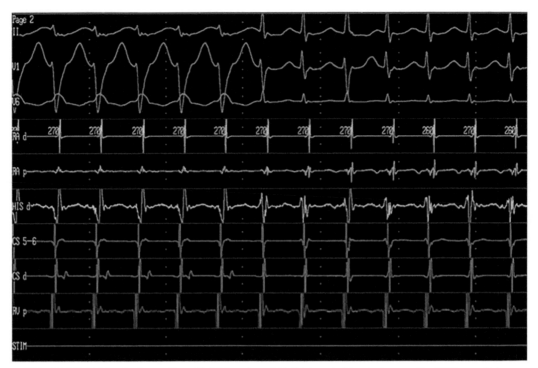

FIG. 16.30 Atrial activation pattern, V–A interval, and H–V interval did not change after QRS morphology change. This pattern is seen in AVNRT.

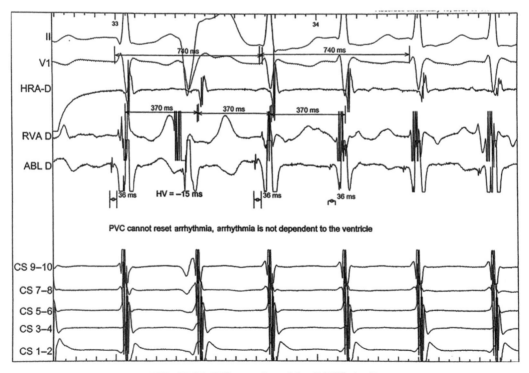

FIG. 16.31 PVC cannot reset the AVNRT circuit.

out ventricular tachycardia, but any atrial cycle length change is after ventricular cycle length variation. Arrhythmia initiation is in the ventricle, but atrial pacing can induce a few ventricular tachycardias such as left septal or outflow tract VTs. Overdrive atrial pacing cannot terminate ventricular tachycardia but transiently normalizes the H–V interval and is a diagnostic maneuver in borderline H–V intervals.

## REFERENCES

1. Lüderitz B. Historical perspectives of cardiac electrophysiology. *Hellenic J Cardiol*. 2009; 50(1):3–16.
2. Mehta D, Ward DE, Wafa S, Camm AJ. Relative efficacy of various physical manoeuvres in the termination of junctional tachycardia. *Lancet*. 1988; 1(8596):1181–1185.
3. Fu D-G. Cardiac arrhythmias: diagnosis, symptoms, and treatments. *Cell Biochem Biophys*. 2015; 73(2):291–296.
4. Sánchez-Quintana D, Yen Ho S. Anatomy of cardiac nodes and atrioventricular specialized conduction system. *Rev Esp Cardiol*. 2003; 56(11):1085–1092.
5. Dhingra RC, Palileo E, Strasberg B, et al. Significance of the HV interval in 517 patients with chronic bifascicular block. *Circulation*. 1981; 64(6):1265–1271.
6. George SA, Faye NR, Murillo-Berlioz A, Lee KB, Trachiotis GD, Efimov IR. At the atrioventricular crossroads: dual pathway electrophysiology in the atrioventricular node and its underlying heterogeneities. *Arrhythm Electrophysiol Rev*. 2017; 6(4):179–185.
7. Efimov IR, Nikolski VP, Rothenberg F, et al. Structure-function relationship in the AV junction. In: *The Anatomical Record Part A: Discoveries in Molecular, Cellular, and Evolutionary Biology*. Wiley; 2004:952–965.
8. Laroussi L, Badhwar N. Atrioventricular conduction disease and block. *Cardiac Electrophysiol Clin*. 2014; 6(3):445–458.
9. Katritsis DG, Wellens HJ, Josephson ME. Mahaim accessory pathways. *Arrhythm Electrophysiol Rev*. 2017; 6(1):29–32.
10. Bohora S, Dora SK, Namboodiri N, Valaparambil A, Tharakan J. Electrophysiology study and radiofrequency catheter ablation of atriofascicular tracts with decremental properties (Mahaim fibre) at the tricuspid annulus. *Europace*. 2008; 10(12):1428–1433.
11. Otomo K, Okamura H, Noda T, et al. Unique electrophysiologic characteristics of atrioventricular nodal reentrant tachycardia with different entriculoatrial block patterns: effects of slow pathway ablation and insights into the location of the reentrant circuit. *Hear Rhythm*. 2006; 3(5):544–554.
12. Knight BP, Ebinger M, Oral H, et al. Diagnostic value of tachycardia features & pacing maneuvers during PSVT. *J Am Coll Cardiol*. 2000; 36(2):574–582.

# CHAPTER 17

# Mechanisms, Diagnosis, and Therapy of Cardiac Arrhythmia

SHABNAM MADADI

Rajaie Cardiovascular, Medical & Research Center, Tehran, Iran

## KEY POINTS

- Mechanisms in impulse formation disorders are automaticity (enhanced normal automaticity and abnormal automaticity) and triggered activity with early afterdepolarization potentials (EADs) and delayed afterdepolarization potentials (DADs).
- Disorders of impulse conduction include block and reflection.
- Patient history, physical examination, electrocardiogram (ECG), exercise test, ambulatory ECG monitoring, and electrophysiology (EPS) study are the most useful for diagnosis of cardiac arrhythmia.
- Classification of antiarrhythmic drugs (AADs) is mostly based on their effect on one of the sodium or potassium or calcium channels or receptors (Vaughan-Williams classification).
- Nonpharmacological treatments of arrhythmia include cardioversion, ablation, and surgical therapy in some cases.

## INTRODUCTION

The known mechanisms for cardiac arrhythmias are disorders of impulse formation, disorders of impulse conduction, or combinations of both. However, in many cases, a combination of mechanisms is responsible for arrhythmia initiation or perpetuation.[1] Sometimes arrhythmia caused by one mechanism could initiate another arrhythmia, such as one PAC with an automaticity mechanism could initiate a macroreentrant atrial tachycardia. The risk of different types of arrhythmia is various; some of them such as VF are very hazardous. AF may be sometimes silent and sometimes cause CVA.[2]

There are different diagnostic approaches for diagnosis of arrhythmia, such as ECG, Holter monitoring, SAECG, and invasive electrophysiologic study (EPS).

Therapy for cardiac arrhythmia includes antiarrhythmic drugs (AADs), electrical cardioversion, radiofrequency ablation of the source of the arrhythmia (RFA), freezing of the culprit site of the arrhythmia, and surgical ablation.

## MECHANISMS OF CARDIAC ARRHYTHMIAS

There are three major mechanisms for cardiac arrhythmia including: (1) disorders of impulse formation; (2) disorders of impulse conduction; and (3) combinations of impulse formation and impulse conduction.[1]

1. **Disorders of impulse formation**: These disorders include an inappropriate rate of the normal pacemaker or abnormal discharge of an ectopic focus and disorders of impulse conduction include block and reflection. Interaction between automatic foci and interactions between automaticity and conduction include both mechanisms of impulse formation and impulse conduction. In impulse formation disorders, the major mechanisms responsible for arrhythmia are automaticity (enhanced normal automaticity and abnormal automaticity) and triggered activity with early afterdepolarization potentials (EADs) and delayed afterdepolarization potentials (DADs).[1-3]

1.1. **Abnormal automaticity**: Abnormal automaticity arises from cells with reduced maximum diastolic potential (positive to $-50$ mv), that is, the threshold potential for the activation of $I_K$ and $I_{ca,L}$ channels. Abnormal automaticity can be seen in normal muscle or Purkinje fibers by reduced diastolic potential.[4-6]

Sinus tachycardia is an example of enhanced normal automaticity and accelerated ventricular rhythm after MI is an example of abnormal automaticity caused by depolarization-induced automaticity in Purkinje myocytes. Other examples of abnormal automaticity are slow atrial, junctional, or ventricular escape rhythm, atrial tachycardia induced by digitalis or atrial tachycardias of the pulmonary veins.[7]

1.2. **Triggered activity**: Triggered activity is initiated by afterdepolarizations. Afterdepolarizations are depolarizing oscillations induced by preceding action potentials. Depolarizations that occur during phases 2 and 3 of the action potential are called EADs. Depolarizations that occur after completion of repolarization (phase 4) are called DADs. If afterdepolarizations reach the threshold potential, they can trigger other afterdepolarizations and initiate arrhythmia.[8–11]

1.2.1. **Delayed afterdepolarizations**: DADs can be seen in Purkinje fibers and pulmonary veins (in dig toxicity), in myocardial cells with Ankyrin-B mutations, and in beta adrenergic stimulation. The mechanism of accelerated idioventricular MI 1 day after MI may be due to DADs. DADs result from activation of calcium sensitive inward currents. Acquired or inherited abnormalities in the SR calcium release channels or SR calcium binding proteins may elicit DADs.[12]

Mutations in the RYR2 and CASQ2, which have been linked to CPVT, can cause an increase in the sensitivity of the RYR2 to luminal $Ca^{2+}$ or adrenergic stimulation and enhance the spontaneous diastolic $Ca^{2+}$ release from the SR and subsequent DAD triggered arrhythmia. DADs may be a cause of arrhythmogenesis in failing hearts, when upregulation of $I_{Na/Ca}$ with downregulation of the inward rectifier $K^+$ current facilitates DAD generation.[13–15]

Short coupling intervals overdrive pacing can induce overdrive acceleration of arrhythmias induced by DADs. A single premature stimulus can both initiate and terminate triggered activity and differentiation from reentry may be difficult, but overdrive acceleration could help in differentiation between triggered arrhythmia and reentrant arrhythmia.[16]

1.2.2. **Early afterdepolarization**: An increase in intracellular positivity due to any cause can cause EADs, such as acquired and congenital forms of long QT syndrome (LQTS). Inherited LQTS causes an abnormally prolonged ventricular action potential duration and increases the risk of SCD from VT and VF. Acquired LQTS and Torsade de Pointes (TdP) from Quinidine, erythromycin, and all class III antiarrhythmic agents may be mediated by EADs. Activators of ATP-dependent potassium channels such as pinacidil and nicorandil can eliminate EADs.[17]

1.3. **Parasystole**: Parasystoles are the function of asynchronously discharging pacemakers that result in a fixed rate, not altered by dominant rhythm. As a result of the complete entrance block, parasystole focus can be protected from surrounding electrical events. Sometimes there is also an exit block that fails to depolarize the excitable myocardium.[18]

2. **Disorders of impulse conduction**: Conduction block can result from bradyarrhythmia or tachyarrhythmia. Some entities associated with conduction block associated arrhythmia are described here:

2.1. **Deceleration-dependent block**: Diastolic depolarization is the cause of conduction block at slow rates. This type of block, which is called phase 4 block, is not always due to diastolic depolarization. Sometimes inactivation of the fast $Na^+$ channels occurs due to reduction in the difference between the membrane potential and threshold potential.[16–18]

2.2. **Tachycardia-dependent block**: This type of block is due to incomplete recovery of refractoriness caused by incomplete recovery of excitability.

2.3. **Decremental conduction**: Decremental conduction occurs due to loss of efficacy of action potential along the length of the fibers.[19]

2.4. **Reentry**: When there is a group of fibers not activated during initial depolarization, these fibers may serve as a link for initiation of reentry with reexcitation and inducing arrhythmia with circus movement, such as atrioventricular nodal reentrant tachycardia (AVNRT), atrioventricular reciprocating tachycardia (AVRT), and reciprocal or echo beat. There is one maneuver for the establishment of the reentry as the mechanism of the arrhythmia, which is called entrainment.[19]

2.5. **Entrainment**: Entrainment means increasing the rate of the tachycardia by pacing with resumption of the intrinsic rate of the tachycardia when the pacing is stopped. Entrainment represent a continuous resetting of the tachycardia.[19]

The criteria of entrainment can be used to determine the mechanism of the arrhythmia and also for localizing the slow conduction zone (isthmus) of the arrhythmia. Arrhythmia caused by reentry includes: atrial flutter, AVNRT, AVRT, and ventricular tachycardia (VT).

## HISTORY AND PHYSICAL EXAM

Patient history, physical examination, electrocardiogram (ECG), exercise test, ambulatory ECG monitoring, and electrophysiology (EPS) study are the most useful manners for diagnosis of cardiac arrhythmia.[20]

1. **Patient history**: Mode of onset and termination, frequency and duration of episodes, and severity of symptoms are important components of the patient's history for differentiation of different subtypes of arrhythmia. For example, palpitations that occur at rest can be caused by vagal tone such as vagotonic atrial fibrillation (AF). Palpitations terminate abruptly by vagal maneuvers are one probably involving the AV node such as AVNRT and AVRT.[21]

2. **Physical examination**: Assessment of the jugular venous pulse can demonstrate a "Cannon" A wave in AV dissociation. Variations in the intensity of S1 and SBP have the same implications. Sometimes facial features are associated with a rhythmic disorder such as low-set ear and micrognathia in the Andersen–Tawil syndrome.[22]

3. **Electrocardiogram**: ECG is very useful for analysis of the arrhythmia. A wide complex tachycardia often arises from the ventricular myocardium and a narrow complex tachycardia almost always has a supraventricular origin.[23]

   The wide complex tachycardia is sometimes supraventricular (SVT) with aberrancy or preexcited SVT. Initiation of tachycardia with a premature P wave, long-short sequences preceding changes in the R-R intervals, QRS contour consistent with aberrant conduction, onset of the QRS to its peak <50 ms, QRS duration ≤140 ms all favor SVT, but initiation with a premature ventricular complex (PVC), tachycardia beats identical to PVCs during sinus rhythm, short-long sequences preceding initiation, and some morphologies such as concordant R wave progression and absence of an "rS" complex in any precordial leads favor VT.[24]

4. **Exercise test**: Exercise test is useful in the induction of various types of SVTs and VTs, and also is useful in evaluation of proarrhythmia of some drugs such as flecainide. Exercise test is also useful in some types of LQTS that are manifest in the recovery phase.[25]

5. **Ambulatory ECG monitoring**: Long-term ECG monitoring and Holter recording are very important for evaluation of some arrhythmia that are not evident in ECG.

6. **SAECG**: Signal average ECG is a method for the detection of late ventricular potentials as follows: (1) filtered QRS duration >114–120 ms, (2) less than 20 µV of the root mean square in the last 40 ms, and (3) terminal filtered QRS <40 µV for longer than 39 ms.

   Heart rate variability and heart rate turbulence are useful for evaluation of the autonomic tone.[25]

7. **Upright tilt table testing**: This test is used for patients who have suspicious neurally mediated syncope. Positive response can be divided into three categories as cardioinhibitory, vasodepressor, and mixed types. Positive tilt test has been reported in two-thirds to three-fourths of patients suspicious to neurally mediated syncope.[23–25]

8. **Electrophysiology study**: Invasive EPS is useful for evaluation of sinus node function conduction properties, intraventricular conduction defect, palpitations, and unexplained syncope.

   In the evaluation of sinus node function, sinus node recovery time (SNRT) and SA conduction times could be evaluated. For determining SNRT, the interval between the last paced high RA beat and the first spontaneous high RA response is measured and minus the basic CL is corrected SNRT (cSNRT). That is normally less than 525 ms. EPS is valuable for evaluation of the AV node and the His-Purkinje system, for AV Wenckebach point evaluation, and HV interval measurement with and without procainamide. In patients with unexplained syncope, EPS could determine the cause of syncope, but the test is falsely negative in 20% of patients. In patients with palpitations, EPS is useful for induction of SVT (AVNRT, AVRT, and monomorphic VT). The complications of EPS are rare and include tamponade, pseudoaneurysms at arterial or venous access sites occurring in less than 0.2%.[26]

## ANTIARRHYTHMIC DRUGS

Classification of AADs is mostly based on their effect on one of the sodium or potassium or calcium channels or receptors (Vaughan-Williams classification). Another classification is based on the effect of the drugs on the mechanism of a particular arrhythmia and was introduced by Sicilian Gambit, but is not widely usable.[27,28]

In the Vaughan-Williams classification, class I drugs act as sodium channel blockers, class II drugs block adrenergic beta-receptors, class III drugs block potassium channels, class IV drugs are calcium channel blockers, and class V drugs include those agents that do not fit cleanly into classes I through IV.[29]

1. **Class I AAD**: Class I is divided into three subclasses of IA, IB, and IC.

    1.1. **Class IA drugs**: Class IA reduces $V_{max}$ and prolongs the action potential duration; it includes: quinidine, procainamide, and disopyramide. These drugs have intermediate rapidity.

    1.1.1. **Quinidine**: Nowadays, there is decreased demand for quinidine. The most common indications for quinidine are prevention of VF storms in the Brugada syndrome and short QT syndrome. Cinchonism is one of the CNS toxicities if the drug and side effects may preclude the long-term administration of the drug in 30%–40% of patients. In 0.5%–2% of patients, it causes TdP.[30] Most episodes of syncope occur during 2–4 days of treatment. Therapy of proarrhythmia is magnesium sulfate as the first line. Then atrial and ventricular pacing for suppression of EADs is recommended. As a bridge to pacing, isoproterenol could be used.

    Phenobarbital and phenytoin could shorten the duration of action of quinidine by increasing the rate of metabolism. In patients with sick sinus syndrome, quinidine could suppress SA node but in normal SA function, due to reflex sympathetic stimulation resulting from alpha adrenergic blockade, it could increase the sinus rate.

    1.1.2. **Procainamide**: Procainamide has the least anticholinergic effects among type IA drugs, but it can depress myocardial contractility through antisympathetic effects on CNS. In patients with CHF and renal failure and in old aged patients, it should be adjusted.

    It could be used for supraventricular and ventricular arrhythmia, but in atrial flutter patients should be coadministered with beta-blockers or calcium channel blockers to prevent acceleration of the ventricular response. It can produce the His-Purkinje block and should be used very cautiously in BBB patients and standby pacemaker facilities should be present. It can be used for provocation of the Brugada sign in suspected patients. In WPW syndrome patients, loss of preexcitation with procainamide is in favor of a long refractory period of the accessory pathway. The dose is 10–15 mg/kg or 1 g (whichever is lower) and should be administered slowly via the intravenous (IV) route. The drug should be discontinued in the case of BP decrease, QRS widening, and termination of the arrhythmia. Rash, myalgia, Reynaud phenomenon, and digital vasculitis are the side effects of procainamide. It could induce a lupus-like syndrome, but the brain and the kidneys are spared. Antinucleotide antibodies may develop in 60%–70% of the patients who received procainamide and clinical symptoms occur in 20%–30%. In the presence of symptoms or positive anti-DNA, the drug should be discontinued.[31]

    1.1.3. **Disopyramide**: Disopyramide can increase the sinus node discharge rate because of the great anticholinergic effects, but in SND could depress the SA node function. The most common indications for disopyramide are neutrally mediated syncope and hypertrophic cardiomyopathy (because of its negative inotropic effect). Disopyramide has potent parasympatholytic properties including urinary retention, constipation, blurred vision, closed-angle glaucoma, and dry mouth.

    It can cause TdP and should be administered in hospital and under cardiac monitoring. Doses are 100 mg q 12 h (in controlled release preparations) up to 600–1200 mg/day.[32]

    1.1.4. **Ajmaline**: It inhibits platelet activity more potently than aspirin. The dose for acute termination of arrhythmia is generally 50 mg IV/1–2 min with a total dose of 1 mg/kg. The indications are: (1) evaluation of the refractory period of the accessory pathway: when delta has disappeared, the ERP of the accessory pathway is longer than 250 ms; (2) evaluation of occult Chagas cardiomyopathy with induction of ST-T abnormalities and IVCD; (3) evaluation of the His-Purkinje disease; (4) provocation of suspected Brugada syndrome ECG abnormalities.

2. **Class IB drugs**: This group shortens the APD and reduces $V_{max}$ with fast onset and offset.

  2.1. **Lidocaine**: Lidocaine has minimal effect on atrial tissue and AV node and accessory pathways. Lidocaine has moderate efficacy against VT and VF, but rarely terminates monomorphic VT. Some conditions increase the effect of lidocaine on the $I_{Na}$ channel: faster stimulation, acidosis, hyperkalemia, and reduced membrane potential. The maintenance dose of lidocaine should be reduced in HF patients by one-third to a half. In patients after coronary revascularization and in those resuscitated from VF, lidocaine is effective but amiodarone has a higher survival rate.[33]

  2.2. **Mexiletine**: Mexiletine is an oral medication for the treatment of VT. In patients with SND, it may cause severe bradycardia. The starting dose is 200 mg TDS, and 50–100 mg may increase every 2–3 days. It is better to use with food. In patients with congenital heart disease, it is very useful. Metabolism of mexiletine is increased by phenytoin and phenobarbital and decreased by cimetidine. In up to 40% patients, it can cause tremor and dizziness.

3. **Class IC drugs**: This group can reduce $V_{max}$, slow conduction velocity, and prolong refractoriness, with slow onset and offset.

  This include flecainide and propafenone. Both of them in IHD could increase the mortality and both of them increase the pacing threshold. Nowadays, it is mostly used for maintenance of NSR in AF patients, but could be used in the treatment of ventricular arrhythmia.

  3.1. **Flecainide**: The starting dose is 100 mg q 12 h with a maximum dose of 400 mg/day. Indications are: paroxysmal AF, some SVTs (such as ATs), some forms of VTs. It is recommended to begin U-E in the hospital. It almost always suppresses PVCs and NSVTs. In proarrhythmic episodes, isoproterenol is effective. In Brugada patients, it can provoke ECG findings. What is more important about flecainide is to be familiar with adverse effects such as sinus arrest in patients with sinus node dysfunction and increase in the pacing threshold. Exercise stress testing is recommended for evaluation about proarrhythmia and occult ischemia. Flecainide is one of the effective drugs in catecholaminergic polymorphic VT.[34]

  3.2. **Propafenone**: The most indication is the treatment of proarrhythmia and some types of ventricular arrhythmia. The dosage is 150–300 mg q 8 h with a maximum dose of 1200 mg. Similar to flecainide, propafenone increases the pacing threshold. Proarrhythmia is more often in patients with reduced EF and sustained VT but is less than flecainide.

4. **Class II AADs**: Beta-blockers are widely used for ventricular and supraventricular arrhythmia. Some of them have particular effects in some disorders. For example, nadolol is very effective in long QT patients and carvedilol is very effective in HF patients (because of the alpha-blocking effects). Beta-blockers have no effect on the normal resting membrane potential, maximum diagnostic potential amplitude, and $V_{max}$ of the atrial, Purkinje, and ventricular muscle cells. They are mostly indicated in the arrhythmia associated with thyrotoxicosis or pheochromocytoma.

  They are also very useful in termination of AVNRT, orthodromic AVRT, inappropriate sinus tachycardia, and rate control of post-MI VT and VF. Beta-blockers are the drug of choice in LQTS. Some of the beta-blockers exert an intrinsic sympathomimetic activity; these types are not associated with reduced mortality in post-MI patients. Adverse effects of beta-blockers are hypotension, bradycardia, CHF, Raynaud phenomenon, mental depression, and hypoglycemia in insulin-dependent patients.

5. **Class III AADs**: These drugs predominantly block potassium channels ($I_{Kr}$) and prolong repolarization. This group includes: sotalol, amiodarone, dronedarone, and ibutilide.

  5.1. **Amiodarone**: Amiodarone blocks all types of channels, in addition to class III effects. Amiodarone depresses conduction at fast rates more than at slow rates (use dependence). Oral Amiodarone slows the sinus rate by 20%–30% and prolongs the QT interval.

    It is a peripheral and coronary vasodilator. Amiodarone is not dialyzable and the terminal half-life of amiodarone is about 100 days. It could suppress a wide spectrum of arrhythmia including supraventricular and ventricular arrhythmia, such as AVNRT, junctional tachycardia, atrial flutter (AFL), AF, VT, and VF.[35–37]

    In hypertrophic cardiomyopathy, post-MI patients, and after resuscitation, amiodarone could improve survival. With oral administration for loading, a dose of 800–1200 mg should be administered for 1–3 weeks, then 400 mg daily for several weeks, and after

2–3 months the dose could be reduced to 300 mg/day. For IV administration, 150 mg stat in 10 min is administered, then 1 mg/min for 6 h, and 0.5 mg/min for 18 h is recommended.

Adverse effects of amiodarone are reported in about 75% of patients. Lung fibrosis due to hypersensitivity reaction or widespread phospholipids is one of the most serious side effects, so chest X-ray and DLCO every 3 months for 1 year and every 6 months for several years are recommended. A rise in LFT up to three times normal is acceptable but in more than that, the drug should be discontinued. Hyperthyroidism is present in 1%–2% and hypothyroidism in 3%–4% of users. The reverse T3 concentration could be used as a marker of drug efficacy. Corneal microdeposits are very common. TdP could be seen in 1%–2% of patients.[38]

5.2. **Dronedarone**: Dronedarone is a noniodinated derivative of amiodarone. In the ANDROMEDA and PALLAS study, dronedarone was associated with increased risk of mortality. It is more potent than amiodarone for $I_{Na}$ blocking. Dronedarone increases the level of dabigatran. It is indicated for facilitation of AF and AFL cardioversion to NSR. In patients with function, class III–IV heart failure is contraindicated. Dronedarone is also prohibited during pregnancy.[39]

5.3. **Sotalol**: Sotalol is a beta-blocker with positive intrinsic sympathetic activity. The dose is 80–160 mg q 12 h with a maximum dose of 320 mg/day. It should be given with an inpatient setting and monitoring of QT, especially in women and AF patients. It is mostly indicated for ventricular arrhythmia and AF. Sotalol decreases ICD discharges and reduces the defibrillation threshold. Proarrhythmia is present in 4% of patients and TdP in 2.5% of them.[40]

5.4. **Ibutilide**: Ibutilide is an agent for AF and AFL termination, with IV infusion of 1 mg over 10 min. It should not be administrated in QT interval longer than 440 ms or in hypokalemia, hypomagnesemia, or bradycardia. Up to 60% of AFL patients convert to NSR with 2 mg ibutilide. Patients should be monitored for 4–6 h after ibutilide.[41]

5.5. **Dofetilide**: Dofetilide is recommended for acute conversion of AF and also chronic suppression of AF. It is recommended as an oral dose of 0.125 mg to 0.5 mg twice daily. It should not be administered in patients with GFR <20 mL/min or QT >440 ms. TdP occurs in 2%–4% of patients. Dofetilide may also decrease DFT.[42]

6. **Class IV AADs**: Verapamil blocks slow calcium channels and reduce $I_{ca,L}$ in cardiac muscle. Verapamil depresses the slope of the diastolic depolarization in SA node and AV node. Peak hemodynamic effects occur 3–5 min after completion of its action. The most known indications are acute termination of SVT or rate control of AF. Diltiazem in IV form is administered at a dose of 0.25 mg/kg over 2 min with a second dose 15 min later.

If significant hypotension occurs with intravenous diltiazem, phenylephrine should be administered. In patients with idiopathic left septal VT, verapamil is the drug of choice. In patients with preexcited AF and antidromic AVRT, verapamil with reflex sympathetic activation could increase the ventricular response over the accessory pathway and is dangerous.

In some patients with sinus node dysfunction, verapamil could depress sinus function or asystole. In such cases, isoproterenol, calcium, glucagon, dopamine, atropine, or temporary pacing may be effective. In hemodynamic deterioration, calcium should be administered, while in bradycardia, isoproterenol is the drug of choice.

7. **Class V AADs**: Include those drugs that do not fit cleanly into categories I through IV.

7.1. **Adenosine**: Adenosine activates K+ channels ($I_{k.Ach}$ and $I_{kAdo}$) similar to acetylcholine. Adenosine blocks conduction in AV node but it rarely blocks conduction in the accessory pathways. Its elimination half-life is 1–6 s. Dipyridamole potentiates its effect. Adenosine is superior to verapamil and beta-blockers in patients with HF or hypotensive or in neonates. In patients with active bronchospasm and inadequate venous access and in patients who receive theophylline, verapamil is the drug of choice. It can cause AF in 12% of patients. Transient side effects are seen in 40% of patients.

7.2. **Digoxin**: Digoxin enhances both central and peripheral vagal tones. It slows the SA nodal discharge rate and AV nodal conduction. Peak effect of IV digoxin occurs after 1.5–3 h. Previously, it was the drug of choice for rate control in AF, but recently it showed that digoxin is not very effective in such situations. Dig toxicity can show general and cardiac manifestation. Halo vision, altered color perception generalized malaise, nausea, and vomiting are general side effects. In situations such as renal failure, hypothyroidism, hypokalemia, and amyloidosis, sensitivity to digoxin increases. In dig toxicity arrhythmia, phenytoin is the drug of choice for supraventricular arrhythmia and lidocaine for ventricular arrhythmia.[43]

7.3. **Ranolazine**: Ranolazine blocks $I_{kr}$ and prolongs atrial and ventricular refractoriness. Its effects are more pronounced in the atrial tissue than in the ventricular tissue. Despite its effect on the QT interval, TdP is rare.[43]

7.4. **Eleclazine**: It blocks late $I_{Na}$ channel and could be used in LQT3 and hypertrophic cardiomyopathy.

7.5. **Vernakalant**: Vernakalant is a potassium and sodium channel blocker. In (ACT1 and ACT3) trials, it was effective in AF conversion. It is available only in Europe.[44]

## NONPHARMACOLOGICAL TREATMENT OF CARDIAC ARRHYTHMIA

1. **D/C cardioversion**: Electrical cardioversion is the method of choice of termination of arrhythmia with reentrant mechanisms, such as AF, AFL, AVRT, most forms of VT, ventricular flutter, and VF. Synchronized cardioversion is done by delivering an electrical shock on with timing on the R wave and is used for all types of cardioversion except in VF and ventricular flutter.

    In SVTs, 25–30 J energy is enough. In AF, energy should not be lower than 100 J. When cardioversion is ineffective, reversing path polarity may be effective. In atrial arrhythmia, anteroposterior position of patches is useful. In patients with AF lasting more than 24 h AFL and AT in congenital heart disease, monitored anticoagulation for 3 weeks, or TEE should be done before cardioversion and should be continued for at least 4 weeks. After cardioversion, transient ST elevation may occur.[45]

2. **Catheter ablation**: Ablation could be done by radiofrequency or by cryoenergy. The purpose of ablation is to destroy myocardial tissue by energy. In focal arrhythmia, the focus is targeted by ablation and in reentrant arrhythmia due to intraatrial macroreentrant or AFL or VT, the narrow portion of the myocardium between unexcitable areas is the target for ablation. RF energy in focal arrhythmia causes initial acceleration of arrhythmia and in reentrant arrhythmia causes slowing and termination of the arrhythmia.[46–48]

2.1. **Accessory pathway ablation**: The target of the ablation is the site of the accessory pathway, which is determined by the earliest onset of ventricular EGM in relation to the onset of delta wave during sinus rhythm showing a QS wave in unipolar EGM or accessory pathway potential on the bipolar electrogram, or earliest site of atrial activation during orthodromic AVRT or ventricular pacing. In patients with septal accessory pathways, cryoablation can be useful. The success rate is about 95%.

2.2. **AVNRT ablation**: A slow pathway is located in the posteroseptal tricuspid annulus close to the CS ostium. In most cases of AVNRT patients, a slow pathway ablation is required. In 40% of patients, the slow pathway is modified after ablation and a residual function is present after ablation, manifested as a persistent dual AN node physiology and single AV node echo. The end point of ablation is noninducibility of AVNRT with and without isoproterenol. In some patients, the ERP of the fast pathway decreases after ablation. In patients with a greatly prolonged PR interval at rest, ablation of the fast pathway could be done, in whom retrograde fast pathway ablation eliminates SVT.

2.3. **Cather ablation of AFL**: In a typical AFL, reentry is in the right atrium, and ablation is done by creating a line across the isthmus of atrial tissue between the IVC and tricuspid annulus. The end point is creation of a line causing a bidirectional block in the isthmus. The success rate is more than 90%.

2.4. **Catheter ablation of VT**: In idiopathic VT, the focal origin of VT is the target and in reentrant VT, the slow conduction zone, or an excitable tissue between two unexcitable tissues, is the target for ablation. This site could be determined by concealed fusion and a short postpacing interval-tachycardia cycle length (PPI-TCL) difference during entrainment maneuvers. This maneuver is for finding a protected region of diastolic activation as a critical part of the reentrant circuit. If the patient was unstable hemodynamically during VT, substrate modification during NSR could be done by defining and ablation of abnormal potentials.

## REFERENCES

1. Boyden PA, Dun W, Robinson RB. Cardiac Purkinje fibers and arrhythmias; the GK Moe Award Lecture 2015. *Heart Rhythm*. 2016;13:1172.
2. Hohendanner F, Walther S, Maxwell JT, et al. Inositol-1,4,5-trisphosphate induced Ca2+ release and excitation-contraction coupling in atrial myocytes from normal and failing hearts. *J Physiol*. 2015;593:1459.

3. Lerman BB. Mechanism, diagnosis, and treatment of outflow tract tachycardia. *Nat Rev Cardiol.* 2015;12:597.

4. Hohendanner F, McCulloch AD, Blatter LA, et al. Calcium and IP3 dynamics in cardiac myocytes: experimental and computational perspectives and approaches. *Front Pharmacol.* 2014;5:35.

5. Jiang W, Lan F, Zhang H. Human induced pluripotent stem cell models of inherited cardiovascular diseases. *Curr Stem Cell Res Ther.* 2016;11(7):533–541.

6. Cashman TJ, Josowitz R, Johnson BV, et al. Human engineered cardiac tissues created using induced pluripotent stem cells reveal functional characteristics of BRAF-mediated hypertrophic cardiomyopathy. *PLoS One.* 2016;11, e0146697.

7. Thavandiran N, Dubois N, Mikryukov A, et al. Design and formulation of functional pluripotent stem cell–derived cardiac microtissues. *Proc Natl Acad Sci USA.* 2013;110: E4698.

8. Schwartz PJ, Woosley RL. Predicting the unpredictable: drug-induced QT prolongation and torsades de pointes. *J Am Coll Cardiol.* 2016;67:1639.

9. Algalarrondo V, Nattel S. Potassium channel remodeling in heart disease. *Card Electrophysiol Clin.* 2016;8:337.

10. Weiss JN, Garfinkel A, Karagueuzian HS, et al. Perspective: a dynamics-based classification of ventricular arrhythmias. *J Mol Cell Cardiol.* 2015;82:136.

11. Qi XY, Diness JG, Brundel BJ, et al. Role of small-conductance calcium-activated potassium channels in atrial electrophysiology and fibrillation in the dog. *Circulation.* 2014;129:430.

12. Tucker NR, Ellinor PT. Emerging directions in the genetics of atrial fibrillation. *Circ Res.* 2014;114:1469.

13. Voigt N, Heijman J, Wang Q, et al. Cellular and molecular mechanisms of atrial arrhythmogenesis in patients with paroxysmal atrial fibrillation. *Circulation.* 2014;129:145.

14. Gemel J, Levy AE, Simon AR, et al. Connexin40 abnormalities and atrial fibrillation in the human heart. *J Mol Cell Cardiol.* 2014;76:159.

15. Chen PS, Chen LS, Fishbein MC, et al. Role of the autonomic nervous system in atrial fibrillation: pathophysiology and therapy. *Circ Res.* 2014;114:1500.

16. Meyers JD, Jay PY, Rentschler S. Reprogramming the conduction system: onward toward a biological pacemaker. *Trends Cardiovasc Med.* 2016;26:14.

17. Priori SG, Wilde AA, Horie M, et al. HRS/EHRA/APHRS expert consensus statement on the diagnosis and management of patients with inherited primary arrhythmia syndromes. Document endorsed by HRS, EHRA, and APHRS in May 2013 and by ACCF, AHA, PACES, and AEPC in June 2013. *Heart Rhythm.* 2013;10:1932.

18. Zhang P, Tung R, Zhang Z, et al. Characterization of the epicardial substrate for catheter ablation of Brugada syndrome. *Heart Rhythm.* 2016;13:2151.

19. Knoebel SB, Crawford MH, Dunn MI, et al. Guidelines for ambulatory electrocardiography. A report of the American College of Cardiology/American Heart Association Task Force on Assessment of Diagnostic and Therapeutic Cardiovascular Procedures (Subcommittee on Ambulatory Electrocardiography). *Circulation.* 1989;79(1):206–215.

20. Crawford MH, Bernstein SJ, Deedwania PC, et al. ACC/AHA guidelines for ambulatory electrocardiography. A report of the American College of Cardiology/American Heart Association Task Force on Practice Guidelines (Committee to Revise the Guidelines for Ambulatory Electrocardiography). Developed in collaboration with the North American Society for Pacing and Electrophysiology. *J Am Coll Cardiol.* 1999;34(3):912–948.

21. Kadish AH, Buxton AE, Kennedy HL, et al. ACC/AHA clinical competence statement on electrocardiography and ambulatory electrocardiography. A report of the ACC/AHA/ACP-ASIM Task Force on Clinical Competence (ACC/AHA Committee to Develop a Clinical Competence Statement on Electrocardiography and Ambulatory Electrocardiography). Endorsed by the International Society for Holter and Noninvasive Electrocardiology. *Circulation.* 2001;104(25):3169–3178.

22. Akhtar M, Fisher JD, Gillette PC, et al. NASPE Ad Hoc Committee on Guidelines for Cardiac Electrophysiological Studies. North American Society of Pacing and Electrophysiology. *Pacing Clin Electrophysiol.* 1985;8 (4):611–618.

23. Zipes DP, DiMarco JP, Gillette PC, et al. Guidelines for clinical intracardiac electrophysiological and catheter ablation procedures. A report of the American College of Cardiology/American Heart Association Task Force on Practice Guidelines (Committee on Clinical Intracardiac Electrophysiologic and Catheter Ablation Procedures). Developed in collaboration with the North American Society of Pacing and Electrophysiology. *J Am Coll Cardiol.* 1995;26(2):555–573.

24. Tracy CM, Akhtar M, DiMarco JP, et al. American College of Cardiology/American Heart Association clinical competence statement on invasive electrophysiology studies, catheter ablation, and cardioversion. A report of the American College of Cardiology/American Heart Association/American College of Physicians–American Society of Internal Medicine Task Force on Clinical Competence. *J Am Coll Cardiol.* 2000;36(5):1725–1736.

25. Tracy CM, Akhtar M, DiMarco JP, et al. American College of Cardiology/American Heart Association 2006 update of the clinical competence statement on invasive electrophysiology studies, catheter ablation, and cardioversion. A report of the American College of Cardiology/American Heart Association/American College of Physicians Task Force on Clinical Competence and Training developed in collaboration with the Heart Rhythm Society. *J Am Coll Cardiol.* 2006;48(7): 1503–1517.

26. Lester RM, Olbertz J. Early drug development: assessment of proarrhythmic risk and cardiovascular safety. *Expert Rev Clin Pharmacol.* 2016;9(12):1611–1618.

27. Rosen MR, Janse MJ. Concept of the vulnerable parameter: the Sicilian Gambit revisited. *J Cardiovasc Pharmacol.* 2010;55(5):428–437.

28. Zaiou M, El Amri H. Cardiovascular pharmacogenetics: a promise for genomically-guided therapy and personalized medicine. *Clin Genet.* 2017;91(3):355–370.

29. Lorberbaum T, Sampson KJ, Chang JB, et al. Coupling data mining and laboratory experiments to discover drug interactions causing QT prolongation. *J Am Coll Cardiol.* 2016;68(16):1756–1764.

30. Wright JM, Page RL, Field ME. Antiarrhythmic drugs in pregnancy. *Expert Rev Cardiovasc Ther.* 2015;13(12): 1433–1444.

31. Frommeyer G, Eckardt L. Drug-induced proarrhythmia: risk factors and electrophysiological mechanisms. *Nat Rev Cardiol.* 2016;13(1):36–47.

32. Liang P, Lan F, Lee AS, et al. Drug screening using a library of human induced pluripotent stem cell–derived cardiomyocytes reveals disease-specific patterns of cardiotoxicity. *Circulation.* 2013;127(16):1677–1691.

33. Marquez MF, Bonny A, Hernandez-Castillo E, et al. Long-term efficacy of low doses of quinidine on malignant arrhythmias in Brugada syndrome with an implantable cardioverter-defibrillator: a case series and literature review. *Heart Rhythm.* 2012;9(12):1995–2000.

34. Mankikian J, Favelle O, Guillon A, et al. Initial characteristics and outcome of hospitalized patients with amiodarone pulmonary toxicity. *Respir Med.* 2014;108(4): 638–646.

35. Hussain N, Bhattacharyya A, Prueksaritanond S. Amiodarone-induced cirrhosis of liver: what predicts mortality? *ISRN Cardiol.* 2013;2013, 617943.

36. Cheng HC, Yeh HJ, Huang N, et al. Amiodarone-associated optic neuropathy: a nationwide study. *Ophthalmology.* 2015;122(12):2553–2559.

37. Epstein AE, Olshansky B, Naccarelli GV, et al. Practical management guide for clinicians who treat patients with amiodarone. *Am J Med.* 2016;129(5):468–475.

38. Qin D, Leef G, Alam MB, et al. Comparative effectiveness of antiarrhythmic drugs for rhythm control of atrial fibrillation. *J Cardiol.* 2016;67(5):471–476.

39. Chatterjee S, Ghosh J, Lichstein E, et al. Meta-analysis of cardiovascular outcomes with dronedarone in patients with atrial fibrillation or heart failure. *Am J Cardiol.* 2012;110(4):607–613.

40. Kpaeyeh Jr JA, Wharton JM. Sotalol. *Card Electrophysiol Clin.* 2016;8(2):437–452.

41. Steinwender C, Honig S, Kypta A, et al. Pre-injection of magnesium sulfate enhances the efficacy of ibutilide for the conversion of typical but not of atypical persistent atrial flutter. *Int J Cardiol.* 2010;141(3):260–265.

42. Malhotra R, Bilchick KC, DiMarco JP. Usefulness of pharmacologic conversion of atrial fibrillation during dofetilide loading without the need for electrical cardioversion to predict durable response to therapy. *Am J Cardiol.* 2014;113(3):475–479.

43. Reiffel JA, Camm AJ, Belardinelli L, et al. The HARMONY trial: combined ranolazine and dronedarone in the management of paroxysmal atrial fibrillation: mechanistic and therapeutic synergism. *Circ Arrhythm Electrophysiol.* 2015;8(5):1048–1056.

44. Kowey PR, Dorian P, Mitchell LB, et al. Atrial Arrhythmia Conversion Trial I. Vernakalant hydrochloride for the rapid conversion of atrial fibrillation after cardiac surgery: a randomized, double-blind, placebo-controlled trial. *Circ Arrhythm Electrophysiol.* 2009;2(6):652–659.

45. Zhang B, Li X, Shen D, et al. Anterior-posterior versus anterior-lateral electrode position for external electrical cardioversion of atrial fibrillation: a meta-analysis of randomized controlled trials. *Arch Cardiovasc Dis.* 2014;107(5):280–290.

46. Houmsse M, Daoud EG. Biophysics and clinical utility of irrigated-tip radiofrequency catheter ablation. *Expert Rev Med Devices.* 2012;9(1):59–70.

47. Andrade JG, Dubuc M, Guerra PG, et al. The biophysics and biomechanics of cryoballoon ablation. *Pacing Clin Electrophysiol.* 2012;35(9):1162–1168.

48. Marchlinski FE, Haffajee CI, Beshai JF, et al. Long-term success of irrigated radiofrequency catheter ablation of sustained ventricular tachycardia: post-approval THERMOCOOL VT trial. *J Am Coll Cardiol.* 2016;67(6):674–683.

# CHAPTER 18

# Hypotension and Syncope

FARZAD KAMALI
Department of Cardiac Electrophysiology, Rajaie Cardiovascular, Medical & Research Center, Iran
University of Medical Sciences, Tehran, Iran

## KEY POINTS

- Syncope is defined as transient loss of consciousness due to cerebral hypoperfusion, characterized by a spontaneous, rapid onset, and short duration event with brief and complete recovery.
- The possible causes of true syncope are generally divided into four major categories: reflex-mediated syncope, orthostatic hypotension, cardiac syncope, and other uncommon causes.
- The history and physical examination are the most important components of the evaluation of syncope. The choice of additional diagnostic testing should be individualized and based on the results of initial evaluation.
- Reflex syncope is the most common cause of syncope resulting from alteration in autonomic system activation. Types of reflex syncope include vasovagal syncope (VVS), situational syncope, and carotid sinus syndrome.
- The postural (orthostatic) tachycardia syndrome (POTS) is one of the most common causes of orthostatic intolerance, characterized by an excessive increase in heart rate that occurs on standing without significant hypotension.
- Pseudosyncope is a conversion disorder that can mimic syncope or seizure.

## DEFINITION

Syncope is a clinical syndrome with an abrupt, transient, complete loss of consciousness that is caused by a period of cerebral hypoperfusion. Recovery from syncope is usually rapid and complete and rarely lasts for more than a few minutes.

Transient loss of consciousness (TLOC) has many potential causes. Syncope is only one of them. Examples of nonsyncopal causes of TLOC include neurological disorders, intoxications, metabolic disorders, and head trauma. On the other hand, we should distinguish true syncope from apparent TLOC conditions such as psychogenic syncope (pseudosyncope), drop attack, and cataplexy (Table 18.1). These conditions are not true loss of consciousness. On some occasions, patients may have warning symptoms (prodromal symptoms), particularly in the case of the vasovagal form of reflex syncope. These symptoms include light-headedness, visual blurring, pallor (reported by an on looker).

Presyncope, or near-syncope, is a manifestation of prodromal symptoms without complete loss of consciousness. Presyncope could progress to syncope, or it could abort without syncope.[1,2]

## PREVALENCE

In a cross section of 1925 randomly selected residents of Olmsted County, Minnesota, with a median age of 62 years (all >45 years of age), the estimated prevalence of syncope was 19%. Females have a higher prevalence, and there is no association of syncope prevalence with age.[1,3] Another observational study including 127,508 patients with the diagnosis of syncope (median age 65 years, 52.6% female) showed that the first episode of syncope commonly occurs around 20, 60, or 80 years of age (trimodal pattern) and the third peak occurs 5–7 years earlier in males.[1,4]

## CLASSIFICATION OF SYNCOPE

The possible causes of TLOC resulting in true syncope are generally divided into several categories. Table 18.2 presents the classification and principal causes of syncope.[1,2]

## DIAGNOSIS

The initial evaluation of suspected syncope should include getting an exact history, physical examination, and obtaining an electrocardiogram (ECG).

**TABLE 18.1**
**Causes of TLOC**

Syncopal causes

Nonsyncopal causes
- True TLOC: seizure disorders, traumatic brain injury, metabolic disorders, intoxications
- Apparent TLOC: psychogenic syncope, drop attacks, cataplexy

**TABLE 18.2**
**Syncope Classification**

1. Reflex, or neurally mediated syncope
   - Vasovagal syncope
   - Situational syncope: (cough, laugh, sneeze, micturition, defecation, swallow, postprandial, etc.)
   - Carotid sinus syndrome

2. Orthostatic hypotension (OH)
   - Autonomic failure
   - Volume depletion
   - Drug induced OH
   - Idiopathic

3. Cardiac syncope
   - Cardiac arrhythmias: [bradycardia (sinus node dysfunction, AV conduction disorder, pacemaker malfunction), tachycardia (supraventricular, ventricular)]
   - Structural cardiac disorders: (aortic stenosis, hypertrophic obstructive cardiomyopathy, acute myocardial ischemia/infarction, pericardial disease/tamponade, cardiac mass, prosthetic valve dysfunction)
   - Cardiopulmonary and great vessels: pulmonary embolus, pulmonary hypertension, acute aortic dissection

4. Other causes: [subclavian steal syndrome, endocrine disorders (pheochromocytoma, carcinoid syndrome), etc.]

Additional diagnostic evaluation should be requested based upon the suspected cause of the syncope. The history and physical examination are the most important components of the evaluation of syncope that can be used to identify the cause in more than 25% of patients.[1,2,5,6]

1. **History:** The comprehensive history should aim to identify the prognosis, diagnosis, comorbidities, medication use, and patient needs. A careful history should be taken from patients and eyewitnesses, in person or through a telephone interview.

   The clinician should not only ascertain whether the collapse was likely true syncope or not, but also determine whether the affected patient should be admitted to the hospital or can be safely managed in the outpatient setting.[1,2,6,7]

   1.1. **Frequency and duration:** The frequency and duration of syncopal events are important. In some patients, frequent syncopal events may result in injury and an impaired quality of life. In addition, patients with TLOC episodes that occur very frequently (such as each day) and episodes lasting many minutes in duration are more likely to have pseudosyncope rather than true syncope.

   1.2. **Onset of syncope:** Benign vasovagal syncope (VVS) is often associated with prodromal symptoms such as lightheadedness, nausea, feeling hot or cold, pallor, and diaphoresis, consistent with increased vagal tone. The sudden onset of syncope without prodromal symptoms is more common among patients with cardiac syncope.

   1.3. **Position of syncope:** Neurally mediated syncope most commonly occurs with an upright standing or sitting position and almost never when supine. In orthostatic hypotension (OH), syncope frequently occurs after changing position from a supine to an upright posture. In comparison, the events that occur when the patient is in supine position suggests a cardiac cause of syncope.

   1.4. **Syncope triggers:** Syncope patients should be asked about situations and circumstances in which the syncope occurred. Situational syncope is a form of neurally mediated syncope that occurs during or immediately after identifiable triggers such as coughing, swallowing, urination, defecation (Table 18.2).

   Syncopal events that occur immediately after exercise, during a prolonged standing position or in association with emotional stress, pain, and dehydration, suggest VVS. However, incidents that occur during exertion or in the supine position may suggest a potentially life-threatening etiology. The syncopal events that occur immediately following abrupt neck movements may suggest the carotid sinus hypersensitivity (CSH) syndrome.

1.5. **Symptoms following syncope:** Patients and eyewitnesses should be asked about any symptoms that occur after syncope. As mentioned earlier, the recovery from true syncope is usually rapid (1–2 min) and complete. However, a prolonged loss of consciousness and long recovery time may indicate a seizure or a pseudosyncope. Note that sometimes following VVS, the symptoms associated with increased vagal tone and fatigue may be persistent.

1.6. **Past medical history:** Patients with syncope should be questioned about a preexisting medical condition, including: structural heart disorders (e.g., prior myocardial infarction, prior cardiac surgery, valvular heart disease, cardiomyopathies, history of pacemaker or ICD implantation, congenital heart disease, etc.), diabetes mellitus, intoxications (e.g., alcohol, narcotics), and neurological and psychiatric disorders.

1.7. **Medications:** Many medications can cause or exacerbate syncope through a variety of mechanisms, including: hypovolemia and hypotension (diuretics and antihypertensive agents), and predisposing to arrhythmia by hypokalemia and/or QT prolongation (e.g., diuretics, antiarrhythmic agents, antiinfective drugs, antipsychotic/antidepressants, etc.)

1.8. **Family history:** Family history of sudden death at a young age (less than 40 years), familial cardiomyopathy (e.g., hypertrophic cardiomyopathy, arrhythmogenic right ventricular cardiomyopathy, etc.) or channelopathy (long/short QT syndrome, Brugada syndrome, etc.) are important elements for risk stratification of patients presenting with syncope.[1,2,6,7]

2. **Physical examination:** A complete and comprehensive cardiac examination is a necessary element in the evaluation of patients with syncope. Physical examination should be focused on the presence of structural heart disease and detecting the significant neurologic abnormalities.

The patients' blood pressure (BP) and heart rate should be obtained while supine and then repeated each minute for 3 min while standing. A drop in systolic BP of ≥20 mmHg or diastolic BP of ≥10 mmHg after changing position from supine to standing is considered as OH. Carotid sinus massage (CSM) is recommended after initial evaluation in patients over age 40 with unknown syncope etiology.

Note that a general examination, guided by patient complaints, may reveal important findings such as

**TABLE 18.3**
**High-Risk ECG Features of Patients With Syncope**

| |
| --- |
| ECG changes consistent with acute MI |
| Persistent sinus bradycardia (<40 bpm) or sinus pauses >3 s in awake patients |
| Mobitz II second- and third-degree AV block |
| Bifascicular block or QRS >120 ms |
| ECG suggestive of ventricular hypertrophic or Q waves consistent with ischemic or nonischemic cardiomyopathy |
| Sustained or nonsustained VT |
| Pacemaker and ICD malfunction with cardiac pauses |
| Brugada ECG pattern |
| QTc >460 ms in repeated ECG indicating LQTS |

gastrointestinal bleeding on rectal exam or a pulsatile abdominal mass.[1,2,6,7]

3. **Electrocardiogram:** The 12-lead ECG is another important element in the workup of patients with syncope. The initial ECG rarely establishes a definite diagnosis. Table 18.3 shows the high-risk ECG findings in patients with syncope, based on the recommendations of the 2018 ESC guideline for the evaluation and management of patients with syncope.[2]

4. **Additional evaluation and diagnostic tests:** For further evaluation of patients with syncope after initial assessment, we do not have a predetermined approach. The choice of testing should be individualized and based on the results of initial assessment.

4.1. **Laboratory testing:** Routine use of laboratory tests (e.g., hematocrit level, electrolytes, cardiac enzymes, blood glucose, etc.) has a low diagnostic value in syncopal patients and is therefore not recommended routinely. Targeted blood tests are reasonable in selected patients when the nature of the syncope presentation or associated comorbidities suggests a diagnostic or prognostic role for laboratory testing.[6,7]

4.2. **Ambulatory ECG monitoring:** If the syncopal events are infrequent, a 24- or 48-h ambulatory ECG monitoring is not likely to be useful in making a diagnosis. Several types of ambulatory cardiac rhythm monitoring are available and provide a variable amount of information. Their selection and usefulness are highly dependent on patient characteristics with regard to the frequency of syncope and the likelihood of an arrhythmic cause of syncope.

4.2.1. **Holter ECG monitoring** records ECG data for a period of 24 or 48 h. It is helpful in syncopal patients with daily or near daily symptoms.

4.2.2. **Event monitors** are small and lightweight devices that are usually utilized for 2–4 weeks. It can be useful for patients with less frequent symptoms (i.e., weekly to monthly).

4.2.3. **Implantable cardiac monitors (ICM)** are subcutaneous monitoring devices for detection of cardiac arrhythmias. A small randomized trial involving 60 patients with syncope of unknown origin was evaluated by conventional testing (event recorder, tilt-table test, and electrophysiology study (EPS)) and ICM with 1 year of monitoring. The diagnosis (primarily bradycardia) made in 55% with ICM compared with a 19% diagnostic yield with conventional testing.[1,6–8]

A systematic review involving a total of 579 participants with unexplained syncope shows an ICM-based diagnostic strategy that does not reduce long-term mortality as compared to a standard diagnostic assessment.[9]

4.3. **Tilt-table test:** An upright tilt-table test is a confirmatory test which can be useful when the diagnosis of a reflex VVS is suspected, but not if the presentation is classical. Furthermore, the upright tilt-table test can be useful for patients with syncope and suspected to delayed OH and postural orthostatic tachycardia syndrome or to establish the diagnosis of pseudosyncope.[1,2]

4.3.1. **Tilt-table test protocol:** Intravenous (IV) access should be obtained at the beginning of the test. The patients should be monitored in the supine position for at least 10 min and the baseline BP and heart rate is measured. IV insertion can cause significant distress for patients; in these circumstances (excess catecholamine states), the initial rest time can be extended to more than 20 min. The upright passive phase (without drug) of the test is generally performed for 20–30 min at an angle between 60 and 80 degrees.

The ECG is recorded continuously during the test. The BP should be monitored noninvasively by beat-to-beat finger arterial monitoring. If no symptoms have developed after the passive phase of the test, the drug provocation phase of the test is considered. The common vasoactive drugs for triggering syncope are intravenous isoproterenol and sublingual nitroglycerin. The infusion rate of the isoproterenol can be increased incrementally 1–3 µg/min to increase average HR by about 20%–25% over baseline. Nitroglycerin is administered sublingually at a fixed dose of 300–400 µg. These two provocative drugs have an equivalent diagnostic accuracy.[10] The choice of the isoproterenol or nitroglycerin is dependent on the local practice and the clinical expertise. However, sublingual nitroglycerin was simpler to use and better tolerated than isoproterenol. After administration of provocative drugs, we will continue the tilt test in an upright position for an additional 15–20 min. Measures that increase test sensitivity include: use of a longer test duration, steeper tilt angle, and use of provocative agents.

Note that the sensitivity and specificity of the test are inversely related. Tilt-table testing should not be performed in patients with severe coronary or cerebrovascular disease in whom hypotension may cause myocardial or cerebral ischemia. It is also not recommended in pregnant woman, if the hypotension and bradycardia may potentially be harmful to the fetus.[1,10–12]

4.4. **Cardiac imaging:** Transthoracic echocardiography can be useful in selected patients presenting with syncope if structural heart disease is suspected (class IIa recommendation in 2017 ACC/AHA guidelines). Other imaging modalities, including CT and MRI, can be helpful in selected patients presenting with syncope, especially when other noninvasive tests are inadequate or inconclusive (class IIb recommendation in 2017 ACC/AHA guidelines).

Routine cardiac imaging is not recommended for the evaluation of patients with syncope (class III recommendation in 2017 ACC/AHA guidelines) unless cardiac etiology is suspected on the basis of an initial evaluation, including history, physical examination, or ECG.[1]

4.5. **Exercise testing:** Generally, exercise stress testing has a low diagnostic value in the evaluation of patients with syncope unless the symptoms occurred during maximum exercise.

Exercise stress testing can be useful to establish the cause of syncope in selected patients who experience syncope or presyncope during exertion (class IIa recommendation in 2017 ACC/AHA guidelines). Exercise testing may be helpful in the following settings: myocardial ischemia or coronary vasospasm, structural heart disease (e.g., hypertrophic obstructive cardiomyopathy, aortic stenosis, interarterial anomalous coronary disease, pulmonary hypertension), and channelopathies (congenital long QT syndrome, catecholaminergic polymorphic ventricular tachycardia).[1,2]

4.6. **Electrophysiology study:** An EPS is indicated in selected patients with unexplained syncope in whom the arrhythmia is suspected for the cause of arrhythmia.

The development of powerful noninvasive methods such as prolonged ECG monitoring with a high diagnostic value has decreased the importance of EPS as a diagnostic test.

In a randomized trial, an implantable loop recorder was applied in 52 patients with BBB and negative EPS during a follow-up of 3–15 months. The syncopal events recurred in 22 patients (42%). The most frequent finding was one or more prolonged asystolic pauses mainly attributable to AV block. So EPS has a low negative predictive value.[13]

During EPS, the SA node function and AV conduction should be assessed primarily. In addition, a complete EPS should also include the SVT and VT induction protocols. Sinus node function is evaluated by determining the sinus node recovery time (SNRT) and corrected SNRT. An abnormal response is defined as $\geq 1.6$ or 2 s for SNRT, or $\geq 525$ ms for corrected SNRT.[1,2,14] AV conduction is assessed by measuring the AH and HV intervals and also by determining the AV conduction response to atrial incremental pacing and atrial extrastimulation. A prolonged HV interval $\geq 70$ ms, or induction of second- or third-degree AV

block by pacing or provoked by pharmacological stress [ajmaline or procainamide (10 mg/kg)], identifies that AV block is the probable cause of the syncope. An HV interval of 100 ms or longer has a higher diagnostic value.[1,2,6]

A sudden onset of brief palpitations before syncopal events suggests SVT or VT as a potential diagnosis. In these settings, an EPS may be indicated to assess the exact mechanism. The isoproterenol infusion can increase the sensitivity of SVT induction during an EP study. An EP study is considered as abnormal and positive for VT when sustained monomorphic VT is induced. The induction of polymorphic VT or VF in patients with ischemic or nonischemic cardiomyopathies cannot be considered a diagnostic finding of the cause of syncope. An EP study is not recommended for syncope evaluation in patients with a normal ECG and normal cardiac structure and function, unless an arrhythmic etiology is suspected. In some patients with syncope and structural heart disease that have an indication for an ICD, an EP study may not be needed.[1,2,6,7]

# 1. CLINICAL PRESENTATION AND TREATMENT OF COMMON CAUSES OF SYNCOPE

1. **Neurally mediated syncope:** Reflex syncope or neurally mediated syncope is a transient loss of consciousness due to cerebral hypoperfusion. It can be caused by autonomic cardioinhibitory and/or vasodilator responses. Types of reflex syncope include VVS, situational syncope, and carotid sinus syndrome (CSS). Alterations in autonomic activation are responsible for reflex syncope.[15,16]

   Reflex syncope has three types of responses:

   – **Cardioinhibitory response:** The cardioinhibitory response is due to an increase in parasympathetic activity. It may be manifested by any or all of the following: sinus bradycardia, PR interval prolongation, AV block, or asystole.

   – **Vasodepressor response:** The vasodepressor response is due to a decrease in sympathetic activity. It is manifested by symptomatic hypotension even in the absence of significant bradycardia.

   – **Mixed response:** The mixed response contains components of both cardioinhibitory and vasodepressor responses.

   1.1. **Vasovagal syncope:** VVS is the most common potential cause of syncope even among athletes and patients with heart disease. It is a frequent reason for emergency department visits. VVS is typically associated with a prodrome of diaphoresis, warmth, and pallor, with fatigue after the event.

The common classic prodromal symptoms associated with VVS include: lightheadedness, feeling of being warm or cold, diaphoresis, pallor (reported by an onlooker), nausea and/or vomiting, palpitation, visual blurring.

The common triggers for typical or classical VVS include: prolonged standing, emotional stress, heat exposure, painful stimuli after physical exercise, dehydration, alcohol, and medications. A typical VVS is more common in young patients. However, in the elderly, the VVS may present as atypical, without an identifiable cause or trigger. As mentioned previously, a comprehensive history, physical examination, and ECG are the first step in risk stratification of syncope. Patients with reflex syncope most often have no evidence of structural heart disease and have a normal baseline ECG.

Patients with a typical presentation do not require future diagnostic tests. For patients with an atypical presentation, the confirmatory tests (upright tilt-table test and ambulatory ECG monitoring) are warranted in order to solidify the diagnosis, or conversely to exclude the diagnosis. Longer term monitoring options (event recorder or ICM) have a higher diagnostic value than shorter monitoring. The patients with situational syncope have the same symptoms as are seen in VVS, but in the setting of a specific scenario or trigger, such as coughing, micturition, defecation, or swallowing (refer to Table 18.2). Situational syncope often does not have prodromal symptoms.[1,2,15,16]

1.1.1. **Treatment:** For most patients with VVS, education and reassurance about the benign nature of the syncope are sufficient, especially in those with infrequent episodes associated with an identifiable precipitant. Patients with vasovagal or situational syncope should be educated to avoid or ameliorate the trigger events (Fig. 18.1).

In patients with a sufficiently long prodrome, physical counterpressure maneuvers (e.g., leg crossing, limb and/or

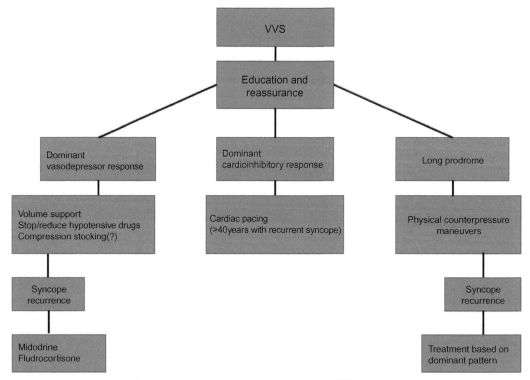

FIG. 18.1 Summary of vasovagal syncope treatments. *VVS*, vasovagal syncope.

abdominal contraction, squatting) are a core management strategy. It may be reasonable to reduce or withdraw medications that cause hypotension (e.g., vasodilators and diuretics), especially in patients with vasodepressor syncope. Evidence for the effectiveness of salt and fluid intake for patients with VVS is limited (class IIb recommendation in 2017 ACC/AHA guidelines). In patients with recurrent VVS and no clear contraindication, such as a history of hypertension, renal disease, HF, or cardiac dysfunction, it may be reasonable to encourage ingestion of 2–3 L of fluid per day and a total of 6–9 g of salt per day, or about 1–2 teaspoonfuls. Orthostatic or tilt training may be a reasonable consideration in patients with frequent syncope recurrences. The training program involves patients instructed to stand against a wall with the heel 25 cm from the wall under supervision of the family members. Standing time should initially be 5 min two times per day with a progressive increase to 40 min twice daily during a period of 2–3 months.

According to the available evidence and 2018 ESC guidelines, beta-blockers are not recommended to treat reflex syncope.[2,16] Regarding the POST trial, beta-blockers might be reasonable in patients 42 years of age or older with recurrent VVS.[1,17] This observation has been included as a IIb recommendation in the 2017 ACC/AHA guidelines. Side effects of beta-blockers occur frequently in children; furthermore, beta-blockers are not beneficial in pediatric patients with VVS (class III recommendation in 2017 ACC/AHA guidelines).

Midodrine is an alpha-1 adrenergic agonist, which is reasonable in patients with recurrent VVS with no history of hypertension, HF, or urinary retention (class IIa recommendation in 2017 ACC/AHA guidelines). In a meta-analysis of five RCTs in adults and children, midodrine was associated with a 43% reduction in syncope recurrence.[1,16]

Fludrocortisone is a very potent mineralocorticoid with high glucocorticoid

activity, resulting in sodium and water retention and potassium excretion, which results in increased blood volume. Fludrocortisone might be reasonable for patients with recurrent VVS and inadequate response to salt and fluid intake, unless contraindicated. Fludrocortisone should not be used in patients with hypertension or heart failure. Fludrocortisone was ineffective in a small randomized double-blind trial in children.[1,2,16]

According to the clinical trials, a pacemaker has a limited role in patients with VVS. A pacemaker can be considered in patients >40 years old age with recurrent syncope and documented spontaneous pauses ≥3 s or asymptomatic pauses ≥6 s. Pacemaker implantation was less beneficial in patients with a positive tilt-table test that induced a vasodepressor response.[1,2,6]

1.2. **Carotid sinus hypersensitivity:** CSH is an exaggerated response of the carotid artery baroreceptors after stimulation that results in a significant drop in the heart rate and blood pressure more than expected. CSH occurs more commonly in men >40 years of age who have atherosclerosis vascular disease. It also may be observed in patients who have acquired neck abnormalities such as carotid sinus tumors and prior neck surgery and/or irradiation.[1,2,6,18]

1.2.1. **Definition:** CSH, most commonly identified as a pause ≥3 s and/or a decrease of systolic pressure ≥50 mmHg occurring upon stimulation of the carotid sinus, may or may not be associated with symptoms.[1,2]

1.2.2. **Carotid sinus massage technique:** The carotid sinus is usually located inferior to the mandibular angle at the level of the thyroid cartilage. CSM should be performed sequentially over the right and left carotid artery sinus in both the supine and upright positions for 5–10 s. Vital signs of all patients should be monitored during and after the maneuver. CSM is recommended after initial evaluation in patients over age 40 with unknown syncope etiology.[1,2,6,18]

Contraindications to performing CSM include auscultation of a carotid bruit and transient ischemic attack, stroke, or myocardial infarction within the prior 3 months, except if the carotid Doppler excludes significant stenosis.[1,2] CSS presents with different symptoms after carotid sinus stimulation such as syncope, lightheadedness, and unexplained falls in older patients.[1,2] In patients with CSS, mechanical stimuli to the neck such as shaving, tie knotting, and head turns can induce syncope.

1.2.3. **Treatment:** Education is an important treatment strategy in CSS, like other reflex syncopes. The patient should be advised to avoid accidental mechanical stimulation of the carotid sinuses. Medications such as vasodilators that may exacerbate the symptoms should be reduced or discontinued, if feasible. Permanent cardiac pacing is reasonable in patients with CSS (symptomatic patients) that is cardioinhibitory or mixed. In asymptomatic patients with a cardioinhibitory response to CSM, permanent pacing in not indicated.[1,2,6,18]

2. **Orthostatic hypotension:** Symptomatic fall in blood pressure after standing and eating is a frequent clinical problem, especially in the elderly. The two major mechanisms for OH are autonomic failure and volume depletion. In neurogenic OH, the impairment of compensatory sympathetic vasoconstriction and inadequate chatecholamine release from sympathetic vasomotor neurones leads to a decline in BP after standing. Several types of neurologic disorders may cause autonomic dysfunction and OH such as Parkinson's disease, dementia with Lewy bodies, multiple system atrophy, and pure autonomic failure. Autonomic peripheral neuropathies such as those due to diabetes mellitus and other systemic diseases can also cause neurogenic OH. Patients with severe volume depletion or significant anemia may experience OH despite normal autonomic reflexes.[1,2,6]

2.1. **Definition:** A drop in systolic BP of $\geq 20$ mmHg or diastolic BP of $\geq 10$ mmHg after changing position from supine to standing is considered as OH.

2.2. **Classification:** OH is subcategorized into three groups: initial, classic, and delayed.

Initial (immediate) OH is characterized by a symptomatic transient BP decrease within 15 s after standing.

Classic OH is characterized by a sustained reduction of systolic BP of $\geq 20$ mmHg or diastolic BP of $\geq 10$ mmHg within 3 min after standing.

Delayed OH is frequently characterized by a sustained reduction of systolic BP of $\geq 20$ mmHg (or 30 mmHg in patients with supine hypertension) or diastolic BP of $\geq 10$ mmHg that takes >3 min of upright posture to develop. The fall in BP is usually gradual until reaching the threshold. Tilt-table testing can be useful for patients with syncope and suspected delayed OH when initial evaluation is not diagnostic.[1,2]

2.3. **Treatment:** The first-line therapy for patients with OH should focus on nonpharmacological interventions. Lowering the dose or discontinuing the exacerbating medications (e.g., diuretics, antihypertensive agents, alpha-adrenergic blockers, nitrates, and antidepressants) is the first step in its management.[19]

The usual practical recommendations for reducing the incidence of OH and postprandial hypotension include: arising slowly from supine to seated and then to standing, avoiding straining, violent coughing, and walking in the hot weather, treatment of constipation and cough, avoiding alcohol intake, maintaining adequate hydration and drinking water before exercise, avoiding large meals and drinking water with meals, and low carbohydrate meals.

Acute water ingestion can temporarily restore orthostatic tolerance. The pressor effect of water is most likely sympathetically driven, with the peak effect occurring 30 min after ingestion of $\geq 240$ mL (an additional benefit was seen with $\geq 480$ mL). Adding sodium or glucose to the water, likely via an increase in fluid osmolality, decreases the magnitude of the gastropressor response, which suggests that a low GI osmolality might be required to trigger the gastropressor response.[1,20,21]

Encouraging increased salt and fluid intake and maintaining adequate hydration may improve blood pressure while decreasing symptoms from OH.[1] In patients with OH, including older adult patients and those with neurogenic etiologies, compression stockings and abdominal binders can improve orthostatic symptoms. The compression stockings should be at least thigh high and preferably include the abdomen, since most peripheral pooling occurs in the splanchnic circulation and shorter stockings have not been proved to be beneficial.

Abdominal binders can relieve symptoms and may be better tolerated than compression stockings. Compression stockings may be contraindicated in patients with evidence of severe peripheral vascular disease, leading to leg ischemia and/or extensive skin lesions on their lower extremities.[22] Raising the head of the bed can relieve symptoms, especially in neurogenic OH. It is also recommended in patients with the concurrent presence of supine hypertension.

A common problem in patients with OH is the concurrent presence of supine hypertension. Supine hypertension does not have a definitive cure. To reduce supine hypertension, it is recommended that the time of lying down during the day should be minimized, especially after taking pressor agents, and if tired, the patient should rest in a seated position. Raising the head of the bed by at least 30–45 degrees during bedtime is recommended. Short acting antihypertensive agents and transdermal nitroglycerin patch during bedtime may be beneficial to reduce supine hypertension. For patients with persistent symptoms despite nonpharmacologic measures, pharmacological treatment in the second step is recommended. Medications such as fludrocortisone, midodrine, or droxidopa may ameliorate symptoms.[1,2,23]

3. **Postural tachycardia syndrome:** The postural (orthostatic) tachycardia syndrome (POTS) is one of the most common causes of orthostatic intolerance. It is more likely to occur in young people (14–45 years) and is more common in women compared with men.[1]

Several studies show hypovolemia and/or redistribution of blood volume may be involved in the etiology of POTS. In some patients, elevation of the arterial norepinephrine level at rest and especially upon standing (>600 ng/mL) suggests that increased sympathetic activity may have an etiological role in POTS.[24,25]

Common symptoms in patients with POTS include dizziness, lightheadedness, palpitation, generalized weakness, blurred vision, exercise intolerance, and fatigue upon standing. In some patients, the onset or exacerbation of symptoms may present following some circumstances such as a viral illness, relative dehydration, or during a menstrual cycle.

Regarding to several investigations diagnostic criteria for POTS is the heart rate increase of ≥30 bpm over the baseline or that of ≥120 bpm within the first 10 min of positional change from supine to standing. In those 12–19 years of age, an increase in heart rate of ≥40 bpm within the first 5 min of tilt is diagnostic.[1,2,25,26] Although syncope occurs in patients with POTS, it is relatively infrequent and most of the patients do not have an OH.[1,27]

3.1. **Treatment:** There is currently no optimal and definitive treatment for POTS. Patients should be educated to avoid exacerbating factors such as dehydration, medications, and physical inactivity. Based on observational studies, exercise training can be associated with attenuated plasma renin and aldosterone, improved quality of life, and improved physical fitness. Some patients may benefit from volume repletion and fludrocortisone (0.05–0.2 mg/day).[1,28,29] Low dose beta-blockers may be effective, especially in those with prominent adrenergic symptoms. In one randomized crossover study, a low dose of beta-blocker was associated with tachycardia attenuation and improvement of symptoms, while a higher dose of beta-blocker was associated with unchanged or exacerbated symptoms.[30] Most patients have a good prognosis.[31]

4. **Pseudosyncope:** Pseudosyncope is believed to be a conversion disorder. It is an involuntary response and should not be confused with malingering.

Psychogenic pseudosyncope should be suspected when patients present with frequent (even daily) symptoms that mimic VVS or seizures. The duration of events is often long (5–20 min). Forced eye closure, prominent jerky muscle movements simulating seizure activity, and lack of pallor and diaphoresis during syncope suggest pseudosyncope. It often does not occur during sleep.[1,2]

Tilt-table testing may be reasonable to establish a diagnosis of pseudosyncope. If the patient appears to suffer from loss of consciousness or is unable to maintain posture, without a significant fall in blood pressure or heart rate, the tilt-table test is considered positive for pseudosyncope.[1]

Psychiatric interventions such as cognitive behavioral therapy are the mainstay of treatment for pseudosyncope, although the response is often incomplete.[32]

## DRIVING RESTRICTIONS

There are limited data on the causes, clinical characteristics, and predictors of syncope while driving. Generally, a symptom-free period of 6 months has been recommended after a syncopal event before resuming driving, but regulations differ geographically. Because of the societal importance of this issue, guidelines have been written to provide recommendations to patients

**TABLE 18.4**
**Recommendations of Driving Restrictions**

| Condition | Driving Restriction Time for Noncommercial Drivers | Driving Restriction Time for Commercial Drivers |
|---|---|---|
| Pacemaker implantation due to nonreflex bradycardia or CSS | 1 week | 4–6 weeks (if the pacemaker analysis is normal) |
| Syncope due to nonreflex bradycardia or CSS without treatment | Not allowed to drive | Not allowed to drive |
| ICD implantation for VT/VF (secondary prevention) | 3–6 months | Permanently bars |
| Prophylactic ICD implantation (primary prevention) | 1 month | Permanently bars |
| Syncope due to arrhythmic causes (SVT or VT/VF), untreated | Not allowed to drive | Not allowed to drive |
| Syncope due to idiopathic VT such as outflow tract VT, untreated | Not allowed to drive | Not allowed to drive |
| Syncope due to idiopathic VT such as outflow tract VT, after catheter ablation | 3 months | 3–6 months (disqualified if incapacity) |
| SVT treated with medication | 1 month | 1–3 months |
| Untreated syncope due to vasovagal, nonreflex bradycardia or cough syncope | Not allowed to drive | Not allowed to drive |
| Treated cough syncope with cough suppression | 1 month | 3 months |
| Frequent VVS (>6 syncope per year) | Not allowed to drive until symptoms resolved | Not allowed to drive unless effective treatment has been established |
| Infrequent VVS (no syncope in prior year) | No restriction | No restriction |
| Restriction after each episode of VVS or OH | 1 month | 1 month |
| Syncope of undetermined etiology | 1 month | After diagnosis and appropriate therapy |

*CSS*, carotid sinus syndrome; *ICD*, implantable cardioverter-defibrillator; *OH*, orthostatic hypotension; *SVT*, supraventricular tachycardia; *VF*, ventricular fibrillation; *VT*, ventricular tachycardia; *VVS*, vasovagal syncope.

who have experienced syncope on the safety and timing of resumption of driving. Many of these recommendations are the consensus of experts.[33,34] Table 18.4 shows the recommendations for resuming driving after the common causes of syncope as well as after pacemaker and ICD implantation.[1,34–36]

## REFERENCES

1. Shen WK, Sheldon RS, Benditt DG, et al. ACC/AHA/HRS guideline for the evaluation and management of patients with syncope: a report of the American College of Cardiology/American Heart Association Task Force on Clinical Practice Guidelines, and the Heart Rhythm Society. *J Am Coll Cardiol.* 2017;17:e39–e110.

2. Bringnole M, Moya A, de Lange FJ, et al. 2018 ESC Guidelines for the diagnosis and management of syncope. *Eur Heart J.* 2018;39:1883.

3. Chen LY, Shen WK, Mahoney DW, et al. Prevalence of syncope in a population aged more than 45 years. *Am J Med.* 2006;119:e1–e7.

4. Ruwald MH, Hansen ML, Lamberts M, et al. The relation between age, sex, comorbidity, and pharmacotherapy and the risk of syncope: Danish nationwide study. *Europace.* 2012;14:1506–1514.

5. Sheldon R, Hersi A, Ritchire D, et al. Syncope and structural heart disease: historical criteria for vasovagal syncope and ventricular tachycardia. *J Cardiovasc Electrophysiol.* 2010;21:1358.

6. Calkins H, Zipes DP. Hypotension and syncope. In: Zipes DP, Libby P, Bonow R, et al., eds. *Braunwald's*

*Heart Disease: A Text Book of Cardiovascular Medicine.* 11th ed. Philadelphia, PA: Elsevier/Saunders; 2019:848–857.

7. Benditt D, Kowey P, Hockberger RS. Syncope in adults: clinical manifestations and diagnostic evaluation. In: Post PK, ed. *UpToDate*. MA: UpToDate; 2020.

8. Krahn AD, Klein GJ, Yee R, Skanes AC. Randomized assessment of syncope trial: conventional diagnostic testing versus a prolonged monitoring strategy. *Circulation*. 2001;104:46.

9. Soliati M, Costantino G, Casazza G, et al. Implantable loop recorder versus conventional diagnostic workup for unexplained recurrent syncope. *Cochrane Database Syst Rev*. 2016;(4):CD011637.

10. Raviele A, Giada F, Bringole M, et al. Comparison of diagnostic accuracy of sublingual nitroglycerin test and low-dose of isoproterenol test in patients with unexplained syncope. *Am J Cardiol*. 2000;85:1194.

11. Benditt D, Kowey P, Downey B. Upright tilt table testing in the evaluation of syncope. In: Post PK, ed. *UpToDate*. MA, Feb: UpToDate;2020.

12. Lemon RB, Clarke E, Gillete P. Significant complications can occur with ischemic heart disease and tilt table testing. *Pacing Clin Electrophysiol*. 1999;22:675.

13. Brignole M, Menozzi C, Moya A, et al. Mechanism of syncope in patients with bundle branch block and negative electrophysiological test. *Circulation*. 2001;104:2045–2050.

14. Dhingra RC. Sinus node dysfunction. *Pacing Clin Electrophysiol*. 1983;6:1062–1069.

15. Morillo CA, Eckberg DL, Ellenbogen KA, et al. Vagal and sympathetic mechanisms in patients with orthostatic vasovagal syncope. *Circulation*. 1997;96:2509.

16. Benditt D, Kowey P, Hockberger RS. Reflex syncope in adults and adolescents: clinical manifestations and diagnostic evaluation. In: Post PK, ed. *UpToDate*. MA: UpToDate; 2020.

17. Sheldon R, Connolly S, Rose S, et al. Prevention of Syncope Trial (POST): a randomized, placebo controlled study of metoprolol in the prevention of vasovagal syncope. *Circulation*. 2006;113:1164.

18. Benditt D, Kowey P, Hockberger RS. Carotid sinus hypersensitivity and carotid sinus syndrome. In: Post PK, ed. *UpToDate*. MA: UpToDate; 2020.

19. Kaufmann H, Aminoff MJ, Wilterdink JL. Mechanism, causes, and evaluation of orthostatic hypotension. In: Post PK, ed. *UpToDate*. MA: UpToDate; 2020.

20. Raj SR, Biaggioni I, Black BK, et al. Sodium paradoxically reduces the gastropressor response in patients with orthostatic hypotension. *Hypertension*. 2006;48:329–334.

21. Lu CC, Li MH, Ho ST, et al. Glucose reduces the effect of water to promote orthostatic tolerance. *Am J Hypertens*. 2008;21:1177–1182.

22. Andriessen A, Apelqvist J, Mosti G, et al. Compression therapy for venous leg ulcers: risk factors for adverse events and complications—a review of present guidelines. *J Eur Acad Dermatol Venereol*. 2017;31:1562.

23. Kaufmann H, Aminoff MJ, Kowey P, Wilterdink JL. Treatment of orthostatic and postprandial hypotension. In: Post PK, ed. *UpToDate*. MA: UpToDate; 2020.

24. Thieben MJ, Sandroni P, Sletten DM, et al. Postural orthostatic tachycardia syndrome: the Mayo clinic experience. *Mayo Clin Proc*. 2007;82:308.

25. Jacob G, Gosta F, Shannon JR, et al. The neuropathic postural tachycardia syndrome. *N Engl J Med*. 2000;343:1008.

26. Jacob G, Biaggoni I. Idiopathic orthostatic intolerance and postural tachycardia syndromes. *Am J Med Sci*. 1999;317:88.

27. Freeman R, Wieling W, Axelrod FB, et al. Consensus statement on the definition of orthostatic hypotension, neurally mediated syncope and the postural tachycardia syndrome. *Auton Neurosci*. 2011;161:46.

28. Winker R, Barth A, Bidmon D, et al. Endurance exercise training in orthostatic intolerance: a randomized controlled trial. *Hypertension*. 2005;45:391.

29. Fu Q, Vangundy TB, Galbreath MM, et al. Cardiac origin of the postural tachycardia syndrome. *J Am Coll Cardiol*. 2010;55:2858.

30. Raj SR, Black BK, Biaggioni I, et al. Propranolol decreases tachycardia and improves symptoms in the postural tachycardia syndrome: less is more. *Circulation*. 2009;120:725.

31. Kimpinski K, Figueroa JJ, Singer W, et al. A prospective, 1-year follow-up study of postural tachycardia syndrome. *Mayo Clin Proc*. 2012;87:746.

32. Kerr MP, Mensah S, Besage F, et al. International consensus clinical practice statements for the treatment of neuropsychiatric conditions associated with epilepsy. *Epilepsia*. 2011;52:2133.

33. Curtis AB, Epstein AE, et al. Syncope while driving. *Circulation*. 2009;120:921–923.

34. Watanabeh E, Abe H, Watanabeh S. Driving restrictions in patients with implantable cardioverter defibrillators and pacemakers. *J Arrhythm*. 2017;33:594.

35. Banning AS, Ng GA. Driving and arrhythmia: a review of scientific basis for interventional guidelines. *Eur Heart J*. 2013;34(3):236–244.

36. Sumiyoshi M. Driving restrictions for patients with reflex syncope. *J Arrhythm*. 2017;33(6):590–593.

# CHAPTER 19

# Preventive Cardiology

MAJID MALEKI[a], ZAHRA HOSSEINI[b]

[a]Rajaie Cardiovascular, Medical & Research Center, Iran University of Medical Sciences, Tehran, Iran,
[b]Assistant Professor of Interventional Cardiology, Cardiovascular Intervention Research Center, Rajaie Cardiovascular, Medical & Research Center, Iran University of Medical Sciences, Tehran, Iran

Cardiovascular diseases (CVDs), which include coronary heart disease (CHD), cerebrovascular disease, and peripheral artery disease, are the leading causes of death in men and women in the United States.[1] In the United States, the rate of CVD mortality has declined since 1975; nearly the half of reduction is attributable to early diagnosis and intensive treatment, and the remaining half is attributable to more aggressive risk factor modification such as blood pressure (BP), lipid control, and smoking cessation.[2] In the Framingham Heart Study, the lifetime risks of CHD in those at age 40 years and free of baseline CVD were 49% and 32% in men and women, respectively,[3] so even in individuals without established CVD, periodic CV risk assessment in those between 20 and 79 years every 3–5 years has been recommended.[4,5] The previous European Society of Cardiology (ESC) preventive guideline recommended that systematic CV assessment may be considered for all men 40 years of age and older and all women 50 years of age and older with no known CV risk factors.

## ASSESSMENT OF CARDIOVASCULAR RISK

Many risk score models have been introduced for predicting first CHD events such as the Framingham Risk Score, SCORE (Systemic Coronary Risk Estimation), Reynolds score, Pooled Cohort Equation (PCE), Joint British Societies (JBS), and Multi-Ethnic Study of Atherosclerosis (MESA). Each model has its own advantages and disadvantages for risk assessment; therefore, the choice of specific risk score should be based on patient characteristics such as age, gender, and ethnicity (Tables 19.1 and 19.2).[6,7]

## HYPERTENSION

Hypertension is an independent risk factor for CHD, stroke, heart failure, renal failure, and peripheral artery disease, and it is more common than cigarette smoking, dyslipidemia, and diabetes. Hypertension is a cause of almost 54% of all strokes and 47% of CHD. The prevalence of hypertension increases as the population ages. In all, 26% of world adults had high BP in 2000. In epidemiologic studies, the risk of CHD, stroke, and CV mortality increase in individuals with BPs higher than 110/75 mmHg.[8,9] In the Second National Health Examination Survey (NHANES II), the baseline BP was associated with a risk of CV mortality and all-cause mortality in 15 years of follow-up in participants between 30 and 74 years old.[10] In the Atherosclerosis Risk in Communities (ARIC) study, individuals with high normal and normal BP had more CV events than those with optimal BP (<120/80 mmHg).[11] Obviously, there is no causal relationship between hypertension and CV mortality; however, elevated BP is a marker of high total CV risk because it often correlates with obesity, diabetes, metabolic syndrome, and dyslipidemia.

Multiple clinical trials revealed that a 10- to 12-mmHg reduction in systolic BP (SBP) and 5- to 6-mmHg drop in diastolic BP (DBP) is correlated with 38% and 16% reductions in stroke and CHD rates, respectively. US Preventive Services Task Force (USPSTF) 2015 guidelines recommend that every adult 18 years of age or older should have his or her BP screened.[12]

The Ambulatory BP monitoring (ABPM), as well as home BP monitoring, seems to be more predictive of CV events than office BP.[13–15] ABPM is recommended in those who are suspected of having white-coat hypertension, resistant hypertension, or episodic hypertension, and those with autonomic dysfunction, especially in people with diabetes or chronic kidney disease (CKD) and older adults.[16,17] ABPM may be used to detect "nondipper" patients (<10% reduction in BP during sleep), which is a strong predictor of the composite outcome of end-stage renal disease and death.[18] Home BP monitoring is a good alternative to ABPM, which improves patients' adherence and BP control.[19,20]

**TABLE 19.1**
**Assessment of Cardiovascular Risk (2019 ACC/AHA Guideline)**

| COR | LOE | Recommendations |
|---|---|---|
| I | B-NR | 1. For adults 40–75 years of age, clinicians should routinely assess traditional cardiovascular risk factors and calculate 10-year risk of ASCVD by using the pooled cohort equations (PCE).[S2 2.1–S2 2.2] |
| IIa | B-NR | 2. For adults 20–39 years of age, it is reasonable to assess traditional ASCVD risk factors at least every 4–6 years.[S2 2.1–S2 2.3] |
| IIa | B-NR | 3. In adults at borderline risk (5% to <7.5% 10-year ASCVD risk) or intermediate risk (≥7.5% to <20% 10-year ASCVD risk), it is reasonable to use additional risk-enhancing factors to guide decisions about preventive interventions (e.g., statin therapy).[S2 2.4–S2 2.14] |
| IIa | B-NR | 4. In adults at intermediate risk (≥7.5% to <20% 10-year ASCVD risk) or selected adults at borderline risk (5% to <7.5% 10-year ASCVD risk), if risk-based decisions for preventive interventions (e.g., statin therapy) remain uncertain, it is reasonable to measure a coronary artery calcium score to guide clinician-patient risk discussion.[S2 2.15–S2 2.31] |

Although isolated systolic hypertension (ISH) (SBP >140 mmHg and DBP <90 mmHg) is more common in older adults, isolated diastolic hypertension (IDH) (SBP <140 mmHg and DBP >90 mmHg) is common in young and obese people.[21] Trials have suggested that both ISH and IDH are correlated with CV events. IDH in youth is more predictive and is associated with mixed systolic and diastolic hypertension thereafter.[22] ISH as well as wide pulse pressure in older adults is suggestive of aortic stiffness and more CV events.[22,23]

White-coat hypertension (i.e., isolated office hypertension), common in older adults, correlates with persistent hypertension,[24,25] and the chance of CV events is higher in these individuals than in those who are persistently normotensive but less than in individuals with sustained hypertension. In a meta-analysis among patients with white-coat HTN, untreated patients were associated with an increased risk for cardiovascular events and all-cause mortality, so out of office BP monitoring is critical in the diagnosis and management of hypertension.[26–28]

Hypertension was traditionally defined as persistent BP of 140/90 mmHg or greater at each of two or more office visits in most guidelines. In the 2013 European Society of Hypertension/European Society of Cardiology (ESH/ESC) guideline, the presence any of the following conditions was the definition of hypertension: 24 h of BP measuring 130/80 mmHg or higher, a daytime average of 135/85 mmHg or higher, and a nocturnal average of 120/70 mmHg or higher.[15] In ESC/ESH 2018 guideline, the definition and treatment threshold of blood pressure is noted in Table 19.3 and below statement, respectively[29]:

**TABLE 19.2**
**Risk-Enhancing Factors for Clinician-Patient Risk Discussion (2019 ACC/AHA Guidelines)**

**Risk-enhancing factors**

Family history of premature ASCVD (males, age <55 years; females, age <65 years)

Primary hypercholesterolemia (IDL-C. 160–189 mg/dL [4.1–4.8 mmol/L]; non-HDL-C 190–219 mg/dL (4.9–5.6 mmol/L])

Metabolic syndrome (increased waist circumference [by ethnically appropriate cutpoints], elevated triglycerides [>150 mg/dL, nonfasting], elevated blood pressure, elevated glucose, and low HDL-C [<40 mg/dL in men; <50 mg/dL in women] are factors; a tally of 3 makes the diagnosis)

Chronic kidney disease (eGFR 15–59 mL/min/1.73 m$^2$ with or without albuminuria; not treated with dialysis or kidney transplantation)

Chronic inflammatory conditions, such as psoriasis, RA, lupus, or HIV/AIDS

History of premature menopause (before age 40 years) and history of pregnancy-associated conditions that increase later ASCVD risk, such as preeclampsia

High-risk race/ethnicity (e.g., South Asian ancestry)

*Continued*

## TABLE 19.2
### Risk-Enhancing Factors for Clinician-Patient Risk Discussion (2019 ACC/AHA Guidelines)—cont'd

Lipids/biomarkers: associated with increased ASCVD risk

Persistently elevated* primary hypertriglyceridemia (≥175 mg/dL, nonfasting)

If measured:

Elevated high-sensitivity C-reactive protein (≥2.0 mg/L)

Elevated Lp(a): A relative indication for its measurement is family history of premature ASCVD. An Lp(a) ≥50 mg/dL or ≥125 nmol/L constitutes a risk-enhancing factor, especially at higher levels of Lp(a)

Elevated apoB (≥130 mg/dL): A relative indication for its measurement would be triglyceride ≥200 mg/dL. A level ≥130 mg/dL corresponds to an LDL-C >160 mg/dL and constitutes a risk-enhancing factor

ABI (<0.9)

## TABLE 19.3
### Classification of Office Blood Pressure (ESC/ESH 2018)

| Category | Systolic (mmHg) | | Diastolic (mmHg) |
|---|---|---|---|
| Optimal | <120 | and | <80 |
| Normal | 120–129 | and/or | 80–84 |
| High normal | 130–139 | and/or | 85–89 |
| Grade 1 hypertension | 140–159 | and/or | 90–99 |
| Grade 2 hypertension | 160–179 | and/or | 100–109 |
| Grade 3 hypertension | ≥180 | and/or | ≥110 |
| Isolated systolic hypertension | ≥140 | and | <90 |

a. **High normal BP (130–139/85–89 mmHg):**

Drug treatment may be considered when cardiovascular (CV) risk is very high due to established cardiovascular disease (CVD), especially coronary artery disease (CAD) (**Recommendation; Class IIb**).

b. **Treatment of low-risk grade 1 hypertension:**

In patients with grade 1 hypertension at low/moderate risk and without evidence of hypertension-mediated organ damage (HMOD), BP-lowering drug treatment is recommended if the patient remains hypertensive after a period of lifestyle intervention (**Recommendation; Class I**).

c. **Older patients:**

BP-lowering drug treatment and lifestyle intervention are recommended in fit older patients (>65 years but not >80 years) when systolic blood pressure (SBP) is in the grade 1, range (140–159 mmHg), provided that treatment is well tolerated (**Recommendation; Class 1**).

In 2019 ACC/AHA preventive guideline, the definition of high BP has been changed and the threshold for nonpharmacological and pharmacological therapy is mentioned in Fig. 19.1.

The target BP should be adjusted based on age, comorbidities, and total CV risk. The absolute benefit of antihypertensive therapy is seen in those with more severe hypertension. Based on the Eighth Joint National Committee (JNC8) guidelines, the treatment goal is SBP less than 140 mmHg and DBP less than 90 mmHg in those 60 years of age and younger[30–32] and SBP less than 150 mmHg and DBP less than 90 mmHg in older individuals.[33–35] It should be considered that if the treatment in older adults leads to SBP less than 140 mmHg without any side effects, the treatment does not need adjustment.[36] Even in patients with diabetes [Action to Control Cardiovascular Risk in Diabetes-Blood Pressure (ACCORD-BP trial)[37]] or chronic kidney disease (CKD) [Modification of Diet in Renal Disease (MDRD), African American Study of Kidney Disease and Hypertension (AASK), and Ramipril Efficacy in Nephropathy-2 (REIN2) trials],[38–40] the target is as in the general population. The exception is patients with proteinuria greater than 3 g/day, in whom the recommended target is BP less than 130/80 mmHg (MDRD trial), which improves only kidney outcomes.[38]

But meta-analyses and RCTs provide evidence for the benefit of BP-lowering medications on ASCVD prevention in adults with moderate to high ASCVD risk and SBP ≥130 mmHg or DBP ≥80 mmHg with significant outcome reductions demonstrated in stroke, heart failure, coronary events, and death. SPRINT (Systolic BP Intervention Trial) trial also has shown that intensive BP treatment (SBP <120 mmHg) in nondiabetic older adults with high CV risk significantly reduced the composite of myocardial infarction (MI), acute coronary syndromes (ACSs), stroke, heart failure, and CV death and reduced mortality

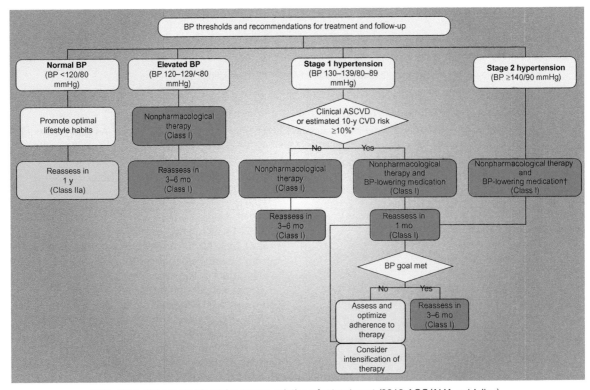

FIG. 19.1 BP thresholds and recommendations for treatment (2019 ACC/AHA guideline).

**TABLE 19.4**
**2018 ESC/ESH Blood Pressure Treatment Target**

| Age Group (Years) | Hypertension (mmHg) | +Diabetes (mmHg) | +CKD (mmHg) | +CAD (mmHg) | +Stroke/TIA (mm Hg) |
|---|---|---|---|---|---|
| 18–65 | Target to 130 or lower if tolerated (not <120) | Target to 130 or lower if tolerated (not <l20) | Target 130–139 if tolerated | Target to 130 or lower if tolerated (not <120) | Target to 130 or lower if tolerated (not <l20) |
| 65–79 | Target 130–139 tolerated | Target 130–139 tolerated | Target 130–139 if tolerated | Target 130–139 if tolerated | Target 130–139 if tolerated |
| >80 | Target 130–139 tolerated | Target 130–139 if tolerated | Target 130–139 if tolerated | Target 130–139 if tolerated | Target 130–139 if tolerated |
| Diastolic blood pressure target (mmHg) | 70–79 | 70–79 | 70–79 | 70–79 | 70–79 |

significantly compared with the less intensive treatment group.[41] So the treatment target in the recent preventive guidelines has become changed (Table 19.4).

In 2019 ACC/AHA preventive guideline, in adult patients with estimated 10 years ASCVD risk of 10% or higher and an average SBP >130 mmHg or DBP >80 mmHg and in those with confirmed hypertension, irrespective of age, CKD or T2DM, the treatment to achieve a BP goal of less than 130/80 mmHg is recommended.[42]

Lifestyle modification is the primary factor in BP control. In prehypertensive or stage 1 hypertension, lifestyle change can control BP, but in those in stage 2 hypertension, antihypertensive treatment is the corner-stone, although lifestyle change is strongly advised. Lifestyle modifications include diet (low salt, DASH [Dietary Approaches to Stop Hypertension] diet; low-fat, high-fiber diet; and high-dose fish oil), weight reduction, smoking cessation, aerobic and resistance exercise, and limited alcohol consumption (see Sections Diet and Supplements, Exercise, and Obesity).

According to recent recommendations [JNC8, American College of Cardiology (ACC)/American Heart Association (AHA) 2013], the important component is controlling BP, not the type of antihypertensive drugs used.[43] All of the four recommended drugs for initial therapy have similar effects in reducing all-cause mortality and CV and kidney outcomes[44,45]; the only exception is heart failure outcomes, for which thiazide-type diuretics are better than calcium channel blockers (CCBs) and angiotensin-converting enzyme (ACE) inhibitors.[46] It appears that CCBs are more effective in stroke reduction in comparison with the other groups. In the general nonblack hypertensive population, the initial antihypertensive drugs should include a thiazide-type diuretics (Chlorthalidone or Indapamide),[47,48] ACE inhibitors or angiotensin II receptor blockers (ARBs), and CCBs. In black hypertensive patients, the initial antihypertensive drugs should include CCBs or thiazide-type diuretics.[46]

Beta-blockers are not recommended for initial anti-hypertensive treatment. In one trial, compared with ARBs, beta-blockers were associated with higher rates of CV death, MI, and stroke,[49] and are less effective in regressing LVH and small vessels remodeling. The Anglo-Scandinavian Cardiac Outcomes Trial (ASCOT) found lower CVD, death and stroke with amlodipine compared with atenolol[50] but some vasodilating beta-blockers such as Carvedilol, Nebivolol, and Labetalol have lower side effects and in some RCTs improve the outcome of heart failure patients.

In nonblack and black CKD patients, it seems better to start antihypertensive treatment with ACE inhibitors or ARBs; this suggestion is based on kidney outcomes only. Otherwise, these classes have no better CV outcomes than other classes.[46,51]

Irrespective of economic status, it appears that only 40% of hypertensive patients receive antihypertensive therapy and among them, only 35% have controlled hypertension. For better adherence of patients, BP control, and cardiovascular outcomes, multiple trials have revealed that single-pill combination (SPC) therapy, especially the combination of CCBs and ACE inhibitors or ARBs and diuretics is superior to monotherapy or combination of diuretics and beta-blockers (which have more metabolic side effects). So based on the last guidelines of hypertension treatment, SPC therapy is superior to maximal dose of monotherapy in the initial phase especially the combination of ACE inhibitors or ARBs with either CCBs or thiazide/thiazide-like diuretics (Fig. 19.2; Table 19.5).[52]

Patients should be followed up 1 month later, and if the goal is not achieved, a third drug should be added and so on, but ACE inhibitors and ARBs should not be used together. If despite three-drug combination therapy, the BP is still uncontrolled (resistant hypertension), other secondary causes of hypertension should be considered. Additional treatment options include the addition of low-dose spironolactone (25–50 mg daily) or another additional diuretic therapy [amiloride 10–20 mg daily, higher dose of thiazide or thiazide-like diuretics, loop diuretics in patients with significant renal impairment (eGFR <45 mL/min/m$^2$)], beta-blockers, alpha-blockers, central acting agents (e.g., clonidine), or minoxidil.

## DYSLIPIDEMIA (Table 19.6)

Coronary heart disease is the leading cause of death all over the world, and although CHD-related mortality has decreased significantly, the event rates have declined slowly, so prevention and screening have important roles.[5] Among the traditional risk factors, one of the most challenging factors is dyslipidemia. There is a log-linear relation between CHD risk and dyslipidemia. About 70% of patients with premature CHD have dyslipidemia. In most trials, total cholesterol and low-density lipoprotein cholesterol (LDL-C) are the primary treatment targets, and the reduction in these factors is proportional to a significant reduction of CV events and mortality. Nonhigh-density lipoprotein cholesterol (HDL-C) and apolipoprotein B are the second treatment targets, especially during hypertriglyceridemia.[53–55] In some studies, non-HDL-C is a better predictor than LDL-C especially in those with high TG combined with diabetes, metabolic syndrome, and CKD; in some others, they have similar values.[53,54] HDL-C is also an independent predictor of CVD, but recent studies have shown that an increase in HDL-C has no athero-protective effects.[55,56] It shows that the presence of non-functional HDL-C is more predictive of adverse events than the low HDL-C level[57,58]; apparently, HDL-C level is not a target of treatment. In some other studies, the ratio of total cholesterol to HDL-C is the primary goal, and its predictive value in decreasing CV events is more than LDL-C.[59] In some studies, high triglyceride (TG)

## Core drug treatment strategy for uncomplicated hypertension—ESC/ESH 2018

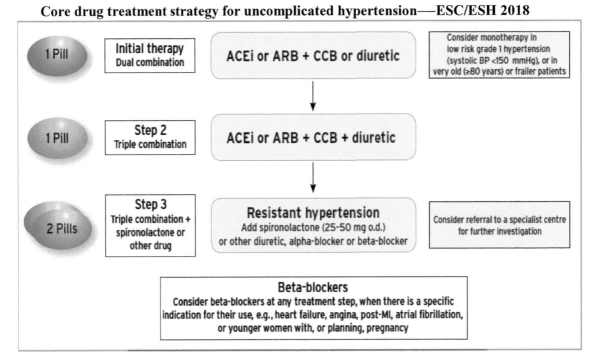

FIG. 19.2 Core drug treatment strategy for uncomplicated hypertension—ESC/ESH 2018.

levels are an independent risk factor of CVD because they are associated with low HDL-C, small dense, and more atherogenic LDL-C (Table 19.6).[60,61]

Lipid screening should be based on total CV risk independent of lipid level. Many risk score systems are available, including the Framingham score,[62] SCORE,[63] pooled cohort equation,[64] and Assessing cardiovascular risk using SIGN guidelines to ASSIGN preventive treatment (ASSIGN) (CV risk estimation model from the Scottish Intercollegiate Guidelines Network).[65] These CV risk scores have included other risk factors such as smoking, hypertension, age, sex, and familial premature CVD. The most relative risk reduction with a statin is seen in those with the lowest absolute risk, and the greatest absolute risk reduction is seen in those with the highest baseline absolute risk.[66] No randomized controlled trials (RCTs) have ever defined a threshold below which the CV risk disappears (Table 19.7).[67]

Recent studies showed no difference between serum level of total cholesterol, LDL-C, and HDL-C in fasting and nonfasting samples, but TGs are affected by food, so the predictive strength of nonfasting lipid levels is similar to fasting levels.[68,69]

The threshold for starting lipid treatment differs among guidelines. SCORE estimates the 10-year cumulative risk of a fatal ASCVD event in contrast to the US Pooled Cohort Equation (US-PCE), which estimates the 10-year risk of a first ASCVD. The European use of CV mortality rather than first ASCVD is preferred because it provides a definite end point in contrast to CV events that vary by definitions, severity, diagnostic tests, each of which limits the ability to relate fatal to total events. Total CVD event risk is about three times higher than the risk for fatal CVD or risk of 5% fatal translates into 15% risk of fatal + nonfatal CVD events; the multiplier is higher in women and lower in the elderly.[70]

### ESC/EAS 2019 Guideline (Table 19.8)

The treatment target in the ESC lipid guideline is based on individual 10-year risk of fatal CVD. A high-intensity statin up to the highest tolerated dose to reach target goals for specific levels of risk. Very high-risk includes documented ASCVD (any clinical CVD/event or imaging), diabetes with end organ damage, or three major risk factors, severe chronic kidney disease (CKD) [estimated

**TABLE 19.5**
2018 ESC/ESH Blood Pressure: Changes in Recommendations

| 2013 | 2018 |
|---|---|
| **Diagnosis** | **Diagnosis** |
| Office BP is recommended for screening and diagnosis of hypertension. | It is recommended to base the diagnosis of hypertension on:<br>• Repeated office BP measurements; or<br>• Out-of-office EP measurement with AMPM and/or HBPM if logistically and economically feasible. |
| **Treatment thresholds**<br>*High-normal BP (130–139/85–89 mmHg):*<br>Unless the necessary evidence is obtained, it is not recommended to initiate antihypertensive drug therapy at high-normal BP. | **Treatment thresholds**<br>*High-normal BP (130–139/85–89 mmHg):*<br>Drug treatment may be considered when CV risk is very high due to established CVD, especially CAD. |
| **Treatment thresholds**<br>*Treatment of low-risk grade 1 hypertension:*<br>Initiation of antihypertensive drug treatment should also be considered in grade 1 hypertensive patients at low–moderate-risk, when BP a within this range at several repeated visits or elevated by elevated by BP criteria, and remains within this range despite a reasonable period of time with lifestyle measures. | **Treatment thresholds**<br>*Treatment of low-risk grade 1 hypertension:*<br>In patients well grade 1 hypertension at low–moderate-risk and without evidence of HMOD, BP-lowering drug treatment is recommended if the patient remains hypertensive after a period of lifestyle intervention. |
| **Treatment thresholds**<br>*Older patients*<br>Antihypertensive drug treatment may be considered m the elderly (at least when younger than 80 years) when SBP is in the 140–159 mmHg range, provided that antihypertensive treatment a well tolerated. | **Treatment thresholds**<br>*Older patients*<br>BP-lowering drug treatment and lifestyle intervention a recommended in fit older patients (>65 years but not >80 years) when SBP is in the grade 1 range (140–159 mmHg), provided that treatment is well tolerated. |
| **BP treatment targets**<br>An SBP goal of <140 is recommended. | **BP treatment targets**<br>• It is recommended that the first objective of treatment should be to lower BP to <140/90 mmHg *in dl* patient and, provided that the treatment is well tolerated, treated BP values should be targeted to 130/80 mmHg or lower in most patients.<br>• In patients <65 years it is recommended that SBP should be lowered to a BP range of 120–129 mmHg in most patients. |

*Continued*

**TABLE 19.5**
2018 ESC/ESH Blood Pressure?: Changes in Recommendations—cont'd

**2013**

**BP treatment targets in older patients (65–80 years)**

An SBP target of between 140 and 150 mmHg is recommended for older patients (65–80 years).

**BP treatment targets in patients aged over 80 years**

An SBP target between 140 and 150 mmHg should be considered if people older than 80 years, with an initial SBP ≥ 160 mmHg, provided that they are in good physical and mental condition.

**DBP targets**

A DBP target of <90 mmHg is always recommended, except in patients with diabetes in whom values <85 mmHg are recommended.

**Initiation of drug treatment**

Initiation of antihypertensive therapy with a two-drug combination may be considered in patients with markedly high baseline BP or at high CV risk.

**Resistant hypertension**

Mineralocorticoid receptor antagonists, amiloride, and the alpha-1 blocker doxazosin should be considered if no contraindication exists.

**Device-based therapy for hypertension**

In case of ineffectiveness of drug treatment, invasive procedures such as renal denervation and baroreceptor stimulation may be considered.

**2018**

**BP treatment targets in older patients (65–80 years)**

In older patients (≥65 years), it is recommended that SBP should be targeted to a BP range of 130–139 mmHg.

**BP treatment targets in patients aged over 80 years**

An SBP target range of 130–139 mmHg is recommended for people older than 80 years, if tolerated.

**DBP targets**

A DBP target of <80 mmHg should be considered for all hypertensive patients, independent of the level of risk and comorbidities.

**Initiation of drug treatment**

It is recommended to initiate an antihypertensive treatment with a two-drug combination, preferably in a SPC. The exceptions are frail in older patients and those at low risk and with grade 1 hypertension (particularly if SBP is <150 mmHg).

**Resistant hypertension**

Recommended treatment of resistant hypertensive is the addition of low-dose spironolactone to existing treatment, or the addition of further diuretic therapy if intolerant so spironolactone, with either eplerenone, amiloride, higher-dose thiazide/thiazide-like diuretic or a loop diuretic, or the addition of bisoprolol or doxazosin.

**Device-based therapy for hypertension**

Use of device-based therapies is not recommended for the routine treatment of hypertensive, unless in the context of clinical studies and RCTs, until further evidence regarding their safety and efficacy becomes available.

**TABLE 19.6**
Recommendations for Lipid Analyses for Screening of CVD Risk

| Recommendations | Class | Level |
|---|---|---|
| TC is recommended to be used for the estimation of total CV risk by means of the SCORE system | I | C |
| LDL-C is recommended to be used as the primary lipid analysis for screening and risk estimation | I | C |
| TG adds information on risk and is indicated for risk estimation | I | C |
| HDL-C is a strong risk factor and is recommended to be used for risk estimation | I | C |
| Non-HDL-C should be considered as an alternative risk marker, especially in combined hyperlipidemias, diabetes, the MetS, or CKD | IIa | C |
| Lp(a) should be recommended in selected cases at high risk and in subjects with a family history of premature CVD | IIa | C |
| Apo B should be considered as an alternative risk marker, especially in combined hyperlipidaemias, diabetes, the MetS, or CKD | IIa | C |
| The ratio apo B/apo A1 combines the risk information of apo B and apo A1 and may be recommended as an alternative analysis for risk screening | IIb | C |
| The ratio non-HDL-C/HDL-C may be recommended as an alternative analysis for risk screening | IIb | C |

glomerular filtration rate (eGFR) <30], heterozygous familial hypercholesterolemia (HeFH) with ASCVD or another major risk factor, or a SCORE ≥ 10% (e.g., annual CV death ≥1%) in which the target is ≥50% reduction in LDL-C with goal <55 mg/dL. High risk is a very high single risk factor (total cholesterol >310 mg/dL, LDL-C > 190 mg/dL, BP 180/110 mmHg), diabetes >10 years or with one major risk factor, moderate CKD (eGFR 30–59), or SCORE 5%–9% in which target LDL-C is <70 mg/dL. Moderate risk is a SCORE 1%–4%, which is not uncommon, and includes type 1 diabetic mellitus

(T1DM) <35 years, type 2 diabetic mellitus (T2DM) <50 years without other risk factors in which target LDL < 100 mg/dL, and low risk a SCORE of <1% where a goal of <116 mg/dL should be considered (Table 19.6).[70]

Treatment of dyslipidemia with statins is recommended for older persons, according to the risk level, in those aged ≤75 years.

Initiation of statin treatment for primary prevention in older people aged ≥75 years may be considered if at high risk or above.[71]

For primary prevention in HeFH patients who are at very high risk, an LDL-C reduction of ≥50% from baseline and an LDL-C goal of <55 mg/dL should be considered (Fig. 19.4).[72]

For patients with an ACS, in whom LDL-C levels are not already at goal despite maximally tolerated statin and ezetimibe, adding a PCSK9 inhibitor early after the event (if possible, during hospitalization for the ACS event) should be considered (Figs. 19.3 and 19.4).[72]

## AHA 2019 Preventive Guideline (Fig. 19.5)

There is no particular age at which the lipid screening program should be stopped. On one hand, age is the most important factor in risk stratification, but on the other hand, the lipid level decreases with aging, so it is likely that even patients older than 75 years may likely benefit from screening and therapy.[73]

In RCTs, the only antilipid agent that can reduce CV events and mortality in secondary and primary prevention in men and women is statin [West of Scotland Coronary Prevention Study (WOSCOPS),[74] Air Force/Texas Coronary Atherosclerosis Prevention Study (AFCAPS/TexCAPS),[75] and Justification for the Use of Statins in Prevention: An Intervention Trial Evaluating Rosuvastatin (JUPITER)[76] in primary prevention and Scandinavian Simvastatin Survival Study (4S),[77] Cholesterol and Recurrent Events (CARE),[78] and Heart Protection Study (HPS)[79] in secondary prevention]. In one study, this effect was also seen when ezetimibe was added to the statin.[80] These trials also suggest that statins are effective in a wide range of baseline lipid profiles, and their efficacy is similar in primary and secondary prevention.[80]

The Fenofibrate Intervention and Event Lowering in Diabetes (FIELD)[81] and Action to Control Cardiovascular Risk in Diabetes (ACCORD)[82] studies failed to show a decrease in cardiac events despite a significant reduction in TGs by fibrates in patients with diabetes, although the subgroup analysis showed the reduction when the high TGs are accompanied by low HDL-C. Therefore, there is no recommendation for TG reduction

**TABLE 19.7**

Intervention Strategies as a Function of Total Cardiovascular Risk and Untreated Low-Density Lipoprotein Cholesterol Levels

| Total C V Risk (SCORE)% | UNTREATED LDL-C LEVELS | | | | | |
|---|---|---|---|---|---|---|
| | <1.4 mmol/L (55 mg/dL) | 1.4 to <1.8 mmol/L (55 to <70 mg/dL) | 1.8 to <2.6 mmol/L (70 to <100 mg/dL) | 2.6 to <3.0 mmol/L (100 to <116 mg/dL) | 3.0 to <4.9 mmol/L (116 to <190 mg/dL) | >4.9 mmol/L (≥190 mg/dL) |
| **Primary prevention** | | | | | | |
| <1 low-risk | Lifestyle advice | Lifestyle advice | Lifestyle advice | Lifestyle advice | Lifestyle intervention. Consider adding drug if uncontrolled | Lifestyle intervention and concomitant drug intervention |
| Class/Level | I/C | I/C | I/C | I/C | IIa/A | IIa/A |
| ≥1 to <5 or moderate risk (see Table 19.4) | Lifestyle advice | Lifestyle advice | Lifestyle advice | Lifestyle intervention, consider adding drug if uncontrolled | Lifestyle intervention, consider adding drug if uncontrolled | Lifestyle intervention and concomitant drug intervention |
| Class/Level | I/C | I/C | I/C | IIa/A | IIa/A | IIa/A |
| ≥5 to <10 or high-risk (see Table 19.4) | Lifestyle advice | Lifestyle advice | Lifestyle intervention, consider adding drug if uncontrolled | Lifestyle intervention and concomitant drug intervention | Lifestyle intervention and concomitant drug intervention | Lifestyle intervention and concomitant drug intervention |
| Class/Level | IIa/A | IIa/A | IIa/A | IIa/A | I/A | I/A |
| ≥10, or at very-high risk due to a risk condition (see Table 19.4) | Lifestyle advice | Lifestyle intervention, consider adding drug if uncontrolled | Lifestyle intervention and concomitant drug intervention | Lifestyle intervention and concomitant drug intervention | Lifestyle intervention and concomitant drug intervention | Lifestyle intervention and concomitant drug intervention |
| Class/Level | IIa/B | IIa/A | IIa/A | I/A | I/A | I/A |
| **Secondary prevention** | | | | | | |
| Very-high-risk | Lifestyle intervention, consider adding drug if uncontrolled | Lifestyle intervention and concomitant drug intervention | Lifestyle intervention and concomitant drug intervention | Lifestyle intervention and concomitant drug intervention | Lifestyle intervention and concomitant drug intervention | Lifestyle intervention and concomitant drug intervention |

**TABLE 19.8**
**New Recommendations, and New and Revised Concepts (2019 ESC/EAS Guidelines)**

| 2016 | UPGRADES / 2019 |
|---|---|
| **Lipid analyses for CVD risk estimation** | **Lipid analyses for CVD risk estimation** |
| ApoB should be considered as an alternative risk marker whenever available, especially in individuals with high TG. | ApoB analysis is recommended for risk assessment, particularly in people with high TG, DM, obesity or metabolic syndrome, or very low LDL-C. It can be used as an alternative to LDL-C, if available, as the primary measurement for screening, diagnosis, and management, and may be preferred over non-HDL-C in people with high TG, DM, obesity, or very low LDL-C. |
| **Pharmacological LDL-C lowering** | **Pharmacological LDL-C lowering** |
| If the LDL goal is not reached, stain combination with a cholesterol absorption inhibitor should be considered. | If the goals are not achieved with the maximum tolerated dose of statin, combination with ezetimibe is recommended. |
| **Pharmacological LDL-C lowering** | **Pharmacological LDL-C lowering** |
| In patients at very-high risk, with persistent high LDL-C despite treatment with maximal tolerated statin dose, in combination with ezetimible or in patients with statin intolerance, a PCSK9 inhibitor may be considered. | For secondary prevention, patients at very-high risk not achieving their goal on a maximum tolerated dose of statin and ezetimibe, a combination with a PCSK9 inhibitor is recommended. |
| | For very-high-risk FH patients (that is, with ASCVD or with another major risk factor) who do not achieve their goals on a maximum tolerated dose of statin and ezetimibe, a combination with a PCSK9 inhibitor is recommended. |
| **Drug treatments of hypertriglyceridemia** | **Drug treatments of hypertriglyceridemia** |
| Statin treatment may be considered as the first drug of choice for reducing CVD risk in high-risk individuals with hypertriglyceridemia. | Statin treatment is recommended as the first drug of choke for reducing CVD risk in high-risk individuals with hypertriglyceridemia [TG >23 mmol/L (200 mg/dL)]. |
| **Treatment of patients with heterozygous FH** | **Treatment of patients with heterozygous FH** |
| Treatment should be considered to aim at reaching an LDL-C <2.6 mmol/L (<100 mg/dL) or in the presence of CVD <1.8 mmol/L (<70 mg/dL). If targets cannot be reached, maximal reduction of LDL-C should be considered using appropriate drug combinations. | For FH patients with ASCVD who are at very-high risk, treatment to achieve at least a 50% reduction from baseline and an LDL-C <1.4 mmol/L (<55 mg/dL) is recommended. If goals cannot be achieved, a drug combination is recommended. |
| **Treatment of patients with heterozygous FH** | **Treatment of patients with heterozygous FH** |
| Treatment with a PCSK9 antibody should be considered in FH patients with CVD or with other factors putting them at very-high risk for CHD, such as other CV risk factors, family history, high Lp(a), or statin intolerance. | Treatment with a PCSK9 inhibitor is recommended in very-high-risk FH patients if the treatment goal is not achieved on maximal tolerated statin plus ezetimibe. |

Continued

**TABLE 19.8**
**New Recommendations, and New and Revised Concepts (2019 ESC/EAS Guidelines)—cont'd**

| UPGRADES | |
|---|---|
| **2016** | **2019** |
| **Treatment of dyslipidemias in older adults** | **Treatment of dyslipidemias in older people** |
| Since older people often have comorbidities and have altered pharmacokinetics, lipid-lowering mediation should be started at a lower dose and then titrated with caution to achieve target lipid levels that arc the same as in younger people. | It is recommended that the statin is started at a low dose if there is significant renal impairment and/or the potential for drug interactions, and then titrated upwards to achieve LDL-C treatment goals. |
| **Lipid-lowering therapy in patients with ACS** | **Lipid-lowering therapy in patients with ACS** |
| If the LDL-C target is not reached with the highest tolerated statin dose and/or ezetimibe. PCSK9 inhibitors may be considered on top of lipid-lowering therapy; or alone or in combination with ezetimibe in statin-intolerant patients or in whom a statin is contraindicated. | If the LDL-C goal is not achieved after 4–6 weeks despite maximal tolerated statin therapy and ezetimibe, addition of a PCSK9 inhibitor is recommended. |
| **Recommendation grading** | |
| Class I          Class IIa | Class IIb          Class III |

# Intensity of lipid lowering treatment

| Treatment | Average LDL-C reduction |
|---|---|
| Moderate intensity statin | ≈30% |
| High intensity statin | ≈50% |
| High intensity statin plus ezetimibe | ≈65% |
| PCSK9 inhibitor | ≈60% |
| PCSK9 inhibitor plus high intensity statin | ≈75% |
| PCSK9 inhibitor plus high intensity statin plus ezetimibe | ≈85% |

FIG. 19.3 ESC 2019.

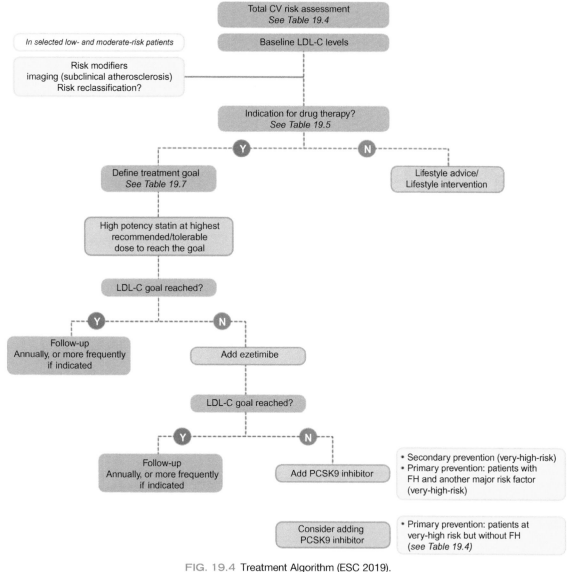

FIG. 19.4 Treatment Algorithm (ESC 2019).

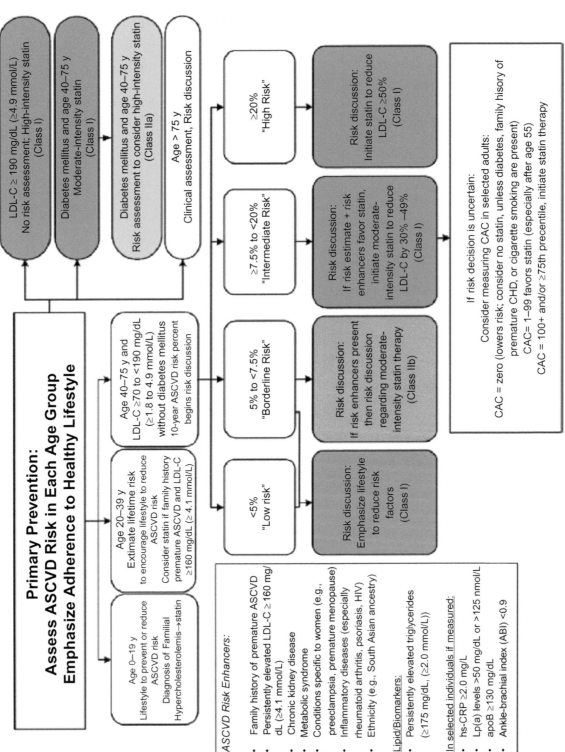

FIG. 19.5 Primary prevention (AHA 2019).

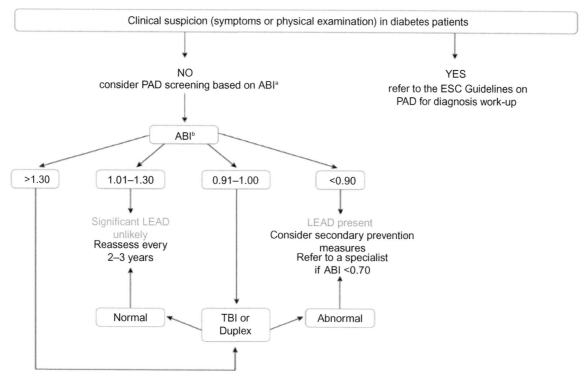

FIG. 19.6 Screening for lower extremity artery disease in patients with DM.

except in patients who are at risk of pancreatitis (Fig. 19.6).

Although HDL-C has a significant inverse relation with CV events and is included in many 10-year risk scores, studies failed to show that any elevation in HDL-C level can reduce CV events. In the Atherothrombosis Intervention in Metabolic Syndrome With Low HDL/High Triglycerides and Impact on Global Health Outcomes (AIM-HIGH)[83] and Heart Protection Study 2-Treatment of HDL to Reduce the Incidence of Vascular Events (HPS2-tHRIVE)[84] studies, no CV event reduction by niacin was detected despite significant HDL-C elevation. Trials that studied the effect of cholesteryl ester transfer protein inhibitors on HDL-C [torcetrapib in the Investigation of Lipid Level Management to Understand its Impact in Atherosclerotic Events (ILLUMINATE),[85] Dalcetrapib in Efficacy and safety of Dalcetrapib in patients with recent acute coronary syndrome study (dal-OUTCOME),[86] and evacetrapib in Impact of the cholesteryl ester transfer protein inhibitor evacetrapib on the cardiovascular outcome (ACCELERATE)[87]] failed to show any reduction in cardiac events, although the elevation in HDL-C level

was significant. Regarding recent studies, it seems that the functional properties of HDL-C are better predictors of CV events.[88] The usage of nonstatin agents in primary and secondary prevention is restricted to special conditions such as patients who cannot tolerate statins at all.

## SMOKING

The most preventable risk factor in CVD is smoking.[89] Although the prevalence of smoking has declined slightly throughout the world in recent decades, about 20% of men and 15.5% of women smoke in the United States.[90] Many smokers do not know that cigarette consumption is the leading cause of CHD and cerebrovascular disease. The World Health Organization estimates that 5.4 million people died from smoking in 2008, and it will reach to 8 million deaths each year to 2030.[91] According to the Surgeon General's Report, smoking is responsible for 20% of US deaths.[92] The smoking rate is higher in low socioeconomic areas and among less educated people. More than 80% of smoking-related deaths occur in developing countries.[93] Smoking increases the risk of all types of cerebrovascular

**TABLE 19.9**
Smoking Effect on Cardiovascular Risk Factors

| Cardiovascular Risk Factors | Increase | Decrease |
|---|---|---|
| Blood pressure | # | |
| Systemic inflammation (CRP) | # | |
| Platelet aggregability | # | |
| LDL-C, VLDL-C, TG | # | |
| HDL-C | | # |
| Oxidative stress | # | |
| Fibrinogen | # | |
| Plasminogen | | # |

events,[94] peripheral artery disease,[95] aortic aneurysms,[96] sudden death,[97] and all-cause mortality.[98] Some recent experimental studies reported that there is a nonlinear relation between exposure and events.[99] Smoking activates the sympathetic nervous system and causes increases in heart rate and arterial vasoconstriction.[100] Smoking induces vascular wall injury and impaired endothelial function (reduced flow-mediated dilatation in systemic arteries) and structure that leads to a decrease in prostacyclin and nitric oxide production and ultimately vascular stiffness.[101–103] Smoking causes hypercoagulable states through increasing platelet activation and aggregation, enhancement of fibrinogen level, tissue factor expression, and serum homocysteine level as well as decreasing plasminogen activator and endogenous fibrinolysis (thrombo-hemostatic dysfunction).[104,105] Smoking enhances inflammatory response [tumor necrosis factor-α, interleukin-1β, and C-reactive protein (CRP)], the cornerstone of atherosclerosis.[105] Smoking elevates total serum cholesterol, LDL-C, very low-density lipoprotein cholesterol (VLDL-C), and TG levels and decreases HDL-C level in a dose–response manner[106] and enhances oxidized LDL-C as well as free radical-mediated oxidative stress (pro-oxidative environment),[105] leading to earlier foam cells and fatty streak formation (Table 19.9).

Smoking elevates matrix metalloproteinase expression (MMP) and decreases the expression of MMP inhibitors in vulnerable plaques that enhance extracellular matrix degradation and plaque rupture.[107] Smoking is an independent risk factor for coronary events and increases the risk of MI six times in women and three times in men.[108] Smokers are usually younger and free of other traditional CV risk factors, but the burden of thrombosis is also higher in smokers because of more procoagulative states, so the response of

smokers to thrombolytic therapy seems to be higher relative to nonsmokers (the "smoker's paradox").[108] Smoking cessation is associated with CV and all-cause mortality reduction in men and women at all ages.[109,110] The risk reduction after cessation is almost equal to the use of aspirin, statins, beta-blockers, and ACE inhibitors,[111] so screening of all patients for cigarette consumption is the most valuable preventive act. After 1 year of smoking cessation, the chance of heart attack reduces about 50%,[112] and after 5 and 15 years, the risk of stroke and MI in former smokers is the same as never smokers, respectively.[92] Only 3%–6% of unassisted quit attempters are still abstinent at 1 year; however, with organized treatment programming, the success rate after one attempt can be greater than 30%.[92,113]

Some believe that smoking is like a chronic disease, so long-term repeated intervention is required for increasing quit rates. It is important to note that complete smoking cessation but not smoking reduction reduces CV mortality. A combination of behavioral counseling and pharmacotherapy has the highest success rate.[98] The essential part of the initial assessment is the model called the five As, which includes ask, advise, assess, assist, and arrange in each clinic visit.[114,115] The first-line pharmacologic agents for quitting are nicotine replacement therapy (NRT), varenicline, and bupropion.[116] ENDS (Electronic Nicotine Delivery Systems) are not recommended as a treatment option, the evidence is unclear whether they are an effective treatment, and even may be potentially harmful. NRT agents eliminate nicotine withdrawal symptoms and increase the quit rate by twofold. Although smoking cessation can cause modest weight gain (3–6 kg),[117] significant improvement in endothelial function offsets the deleterious effect of weight gain.

## DIABETES AND METABOLIC SYNDROME

Coronary heart disease is the leading cause of morbidity and mortality in patients with diabetes.[118] The prevalence of diabetes in adults is about 6.4% (285 million) all over the world. The rate of undiagnosed diabetes is around 50% in some areas.[119] Data analysis from the National Health Interview Survey showed doubling of the prevalence of diabetes from 1990 to 2008 but no change from 2008 to 2012.[120] With a growing obesity rate in children and with population aging, it is expected that the prevalence of diabetes will increase in the next decade. Type 2 diabetes increases the risk of CHD two times in men and three times in women.[121] One-third of patients with ACS, peripheral artery disease, or stroke have diabetes; these patients have a worse prognosis compared with their nondiabetic counterparts.[122–124]

**TABLE 19.10**
**Stratification of Cardiovascular Risk in Individuals With Diabetes (ESC 2019)[a]**

| | |
|---|---|
| Very high risk | Patients with DM *and* established CVD *or* other target organ damage[b] *or* three or more major risk factors[c] *or* early onset T1DM of long duration (>20 years) |
| High risk | Patients with DM duration ≥10 years without target organ damage plus any other additional risk factor |
| Moderate risk | Young patients (T1DM aged <35 years or T2DM aged <50 years) with DM duration <10 years, without other risk factors |

*CV*, cardiovascular; *CVD*, cardiovascular disease; *DM*, diabetes mellitus; *T1DM*, type 1 diabetes mellitus; *T2DM*, type 2 diabetes mellitus.
[a]Modified from the 2016 European Guidelines on cardiovascular disease prevention in clinical practice.
[b]Proteinuria, renal impairment defined as eGFR ≥30 mL/min/1.73 m², left ventricular hypertrophy, or retinopathy.
[c]Age, hypertension, dyslipidemia, smoking obesity.

Diabetes has a long asymptomatic period (≈10 years), and the atherosclerosis process starts years before overt diabetes has been detected.[125] In the Nurses' Health Study, in women who eventually developed diabetes, the risk of CV events was similar to patients who had clinical diabetes at study entry.[126] But the 2016 ESC preventive guideline states that at diagnosis or in those with a short duration of disease, diabetes is not a CAD risk equivalent state. In general, risk levels approach CAD risk equivalence after about a decade or in those with proteinuria or low eGFR (Table 19.10).[127]

The American Diabetes Association (ADA) has recommended at least annual testing in patients with prediabetes and use of metformin in patients with prediabetes, especially those with body mass indexes (BMIs) of 35 or more and prior gestational diabetes.[128] Diabetes self-management education is helpful for patients with prediabetes to receive education and support to develop and maintain behaviors that can delay the onset of diabetes.

Although no trials have proved a reduction in diabetes morbidity and mortality rates by screening in patients with prediabetes or even by lifestyle change and pharmacologic therapy in patients with overt diabetes, many expert opinions have recommended these modalities because of significant benefits.[128]

There are many controversies in guidelines for diabetes screening, but according to the recent ADA guideline, all adults should start undergoing testing at age 45 years; if the test result is normal, it should be repeated at 3-year intervals. Also, screening should be considered in all adults who are overweight (BMI >25 kg/m²) and have other risk factors, including physical inactivity, first-degree relatives with diabetes, women with gestational diabetes, women with gestational hypertension or who have delivered a baby weighing more than 9 lb, HDL-C less than 35 mg/dL or TG level greater than 250 mg/dL, women with polycystic ovary syndrome, HbA1c greater than 5.7%, impaired fasting glucose or impaired glucose test result, or history of CVD.[128]

Criteria for the diagnosis of diabetes are noted in Table 19.11 (ADA 2019).[129]

**TABLE 19.11**
**ADA 2019**

| Diagnosis/ Measurement | WHO 2006[3]/ 2011[4] | ADA 2019[5] |
|---|---|---|
| *DM* | | |
| | *Can be used* | *Recommended* |
| HbA1c | If measured, ≥6.5% (48 mmol/ mol) | ≥6.5% (48 mmol/mol) |
| | *Recommended* | |
| FPG | ≥7.0 mmol/L (126 mg/dL) | ≥7.0 mmol/L (126 mg/dL) |
| | *or* | *or* |
| 2hPG | ≥11.1 mmol/L (≥200 mg/dL) | ≥11.1 mmol/L (≥200 mg/dL) |
| RPG | Symptoms plus ≥11.1 mmol/L (≥200 mg/dL) | Symptoms plus ≥11.1 mmol/L (≥200 mg/dL) |
| *IGT* | | |
| FPG | <7.0 mmol/L (<126 mg/dL) | <7.0 mmol/L (<126 mg/dL) |
| 2hPG | ≥7.8 to <11.1 mmol/L (≥140–200 mg/ dL) | ≥7.8 to <11.0 mmol/L (≥140–199 mg/ dL) |
| *IFG* | | |
| FPG | 6.1–6.9 mmol/L (110–125 mg/dL) | 5.6–6.9 mmol/L (100–125 mg/dL) |
| 2hPG | <7.8 mmol/L (<140 mg/dL) | <7.8 mmol/L (<140 mg/dL) |

*2hPG*, 2 h plasma glucose; *ADA*, American Diabetes Association; *DM*, diabetes mellitus; *FPG*, fasting plasma glucose; *IFG*, impaired fasting glycaemia; *IGT*, impaired glucose tolerance; *HbA1c*, hemoglobin A1c; *RPG*, random plasma glucose; *WHO*, World Health Organization.
[3]Guideline of 2006.
[4]Revised guideline.
[5]Last recommendation of ADA guideline.

So, it is recommended that for the screening of DM in patients with CVD, first Hb1Ac and FPG being checked, then if they are inconclusive or suspected, IGF or OGTT is added.[130,131] In ACS, the OGTT should not be performed earlier than 4‒5 days, to minimize false-positive results.[132] The Swedish National Diabetes Register has provided important insights into the prevalence of CVD and CV death in both type 1 DM (T1DM) and T2DM. The most important risk factors were age at DM diagnosis, glycemic control, and renal complications. Although T2DM is far more common than T1DM, these results confirm the loss of years of life in both populations, which is particularly severe in the young in general and perhaps in young-onset female individuals with T1DM, emphasizing the need for intensive risk factor management in these groups.[133]

a. Routine assessment of microalbuminuria should be carried out to identify patients at risk of developing renal dysfunction and/or CVD.
b. A resting electrocardiogram (ECG) is indicated in patients with DM and hypertension, or if CVD is suspected.
c. Other tests, such as transthoracic echocardiography, coronary artery calcium (CAC) score, and ankle-brachial index (ABI), may be considered to test for structural heart disease or as risk modifiers in those at moderate or high risk of CVD.

A meta-analysis of five RCTs with 329 asymptomatic subjects with DM showed that noninvasive imaging for CAD did not significantly reduce event rates of nonfatal MI and hospitalization for HF, accordingly, routine screening of CAD in asymptomatic DM is not recommended.[134] However, stress testing or CTCA (Coronary Tomography CT Angiography) may be indicated in very high-risk asymptomatic individuals (with peripheral arterial disease, a high CAC score, proteinuria, or renal failure) (Table 19.12).

## Prevention of CVD in Diabetic Patients

Diabetes is a complex disorder. It is associated with other CV risk factors; more than 50% of patients with diabetes are obese, and about 75% have hypertension or dyslipidemia. Therefore, lifestyle modification is a principal part of the management and treatment of patients with prediabetes and diabetes. Body weight reduction as low as 7% is recommended by high intake of vegetables and fruits, a low-salt DASH diet (see Diet section), Mediterranean diet, limited saturated and trans-fatty acid intake, and moderate to intense physical activity (a combination of aerobic and resistant exercise; at least 150 min/week). A recent meta-analysis of 63 studies ($n = 17,272$, mean age 49.7 years) showed

**TABLE 19.12**

**Recommendation for Imaging Tests for CVD Risk Assessment in Asymptomatic Diabetic Patients (ESC 2019)**

| | | |
|---|---|---|
| CAC score with CT may be considered as a risk modifier in the CV risk assessment of asymptomatic patients with DM at moderate risk.[63] | IIb | B |
| CTCA or functional imaging (radionuclide myocardial perfusion imaging, stress cardiac magnetic resonance imaging, or exercise or pharmacological stress echocardiography) may be considered in asymptomatic patients with DM for screening of CAD.[47,48,64,65,67–70] | IIb | B |
| ABI may be considered as a risk modifier in CV risk assessment.[76] | IIb | B |
| Detection of atherosclerotic plaque of carotid or femoral arteries by CT, or magnetic resonance imaging, may be considered as a risk modifier in patients with DM at moderate or high risk CV.[c 75,77] | IIb | B |
| Carotid ultrasound intima–media thickness screening for CV risk assessment is not recommended.[62,73,78] | III | A |
| Routine assessment of circulating biomarkers is not recommended for CV risk stratification.[27,31,35–37] | III | A |
| Risk scores developed for the general population are not recommended for CV risk assessment in patients with DM. | III | C |

that each additional kilogram loss was associated with 43% lower odds of T2DM.[135] In the Look AHEAD study,[136] interestingly, in patients with diabetes with significant weight reduction by intensive lifestyle intervention via diet control and increased physical activities (average 8.6%), weight loss was associated with a significant reduction in HbA1c and CVRFs. Although these benefits were sustained for 4 years, there was no difference in CV events between groups. The Diabetes Remission Clinical Trial (Di-RECT) nonopen-label, cluster-randomized trial—assigned practices to provide either a weight management program (intervention) or best-practice care by guidelines (control). The results showed that at 12 months, almost one-half of the participants achieved remission to a nondiabetic state and were off glucose-lowering drugs.[137] Sustained remissions at 24 months for over one-third of people with T2DM have been confirmed recently, no reduction in CV events during 10 years of follow-up was reported. This finding may be related to the inability of participants to maintain their weight in the long term.

## Glycemic, Blood Pressure, and Lipid Targets in Patients With Diabetic Mellitus

The combined reduction in HbA1c, SBP, and lipids decreases CV events by 75%. The goal of blood sugar is varied in different guidelines. In the UK Prospective Diabetes Study (UKPDS), intensive blood sugar control decreased all diabetes-related complications, especially microvascular diseases, and a trend toward a decrease in the risk of MI was seen.[138] An ACCORD study showed an increase in all-cause mortality in the intensively treated group and no significant difference in CV death, MI, and stroke.[139] The Action in Diabetes and Vascular Disease: Preterax and Diamicron MR Controlled Evaluation (ADVANCE) and Veterans Affairs Diabetes Trial (VADT) studies failed to show any improvement in CV outcomes in the intensively treated group.[140,141] The recent meta-analysis of intensive blood sugar control has revealed a significant reduction in nonfatal MI but no effect on all-cause mortality.[142] So, it appears that the blood sugar target should be individualized in patients with diabetes according to their total CV risk.[143] The ESC 2019 has been recommended, more stringent goals (6.0–6.5) in younger patients with a short duration of DM and no evidence of CVD, if achieved without significant hypoglycemia. Less stringent HbA1c goals (e.g., <8% or ≤9%) may be adequate for elderly patients with long-standing DM and limited life expectancy, and frailty with multiple comorbidities, including hypoglycemic episodes.[144] The lipid profiles in patients with diabetes usually show high TG level, low HDL-C level, small and denser LDL-C. The lipid target in patients with diabetes is mentioned in the lipid section. Although hypertriglyceridemia and low HDL-C is the most abnormal lipid profile in patients with diabetes, no studies have shown that a decrease in TG level by fibrates (ACCORD[82] and FIELD[145]) or an increase in HDL-C level by niacin (AIM-HIGH[83] and HPS2THRIVE[146]) leads to CVD protection. Therefore, statins are the cornerstone treatment in patients with diabetes as in those without diabetes (in primary and secondary prevention).

**Statins** are safe and generally well tolerated. Adverse events, except for muscle symptoms, are rare. Patients who are taking statin therapy, frequently report muscle symptoms so-called "statin-associated muscle symptoms" (SAMS), and in nonrandomized, observational studies, statins are associated with muscular pain and tenderness (myalgia) without CK elevation or major functional loss, with the reported frequency of SAMS in such studies varying between 10% and 15%

among statin-treated individuals. In the majority cases of myopathy or rhabdomyolysis, there are drug interactions with a higher than the standard dose of statin or combination with gemfibrozil. Statin therapy has been associated with new-onset DM: for every 40 mmol/L (mg/dL) reduction of LDL-C by statins, conversion to DM is increased by 10%.[147] The risk of new-onset DM increases with age and is confined to those already at risk of developing DM. Nevertheless, the benefits in terms of CV event reduction greatly exceed the risks of statin therapy, and this has been confirmed in patients at low CV risk. Further LDL-C reduction occurs by adding *Ezetimibe* to the statins. Ezetimibe by inhibiting cholesterol absorption in the intestine, reduce LDL-C about 15%–22%. Combination of Statin with Ezetimibe has been proved to improve outcomes in DM patients with recent ACS, especially in those with recent ACS and LDL-C more than 55 mg/dL despite the maximum dose of Statin (Table 19.13).[148]

**Proprotein convertase subtilisin/kexin type 9 inhibitors (PCSK-9 inhibitors)** are new LDL-C reduction categories which reduce LDL-C with or without statins about 60%, also they reduce LP(a) about 30%–40%.[149] In the Efficacy and Safety of Alirocumab in Insulin-treated Individuals with Type 1 or Type 2 Diabetes and High Cardiovascular Risk (ODYSSEY DM-INSULIN) trial,[150] alirocumab, compared with placebo, reduced LDL-C by 50% in patients with DM after 24 weeks of treatment. In the Further Cardiovascular Outcomes Research with PCSK9 Inhibition in Subjects with Elevated Risk (FOURIER) trial,[151] patients with atherosclerotic CVD on statin therapy were randomly assigned to a fixed dose of Evolocumab or placebo. The results demonstrated that the primary composite endpoint (CV death, MI, stroke, hospital admission for unstable angina, or coronary revascularization) was significantly reduced. Similar results were obtained from the ODYSSEY OUTCOMES (Evaluation of Cardiovascular Outcomes After an Acute Coronary Syndrome During Treatment With Alirocumab) trial, which randomly assigned patients with CVD and LDL-C -> 1.8 mmol/L (70 mg/dL), despite high-intensity statins, to alirocumab or placebo, with dose titration of the active drug targeting an LDL-C level of 0.6–1.3 mmol/L (25–50 mg/dL). Alirocumab significantly reduced the risk of the primary composite end point (CV death, MI, stroke, or hospital admission for unstable angina) compared with placebo, with the greatest absolute benefit of alirocumab seen in patients with baseline LDL-C levels >2.6 mmol/L (100 mg/dL). But this group of LDL-C reducing agents has no effects on all-cause mortality in long-term outcomes trials.

**TABLE 19.13**

**Recommendations for the Management of Dyslipidemia With Lipid-Lowering Drugs in Diabetic Patients (ESC 2019)**

| Recommendations | Class | Level |
|---|---|---|
| *Targets* | | |
| In patients with T2DM at moderate CV risk, an LDL-C target of <2.5 mmol/L (<100 mg/dL) is recommended.[210-212] | I | A |
| In patients with T2DM at high CV risk, an LDL-C target of <1.8 mmol/L (<70 mg/dL) or an LDL-C reduction of at least 50% is recommended.[210-212] | I | A |
| In patients with T2DM at very high CV risk, an LDL-C target of <1.4 mmol/dL (<55 mg/dL) or an LDL-C reduction of at least 50% is recommended.[200,201,210] | I | B |
| In patients with T2DM, a secondary goal of a non-HDL-C target of <22 mmol/L (<85 mg/dL) in very high CV-risk patients, and <2.6 mmol/L (<100 mg/dL) in high CV-risk patients, is recommended.[213,214] | I | B |
| *Treatment* | | |
| Statins are recommended as the first-choice lipid-lowering treatment in patients with DM and high LDL-C levels: administration of statins is defined based on the CV risk profile of the patient and the recommended LDL-C (or non-HDL-C) target levels.[187] | I | A |
| If the target LDL-C is not reached, combination therapy with ezetimobe is recommended.[200,201] | I | B |
| In patients at very high CV risk, with persistent high LDL-C despite treatment with a maximum tolerated statin dose, in combination with ezetimibe, or in patients with statin intolerance a PCSK9 inhibitor is recommended.[203-206] | I | A |
| Lifestyle intervention (with a focus on weight reduction, and decreased consumption of fast-absorbed carbohydrates and alcohol) and fibrates should be considered in patients with low HDL-C and high triglyceride levels.[191,207] | IIa | B |
| Intensification of statin therapy should be considered before the introduction of combination therapy. | IIa | C |
| Statins should be considered in patients with T1DM at high CV risk, irrespective of the baseline LDL-C level.[187,215] | IIa | A |
| Statins may be considered in asymptomatic patients with T1DM beyond the age of 30 years. | IIb | C |
| Statins are not recommended in women of childbearing potential.[189,190] | III | A |

*Fibrates*, both the Fenofibrate Intervention and Event Lowering in Diabetes (FIELD) and ACCORD studies demonstrated that administration of fenofibrate on top of statins significantly reduced CV events, but only in patients who had both elevated triglyceride and reduced HDL-C levels. Gemfibrozil should be avoided because of the risk of myopathy. A meta-analysis of fibrate trials reported a significant reduction in nonfatal MI, with no effect on mortality.[152] Fibrates may be administered in patients with DM who are statin-intolerant and have high triglyceride levels. If triglycerides are not controlled by statins or fibrates, high-dose omega-3 fatty acids (4 g/day) of icosapent ethyl may be used.

The initial hypertension treatment drugs in patients with diabetes are the same as in hypertensive patients without diabetes, but it is reasonable to start with renin–angiotensin–aldosterone inhibitors, especially in those with proteinuria (Table 19.14).[153]

For blood sugar control, there are many oral and injected types of medications such as Metformin, Sulfonylurea, Thiazolidinediones, Insulins, and much newer oral glucose-lowering agents. Each one has its own benefits and side effects and is evaluated in many trials. Dipeptidyl peptidase-4 inhibitors (DPP-4) such as Saxagliptin, Alogliptin, Sitagliptin, and Linagliptin, However, none of the DPP4 inhibitors was associated with significant CV benefits in their trials populations, which comprised patients with a long history of DM and CVD, or clustered CVD risk factors.

Glucagon-like peptide-1 receptor agonists (GLP-RAs) like Lixisenatide, Exenatide, Liraglutide, Semaglutide,

**TABLE 19.14**

**Recommendations for the Management of Blood Pressure in Patients With Diabetes and Prediabetes (ESC 2019)**

| Recommendations | Class | Level |
|---|---|---|
| *Treatment targets* | | |
| Antihypertensive drug treatment is recommended for people with DM when office BP is >140/90 mmHg.[155,178–180] | I | A |
| It is recommended that patients with hypertension and DM are treated in an individual manner. The BP goal is to target SBP to 130 mmHg and <130 mmHg if tolerated, but not <120 mmHg. In older people (aged >65 years), the SBP goal is to a range of 130–139 mmHg.[155,159,160,181–183] | I | A |
| It is recommended that target DBP is targeted to <80 mmHg, but not <70 mmHg.[160] | I | C |
| An on-treatment SBP of <130 mmHg may be considered in patients at particularly high risk of a cerebrovascular event, such as those with a history of stroke.[154–157,173] | IIb | C |
| *Treatment and evaluation* | | |
| Lifestyle changes [weight loss if overweight, physical activity, alcohol restriction, sodium restriction, and increased consumption of fruits (e.g., 2–3 servings), vegetables (e.g., 2–3 servings), and low-fat dairy products] are recommended in patients with DM and pre-DM with hypertension.[161–163,166] | I | A |
| A RAAS blocker (ACEI or ARB) is recommended in the treatment of hypertension in patient with DM, particularly in the presence of microalbuminuria, albuminuria, proteinuria, or LV hypertrophy.[167–170] | I | A |
| It is recommended that treatment is initiated with a combination of a RAAS blocker with a calcium channel blocker or thiazide/thiazide-like diuretic.[167–171] | I | A |
| In patients with IFG or IGT, RAAS blockers should be preferred to beta-blockers or diuretics to reduce the risk of new-onset DM.[173–175] | IIa | A |
| The effects of GLP1-RAs and SGLT2 inhibitors on BP should be considered. | IIa | C |
| Home BP self-monitoring should be considered in patients with DM on antihypertensive treatments to check that their BP is appropriately controlled.[184] | IIa | C |
| 24-h ABPM should be considered to assess abnormal 24-h BP patterns and adjust antihypertensive treatment.[185] | IIa | C |

and Albiglutide, each one has investigated in diabetic patients. Although the mechanisms through which some of these GLP-RAs reduced CV outcomes have not been established, their long half-lives may be contributing to their CV benefits. In addition, GLP1-RAs improve several CV parameters, including a small reduction in SBP and weight loss, and have direct vascular and cardiac effects that may contribute to the results. The gradual divergence of the event curves in the trials suggests that the CV benefit is mediated by a reduction in atherosclerosis-related events.[154]

Sodium-glucose-cotransporter-2 inhibitors: Four CVOTs with SGLT2 inhibitors [Empagliflozin Cardiovascular Outcome Event Trial in Type 2 Diabetes Mellitus Patients-Removing Excess Glucose (EMPA-REG OUTCOME),[155] Canagliflozin Cardiovascular Assessment Study (CANVAS)[156] Program, Dapagliflozin Effect on Cardiovascular Events-Thrombolysis In Myocardial

Infarction (DECLARE-TIMI 58),[157] and the Canagliflozin and Renal Events in Diabetes with Established Nephropathy Clinical Evaluation (CREDENCE trial)[158] have been published. Empagliflozin significantly reduced the risk of the three-point composite primary outcome (CV death, nonfatal MI, or nonfatal stroke) by 14% compared with placebo. This reduction was driven mainly by a highly significant 38% reduction in CV death. Empagliflozin was associated with a 35% reduction in hospitalization for HF, with separation of the empagliflozin and placebo groups evident almost immediately after treatment initiation, suggesting a very early effect on HF risk. Empagliflozin also reduced the overall mortality by 32%.[159] The CV benefits of SGLT2 inhibitors are mostly unrelated to the extent of glucose-lowering and occur too early to be the result of weight reduction. The rapid separation of placebo and active arms in the four studies in terms of reduction in HF

**TABLE 19.15**
**Recommendations for Glucose-Lowering Treatment for Patients With Diabetes (ESC 2019)**

| Recommendations | Class | Level |
|---|---|---|
| *SGLT2 inhibitors* | | |
| Empagliflozin, canagliflozin, or dapagliflozin are recommended in patients with T2DM and CVD, or at very high/high CV risk,[c] to reduce CV events. | I | A |
| Empagliflozin is recommended *n* patients with T2DM and CVD to reduce the risk of death.[306] | I | B |
| *GLPI-RAs* | | |
| Liraglutide, semaglutide, or dulaglutide are recommended in patterns with T2DM and CVD, or at very high/high CV risk,[c] to reduce CV events.[176] | I | A |
| Liraglutide is recommended in patients with T2DM and CVD or at very high/high CV risk,[c] to reduce the risk of death.[176] | I | B |
| *Biguanides* | | |
| Metformin should be considered in overweight patients with TCDM without CVD and at moderate CV risk.[146,149] | IIa | C |
| *Insulin* | | |
| Insulin-based glycemic control should be considered in patients with ACS with significant hyperglycemia (>10 mmol/L or >180 mg/dL), with the target adapted according to comorbidities. | IIa | C |
| *Thiazolidinediones* | | |
| Thiazolidinediones are not recommended in patients with HF. | III | A |
| *DPP4 inhibitors* | | |
| Saxagliptin is not recommended in patients with TCDM and a high risk of HF. | III | B |

hospitalizations indicates that the beneficial effects achieved in these trials are more likely the result of a reduction in HF-associated events. They could involve effects on hemodynamic parameters, such as reduced plasma volume, direct effects on cardiac metabolism and function, or other CV effects (Tables 19.15 and 19.16).[160]

Although there is no doubt about the effect of aspirin in reducing mortality and nonfatal CV events in secondary prevention, its benefit in primary prevention is not established. A meta-analysis in primary prevention with aspirin showed a statistically significant reduction in nonfatal MI and total CV events but no significant reduction in stroke, CV, and all-cause mortality (Table 19.17).

Studies failed to show any benefit of aspirin for primary prevention in patients with diabetes without CVD.[161] But the recommendation of the last ESC guideline is as below (Tables 19.15 and 19.16)[162]:

Lower extremity arterial disease (LEAD): In patients with DM, LEAD more frequently affects arteries below the knee, as a consequence, the revascularization options, as well as their chances of success, are reduced. In patients with DM, LEAD is often diagnosed at a later

stage (e.g., a nonhealing ulcer), because of concomitant neuropathy with decreased pain sensitivity. All of these factors increase the risk of limb infection. Clinically these patients have atypical symptoms. About 50%–70% of patients with critical limb ischemia have DM (Tables 19.15 and 19.16).[163]

Patients with intermittent claudication should take part in exercise training programs (>30–45 min, at least three times per week) as regular intensive exercise improves walking distance although with less pronounced benefits in patients with DM.[164] In patients with CLI, strict glycemic control is associated with improved limb outcomes. However, revascularization must be attempted when possible, and amputation only considered when revascularization options fail. Revascularization should also be considered in severe/disabling claudication. There has not been a specific trial on revascularization strategies in patients with DM; however, a review of 56 studies including patients with DM suggested higher limb salvage rates after revascularization (78%–85% at 1 year).[165] In patients with DM and chronic symptomatic LEAD without high bleeding risk, a combination of low-dose rivaroxaban (2.5 mg b.i.d.)

**TABLE 19.16**

**Recommendations for the Treatment of Patients With Diabetes to Reduce Heart Failure Risk (ESC 2019)**

| Recommendations | Class | Level |
|---|---|---|
| SGLT2 inhibitors (empagliflozin, canagliflozin, and dapagliflozin) are associated with a lower risk of HF hospitalization in patients with DM, and are recommended. | I | A |
| Metformin should be considered for DM treatment In patients with HF, If the eGFR is stable and >30 mL/min/1.73 m². | IIa | C |
| GLP1-RAs (lixisenatide, liraglutide, semaglutide, exenatide, and dulaglutide) have a neutral effect on the risk of HF hospitalization, and may be considered for DM treatment in patients with, HF.[158,176] | IIb | A |
| The DPP4 inhibitors sitagliptin and linagliptin have a neutral effect on the risk of HF hospitalization, and may be considered for DM treatment in patients with HF. | IIb | B |
| Insulin may be considered in patients with, advanced systolic HFrEF. | IIb | C |
| Thiazolidinediones (pioglitazone and rosiglitazone) are associated with, an increased risk of incident HF in patients with, DM, and are not recommended for DM treatment in patients at risk of HF (or with previous HF). | III | A |
| The DPP4 inhibitor saxagliptin is associated with, an increased risk of HF hospitalization, and is not recommended for DM treatment in patients at risk of HF (or with, previous HF). | III | B |

**TABLE 19.17**

**Recommendations for the Use of Antiplatelet Therapy in Primary Prevention in Patients With Diabetes (ESC 2019)**

| Recommendations | Class | Level |
|---|---|---|
| In patients with DM at high/very high risk, aspirin (75–100 mg/day) may be considered in primary prevention in the absence of clear contraindications.[231] | IIb | A |
| In patients with DM at moderate CV risk, aspirin for primary prevention is not recommended. | III | B |
| *Gastric protection* | | |
| When low-dose aspirin is used, proton pump inhibitors should be considered to prevent gastrointestinal bleeding. | IIIa | A |

and aspirin (100 mg OD) should be considered (IIa) (Table 19.17).[166]

### Chronic kidney disease in DM

CKD is defined as a reduction in eGFR to <60 mL/min/ 1.73 m² and/or persistent proteinuria (e.g., urinary albumin:creatinine ratio >3 mg/mmol), sustained over ≥90 days.[167] Approximately 30% of patients with T1DM and 40% with T2DM will develop CKD. ACEIs and ARBs are the preferred antihypertensive drugs in patients with albuminuria. Data from recent CVOTs suggest that SGLT2 inhibitors and GLP1-RAs may confer renoprotection. In the CREDENCE trial, canagliflozin reduced the relative risk of the primary renal outcome by 30% compared with placebo (Table 19.18).[168]

**TABLE 19.18**

**Recommendations for the Prevention and Management of Chronic Kidney Disease in Patients With Diabetes (ESC 2019)**

| | | |
|---|---|---|
| Treatment with an SGLT2 inhibitor (empagliflozin, canagliflozin, or dapagliflozin) is associated with a lower risk of renal endpoints and is recommended if eGFR is 30 to <90 mL/min/1.73 m². | I | B |
| Treatment with the GLP1-RAs liraglutide and semaglutide is associated with a lower risk of renal endpoints, and should be considered for DM treatment if eGFR is >30 mL/min/1.73 m².[176] | IIa | B |

## METABOLIC SYNDROME (SYNDROME X)

Insulin resistance is an independent risk factor for atherosclerosis and increases the risk of CV and all-cause mortality.[169] According to the previous studies, metabolic syndrome is a complex disorder that includes most CV risk factors (obesity, hypertension, diabetes, and sleep apnea). The definition of this syndrome varies in different nations. The most popular definition according to the National Cholesterol Education Program Adult Treatment Panel is the presence of at least three of these criteria: waist circumference 102 cm or greater in men and 88 cm or greater in women, serum TG level 150 mg/dL or greater, HDL-C less than 40 mg/dL in men and less than 50 mg/dL in women, BP 130/85 mmHg or greater, and fasting plasma glucose 110 mg/dL or greater. In studies, metabolic syndrome is a kind of inflammatory disease, and inflammatory markers, such as high sensitivity C-reactive protein (hsCRP), are included in some definitions.[170] Some cardiologists use the term "syndrome Z" for the combination of syndrome X and sleep apneas, which together increases the CV risk more powerfully.[171] Treatment of metabolic syndrome is based on lifestyle changes and weight reduction as in patients with diabetes.

## OBESITY

Obesity is a chronic disease that is an epidemic around the world. The prevalence of obesity is increasing in adults, adolescents, and children. The prevalence of obesity is 34.9% in the United States and seems to have stabilized in the recent decade.[157] Worldwide, 36.9% of men and 38% of women have BMIs of 25 kg/m$^2$ or greater.[172] Obesity is a disorder that has a close relationship with hypertension, dyslipidemia, diabetes, prothrombotic state, inflammation, and metabolic syndrome. It is an independent risk factor of all-cause mortality.[173] The obesity-related risk is especially prominent in those who have started to gain weight before 40 years of age.[174] BMI is generally used for classification of obesity severity (Table 19.19).[175]

Waist circumference is another surrogate that helps to estimate abdominal fat. Although BMI is a good predictor of CVD, more important is the distribution of body fat. Abdominal obesity (centripetal–visceral obesity) is an independent risk factor for vascular events.[176] Waist circumference especially is helpful in risk stratification of those with BMIs between 25 and 35 kg/m$^2$.

The ESC 2016 guideline has recommended that a waist circumference of 102 cm or greater in men and 88 cm or greater in women is a threshold at which

**TABLE 19.19**
**Body Mass Index**

| Classification | Body Mass Index (kg/m$^2$) |
|---|---|
| Normal weight | 18.5–24.9 |
| Overweight | 25–29.9 |
| Obesity class I | 30–34.9 |
| Obesity class II | 35–39.9 |
| Obesity class III | ≥40 |

weight reduction should be considered; a waist circumference less than 94 cm in men and less than 80 cm in women are the targets.[177] Weight reduction as low as 5%–10% can reduce BP and insulin resistance, decrease TG level, and increase HDL-C level.[178]

There is no agreement about obesity screening, but ACC/AHA guidelines recommend the measurement of BMI annually.

The management of obese patients focuses on risk factors (hypertension, diabetes, and dyslipidemia), controlling and finding the underlying causes.

Patients who need interventions are those with BMIs of 30 kg/m$^2$ or greater and those who have BMIs between 24.9 and 30 kg/m$^2$ with one or more CVD risk factors (hypertension, diabetes, and dyslipidemia).[178] Those with BMIs between 24.9 and 30 kg/m$^2$ and no other CV risk factors should be advised to prevent weight gain and try to improve their lifestyle. Interventions for weight loss in the mentioned groups include dietary management, physical activities, pharmacologic treatment, and bariatric surgery.

Many dietary patterns are suggested by nutritionists, including low-fat diets, low-carbohydrate diets, high-protein diets, the Mediterranean diet, and balanced low-calorie diets. Most trials have found that the rate of weight reduction is not significantly different in varied dietary patterns[179] (although low-carbohydrate diets had more weight reduction in the short term but not in the long term); the most important factors are total calories intake and diet adherence independent of diet macronutrient composition.[180] According to the 2019 ACC/AHA preventive guideline, adults with obesity are typically prescribed a diet designed to reduce caloric intake by ≥500 kcal/day from baseline, which often can be attained by limiting women to 1200–1500 kcal/day and men to 1500–1800 kcal/day, also increased physical activity, preferably aerobic physical activity (e.g., brisk walking) for ≥150 min/week (equal to ≥30 min/day on most days of the week), is recommended for initial weight loss. Higher levels of physical activity, approximately 200–300 min/week, are recommended to maintain weight loss or minimize weight regain after 1 year. Antiobesity drugs are considered for those with BMIs of 30 kg/m$^2$ or greater who have failed to lose weight despite dietary adherence and physical activity (<5% at 3–6 months) and those with BMIs between 27 and 29.9 kg/m$^2$ with comorbidities.[181] These drugs include orlistat, lorcaserin, phentermine, extended-release topiramate, bupropion, naltrexone, and many others. Trials have confirmed the efficacy and safety of orlistat.[182]

Bariatric surgery should be considered for those with BMIs of 40 kg/m$^2$ or greater and may be considered for those with BMIs greater than 35 kg/m$^2$ who have comorbidities and have failed in losing weight with behavior change and pharmacologic therapy.[183] Bariatric surgeries include restrictive and malabsorptive procedures. A recent meta-analysis has shown that bariatric surgery reduced the risk of MI, stroke, and mortality compared with control participants.[184] In one systematic review, the average weight reduction, improvement in BP, and dyslipidemia were about 54%, 63%, and 65%, respectively. The review also showed a reduction in left ventricular mass and an increase in right ventricular systolic function after bariatric surgery at a mean 57.8 months of follow-up.[185]

## DIET AND SUPPLEMENTS

The Mediterranean diet includes high intake of fruits, vegetables, whole grains, fatty fish, oil (canola or olive), and nuts and low intake of red meat and fat dairy food. A diet that is moderate in total fat (32%–35% of total calorie), high in fiber, and high in PUFAs is recommended.[186] The AHA 2013 guideline assessed the strength of evidence as being low for hypertension and dyslipidemia in the Mediterranean diet. But one recent RCT has suggested that 5 years of Mediterranean diet adherence reduces the risk of CVD by 29%.[186]

The DASH focuses on high intake of fruits, vegetables, whole grain, nuts, and fish and low intake of sweets, sugar-sweetened beverages, and red meat. It includes low saturated FAs, total fat, and cholesterol but is rich in potassium, magnesium, calcium, and fiber.[187] The AHA 2013 guideline assessed the strength of evidence as being high for hypertension and dyslipidemia in the DASH diet.[188]

High sodium intake increases the risk of stroke, stroke mortality, and CHD mortality.[189] The AHA 2013 recommends "no more than 2400 mg/day sodium intake and further reduction to 1500 mg/day,"[190] but the Institute of Medicine reports that although high sodium intake increases CV risk, a very stringent salt restriction may increase all health risk, especially in heart failure patients.[191] The recent 2016 ESC guideline recommends less than 5 g/day of salt intake[192]; further studies are needed to establish the sodium level target.

In observational studies, there is an inverse relationship between potassium intake and BP, especially in patients with high sodium intake. It seems that a high-potassium diet reduces CVD, especially stroke rate.[193] Further studies are needed for recommendations on potassium supplementation.

## ALCOHOL CONSUMPTION

Alcohol has a complex effect on the CV and hemostatic system. There is a J-shaped curve between alcohol consumption and CV events. Low to moderate alcohol consumption irrespective of alcohol type decreases the risk of coronary events, stroke, peripheral vascular disease, and all CV death.[194] These favorable effects may be related to increasing baroreflex sensitivity, insulin sensitivity,[195] improvement in endogenous fibrinolysis,[196] decreased inflammatory responses,[197] increased HDL-C and plasminogen[198] and adiponectin levels, decreased lipoprotein a (LPa) and fibrinogen levels, and finally by the antioxidant effect of alcohol. On the other hand, heavy alcohol consumption increases the risk of hypertension,[199] CHD,[200] stroke,[201] heart failure,[202] all-cause mortality, and sudden death.[203] Therefore, the recommended dose is up to one drink per day in women and up to two drinks per day in men. Alcohol consumption cannot be recommended only for the reduction of CV risk.

## VITAMIN D

Vitamin D has a crucial role in mineral homeostasis and skeletal systems. There is no established level for explaining vitamin D deficiency.

Epidemiologic studies have suggested an inverse relationship between vitamin D level and cardiometabolic risk factors such as hypertension, DM, metabolic syndrome, and CHD in a dose–response fashion.[204] A recent population-based study found that vitamin D deficiency has a significant relationship with all-cause mortality but not CV mortality.[205] Vitamin D regulates insulin secretion[206] and the renin–angiotensin system,[207] decreases inflammation and vascular calcification,[208] and induces prothrombotic states. The meta-analysis failed to show a decrease in CVD risk with vitamin D supplements,[209] so they are not recommended for this purpose.

## COENZYME Q10

Coenzyme Q10 (CQ10) is a fat-soluble quinone in the mitochondria of the liver, heart, and kidney with antioxidant and membrane-stabilizing effects. There is controversy about the effect of CQ10 in heart failure patients; some studies have found a reduction in CV and all-cause mortality in advanced heart failure patients, but the others failed to show any benefits.[210] The ACC/AHA 2013 guidelines do not recommend the use of CQ10 in heart failure patients.[211] This controversy is also seen in the role of CQ10 in statin myopathy; the 2015 meta-analysis has not found any benefit in reducing statin myopathy by CQ10.[212]

## INFLAMMATORY MARKERS

Inflammation is the basis of atherosclerosis process and plaque formation. During fatty streak formation, the recruitment of leukocytes and foam cell formation predispose the stable plaques to the vulnerable ones. In studies, the vulnerable plaques have more inflammatory cells, so in recent trials, the inflammatory markers are the reasonable surrogate for CVD risk stratification. The most studied marker is hsCRP, an acute phase reactant that synthesizes in the liver. CRP has a direct correlation with age, diabetes, metabolic syndrome, and hypertension.[213]

Whether CRP is an independent risk factor for CVD in the general population is controversial. In several large studies in asymptomatic low-risk people, the baseline hsCRP is predictive of long-term risk of hypertension, first MI, stroke, and all-cause mortality.[214] CRP improves the prediction value of Framingham risk score, especially in intermediate-risk men and high-risk women.[215] Several meta-analyses have suggested that it appears to have an independent CVD risk prediction, especially in those with intermediate CVD risk but modestly added to traditional risk factors' predictive value.[216]

The 2003 Centers for Disease Control and Prevention/AHA guidelines define low-, intermediate-, and high-risk CRP values as less than 1 mg/L, 1–3 mg/L, and greater than 3 mg/L, respectively, and suggest that in those with intermediate Framingham risk scores, CRP may help further evaluation and treatment in primary prevention. However, in those with CVD, the measurement of CRP is helpful only for prognosis.[217] In 2009, the Canadian Cardiovascular Society recommended measurement of hsCRP in men older than 50 years and women older than 60 years with intermediate Framingham risk scores with no indication for statin therapy (LDL-C <135 mg/dL) because of the potential effect of statin in reducing hsCRP in those with elevated levels.[218]

The JUPITER trial showed that in those with LDL-C levels less than 130 mg/dL and hsCRP of 2 mg/L or greater, rosuvastatin reduced all vascular events and all-cause mortality, and those with both LDL-C less than 70 mg/dL and hsCRP less than 1 mg/L had an 80% reduction in CV risk.[76]

The normal level of hsCRP varies depending on ethnicity and gender.[219] CRP is a nonspecific marker that rises in almost all inflammatory processes, so if its level is greater than 10 mg/L, another inflammatory disease should be considered, and it should be rechecked at least 2 weeks later. So, for CV risk stratification, it is better to measure fasting or nonfasting CRP level twice at least 2 weeks apart.

In trials, after statin initiation, the hsCRP level declines 15%–25% as early as 2 weeks.[220] The magnitude of hsCRP reduction is independent of the magnitude of LDL-C reduction.

Other inflammatory markers that may have prognostic values are IL-1, IL-6, myeloperoxidase, pregnancy-associated plasma protein A, and Lp-PLA2. The benefit of new antiinflammatory agents such as Canakinumab (anti-IL-1β) has evaluated in a randomized controlled trial (CANTOS), which demonstrated a significant lower rate of recurrent cardiovascular events than placebo, independent of lowering of the lipid level.[221] The role of other agents such as Darapladib (LpPLA2 inhibitor), colchicine, and methotrexate are not yet clear, and more studies are needed.

## CARDIAC REHABILITATION

Cardiac rehabilitation (CR) includes comprehensive long-term services such as CVD risk factor education, exercise training, psychological support, and medication adherence. Exercise training is the cornerstone of CR in CHD patients, but in one meta-analysis, the rate of mortality and recurrent MI reduction was similar in each component of CR.[222]

Many trials in stable CHD, ACS, and postcoronary bypass surgery patients suggested lower rates of all-cause mortality and recurrent MI in exercise-based CR.[223] A large 2016 meta-analysis in patients with exercise-based CR has shown lower risk of CV death and hospitalization with no significant effect on rates of all-cause death, MI, or revascularization.[224]

The benefit of exercise rehabilitation is attributed to behavior change, control of risk factors (hypertension, obesity, and smoking), endothelial function improvement,[225] decline in inflammation,[226] and improvement in aerobic capacity via an increase in $VO_{2max}$ (maximal oxygen consumption), which leads to lower myocardial oxygen consumption. In post-MI patients, early CR seems to reduce left ventricle remodeling.[227]

The major concern in CR is underutilization; only 20% of eligible patients are referred for CR.[228]

Recent guidelines strongly recommend CR for patients with stable angina, recent MI, postpercutaneous coronary intervention, or coronary bypass surgery and heart failure. Some consider CR for those with heart or heart–lung transplantation or valve surgery.[229]

The risk of CV events should be assessed before participation in an exercise program. The AHA classified patients into four groups based on clinical characteristics[230]:

- Class A includes individuals with no clinical evidence of CV risk of exercise.
- Class B includes individuals with a low risk of CV risk of exercise, including those with stable CHD.
- Class C includes individuals with a moderate or high risk of cardiac events during exercise, including those with recurrent MI, aborted sudden death, exercise capacity less than six metabolic equivalents, or severe ischemia on the exercise test.
- Class D includes individuals with unstable conditions, so exercise is contraindicated.

Most patients who are referred for CR are in categories B and C. Before initiating exercise training, symptom-limited exercise should be performed to address the baseline fitness level and maximum heart rate.[231]

The intensity of exercise generally should begin at a lower percentage of capacity, usually at 60%–70% of maximal heart rate. The progression rate should be individualized based on fitness, symptoms, and motivation.

Patients in class C should participate in a supervised program with ECG monitoring for 2–3 months until the safety of the program has been documented.[230] Those in class B should be supervised for 2–4 weeks, although self-monitored, home-based exercise is also safe in these patients.[230]

The frequency of exercise should be at least three times a week for 3 months minimally. Each exercise session should consist of three phases (1): the warm-up phase for 5–10 min, which includes stretching and aerobic activities; (2) the training phase for at least 20 min of continuous or discontinuous aerobic and resistance exercise; and (3) the cool-down phase for 5–10 min.

The other components of CR are risk factors education and psychological support by CR personnel.

# REFERENCES

1. Lopez AD, Mathers CD, Ezzati M, et al. Global and regional burden of disease and risk factors, 2001: systematic analysis of population health data. *Lancet.* 2006;367:1747.
2. Capewell S, Beaglehole R, Seddon M, Mcmurray J. Explanation for the decline in coronary heart disease mortality rates in Auckland, New Zealand, between 1982 and 1993. *Circulation.* 2000;102:1511.
3. Lioyd-Jones DM, Larson MG, Beiser A, Levy D. Lifetime risk of developing coronary heart disease. *Lancet.* 1999;353:89.
4. Graham I, Attar D, Borch-Johnsen K, et al. European guidelines on cardiovascular disease prevention in clinical practice: executive summary: Fourth Joint Task Force of the European society of Cardiology and Other Societies on Cardiovascular Disease prevention in Clinical practice (constituted by representatives of nine societies and by invited experts). *Eur Heart J.* 2007; 28:2375.
5. DeFilipps AP, Young R, Carrubba CJ, et al. An analysis of calibration and discrimination among multiple cardiovascular risk scores in a modern multiethnic cohort. *Ann Intern Med.* 2015;162:266.
6. Piepoli Massimo F, Hoes Arno W, Stefan A, et al. European guidelines on cardiovascular disease prevention in clinical practice: the Sixth Joint Task Force of the European Society of Cardiology and Other Societies on Cardiovascular Disease Prevention in Clinical Practice (constituted by representatives of 10 societies and by invited experts) Developed by the special contribution of the European Association for Cardiovascular Prevention and Rehabilitation (EACPR). *Eur Heart J.* 2016;37:2322.
7. Bazo-Alvarez JC, Quispe R, Peralta F, et al. Agreement between cardiovascular disease risk scores in resource-limited settings: evidence from 5 Peruvian sites. *Crit Pathw Cardiol.* 2015;14:74.
8. Chobanian AV, Bakris GL, Black HR, et al. The Seventh Report of the Joint National Committee on Prevention, Detection, Evaluation, and Treatment of High Blood Pressure: the JNC 7 report. *JAMA.* 2003;289:2560.
9. Lewington S, Clarke R, Qizilbash N, et al. Age-specific relevance of usual blood pressure to vascular mortality: a meta-analysis of individual data for one million adults in 61 prospective studies. *Lancet.* 2002;360:1903.
10. Pastor-Barriuso R, Banegas JR, Damian J, et al. Systolic blood pressure, diastolic blood pressure, and pulse pressure: an evaluation of their joint effect on mortality. *Ann Intern Med.* 2003;139:731.
11. Kshirsagar AV, Carpenter M, Bang H, et al. Blood pressure usually considered normal is associated with an elevated risk of cardiovascular disease. *Am J Med.* 2006;119:133.
12. Siu AL, U.S. Preventive Services Task Force. Screening for high blood pressure in adults: U.S. Preventive Services Task Force recommendation statement. *Ann Intern Med.* 2015;163:778.
13. Fann HQ, Li Y, Thijs L, et al. Prognostic value of isolated nocturnal hypertension on ambulatory measurement in

8711 individuals from 10 populations. *J Hypertens.* 2010;28:2036.

14. Hansen TW, Jeppesen J, Rasmussen S, et al. Ambulatory blood pressure and mortality: a population based study. *Hypertension.* 2005;45:499.

15. White WB. Relating cardiovascular risk to out-of-office blood pressure and the importance of controlling blood pressure 24 hours a day. *Am J Med.* 2008;121:S2.

16. Hemmelgen BR, McAllister FA, Myers MG, et al. The 2005 Canadian Hypertension Education Program recommendation for the management of hypertension: part 1—blood pressure measurement diagnosis and assessment of risk. *Can J Cardiol.* 2005;21:645.

17. Weber MA, Schiffrin EL, White WB, et al. Clinical practice guidelines for the management of hypertension in the community a statement by the American Society of Hypertension and the International Society of Hypertension. *J Hypertens.* 2014;32:3.

18. Agarwal R, Andersen MJ. Prognostic importance of ambulatory blood pressure recordings in patients with chronic kidney disease. *Kidney Int.* 2006;69:1175.

19. Uhlig K, Patel K, Ip S, et al. Self-measured blood pressure monitoring in the management of hypertension: a systematic review and meta-analysis. *Ann Intern Med.* 2013;159:185.

20. Agarwal R, Bills JE, Hecht TJ, Light RP. Role of home blood pressure monitoring in overcoming therapeutic inertia and improving hypertension control: a systematic review and meta-analysis. *Hypertension.* 2011;57:29.

21. Franklin SS, Larson MG, Khan SA, et al. Does the relation of blood pressure to coronary heart disease risk change with aging? The Framingham Heart Study. *Circulation.* 2001;103:1245.

22. Chirinos JA, Franklin SS, Townsend RR, Raij L. Body mass index and hypertension hemodynamic subtypes in the adult US population. *Arch Intern Med.* 2009;169:580.

23. Franclin SS, Pio JR, Wong ND, et al. Predictors of new onset diastolic and systolic hypertension: the Framingham Heart Study. *Circulation.* 2005;111:1121.

24. Bidlingmeyer I, Burnier M, Bidlingmey M, et al. Isolated office hypertension: a prehypertension state? *J Hypertens.* 1996;118:833.

25. Pierdomenico SD, Cuccurullo F. Prognostic value of white-coat and masked hypertension diagnosed by ambulatory monitoring in initially untreated subjects: an updated meta-analysis. *Am J Hypertens.* 2011;24:52.

26. Manica G, Bombelli M, Brambilla G, et al. Long term prognostic value of white coat hypertension: an insight from diagnostic use of both ambulatory and home blood pressure measurements. *Hypertension.* 2013;62:168.

27. Verdecchia P, Reboldi GP, Angeli F, et al. Short and long term incidence of stroke in white coat hypertension. *Hypertension.* 2005;45:203.

28. Cohen JB, et al. Cardiovascular events and mortality in white coat hypertension: a systematic review and meta-analysis. *Ann Intern Med.* 2019;170(12):853–862.

29. 2018 ESC/ESH Guidelines for the management of arterial hypertension. *Eur Heart J.* 2018;39:3021–3104.

30. MRC trial of treatment of mild hypertension: principal results. Medical Research Council Working Party. *Br Med J (Clin Res Ed).* 1985;291:97.

31. The effect of treatment on mortality in mild hypertension: results of the hypertension detection and follow up program. *N Engl J Med.* 1982;307:976.

32. Liu L, Zhang Y, Liu G, et al. The Felodipine Event Reduction (FEVER) Study: a randomized long term placebo controlled trial in Chinese hypertensive patients. *J Hypertens.* 2005;23:2157.

33. Staessen JA, Fagard R, Thijs L, et al. Randomised double-blind comparison of placebo and active treatment for older patients with isolated systolic hypertension. The Systolic Hypertension in Europe (Syst-Eur) Trial Investigators. *Lancet.* 1997;350(9080):757–764.

34. SHEP Cooperative Research Group. Prevention of stroke by antihypertensive drug treatment in older persons with isolated systolic hypertension: final results of the Systolic Hypertension in the Elderly Program (SHEP). *JAMA.* 1991;265(24):3255–3264.

35. Verdecchia P, Staessen JA, Angeli F, et al. Cardio-Sis investigators. Usual versus tight control of systolic blood pressure in non-diabetic patients with hypertension (Cardio-Sis): an open-label randomised trial. *Lancet.* 2009;374(9689):525–533.

36. Beckett NS, Peters R, Fletcher AE, et al. HYVET Study Group. Treatment of hypertension in patients 80 years of age or older. *N Engl J Med.* 2008;358(18):1887–1898.

37. Cushman WC, Evans GW, Byington RP, et al. ACCORD Study Group. Effects of intensive blood-pressure control in type 2 diabetes mellitus. *N Engl J Med.* 2010;362 (17):1575–1585.

38. Ruggenenti P, Perna A, Loriga G, et al. REIN-2 Study Group. Blood-pressure control for renoprotection in patients with non-diabetic chronic renal disease (REIN2): multicentre, randomised controlled trial. *Lancet.* 2005;365 (9463):939–946.

39. Wright Jr. JT, Bakris G, Greene T, et al. Effect of blood pressure lowering and antihypertensive drug class on progression of hypertensive kidney disease: results from the AASK trial. *JAMA.* 2002;288(19):2421–2431.

40. Klahr S, Levey AS, Beck GJ, et al. The effects of dietary protein restriction and blood-pressure control on the progression of chronic renal disease. Modification of Diet in Renal Disease Study Group. *N Engl J Med.* 1994;330(13):877–884.

41. SPRINT Research Group, Wright Jr. JT, Williamson JD, et al. A randomized trial of intensive versus standard blood pressure control. *N Engl J Med.* 2015;373:2103.

42. Rubenfire M, Arnett DK, Blumenthal RS, et al. 2019 ACC/AHA guideline on the primary prevention of cardiovascular disease. *Circulation.* 2019;140:e563–e595.

43. Law MR, Morris JK, Wald NJ. Use of blood pressure lowering drugs in the prevention of cardiovascular disease: meta-analysis of 147 randomized trials in the

context of expectations from prospective epidemiological studies. *BMJ.* 2009;338:1665.

44. Staessen JA, Wang JG, Thijs L. Cardiovascular prevention and blood pressure reduction: a quantitative overview updated until 1 March 2003. *J Hypertens.* 2003;21:1055.

45. Nissen SE, Tuzcu EM, Libby P, et al. Effect of antihypertensive agents on cardiovascular events in patients with coronary disease and normal blood pressure: the CAMELOT study: a randomized controlled trial. *JAMA.* 2004;292:2217.

46. ALLHAT Officers and Coordinators for the ALLHAT Collaborative Research Group. The Antihypertensive and Lipid-Lowering Treatment to Prevent Heart Attack Trial. Major outcomes in high risk hypertensive patients randomized to angiotensin-converting enzyme inhibitor or calcium channel blocker vs diuretic: the Antihypertensive and Lipid Lowering Treatment to Prevent Heart Attack Trial (ALLHAT). *JAMA.* 2002;288:2981.

47. Sica DA. Chlorthalidone: has it always been the best thiazide-type diuretic? *Hypertension.* 2006;47:321.

48. Ernst ME, Carter BL, Basile JN. All thiazide like diuretics are not chlorthalidone: putting the ACCOMPLISH study into perspective. *J Clin Hypertens (Greenwich).* 2009;51:9.

49. Dahlöf B, Devereux RB, Kjeldsen SE, et al. Cardiovascular morbidity and mortality in the Losartan Intervention for Endpoint reduction in hypertension study (LIFE): a randomised trial against atenolol. *Lancet.* 2002;359 (9311):995–1003.

50. Dahlof B, Sever PS, Poulter NR, et al. Prevention of cardiovascular events with an antihypertensive regimen of amlodipine adding perindopril as required versus atenolol adding bendroflumethiazide as required, in the Anglo-Scandinavian Cardiac Outcomes Trial Blood Pressure Lowering Arm (ASCOT-BPLA): a multicenter randomized controlled trial. *Lancet.* 2005;366:895.

51. Lewis EJ, Hunsicker LG, Clarke WR, et al. Renoprotective effect of the angiotensin-receptor antagonist irbesartan in patients with nephropathy due to type 2 diabetes. *N Engl J Med.* 2001;345(12):851–860.

52. Jamerson K, Weber MA, Bakris GL, et al. Benazepril plus amlodipine or hydrochlorothiazide for hypertension in high-risk patients. *N Engl J Med.* 2008;359:2417–2428.

53. Emerging Risk Factors Collaboration. Di Angelantonio E, Gao P, et al. Lipid-related markers and cardiovascular disease prediction. *JAMA.* 2012;307:24.

54. Boekholdt SM, Arsenault BJ, Mora S, et al. Association of LDL cholesterol, non-HDL cholesterol, and apolipoprotein B levels with risk of cardiovascular events among patients treated with statins: a meta-analysis. *JAMA.* 2012;307:1302–1309.

55. Robinson JG, Wang S, Jacobson TA. Meta-analysis of comparison of effectiveness of lowering apolipoprotein B versus low-density lipoprotein cholesterol and nonhigh-density lipoprotein cholesterol for cardiovascular risk reduction in randomized trials. *Am J Cardiol.* 2012;110:1468–1476.

56. Haase CL, Tybjærg-Hansen A, Grande P, Frikke-Schmidt R. Genetically elevated apolipoprotein A-I, high-density lipoprotein cholesterol levels, and risk of ischemic heart disease. *J Clin Endocrinol Metab.* 2010;95:E500–E510.

57. Khera AV, Cuchel M, de la Llera-Moya M, et al. Cholesterol efflux capacity, high-density lipoprotein function, and atherosclerosis. *N Engl J Med.* 2011;364:127–135.

58. Li XM, Tang WH, Mosior MK, et al. Paradoxical association of enhanced cholesterol efflux with increased incident cardiovascular risks. *Arterioscler Thromb Vasc Biol.* 2013;33:1696–1705.

59. Arsenault BJ, Boekholdt SM, Kastelein JJ. Lipid parameters for measuring risk of cardiovascular disease. *Nat Rev Cardiol.* 2011;8:197.

60. Sarwar N, Danesh J, Eiriksdottir G, et al. Triglycerides and the risk of coronary heart disease: 10,158 incident cases among 262,525 participants in 29 Western prospective studies. *Circulation.* 2007;115:450–458.

61. Hokanson JE, Austin MA. Plasma triglyceride level is a risk factor for cardiovascular disease independent of high-density lipoprotein cholesterol level: a meta-analysis of population-based prospective studies. *J Cardiovasc Risk.* 1996;3:213–219.

62. D'agostino Sr. RB, Vasan RS, Pencina MJ, et al. General cardiovascular risk profile for use in primary care: the Framingham Heart Study. *Circulation.* 2008;117:743–753.

63. Conroy RM, Pyorala K, Fitzgerald AP, et al. Estimation of ten-year risk of fatal cardiovascular disease in Europe: the SCORE project. *Eur Heart J.* 2003;24:987–1003.

64. Goff Jr. DC, Lloyd-Jones DM, Bennett G, et al. 2013 ACC/AHA guideline on the assessment of cardiovascular risk: a report of the American College of Cardiology/American Heart Association Task Force on Practice Guidelines. *J Am Coll Cardiol.* 2014;63(25 pt. B):2935–2959.

65. Woodward M, Brindle P, Tunstall-Pedoe H. Adding social deprivation and family history to cardiovascular risk assessment: the ASSIGN score from the Scottish Heart Health Extended Cohort (SHHEC). *Heart.* 2007;93:172–176.

66. Mann Douglas L, Douglas Z, Peter L, Robert B, Eugene B. *Braunwald's Heart Disease: A Text Book of Cardiovascular Medicine.* 10th ed. Philadelphia: Elsevier; 2015899.

67. Stamler J, Wentworth D, Neaton JD. Is relationship between serum cholesterol and risk of premature death from coronary heart disease continuous and graded? Findings in 356, 222 primary screens of the Multiple Risk Factor Intervention Trial (MRFIT). *JAMA.* 1986;256:2823.

68. Kolovou GD, Mikhailidis DP, Kovar J, et al. Assessment and clinical relevance of non-fasting and postprandial triglycerides: an expert panel statement. *Curr Vasc Pharmacol.* 2011;9:258–270.

69. Mihas C, Kolovou GD, Mikhailidis DP, et al. Diagnostic value of postprandial triglyceride testing in healthy subjects: a meta-analysis. *Curr Vasc Pharmacol.* 2011;9:271–280.

70. Mach F, et al. 2019 ESC/EAS guidelines for the management of dyslipidemias: lipid modification to

reduce cardiovascular risk: The Task Force for the management of dyslipidaemias of the European Society of Cardiology (ESC) and European Atherosclerosis Society (EAS). *Eur Heart J.* 2020;41:111–188.

71. Cholesterol Treatment Trialists Collaboration. Efficacy and safety of statin therapy in older people: a meta-analysis of individual participant data from 28 randomised controlled trials. *Lancet.* 2019;393:407–415.

72. Schmidt AF, Pearce LS, Wilkins JT, Overington JP, Hingorani AD, Casas JP. PCSK9 monoclonal antibodies for the primary and secondary prevention of cardiovascular disease. *Cochrane Database Syst Rev.* 2017;4:CD011748.

73. Waheed S, Pollack S, Roth M, et al. Collective impact of conventional cardiovascular risk factors and coronary calcium score on clinical outcomes with or without statin therapy: the St Francis Heart Study. *Atherosclerosis.* 2016;255:193–199.

74. Shepherd J, Cobbe SM, Ford I, et al. Prevention of coronary heart disease with paravastatin in men with hypercholesterolemia. West of Scotland Coronary Prevention Study Group. *N Engl J Med.* 1995;333:1301.

75. Downs JR, Clearfeild M, Weis S, et al. Primary prevention of acute coronary events with lovastatin in men and women with average cholesterol levels: results of AFCAPS/TexCAPS. Air Force/Texas Coronary Atherosclerosis Prevention Study. *JAMA.* 1998;279:1615.

76. Ridker PM, Danielson E, Fonseca FA, et al. Rosuvastatin to prevent vascular events in men and women with elevated C-reactive protein. *N Engl J Med.* 2008;359:2195.

77. Randomised trial of cholesterol lowering in 4444 patients with coronary heart disease: the Scandinavian simvastatin survival study (4S) of cholesterol lowering. *Am Cardiol.* 2000;86:257.

78. Plehn JF, Davis BR, Sacks FM, et al. Reduction of stroke incidence after myocardial infarction with paravastatin: the cholesterol and recurrent events (CARE) study. The Care investigators. *Circulation.* 1999;99:216.

79. Heart Protection Study Collaborative Group. MRC/BHF Heart Protection Study of cholesterol lowering with simvastatin in 20,536 high-risk individuals: a randomized placebo-controlled trial. *Lancet.* 2002;360:7.

80. Cannon CP, Blazing MA, Giugliano RP, et al. Ezetimibe added to statin therapy after acute coronary syndromes. *N Engl J Med.* 2015;372:2387.

81. Keech A, Simes RJ, Barter P, et al. Effects of long term fenofibrate therapy on cardiovascular events in 9795 people with type 2 diabetes mellitus (the FIELD study): randomized controlled trial. *Lancet.* 2005;366:1849.

82. ACCORD Study Group, Ginsberg HN, Elam MB, et al. Effects of combination lipid therapy in type 2 diabetes mellitus. *N Engl J Med.* 2010;362:1563.

83. AIM-HIGH Investigators, Boden WE, Probstfield JL, et al. Niacin in patients with low HDL cholesterol levels receiving intensive statin therapy. *N Engl Med.* 2011;365:2255.

84. HPS2-THRIVE Collaborative Group. Landray MJ, Haynes R, et al. Effects of extended release niacin with laropiprant in high risk patients. *N Engl J Med.* 2014;371:203.

85. Barter PJ, Caulfield M, Eriksson M, et al. Effects of torcetrapib in patients at high risk for coronary events. *N Engl J Med.* 2007;356:1620.

86. Schwatz GG, Olsson AG, Abt M, et al. Effects of dalcetrapib in patients with a recent acute coronary syndromes. *N Engl J Med.* 2012;367:2089.

87. Nicholls SJ, Brewer HB, Kastelein JJ, et al. Effects of the CETP inhibitor evacetrapib administered as monotherapy or in combination with statin on HDL and LDL cholesterol: a randomized controlled trial. *JAMA.* 2011;306:2099.

88. Rohatgi A, Khera A, Berry JD, et al. HDL cholesterol efflux capacity and incident cardiovascular events. *N Engl J Med.* 2014;371:2383.

89. *World Health Organization Report on the Global Tobacco Epidemic, 2011: Warning About the Dangers of Tobacco.* Geneva: World Health Organization; 2011.

90. Mozaffarian D, Benjamin EJ, Go AS, et al. Heart disease and stroke statistics—2015 update: a report from the American Heart Association. *Circulation.* 2015;131:e29.

91. Centers for Disease Control and Prevention (CDC). Smoking–attributable mortality, years of potential life lost, and productivity losses—United States, 2000–2004. *MMWR Morb Mortal Wkly Rep.* 2008;57:1226–1228.

92. Mann Douglas L, Douglas Z, Peter L, Robert B, Eugene B. *Braunwald's Heart Disease: A Text Book of Cardiovascular Medicine.* 10th ed. Philadelphia: Elsevier; 2015894.

93. Kawachi I, Coldtiz GA, Stampfer MJ, et al. Smoking cessation and decreased risk of stroke in women. *JAMA.* 1993;269:232.

94. Gornik HL, Creager MA. Medical treatment of peripheral artery disease. In: Creger MA, Beckman JA, Loscalzo J, eds. *Vascular Medicine: A Companion to Braunwald's Heart Disease.* 2nd ed. Philadelphia: Elsevier; 2013:242–248.

95. Mann Douglas L, Douglas Z, Peter L, Robert B, Eugene B. *Braunwald's Heart Disease: A Text Book of Cardiovascular Medicine.* 10th ed. Philadelphia: Elsevier; 20151279.

96. Hurt RD, Weston SA, Ebbert JO, et al. Myocardial infarction and sudden cardiac death in Olmsted County, Minnesota, before and after smoke free workplace laws. *Arch Intern Med.* 2012;172:1635.

97. Qiao Q, Tervahauta M, Nissinen A, Tuomilehto J. Mortality from all causes and from coronary heart disease related to smoking and changes in smoking during a 35 year follow up of middle-aged Finnish men. *Eur Heart J.* 2000;21:1621.

98. Jha P, Ramasundarahettige C, Lasndsman V, et al. 21st-Century hazards of smoking and benefits of cessation in the United States. *N Engl J Med.* 2013;368:341.

99. Narkiewicz K, van de Borne PJ, Hausberg M, et al. Cigarette smoking increases sympathetic outflow in humans. *Circulation.* 1998;98:528.

100. Stefanadis C, Tsiamis E, Vlachopoulos C, et al. Unfavorable effect of smoking on the elastic properties of the human aorta. *Circulation.* 1997;95:31.

101. Celermajer DS, Sorensen KE, Georgakopoulos D, et al. Cigarette smoking is associated with dose-related and potentially reversible impairment of endothelium-dependent vasodilation. *Circulation.* 2001;104:1905.

102. Messner B, Bernhald D. Smoking and cardiovascular disease: mechanism of endothelial dysfunction and early atherogenesis. *Arterioscler Thromb Vasc Biol.* 2014;34:509.
103. Newby DE, Wright RA, Labinjoh C, et al. Endothelial dysfunction, impaired endogenous fibrinolysis, and cigarette smoking: a mechanism for arterial thrombosis and myocardial infarction. *Circulation.* 1999;99:1411.
104. Fusegawa Y, Goto S, Handa S, et al. Platelet spontaneous aggregation in platelet rich plasma is increased in habitual smokers. *Thromb Res.* 1999;93:271.
105. Bazzano LA, He J, Muntner P, et al. Relationship between cigarette smoking and novel risk factors for cardiovascular disease in the United States. *Ann Intern Med.* 2003;138:891.
106. Craig WY, Palomaki GE, Haddow JE. Cigarette smoking and serum lipid and lipoprotein concentrations: an analysis of published data. *BMJ.* 1989;298:784.
107. Prescott E, Hippe M, Schnohr P, et al. Smoking and risk of myocardial infarction in women and men: longitudinal population study. *BMJ.* 1998;316:1043.
108. de Chillou C, Riff P, Sadoul N, et al. Influence of cigarette smoking on rate of reopening of the infarct-related coronary artery after myocardial infarction: a multivariable analysis. *J Am Coll Cardiol.* 1996;27:1662.
109. Kenfield SA, Stampfer MJ, Rosner BA, Colditz GA. Smoking and smoking cessation in relation to mortality in women. *JAMA.* 2008;21:416.
110. Cao Y, Kenfield S, Song Y, et al. Cigarette smoking cessation and total and cause-specific mortality: a 22-year follow-up study among US male physicians. *Arch Intern Med.* 1956;2011:171.
111. Mann Douglas L, Douglas Z, Peter L, Robert B, Eugene B. *Braunwald's Heart Disease: A Text Book of Cardiovascular Medicine.* 10th ed. Philadelphia: Elsevier; 2015895.
112. Mann Douglas L, Douglas Z, Peter L, Robert B, Eugene B. *Braunwald's Heart Disease: A Text Book of Cardiovascular Medicine.* 10th ed. Philadelphia: Elsevier; 2015893.
113. Rigotti NA. Strategies to help a smoker who is struggling to quit. *JAMA.* 2012;308:1573.
114. Stead LF, Koilpillai P, Lancaster T. Additional behavioural support as an adjunct to pharmacotherapy for smoking cessation. *Cochrane Database Syst Rev.* 2015;10: CD009670.
115. Fiore MC, Jaen C, Baker T, et al. *Treating Tobacco Use and Dependence: 2008 Update. Clinical Practice Guideline.* Rockville, MD: US Department of Health and Human Services; 2008.
116. Siu AL, U. S. Preventive Services Task Force. Behavioral and pharmacotherapy interventions for tobacco smoking cessation in adults, including pregnant women: U.S. preventive services task forces recommendation statement. *Ann Intern Med.* 2015;163:622.
117. Flegal KM, Troiano RP, Pamuk ER, et al. The influence of smoking cessation on the prevalence of overweight in the United States. *N Engl J Med.* 1995;333:1165.
118. Buse JB, Ginsberg HN, Bakris GL, et al. Primary prevention of cardiovascular disease in people with diabetes mellitus: a scientific statement from the American Heart Association and the American Diabetes Association. *Diabetes Care.* 2007;30:162–172.
119. Yang W, Lu Weng J, et al. Prevalence of diabetes among men and women in China. *N Engl J Med.* 2010;362:1090.
120. Giessi LS, Wang J, Cheng YJ, et al. Prevalence and incidence trends for diagnosed diabetes among adults aged 20 to 79 years, United States, 1980-2012. *JAMA.* 2014;312(12):1218–1226.
121. Huxley R, Barzi F, Woodward M. Excess risk of fatal coronary heart disease associated with diabetes in men and women: meta-analysis of 37 prospective cohort studies. *BMJ.* 2006;332:73.
122. Fang J, Alderman MH. Impact of the increasing burden of diabetes on acute myocardial infarction in New York City: 1990-2000. *Diabetes.* 2006;55:768.
123. Wiviott SD, Braunwald E, Angiolillo DJ, et al. Greater clinical benefit of more intensive oral antiplatelet therapy with prasugrel in patients with diabetes mellitus in the trial to assess improvement in therapeutic outcomes by optimizing platelet inhibition with prasugrel—Thrombolysis in Myocardial Infarction 38. *Circulation.* 2008;118:1626.
124. Martini SR, Kent TA. Hyperglycemia in acute ischemic stroke. A vascular perspective. *J Cereb Blood Flow Metab.* 2007;27:435.
125. Levitan EB, Song Y, Ford ES, Liu S. Is nondiabetic hyperglycemia a risk factor for cardiovascular disease? A meta-analysis of prospective studies. *Arch Intern Med.* 2004;164:2147.
126. Hu FB, Stampfer MJ, Haffner SM, et al. Elevated risk of cardiovascular disease prior to clinical diagnosis of type 2 diabetes. *Diabetes Care.* 2002;25:1129.
127. Piepoli Massimo F, Hoes Arno W, Stefan A, et al. European guidelines on cardiovascular disease prevention in clinical practice: the Sixth Joint Task Force of the European Society of Cardiology and other societies on cardiovascular disease prevention in clinical practice (constituted by representatives of 10 societies and by invited experts) developed by the special contribution of the European Association for Cardiovascular Prevention and Rehabilitation (EACPR). *Eur Heart J.* 2016;37:2356.
128. Modified from American Diabetes Association. Classification and diagnosis of diabetes. *Diabetes Care.* 2016;39(suppl. 1):S14.
129. Cosentino F, Grant PJ, Aboyans V, et al. 2019 ESC guidelines on diabetes, pre-diabetes, and cardiovascular diseases developed in collaboration with the EASD. *Eur Heart J.* 2020;41:255–323.
130. Barry E, Roberts S, Oke J, Vijayaraghavan S, Normansell R, Greenhalgh T. Efficacy and effectiveness of screen and treat policies in prevention of type 2 diabetes: systematic review and meta-analysis of screening tests and interventions. *BMJ.* 2017;356:i6538.
131. Cosson E, Hamo-Tchatchouang E, Banu I, et al. A large proportion of prediabetes and diabetes goes undiagnosed when only fasting plasma glucose and/or

HbA1c are measured in overweight or obese patients. *Diabetes Metab*. 2010;36:312318.

132. Opie LH. Metabolic management of acute myocardial infarction comes to the fore and extends beyond control of hyperglycemia. *Circulation*. 2008;117:2172–2177.

133. Rawshani A, Sattar N, Franzen S, et al. Excess mortality and cardiovascular disease in young adults with type 1 diabetes in relation to age at onset: a nationwide, register-based cohort study. *Lancet*. 2018;392:477486.

134. Clerc OF, Fuchs TA, Stehli J, et al. Non-invasive screening for coronary artery disease in asymptomatic diabetic patients: a systematic review and meta-analysis of randomised controlled trials. *Eur Heart J Cardiovasc Imaging*. 2018;19:838846.

135. Galaviz KI, Weber MB, Straus A, Haw JS, Narayan KMV, Ali MK. Global diabetes prevention interventions: a systematic review and network meta-analysis of the real-world impact on incidence, weight, and glucose. *Diabetes Care*. 2018;41:15261534.

136. Look AHEAD Research Group, Wing RR, Bolin P, et al. Cardiovascular effects of intensive lifestyle intervention in type 2 diabetes. *N Engl J Med*. 2013;369:145–154.

137. Lean ME, Leslie WS, Barnes AC, et al. Primary care-led weight management for remission of type 2 diabetes (DiRECT): an open-label, cluster-randomised trial. *Lancet*. 2018;391:541551.

138. Holman RR, Paul SK, Bethel MA, et al. Effects of intensive glucose lowering in type 2 diabetes. *N Engl J Med*. 2008;359:1577.

139. Accord Study Group, Gerstein HC, Miller ME, et al. Long-term effects of intensive glucose lowering on cardiovascular outcomes. *N Engl J Med*. 2011;364:818.

140. Patel A, MacMahon S, Chalmers J, et al. Intensive blood glucose control and vascular outcomes in patients with type 2 diabetes. *N Engl J Med*. 2008;358:2560.

141. Duckworth W, Abraira C, Mortiz T, et al. Glucose control and vascular complication in veterans with type 2 diabetes. *N Engl J Med*. 2009;360:129.

142. Ray K, Seshasai SR, Wijesuriya S, et al. Effect of intensive control of glucose on cardiovascular outcomes and death in patients with diabetes mellitus: a meta-analysis of randomized controlled trails. *Lancet*. 2009;373:1765–1772.

143. American Diabetes Association. Glycemic targets. *Diabetes Care*. 2016;39(suppl. 1):S39.

144. Doucet J, Verny C, Balkau B, Scheen AJ, Bauduceau B. Haemoglobin A1c and 5-year all-cause mortality in French type 2 diabetic patients aged 70 years and older: the GERODIAB observational cohort. *Diabetes Metab*. 2018;44:465472.

145. Keech A, Simes RJ, Barter P, et al. Effects of long term fenofibrate therapy on cardiovascular events in 9795 people with type 2 diabetes mellitus: randomised controlled trial. *Lancet*. 2005;366:1849.

146. HPS-THRIVE Collaborative Group. HPS2-THRIVE randomized placebo-controlled trial in 25673 high-risk patients of ER niacin/laropiprant: trial design, Pre-specified muscle and liver outcomes, and reasons for stopping study treatment. *Eur Heart J*. 2013;34:1279.

147. Preiss D, Seshasai SR, Welsh P, et al. Risk of incident diabetes with intensive-dose compared with moderate-dose statin therapy: a meta-analysis. *JAMA*. 2011;305:25562564.

148. Cannon CP, Blazing MA, Giugliano RP, et al. Ezetimibe added to statin therapy after acute coronary syndromes. *N Engl J Med*. 2015;372:23872397.

149. Robert S. Rosenson, Robert A, et al. Cholestrol-Lowering Agents. PCSK9 Inhibitors Today and Tomorrow. *Circ Res*. 2019;124:364–385

150. Leiter LA, Cariou B, Muller-Wieland D, et al. Efficacy and safety of alirocumab in insulin-treated individuals with type 1 or type 2 diabetes and high cardiovascular risk: the ODYSSEY DM-INSULIN randomized trial. *Diabetes Obes Metab*. 2017;19:17811792.

151. Sabatine MS, Giugliano RP, Keech AC, et al. Evolocumab and clinical outcomes in patients with cardiovascular disease. *N Engl J Med*. 2017;376:17131722.

152. Saha SA, Arora RR. Fibrates in the prevention of cardiovascular disease in patients with type 2 diabetes mellitus—a pooled meta-analysis of randomized placebo-controlled clinical trials. *Int J Cardiol*. 2010;141:157166.

153. Niskanen L, Hedner T, Hansson L, Lanke J, Niklason A. CAPPP Study Group Reduced cardiovascular morbidity and mortality in hypertensive diabetic patients on first-line therapy with an ACE inhibitor compared with a diuretic/beta-blocker-based treatment regimen: a subanalysis of the Captopril Prevention Project. *Diabetes Care*. 2001;24:20912096.

154. Nauck MA, Meier JJ, Cavender MA, Abd El Aziz M, Drucker DJ. Cardiovascular actions and clinical outcomes with glucagon-like peptide-1 receptor agonists and dipeptidyl peptidase-4 inhibitors. *Circulation*. 2017;136:849870.

155. Zinman B, Inzucchi SE, Lachin JM, et al. Rationale, design, and baseline characteristics of a randomized, placebo-controlled cardiovascular outcome trial of empagliflozin (EMPA-REG OUTCOME). *Cardiovasc Diabetol*. 2014;13:102.

156. Neal B, Perkovic V, Matthews DR, et al. Rationale, design and baseline characteristics of the CANagliflozin cardioVascular Assessment Study-Renal (CANVAS-R): a randomized, placebo-controlled trial. *Diabetes Obes Metab*. 2017;19:387393.

157. Wiviott SD, Raz I, Bonaca MP, et al. Dapagliflozin and cardiovascular outcomes in type 2 diabetes. *N Engl J Med*. 2019;380:347357.

158. Perkovic V, Jardine MJ, Neal B, et al. Canagliflozin and renal outcomes in type 2 diabetes and nephropathy. *N Engl J Med*. 2019;380:22952306.

159. Zinman B, Wanner C, Lachin JM, et al. Empagliflozin, cardiovascular outcomes, and mortality in type 2 diabetes. *N Engl J Med*. 2015;373:21172128.

160. Verma S, McMurray JJV, Cherney DZI. The metabolodiuretic promise of sodium-dependent glucose cotransporter 2 inhibition: the search for the sweet spot in heart failure. *JAMA Cardiol.* 2017;2:939940.

161. Bartolucci AA, Tendera M, Howard G. Meta-analysis of multiple primary prevention trials of cardiovascular events using aspirin. *Am J Cardiol.* 2011;107:1796.

162. ASCEND Study Collaborative Group. Bowman L, Mafham M, et al. Effects of aspirin for primary prevention in persons with diabetes mellitus. *N Engl J Med.* 2018;379:15291539.

163. Uccioli L, Gandini R, Giurato L, et al. Long-term outcomes of diabetic patients with critical limb ischemia followed in a tertiary referral diabetic foot clinic. *Diabetes Care.* 2010;33:977982.

164. Lyu X, Li S, Peng S, Cai H, Liu G, Ran X. Intensive walking exercise for lower extremity peripheral arterial disease: a systematic review and meta-analysis. *J Diabetes.* 2016;8:363377.

165. Hinchliffe RJ, Brownrigg JR, Andros G, et al. Effectiveness of revascularization of the ulcerated foot in patients with diabetes and peripheral artery disease: a systematic review. *Diabetes Metab Res Rev.* 2016;32:136144.

166. Belch J, MacCuish A, Campbell I, et al. The prevention of progression of arterial disease and diabetes (POPADAD) trial: factorial randomised placebo controlled trial of aspirin and antioxidants in patients with diabetes and asymptomatic peripheral arterial disease. *BMJ.* 2008;337:a1840.

167. Kidney Disease: Improving Global Outcomes (KDIGO) CKD Work Group. KDIGO 2012 Clinical Practice Guideline for the evaluation and management of chronic kidney disease. *Kidney Int Suppl.* 2013;3:1150.

168. Jardine MJ, Mahaffey KW, Neal B, et al. The Canagliflozin and Renal Endpoints in Diabetes with Established Nephropathy Clinical Evaluation (CREDENCE) study rationale, design, and baseline characteristics. *Am J Nephrol.* 2017;46:462472.

169. Ford ES. Risks for all-cause mortality, cardiovascular disease, and diabetes associated with metabolic syndrome: a summary of the evidence. *Diabetes Care.* 2005;28:1769.

170. Ridker PM, Buring JE, Cook NR, Rifai N. C-reactive protein, the metabolic syndrome, and risk of incident cardiovascular events: an 8 year follow up of 14719 initially healthy American women. *Circulation.* 2000;102:42.

171. Wilcox I, McNamara SG, Collins FL, et al. Syndrome Z: the interaction of sleep apnea, vascular risk factors and heart disease. *Thorax.* 1998;53(suppl. 3):S25–S28.

172. Ogden CL, Carroll MD, Kit BK, Flefal KM. Prevalence of childhood and adult obesity in the United States, 20112012. *JAMA.* 2014;311:806.

173. Berrington de Gonzalez A, Hartge P, Cerhan JR, et al. Body-mass index and mortality among 1.46 million white adults. *N Engl J Med.* 2010;363:2211.

174. Fontaine KR, Redden DT, Wang C, et al. Years of life lost due to obesity. *JAMA.* 2003;289:187.

175. Obesity: preventing and managing the global epidemic. Report of the WHO Consultation. *World Health Organ Tech Rep Ser.* 2000;894:i.

176. Janssen I, Katzmarzyk PT, Ross R. Waist circumference and not body mass index explains obesity-related health risk. *Am J Clin Nutr.* 2004;79:379.

177. Piepoli Massimo F, Hoes Arno W, Stefan A, et al. European guidelines on cardiovascular disease prevention in clinical practice: the Sixth Joint Task Force of the European Society of Cardiology and Other Societies on Cardiovascular Disease Prevention in Clinical Practice: the Sixth Joint Task Force of the European Society of Cardiology and Other Societies on Cardiovascular Disease Prevention in Clinical Practice Douketis JD, Macie C, Thabane L, Williamson DF. Systematic review of long-term weight loss studies in obese adults: clinical significance and applicability to clinical practice. *Int J Obes (Lond).* 2005;29:1153.

178. Jensen MD, Ryan DH, Apovian CM, et al. 2013 AHA/ACC/TOS guideline for management of overweight and obesity in adults: a report of the American College of Cardiology/American Heart Association Task Force on practice guidelines and the obesity society. *Circulation.* 2014;129:S102.

179. Del Corral P, Chandler-Laney PC, Casazza K, et al. Effect of dietary adherence with or without exercise on weight loss: a mechanistic approach to a global problem. *J Clin Endocrinol Metab.* 2009;94:1602.

180. Sacks FM, Bray GA, Carey VJ, et al. Comparison of weight-loss diets with different compositions of fat, protein, and carbohydrates. *N Engl J Med.* 2009;360:859.

181. Apovian CM, Aronne LJ, Bessesen DH, et al. Pharmacological management of obesity: an Endocrine Society clinical practice guideline. *J Clin Endocrinol Metabol.* 2015;100:342.

182. Heck AM, Yanovski JA, Calis KA. Orlistat, a new lipase inhibitor for the management of obesity. *Pharmacotherapy.* 2000;20:270.

183. Maggard MA, Shugarman LR, Suttorp M, et al. Meta-analysis: surgical treatment of obesity. *Ann Intern Med.* 2005;142:547.

184. Yermilov I, McGory ML, Shekelle PW, et al. Appropriateness criteria for bariatric surgery: beyond the NIH guidelines. *Obesity (Silver Spring).* 2009;17:1521.

185. Kwok CS, Pradhan A, Khan MA, et al. Bariatric surgery and its impact on cardiovascular disease and mortality: a systematic review and meta-analysis. *Int J Cardiol.* 2014;173:20–28.

186. Estruch R, Ros E, Salas-Salvado J, et al. Primary prevention of cardiovascular disease with a Mediterranean diet. *N Engl J Med.* 2013;368:1279–1290.

187. Aburto NJ, Ziolkovaska A, Hooper L, et al. Effects of lower sodium intake on health: systematic review and meta-analysis. *BMJ.* 2013;346:f1326.

188. Eckel RH, Jakicic JM, Ard JD, et al. 2013 AHA/ACC guideline on lifestyle management to reduce cardiovascular risk: a report of the American College of Cardiology/American Heart Association Task Force on Practice Guidelines. *Circulation.* 2014;129(suppl. 2):S84.

189. Eckel RH, Jakicic JM, Ard JD, et al. 2013 AHA/ACC guideline on lifestyle management to reduce cardiovascular risk: a report of the American College of Cardiology/American Heart Association Task Force on Practice Guidelines. *Circulation.* 2014;129(suppl. 2):S88.

190. *Institute of Medicine: Sodium Intake in Populations: Assessment of Evidence.* Washington, DC: National Academy Press; 2013.

191. Piepoli Massimo F, Hoes Arno W, Stefan A, et al. European guidelines on cardiovascular disease prevention in clinical practice: the Sixth Joint Task Force of the European Society of Cardiology and Other Societies on Cardiovascular Disease Prevention in Clinical Practice (constituted by representatives of 10 societies and by invited experts) Developed by the special contribution of the European Association for Cardiovascular Prevention and Rehabilitation (EACPR). *Eur Heart J.* 2016;37:2347.

192. Mann Douglas L, Douglas Z, Peter L, Robert B, Eugene B. *Braunwald's Heart Disease: A Text Book of Cardiovascular Medicine.* 10th ed. Philadelphia: Elsevier; 20151009.

193. D'Elia L, Barba G, Cappuccio FP, Strazzullo P. Potassium intake, stroke and cardiovascular disease: a meta-analysis of prospective studies. *J Am Coll Cardiol.* 2011;57:1210.

194. Ronksley PE, Brien SE, Turner BJ, et al. Association of alcohol consumption with selected cardiovascular disease outcomes: a systematic review and meta-analysis. *BMJ.* 2011;342:d671.

195. Davies MJ, Baer DJ, Judd JT, et al. Effects of moderate alcohol intake on fasting insulin and glucose concentrations and insulin sensitivity in postmenopausal women: a randomized controlled trial. *JAMA.* 2002;287:2559.

196. Mukamal KJ, Jadhav PP, D'Agostino RB, et al. Alcohol consumption and hemostatic factors: analysis of the Framingham Offspring cohort. *Circulation.* 2001;104:1367.

197. Albert MA, Glynn RJ, Ridker PM. Alcohol consumption and plasma concentration of C-reactive protein. *Circulation.* 2003;107:443.

198. Gaziano JM, Buring JE, Breslow JL, et al. Moderate alcohol intake, increased levels of high density lipoprotein and its subfractions, and decreased risk of myocardial infarction. *N Engl J Med.* 1993;329:1829.

199. Fuchs FD, Chambless LE, Whelton PK, et al. Alcohol consumption and the incidence of hypertension: the Atherosclerosis Risk in Communities Study. *Hypertension.* 2001;37:1242.

200. Ruidavets JB, Ducimetiere P, Evans A, et al. Patterns of alcohol consumption and ischemic heart disease in culturally divergent countries: the Prospective Epidemiological Study of Myocardial Infarction (PRIME). *BMJ.* 2010;341:c6077.

201. Reynolds K, Lewis B, Nolen JD, et al. Alcohol consumption and risk of stroke: a meta-analysis. *JAMA.* 2003;289:579.

202. Walsh CR, Larson MG, Evans JC, et al. Alcohol consumption and risk of congestive heart failure in the Framingham Heart Study. *Ann Intern Med.* 2002;136:181.

203. Chiuve S, Albert C, Conen D. Arrhythemias in women: atrial fibrillation and sudden cardiac death. In: Goldman MB, Troisi R, Rexrode KM, eds. *Women and Health.* 2nd ed. San Diego: Academic Press; 2013:1039–1053.

204. Kim DH, Sabour S, Sagar UN, et al. Prevalence of hypovitaminosis D in cardiovascular disease (from the National Health and Nutrition Examination Survey 2001 to 2004). *Am J Cardiol.* 2008;102:1540.

205. Melmed ML, Michos ED, Post W, et al. 25-Hydroxyvitamin D levels and the risk of mortality in the general population. *Arch Intern Med.* 2008;168:1629.

206. Norman AW, Frankel JB, Heldt AM, et al. Vitamin D deficiency inhibits pancreatic secretion of insulin. *Science.* 1980;209:823.

207. Qiao G, Kong J, Uskokovic M, et al. Analogs of 1alpha,25-dihydroxyvitamin D3 as novel inhibitors of renin biosynthesis. *J Steroid Biochem Mol Biol.* 2005;96:59.

208. Zittermann A, Schleithoff SS, Koerfer R. Vitamin D and vascular calcification. *Curr Opin Lipidol.* 2007;18:41.

209. Lacroix AZ, Kotchen J, Anderson G, et al. Calcium plus vitamin D supplementation and mortality in postmenopausal women: the Women's Health Initiative calcium-vitamin D randomized controlled trial. *J Gerontol A Biol Sci Med Sci.* 2009;64:559.

210. Mortensen SA, Rosenfeldt F, Kumar A, et al. The effect of coenzyme Q10 on morbidity and mortality in chronic heart failure: results from Q-SYMBIO: a randomized double-blind trial. *JACC Heart Fail.* 2014;2:641.

211. Yancy CW, Jessup M, Bozkurt B, et al. 2013 ACCF/AHA guideline for the management of heart failure: a report of the American College of Cardiology Foundation/American Heart Association Task Force on practice guidelines. *J Am Coll Cardiol.* 2013;62:e147.

212. Banach M, Serban C, Sahebkar A, et al. Effects of coenzyme Q10 on statin-induced myopathy: a meta-analysis of randomized controlled trials. *Mayo Clin Proc.* 2015;90:24.220.

213. Ridker PM, Buring JE, Cook NR, Rifai N. C-reactive protein, the metabolic syndrome, and risk of incident cardiovascular events: an 8-year follow up of 14719 initially healthy American women. *Circulation.* 2003;107:391.

214. Mendall MA, Strachan DP, Butland BK, et al. C-reactive protein: relation to total mortality, cardiovascular mortality and cardiovascular risk factors in men. *Eur Heart J.* 2000;21:1584.

215. Wilson PW, Pencina M, Jacques P, et al. C-reactive protein and reclassification of cardiovascular risk in Framingham Heart Study. *Circ Cardiovasc Qual Outcomes.* 2008;1:92.

216. Emerging Risk Factors Collaboration. Kaptoge S, Di Angelantonio E, et al. C-reactive protein, fibrinogen, and cardiovascular disease prediction. *N Engl J Med.* 2012;367:1310.

217. Pearson TA, Mensah GA, Alexander RW, et al. Markers of inflammation and cardiovascular disease: application to clinical and public health practice: a statement for healthcare professionals from the Centers for Disease Control and Prevention. *Circulation.* 2003;107:499.

218. Genest J, McPherson R, Frohlich J, et al. 2009 Canadian Cardiovascular Society/Canadian guidelines for the diagnosis and treatment of dyslipidemia and prevention of cardiovascular disease in the adult-2009 recommendations. *Can J Cardiol.* 2009;25:567.

219. Shah T, Newcombe P, Smeeth L, et al. Ancestry as a determinant of mean population C-reactive protein values: implications for cardiovascular risk prediction. *Circ Cardiovasc Genet.* 2010;3:436.

220. Plenge JK, Hernandez TL, Weil KM, et al. Simvastatin lowers C-reactive protein within 14 days: an effect independent of low-density lipoprotein cholesterol reduction. *Circulation.* 2002;106:1447.

221. Ridker PM, Everett BM, et al. Antiinflammatory therapy with canakinumab for atherosclerotic disease. *N Engl J Med.* 2017;1119–1131.

222. Goel K, Lennon RJ, Tilbury RT, et al. Impact of cardiac rehabilitation on mortality and cardiovascular events after percutaneous coronary intervention in the community. *Circulation.* 2011;123:2344.

223. Pack QR, Goel K, Lahr BD, et al. Participation in cardiac rehabilitation and survival after coronary artery bypass graft surgery: a community-based study. *Circulation.* 2013;128:590.

224. Anderson L, Oldridge N, Thompson DR, et al. Exercise-based cardiac rehabilitation for coronary heart disease: Cochrane Systematic Review and Meta-Analysis. *J Am Coll Cardiol.* 2016;67:1.

225. Gielen S, Schuler G, Adams V. Cardiovascular effects of exercise training: molecular mechanisms. *Circulation.* 2010;122:1221.

226. Milani RV, Lavie CJ, Mehra MR. Reduction in C-reactive protein through cardiac rehabilitation and exercise training. *J Am Coll Cardiol.* 2004;43:1056.

227. Haykowsky M, Scott J, Esch B, et al. A meta-analysis of the effects of exercise training on left ventricular remodeling following myocardial infarction: start early and go longer for greatest exercise benefits on remodeling. *Trials.* 2011;12:92.

228. Smith Jr. SC, Benjamin EJ, Bonow RO, et al. AHA/ACCF secondary prevention and risk reduction therapy for patients with coronary and other atherosclerotic vascular disease: 2011 update: a guideline from the American Heart Association and American College of Cardiology Foundation. *Circulation.* 2011;124:2458.

229. Fletcher GF, Balady GL, Amsterdam EA, et al. Exercise standards for testing and training: a statement for healthcare professionals from the American Heart Association. *Circulation.* 2001;104:1694.

230. Fletcher GF, Ades PA, Kligfield P, et al. Exercise standards for testing and training: a scientific statement from the American Heart Association. *Circulation.* 2013;128:873.

231. Ades PA, Pashkow FJ, Fletcher G, et al. A controlled trial of cardiac rehabilitation in the home setting using electrocardiographic and voice transtelephone monitoring. *Am Heart J.* 2000;139:543.

# CHAPTER 20

# Hypertension

ALI ZAHED MEHR

Cardiovascular Intervention Research Center, Rajaie Cardiovascular, Medical & Reasrch Center, Iran University of Medical Sciences, Tehran, Iran

## KEY POINTS

- Arterial hypertension is very common and acts as a major risk factor for many cardiac, cerebral, and renal morbidities and mortalities.
- Neural, renal, hormonal, and vascular mechanisms are involved in the pathogenesis of hypertension.
- Fewer than 10% of hypertension cases have an identifiable cause, so they are considered secondary hypertension.
- Hypertension management includes lifestyle modification and antihypertensive drugs.
- Acute blood pressure elevations are common among patients who present to emergency departments and need special attendance.

## INTRODUCTION

Arterial hypertension is a very common disease and affects about 1 billion people around the world. It is a major risk factor for coronary artery disease (CAD), stroke, aortic dissection, heart failure, atrial fibrillation, chronic kidney disease (CKD), and peripheral arterial disease (PAD). Therefore, it has the biggest role in the burden of diseases and global mortality.[1, 2]

The diagnosis of hypertension is not so easy because hypertension is usually asymptomatic, and the cut-off point between the existence and the absence of hypertension is not clear. Some of the adverse effects of hypertension occur in blood pressures (BPs) lower than 140/90 mmHg; there are some evidences which show benefits of initiating antihypertensive medications in some high-risk patients with BPs lower than 140/90 mmHg.[3, 4]

In more than 90% of patients, there is not a single cause for arterial hypertension; this group has essential or primary hypertension. In the remaining minority, which is known as secondary hypertension, a certain cause can be found that is somehow correctable.

Systolic BP (SBP) increases with aging, although the diastolic BP (DBP) normally decreases after 55–60 years of age because of arterial wall stiffening. In young people, hypertension is more frequent among men, but women have an accelerating occurrence after menopause. Therefore, hypertension is more common in older women than men.[1]

Many genetic and environmental factors have roles in hypertension development. Smoking, heavy drinking, obesity, lack of physical activity, and high salt and calorie intake are some behavioral factors.[1]

## MECHANISMS OF HYPERTENSION

Mechanisms involved in hypertension development are classified as neural, renal, hormonal, and vascular.

Due to Ohm's law, BP is the result of multiplying cardiac output and systemic vascular resistance (SVR). These mechanisms can be explained by these formulas.

$$\text{Voltage} = \text{flow} \times \text{resistance}$$
$$\text{Blood pressure} = \text{flow} \times \text{SVR}$$

For example, stress increases the sympathetic tone; the resultant arterial wall smooth muscle contraction leads to higher SVR. This high SVR translates to high BP in the long term. Carotid baroreceptors also become desensitized and reset by repeated high BPs.

In obese persons, to burn fat, sympathetic tone is increased. This results in elevated SVR.[5]

In sleep apnea syndrome, nocturnal hypoxic episodes sensitize chemoreceptors, and these receptors remain active even in the daytime when the person is not hypoxic. These chemoreceptors increase heart rate and contractility through neural reflexes.

Another example from renal and hormonal mechanisms is the effect of salt ingestion on BP. High amounts of salt consumption in modern life requires extrarenal

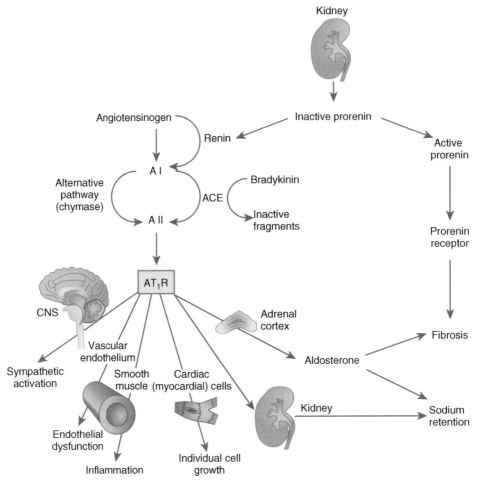

FIG. 20.1 The renin–angiotensin–aldosterone system. *ACE*, angiotensin-converting enzyme; *AT₁R*, angiotensin receptor type 1; *CNS*, central nervous system. (From Victor RG. Systemic hypertension: mechanisms and diagnosis. In: Mann DL, Zipes DP, Libby P, et al., eds. *Braunwald's Heart Disease: A Textbook of Cardiovascular Medicine.* 10th ed. Philadelphia: Saunders; 2015, with permission.)

work to excrete Na. This can increase cardiac output repeatedly. SVR increases to protect the vital organs from high blood flow. However, we expect inhibition of the renin–angiotensin–aldosterone (RAS) pathway (Fig. 20.1) when someone has high salt intake, but in some patients, increased sympathetic tone leads to renin release from the kidneys and persistence of RAS system activity.

## DIAGNOSIS OF HYPERTENSION

Arterial hypertension typically has no symptoms; so, BP should be measured in every patient who presents to the clinic with any complaint.

The patient must be seated in a chair for about 5 min. The cuff size should be appropriate, and the arm must be held at the heart level. BPs in both arms need to be measured. To increase the accuracy of the assessment, a measurement repetition is advised.[4]

If the average of measurements is more than 140/90 mmHg or evidence of target organ damage exists, ambulatory BP monitoring (ABPM) is suggested.[6] Target organ damage includes retinopathy, left ventricular hypertrophy (LVH), encephalopathy, cerebrovascular accidents, acute aortic syndromes, renal disease, and so on. If ABPM is not available, another option is home BP monitoring at least twice a day for 4–7 days. Those who cannot afford ABPM or home BP monitoring must have their office BP rechecked 1–2 months later.

Patients with BP above 180/110 mmHg in the first visit can be considered hypertensive and receive drug therapy.[6]

The criteria for hypertension diagnosis in ABPM are average 24-h BP greater than 130/80 mmHg, average daytime BP greater than 135/85 mmHg, and average nighttime BP greater than 120/70 mmHg.[1]

It has been shown that ABPM, especially nighttime BP monitoring, has better prognostic value than office BP in predicting cardiovascular outcomes.[7, 8]

For home BP monitoring, average BPs greater than 135/85 are considered hypertension. It is better to omit the first-day measurements.[5]

In some patients, average BPs at home or in ABPM are normal, but high pressures are detected in the office. This phenomenon is called *white coat hypertension*. These patients are not truly hypertensive but need to be followed.[1]

On the other hand, some patients have normal clinic BPs but high pressures at home or on ABPM. This situation is known as *masked hypertension*. These individuals need to be regarded as hypertensive and treated appropriately.[1]

### Initial Evaluation

When taking the patient history, it is important to ask about drugs that can increase BP such as glucocorticoids, nonsteroidal antiinflammatory drugs, antineoplastics, antidepressants, immunosuppressive agents, licorice derivatives, sex hormones, oral decongestants, yohimbine, and ergotamine.[9, 10]

During the physical examination, evaluating limb pulses and investigating the neck and abdomen for possible bruits are important.

Other tests that are recommended in every patient with a possible diagnosis of hypertension are hemoglobin, fasting blood glucose, lipid profile, Na, K, Ca, uric acid, blood urea, creatinine, urinalysis, thyroid-stimulating hormone, and electrocardiography.[4, 11]

### Secondary Hypertension

In the initial evaluation of hypertension, some clues may be found to suggest secondary hypertension (e.g., azotemia, hypokalemia). Other characteristics that need screening for secondary hypertension include hypertension diagnosis before 30 years of age, severe or resistant hypertension, sudden initiation, or worsening of hypertension, target organ damages inappropriate for the duration of hypertensive period, and adrenal incidentaloma.[11]

- Renal parenchymal disease is the most common cause of secondary hypertension. Acute or chronic kidney injuries can increase BP. As discussed earlier, hypertension is a major risk factor for CKD, and CKD is one of the main features of secondary hypertension.
- Renovascular hypertension: Stenosis of the main stem of renal arteries or even a branch or accessory renal artery can decrease glomerular perfusion of the affected area. The results are increased renin secretion and high BP.

There are some situations in which we must consider renovascular hypertension in the differential diagnosis. These include the absence of a family history of hypertension, initiation of hypertension before age 30 years or after 50 years, resistant hypertension, episodes of flash pulmonary edema, creatinine rise with consumption of RAS inhibitors, audible abdominal bruits, or significant difference between right and left kidney sizes.[1, 11]

For renovascular hypertension screening, computed tomography angiography and magnetic resonance angiography are first choices.[1] The latter is not safe in those with CKD. Another option is duplex sonography of the renal arteries.[1]

In women younger than 60 years old, the cause is often fibromuscular dysplasia, which affects the distal two-thirds of the renal arteries with a beading pattern. These lesions are best treated by balloon angioplasty.[1]

In older adult patients, especially men, the cause is mostly atherosclerosis. It usually affects the proximal third of the renal arteries. Regarding randomized controlled trials, there are insufficient data to support renal artery stenting in every patient with severe hypertension[12, 13]; therefore, except in very resistant cases or confirmed renal ischemia, medical therapy is recommended. Tight bilateral renal stenoses more possibly need interventional treatment.

- Mineralocorticoid excess: Adrenal adenomas or carcinomas, bilateral adrenal hyperplasia, Cushing syndrome, and some enzyme deficiencies are some examples of secondary hypertension caused by aldosteronism. We should suspect these conditions in hypokalemic patients. The screening test is the aldosterone–renin ratio.[1]
- Pheochromocytoma: see Chapter 36.
- Aortic coarctation: see Chapter 26.

## HYPERTENSION MANAGEMENT
### Lifestyle Modification

It is recommended that all patients with hypertension or prehypertension (SBP, 120–139 mmHg; DBP, 80–89 mmHg) be encouraged to consume less salt, do regular exercise, and use diets that lower BP.[14]

Dietary Approaches to Stop Hypertension, known as the DASH diet, includes almost every dietary change with confirmed evidence to lower BP:

- High amounts of fruits and vegetables
- Low-fat dairy products
- Fish and poultry
- Whole grains and nuts
- Foods rich in potassium, calcium, magnesium, protein, and fiber
- Foods with lower amounts of red meat, cholesterol, total fat, saturated fat, sweets, and sugar-sweetened beverages

Stopping smoking and maintaining a body mass index lower than 25 can delay the occurrence of hypertension and decrease the dose of antihypertensive drugs.[1]

## Drug Therapy

Many classes of drugs have antihypertensive characteristics (Table 20.1). Some classes can better prevent cardiovascular and cerebral adverse events, so they are considered first choices.

### First-class drugs

Three drug classes are considered first choices to begin hypertension drug therapy: calcium channel blockers (CCBs), RAS inhibitors, and thiazide-type diuretics. These drugs have synergistic effects, so even in mild hypertension, an acceptable approach is to begin therapy with low-dose combinations of them. However, this strategy lowers the possibility of side effects related to higher doses of one drug.[11]

**Calcium Channel Blockers.** Nondihydropyridines such as diltiazem and verapamil are weak antihypertensive drugs (verapamil is weaker); however, they are good options in patients with hypertrophic obstructive cardiomyopathy.

Dihydropyridines are among the best antihypertensive drugs that can prevent stroke more than any other drug. Nifedipine has the side effect of reflex tachycardia, so its use is somehow restricted to the patients with severe aortic insufficiency and pregnant women.

Another dihydropyridine, amlodipine, is the most frequently prescribed drug in this class. It can effectively reduce the probability of adverse cardiovascular events and stroke. It can be used once daily. Its combination with RAS inhibitors is one of the best combination therapies.[1]

According to some guidelines, CCBs such as amlodipine are the first choice in patients older than 55 years,[5] but American College of Cardiology/American Heart

### TABLE 20.1
### Oral Antihypertensive Drugs

| Drug | Dose Range, Total mg/day (Doses Per Day) |
|---|---|
| **DIURETICS** | |
| **THIAZIDE AND THIAZIDE-TYPE DIURETICS** | |
| Chlorthalidone | 6.25–50 (1) |
| HCTZ | 6.25–50 (1) |
| Indapamide | 1.25–5 (1) |
| Metolazone | 2.5–5 (1) |
| **LOOP DIURETICS** | |
| Furosemide | 20–160 (2) |
| Torsemide | 2.5–0 (1–2) |
| Bumetanide | 0.5–2 (2) |
| Ethacrynic acid | 25–100 (2) |
| **POTASSIUM-SPARING DIURETICS** | |
| Amiloride | 5–20 (1) |
| Triamterene | 25–100 (1) |
| Spironolactone | 12.5–400 (1–2) |
| Eplerenone | 25–100 (1–2) |
| **BETA BLOCKERS** | |
| **STANDARD BETA BLOCKERS** | |
| Acebutolol | 200–800 (2) |
| Atenolol | 25–100 (1) |
| Betaxolol | 5–20 (1) |
| Bisoprolol | 2.5–20 (1) |
| Carteolol | 2.5–10 (1) |
| Metoprolol | 50–450 (2) |
| Metoprolol XL | 50–200 (1–2) |
| Nadolol | 20–320 (1) |
| Penbutolol | 10–80 (1) |
| Pindolol | 10–60 (2) |
| Propranolol | 40–180 (2) |
| Propranolol LA | 60–180 (1–2) |
| Timolol | 20–60 (2) |
| **VASODILATING BETA BLOCKERS** | |
| Carvedilol | 6.25–50 (2) |
| Carvedilol CR | 10–40 (1) |
| Nebivolol | 5–40 (1) |
| Labetalol | 200–2400 (2) |

*Continued*

**TABLE 20.1**
**Oral Antihypertensive Drugs—cont'd**

| Drug | Dose Range, Total mg/day (Doses Per Day) |
|---|---|
| **CALCIUM CHANNEL BLOCKERS** | |
| **DIHYDROPYRIDINES** | |
| Amlodipine | 2.5–10 (1) |
| Felodipine | 2.5–20 (1–2) |
| Isradipine CR | 2.5–20 (2) |
| Nicardipine SR | 30–120 (2) |
| Nifedipine XL | 30–120 (1) |
| Nisoldipine | 10–40 (1–2) |
| **NONDIHYDROPYRIDINES** | |
| Diltiazem CD | 120–540 (1) |
| Verapamil HS | 120–480 (1) |
| **ANGIOTENSIN-CONVERTING ENZYME INHIBITORS** | |
| Benazepril | 10–80 (1–2) |
| Captopril | 25–150 (2) |
| Enalapril | 2.5–40 (2) |
| Fosinopril | 10–80 (1–2) |
| Lisinopril | 5–80 (1–2) |
| Moexipril | 7.5–30 (1) |
| Perindopril | 4–16 (1) |
| Quinapril | 5–80 (1–2) |
| Ramipril | 2.5–20 (1) |
| Trandolapril | 1–8 (1) |
| **ANGIOTENSIN RECEPTOR BLOCKERS** | |
| Candesartan | 8–32 (1) |
| Eprosartan | 400–800 (1–2) |
| Irbesartan | 150–300 (1) |
| Losartan | 25–100 (2) |
| Olmesartan | 5–40 (1) |
| Telmisartan | 20–80 (1) |
| Valsartan | 80–320 (1–2) |
| **DIRECT RENIN INHIBITOR** | |
| Aliskiren | 75–300 (1) |
| **ALPHA BLOCKERS** | |
| Doxazosin | 1–16 (1) |
| Prazosin | 1–40 (2–3) |
| Terazosin | 1–20 (1) |

*Continued*

**TABLE 20.1**
**Oral Antihypertensive Drugs—cont'd**

| Drug | Dose Range, Total mg/day (Doses Per Day) |
|---|---|
| Phenoxybenzamine | 20–120 (2) for pheochromocytoma |
| **CENTRAL SYMPATHOLYTICS** | |
| Clonidine | 0.2–1.2 (2–3) |
| Clonidine patch | 0.1–0.6 (weekly) |
| Guanabenz | 2–32 (2) |
| Guanfacine | 1–3 (1) (qhs) |
| Methyldopa | 250–1000 (2) |
| Reserpine | 0.05–0.25 (1) |
| **DIRECT VASODILATORS** | |
| Hydralazine | 10–200 (2) |
| Minoxidil | 2.5–100 (1) |
| **FIXED-DOSE COMBINATIONS** | |
| Aliskiren–HCTZ | 75–300/12.5–25 (1) |
| Amiloride–HCTZ | 5/50 (1) |
| Amlodipine–benazepril | 2.5–5/10–20 (1) |
| Amlodipine–valsartan | 5–10/160–320 (1) |
| Amlodipine–olmesartan | 5–10/20–40 (1) |
| Atenolol–chlorthalidone | 50–100/25 (1) |
| Benazepril–HCTZ | 5–20/6.25–25 (1) |
| Bisoprolol–HCTZ | 2.5–10/6.25–25 (1) |
| Candesartan–HCTZ | 16–32/12.5–25 (1) |
| Enalapril–HCTZ | 5–10/25 (1–2) |
| Eprosartan–HCTZ | 600/12.5–25 (1) |
| Fosinopril–HCTZ | 10–20/12.5 (1) |
| Irbesartan–HCTZ | 15–30/12.5–25 (1) |
| Losartan–HCTZ | 50–100/12.5–25 (1) |
| Olmesartan–amlodipine | 20–40/5–10 (1) |
| Olmesartan–HCTZ | 20–40/12.5–25 (1) |
| Olmesartan–amlodipine–HCTZ | 20–40/5–10/12.5–25 (1) |
| Spironolactone–HCTZ | 25/25 (1/2–1) |

*Continued*

**TABLE 20.1**
**Oral Antihypertensive Drugs—cont'd**

| Drug | Dose Range, Total mg/day (Doses Per Day) |
|---|---|
| Telmisartan–HCTZ | 40–80/12.5–25 (1) |
| Trandolapril–verapamil | 2–4/180–240 (1) |
| Triamterene–HCTZ | 37.5/25 (1/2–1) |
| Valsartan–HCTZ | 80–160/12.5–25 (1) |
| Valsartan–amlodipine–HCTZ | 80–160/5–10/12.5–25 (1) |

*HCTZ*, hydrochlorothiazide; *qhs*, at bedtime.
From Victor RG. Systemic hypertension: mechanisms and diagnosis. In: Mann DL, Zipes DP, Libby P, et al., eds. *Braunwald's Heart Disease: A Textbook of Cardiovascular Medicine*. 10th ed. Philadelphia: Saunders; 2015, with permission.

Association guidelines emphasize using thiazide-type diuretics for older adults.[15]

Ankle edema is a well-known side effect of amlodipine, especially with doses more than 10 mg/day. Adding RAS inhibitors can dissipate this problem.

Gingival hyperplasia is a rare CCB side effect; drug discontinuation is necessary in such cases.[1]

**RAS Inhibitors.** Although many recent guidelines accept all three first-class drugs to initiate hypertension therapy in patients with diabetes, there is a lot of evidence that favors RAS inhibitors. They can postpone the occurrence of diabetes in glucose-intolerance patients, too.[1]

Angiotensin-converting enzyme (ACE) inhibitors and angiotensin receptor blockers (ARBs) are also first choices in patients with heart failure or CKD, especially those with proteinuric CKD.[11,16]

The third group of RAS inhibitors is direct renin inhibitors; the prototype drug in this group is aliskiren. Using this drug in combination with ACE inhibitors or ARBs is contraindicated, so its use is perhaps restricted to patients who cannot tolerate ACE inhibitors or ARBs. For patients younger than 55 years of age, ACE inhibitors or ARBs are the preferred drugs[5]; then a CCB or a diuretic can be added. In contrast with ACE inhibitors, ARBs do not induce cough; ARBs are also the best drugs for LVH regression.[17]

All of the RAS inhibitors are contraindicated in pregnancy. Important side effects of ACE inhibitors are cough and angioedema. Another problem with RAS inhibitors is hyperkalemia. Creatinine increases up to 30% above baseline are acceptable in CKD patients receiving RAS inhibitors and do not require drug discontinuation.[1]

Combination therapy with ACE inhibitors and ARBs is contraindicated.[11,18]

**Thiazide-Type Diuretics.** These are very effective drugs, especially when combined with the abovementioned classes. As said before, these drugs can be the first choice in older adults. The diuretic role is so important that without administering them, we cannot consider someone a resistant hypertension case.

In this group, hydrochlorothiazide is somewhat weak with many side effects, and its effect does not last for 24 h. Chlorthalidone and indapamide are the first choices.

Despite the common misconception, thiazide-type diuretics, especially chlorthalidone, can be used in advanced CKD.[18] Loop diuretics are also good options in severe CKD.

Important side effects are precipitating gout; erectile dysfunction; dyslipidemia; and metabolic derangements such as hypokalemia, hypomagnesemia, and hyponatremia. They can worsen glucose intolerance when used in combination with beta blockers.[1]

### Add-On Drugs

When combination therapy with all three first-class drugs fails to control hypertension, other antihypertensive classes can be used. These drugs may be added earlier if a patient cannot tolerate one of the first classes.

**Aldosterone Antagonists.** Spironolactone is one of the best add-on drugs, and it has shown much success in controlling resistant hypertension; however, it has some side effects such as gynecomastia, erectile dysfunction, uterine bleeding, and hyperkalemia.[1,19–21]

Eplerenone is more specific without antiadrenergic side effects, but the evidence of its effectiveness in resistant hypertension is not confirmed.[20]

Aldosterone antagonists should be avoided in patients with advanced CKD.[11]

**Beta Blockers.** This class of drugs can be used as add-on drugs in isolated hypertension cases, but CAD, heart failure, atrial fibrillation rhythm, aortic aneurysm, and hypertrophic cardiomyopathy (HCM) are some conditions that need beta blockers to be started earlier. In such hypertensive cases, a vasodilator beta blocker must be used. Carvedilol and labetalol have alpha blocker characteristics, and nebivolol induces nitric oxide release.

It is better to avoid atenolol, metoprolol, and propranolol in hypertension.

The side effects of beta blockers include fatigability, bronchospasm, bradycardia, conduction disturbances, and glucose intolerance.[1]

**Alpha Blockers.** Drugs such as prazosin and terazosin, which are used for prostatism, are good add-on drugs for controlling hypertension. Phentolamine and phenoxybenzamine have important roles in pheochromocytoma.[1]

**Central Sympatholytics.** These are effective drugs as add-on drugs or oral agents used in hypertension urgencies. They can be helpful in patients with HCM if beta blockers and CCBs fail to control hypertension. Methyldopa is used in pregnancy.

These drugs have many central nervous system symptoms. Another problem with them is rebound hypertension, which is especially seen with clonidine.

**Direct Vasodilators.** Hydralazine is a good choice in pregnancy and is effective in patients with heart failure when combined with nitrates. Minoxidil's main usage is in CKD-resistant hypertension. It should be used with loop diuretics and beta blockers because its major side effect is reflex tachycardia.[1]

## RESISTANT HYPERTENSION

Resistant hypertension is uncontrolled hypertension (BP >140/90 mmHg) despite maximal doses of three antihypertensive agents of which one is a diuretic.[22]

First, we should rule out pseudoresistance in which the below conditions may spuriously show resistance:
* Inaccurate measurements
* White coat phenomenon
* Agents that increase BP
* Medication noncompliance
* Some low-quality generic drugs

In resistant hypertension, we should encourage lifestyle changes and search for probable secondary causes of hypertension. Then we need to maximize antihypertensive agents' doses and use add-on drugs.

Despite all of these measures, some refractory patients still show resistance in ABPM and have SBPs more than 160 mmHg in the clinic. There may be some place for percutaneous intervention procedures in such challenging cases.[1]

Renal denervation, which is actually renal artery sympathetic nerve ablation, was a very attractive field of intervention, until publication of discouraging results of some blinded sham-controlled trials.[23, 24] Therefore, we should wait for larger and more accurate trials, possibly with better devices.

Another intervention is to deploy a carotid baroreceptor pacemaker, which has been promising in controlling resistant hypertension.[25, 26]

## HYPERTENSION IN PREGNANCY

Chronic hypertension can extend into the pregnancy period. The problem is that it can be superimposed by preeclampsia (see later).

Gestational hypertension is initiation of hypertension (BP >140/90 mmHg) after 20 weeks of gestation without preeclampsia features.

Preeclampsia is the same as gestational hypertension, but with one of the below conditions:
* Proteinuria (>300 mg/day)
* Thrombocytopenia (<100,000/μL)
* Renal failure
* Liver function impairment (doubling of hepatic enzymes)
* Pulmonary edema
* Visual or cerebral symptoms[27]

Patients with chronic or gestational hypertension should be followed closely. Their BPs must be checked twice per week and their platelets and hepatic enzymes and urinalysis checked weekly.[1] Hypertension in the third trimester should be considered serious, and drug therapy is of paramount importance in those with BPs above 160/110 mmHg. It is even suggested to give magnesium sulfate to these patients to prevent eclampsia.[28] The side effects of magnesium sulfate include motor paralysis, absence of reflexes, arrhythmia, and respiratory depression, which need calcium gluconate injection as an antidote.[29]

In preeclampsia, termination of pregnancy may be curative. If it is not possible, magnesium sulfate and labetalol are recommended, and some guidelines suggest nitroprusside.[11] More stable patients can receive oral agents such as labetalol, nifedipine, or methyldopa. In pulmonary edema, intravenous (IV) nitroglycerine is effective. For prevention of preeclampsia, it is suggested that pregnancy be avoided before 20 years of age. Low-dose aspirin is recommended for those with risk factors for preeclampsia.

After childbirth, there is still some risk, so the hypertensive mother should remain admitted for 3 days. If the mother takes high doses of propranolol and nifedipine, the secreted drugs in milk may be hazardous to the infant.[1]

## PERIOPERATIVE HYPERTENSION MANAGEMENT

Uncontrolled hypertension may be a risk factor in anesthesia and major surgeries. Severe hypertension (>180/110 mmHg) with symptoms of target organ damage can be an indication to postpone an elective surgery. The delay should be for 4–6 weeks. In other situations, hypertension can be controlled with oral and then IV agents and appropriate anesthesia during surgery.[30]

In the postoperative period, especially after cardiac surgeries, hypertension crises can occur, which need proper management.

## THERAPEUTIC GOALS IN HYPERTENSION

Maintaining BPs under 140/90 mmHg can be an appropriate goal in most hypertensive patients. Older adults with low BPs, regarding the J-curve hypothesis, could be at higher risk for adverse outcomes, orthostatic hypotension, and fallings. A controversial recommendation from the Joint National Committee on Prevention, Detection, Evaluation, and Treatment of High Blood Pressure 8 guideline (JNC 8) was to consider SBP less than 150 mmHg as the goal in patients older than 60 years (except patients with diabetes and CKD).[16] Newer guidelines assume 140/90 mmHg for 60- to 80-year-old patients unless they are fragile and SBP below 150 mmHg as the goal in patients older than 80 years of age.[3, 4] In patients with diabetes, DBP lower than 80–85 mmHg is advisable.[11, 31, 32]

When the Systolic Blood Pressure Intervention Trial (SPRINT) was published in 2015, it was shown that for patients with higher risk of cardiovascular events such as old age, CKD, or ischemic heart disease, SBP below 120 mmHg is beneficial.[33, 34]

## ACUTE BLOOD PRESSURE ELEVATIONS

Some situations can precipitate acute BP elevation:
- Treatment noncompliance
- High-salt food
- Infections
- Cardiovascular or cerebral events
- Seasonal changes (often patients need higher drug doses in winter)[35]
- Stress
- Natural course of a disease (e.g., pheochromocytoma, glomerulonephritis, preeclampsia)

There are three categories of acute BP rises:
1. Hypertension crises or emergencies: acute BP elevations often greater than 220/130 mmHg accompanied by target organ damage

2. Hypertensive urgencies: same as previous, but target organ damage does not exist
3. Severe hypertension: BPs 180/110 mmHg to 220/130 mmHg without target organ damage or symptoms

The first group needs IV antihypertensive agents, but the second and third groups can be managed with oral drugs.[1]

In hypertension emergencies, the rapidity of pressure rise is more important than the absolute number of the pressure. In some situations such as preeclampsia or glomerulonephritis, the crisis occurs with lower pressures. A full-blown hypertension crisis is often associated with retinopathy. The first stage of retinopathy is arterial diffuse narrowing. Then, arteriovenous nicking occurs. The third stage includes exudates and hemorrhages. Finally, papilledema occurs. Other features are nausea and vomiting, cardiac or renal failure, schistocytes in the peripheral blood smear, and hypertensive encephalopathy. This latter condition includes mental and cognitive disturbances with evidence of cerebral edema in imaging studies. Rarely, transient focal symptoms may occur. It shows that the BP is more than cerebral autoregulation tolerance. Cyclosporine and tacrolimus can cause such high pressures in heart transplant recipients. (The first-choice drugs are CCBs with diuretics and central sympatholytics.)

Generally, the drug of choice for hypertension crisis, especially hypertensive encephalopathy, is labetalol (Table 20.2). The rule of thumb is about 10% BP reduction in the first hour and then another 15% in the next 12 h to about 160/110 mmHg. Normal saline is recommended with antihypertensive drugs.[1] In some hypertensive emergencies, the BP must be lowered much more rapidly. Examples are aortic dissection, preeclampsia, and bleeding from suture lines after surgeries.

In acute ischemic strokes, if there is an indication to administer thrombolytics, the BP should be lowered to under 185/110 mmHg. If there is no indication to administer thrombolytics, antihypertensive drugs must be reserved only for those with pressures more than 220/120 mmHg.[1, 11] Labetalol is the first-choice drug.

In hemorrhagic strokes, labetalol or nicardipine are preferred. It is better to avoid nitroprusside and hydralazine.

In acute coronary syndromes, IV nitroglycerine and beta blockers are helpful, and in acute heart failure, nitroprusside with loop diuretics is recommended.

In pheochromocytoma, phentolamine administration must precede beta blockers.

In hypertension urgencies, some recommended oral drugs are as follows:

**TABLE 20.2**
**Intravenous Drugs for Treatment of Hypertensive Emergencies**

| Drug | Onset of Action | Half-Life | Dose | Contraindications and Side Effects |
|------|-----------------|-----------|------|-------------------------------------|
| Labetalol | 5–10 min | 3–6 h | 0.25–0.5 mg/kg; 2–4 mg/min until goal BP is reached; thereafter 5–20 mg/h | Second- or third-degree AV block, systolic heart failure, COPD (relative), bradycardia |
| Nicardipine | 5–15 min | 30–40 min | 5–15 mg/h as continuous infusion; starting dose of 5 mg/h; increase q15–30 min with 2.5 mg until goal BP achieved; thereafter decrease to 3 mg/h | Liver failure |
| Nitroprusside | Immediate | 1–2 min | 0.3–10 µg/kg/min; increase by 0.5 µg/kg/min q5 min until goal BP achieved | Liver or kidney failure (relative), cyanide toxicity |
| Nitroglycerin | 1–5 min | 3–5 min | 5–200 µg/min, 5 µg/min increase q5 min | |
| Urapidil | 3–5 min | 4–6 h | 12.5–25 mg as bolus injections; 5–40 mg/h as continuous infusion | |
| Esmolol | 1–2 min | 10–30 min | 0.5–1.0 mg/kg as bolus; 50–300 µg/kg/min as continuous infusion | Second- or third-degree AV block, systolic heart failure, COPD (relative), bradycardia |
| Phentolamine | 1–2 min | 3–5 min | 1–5 mg; repeat after 5–15 min until goal BP is reached; 0.5–1 mg/h as continuous infusion | Tachyarrhythmia, angina pectoris |

*AV*, atrioventricular; *BP*, blood pressure; *COPD*, chronic obstructive pulmonary disease.
Modified from van den Born BJ, Beutler JJ, Gaillard CA, et al. Dutch guideline for the management of hypertensive crisis—2010 revision. *Neth J Med.* 2011;69:248.

- Oral labetalol: 200–300 mg, repeated after 2–3 h and then twice daily
- Clonidine (if beta blockers are contraindicated): 0.1–0.2 mg; then 0.1 mg hourly
- Captopril: 25 mg, repeated after 1–2 h and then twice daily

## REFERENCES

1. Victor RG, Libby P. Systemic hypertension. In: Zipes DP, Libby P, Bonow RO, Mann DL, Tomaselli GF, Braunwald E, eds. *Braunwald's Heart Disease: A Textbook of Cardiovascular Medicine.* 11th ed. Philadelphia: WB Saunders; 2019:910–959.
2. Lim SS, Vos T, Flaxman AD, et al. A comparative risk assessment of burden of disease and injury attributable to 67 risk factors and risk factor clusters in 21 regions, 1990–2010: a systematic analysis for the Global Burden of Disease Study 2010. *Lancet.* 2012;380:2224–2260.
3. Whelton PK, Carey RM, et al. 2017 ACC/AHA/AAPA/ABC/ACPM/AGS/APhA/ASH/ASPC/NMA/PCNA guideline for the prevention, detection, evaluation, and management of high blood pressure in adults. *Hypertension.* 2018;71(6):e13–e115.
4. Williams B, Mancia G, et al. 2018 ESC/ESH guideline for the management of arterial hypertension of the European Society of Cardiology (ESC) and the European Society of Hypertension (ESH). *Eur Heart J.* 2018;39:3021–3104.
5. Jordana J, Yumukb V, Schlaichc M, et al. Joint statement of the European Association for the Study of Obesity and the European Society of Hypertension: obesity and difficult to treat arterial hypertension. *J Hypertens.* 2012;30:1047–1055.
6. Cloutier L, Daskalopoulou SS, Padwal RS, et al. A new algorithm for the diagnosis of hypertension in Canada. *Can J Cardiol.* 2015;31:620–630.
7. Dolan E, Stanton A, Thijs L, et al. Superiority of ambulatory over clinic blood pressure measurement in predicting mortality. The Dublin Outcome Study. *Hypertension.* 2005;46:156.
8. Hansen TW, Kikuya M, Thijs L, et al. Prognostic superiority of daytime ambulatory over conventional blood pressure in four populations: a meta-analysis of 7030 individuals. *J Hypertens.* 2007;25:1554–1564.
9. Grossman A, Messerli FH, Grossman E. Drug induced hypertension—an unappreciated cause of secondary hypertension. *Eur J Pharmacol.* 2015;763:15–22.
10. Kassel LE, Odum LE. Our own worst enemy: pharmacologic mechanisms of hypertension. *Adv Chronic Kidney Dis.* 2015;22(3):245–252.
11. Mancia G, Fagard R, et al. 2013 ESH/ESC guidelines for the management of arterial hypertension. The task force for the management of arterial hypertension of the European

Society of Hypertension (ESH) and of the European Society of Cardiology (ESC). *J Hypertens.* 2013;31: 1281–1357.

12. Ritchie J, Green D, Kalra PA. Current views on the management of atherosclerotic renovascular disease. *Ann Med.* 2012;44(suppl. 1):S98.

13. Wheatley K, Ives N, Gray R, et al. Revascularization versus medical therapy for renal-artery stenosis. *N Engl J Med.* 1953;361:2009.

14. Eckel RH, Jakicic JM, Ard JD, et al. 2013 AHA/ACC guideline on lifestyle management to reduce cardiovascular risk: a report of the American College of Cardiology/American Heart Association Task Force on Practice Guidelines. *J Am Coll Cardiol.* 2014;63 (25_PA):2960–2984.

15. Aronow WS, Fleg JL, Pepine CJ, et al. ACCF/AHA 2011 expert consensus document on hypertension in the elderly: a report of the American College of Cardiology Foundation Task Force on Clinical Expert Consensus Documents developed in collaboration with the American Academy of Neurology, American Geriatrics Society, American Society for Preventive Cardiology, American Society of Hypertension, American Society of Nephrology, Association of Black Cardiologists, and European Society of Hypertension. *J Am Soc Hypertens.* 2011;5:259.

16. James PA, Oparil S, Carter BL, et al. Evidence-based guideline for the management of high blood pressure in adults. Report from the panel members appointed to the Eighth Joint National Committee (JNC 8). *JAMA.* 2014; (2014). https://doi.org/10.1001/jama.2013.284427.

17. Fagard RH, Celis H, Thijs L, et al. Regression of left ventricular mass by antihypertensive treatment: a meta-analysis of randomized comparative studies. *Hypertension.* 2009;54:1084.

18. Argulian E, Grossman E, Messerli FH. Misconceptions and facts about treating hypertension. *Am J Med.* 2015;128:450–455.

19. Oliverasa A, Armariob P, Clara A, et al. Spironolactone versus sympathetic renal denervation to treat true resistant hypertension: results from the DENERVHTA study: a randomized controlled trial. *J Hypertens.* 2016;34:1863–1871.

20. Colussi GL, Catena C, Sechi LA. Spironolactone, eplerenone and the new aldosterone blockers in endocrine and primary hypertension. *J Hypertens.* 2013;31:3–15.

21. Williams B, MacDonald TM, Morant S, et al. Spironolactone versus placebo, bisoprolol, and doxazosin to determine the optimal treatment for drug-resistant hypertension (PATHWAY-2): a randomised, double-blind, crossover trial. *Lancet.* 2015;386: 2059–2068.

22. Calhoun DA, Jones D, Textor S, et al. Resistant hypertension: diagnosis, evaluation, and treatment. A scientific statement from the American Heart Association Professional Education Committee of the Council for High Blood Pressure Research. *Hypertension.* 2008;51:1403–1419.

23. Bhatt DL, Kandzari DE, O'Neill WO. A controlled trial of renal denervation for resistant hypertension. *N Engl J Med.* 2014;370:1393–1401.

24. Mathiassena ON, Vasea H, Bech JN, et al. Renal denervation in treatment-resistant essential hypertension. A randomized, SHAM-controlled, double-blinded 24-h blood pressure-based trial. *J Hypertens.* 2016;34:1639–1647.

25. Bisognano JD, Bakris G, Nadim MK, et al. Baroreflex activation therapy lowers BP in patients with resistant hypertension: results from the double-blind, randomized, placebo controlled Rheos pivotal trial. *J Am Coll Cardiol.* 2011;58:765.

26. Hoppe UC, Brandt MC, Wachter R. Minimally invasive system for baroreflex activation therapy chronically lowers blood pressure with pacemaker-like safety profile: results from the Barostim neo trial. *J Am Soc Hypertens.* 2012;6(4):270–276.

27. Roberts JM, August PA, Bakris G, et al. Hypertension in pregnancy. Report of the American College of Obstetricians and Gynecologists' Task Force on Hypertension in Pregnancy. *Obstet Gynecol.* 2013;122:1122.

28. Dennis AT, Chambers E, Serang K. Blood pressure assessment and first-line pharmacological agents in women with eclampsia. *Int J Obstet Anesth.* 2015;24:247–251.

29. McCarthy F, Kenny LC. Hypertension in pregnancy. *Obstet Gynaecol Reprod Med.* 2015;25:8.

30. James MFM, Dyer RA, Rayner BL. A modern look at hypertension and anaesthesia. *S Afr J Anaesth Analg.* 2011;17(2):168–173.

31. Canadian Hypertension Education Program (CHEP): 2013 Recommendations. (2013). http://www.hypertension.ca/ chep; 2013.

32. American Diabetes Association. Standards of medical care in diabetes 2013. *Diabetes Care.* 2013;36(suppl. 1):S11.

33. Wright Jr. JT, Williamson JD, Whelton PK. A randomized trial of intensive versus standard blood-pressure control. *N Engl J Med.* 2015;373:2103–2116.

34. Leung AA, Nerenberg K, Daskalopoulou SS, et al. Hypertension Canada's 2016 Canadian Hypertension Education Program guidelines for blood pressure measurement, diagnosis, assessment of risk, prevention, and treatment of hypertension. *Can J Cardiol.* 2016;32 (5):569–588.

35. Lewington S. Seasonal variation in blood pressure and its relationship with outdoor temperature in 10 diverse regions of China: the China Kadoorie Biobank. *J Hypertens.* 2012;30:1383–1391.

# Dyslipidemia

REZA KIANI

Cardiovascular Intervention Research Center, Rajaei Cardiovascular, Medical and Research Center, Iran University of Medical Sciences, Tehran, Iran

## KEY POINTS

- Lipoproteins play a major role in the metabolism of all types of tissues and are critical for normal function of various organs such as liver, brain, and heart muscle.
- Abnormal handling of lipoprotein metabolism contributes to atherosclerotic changes in the vascular endothelium and serious conditions such as cardiovascular events.
- Better understanding of lipid metabolism has led to the development of effective medications that have significantly changed blood lipid profile and outcome of patients.
- The field is continuously evolving and novel approaches such as gene therapy are expected to result in major new breakthroughs in the near future.

## INTRODUCTION

Abnormal lipid metabolism plays a major role in the early development of atherosclerotic disease in the cardiovascular system. Excessive cholesterol deposition in the endothelial cell membrane and its oxidation signal an inflammatory response by provoking migration of leukocytes and accumulation of foam cells in the endothelium. The resultant fatty streak is the early stage of the atherosclerotic process leading finally to stenotic and vulnerable plaques and its complications such as ischemia and infarction. Numerous studies have demonstrated the negative impact of high blood cholesterol level on cardiovascular health. On the other hand, primitive human societies with low-fat diets have much lower rates of atherosclerotic cardiovascular problems compared with modern societies.

## BIOCHEMISTRY AND METABOLISM OF LIPIDS

Lipidic molecular structures have many critical roles in a wide variety of cells and organs. Lipids are an important source of energy, function as an essential part of the cell membrane, and are used for the production of steroid hormones and bile acids. Major components of lipids are sterols (including cholesterol and cholesteryl ester), triglycerides, and phospholipids. Triglycerides are composed of three fatty acids attached to the three hydroxyl groups of one molecule of glycerol. The three fatty acids could be the same but usually are of different chain lengths, creating numerous possibilities of combinations and different structures of triglycerides. In phospholipids, the third hydroxyl position of glycerol contains a phosphate group attached to basically four different molecules: choline, serine, inositol, and ethanolamine. So, there are four major phospholipids: phosphatidylcholine (lecithin), phosphatidylethanolamine, phosphatidylserine, and phosphatidylinositol. There are also other structurally related molecules to phospholipids such as sphingomyelin, which has important functions in neural signal transmission and also in specialized structures of cell membrane such as lipid rafts.

Lipoproteins are composed of various types of lipids and proteins. They are assembled in the intestine and liver and are the major mode of transportation of lipids in the aqueous environment of plasma. The basic structure of lipoproteins is composed of a bilayer membrane enveloping a nearly spherical core.[1] Hydrophilic components such as cholesterol, phospholipids, and proteins including apolipoproteins are part of the membrane, while hydrophobic cholesteryl ester and triglycerides constitute the core. Apolipoproteins have various functions. They may act as a ligand for receptors in target cells or as a cofactor for activation or inhibition of different enzymes (Fig. 21.1).

There are five major types of lipoproteins: chylomicron, VLDL (very low-density lipoprotein), IDL

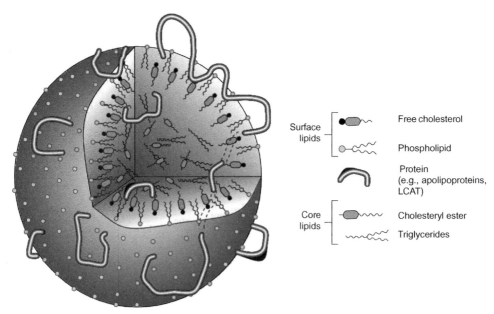

Surface lipids
- ⬤〜 Free cholesterol
- ◯〜 Phospholipid

〜 Protein (e.g., apolipoproteins, LCAT)

Core lipids
- ⬭〜 Cholesteryl ester
- 〜〜 Triglycerides

FIG. 21.1 Basic structure of lipoprotein particle. It is composed of a bi-layer membrane of hydrophilic components and a lipophilic core.

(intermediate-density lipoprotein), LDL (low-density lipoprotein), and HDL (high-density lipoprotein). The size of the particle has an inverse relationship with its density. So, HDL is the smallest particle while chylomicron and VLDL are the largest.

### Intestinal Pathway

Chylomicron is assembled in the intestinal epithelium. Absorbed fatty acids are reesterified to form triglycerides and they are added to apo B48 to form chylomicrons.[2] Apo B48 is derived from apo B100 by apo B48 editing enzyme complex (ApoBec). Apo B48 contains the first 48% of apo B100's amino acids and is only produced in the intestine. Chylomicrons enter the portal system and could interact with lipoprotein lipase (LPL) on the surface of muscle cells or adipose cells. LPL separates all three fatty acids from glycerol. Fatty acids could be used as a source of energy by muscle cells or be stored in adipose tissue in the form of triglyceride. Apo C-II, an apolipoprotein mainly present in chylomicron and VLDL, activates LPL while another apo, apo C-III inhibits its activity. The process of fatty acid uptake is also insulin-dependent and could be impaired in diabetes with resultant hypertriglyceridemia.

### Hepatic Pathway

Hepatic pathway serves as a provider of triglycerides and cholesterol during fasting. It begins with the production of VLDL in the liver. VLDL has apo B100 as its main apolipoprotein.[3] Microsomal triglyceride transfer protein (MTP) is pivotal for assembly of triglycerides to apo B100 and production of primordial VLDL or VLDL1. Further lipidation and attachment of other lipoproteins produce mature VLDL or VLDL2 which can enter the circulation. VLDL can have the same interactions with LPL as chylomicron. VLDL also has many interactions with HDL particle. HDL transfers apo C's and apo E to VLDL. There is also an exchange of triglyceride and cholesteryl ester by cholesteryl ester transferase protein (CETP). Another enzyme, phospholipid transferase protein transfers phospholipids from VLDL to HDL. This process of losing triglyceride and phospholipid and increased content of cholesteryl ester leads to a smaller and denser lipoprotein called IDL. IDL can be absorbed by the liver or continue the same catabolic process of VLDL to become an even denser particle called LDL. LDL is the main source of circulating cholesterol in humans. There is a strict regulation of cholesterol content in cells. It can be regulated by modifying the process of cholesterol synthesis within cells or its uptake by LDL receptor which binds to apo B100. Accordingly, there is an upregulation of LDL receptor when there is a shortage of cholesterol and vice versa.[4]

LDL's core contains mainly cholesteryl ester. Its triglyceride content can be influenced by the level of plasma triglyceride. In hypertriglyceridemia, LDL's core will contain more triglyceride and becomes denser and smaller. This form of LDL is more atherogenic because of its increased half-life and is partly responsible for the increased risk of atherosclerotic disease in diabetes and metabolic syndrome.

## Reverse Cholesterol Transport

HDL is produced in the liver and intestine. ATP-binding cassette A-1 (ABCA1) adds phospholipids and some cholesterol to apo A1. This forms a primordial or nascent HDL which has very low cholesterol. Upon reaching cell membrane, nascent HDL interacts with SR-B1, ABCG1, and ABCA1 which mediate the transport of cholesterol from cell membrane to the HDL.[5] Lecithin cholesterol acyltransferase (LCAT) esterifies cholesterol into cholesteryl ester and it is stored in the HDL core. This mature HDL then transports cholesterol to the liver where it can be used to form new VLDL particles or further metabolized for bile acid production.

HDL particle acts as a pivotal player in reverse transport of cholesterol from the cell membrane into the liver. It promotes cholesterol efflux from cell membrane and as a result, the cholesterol content of the cell is decreased. In the vascular endothelium, this cholesterol uptake will decrease LDL oxidation and therefore, exerts antiinflammatory and antiatherogenic effects.[6]

## LIPOPROTEIN DISORDERS

Lipoprotein abnormalities are very common. It affects nearly half of the adult population in the United States.[7] Lipid disorders could be classified as primary or secondary. The vast majority of lipoprotein disorders are secondary to other metabolic disorders such as diabetes mellitus, obesity, and metabolic syndrome. Other medical conditions with significant impact on lipid profile include hypothyroidism, nephrotic syndrome, chronic renal failure, primary biliary cirrhosis, and use of medications. Primary disorders are caused by defective expression of genes related to important steps in production or metabolism of lipoproteins. They could be due to monogenic mutations such as familial hypercholesterolemia (FH) or familial dysbetalipoproteinemia or could be polygenic. The old classification of primary lipid disorders (type I to type V) has been outdated as it does not specify the etiology and it does not include many newly discovered disorders such as genetic abnormalities of HDL.

### Primary Lipid Disorders
#### Familial hypercholesterolemia
FH is an autosomal codominant disorder. Its heterozygote phenotype has a prevalence of about 1:500. It is

caused by mutations in LDL receptor, so the clearance of LDL is impaired. It is characterized by high LDL level, premature cardiovascular disease, and peripheral phenomena such as tendinous xanthoma, xanthelasma, and corneal arcus.[8] Cardiovascular involvement in homozygous form occurs in childhood. Many nonfunctional mutations of LDL-R have been identified and have been correlated to FH. There are also genetic abnormalities other than LDL-R mutations which are clinically indistinguishable from FH. These include familial defective apo B100 which is caused by mutations in LDL-R ligand (apo B100), or gain-of-function mutations in PCSK9, which is a convertase related to downregulation of LDL-R. There are also polygenic forms of hypercholesterolemia which are due to a combination of increased apo B production and decreased expression of LDL-R.

#### Familial hypertriglyceridemia
It is a common, polygenic disorder with high fasting and postprandial plasma triglyceride levels.[9] LDL level is usually within normal limits. It is not associated with atherosclerosis or peripheral manifestations such as xanthomas. The etiology is probably overproduction of TG-reach VLDL; however, production of apo B may not be increased. Familial hyperchylomicronemia is associated with more severe hypertriglyceridemia than familial hypertriglyceridemia. It is usually caused by single nonfunctional mutations of LPL or its cofactor, apo C-II. It is also associated with eruptive xanthoma and a higher risk of pancreatitis.

#### Dysbetalipoproteinemia
It is a rare, autosomal recessive disorder related to mutation of apo E and defective clearance of apo E-containing particles such as chylomicron, VLDL, and IDL.[9] Laboratory measurement shows elevated levels of both cholesterol and TG; however, the ratio of VLDL:TG is higher than familial hypertriglyceridemia and other combined lipid disorders. These patients have a higher risk of CAD and could also manifest pathognomonic forms of xanthomas such as tuberoeruptive and palmar striated xanthoma.

#### Familial combined hyperlipidemia
It is the most common hereditary lipid disorder. It is characterized by an increased level of LDL cholesterol, triglyceride, and apo B100.[10] There is an increased risk of premature CVD and the phenotype should also be present in at least one first-degree relative. The underlying metabolic defect is the overproduction of apo B100 in the liver combined with decreased activity of LPL.

Metabolic syndrome has many features in common with familial combined hyperlipidemia; however, the metabolic syndrome does not follow a distinctive hereditary pattern.

### Genetic HDL abnormalities

HDL has complex functions in lipid metabolism and currently many aspects of its function are not fully understood. A wide range of genetic mutations affecting HDL production and function have been detected; however, many of them do not have a significant correlation with cardiovascular disease.[11] For example, the loss-of-function mutation of LCAT leads to very low HDL levels because cholesterol esterification and HDL maturation are impaired. Interestingly, the risk of CVD is not increased in patients with LCAT deficiency. Another example is a Tangier disease in which ABCA1 is non-functional and very low HDL level is observed; again, risk of CVD does not appear to be increased. In CETP deficiency, HDL level is dramatically high because of deficient transport of cholesteryl ester from HDL to other lipoproteins. However, this does not have a protective effect against CVD. In familial hypoalphalipoproteinemia, mutations in apo A-I results in a decreased level of HDL. Some of these mutations are associated with premature CVD and xanthomas. Apo A-I Milano is caused by a single amino acid substitution in Apo A-I (cysteine for arginine). This mutant HDL seems to be very efficient in promoting cholesterol efflux from the cell membrane and in some animal models, infusion of apo A-I Milano had promising results in regression of atherosclerosis.

## IMPACT OF LIPOPROTEIN DISORDERS ON CARDIOVASCULAR RISK

Many observational studies have confirmed the positive association between increased total cholesterol or LDL-C level and the incidence of CVD-related outcomes. The proportional effects of increased cholesterol on CVD is greater in younger ages, as the individual is exposed to higher cholesterol levels for a longer time; however, the absolute effects on CVD mortality increase sharply with age. There is also plenty of evidence showing that interventions aimed at reducing LDL-C levels significantly reduce CVD-related outcomes in both short term and long term.[12,13] In some studies, this positive effect is even observed in individuals with normal baseline cholesterol levels.[14]

Triglyceride level has not been consistently associated with increased risk of cardiovascular disease; however, there is increasing evidence that plasma TG levels,[15] especially postprandial TG levels, may have

significant predictive value for adverse outcomes of cardiovascular disease. Currently, interventions to reduce TG levels have not shown to improve outcome independent of LDL-lowering effects of medications. HDL-C level has a significant inverse relationship with the occurrence of cardiovascular disease.[16] Furthermore, it has been shown that addition of HDL-C to total cholesterol (as a surrogate of LDL-C) improves its predictive power, so the ratio of total cholesterol to HDL-C has emerged as a strong prognostic factor. Like triglyceride, interventions to improve HDL-C levels have not been associated with a better outcome.

Apo B100 particle size and number measurement have been proposed as an alternative for conventional lipid markers. Especially, small dense LDL particle has been the focus of attention as it is strongly related to increased incidence of CVD in diabetics and individuals with metabolic syndrome. However, LDL particle measurement has not been superior to LDL-C or total cholesterol/HDL-C ratio.

HDL particle number has been shown to be as useful as HDL-C for prediction of CVD-related outcomes.[17] However, unlike HDL-C, it is independent of other markers such as LDL-C or triglyceride-rich particles.

## MANAGEMENT OF LIPOPROTEIN DISORDERS

Nonpharmacologic management of hyperlipidemia generally includes control of other risk factors, regular exercise, weight loss, and a healthy diet. Low-fat diet is not necessarily associated with a better control of hyperlipidemia or lower cardiovascular adverse events. Instead, adoption of a dietary pattern low in saturated fat, cholesterol, and refined carbohydrate dramatically improves these endpoints.

### Statins

Statins block the formation of mevalonate by inhibiting hydroxymethylglutaryl–coenzyme-A reductase (HMG-CoA) which is pivotal in the production of cholesterol in the liver. Decreased cholesterol content of cells leads to upregulation of LDL-R and increased clearance of LDL from plasma. Statins also have complex effects on the metabolism of TG and HDL which is partly explained by modifying signaling proteins in cell membrane and phosphorylation of peroxisome proliferator-activated receptor alpha (PPAR alpha).

Statins have also antiinflammatory and antithrombotic properties which add to their beneficial effects in the cardiovascular system.

Statins have been the subject of numerous randomized clinical trials. These trials show a significant risk reduction in patients with cardiovascular disease.[12,13] The degree of risk reduction has a linear relationship with an absolute decrease in LDL-C level; a 1 mmol/L (about 39 mg/dL) decrease in LDL-C level was associated with about 20% reduction in cardiovascular events.

Statins are very effective in LDL cholesterol lowering. An intermediate dose of most statins will reduce cholesterol by 30%–50%. High doses provide an additional 6% decrease in LDL-C level. Statins are generally safe and serious side effects are very rare.[18] Most notable side effects include new-onset diabetes (0.1%–0.3%) and rhabdomyolysis (0.01%). Statin use has also been associated with minimal increased risk of intracranial hemorrhage (0.01%). Hepatic enzyme elevation is common but hepatotoxicity and hepatic failure are very unusual and are commonly due to drug interactions or other medical conditions. Overall, the discontinuation of statins due to intolerance is observed in less than 1% of patients.

Myalgia occurs frequently (10% of patients) but is benign and alleviates with dose reduction. Myalgia and the risk of myositis increase in patients with preexisting musculoskeletal problems such as polymyalgia rheumatica and myopathies. Hypothyroidism also predisposes to statin-induced muscle symptoms. In case of persistent muscle symptoms in patients taking statins, it is recommended to stop the drug, check plasma creatine kinase level for the possibility of rhabdomyolysis and search for possible coexisting musculoskeletal problems. After alleviation of the symptoms, low-dose statin could be initiated and uptitrated slowly.

## Ezetimibe

Ezetimibe interferes with intestinal cholesterol absorption by inhibition of Niemann–Pick C1-Like 1 (NPC1L1). NPC1L1 promotes the absorption of cholesterol and other plant sterols. Effects of ezetimibe are additive to statins, so it can be used in patients already on statins to reduce LDL-C level further. Recently, it has been shown that addition of ezetimibe to statins also improves outcome in patients with cardiovascular disease.[19] Ezetimibe is the drug of choice in the treatment of sitosterolemia, a rare disorder resembling FH which is due to increased absorption of plant sterols in the intestine.

## Fibrates

Fibrates modify transcription of PPAR alpha. PPAR alpha is a nuclear receptor which is important in the metabolism of triglyceride-rich lipoproteins and HDL. As a result, fibrates increase HDL-C level and reduce TG level. Its effect on LDL is minimal or it may increase LDL-C level by induction of VLDL lipolysis. Earlier studies on fibrates in cardiovascular patients reported benefits in the outcome; however, major recent studies have not shown any improvement when fibrates are added to statins. There may be implications for statin use in severe hypertriglyceridemia but it is not clear whether it is superior to weight reduction and lifestyle modification. Indeed, lowering the TG level has not been associated with a net clinical benefit in cardiovascular or diabetic patients.[20] Fibrates especially gemfibrozil interferes with the metabolism of statins and the combination of gemfibrozil and statins should be avoided.

## Niacin

Nicotinic acid or niacin increases HDL and decreases TG levels. The mechanism of action of niacin is not completely understood. It is particularly effective in raising HDL-C level.[21] However, like fibrates, adding niacin to statins was not associated with an increased clinical benefit. Side effects are common including flushing, GI upset, hepatotoxicity, impaired glucose tolerance, and hyperuricemia. Not surprisingly, patient adherence to treatment is low.

## Bile Acid Sequestrants

Bile acid sequestrants (BASs) bind to bile acids in the intestine and inhibit their absorption. Bile acids are derived from cholesterol and increased bile excretion significantly lowers the cholesterol content of the body. It is an effective cholesterol-lowering agent without any serious side effect.[22] It could be used as an adjunct to statins if the target LDL-C levels could not be achieved with high-dose statins. It is considered safe in children and is an important part of the treatment of FH in young patients. BAS interferes with the absorption of drugs and should not be used at the same time with other medications. Since BAS may induce hepatic production of VLDL, it is prohibited in patients with severe hypertriglyceridemia including dysbetalipoproteinemia.

## Fish Oil

Fish oil contains omega-3 fatty acids. These polyunsaturated fatty acids decrease VLDL secretion in the liver and have been used successfully in patients with severe hypertriglyceridemia. Omega-3 fatty acids had promising results in the primary prevention of cardiovascular disease.[23] However, clinical benefits in diagnosed CVD patients are less clear.

## Plant Sterols/Stanols

Plant sterols and stanol esters decrease the intestinal absorption of cholesterol and bile acids. It has been effective in lowering LDL-C level when used alone or in combination with statins. Like fish oil, plant sterol/stanols are currently recommended for primary prevention but data is lacking on its efficacy for secondary prevention.

### Mipomersen

Mipomersen inhibits apo B100 production by blocking its messenger RNA in the liver. It has been used as adjunctive therapy in homozygous FH.[24] There is currently limited data about the safety profile of the drug.

### Lomitapide

Lomitapide is another novel adjunctive agent for the management of FH.[25] It is an MTP inhibitor and prevents the production of VLDL in hepatic cells. Most frequent side effects include increased liver enzyme levels and some degrees of gastrointestinal upset.

### PCSK9 Inhibitors

Proprotein convertase subtilisin/kexin type 9 (PCSK9) is a convertase protein which binds to LDL-R and renders it nonfunctional. So, inhibition of PCSK9 upregulates LDL-R and increases the clearance of LDL from plasma. PCSK9 inhibitors have been very effective in LDL-C lowering.[26] In patients who cannot tolerate statins, PCSK9 inhibitors have been shown to be more effective than ezetimibe in terms of lowering LDL plasma levels.[27] These agents improved all-cause mortality but not cardiovascular death or MI in short-term follow-up; however, their long-term impact on cardiovascular outcomes are not clear yet.[28,29] PCSK9 inhibitors have been approved for the treatment of statin-intolerant patients and as an adjunctive agent in FH.

### LDL Apheresis

LDL apheresis is very effective in lowering cholesterol level and cardiovascular outcome in FH. It is the first line of treatment in homozygous FH and is recommended for heterozygous FH if cholesterol level could not be controlled by current medications.[30] It is a costly treatment and there is no consensus on selecting patients for apheresis.

## TREATMENT GOALS IN LIPOPROTEIN DISORDERS

There has been debate over optimal cholesterol level for patients receiving lipid-lowering therapy. In 2018, the American College of Cardiology/American Heart Association issued a guideline for the management of hyperlipidemia.[31] For secondary prevention, it recommends high-intensity treatment to achieve an LDL-C level

decrease of at least 50%. This could be achieved by high-dose statin alone or in combination with other agents. In very high-risk settings such as recent acute coronary syndrome, history of myocardial infarction or stroke, the guideline suggests a more aggressive approach to reach an LDL-C level of less than 70 mg/dL. If the goal cannot be achieved by statins, it is recommended to add ezetimibe or PCSK9 inhibitors. For primary prevention, projected risk assessment of the individual will guide the intensity of treatment. Individuals with an estimated 10-year risk of atherosclerosis of more than 20% need high-intensity treatment to reach 50% reduction of LDL-C level. High-risk diabetics and patients with a baseline LDL-C level higher than 190 mg/dL also fall into this category. For individuals with a projected risk of 7.5%–20%, moderate-intensity therapy to achieve a 30%–50% decrease in LDL-C level is recommended.

European Society of Cardiology recommends a target LDL-C level of 55–70 mg/dL for patients with cardiovascular involvement.[32] For FH patients or diabetes at very high risk of future events, drug therapy to reach a level of less than 55 mg/dL was also suggested. For lower risk subjects, higher LDL-C levels may be accepted.

Regardless of which guideline is used for clinical practice, the presence of atherosclerotic cardiovascular disease, diabetes, and the estimated risk of future cardiovascular events are important factors to consider before initiation of medications and deciding about the intensity of treatment or setting target levels for individuals with hyperlipidemia.

## REFERENCES

1. Ginsberg HN. Lipoprotein physiology. *Endocrinol Metab Clin North Am.* 1998;27:503–519.
2. Williams KJ. Molecular processes that handle—and mishandle—dietary lipids. *J Clin Invest.* 2008;118:3247–3259.
3. Fisher EA, Ginsberg HN. Complexity in the secretory pathway: the assembly and secretion of apolipoprotein B-containing lipoproteins. *J Biol Chem.* 2002;277:17377–17380.
4. Brown MS, Goldstein JL. A receptor-mediated pathway for cholesterol homeostasis. *Science.* 1986;232:34.
5. Tall AR, Yvan-Charvet L, Terasaka N, Pagler T, Wang N. HDL, ABC transporters, and cholesterol efflux: implications for the treatment of atherosclerosis. *Cell Metab.* 2008;7:365–375.
6. Khera AV, Cuchel M, de la Llera-Moya M, et al. Cholesterol efflux capacity, high-density lipoprotein function, and atherosclerosis. *N Engl J Med.* 2011;364:127.

CHAPTER 21  Dyslipidemia  **393**

7. Wong ND, Lopez V, Tang S, Williams GR. Prevalence, treatment, and control of combined hypertension and hypercholesterolemia in the United States. *Am J Cardiol.* 2006;98(2):204–208.

8. Humphries SE. Guidelines for the identification and management of patients with familial hypercholesterolaemia (FH): are we coming to a consensus? *Atheroscler Suppl.* 2011;12:217.

9. Hachem SB, Mooradian AD. Familial dyslipidaemias: an overview of genetics, pathophysiology and management. *Drugs.* 2006;66:1949–1969.

10. deGraaf J, Veerkamp MJ, Stalenhoef AF. Metabolic pathogenesis of familial combined hyperlipidaemia with emphasis on insulin resistance, adipose tissue metabolism and free fatty acids. *J R Soc Med.* 2002;95(suppl. 42):46–53.

11. Voight BF, Peloso GM, Orho-Melander M, et al. Plasma HDL cholesterol and risk of myocardial infarction: a mendelian randomisation study. *Lancet.* 2012;380:572.

12. LaRosa JC, Grundy SM, Waters DD, et al. Intensive lipid lowering with atorvastatin in patients with stable coronary disease. *N Engl J Med.* 2005;352:1425–1435.

13. Cannon CP, Braunwald E, McCabe CH, et al. Intensive versus moderate lipid lowering with statins after acute coronary syndromes. *N Engl J Med.* 2004;350:1495–1504.

14. Ridker PM, Danielson E, Fonseco FAH, et al. Rosuvastatin to prevent vascular events in men and women with elevated C-reactive protein. *N Engl J Med.* 2008;359:2195–2207.

15. Miller M, Stone NJ, Ballantyne C, et al. Triglycerides and cardiovascular disease: a scientific statement from the American Heart Association. *Circulation.* 2011;123:2292–2333.

16. Boekholdt SM, Arsenault BJ, Mora S, et al. Association of LDL cholesterol, non-HDL cholesterol, and apolipoprotein B levels with risk of cardiovascular events among patients treated with statins: a meta-analysis. *JAMA.* 2012;307:1302.

17. El Harchaoui K, Arsenault BJ, Franssen R, et al. High-density lipoprotein particle size and concentration and coronary risk. *Ann Intern Med.* 2009;150:84–93.

18. Stone NJ, Robinson J, Lichtenstein AH, et al. 2013 ACC/AHA guideline on the treatment of blood cholesterol to reduce atherosclerotic cardiovascular risk in adults: a report of the American College of Cardiology/American Heart Association Task Force on Practice Guidelines. *Circulation.* 2014;129:S1–S45.

19. Cannon CP, Blazing MA, Giugliano RP, et al. Ezetimibe added to statin therapy after acute coronary syndromes. *N Engl J Med.* 2015;372:2387–2397.

20. Keech A, Simes RJ, Barter P, et al. Effects of long-term fenofibrate therapy on cardiovascular events in 9795 people with type 2 diabetes mellitus (the FIELD study): randomised controlled trial. *Lancet.* 2005;366:1849–1861.

21. Brown BG, Zhao XQ. Nicotinic acid, alone and in combinations, for reduction of cardiovascular risk. *Am J Cardiol.* 2008;101:58B–62B.

22. Einarsson K, Ericsson S, Ewerth S, et al. Bile acid sequestrants: mechanisms of action on bile acid and cholesterol metabolism. *Eur J Clin Pharmacol.* 1991;40(suppl. 1):S53–S58.

23. Yokoyama M, Origasa H. Effects of eicosapentaenoic acid on cardiovascular events in Japanese patients with hypercholesterolemia: rationale, design, and baseline characteristics of the Japan EPA Lipid Intervention Study (JELIS). *Am Heart J.* 2003;146:613–620.

24. Agarwala A, Jones P, Nambi V. The role of antisense oligonucleotide therapy in patients with familial hypercholesterolemia: risks, benefits, and management recommendations. *Curr Atheroscler Rep.* 2015;17:467.

25. Cuchel M, Meagher EA, du Toit Theron H, et al. Efficacy and safety of a microsomal triglyceride transfer protein inhibitor in patients with homozygous familial hypercholesterolaemia: a single-arm, open-label, phase 3 study. *Lancet.* 2013;381(9860):40–46.

26. Raal FJ, Stein E, Dufour R, et al. PCSK9 inhibition with evolocumab (AMG 145) in heterozygous familial hypercholesterolaemia (RUTHERFORD-2): a randomised, double-blind, placebo-controlled trial. *Lancet.* 2014;385:331–340.

27. Moriarty PM, Thompson PD, Cannon CP, et al. Efficacy and safety of alirocumab vs ezetimibe in statin-intolerant patients, with a statin rechallenge arm: the odyssey alternative randomized trial. *J Clin Lipidol.* 2015;9(6):758–769.

28. Sabatine MS, Giugliano RP, Keech AC, et al. Evolocumab and clinical outcomes in patients with cardiovascular disease. *N Engl J Med.* 2017;376:1713–1722.

29. Schwartz GG, Steg PG, Szarek M, et al. Alirocumab and cardiovascular outcomes after acute coronary syndrome. *N Engl J Med.* 2018;379:2097–2107.

30. Thompsen J, Thompson PD. A systematic review of LDL apheresis in the treatment of cardiovascular disease. *Atherosclerosis.* 2006;189(1):31–38.

31. Grundy SM, Stone NJ, Bailey AL, et al. AHA/ACC/AACVPR/AAPA/ABC/ACPM/ADA/AGS/APhA/ASPC/NLA/PCNA guideline on the management of blood cholesterol: executive summary: a report of the American College of Cardiology/American Heart Association Task Force on Clinical Practice Guidelines. *J Am Coll Cardiol.* 2019;73:3168–3209.

32. Mach FO, Colin Baigent C, Catapano AL, et al. 2019 ESC/EAS guidelines for the management of dyslipidaemias: lipid modification to reduce cardiovascular risk. The Task Force for the management of dyslipidaemias of the European Society of Cardiology (ESC) and European Atherosclerosis Society (EAS). *Eur Heart J.* 2020;41:111–188. https://doi.org/10.1093/eurheartj/ehz455.

# CHAPTER 22

# ST-Segment Elevation Myocardial Infarction

BAHRAM MOHEBBI

Cardiovascular Intervention Research Center, Cardio-Oncology Research Center, Rajaie Cardiovascular, Medical & Research Center, Iran University of Medical Sciences, Tehran, Iran

## KEY POINTS

- A clinical or pathologic event caused by myocardial ischemia when there is evidence of myocardial injury or necrosis is explained as myocardial infarction (MI).
- Chest discomfort, dyspnea, palpitation, and syncope are common manifestations of ST-segment elevation myocardial infarction (STEMI).
- Electrocardiography is used in the early diagnosis of patients with suspected STEMI with a special focus on ST-segment elevation or new left bundle branch block.
- Different biomarkers are used to evaluate patients with suspected acute MI. The cardiac troponins (cTn) I and T (preferred biomarkers) and the MB isoenzyme of creatine kinase (CK-MB), if a cardiac-specific troponin assay is not available, are used.
- The reperfusion strategy of the infarcted artery with primary percutaneous coronary intervention or fibrinolytic therapy improves myocardial recovery and reduces mortality compared with no reperfusion.
- Major complications in STEMI include conduction abnormalities after MI, ventricular arrhythmia during acute MI, mechanical complications of STEMI, and pericardial complications of MI.

## DEFINITION

A clinical or pathologic event caused by myocardial ischemia when there is evidence of myocardial injury or necrosis is named as myocardial infarction (MI).[1,2] Diagnosis is made when there is a rise and/or fall of cardiac biomarkers [preferably cardiac troponin (cTn) with at least one value above the 99th percentile upper reference limit (URL) and at least one of the following: symptoms of ischemia, electrocardiographic (ECG) changes including pathologic Q waves, new or presumed new significant ST-segment–T wave (ST-T) changes or new left bundle branch block (LBBB), identification of an intracoronary thrombus by angiography or autopsy, or imaging evidence of new loss of myocardial viability or new regional wall motion abnormality].

According to the assumed cause of myocardial ischemia, the clinical classification is as follows:

- Type 1 (spontaneous MI): MI caused by a pathologic process in the wall of the coronary artery such as plaque erosion or rupture, fissuring, or dissection, resulting in intraluminal thrombus.

- Type 2 (MI secondary to an ischemic imbalance): MI consequent to enhanced oxygen demand or decreased supply such as coronary endothelial dysfunction, coronary artery spasm, coronary artery embolus, tachy- or bradyarrhythmias, anemia, respiratory failure, hypertension, or hypotension.
- Type 3 (MI resulting in death because of the unavailability of biomarker values): Sudden unexpected cardiac death before checking biomarkers to assess the change or before cardiac biomarkers could increase.
- Type 4a [MI related to percutaneous coronary intervention (PCI)]: When elevation of biomarker values (cTn is preferred) is greater than 5 × 99th percentile URL in patients with normal baseline values (<99th percentile URL) or a rise of values more than 20% if the baseline values are elevated but stable or falling, PCI-related MI occurred. Besides (1) symptoms of myocardial ischemia, (2) new pathologic Q waves or new LBBB, (3) patency loss of major coronary artery or a side branch or no flow/slow flow or embolization, or (4) imaging facts of new loss of viable

myocardium or new regional wall motion abnormality is required.

- Type 4b (MI related to stent thrombosis): Stent thrombosis-associated MI is detected by coronary angiography/autopsy in the presence of myocardial ischemia and with typical rise and/or fall in cardiac biomarkers, at least one value above the 99th percentile URL.
- Type 5 [MI related to coronary artery bypass graft (CABG) surgery]: CABG-associated MI explained by elevation of cardiac biomarker values greater than $10 \times$ 99th percentile URL in patients with normal baseline cTn values. Also (1) new pathologic Q waves or new LBBB, (2) angiography-documented new graft or native coronary artery occlusion, or (3) imaging evidence of new loss of viable myocardium or new regional wall motion abnormality.

In patients with an acute ST-segment elevation myocardial infarction (STEMI), immediate diagnosis is crucial. It can be more highlighted in which reperfusion therapy consider as soon as possible after diagnosis. Relieving ischemic pain, hemodynamic assessment, starting reperfusion therapy with PCI or using fibrinolysis agents, and antithrombotic therapy to prevent rethrombosis or acute stent thrombosis must be considered as initials goals after acute STEMI diagnosis. The next step in risk reduction of recurrent coronary artery thrombosis is antiplatelet therapy. In terms of existing left ventricular (LV) thrombus or chronic atrial fibrillation, anticoagulation therapy must be started.

Some patients are diagnosed with STEMI when hospitalized for other problems. In respect to their specific issues, the approach is similar to that used in patients referred to emergency units with STEMI. But evidence has revealed that the diagnosis of STEMI in inpatients is not timely and even longer than patients referred to emergency units for cardiac problems, which can result in lower survival rates.[3]

### ST-Segment Elevation Myocardial Infarction in Special Groups

Some special groups such as older adults (especially those with hypertension, chronic kidney disease, cerebrovascular events, and more complex STEMI that may appear as cardiac arrest and cardiogenic shock), women, and patients with cocaine-associated MI may have poor outcomes, so they need more attention in terms of STEMI. Although STEMI is common in older adults, ECG may reveal ST-segment depression or may be nondiagnostic for STEMI.[4] Approximately 60%–65% of STEMIs happen in patients 65 years of age or older and 28%–33% occur in patients 75 of age or

older.[4–6] Patients 75 years of age or older have higher inhospital mortality rates from electrical and mechanical complications.[4] Primary PCI can lead to better outcomes than fibrinolysis in older adults who need more attention to prevent severe bleeding resulting from the use of fibrinolysis and antithrombotic therapy.[4]

Although women present with more atypical symptoms (being older and more hypertensive, having a higher risk of bleeding, and having a greater delay to show symptoms), the approach is the same as in other patients. Acute plaque rupture followed by thrombosis causes STEMI in the majority of women, but STEMI may be caused by coronary artery dissection in young or peripartum individuals. On the other hand, myocarditis, aortic dissection, or stress-induced cardiomyopathy should be considered in women with clinical diagnosis of acute coronary syndromes (ACSs).

STEMI also can be a complication of cocaine-induced ischemia. However, there are two points to consider in these kinds of patients. First, due to the possibility of exacerbation of coronary artery vasoconstriction, benzodiazepines should be administered early because benzodiazepines may improve chest discomfort and have beneficiary effects on hemodynamic. Second, beta-blockers should not be used in patients with acute cocaine intoxication accompanied by chest pain.[7]

An important issue to note is that death in patients with STEMI is higher among those with coronary artery stent thrombosis as opposed to ruptured plaque. The treatment choice is similar to that in spontaneous STEMI. Also, thrombolytic therapy could be used in STEMI patients with coronary artery stent thrombosis.

There is a need to pay close attention to assess specific groups in the ACS setting to implement timely and appropriate intervention procedures to achieve better outcomes.

### CLINICAL EVALUATION

When patients with a possible ACS come to the emergency unit and then the coronary care unit, assessment should be initiated based on accurate principles. Special attention should be paid to check responsiveness, airway, breathing, and circulation, and in the case of respiratory or cardiorespiratory arrest, appropriate resuscitation algorithms should be done. Evidence of systemic hypoperfusion such as hypotension; tachycardia; impaired cognition; and cool, clammy, and pale skin should be recognized immediately, and in the case of cardiogenic shock, which can complicate acute MI, appropriate and timely management should be considered. Patients who develop left heart failure and present with dyspnea, hypoxia, pulmonary edema, or impending respiratory compromise need forceful oxygenation therapy, stabilization of the airway, diuretic therapy, and afterload reduction as well as standard treatments. Prompt treatment of ventricular tachyarrhythmias is of great importance because of its harmful effect on cardiac output, possible exacerbation of myocardial ischemia, and the risk of deterioration into ventricular fibrillation (VF). Patients with old age, low blood pressure, tachycardia, heart failure, and anterior MI are at greater risk for complications.[8,9]

In a patient presenting with an acute MI, the characteristics of the chest pain and the ECG findings can help with early risk stratification. An ECG and a brief history and physical examination should be performed within 10 min of patient arrival.[10] The history should be focused on pain duration, its character and previous episodes, and precipitating factors, as well as past history of coronary disease risk factors. The physical examination should consist of heart and lung auscultation, blood pressure measurement of both arms, and heart failure or circulatory compromise assessment. Prompt reperfusion therapy should be considered for patients with a strong clinical history and ST-segment elevation or new LBBB.

### Electrocardiography

Electrocardiography is used in the early diagnosis of patients with suspected ACS with special focus on ST-segment elevation or new LBBB. Development of a hyperacute or peaked T wave that reflects localized hyperkalemia is the earliest change in a STEMI. The ST segment rises in the leads based on the electrical activity of the involved region of the myocardium. First, it reveals elevation of the J point, and the ST segment retains its concave configuration. Then, the ST-segment elevation becomes more easily detected, and the ST segment becomes more convex or rounded upward. Finally, the ST segment may ultimately merge with the T wave, so the QRS–T-wave complex can actually resemble a monophasic action potential. In addition to ST-segment elevation, special attention should be paid to new or presumably new LBBB and also on those with a true posterior MI to prompt diagnosis of STEMI.

Patients with the absence of Q waves with early ST-segment elevation are treated for a STEMI with a better prognosis because of higher probability of reperfusion; less severe infarction; and, at follow-up, better LV function and improved survival rate than others with Q-wave development.

Electrocardiography can be used to diagnose the location of MI. Inferior wall MI reveals ST elevation in leads II, III, and aVF. In addition, right ventricular infarction results in ST elevation on the right-sided leads V3R, V4R, V5R, and V6R. ST elevation in posterior leads (V7–V9) is usually associated with ST-segment depression in V1–V3 leads and an abnormal R wave in V1 reveals posterior infarction.[11]

The early ECG may be nondiagnostic in patients with MI. In these cases, in terms of suspicion of acute MI, obtaining ECG with 20–30-min intervals for any patient with ongoing pain is recommended. In some patients, ECG changes progress to ST-segment elevation or ST-segment depression.[12,13]

### Cardiac Biomarkers

Different biomarkers are used to evaluate patients with a suspected acute MI. The cardiac troponins (cTn) I and T (preferred biomarkers) and the MB isoenzyme of creatine kinase (CK-MB), if a cardiac-specific troponin assay is not available, are used. Values above the 99th percentile of the URL should be considered abnormal.[2] This value for troponin and CK-MB will be different depending on its use. Troponin is the preferred marker to detect myocardial injury for all diagnostic categories compared with CK-MB because of its specificity and sensitivity.[1,2,10]

CTnI elevation may continue for 7–10 days after MI, whereas cTnT elevation may continue for 10–14 days. It is important to consider that any interpretation of elevation of troponins must be based on clinical history and ECG findings. Cardiac injury should be applied to a situation in which elevation of cTn is associated with no ischemia, including heart failure, rapid atrial fibrillation, myocarditis, anthracycline cardiotoxicity, subendocardial wall stress, myopericarditis, sepsis, and so on.[14,15] Troponin also increases in chronic kidney disease.

High-sensitivity methods provide more accurate detection of very low concentration of cardiac troponin. High-sensitivity troponin (hsTn) can measure troponin earlier than previous methods. Such methods have higher sensitivity than previous assays, but have less clinical specificity for MI because these methods could discover myocardial injury in many other clinical situations. Conventional troponin methods provide diagnosis of MI by measuring at initial assessment and 3–6 h after that. The use of hsTn methods decreases time interval between sampling to 1–2 h due to lack of diagnosing ECG changes. It can be suggested that an initially measured hsTn less than the detection limit might prepare sufficient sensitivity and negative predictive value to provide discharge. Later sampling may be necessary if there is any suspicion of the pain or when there are symptom fluctuation. Patients who have been evaluated less than 2 h after onset of symptoms, also need sampling after 2 h from arrival in hospital.[16] Measuring of both CK-MB and cardiac-specific troponin is not necessary but if there is dearth of cardiac-specific troponin measurement, CK-MB assessment is an appropriate alternative. Although in the majority of patients MI can be ruled out after 6 h with cTn check, a 12-h sample should be gained in a high degree of doubt in ACSs,[1,2,10] but in a small number of patients, cTn becomes positive after 8 h.[17] Critical causes of chest pain associated with cTn elevation in the absence of coronary artery stenosis include acute pulmonary emboli (troponin elevation can occur from acute pressure overload of right heart), myocarditis,[18] and stress-induced cardiomyopathy. Some patients with STEMI who were quickly reperfused did not experience cardiac biomarker elevation (aborted MIs) using older tests. In terms of new troponin tests, this does not occur or is very uncommon.[19] Using the characteristics of cTn, which remains high 1–2 weeks after acute MI and usually does not rise or fall fast during this interval, one is able to discriminate acute from chronic events.[2,20,21]

In patients who are suspicious for reinfarction after initial infarction according to the clinical sign and symptoms, CK-MB can discover it. Measurement of troponin levels immediately followed by another measurement 3–6 h later can detect reinfarction if at least 20% increment in the second measurement was seen.[2]

## Treatment

Patients with acute STEMI need cardiac monitoring, oxygen (if arterial oxygen saturation <90%), and intravenous (IV) access. Initial therapy should focus on relieving ischemic pain, stabilizing the hemodynamic situation, and reducing ischemia as well as patient assessment and selection for fibrinolytic therapy or primary PCI. Other usual hospital care such as anxiolytics, monitoring of blood pressure, and serial ECGs should be provided.

- Supplemental oxygen is recommended for patients who have arterial saturation below 90% and patients experiencing respiratory distress. Some evidence supports using supplemental oxygen in normoxic patients with acute MI, but it is a weak recommendation and is not used in most cases.
- Restoration of myocardial blood flow without any delay is essential to gain optimal myocardial salvage to reduce mortality rates.[22] Reperfusion strategy of the infarct-related artery with PCI or fibrinolytic therapy improves myocardial recovery and reduces the mortality rate compared with no reperfusion. So as

soon as possible, reperfusion method should be selected between fibrinolytic agents and primary PCI.
- If a patient with an acute STEMI arrives at a PCI-capable hospital, primary PCI should be performed and first medical contact (FMC) to reperfusion (wire crossing) time should be less than 60 min.
- If the STEMI patient arrives at a non-PCI-capable hospital, emergency interhospital transfer to PCI-capable hospital should be considered if FMC to reperfusion (wire crossing) time is equal to or less than 120 min. If it last greater than 120 min, fibrinolytic therapy should be started in non-PCI-capable hospital in less than 10 min of STEMI diagnosis. After that, all the patients should be transferred to PCI-capable hospital for coronary angiography, which in case of fibrinolytic therapy failure (<50% ST-segment resolution at 60–90 min following fibrinolytic administration), hemodynamic or electrical instability, worsening ischemia, or persistent chest pain, coronary angiography and PCI should be done without delay (rescue PCI) and in case of successful fibrinolytic therapy, this should be performed 2–24 h later (pharmacoinvasive strategy).[23,24]
- It is important to note that in some patients coronary angiography with PCI if indicated is preferred, including when diagnosis of STEMI is doubted (when signs and symptoms exactly do not match the diagnostic findings for STEMI, e.g., pericarditis), high bleeding risk (possibility of intracranial hemorrhage risk ≥4% caused by fibrinolytic therapy),[23–26] and high risk of death like patients present with cardiogenic shock.[27–32]
- In patients with symptoms starting >12 h, a primary PCI strategy should be selected with persistent symptoms of ischemia, ECG finding of persistent ischemia, hemodynamic instability, or life-threatening arrhythmias. Although some evidence has revealed improvement of LV function with late PCI, clinical end point improvement was not confirmed.[27,28,33–36]

## Coronary Artery Bypass Graft Surgery

Conduction of CABG surgery in patients with STEMI is uncommon. Emergency CABG surgery could be considered in STEMI patients with inappropriate anatomy of infarct-related artery for PCI, and either a large area of myocardium is at risk or with cardiogenic shock.

Emergency CABG is infrequently done in STEMI patients with coronary obstruction not suitable for PCI or unsuccessful PCI, because the benefits of surgical revascularization in STEMI patients are uncertain. Since there is a long delay to reperfusion, the possibility of myocardial saving which affects the prognosis is low and the surgical risks are elevated. In patients with mechanical complication of MI who require coronary revascularization, CABG is performed at the time of surgery.[23,24]

## Medications

Some specific agents with their usual dosing regimens that should be considered as medication therapy are listed here:

- Aspirin must be started as soon as possible for all patients. A potent P2Y12 inhibitor (ticagrelor or prasugrel) or clopidogrel, if ticagrelor and prasugrel are unavailable or are contraindicated, is recommended before primary PCI and continued for 12 months. Glycoprotein (GP) IIb/IIIa inhibitors should be considered as bailout if there is evidence of no-reflow or a thrombotic complication during primary PCI procedure.

The dosing regimen includes ASA 150–300 mg orally (should be chewed) with a maintenance dose of 75–100 mg/day, ticagrelor loading dose of 180 mg orally with a maintenance dose of 90 mg every 12 h, and prasugrel loading dose of 60 mg orally, with a maintenance dose of 10 mg/day (if the patient body weight is equal to or less than 60 kg the maintenance dose is 5 mg/day). In patients aged 75 years or older, prasugrel is not recommended but if the treatment seems to be mandatory a dose of 5 mg/day could be used. Prasugrel should not be given to patients with a history of stroke. For patients with high bleeding risk of gastrointestinal bleeding, a proton pump inhibitor is recommended with dual antiplatelet therapy (DAPT).[23,37,38]

- When patients receive fibrinolytic therapy, clopidogrel in addition to ASA is suggested (prasugrel and ticagrelor have not been studied as adjuncts to fibrinolysis). For patients who receive fibrinolysis, the suggested loading dose of clopidogrel is 300 mg with a maintenance dose 75 mg/day for those who are younger than 75 years of age; for patients aged 75 years and older, a loading dose of 75 mg of clopidogrel with maintenance dose of 75 mg/day is sufficient. However, for patients with STEMI who undergo primary PCI, the recommended loading dose of clopidogrel is 600 mg.[23,39,40]
- For STEMI patients treated with primary PCI who are not at high bleeding risk and who do not have

noncardiac surgery planned within 1 year, DAPT for at least 12 months rather than a shorter treatment duration is recommended. For most patients undergoing primary PCI and who receive early antiplatelet therapy with aspirin and a P2Y12 inhibitor, routine use of a GP IIb/IIIa inhibitor is not recommended.[41-43] In patients who have not received fibrinolytic therapy and primary PCI, ticagrelor is recommended in preference to clopidogrel or prasugrel.[27,28,44]

- Anticoagulation therapy in primary PCI includes unfractionated heparin (UFH), enoxaparin, and bivalirudin. Some studies have shown that the use of fondaparinux in the context of primary PCI was associated with potential harm and is not recommended. Routine use of UFH is recommended (class of recommendation: I), also routine use of enoxaparin or bivalirudin could be considered (class of recommendation: IIa). Bivalirudin is recommended for patients with heparin-induced thrombocytopenia, as anticoagulant agent during primary PCI. Dosing regimen includes UFH 70–100 U/kg intravenous bolus and enoxaparin 0.5 mg/kg intravenous bolus.

Postprocedural anticoagulation therapy following primary PCI is not recommended unless there is a separate indication for anticoagulation therapy including mechanical heart valve, atrial fibrillation, left ventricle thrombosis, or prevention of venous thromboembolism in patients who need prolonged bed rest.[23]

- In patients with chest pain after three sublingual nitroglycerin tablets and in patients with hypertension or heart failure, IV nitroglycerin therapy is valuable. In the case of right ventricular infarction or severe aortic stenosis, nitrates must be used with caution or avoided because of serious hemodynamic decompensation. In patients who have used a phosphodiesterase type 5 inhibitor for erectile dysfunction or pulmonary hypertension within the previous 48 h, nitrates are contraindicated.
- To relieve chest pain in acute MI, morphine may be prescribed. Morphine is recommended for patients with an unacceptable level of pain. IV morphine sulfate is administered at an initial dose of 2–4 mg, with increments of 2–8 mg repeated at 5–15-min intervals.
- Early prescription of intravenous beta-blockers at the presentation of STEMI followed by oral beta-blockers is recommended in hemodynamically stable STEMI patients undergoing primary PCI.[23,27,28]

Contraindications to oral beta-blockers consist of heart failure, signs of low output, high risk for cardiogenic shock, bradycardia, heart block, and reactive airway disease.

- High-intensity statin therapy is recommended as early as possible in all patients with STEMI.[23,45,46] Most patients should have a lipid profile test early in their initial hospitalization; however, some patients have had their lipid profile checked recently. When statin therapy is started in ACSs, lipid profile response should be evaluated after 2 months because acute-phase response, in addition to other factors, can reduce low-density lipoprotein cholesterol by up to 50%, and this can result in virtually normal levels after an ACS episode. The treatment goal is an LDL-C concentration of less than 70 mg/dL or at least 50% decrease in LDL-C if the baseline LDL-C level is 70–135 mg/dL.
- Treatment with ACE inhibitors should be considered in patients with systolic LV dysfunction (LV EF equal or less than 40%) or heart failure, diabetes, or hypertension, and should be prescribed in all STEMI patients. Angiotensin II receptor blocker should be prescribed if the patient does not tolerate an ACE inhibitor.
- Even though there is no clinical evidence that proves the benefits of electrolyte replacement in acute MI, maintaining the serum potassium concentration above 4.0 mEq/L and serum magnesium concentration above 2.0 mEq/L (2.4 mg/dL or 1 mmol/L) is recommended.[47]
- Both atrial (atrial fibrillation or flutter) and ventricular [ventricular tachycardia (VT) or VF] arrhythmias can be seen during and after the acute phase of STEMI. Arrhythmia management is vital. Prophylactic IV or intramuscular lidocaine to prevent VT and VF in acute MI patients is not recommended.[48] Sinus bradycardia, especially in inferior wall involvement, can occur in patients with STEMI and often require no treatment. If sinus bradycardia accompanied by severe hypotension, it should be treated with intravenous atropine. If sinus bradycardia remains, temporary pacing may be needed. Atrioventricular (AV) nodal and intraventricular conduction abnormalities can occur in STEMI. Second-degree Mobitz I (Wenckebach) AV block is usually associated with inferior wall MI and rarely results in adverse hemodynamic effects. If so, initially atropine should be prescribed; if failure of treatment occurs, pacing should be used. Complete AV block and also second-degree Mobitz II AV block may be indications for pacing.
- Based on the evidence, use of IV glucose–insulin–potassium to improve outcomes in patients with suspected or diagnosed acute MI is not recommended.[49]

- Use of erythropoietin as a cardioprotective agent derived from experimental evidence that revealed erythropoietin's nonerythropoietic effects, including antiinflammatory, antiapoptotic, and angiogenic properties, which may be helpful. However, significantly increased risk of death, recurrent MI, stroke, or stent thrombosis in erythropoietin-treated patients suggested an increased thrombotic risk caused by erythropoietin in patients with STEMI.[50–52]

In the face of STEMI, somehow angiography reveals normal results. In 7% of patients with acute STEMI, there is no critical coronary artery lesion,[53] and approximately 3% have normal epicardial coronary arteries.[54–56] This event is more prevalent in younger patients and in women.[53] The probable mechanisms may include coronary spasm, acquired or inherited coagulation disorders, toxins such as cocaine, collagen vascular disease, embolism, myocarditis, and microvascular disease.[55]

Stress-induced cardiomyopathy (takotsubo cardiomyopathy) is an increasingly reported syndrome. The syndrome is recognized by transient systolic dysfunction of the apical or mid segments of the LV that resembles MI but without significant coronary artery disease (CAD).

## Fibrinolysis for Acute ST-Segment Elevation Myocardial Infarction

The majority of cases of STEMI are caused by atherosclerotic plaque rupture followed by thrombus formation and total occlusion of the coronary artery. STEMI patients can receive reperfusion by either primary PCI or fibrinolysis. Although primary PCI is the reperfusion method of choice in most STEMI patients, if it is not available in a timely manner, fibrinolytic (thrombolytic) therapy should be used within 12 h of symptom onset in patients without contraindications. Major benefit has been observed in patients at highest risk, including the elderly patients, and when treatment is started less than 2 h after onset of symptom. After fibrinolysis, the patient should be transferred to PCI-capable hospital for coronary angiography, which in case of fibrinolytic therapy failure should be done without delay (rescue PCI) and in case of successful fibrinolytic therapy, this should be performed 2–24 h after pharmacoinvasive strategy.[23,24]

### Indications

Chest pain due to myocardial infarction could be evident by the following ECG changes: at least two contiguous leads with ST-segment elevation ≥2.5 mm in men <40 years, ≥2 mm in men ≥40 years, or ≥1.5 mm in women in leads V2–V3 and/or ≥1 mm in the other leads (in the absence of left ventricular hypertrophy or left bundle branch block), and also patients with ischemic symptoms in addition to new or probably new left bundle branch block or true posterior MI are candidates for reperfusion therapy either by primary PCI or by fibrinolytic therapy. Although primary PCI is the reperfusion method of choice in most STEMI patients, if it is not available in a timely manner, fibrinolytic (thrombolytic) therapy should be used within 12 h of symptom onset in patients without contraindications.[27,28]

In patients with an acute STEMI, fibrinolytic therapy should not await the availability of results of cardiac biomarkers.[23,27,28,44] The benefit from therapy reduces as time interval between symptom onset and starting of fibrinolytic (thrombolytic) therapy increases. The greatest survival benefit is when thrombolytic therapy is administered within the first 2 h after symptom onset[23,35,57,58] and particularly within the first 70 min.[59,60] So when fibrinolysis is chosen as reperfusion strategy, it is important to initiate the therapeutic regimen as soon as possible after STEMI diagnosis was made, even in the prehospital setting. A fibrin-specific agent (i.e., reteplase, alteplase, or tenecteplase) should be an option. A half-dose of tenecteplase should be used in STEMI patients equal or older than 75 years old.[23]

### Contraindications

The contraindications for fibrinolytic therapy include previous intracranial hemorrhage, malignant intracranial neoplasm, known structural cerebrovascular lesion (e.g., arteriovenous malformation), ischemic stroke within 3 months except for acute ischemic stroke within 4.5 h, significant facial trauma or closed-head trauma within 3 months, intracranial and intraspinal surgery within 2 months, suspicious to aortic dissection, active bleeding (except for menstrual period) or bleeding diathesis, severe uncontrolled hypertension unresponsive to emergency therapy, and for streptokinase, previous treatment in less than previous 6 months. Also relative contraindications consist of history of poorly controlled, chronic, and severe hypertension, significant hypertension at initial evaluation (systolic blood pressure >180 mm Hg or diastolic blood pressure >110 mm Hg), ischemic stroke in more than previous 3 months, major surgery (within <3 weeks), dementia, known intracranial pathology not covered in absolute contraindications, recent (within 2–4 weeks) internal bleeding, traumatic, or prolonged cardiopulmonary resuscitation (>10 min), pregnancy, active peptic ulcer, noncompressible vascular puncture, and oral anticoagulant therapy.

Intraocular hemorrhage from fibrinolytic therapy in patients with diabetes is rare, and diabetic retinopathy should not be considered as a contraindication to fibrinolytic therapy in acute MI.[23,61–64]

The most important complication of fibrinolytic therapy is bleeding, and among the bleeding complications, hemorrhagic stroke has great concern. Predictors of intracranial hemorrhage include age 75 years or older, black race, female sex, prior history of stroke, systolic blood pressure 160 mmHg or greater, weight 65 kg or less for women or 80 kg or less for men, international normalized ratio greater than 4 or prothrombin time greater than 24 s, and use of alteplase (vs another fibrinolytic agent).[23,24,61,65,66]

## COMPLICATIONS OF ST-SEGMENT ELEVATION MYOCARDIAL INFARCTION

Major complication groups in STEMI include conduction abnormalities after MI, ventricular arrhythmia during acute MI, mechanical complications of STEMI, and pericardial complications of MI.

### Conduction Abnormalities After Myocardial Infarction

Conduction abnormalities are known as complications of acute MI. They may result from autonomic imbalance or ischemia of the conduction system. Bradycardia is a common frequent feature and complete heart block with a slow escape rhythm is a potentially lethal complication if it is not diagnosed and treated appropriately. Conduction abnormalities can be classified as right bundle branch block (RBBB), LBBB, first-degree heart block, second-degree heart block, high-degree heart block, or third-degree (complete) heart block.[67,68] In inferior MI, conduction disturbance may occur acutely or after hours or days. Sinus bradycardia, second-degree AV block, and complete heart block also can be seen because the sinoatrial node, AV node, and His bundle are mainly supplied by the right coronary artery.[69] Conduction abnormalities, which happen with anteroseptal MI, are less common but more complicated, and the degree of arrhythmic complications is usually directly related to the extent of MI. Complete heart block with anterior MI may happen in the first 24 h. It may happen without warning or may be heralded by the occurrence of RBBB with either a left anterior fascicular block or left posterior fascicular block. Heart block in this situation seems to result from extensive infarction that involves the bundle branches traveling within the septum.[70] In patients with anterior or inferior MI, high (second- or third-) degree AV block is associated with an increased mortality rate. In inferior MI, high-grade AV block is usually transient, and it is associated with a higher inhospital mortality rate.[71,72]

### Management of atrioventricular block

An important item in the management of AV block in the setting of an acute MI is that bradycardia, even if asymptomatic or transient, can reduce coronary blood flow and myocardial perfusion. The most frequently used therapies for symptomatic bradycardia in the setting of acute MI include atropine or temporary transcutaneous or right ventricular pacing.[69,73]

### Ventricular arrhythmia during acute myocardial infarction

Ventricular arrhythmia, ranging from isolated ventricular premature beats to VT or VF, is frequent in the immediate postinfarction period.[74,75] In typical form, the arrhythmia presents as unstable, mainly polymorphic, and relatively rapid VT, often degenerating into VF.[23] In the era of primary PCI, VT (especially nonsustained VT) remains relatively frequent.[76] The incidence of ventricular arrhythmias seems to be greater with ST-segment elevation than NSTEMI.

### Sustained Ventricular Tachycardia

Sustained monomorphic VT in the peri-infarction period (within 48 h after MI) happens in about 2%–3% of STEMI patients[77,78] and fewer than 1% with non-STEMI or unstable angina.[79] Sustained monomorphic VT is associated with larger infarction size.[78]

**Treatment.** Patients with sustained polymorphic VT, very rapid VT, or pulseless monomorphic VT should be treated with unsynchronized electrical shock (defibrillation). A biphasic waveform defibrillator is optional because the success rate for defibrillation is greater than for monophasic waveform. For a biphasic defibrillator, the initial shock should be at 120–200 J. For monophasic defibrillation, shocks start at 360 J.

Patients with sustained monomorphic VT associated with angina, pulmonary edema, or hypotension (systolic blood pressure <90 mmHg) should be treated with immediately synchronized electrical cardioversion with an initial energy of 100 J.

Stable monomorphic VT in the peri-MI period, even when hemodynamically tolerated, should be treated urgently because of its adverse effect on cardiac output, precipitation of ischemia, and risk of progression to VF. In hemodynamically stable and asymptomatic patients, cardioversion may be postponed for several minutes and IV amiodarone started. In case of contraindications to amiodarone, lidocaine may be considered. Synchronized electrical cardioversion should be performed if VT persists after administration of the initial dose of medication.[23,80,81]

### Ventricular fibrillation

Ventricular fibrillation is the most common mechanism of sudden cardiac death. Most episodes of VF happen within the first 48–72 h after onset of symptoms.[77,81,82] It is a manifestation of ischemia and is associated with lack of reperfusion in the infarct-related artery.

The predictive role of early VT/VF (within the first 48 h of STEMI) for prognosis remained controversial. Patients with early VT/VF may have high 30-day mortality but long-term arrhythmic risk does not increase. VF is more frequent in patients with MI complicated by heart failure or recurrent ischemia.

Ventricular fibrillation is lethal if not treated. Defibrillation is the definitive therapy for VF. A biphasic waveform defibrillator, with an initial shock of 120–200 J, is optional because the success rate for defibrillation is greater than with a monophasic waveform.[23,83,84]

### Mechanical Complications of ST-Segment Elevation Myocardial Infarction

Three major mechanical complications of STEMI are LV free wall rupture, interventricular septum rupture, and development of mitral regurgitation (MR).

### Left ventricular free wall rupture

A serious and often lethal complication of STEMI is myocardial perforation.[85] In about half of STEMI cases, myocardial perforation occurs within 5 days after STEMI, and more than 90% of cases occur within 2 weeks after STEMI.[86–89] Features associated with rupture include female gender, older age, hypertension, reperfusion with a fibrinolytic agent vs PCI, single-vessel disease without collateral circulation, and an anterior or first MI. The findings in early-phase (<72 h) and late (>4 days) perforations were different. Early perforation, which is more common in anterior infarction sites, is characterized by a sudden slit-like tear in the infarcted myocardium. Late perforation with no preferential infarction site is characterized by infarct expansion, and there is a low incidence in patients with successful reperfusion. Myocardial perforation more frequently affects the LV than the right ventricle and rarely affects the atria.[89–91] The perforation commonly involves the anterior or lateral walls of the LV, and tear frequently occurs near the junction of the infarcted and normal myocardium. The rate of myocardial perforation has decreased over time; this reduction is associated with increased use of reperfusion therapies; better control of blood pressure; and use of aspirin, beta-blockers, and angiotensin-converting enzyme inhibitors. The incidence of myocardial perforation may be lower in patients treated with PCI than in those who received thrombolytic therapy.[92] Other risk factors for rupture include age older than 70 years, female sex, and anterior STEMI.[92,93] However, beta-blockers, which are routinely administered to patients with acute MI, decrease the rate of death from free wall perforation compared with placebo.[94]

### Effect of reperfusion

Myocardial perforation after MI is less frequent in patients with a patent infarct-related coronary artery.[95,96] Perforation usually develops in an area that had been infarcted without successful reperfusion. PCI may decrease the risk of cardiac perforation if successful reperfusion is obtained.[96] Some studies have revealed that thrombolytic therapy after MI rarely improves survival and reduces the cardiac perforation risk.[97–99] Conversely, thrombolytic therapy may accompany with a significant increment in free wall perforation in patients older than 75 years old.[100–102] Late primary PCI may reduce the free wall perforation. It has been shown that delayed primary PCI (after 24 h) of a totally occluded artery may improve clinical outcomes.[103]

**Clinical presentation.** Perforation can present as unexpected death in a case of silent MI. With a known MI, complete or incomplete perforation can occur.[104] Complete perforation of the LV free wall can result in death from tamponade. Early suggestion of myocardial perforation could be the occurrence of sudden severe heart failure and shock, which can progress rapidly to pulseless electrical activity and death. Some studies have reported that pulseless electrical activity in a patient with MI and without heart failure had a great accuracy in predicting the diagnosis of LV free wall perforation.[104,105] Emergency pericardiocentesis confirms the diagnosis and temporarily improves tamponade. Transthoracic echocardiography also can confirm the diagnosis.[95] Incomplete perforation of the LV free wall can result when organized thrombus and pericardium seal the ventricular perforation. This situation may progress

to frank perforation with cardiac tamponade and hemodynamic impairment to create a false aneurysm surrounded by pericardial tissue and communication with the LV through the perforation or to the formation of an LV diverticulum.[87–89,106] Clinical manifestations of incomplete perforation may include chest pain, particularly pericardial pain; nausea; agitation; temporary hypotension; and ECG features of pericarditis.[87–89] The diagnosis of incomplete perforation is approved by transthoracic echocardiography.[104]

**Management.** Immediate surgery is indicated and surgical repair is indicated for LV false aneurysm.[89] Medical therapies to stabilize the hemodynamic should be conducted, and this includes fluid therapy, inotropic support, and vasopressors.[87–89,97,99,107,108] Rapid implantation of the named regimen can result in an appropriate survival rate, particularly in subacute rupture.[89]

### Rupture of the interventricular septum

Septal rupture usually occurs 3–5 days after STEMI, but it may occur as soon as within 24 h or as late as 2 weeks. Septal rupture risk may increase in patients with single-vessel involvement [especially the left anterior descending coronary artery (LAD)], widespread myocardial damage, and reduced septal collaterals, advanced age, female sex, and chronic kidney disease.[109–114] Septal rupture has greater frequency in a first infarction. STEMI caused by obstruction of a wraparound LAD seems to have a higher risk of septal rupture. Because previous ischemia may result in myocardial preconditioning and reducing the likelihood of transmural MI and septal rupture, patients with chronic angina, previous MI, hypertension, or diabetes mellitus are less likely to experience rupture.[115,116] The presence of ST-segment elevation in numerous leads may portend a large MI irrespective of coronary anatomy, so these patients are at high risk for septal rupture.

Without reperfusion, septal rupture can occur in 2% of cases of acute MI and may be responsible for nearly 10% of total cardiac ruptures.[85,117] In patients treated with thrombolytic therapy, the incidence of septal rupture is lower than in conservatively treated patients.[118] The perforation usually occurs at the border between the necrotic and nonnecrotic myocardium.[114,119]

Patients with septal perforation usually develop a rapid onset of hemodynamic compromise associated with hypotension; heart failure (especially right heart failure); and a loud, harsh holosystolic murmur.[85,114,120] Septal perforation probability is increased in patients with right ventricular MI.[119,121]

The septal perforation can be diagnosed by two-dimensional and color-flow Doppler transthoracic echocardiography.[85,114,122–124] The diagnosis is usually confirmed by a pulmonary artery balloon catheter to document the left-to-right shunt.[85,114] Transesophageal echocardiography sometimes is required to determine the extent of the rupture.[125]

The therapeutic approach depends on the clinical features. When the patient is in cardiogenic shock, death is inevitable without urgent surgery. The patient should be stabilized with vasodilators to reduce the afterload and hence reduce the left-to-right shunt, inotrope agents to increase the cardiac output, diuretics, and intraaortic balloon pump (IABP) counterpulsation with a role similar to vasodilators. This is followed by cardiac catheterization and coronary angiography and then surgical repair. The surgical mortality rate is high, but in survivors, the final results are good.[118,125–127] Late elective surgery could be done in patients with heart failure with a lack of cardiogenic shock; however, the risk for rapid and unexpected deterioration is always present. Advanced age and a long delay between septal perforation and surgical repair are associated with poor outcomes.[127–129] Bypassing the associated CAD can improve long-term survival rates.[130] Septal perforation closure with a transcatheter approach is another therapeutic option.[131] This approach is of great value in the treatment of septal perforation when other surgical options (e.g., coronary bypass or valve replacement) are not indicated.

### Mitral regurgitation

The development of MR after acute MI could be attributable to ischemic papillary muscle dysfunction, LV dilation or true aneurysm, and papillary muscle or chordal perforation.[85,114,132–134]

Some patients with equal or more than moderate MR, except for patients with papillary muscle dysfunction, can be hemodynamically stable. They may improve with medical therapy and revascularization, including thrombolytic therapy or primary PCI. Some patients may finally require mitral valve replacement or repair associated with CABG surgery.[132,135]

Papillary muscle rupture is a lethal problem after acute MI. It usually appears 2–7 days after MI.[132,135] There are two types of ruptures: partial (occurring at one of the muscle heads) and complete.

Rupture of the posteromedial papillary muscle develops 6–12 times more commonly than rupture of the anterolateral papillary muscle, and this could be attributable to differences in blood supply. The posteromedial papillary muscle has a single blood supply,

which is via the posterior descending artery, but the anterolateral papillary muscle perfusion is via a dual blood supply from the LAD and left circumflex arteries.[85,114,132,136]

Both ST-segment elevation and STEMI can result in rupture of papillary muscle. The majority of patients have relatively small areas of necrosis with poor collaterals, and about 50% of patients have single-vessel disease.[85,132] Some studies suggest that papillary muscle rupture after MI may be more common in patients with a first MI.[137]

The diagnosis of papillary muscle rupture is made by echocardiography and cardiac catheterization. Transthoracic echocardiography may reveal a flail part of the mitral valve, and frequently a damaged papillary muscle or chordae can be found moving freely within the LV cavity. In some patients, transesophageal echocardiography may be required to make the diagnosis.[124] The pulmonary capillary pressure may show giant V waves. Because the LV contracts against the low resistant left atrium, the function of LV function seems hyperdynamic.[85,132,137,138]

Early diagnosis, administration of medical therapy, and emergency surgery are all required in the treatment plan. Medical therapy consists of reducing the afterload, usually by means of nitrates, sodium nitroprusside, diuretics, and IABP counterpulsation. Afterload reduction decreases the regurgitant volume, thereby increasing the forward flow.

Emergency surgery still is the optional modality of treatment for papillary muscle perforation. Although the operative mortality rate is high (20%–25%), survival in medically treated patients is very low.[139] Mitral valve repair rather than replacement should be considered when sufficient experience in performing this procedure is present.[132,135] Risk factors for a worse prognosis after surgery consist of old age, female gender, and poor LV systolic function.[140]

When papillary muscle perforation is partial, some surgeons prefer to stabilize the patient and delay surgery for 6–8 weeks after MI to avoid surgery on the necrotic myocardium. However, the majority of patients cannot be stabilized, and acute surgery must be considered.

### Pericardial Complications of Myocardial Infarction

There are three types of pericardial complications after MI:

- Early infarct-associated pericarditis (often termed *peri-infarction pericarditis*)
- Pericardial effusion (with or without tamponade)

- Dressler syndrome (postmyocardial infarction syndrome)

### Peri-infarction pericarditis

Acute pericarditis, diagnosed by a pericardial friction rub with or without chest discomfort, may complicate MI. Peri-infarction pericarditis usually happens early after the MI and is temporary. It may produce pain as early as the first day and as late as 8 weeks after STEMI.[141]

The incidence of peri-infarction pericarditis has decreased since the use of fibrinolytics and primary PCI became widespread. Studies have shown that pericarditis occurs in approximately 5% of patients treated with thrombolytic therapy vs 12%–20% in those not receiving fibrinolytic therapy.[141–143]

Pleuritic-type chest pain, especially pain in the trapezius ridges, and the presence of a pericardial friction rub are compatible with the diagnosis. Echocardiography should be performed in patients suspected for peri-infarction pericarditis to assess for pericardial effusion.[144–147]

The treatment of peri-infarction pericarditis is supportive because most cases are self-limited.[27] In patients who remain symptomatic after the initial 7–10 days, aspirin is recommended at higher doses (650–1000 mg three times daily) rather than other nonsteroidal antiinflammatory drugs or glucocorticoids. There is insufficient data for routine coadministration of colchicine (along with aspirin) in this situation.[27]

### Pericardial Effusion (With or Without Tamponade)

Pericardial effusion without tamponade is frequent in the early course of transmural MI. The majority of pericardial effusions are minimal or mild and most pericardial effusions following myocardial infarction do not result in hemodynamic compromise. Effusions are more common in patients with anterior or lateral STEMI, more microvascular obstructive disease, greater infarct size, more LV dysfunction, no reperfusion, and higher rate of heart failure.[148,149]

The mechanisms of tamponade in acute MI are pericardial involvement with hemorrhagic pericarditis and transmural free wall rupture caused by transmural MI. In addition, in MI patients treated with PCI, an uncommon reason for tamponade is an iatrogenic perforation of the coronary artery.

Predictors of tamponade are increasing age, anterior wall MI, female sex, and increased time from symptom onset to therapy. Tamponade was associated with a higher 30-day mortality rate. If the patient survived for 30 days, there would be no increase in 1-year mortality risk.[147,150,151]

Post-MI pericardial effusion may be a marker for greater myocardial damage, and the effusion is usually asymptomatic. An effusion does not necessarily show pericarditis; although effusion and pericarditis may coexist, most effusions develop without other evidence of pericarditis. The reabsorption rate of a post-MI pericardial effusion is slow, and resolution of effusion may take several months. Rarely, large effusions may happen and cause tamponade. Such patients should be evaluated carefully for evidence of LV free wall rupture.[151]

### Dressler Syndrome (Postmyocardial Infarction Syndrome)

Dressler syndrome usually occurs 1–8 weeks after MI. The clinical features consist of pleuritic-type chest pain, pericardial friction rub, fever, malaise, leukocytosis, elevated erythrocyte sedimentation rate, and pericardial effusion. The etiology of Dressler syndrome is not clearly established, but an immune pathologic process is suggested based on the detection of antibodies to cardiac tissue. Treatment is with aspirin, 650 mg every 4 h, may be effective. Glucocorticosteroids and nonsteroidal antiinflammatory drug should be avoided in patients with Dressler syndrome who are within 4 weeks of MI, since they may impair healing process, and may cause ventricular rupture. Some patients may experience recurrences; colchicine may be helpful in these cases.[152,153]

### REFERENCES

1. Alpert JS, Thygesen K, Antman E, Bassand JP. Myocardial infarction redefined—a consensus document of The Joint European Society of Cardiology/American College of Cardiology Committee for the redefinition of myocardial infarction. *J Am Coll Cardiol*. 2000;36:959.
2. Thygesen K, Alpert JS, White HD. Joint ESC/ACCF/AHA/WHF Task Force for the Redefinition of Myocardial Infarction. Universal definition of myocardial infarction. *Eur Heart J*. 2007;28:2525.
3. Garberich RF, Traverse JH, Claussen MT, et al. ST-elevation myocardial infarction diagnosed after hospital admission. *Circulation*. 2014;129:1225.
4. Alexander KP, Newby LK, Armstrong PW, et al. Acute coronary care in the elderly, part II: ST-segment-elevation myocardial infarction: a scientific statement for healthcare professionals from the American Heart Association Council on Clinical Cardiology: in collaboration with the society of geriatric cardiology. *Circulation*. 2007;115:2570.

5. Goldberg RJ, McCormick D, Gurwitz JH, et al. Age-related trends in short- and long-term survival after acute myocardial infarction: a 20-year population-based perspective (1975-1995). *Am J Cardiol*. 1998;82:1311.

6. Roger VL, Jacobsen SJ, Weston SA, et al. Trends in the incidence and survival of patients with hospitalized myocardial infarction, Olmsted County, Minnesota, 1979 to 1994. *Ann Intern Med*. 2002;136:341.

7. McCord J, Jneid H, Hollander JE, et al. Management of cocaine-associated chest pain and myocardial infarction: a scientific statement from the American Heart Association Acute Cardiac Care Committee of the Council on Clinical Cardiology. *Circulation*. 2008;117:1897.

8. Morrow DA, Antman EM, Parsons L, et al. Application of the TIMI risk score for ST-elevation MI in the National Registry of Myocardial Infarction 3. *JAMA*. 2001;286:1356.

9. Wu AH, Parsons L, Every NR, et al. Hospital outcomes in patients presenting with congestive heart failure complicating acute myocardial infarction: a report from the Second National Registry of Myocardial Infarction (NRMI-2). *J Am Coll Cardiol*. 2002;40:1389.

10. Levine GN, Bates ER, Blankenship JC, et al. 2015 ACC/AHA/SCAI focused update on primary percutaneous coronary intervention for patients with ST-elevation myocardial infarction: an update of the 2011 ACCF/AHA/SCAI guideline for percutaneous coronary intervention and the 2013 ACCF/AHA guideline for the management of ST-elevation myocardial infarction [published correction appears in J Am Coll Cardiol. 2016 Mar 29;67(12):1506]. *J Am Coll Cardiol*. 2016;67 (10):1235–1250. https://doi.org/10.1016/j.jacc.2015.10.005.

11. Kulkarni AU, Brown R, Ayoubi M, Banka VS. Clinical use of posterior electrocardiographic leads: a prospective electrocardiographic analysis during coronary occlusion. *Am Heart J*. 1996;131:736.

12. Fesmire FM, Percy RF, Bardoner JB, et al. Usefulness of automated serial 12-lead ECG monitoring during the initial emergency department evaluation of patients with chest pain. *Ann Emerg Med*. 1998;31:3.

13. Kudenchuk PJ, Maynard C, Cobb LA, et al. Utility of the prehospital electrocardiogram in diagnosing acute coronary syndromes: the Myocardial Infarction Triage and Intervention (MITI) Project. *J Am Coll Cardiol*. 1998;32:17.

14. Guest TM, Ramanathan AV, Tuteur PG, et al. Myocardial injury in critically ill patients. A frequently unrecognized complication. *JAMA*. 1995;273:1945.

15. Babuin L, Vasile VC, Rio Perez JA, et al. Elevated cardiac troponin is an independent risk factor for short- and long-term mortality in medical intensive care unit patients. *Crit Care Med*. 2008;36:759.

16. Morrow DA. Evidence-based algorithms using high-sensitivity cardiac troponin in the emergency department. *JAMA Cardiol*. 2016;1:379–381.

17. Newby LK, Christenson RH, Ohman EM, et al. Value of serial troponin T measures for early and late risk stratification in patients with acute coronary syndromes. The GUSTO-IIa Investigators. *Circulation*. 1998;98:1853.

18. Jaffe AS, Babuin L, Apple FS. Biomarkers in acute cardiac disease: the present and the future. *J Am Coll Cardiol*. 2006;48:1.

19. Vasile VC, Babuin L, Ting HH, et al. Aborted myocardial infarction: is it real in the troponin era? *Am Heart J*. 2009;157:636.

20. Hollander JE, Than M, Mueller C. State-of-the-art evaluation of emergency department patients presenting with potential acute coronary syndromes. *Circulation*. 2016;134:547–564.

21. Jaffe AS. Chasing troponin: how low can you go if you can see the rise? *J Am Coll Cardiol*. 2006;48:1763.

22. Anderson JL, Karagounis LA, Califf RM. Metaanalysis of five reported studies on the relation of early coronary patency grades with mortality and outcomes after acute myocardial infarction. *Am J Cardiol*. 1996;78:1.

23. Ibanez B, James S, Agewall S, et al. 2017 ESC Guidelines for the management of acute myocardial infarction in patients presenting with ST-segment elevation: The Task Force for the management of acute myocardial infarction in patients presenting with ST-segment elevation of the European Society of Cardiology (ESC). *Eur Heart J*. 2018;39(2):119–177. https://doi.org/10.1093/eurheartj/ehx393.

24. Neumann FJ, Sousa-Uva M, Ahlsson A, et al. 2018 ESC/EACTS Guidelines on myocardial revascularization [2018 ESC/EACTS Guidelines on myocardial revascularization]. *Kardiol Pol*. 2018;76(12):1585–1664. https://doi.org/10.5603/KP.2018.0228 25.

25. Grzybowski M, Clements EA, Parsons L, et al. Mortality benefit of immediate revascularization of acute ST-segment elevation myocardial infarction in patients with contraindications to thrombolytic therapy: a propensity analysis. *JAMA*. 2003;290:1891.

26. Antman EM, Anbe DT, Armstrong PW, et al. ACC/AHA Guidelines for the Management of Patients With ST-Elevation Myocardial Infarction. (2015). www.acc.org/qualityandscience/clinical/statements.htm; 2015. Accessed 23 June 2015.

27. O'Gara PT, Kushner FG, Ascheim DD, et al. 2013 ACCF/AHA guideline for the management of ST-elevation myocardial infarction: a report of the American College of Cardiology Foundation/American Heart Association Task Force on Practice Guidelines. *Circulation*. 2013;127: e362.

28. O'Gara PT, Kushner FG, Ascheim DD, et al. 2013 ACCF/AHA guideline for the management of ST-elevation myocardial infarction: executive summary: a report of the American College of Cardiology Foundation/American Heart Association Task Force on Practice Guidelines. *Circulation*. 2013;127:529.

29. Van de Werf F, Ardissino D, Betriu A, et al. Management of acute myocardial infarction in patients presenting with

ST-segment elevation. The Task Force on the Management of Acute Myocardial Infarction of the European Society of Cardiology. *Eur Heart J.* 2003;24:28.

30. Thune JJ, Hoefsten DE, Lindholm MG, et al. Simple risk stratification at admission to identify patients with reduced mortality from primary angioplasty. *Circulation.* 2005;112:2017.

31. Kent DM, Schmid CH, Lau J, Selker HP. Is primary angioplasty for some as good as primary angioplasty for all? *J Gen Intern Med.* 2002;17:887.

32. Morrow DA, Antman EM, Charlesworth A, et al. TIMI risk score for ST-elevation myocardial infarction: a convenient, bedside, clinical score for risk assessment at presentation: an intravenous nPA for Treatment of Infarcting Myocardium Early II trial substudy. *Circulation.* 2000;102:2031.

33. Rogers WJ, Bowlby LJ, Chandra NC, et al. Treatment of myocardial infarction in the United States (1990 to 1993). Observations from the National Registry of Myocardial Infarction. *Circulation.* 1994;90:2103.

34. Goodman SG, Menon V, Cannon CP, et al. Acute ST-segment elevation myocardial infarction: American College of Chest Physicians Evidence-Based Clinical Practice Guidelines (8th Edition). *Chest.* 2008;133:708S.

35. The GUSTO investigators. An international randomized trial comparing four thrombolytic strategies for acute myocardial infarction. *N Engl J Med.* 1993;329:673.

36. Ross AM, Coyne KS, Moreyra E, et al. Extended mortality benefit of early postinfarction reperfusion. GUSTO-I Angiographic Investigators. Global Utilization of Streptokinase and Tissue Plasminogen Activator for Occluded Coronary Arteries Trial. *Circulation.* 1998;97:1549.

37. CURRENT-OASIS 7 Investigators, Mehta SR, Bassand JP, et al. Dose comparisons of clopidogrel and aspirin in acute coronary syndromes. *N Engl J Med.* 2010;363:930.

38. Xian Y, Wang TY, McCoy LA, et al. Association of discharge aspirin dose with outcomes after acute myocardial infarction: insights from the treatment with ADP receptor inhibitors: longitudinal assessment of treatment patterns and events after acute coronary syndrome (TRANSLATE-ACS) study. *Circulation.* 2015;132:174.

39. http://www.fda.gov/NewsEvents/Newsroom/PressAnnounce-ments/ucm452172.htm (Accessed on June 23, 2015).

40. http://accessdata.fda.gov/drugsatfda_docs/appletter/2015/204958Orig1s000ltr.pdf (Accessed on June 23, 2015).

41. Chen ZM, Jiang LX, Chen YP, et al. Addition of clopidogrel to aspirin in 45,852 patients with acute myocardial infarction: randomized placebo-controlled trial. *Lancet.* 2005;366:1607.

42. Fox KA, Mehta SR, Peters R, et al. Benefits and risks of the combination of clopidogrel and aspirin in patients undergoing surgical revascularization for non-ST-elevation acute coronary syndrome: the Clopidogrel in

Unstable angina to prevent Recurrent ischemic Events (CURE) trial. *Circulation.* 2004;110:1202.

43. Chu MW, Wilson SR, Novick RJ, et al. Does clopidogrel increase blood loss following coronary artery bypass surgery? *Ann Thorac Surg.* 2004;78:1536.

44. Task Force on the Management of ST-segment elevation acute myocardial infarction of the European Society of Cardiology (ESC), Steg PG, James SK, et al. ESC Guidelines for the management of acute myocardial infarction in patients presenting with ST-segment elevation. *Eur Heart J.* 2012;33:2569.

45. Cannon CP, Braunwald E, McCabe CH, et al. Intensive versus moderate lipid lowering with statins after acute coronary syndromes. *N Engl J Med.* 2004;350:1495.

46. Schwartz GG, Olsson AG, Ezekowitz MD, et al. Effects of atorvastatin on early recurrent ischemic events in acute coronary syndromes: the MIRACL study: a randomized controlled trial. *JAMA.* 2001;285:1711.

47.

48. Martí-Carvajal AJ, Simancas-Racines D, Anand V, Bangdiwala S. Prophylactic lidocaine for myocardial infarction. *Cochrane Database Syst Rev.* 2015;CD008553.

49. Grossman AN, Opie LH, Beshansky JR, et al. Glucose-insulin-potassium revived: current status in acute coronary syndromes and the energy-depleted heart. *Circulation.* 2013;127:1040.

50. Singh AK, Szczech L, Tang KL, et al. Correction of anemia with epoetin alfa in chronic kidney disease. *N Engl J Med.* 2006;355:2085.

51. Bennett CL, Silver SM, Djulbegovic B, et al. Venous thromboembolism and mortality associated with recombinant erythropoietin and darbepoetin administration for the treatment of cancer-associated anemia. *JAMA.* 2008;299:914.

52. Bohlius J, Wilson J, Seidenfeld J, et al. Recombinant human erythropoietins and cancer patients: updated meta-analysis of 57 studies including 9353 patients. *J Natl Cancer Inst.* 2006;98:708.

53. Hochman JS, Tamis JE, Thompson TD, et al. Sex, clinical presentation, and outcome in patients with acute coronary syndromes. Global Use of Strategies to Open Occluded Coronary Arteries in Acute Coronary Syndromes IIb Investigators. *N Engl J Med.* 1999;341:226.

54. Raymond R, Lynch J, Underwood D, et al. Myocardial infarction and normal coronary arteriography: a 10 year clinical and risk analysis of 74 patients. *J Am Coll Cardiol.* 1988;11:471.

55. Da Costa A, Isaaz K, Faure E, et al. Clinical characteristics, aetiological factors and long-term prognosis of myocardial infarction with an absolutely normal coronary angiogram; a 3-year follow-up study of 91 patients. *Eur Heart J.* 2001;22:1459.

56. Alpert JS. Myocardial infarction with angiographically normal coronary arteries. A personal perspective. *Arch Intern Med.* 1994;154:245.

57. Indications for fibrinolytic therapy in suspected acute myocardial infarction: collaborative overview of early

mortality and major morbidity results from all randomised trials of more than 1000 patients. Fibrinolytic Therapy Trialists' (FTT) Collaborative Group. *Lancet*. 1994;343:311.

58. Gibson CM, Murphy SA, Kirtane AJ, et al. Association of duration of symptoms at presentation with angiographic and clinical outcomes after fibrinolytic therapy in patients with ST-segment elevation myocardial infarction. *J Am Coll Cardiol*. 2004;44:980.

59. Boersma E, Maas AC, Deckers JW, Simoons ML. Early thrombolytic treatment in acute myocardial infarction: reappraisal of the golden hour. *Lancet*. 1996;348:771.

60. Weaver WD, Cerqueira M, Hallstrom AP, et al. Prehospital-initiated vs hospital-initiated thrombolytic therapy. The Myocardial Infarction Triage and Intervention Trial. *JAMA*. 1993;270:1211.

61. Aylward PE, Wilcox RG, Horgan JH, et al. Relation of increased arterial blood pressure to mortality and stroke in the context of contemporary thrombolytic therapy for acute myocardial infarction. A randomized trial GUSTO-I Investigators. *Ann Intern Med*. 1996;125:891.

62. Krumholz HM, Pasternak RC, Weinstein MC, et al. Cost effectiveness of thrombolytic therapy with streptokinase in elderly patients with suspected acute myocardial infarction. *N Engl J Med*. 1992;327:7.

63. Mahaffey KW, Granger CB, Toth CA, et al. Diabetic retinopathy should not be a contraindication to thrombolytic therapy for acute myocardial infarction: review of ocular hemorrhage incidence and location in the GUSTO-I trial. Global Utilization of Streptokinase and t-PA for Occluded Coronary Arteries. *J Am Coll Cardiol*. 1997;30:1606.

64. Ward H, Yudkin JS. Thrombolysis in patients with diabetes. *BMJ*. 1995;310:3.

65. Gurwitz JH, Gore JM, Goldberg RJ, et al. Risk for intracranial hemorrhage after tissue plasminogen activator treatment for acute myocardial infarction. Participants in the National Registry of Myocardial Infarction 2. *Ann Intern Med*. 1998;129:597.

66. Barron HV, Rundle AC, Gore JM, et al. Intracranial hemorrhage rates and effect of immediate beta-blocker use in patients with acute myocardial infarction treated with tissue plasminogen activator. Participants in the National Registry of Myocardial Infarction-2. *Am J Cardiol*. 2000;85:294.

67. Go AS, Barron HV, Rundle AC, et al. Bundle-branch block and in-hospital mortality in acute myocardial infarction. National Registry of Myocardial Infarction 2 Investigators. *Ann Intern Med*. 1998;129:690.

68. Stenestrand U, Tabrizi F, Lindbäck J, et al. Comorbidity and myocardial dysfunction are the main explanations for the higher 1-year mortality in acute myocardial infarction with left bundle-branch block. *Circulation*. 2004;110:1896.

69. Feigl D, Ashkenazy J, Kishon Y. Early and late atrioventricular block in acute inferior myocardial infarction. *J Am Coll Cardiol*. 1984;4:35.

70. Hindman MC, Wagner GS, JaRo M, et al. The clinical significance of bundle branch block complicating acute myocardial infarction. 1. Clinical characteristics, hospital mortality, and one-year follow-up. *Circulation*. 1978;58:679.

71. Aplin M, Engstrøm T, Vejlstrup NG, et al. Prognostic importance of complete atrioventricular block complicating acute myocardial infarction. *Am J Cardiol*. 2003;92:853.

72. Goldberg RJ, Zevallos JC, Yarzebski J, et al. Prognosis of acute myocardial infarction complicated by complete heart block (the Worcester Heart Attack Study). *Am J Cardiol*. 1992;69:1135.

73. Zimetbaum PJ, Josephson ME. Use of the electrocardiogram in acute myocardial infarction. *N Engl J Med*. 2003;348:933.

74. Bigger Jr. JT, Dresdale FJ, Heissenbuttel RH, et al. Ventricular arrhythmias in ischemic heart disease: mechanism, prevalence, significance, and management. *Prog Cardiovasc Dis*. 1977;19:255.

75. O'Doherty M, Tayler DI, Quinn E, et al. Five hundred patients with myocardial infarction monitored within one hour of symptoms. *Br Med J (Clin Res Ed)*. 1983;286:1405.

76. Harkness JR, Morrow DA, Braunwald E, et al. Myocardial ischemia and ventricular tachycardia on continuous electrocardiographic monitoring and risk of cardiovascular outcomes after non-ST-segment elevation acute coronary syndrome (from the MERLIN-TIMI 36 Trial). *Am J Cardiol*. 2011;108:1373.

77. Newby KH, Thompson T, Stebbins A, et al. Sustained ventricular arrhythmias in patients receiving thrombolytic therapy: incidence and outcomes. The GUSTO Investigators. *Circulation*. 1998;98:2567.

78. Mont L, Cinca J, Blanch P, et al. Predisposing factors and prognostic value of sustained monomorphic ventricular tachycardia in the early phase of acute myocardial infarction. *J Am Coll Cardiol*. 1996;28:1670.

79. Al-Khatib SM, Granger CB, Huang Y, et al. Sustained ventricular arrhythmias among patients with acute coronary syndromes with no ST-segment elevation: incidence, predictors, and outcomes. *Circulation*. 2002;106:309.

80. Field JM, Hazinski MF, Sayre MR, et al. Part 1: executive summary: 2010 American Heart Association Guidelines for Cardiopulmonary Resuscitation and Emergency Cardiovascular Care. *Circulation*. 2010;122:S640.

81. Neumar RW, Otto CW, Link MS, et al. Part 8: adult advanced cardiovascular life support: 2010 American Heart Association Guidelines for Cardiopulmonary Resuscitation and Emergency Cardiovascular Care. *Circulation*. 2010;122:S729.

82. Volpi A, Cavalli A, Santoro L, Negri E. Incidence and prognosis of early primary ventricular fibrillation in acute myocardial infarction—results of the Gruppo Italiano per lo Studio della Sopravvivenza nell'Infarto

Miocardico (GISSI-2) database. *Am J Cardiol.* 1998;82:265.

83. Berger PB, Ruocco NA, Ryan TJ, et al. Incidence and significance of ventricular tachycardia and fibrillation in the absence of hypotension or heart failure in acute myocardial infarction treated with recombinant tissue-type plasminogen activator: results from the Thrombolysis in Myocardial Infarction (TIMI) Phase II trial. *J Am Coll Cardiol.* 1993;22:1773.

84. Gheeraert PJ, Henriques JP, De Buyzere ML, et al. Preinfarction angina protects against out-of-hospital ventricular fibrillation in patients with acute occlusion of the left coronary artery. *J Am Coll Cardiol.* 2001;38:1369.

85. Reeder GS. Identification and treatment of complications of myocardial infarction. *Mayo Clin Proc.* 1995;70:880.

86. Purcaro A, Costantini C, Ciampani N, et al. Diagnostic criteria and management of subacute ventricular free wall rupture complicating acute myocardial infarction. *Am J Cardiol.* 1997;80:397.

87. Batts KP, Ackermann DM, Edwards WD. Postinfarction rupture of the left ventricular free wall: clinicopathologic correlates in 100 consecutive autopsy cases. *Hum Pathol.* 1990;21:530.

88. Oliva PB, Hammill SC, Edwards WD. Cardiac rupture, a clinically predictable complication of acute myocardial infarction: report of 70 cases with clinicopathologic correlations. *J Am Coll Cardiol.* 1993;22:720.

89. López-Sendón J, González A, López de Sá E, et al. Diagnosis of subacute ventricular wall rupture after acute myocardial infarction: sensitivity and specificity of clinical, hemodynamic and echocardiographic criteria. *J Am Coll Cardiol.* 1992;19:1145.

90. Becker RC, Gore JM, Lambrew C, et al. A composite view of cardiac rupture in the United States National Registry of Myocardial Infarction. *J Am Coll Cardiol.* 1996;27:1321.

91. Woldow AB, Mattleman SJ, Ablaza SG, Nakhjavan FK. Isolated rupture of the right ventricle in a patient with acute inferior wall MI. *Chest.* 1990;98:484.

92. Moreno R, López-Sendón J, García E, et al. Primary angioplasty reduces the risk of left ventricular free wall rupture compared with thrombolysis in patients with acute myocardial infarction. *J Am Coll Cardiol.* 2002;39:598.

93. Becker RC, Hochman JS, Cannon CP, et al. Fatal cardiac rupture among patients treated with thrombolytic agents and adjunctive thrombin antagonists: observations from the Thrombolysis and Thrombin Inhibition in Myocardial Infarction 9 Study. *J Am Coll Cardiol.* 1999;33:479.

94. ISIS-1 (First International Study of Infarct Survival) Collaborative Group. Mechanisms for the early mortality reduction produced by beta-blockade started early in acute myocardial infarction: ISIS-1. *Lancet.* 1988;1:921.

95. Cheriex EC, de Swart H, Dijkman LW, et al. Myocardial rupture after myocardial infarction is related to the perfusion status of the infarct-related coronary artery. *Am Heart J.* 1995;129:644.

96. Morishima I, Sone T, Mokuno S, et al. Clinical significance of no-reflow phenomenon observed on angiography after successful treatment of acute myocardial infarction with percutaneous transluminal coronary angioplasty. *Am Heart J.* 1995;130:239.

97. Honan MB, Harrell Jr. FE, Reimer KA, et al. Cardiac rupture, mortality and the timing of thrombolytic therapy: a meta-analysis. *J Am Coll Cardiol.* 1990;16:359.

98. Gertz SD, Kragel AH, Kalan JM, et al. Comparison of coronary and myocardial morphologic findings in patients with and without thrombolytic therapy during fatal first acute myocardial infarction. The TIMI Investigators. *Am J Cardiol.* 1990;66:904.

99. Becker RC, Charlesworth A, Wilcox RG, et al. Cardiac rupture associated with thrombolytic therapy: impact of time to treatment in the Late Assessment of Thrombolytic Efficacy (LATE) study. *J Am Coll Cardiol.* 1995;25:1063.

100. Keeley EC, de Lemos JA. Free wall rupture in the elderly: deleterious effect of fibrinolytic therapy on the ageing heart. *Eur Heart J.* 2005;26:1693.

101. Bueno H, Martínez-Sellés M, Pérez-David E, López-Palop R. Effect of thrombolytic therapy on the risk of cardiac rupture and mortality in older patients with first acute myocardial infarction. *Eur Heart J.* 2005;26:1705.

102. Maggioni AP, Maseri A, Fresco C, et al. Age-related increase in mortality among patients with first myocardial infarctions treated with thrombolysis. The Investigators of the Gruppo Italiano per lo Studio della Sopravvivenza nell'Infarto Miocardico (GISSI-2). *N Engl J Med.* 1993;329:1442.

103. Nakatani D, Sato H, Kinjo K, et al. Effect of successful late reperfusion by primary coronary angioplasty on mechanical complications of acute myocardial infarction. *Am J Cardiol.* 2003;92:785.

104. McMullan MH, Maples MD, Kilgore Jr. TL, Hindman SH. Surgical experience with left ventricular free wall rupture. *Ann Thorac Surg.* 2001;71:1894.

105. Figueras J, Curós A, Cortadellas J, Soler-Soler J. Reliability of electromechanical dissociation in the diagnosis of left ventricular free wall rupture in acute myocardial infarction. *Am Heart J.* 1996;131:861.

106. Frances C, Romero A, Grady D. Left ventricular pseudoaneurysm. *J Am Coll Cardiol.* 1998;32:557.

107. Figueras J, Cortadellas J, Soler-Soler J. Left ventricular free wall rupture: clinical presentation and management. *Heart.* 2000;83:499.

108. Nakatsuchi Y, Minamino T, Fujii K, Negoro S. Clinicopathological characterization of cardiac free wall rupture in patients with acute myocardial infarction: difference between early and late phase rupture. *Int J Cardiol.* 1994;47:S33.

109. Figueras J, Alcalde O, Barrabés JA, et al. Changes in hospital mortality rates in 425 patients with acute ST-elevation myocardial infarction and cardiac rupture over a 30-year period. *Circulation.* 2008;118:2783.

110. Radford MJ, Johnson RA, Daggett Jr. WM, et al. Ventricular septal rupture: a review of clinical and physiologic features and an analysis of survival. *Circulation.* 1981;64:545.

111. Skehan JD, Carey C, Norrell MS, et al. Patterns of coronary artery disease in post-infarction ventricular septal rupture. *Br Heart J.* 1989;62:268.

112. Prêtre R, Rickli H, Ye Q, et al. Frequency of collateral blood flow in the infarct-related coronary artery in rupture of the ventricular septum after acute myocardial infarction. *Am J Cardiol.* 2000;85:497.

113. Birnbaum Y, Wagner GS, Gates KB, et al. Clinical and electrocardiographic variables associated with increased risk of ventricular septal defect in acute anterior myocardial infarction. *Am J Cardiol.* 2000;86:830.

114. Pasternak RC, Braunwald E, Sobel BE. Acute myocardial infarction. In: Braunwald EB, ed. *Heart Disease.* 4th ed. Philadelphia: Saunders; 1992:200.

115. Hayashi T, Hirano Y, Takai H, et al. Usefulness of ST-segment elevation in the inferior leads in predicting ventricular septal rupture in patients with anterior wall acute myocardial infarction. *Am J Cardiol.* 2005;96:1037.

116. Sasaki K, Yotsukura M, Sakata K, et al. Relation of ST-segment changes in inferior leads during anterior wall acute myocardial infarction to length and occlusion site of the left anterior descending coronary artery. *Am J Cardiol.* 2001;87:1340.

117. Pierli C, Lisi G, Mezzacapo B. Subacute left ventricular free wall rupture. Surgical repair prompted by echocardiographic diagnosis. *Chest.* 1991;100:1174.

118. Crenshaw BS, Granger CB, Birnbaum Y, et al. Risk factors, angiographic patterns, and outcomes in patients with ventricular septal defect complicating acute myocardial infarction. GUSTO-I (Global Utilization of Streptokinase and TPA for Occluded Coronary Arteries) Trial Investigators. *Circulation.* 2000;101:27.

119. Mann JM, Roberts WC. Acquired ventricular septal defect during acute myocardial infarction: analysis of 38 unoperated necropsy patients and comparison with 50 unoperated necropsy patients without rupture. *Am J Cardiol.* 1988;62:8.

120. Perloff JK, Talano JV, Ronan Jr. JA. Noninvasive techniques in acute myocardial infarction. *Prog Cardiovasc Dis.* 1971;13:437.

121. Vargas-Barrón J, Molina-Carrión M, Romero-Cárdenas A, et al. Risk factors, echocardiographic patterns, and outcomes in patients with acute ventricular septal rupture during myocardial infarction. *Am J Cardiol.* 2005;95:1153.

122. Bishop HL, Gibson RS, Stamm RB, et al. Role of two-dimensional echocardiography in the evaluation of patients with ventricular septal rupture postmyocardial infarction. *Am Heart J.* 1981;102:965.

123. Smyllie JH, Sutherland GR, Geuskens R, et al. Doppler color flow mapping in the diagnosis of ventricular septal rupture and acute mitral regurgitation after myocardial infarction. *J Am Coll Cardiol.* 1990;15:1449.

124. Moursi MH, Bhatnagar SK, Vilacosta I, et al. Transesophageal echocardiographic assessment of papillary muscle rupture. *Circulation.* 1996;94:1003.

125. Jones MT, Schofield PM, Dark JF, et al. Surgical repair of acquired ventricular septal defect. Determinants of early and late outcome. *J Thorac Cardiovasc Surg.* 1987;93:680.

126. Davies RH, Dawkins KD, Skillington PD, et al. Late functional results after surgical closure of acquired ventricular septal defect. *J Thorac Cardiovasc Surg.* 1993;106:592.

127. Lemery R, Smith HC, Giuliani ER, Gersh BJ. Prognosis in rupture of the ventricular septum after acute myocardial infarction and role of early surgical intervention. *Am J Cardiol.* 1992;70:147.

128. Nishimura RA, Schaff HV, Gersh BJ, et al. Early repair of mechanical complications after acute myocardial infarction. *JAMA.* 1986;256:47.

129. Litton TC, Sutton JP, Smith CW, et al. Surgical treatment of ventricular septal rupture complicating myocardial infarction. *Am J Surg.* 1988;155:587.

130. Muehrcke DD, Daggett Jr. WM, Buckley MJ, et al. Postinfarct ventricular septal defect repair: effect of coronary artery bypass grafting. *Ann Thorac Surg.* 1992;54:876.

131. Benton JP, Barker KS. Transcatheter closure of ventricular septal defect: a nonsurgical approach to the care of the patient with acute ventricular septal rupture. *Heart Lung.* 1992;21:356.

132. Lavie CJ, Gersh BJ. Mechanical and electrical complications of acute myocardial infarction. *Mayo Clin Proc.* 1990;65:709.

133. Tcheng JE, Jackman Jr. JD, Nelson CL, et al. Outcome of patients sustaining acute ischemic mitral regurgitation during myocardial infarction. *Ann Intern Med.* 1992;117:18.

134. Levine RA, Schwammenthal E. Ischemic mitral regurgitation on the threshold of a solution: from paradoxes to unifying concepts. *Circulation.* 2005;112:745.

135. David TE. Techniques and results of mitral valve repair for ischemic mitral regurgitation. *J Card Surg.* 1994;9:274.

136. James TN. Anatomy of the coronary arteries in health and disease. *Circulation.* 1965;32:1020.

137. Barbour DJ, Roberts WC. Rupture of a left ventricular papillary muscle during acute myocardial infarction: analysis of 22 necropsy patients. *J Am Coll Cardiol.* 1986;8:558.

138. Nishimura RA, Shub C, Tajik AJ. Two dimensional echocardiographic diagnosis of partial papillary muscle rupture. *Br Heart J.* 1982;48:598.

139. Kishon Y, Oh JK, Schaff HV, et al. Mitral valve operation in postinfarction rupture of a papillary muscle:

immediate results and long-term follow-up of 22 patients. *Mayo Clin Proc.* 1992;67:1023.

140. DiSesa VJ, Cohn LH, Collins Jr. JJ, et al. Determinants of operative survival following combined mitral valve replacement and coronary revascularization. *Ann Thorac Surg.* 1982;34:482.

141. Tofler GH, Muller JE, Stone PH, et al. Pericarditis in acute myocardial infarction: characterization and clinical significance. *Am Heart J.* 1989;117:86.

142. Correale E, Maggioni AP, Romano S, et al. Comparison of frequency, diagnostic and prognostic significance of pericardial involvement in acute myocardial infarction treated with and without thrombolytics. Gruppo Italiano per lo Studio della Sopravvivenza nell'Infarto Miocardico (GISSI). *Am J Cardiol.* 1993;71:1377.

143. Wall TC, Califf RM, Harrelson-Woodlief L, et al. Usefulness of a pericardial friction rub after thrombolytic therapy during acute myocardial infarction in predicting amount of myocardial damage. The TAMI Study Group. *Am J Cardiol.* 1990;66:1418.

144. Oliva PB, Hammill SC, Edwards WD. Electrocardiographic diagnosis of postinfarction regional pericarditis. Ancillary observations regarding the effect of reperfusion on the rapidity and amplitude of T wave inversion after acute myocardial infarction. *Circulation.* 1993;88:896.

145. Oliva PB, Hammill SC, Talano JV. T wave changes consistent with epicardial involvement in acute myocardial infarction. Observations in patients with a postinfarction pericardial effusion without clinically recognized postinfarction pericarditis. *J Am Coll Cardiol.* 1994;24:1073.

146. Figueras J, Juncal A, Carballo J, et al. Nature and progression of pericardial effusion in patients with a first myocardial infarction: relationship to age and free wall rupture. *Am Heart J.* 2002;144:251.

147. Figueras J, Barrabés JA, Serra V, et al. Hospital outcome of moderate to severe pericardial effusion complicating ST-elevation acute myocardial infarction. *Circulation.* 2010;122:1902.

148. Galve E, Garcia-Del-Castillo H, Evangelista A, et al. Pericardial effusion in the course of myocardial infarction: incidence, natural history, and clinical relevance. *Circulation.* 1986;73:294.

149. Belkin RN, Mark DB, Aronson L, et al. Pericardial effusion after intravenous recombinant tissue-type plasminogen activator for acute myocardial infarction. *Am J Cardiol.* 1991;67:496.

150. Sugiura T, Iwasaka T, Tarumi N, et al. Clinical significance of pericardial effusion in Q-wave inferior wall acute myocardial infarction. *Am J Cardiol.* 1994;73:862.

151. Widimský P, Gregor P. Pericardial involvement during the course of myocardial infarction. A long-term clinical and echocardiographic study. *Chest.* 1995;108:89.

152. Khan AH. The postcardiac injury syndromes. *Clin Cardiol.* 1992;15:67.

153. Madsen SM, Jakobsen TJ. Colchicine treatment of recurrent steroid-dependent pericarditis in a patient with post-myocardial-infarction syndrome (Dressler's syndrome). *Ugeskr Laeger.* 1992;154:3427.

# CHAPTER 23

# Non-ST-Elevation Acute Coronary Syndromes

SAMAD GHAFFARI*

Cardiovascular Research Center, Tabriz University of Medicine, Tabriz, Iran

---

## KEY POINTS

- The majority of NSTE-ACS cases are atherosclerotic in origin. In some, vasoconstriction is the dominant cause. Increased myocardial demand or decreased myocardial supply can participate in the development of NSTE-ACS.
- Patients often present with chest discomfort typical of angina, which is usually more severe, occurs at rest, and lasts longer.
- The initial electrocardiogram (ECG) may be normal in more than one-third of patients. Characteristic abnormalities include ST depression, transient ST elevation, and T-wave changes.
- Cardiac troponins (cTns) are the preferred biomarkers for the diagnosis of myocardial necrosis and the MB isoenzyme of creatine kinase (CK-MB) is an alternative option. An increasing number of emergency departments are using highly sensitive troponin (hsTn) assays for the rapid diagnosis of myocardial necrosis.
- NSTE-ACS include a wide spectrum of population from low-risk patients who are candidates for medical treatment to very high-risk patients who need immediate angiography and revascularization.
- Nitrates, beta-blockers, and calcium blockers are usual selections to alleviate ischemia and related symptoms while antiplatelet and anticoagulants are used to prevent adverse cardiac events including myocardial infarction, heart failure, and death. Invasive approaches and revascularization help to achieve both therapeutic goals.
- Patients are advised to participate in cardiac rehabilitation and secondary prevention programs to ensure medication adherence and lifestyle changes including smoking cessation, regular physical activity, and a healthy diet.

---

## INTRODUCTION

Acute coronary syndrome (ACS) is a constellation of symptoms and signs resulting from acute myocardial ischemia caused by obstruction of blood flow in coronary arteries. Most commonly, this is the result of atherosclerotic plaque rupture; however, plaque erosion or a combination of both mechanisms with superimposed intracoronary thrombosis may be involved and result in heart muscle necrosis and death.[1] ACS can manifest as a clinical spectrum from unstable angina (UA) and *non-ST-segment elevation myocardial infarction* (NSTEMI) to *ST-segment elevation myocardial infarction* (STEMI).

Patient history, electrocardiogram (ECG), and the level of specific serum biomarkers are cornerstones of the diagnosis and classification of ACS. Patients with

new ST elevation in the first ECG are labeled as having STEMI and are usually referred to receive reperfusion therapy. In those without ST elevation, an elevated level of specific biomarkers differentiates patients with detectable myonecrosis (NSTEMI) from patients without evidence of heart muscle necrosis (UA). The distinction between these two entities is often difficult or even impossible at the time of presentation and depends on subsequent analysis of cardiac biomarkers. So, the term *non-ST-elevation acute coronary syndrome* (NSTE-ACS) is used in initial identification of both conditions, which together constitute the largest group of patients with ACS.[2]

NSTEMI that is associated with myocardial necrosis usually progresses to non-Q-wave MI (NQWMI) and in a very small subset of patients to Q-wave MI (QWMI) (Fig. 23.1). Currently, with the advent of high-sensitivity cardiac troponin measurements, the detection of cases with NSTEMI has been increased.[3,4]

---

*The author is grateful to Dr. Hamidreza Sanati for contribution to previous edition of this chapter.

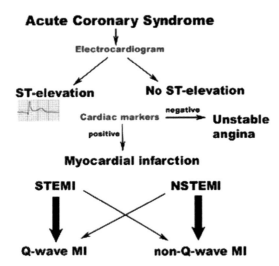

**FIG. 23.1** Definition of the acute coronary syndromes. Based on the first electrocardiogram, patients are divided into STEMI and NSTE-ACS. The latter group is further subcategorized by the presence or absence of an elevated cardiac biomarkers into unstable angina and NSTEMI. (From Alpert JS, Thygesen K, Antman E, Bassand JP. Myocardial infarction redefined—a consensus document of The Joint European Society of Cardiology/American College of Cardiology Committee for the redefinition of myocardial infarction. *J Am Coll Cardiol.* 2000;36(3):959–969. https://doi.org/10.1016/S0735-1097(00)00804-4. PMID 10987628.)

## PATHOPHYSIOLOGY

The majority of NSTE-ACS cases are atherosclerotic in origin. Plaque rupture or erosion results in the formation of superimposed thrombus, reduction in myocardial supply, ischemia, and finally myocardial necrosis in some cases. Concurrent vasoconstriction derived from vasoconstrictors released by platelets, endothelial dysfunction, or adrenergic stimuli contributes to the process. In some cases, vasoconstriction is the dominant cause, as the vasoconstriction of small intramural coronary arteries. Increased myocardial demand (e.g., tachycardia, fever, thyrotoxicosis, severe left ventricular hypertrophy, and aortic stenosis) or decreased myocardial supply (e.g., anemia and hypotension) can participate in the development of NSTE-ACS or even cause myocardial ischemia and necrosis in the absence of obstructive coronary artery disease (CAD). Progressive intraluminal narrowing caused by atherosclerosis or in-stent restenosis might present as NSTE-ACS. Any combinations of these processes might be occurring simultaneously. Targeting, inhibition, and reversal of these processes using pharmacologic and mechanical interventions are pivotal in the treatment of NSTE-ACS.

## INITIAL ASSESSMENT

### History

Patients with NSTE-ACS often present with chest discomfort typical of angina. They usually describe it as retrosternal heaviness, compression, or frank pain. Although the quality of discomfort is similar to chronic stable ischemic pain, it is usually more severe, occurs at rest and lasts longer. The discomfort is exacerbated by activity or emotional stress and is less likely to be completely resolved with sublingual nitroglycerin (NTG). The typical location of the pain is substernal (sometimes epigastrium) but frequently radiates to either shoulder, left arm, jaw, or neck. Some patients may suffer from dyspnea, nausea and vomiting, diaphoresis, and unexplained fatigue as "anginal equivalents."[5]

Clinical severity of NSTE-ACS can be categorized according to the Braunwald's unstable angina classification from Grade I; defined as new onset of severe angina or accelerated angina in the absence of resting pain to Grade II with angina at rest within past month but not within preceding 48 h (subacute) and Grade III with resting angina within last 48 h (acute).[6] This clinical classification has prognostic and therapeutic implications. While accelerated angina is more probably associated with a fixed coronary atherosclerotic stenosis, resting angina commonly reflects a ruptured and thrombotic coronary plaque.

Atypical symptoms such as isolated dyspnea, epigastric pain, indigestion, unusual locations of pain, altered mental status, and syncope always should be taken into consideration. These atypical symptoms are more common in older patients, women, diabetics, dementia, and those with chronic renal insufficiency and are associated with a worse prognosis.[7,8] The presence of risk factors for CAD, history of previous symptomatic CAD, peripheral artery disease, percutaneous coronary intervention (PCI), and coronary artery bypass graft surgery (CABG) increases the possibility of NSTE-ACS in a patient with acute chest pain.

In younger people, especially women, and in the absence of familial hypercholesterolemia and premature CAD, acute chest pain resulting from atherosclerotic CAD is a relatively uncommon finding. Cocaine use should always be considered in this group. In all patients with acute ischemic chest pain, secondary exacerbating or participating conditions such as anemia, fever, infection, metabolic disorders, and hyperthyroidism need to be evaluated.

### Physical Examination

In the systemic physical examination of patients with suspected NSTE-ACS, precipitating factors such as anemia, fever, thyroid disease, and the evidence of other serious conditions like pulmonary embolism and aortic dissection should be evaluated. Findings in the cardiovascular system depend on the extent of ischemic myocardium. Most patients have unremarkable findings but in those with extensive ischemia, signs of heart failure such as S3, cold sweating, and pulmonary rales may be present. The transient systolic murmur of mitral regurgitation may be audible during the acute phase and suggests papillary muscle ischemia.

## Electrocardiography

Electrocardiography is the first-line diagnostic modality in patients with suspected ACS. While the initial electrocardiogram (ECG) in the setting of NSTE-ACS may be normal in more than one-third of patients, characteristic abnormalities include ST depression, transient ST elevation, and T-wave changes.[9] Serial ECGs, especially when recorded in the symptomatic phase, could increase the chance of recording abnormal findings and may show dynamic ST-T changes and high-risk patients. Dynamic ST-segment depression $\geq$0.5 mm is a sensitive but not specific marker for NSTE-ACS. Greater degrees of ST-segment depression and larger number of involved leads predict poorer outcomes. T-wave inversions more than 2 mm are compatible with, but not necessarily diagnostic of NSTE-ACS.[10] This deep and symmetrical T-wave inversions in the anterior precordial leads may be part of so-called Wellens syndrome indicating critical stenosis of the proximal left anterior descending artery (LAD) (Fig. 23.2). Lesser degrees of isolated T-wave inversions have low specificity.

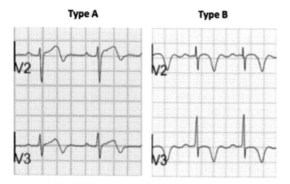

FIG. 23.2 There are two patterns of T-wave changes in Wellens syndrome. Type A: Biphasic T waves with initial positivity and terminal negativity (25% of cases), and Type B: Deeply and symmetrically inverted T waves (75% of cases). (Modified from https://www.grepmed.com/images/1677/cardiology-diagnosis-syndrome-wellens-typeb-typea-ekg.)

Diffuse ST depression associated with ST-elevation $\geq$1 mm in lead aVR/V1 may indicate a high-risk group of patients with either left main coronary artery as the culprit lesion or proximal occlusion of the left anterior descending coronary artery in the presence of severe three-vessel CAD.[9]

Ischemia in some territories might not be reflected on the standard 12-lead ECG. Recording the additional ECG leads including V7–V9 and V3R/V4R might help to diagnose culprit lesions in the left circumflex and acute marginal branch of the right coronary artery, respectively.[11] Continuous ECG monitoring is not generally recommended for initial diagnosis when the changes are nonspecific, but ST depressions detected in the early post-MI period are associated with an increased risk of future major events.

## Cardiac Biomarkers

Heart-specific biomarkers have diagnostic and prognostic value in patients with suspected or confirmed NSTE-ACS. Cardiac troponins (cTns) are the preferred biomarkers for the diagnosis of myocardial necrosis and the MB isoenzyme of creatine kinase (CK-MB) is an alternative option when troponin is not available.[11] Both types of cardiac troponins (cTnT and cTnI) are very specific for the heart muscle. An elevated cTn level is defined as values of cTnI or cTnt above the 99th percentile of the normal range defined for any specific test.[11] Even minor troponin elevations are independently associated with adverse events in patients with NSTE-ACS. CK-MB levels may be normal in most of these patients.[12]

Various cardiac and noncardiac conditions may be associated with elevated levels of cTns (Table 23.1). An elevated cTn could be attributed to ACS only in the presence of clinical background supporting this diagnosis. Elevations caused by ACS are usually of a greater magnitude and should demonstrate a dynamic pattern. Demonstration of a transient increase or decrease in cTn level with serial measurements improves the specificity for ACS diagnosis.[13]

With conventional cTn assays, we need two measurements with at least 6 h apart to exclude clinically significant myocardial necrosis. In recent years an increasing number of emergency departments are using high-sensitive troponin (hsTn) assays for rapid diagnosis of myocardial necrosis. Clinicians using these rapid tests should pay more attention than before to the clinical background of the patients to avoid misdiagnosis. Some centers have a 1-h protocol combining patient history, ECG, and hsTn allowing fast rule-out and rule-in of 30-day major adverse cardiac events (MACE) that performed better than the troponin-alone algorithm.[14]

**TABLE 23.1**
Selected Cardiac and Non-Cardiac Causes of Elevated Cardiac Troponin Level

| Primary Cardiac Conditions | Non-Cardiac Conditions |
| --- | --- |
| Myocardial Infarction | End stage renal disease |
| Congestive heart failure | Pulmonary embolism |
| Cardiomyopathies | Intense exercise |
| Myocarditis | Sepsis |
| Procedural (heart surgery, angioplasty, defibrillation, radiofrequency ablation) | Stroke and subarachnoid hemorrhage |
| Tachyarrhythmia | Critical illness |
| Chest trauma and cardiopulmonary resuscitation | Drug toxicity |

Besides heart-specific markers, some other biomarkers may help to risk stratify NSTE-ACS population further. Increased C-reactive peptide levels are associated with a higher risk of adverse events and a similar graded correlation has been reported for brain natriuretic peptides (BNP). Combining BNP, CRP, and cTnI provides a multimarker approach for risk stratification of NSTE-ACS patients.[15]

### Noninvasive Testing

In patients with NSTE-ACS who are managed with an initial conservative approach, in the absence of high-risk criteria and after stabilization with medical therapy, a noninvasive test may be needed for further risk stratification. In the absence of hemodynamic and electrophysiologic abnormality, the test can be safely performed at least 24 h after symptoms have subsided.[16] If the resting ECG lacks significant baseline abnormality, a symptom-limited exercise stress testing is usually recommended. If significant baseline ECG abnormalities are present or the patient cannot tolerate the exercise, stress echocardiography or stress myocardial perfusion imaging can be used. Those with evidence of severe ischemia in mentioned noninvasive tests (e.g., ST depression $\geq 2$ mm in low workload, large ischemic territory, hypotension, malignant arrhythmia, LV dilation with reduced function, and pulmonary uptake of a radioisotope) are candidates of early inhospital angiography and revascularization.

Coronary CT angiography (CTA) is another useful modality in chest pain units. Randomized trials have shown that it can shorten hospital stay and reduce costs and may be more widely accepted by the patients.[17,18] In the multicenter randomized (SCOT-HEART) study,

the addition of coronary CTA to standard clinical care increased the need for invasive coronary angiography but reduced the need for further stress testing and changed treatment regimens in a direction that might be associated with a trend of reduced rate of myocardial infarction.[19] In the absence of contraindications like documented ACS or significant nephropathy, the most appropriate indications to use CTA in chest pain units include low to moderate risk patients, normal or indeterminate ECG, and $\geq 1$ negative troponin test.[20]

### Invasive Coronary Angiography

Using coronary angiography, about 85% of patients with NSTE-ACS have at least one major coronary artery lesion with a diameter stenosis of $\geq 50\%$. The left main stem is involved in about 10% and almost equal numbers (25%) have one-, two-, and three-vessel CAD. About 15% of patients, mostly women, have no significant angiographic CAD and in the absence of discernible noncardiac causes, cardiac X syndrome or variant angina should be considered in this population.[13] Angiographic feature of culprit plaque is usually characterized by its eccentricity and hazy appearance due to the presence of thrombosis and this helps to differentiate it from nonculprit plaques. Histologically these vulnerable plaques are characterized by high lipid core content and calcification compared with higher fibrotic tissue in nonculprit plaques.[21]

### RISK STRATIFICATION

NSTE-ACS include a wide spectrum of population from low-risk patients who are candidates for medical treatment to very high-risk patients who need immediate angiography and revascularization. Various clinical, electrocardiographic, and paraclinical factors are associated with the risk of adverse events in the future. The presence of resting chest pain, pain in the first 2 weeks following STEMI, pain with minimal exercise, evidence of clinical heart failure, advanced age, the presence of comorbidities such as chronic kidney disease (CKD), diabetes, and known atherosclerotic vascular disease are among important factors indicating a higher risk and a poor outcome. Electrocardiographic evidence of dynamic ST-T changes, transient ST-segment elevation, and cardiac arrhythmias also predict a group of high-risk patients. Echocardiography may help to risk stratify patients by determining LV dysfunction and evidence of ischemic mitral regurgitation. Levels of serum biomarkers and findings of noninvasive tests and coronary angiography are also among important prognostic factors that were discussed earlier in this chapter. Several risk-scoring models have been described based on clinical trials (TIMI and PURSUIT) or registry data (GRACE).[22–24] Among these, TIMI risk score is simpler and can be calculated at the bedside without a calculator and might be used to guide treatment (Fig. 23.3).

## MANAGEMENT

Patients with atypical or mild symptoms, negative admission ECG, and normal initial cTn level should be observed in a chest pain unit. If the patient has no

continuing angina and serial ECG and troponin assays are normal, a noninvasive test (exercise test, stress myocardial perfusion imaging, and stress echocardiography) could be performed before or early after discharge to decide for specific treatments. Some centers have specific protocols using hsTn or coronary CTA as discussed earlier. Other patients with no high-risk features such as ongoing or recurrent chest pain, new ST-T changes or elevated biomarkers in serial assessments, could be admitted to a step-down or regular unit. Patients with any of these high-risk criteria or those in a moderate to high-risk category based on risk stratification protocols should be admitted to an intensive coronary unit. General considerations in patients with possible or definite NSTE-ACS are summarized in Table 23.2.

Specific treatments in the acute phase of NSTE-ACS are directed either to alleviate ischemia and related symptoms or to prevent adverse cardiac events including myocardial infarction, heart failure, and death. Nitrates, beta-blockers, and calcium blockers are usual selections to achieve the first goal while antiplatelet and anticoagulants are used to target the second aim. Invasive approaches and revascularization help to achieve both therapeutic goals.

In addition to acute-phase treatments, after hospital discharge, all measures should be taken to control risk factors and prevent further events. Statins not only have an important therapeutic value in the acute phase but also have a pivotal role in reducing recurrent events.

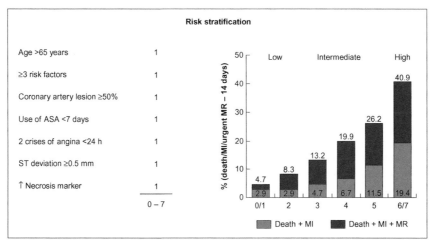

FIG. 23.3 TIMI risk score of 0–2 are usually classified as low risk, TIMI score of 3–4 intermediate, and ≥5 as high risk. *ASA*, acetylsalicylic acid; *MI*, myocardial infarction; *MR*, myocardial revascularization. (Feitosa-Filho GS, Baracioli LM, Barbosa CJ, et al. SBC Guidelines on unstable angina and non-ST-elevation myocardial infarction: executive summary. *Arq Bras Cardiol*. 2015;105(3):214–227.)

**TABLE 23.2**

**General Considerations in the Management of Patients With Non-ST-Segment Elevation Acute Coronary Syndrome**

*Admission*

- Patients with atypical symptoms who are deemed to be at low risk might be observed in the ED
- Patients with UA without ECG changes should be admitted in regular ward or step-down unit ± continuous ECG monitoring
- Patients with new ECG changes or elevated cardiac enzymes should be monitored in an intensive care unit or coronary care unit
- Initial bed rest and ambulation after 12–24 h if the patient is stable without ongoing chest pain or ECG changes
- Administer supplemental oxygen if $O_2$ saturation is <90% and in those with heart failure and pulmonary rales

*Electrocardiography*

- Obtain an initial 12-lead ECG within 10 mm of arrival
- Obtain serial ECGs at 15- to 30-min intervals during the first hour if the initial ECG is nondiagnostic
- Consider additional ECG leads ($V_7$–$V_9$, and $V_3R$–$V_4R$)

*Cardiac biomarkers*

- Obtain a sample for cTn at presentation
- Obtain serial cTn measurements at 3–6 h after symptom onset
- Consider a delayed cTn sample after 6 h if the serial measurements are negative

*cTn*, cardiac troponin; *ED*, emergency department; *ECG*, electrocardiography; *UA*, unstable angina.

## ANTI-ISCHEMIC DRUGS

### Nitrates

Nitrates decrease myocardial $O_2$ demand by reducing preload (ventricular wall stress) and afterload and by increasing supply through coronary vasodilation. In the absence of contraindications and especially in the prehospital phase, sublingual nitroglycerin is preferred and could be substituted with IV infusion in those with continuing symptoms, hypertension, and pulmonary congestion.

Clinical trials do not support the role of nitrates in reducing tight endpoints of ACS and long-term nitrate prescription is limited to patients with recurrent symptoms.[25] Nitrates should be used with caution or not to be used in those with left ventricular (LV) outflow obstruction or right ventricular infarction and they

are contraindicated in patients with hypotension (SBP < 90 mmHg) or recent use of a phosphodiesterase type 5 (PDE-5) inhibitors like sildenafil or tadalafil.

### Beta-Blockers

By decreasing heart rate, blood pressure, and myocardial contractility, beta-blockers reduce myocardial $O_2$ demand and ischemia. Most of our data regarding this group of drugs come from studies performed decades ago as well as studies on STEMI, which overall are in favor of a survival benefit. In the absence of known contraindications (Chapter 22) latest guidelines of both AHA/ACC and ESC recommend early initiation of beta-blockers preferably in the first 24 h of admission in patients with NSTE-ACS.[9,16] It is recommended to continue beta-blocker therapy for a longer period especially in those with reduced LV function. Patients with evidence of heart failure or high risk for developing cardiogenic shock (older age, tachycardia, and hypotension) are at increased risk of shock and mortality with early beta-blocker therapy and it is recommended to avoid early initiation of beta-blockers in this situation. This group of patients and those with initial contraindications should be reevaluated in the following days to determine their subsequent eligibility.[26] Patients with stabilized heart failure benefit from beta-blockers, especially products with proven efficacy in heart failure, including sustained-release metoprolol succinate, carvedilol, or bisoprolol.[27]

### Calcium Channel Blockers

By targeting smooth muscle cells of vessels wall, calcium channel blockers (CCBs) exert a vasodilatory effect. Nondihydropyridines (verapamil and diltiazem) have dominant cardiac effects and reduce contractility, heart rate, and AV nodal conduction. Conversely, the dihydropyridines (e.g., amlodipine and nifedipine) have predominant vasodilatory effects and have minimal effect on the conduction system. Patients with contraindications to beta-blockers, those with refractory chest pain despite treatment with beta-blockers and nitrates, and those with refractory hypertension are good candidates for treatment with CCBs. Nondihydropyridine CCBs are preferred, but long-acting dihydropyridines also might be safe. Long-acting CCBs are especially efficacious in cases with vasospastic angina, alone or in combination with nitrates, and seem to be safe in patients with LV dysfunction.[16,28] Nifedipine that is an immediate-release CCB should be avoided in patients with NSTE-ACS, especially without concurrent administration of a beta-blocker. It can cause a rapid increase in heart rate and decrease in blood pressure, which is harmful to these patients. Nondihydropyridine CCBs should not be used in patients with slow heart rate, PR interval >0.24 s, high-grade AV blocks, heart failure, and LV dysfunction.

### Analgesics

Intravenous morphine is the most widely used analgesic, followed by meperidine. In patients with persistent chest pain after initiation of nitrates and beta-blockers, repeated IV injection of 1–5 mg morphine is recommended. Other than analgesic effects, it reduces anxiety of the patient and sympathetic overactivity. In patients with heart failure, its venodilatory effects are useful in reducing pulmonary congestion and cardiac workload. In recent years there have been some concerns regarding delayed absorption of P2Y12 inhibitors following morphine injection because of reduced intestinal motility.[29]

## ANTIPLATELET THERAPY

### Aspirin

By irreversible inhibition of cyclooxygenase-1 (COX-1) through acetylation in platelets, aspirin (ASA) prevents thromboxane A2 production that is a potent platelet activator and vasoconstrictor. ASA use in NSTE-ACS is associated with a significant reduction in the rate of major events and mortality. It should be started with a dose of 160 or 325 mg, and continued indefinitely with a reduced dose of 75–100 mg.[9,16] The loading dose of ASA should be chewed in order to rapidly achieve the desired serum level, and enteric-coated products should be avoided because of their slow and unreliable absorption.[30] Higher maintenance dosages were no more preventive than the recommended dose but were associated with a higher rate of gastrointestinal bleeding.[31] Lower doses of ASA also are necessary when used in combination with ticagrelor. Nonsteroidal antiinflammatory drugs (NSAIDs) are associated with a higher rate of major events in NSTE-ACS and their reversible binding to COX-1 impairs ASA efficacy.[16]

### Oral P2Y12 Inhibitors

This group of antiplatelet agents includes thienopyridines, with irreversible P2Y12 receptor binding capability (ticlopidine, clopidogrel, and prasugrel) and ticagrelor, a reversible P2Y12 inhibitor. Inhibiting this receptor prevents ADP-induced platelet activation and aggregation. In recent years ticlopidine use is limited because of its poor safety profile, especially in terms of increased risk of neutropenia and thrombotic thrombocytopenic purpura. Since ASA and various P2Y12 inhibitors use

different pathways to inhibit platelets, the combined use of these drugs has been considered by many investigators, and it is known as dual antiplatelet therapy (DAPT). The first randomized clinical trial for establishing the superiority of DAPT over ASA alone was conducted on patients undergoing PCI in 1996.[32] Since that time, many studies, including over 35 randomized clinical trials, have investigated DAPT in a wide range of cardiovascular medicine.[33] In the absence of contraindications such as high bleeding risk, a P2Y12 inhibitor is recommended for 12 months in addition to aspirin.

### Clopidogrel

In the Clopidogrel in Unstable Angina to Prevent Recurrent Ischemic Events (CURE) randomized trial, conducted on patients with UA/NSTEMI, those received a combination of ASA and clopidogrel for average 9 months had a significantly lower rate of CV death, MI, or stroke compared with those received ASA alone. This benefit was also observed in patients treated medically without revascularization.[34] The risk of major bleeding was significantly higher in the clopidogrel arm and was more remarkable in patients who underwent CABG surgery within the first 5 days of stopping clopidogrel. It is recommended that whenever possible, clopidogrel be discontinued at least 5 days before major surgery.

The recommended dose of clopidogrel in NSTE-ACS patients is an initial loading dose of 300–600 mg, followed by a maintenance dose of 75 mg daily for at least 12 months. Similar to the other thienopyridines, clopidogrel is a prodrug and needs hepatic cytochrome P-450 (CYP) system to be converted to its active metabolites. Certain genetic polymorphisms of the CYP system may render the patient clopidogrel-hyporesponsive. Also, other drugs' competition for cytochrome P-450 enzymes may interfere with the activation of clopidogrel. Higher loading dose (600 mg clopidogrel) is preferred in high-risk patients who are candidates of urgent PCI and need more rapid achievement to therapeutic blood level.[35]

### Prasugrel

Prasugrel is a thienopyridine that is similar to clopidogrel, requires conversion to its active metabolite by CYP system. However, prasugrel needs only one-step hepatic metabolism, and this results in a rapid onset of more potent antiplatelet activity of this drug.

In the TRITON-TIMI-38 trial, prasugrel (60 mg loading; then 10 mg/day) was compared with clopidogrel (300 mg load; 75 mg/day). The composite rate of CV death, MI, and stroke was significantly lower in the prasugrel group, mostly own to a reduced rate of nonfatal procedural MI especially in diabetic patients. There was also a significant reduction in the rate of stent thrombosis.[36] Patients in the prasugrel group had a significantly higher rate of major bleeding. In those with prior stroke or transient ischemic attack, net harm was detected, and prasugrel is contraindicated in this group. Patients older than 75 years and those with body weight <60 kg were more susceptible to bleeding, and prasugrel, either should be avoided in these groups or be considered with a lower maintenance dose of 5 mg/day if the risk of thrombosis is high.

In two other next studies, the benefit of prasugrel over clopidogrel was not reported, and a similar or higher rate of bleeding was detected with the former.[37,38] In the absence of contraindications and preferentially high-risk features (age ≥75, body weight <60 kg), prasugrel (60-mg loading dose and 10-mg daily dose) is recommended in patients who are proceeding to PCI. This drug is contraindicated in NSTE-ACS patients in whom coronary anatomy is not known. It is recommended that prasugrel be discontinued at least 7 days before major nonemergency surgery.[9]

### Ticagrelor
Ticagrelor is a nonthienopyridine and reversible P2Y12 inhibitor. The drug is in active form, and CYP system is not necessary for its conversion to an active metabolite. This leads to a more rapid and more potent platelet inhibition not affected by CYP system polymorphism. Nearly 40% inhibition of platelet aggregation in the first 30 min after a loading dose of 180 mg (compared with 8% for clopidogrel) is expected, and the drug achieves full activity at 2 h.[39]

In the NSTE-ACS subgroup of patients enrolled in PLATO trial, comparing ticagrelor with clopidogrel, significantly reduced rate of the primary end point (CV death, MI, or stroke) and stent thrombosis was observed with ticagrelor. This benefit also was reported in patients managed noninvasively and even in elderly patients with a history of TIA or stroke or those with body weight <60 kg. Non-CABG major bleeding was increased significantly but this was not the case for CABG-related bleeding.[40]

Several unique side effects have been observed with ticagrelor, which may be adenosine mediated. These include dyspnea, ventricular pauses, and bradycardia without an increased need for a pacemaker. Most of these side effects are limited to the first week of treatment and decrease in frequency over time. An increased level of serum uric acid and creatinine, mostly in elderly people is reported.[40]

Ticagrelor should be started with a loading dose of 180 mg and continued with 90 mg twice daily for at least 12 months except in those at higher risk for bleeding. Despite reversible P2Y12 inhibition, it should be discontinued 5 days before major surgery because of its higher level of platelet inhibition. Different results of PLATO trial in the United States and non-US countries may be related to high ASA dosages prescribed in the former, and it is recommended that the dose of ASA in combination with ticagrelor be restricted to 80 mg and high dose ASA be avoided.[41] Unlike ESC guidelines, preference for ticagrelor over clopidogrel in NSTE-ACS based on AHA/ACC guidelines has a class IIa recommendation in both medical alone and PCI groups.[35]

There is some evidence supporting short-term DAPT in patients at high bleeding risk. The TWILIGHT trial showed that among a subgroup of high-risk NSTE-ACS patients undergoing PCI with a DES, short-duration DAPT (3 months), followed by ticagrelor monotherapy for 12 months, is associated with less bleeding compared with longer-duration DAPT, with no higher risk of death, myocardial infarction, or stroke.[42]

### Intravenous Antiplatelet Agents
#### Cangrelor
Cangrelor directly and reversibly inhibits ADP binding to the P2Y12 receptor. It is an intravenous ATP analog with a very short plasma half-life of about 3–6 min and is deactivated through dephosphorylation. After discontinuation of cangrelor infusion, platelet function recovery occurs rapidly in about 60 min.[43] This unique rapid onset and offset features of antiplatelet activity has made cangrelor as an attractive agent during PCI in patients not pretreated with oral P2Y12 inhibitors or those with doubtful absorption of drugs because of vomiting and those with a possible immediate need to major surgery in less than next 5–7 days.

In a pooled analysis of three CHAMPION trials enrolling 25,000 patients, of whom 57.4% were NSTE-ACS patients, cangrelor, compared to control (clopidogrel or placebo), lowered the rate of primary composite efficacy end point of death, MI, ischemia-driven revascularization, or stent thrombosis at 48 h. Mild bleeding was higher in the cangrelor group, but moderate to large bleedings and need for transfusion were not different.[44]

#### Glycoprotein IIb–IIIa inhibitors
By interfering in the process of fibrinogen binding to glycoprotein IIb–IIIa (GP IIb–IIIa) receptors, these agents

**TABLE 23.3**
Characteristics of the Glycoprotein IIb/IIIa Inhibitors

|  | Abciximab | Eptifibatide | Tirofiban |
|---|---|---|---|
| Molecule | Fab 7E3 | Synthetic peptide | Nonpeptide mimetic |
| Molecular weight | ~50,000 | ~800 | ~500 |
| Stoichiometry (drug to GP IIb/IIIa) | ~1.5:1 | ≫100:1 | ≫100:1 |
| Binding | Noncompetitive | Competitive | Competitive |
| Half-life | Plasma: 10–15 h<br>Biologic: 12–24 h | Plasma: 2–2.5 h<br>Biologic = plasma | Plasma: 2–2.5 h<br>Biologic = plasma |
| PCI dosing | Bolus: 0.25 mg/kg (10–60 min)<br>Infusion: 0.125 µg/kg/min (12 h) | Bolus: 180 µg/kg (10 min) + 180 µg/kg<br>Infusion: 2 µg/kg/min (24–48 h) | Bolus: 25 µg/kg (30 min)<br>Infusion: 0.10 µg/kg/min (48 h) |
| Renal adjustment | No | Bolus: 180 µg/kg<br><br>Infusion: 1 µg/kg/min (24–48 h) | Bolus: 12.5 µg/kg (30 min)<br>Infusion: 0.10 µg/kg/min (48 h) |

*Fab*, fragment antigen binding; *GP*, glycoprotein; *PCI*, percutaneous coronary intervention.
From Price MJ, Angiolillo DJ. Platelet inhibitor agents. In: Topol EJ, Terstein PS, eds. *Textbook of Interventional Cardiology*. 7th ed. Philadelphia: Elsevier; 2016:165.

impair the final common pathway of platelet aggregation. Pharmacologic characteristics of three available GP IIb–IIIa inhibitors are listed in (Table 23.3). Eptifibatide and tirofiban are small molecules with reversible binding capability that have short half-lives (2 h) and are approved for both medical and invasive management strategies. Abciximab is a monoclonal antibody with a longer half-life (12 h) and is approved only in patients undergoing PCI. Upstream usage of eptifibatide was compared with provisional use in NSTE-ACS patients undergoing invasive approach in the EARLY ACS trial.[45] There was no significant difference in the rate of ischemic end points between two groups; however, the rate of bleeding and need for transfusion was significantly higher in those received upstream eptifibatide. Currently, with the availability of more potent oral P2Y12 inhibitors, the overall usage of these agents has been reduced and is limited to bailout situations or thrombotic complications during PCI of high-risk patients. These agents are not recommended to administer in patients in whom coronary anatomy is not known.[9]

## ANTICOAGULANT THERAPY

In the absence of absolute contraindications, parenteral anticoagulants should be administered in all patients with NSTE-ACS regardless of the initial therapeutic strategy. Anticoagulants inhibit thrombus formation and reduce thrombus-related ischemic events, especially when used in combination with antiplatelets. In patients undergoing PCI, anticoagulants reduce the risk of intracoronary and catheter-related thrombus formation. A general guide for anticoagulant therapy in NSTE-ACS is presented in Table 23.4.

### Unfractionated Heparin

Unfractionated heparin (UFH) binds to the antithrombin III to activate it. This activated antithrombin blocks thrombin (IIa) and factor Xa to exert an anticoagulant effect. UFH is widely available, has a short half-life (1–1.5 h), is almost completely and quickly reversible by protamine in case of bleeding or PCI complications, does not need adjustment in patients with renal insufficiency, and can be easily monitored during PCI. Therefore, it serves as a good option in many patients in current practice, especially in those who are candidates for an early invasive strategy. A weight-adjusted loading dose of 60 IU/kg (maximum, 4000 IU) with an initial infusion of 12 IU/kg/h (maximum 1000 IU/h) is recommended to maintain activated partial thromboplastin time (aPTT) between 50 and 70 s. Frequent monitoring of the aPTT every 6 h until the target range is reached, and every 12–24 h

**TABLE 23.4**
**Anticoagulant Therapy in Patients With NSTE-ACS**

*Anticoagulant therapy*

Enoxaparin is recommended at presentation (COR I, LOE: A); other options include unfractionated heparin (UFH) (COR I, B) and fondaparinux (COR I, LOE: B). If an early invasive strategy is planned, bivalirudin (COR I, LOE: B) is also an option

If fondaparinux is used initially, add UFH or bivalirudin just before or during PCI to prevent catheter-related thrombosis (COR I, LOE: B)

Bivalirudin is preferred over UFH plus GP IIb/IIIa inhibitor in patients undergoing PCI who are at high risk of bleeding (COR IIa, LOE: B)

It is reasonable to use enoxaparin during PCI if it was used as the initial anticoagulant (COR IIb, LOE: B)

*COR*, class of recommendation; *LOE*, level of evidence; *PCI*, percutaneous coronary intervention.
From Giugliano RP, Braunwald E. Non-ST elevation acute coronary syndromes. In: Zipes DP, Libby P, Bonow RO, Mann DL, Tomaselli GF, eds. Braunwald's Heart Disease: A Textbook of Cardiovascular Medicine. 11th ed. Philadelphia, PA: Elsevier/Saunders; 2019:1181–1202.

thereafter for possible dose adjustment is necessary.[16] During the PCI, activated clotting time is commonly used for monitoring the anticoagulant effect of UFH, and additional doses might be administered. A reduced dose is usually considered with a concomitant infusion of GP IIb–IIIa inhibitors. Extreme care should be taken to heparin-induced thrombocytopenia (HIT), which is an infrequent but potentially lethal complication of UFH. Treatment with a nonheparin anticoagulant is recommended in case of documented or suspected HIT.[9]

### Low-Molecular-Weight Heparin

Enoxaparin is the most widely studied drug of this group in ACS. It has a more predictable dose–response relationship that allows subcutaneous (SC) administration without the need for monitoring. Enoxaparin exerts more great inhibition of factor Xa compared with IIa, and less frequently causes HIT, but should not be used in patients with such history.[9] Meta-analysis of trials comparing enoxaparin with UFH has shown a significant reduction of ischemic events in favor of enoxaparin with no significant difference in the rate of bleeding.[46] Enoxaparin is usually administered 1 mg/kg SC twice daily and needs to be adjusted in patients with a glomerular filtration rate

(GFR) below 30 mL/min to 1 mg/kg SC once daily and should not be administered in patients with a GFR below 15 mL/min. In patients with NSTE-ACS who have previously pretreated with SC enoxaparin within the last 12 h, crossing over to another anticoagulant during the PCI could be harmful and should not be performed.[47] In pretreated patients, additional enoxaparin is not recommended at the time of PCI if the last SC dose was injected 8 h before PCI. In patients who have received the last dose of SC enoxaparin 8–12 h before PCI, an additional IV bolus dose of 0.3 mg/kg enoxaparin should be administered at the time of PCI. If the patient has received enoxaparin more than 12 h before PCI, conventional anticoagulant therapy is indicated.[48]

### Bivalirudin

Bivalirudin is the most widely used direct thrombin inhibitor, and with reversible binding to thrombin, it impairs fibrinogen conversion to fibrin. Bivalirudin has a more predictable anticoagulant effect and does not need monitoring. Thrombocytopenia does not happen with bivalirudin, and it is the best anticoagulant agent in patients with a history of HIT. Studies comparing bivalirudin with UFH- or LMWH-based strategies generally have shown a similar efficacy end point with a reduced bleeding rate with bivalirudin.[49–51] This makes bivalirudin as an attractive anticoagulant in patients with high bleeding risk who are candidates for invasive treatment. In patients with NSTE-ACS before angiography, the recommended dose of bivalirudin is 0.10-mg/kg IV bolus followed by an infusion of 0.25 mg/kg/h. During the angiography and PCI of such patients, an additional loading dose of 0.5 mg/kg is recommended with an increased infusion rate to 1.75 mg/kg/h during PCI. For patients who have not received prior anticoagulant therapy, 0.75-mg/kg loading dose, and 1.75 mg/kg/h IV infusion rate are recommended.[16]

### Fondaparinux

Fondaparinux is a selective factor Xa inhibitor that binds to antithrombin and blocks prothrombin to thrombin conversion. Its more predictable anticoagulant effect allows single-dose injection without the need for monitoring or dose adjustment. The recommended dose is 2.5 mg/day through SC injection. HIT is not a concern with fondaparinux, but because of renal elimination, fondaparinux is contraindicated if eGFR is $<20$ mL/min/1.73 m$^2$.[9]

In the large OASIS-5 study enrolled 20,078 patients with NSTE-ACS, the fondaparinux group had similar ischemic event rates with significantly reduced inhospital major bleeding and 1-month mortality, compared with those treated with enoxaparin.[52] However, in a subgroup of patients undergoing PCI, despite a significantly lower rate of major bleeding, a higher rate of catheter-associated thrombus was detected. This risk was abolished by the injection of a bolus dose of UFH at the time of PCI.[53] This efficacy–safety profile of fondaparinux has made it an ideal alternative to heparin-based treatments for patients with NSTE-ACS at high bleeding risk, especially in those managed noninvasively.

## LIPID-LOWERING AGENTS

High-intensity statin therapy should be initiated as soon as possible after admission to achieve an LDL-cholesterol (LDL-C) concentration of <1.8 mmol/L (<70 mg/dL) or at least 50% reduction in LDL-C. In patients already receiving lower doses of statins, in the absence of contraindications and/or intolerance, the dose should be increased to high-intensity dosages and continued indefinitely.[9,54] Using this high-intensity statin therapy, a 19% decrease in the rate of death and CV events over 2 years of follow-up has been reported in a meta-analysis of RCTs.[55] Also, early initiation of statins before coronary angiography provides a protective effect against contrast-induced nephropathy (CIN).[56] In a recent trial (IMPROVE-IT), adding ezetimibe to a background of statin therapy was associated with a more significant decrease in the rate of CV death and vascular events compared with high-intensity statin alone.[57] Adding ezetimibe to statin therapy also may be considered in patients intolerant to high-intensity statin treatment. Based on AHA/ACC guidelines in very high-risk patients, it is reasonable to add ezetimibe to the maximally tolerated statin therapy when the LDL-C level remains ≥70 mg/dL. If the target level is not achieved with this combined regimen, adding a PCSK9[a] inhibitor is reasonable.[58] More recent ESC guidelines have even considered lower target levels; <55 mg/dL for very-high-risk patients and <40 mg/dL for very high-risk patients who have suffered a second vascular event within 2 years while taking the maximally tolerated statin therapy.[59]

## EARLY INVASIVE VS CONSERVATIVE STRATEGIES

The early invasive strategy is defined as coronary angiography within the first 48–72 h after presentation followed by PCI, CABG, or medical therapy alone, depending on the coronary anatomy, LV function, and comorbidities. On the other hand, in conservative or

ischemic-guided strategy, patients receive appropriate medical therapy and the decision regarding any invasive intervention is made depending on the response to anti-ischemic therapy, the presence of hemodynamic instability or recurrent ischemia, and evidence of ischemia on a noninvasive test.[9,16] According to a meta-analysis of 7 RCTs in 8375 NSTE-ACS patients with NSTE-ACS, a routine invasive strategy was associated with a significantly lower risk of death, MI, and rehospitalization in a mean follow-up period of 2 years.[60] Further studies have shown that the benefit of an early invasive strategy on tight end points is considered only in high-risk patients including those with ST changes, elevated cTn level, recurrent angina, and heart failure.[16,61] However, trans-radial approach, new-generation DES, and more effective P2Y12 inhibitors were not available or broadly implemented in these trials, and it seems that in the current era of interventional cardiology, the magnitude of this beneficial effect, especially in frail patients is even more prominent.[61] Overall, based on current knowledge and data obtained through the meta-analysis of randomized trials, it seems that an early invasive approach is safe and associated with a lower risk of recurrent or refractory ischemia and a shorter duration of hospital stay compared with a strategy of a conservative approach. Optimal timing of invasive coronary angiography should be guided by individual risk stratification. For practical purposes, ESC guidelines[9] has categorized the NSTE-ACS patients in different risk categories and has suggested an optimum time period for invasive approach in each group. An ACE inhibitor (or ARB as an alternative) is recommended as class I indication in patients with LVEF ≤40% or heart failure, hypertension or diabetes, unless contraindicated. In the absence of contraindications, beta blockers are class I indication in those with LVEF ≤40%. In patients with LVEF ≤35% and either heart failure or diabetes and in the absence of significant renal dysfunction (serum creatinine <2.5 mg/dL for men and <2.0 mg/dL for women) or hyperkalaemia (serum potassium concentration <5.0 mmol/L), mineralocorticoid receptor antagonists, preferably eplerenone are recommended.[9]

Either PCI or CABG may be indicated for revascularization. PCI is the commonly used strategy and new-generation drug-eluting stents (DESs) are preferred even in those patients who cannot tolerate more than 1 month of DAPT. Recurrent ischemia is the major drawback of PCI. CABG is indicated in about 5%–10% of patients and optimal timing should be determined individually. In the absence of randomized trials to compare PCI and CABG in patients with NSTE-ACS, available guidelines recommend the same strategy as in patients with

---

[a]PCSK9, proprotein convertase subtilisin/kexin type 9.

stable angina. According to current ESC/EACTS guidelines on myocardial revascularization, in patients with 1 and 2 VD in the absence of proximal LAD lesion, PCI is preferred over CABG, while in those with proximal LAD lesion, both strategies have a class I recommendation. In patients with three-vessel disease, the presence of diabetes or a SYNTAX score >22 are in favor of CABG; moreover, a similar recommendation is applied for patients with complex CAD and left main (LM) lesion with SYNTAX score >32 or severe LV dysfunction. In patients with LM lesion with low SYNTAX score 0–22, a strategy of either CABG or PCI may be selected.[61]

## LONG-TERM MANAGEMENT

Patients are advised to participate in cardiac rehabilitation and secondary prevention programs to ensure medication adherence and lifestyle changes including smoking cessation, regular physical activity (at least 30 min and three or more times a week) and a healthy diet. High-intensity statin therapy started in the acute phase should be continued in the absence of contraindications and intolerance. For patients, not at high bleeding risk, DAPT is recommended for at least 12 months and can be continued longer in high-risk groups. Based on the results of ATLAS ACS 2-TIMI 51 trial, in patients with no prior stroke/TIA and at high ischemic and low bleeding risk, low-dose rivaroxaban (2.5 mg twice daily for approximately 1 year) may be considered and added to DAPT regimen.[62] Currently, this recommendation has a class IIb indication in ESC guidelines for the management of NSTE-ACS patients.[9] Proton pump inhibitors (PPI) should be added in this group and those at high risk for GI bleeding. An ACE inhibitor (or ARB as an alternative) is recommended as class I indication in patients with LVEF ≤40% or heart failure, hypertension or diabetes, unless contraindicated. In the absence of contraindications, beta blockers are class I indication in those with LVEF ≤40%. In patients with LVEF ≤35% and either heart failure or diabetes and in the absence of significant renal dysfunction (serum creatinine <2.5 mg/dL for men and <2.0 mg/dL for women) or hyperkalaemia (serum potassium concentration <5.0 mmol/L), mineralocorticoid receptor antagonists, preferably eplerenone are recommended.[9]

## MANAGEMENT OF NSTE-ACS IN SPECIAL SUBGROUPS

### Elderly

As discussed earlier, atypical symptoms, presentation with angina equivalents, and nondiagnostic ECG changes are more common in the elderly. The presence of multiple risk factors, comorbidities, impaired renal function, and polypharmacy are important features that should be considered in the management of elderly patients. Extensive CAD is more common and considering the high-risk profile of the elderly people, the benefit of guideline-recommended treatments in this age group is even higher than young patients. A meta-analysis of RCTs showed the efficacy of early invasive strategy in this age group in reducing the rate of death or MI.[63] Advanced age per se, is not a contraindication for invasive strategies, and the presence of comorbidities and frailty are more important.[10] Avoiding prasugrel, high dose aspirin, and abciximab and replacing them with the safer alternatives, emphasis on PPIs, using fondaparinux in medical management and bivalirudin during PCI, adjusting the dose of all prescribed medications with kidney function, and more attention to drug–drug interactions are some of the important precautions in the management of elderly people with ACS.

### Chronic Kidney Disease

Patients with NSTE-ACS and renal dysfunction are older, have higher rates of comorbidities including diabetes, and more frequent silent ischemia and LV dysfunction. An elevated level of high-sensitive cTns above the 99th percentile of normal is common in CKD. In evaluating acute chest pain in patients with CKD, cTnI is preferred over CTnT, the latter being more prognostic in chronic stable angina and reflecting heart and kidney function. Considering higher basal troponin levels in patients with CKD or ESRD, the diagnosis of MI in this situation should rely on serial measurements.[64] Uremia-induced excess thrombin generation and platelet dysfunction result in both higher rate of hemorrhagic and thrombotic complications (including stent thrombosis). Data regarding the management of patients with NSTE-ACS and CKD is scarce since most studies have excluded these patients. In a meta-analysis of five RCTs, an early invasive strategy was associated with nonsignificant reductions in all-cause mortality, nonfatal MI, and a composite of death or nonfatal MI with a significant reduction in the rate of rehospitalization.[65] Coronary angiography should be considered in patients with CKD with adequate hydration to reduce the rate of CIN. The decision for selecting the type of revascularization should be made based on patient risk profile and life expectancy. In patients with multivessel CAD and acceptable surgical risk profile and life expectancy >1 year, CABG should be considered over PCI. On the other hand, PCI should be considered over CABG in patients with multivessel CAD, high surgical risk profile or life expectancy <1 year.[9] All medications should be prescribed for patients with CKD considering possible renal clearance and with dose adjustments if necessary (Chapter 36).

## Diabetes

About one-third of patients admitted with NSTE-ACS have a history of known diabetes. Previously undetected diabetes is also common and both of these conditions are independent predictors of increased mortality in NSTE-ACS. Hence, it is recommended to screen all patients with NSTE-ACS for diabetes and to monitor blood glucose levels frequently in patients with known diabetes or admission hyperglycemia.[9] Considering the U-shaped relationship between blood glucose level and outcome in patients with ACS, it is recommended to initiate glucose-lowering therapy with blood glucose levels >180 mg/dL (or >10 mmol/L), while avoiding episodes of hypoglycemia (glucose level <90 mg/dL or 5 mmol/L).[9,10] In patients with diabetes, general medical management in the acute phase of NSTE-ACS, decisions to perform stress testing, angiography, and revascularization should be similar to the nondiabetics.[16] However, in RCTs, the benefit of potent P2Y12s like ticagrelor, prasugrel, and intravenous GP IIb–IIIa inhibitors have been more prominent in the diabetic subgroup of patients with ACS.[36,41] Overall, an invasive strategy is preferred and it is recommended to monitor renal function for 2–3 days after coronary angiography or PCI in patients on metformin or those with impaired baseline kidney function.[9] According to the current ESC/EACTS guidelines on myocardial revascularization in patients with three-vessel disease in the presence of diabetes, CABG is preferred over PCI.[61] However, these guidelines are based on trials performed at the era of first-generation DESs.

## PRINZMETAL VARIANT ANGINA

Prinzmetal variant angina (PVA) is a syndrome of resting angina with transient ST-segment elevation first described in 1959 by Myron Prinzmetal. In contrast to the classic definition of Heberden angina, episodes of severe angina occur without exertion and are clustered in the early morning hours. The attacks may be associated with ventricular arrhythmia and AV block resulting in syncope. MI and sudden cardiac death also might occur. Coronary angiography reveals focal coronary artery spasm as the leading cause of this syndrome.[13] Patients are usually younger than those with classic atherosclerotic NSTE-ACS with fewer traditional cardiovascular risk factors except for smoking that is more common in those with PVA. Also, they have lower TIMI risk scores and higher left ventricular ejection fraction compared with the obstructive CAD group.[66,67] The incidence of PVA is greater in Japan than in Western countries and in a multicenter study from Japan, 79.2% of patients with NSTE-ACS without a culprit lesion, who underwent a provocative test with acetylcholine, had a positive test for spasm.[66] History of migraine headaches and Raynaud phenomenon is more common in PVA. Endothelial dysfunction and impaired nitric oxide activity may be involved in the pathophysiology of the spasm.[13]

Patient history and ECG changes are very important to make the correct diagnosis. Ambulatory ECG monitoring or an event monitor might help to confirm it. In approximately one-third of patients, exercise testing provokes angina with ST-segment elevation. All patients with PVA should undergo coronary angiography unless an absolute contraindication is present.[13] After ruling out significant obstructive coronary lesions during coronary angiography, three provocative tests (hyperventilation, intracoronary ergonovine, and intracoronary acetylcholine injection) may be used to confirm the diagnosis, the latter being the most preferred method.

Smoking cessation is strongly recommended in the management of patients with PVA. Sublingual NTG relieves variant angina attacks within minutes. Calcium blockers are the cornerstone of the therapy. Usually, high doses of calcium blockers or a combination of them are necessary and might be used in combination with long-acting nitrates to prevent future attacks. No beneficial effect of low-dose aspirin has yet been proven and higher doses may even be detrimental. Statins are useful in reducing cardiovascular events and are recommended in the absence of contraindications. Current guidelines do not support the routine use of alpha 1 adrenergic receptor blockers to prevent attacks. Considering the risk of recurrent spasm in different coronary territories, revascularization is not recommended. For secondary prevention, ICD implantation is indicated in patients who have suffered malignant arrhythmic events and continue to have ischemic events despite maximal medical therapy.[67]

## REFERENCES

1. Fuster V, Moreno PR, Fayad ZA, Corti R, Badimon JJ. Atherothrombosis and high-risk plaque: part I: evolving concepts. *J Am Coll Cardiol.* 2005;46:937–954.
2. Baber U, Holmes D, Halperin J, Fuster V. Definitions of acute coronary syndromes. In: Fuster F, Harrington RA, Narula J, Eapen JZ, eds. *Hurst's the Heart.* 14th ed. New York: McGraw-Hill; 2017:946.

3. Reichlin T, Twerenbold R, Maushart C, et al. Risk stratification in patients with unstable angina using absolute serial changes of 3 high-sensitive troponin assays. *Am Heart J.* 2013;165(3). 371–378.e3.

4. Reichlin T, et al. Introduction of high-sensitivity troponin assays: impact on myocardial infarction incidence and prognosis. *Am J Med.* 2012;125(12). 1205–1213.e1.

5. Kumar A, Cannon CP. Acute coronary syndromes: diagnosis and management, part I. *Mayo Clin Proc.* 2009;84(10):917–938. https://doi.org/10.1016/S0025-6196(11)60509-0.

6. Scirica BM, Cannon CP, McCabe CH, et al. Prognosis in the thrombolysis in myocardial ischemia III registry according to the Braunwald unstable angina pectoris classification. *Am J Cardiol.* 2002;90(8):821–826.

7. Canto JG, Fincher C, Kiefe CI, et al. Atypical presentations among medicare beneficiaries with unstable angina pectoris. *Am J Cardiol.* 2002;90(3):248–253.

8. Canto JG, Shlipak MG, Rogers WJ, et al. Prevalence, clinical characteristics, and mortality among patients with myocardial infarction presenting without chest pain. *JAMA.* 2000;283(24):3223–3229.

9. Roffi M, Patrono C, Collet JP, et al. 2015 ESC guidelines for the management of acute coronary syndromes in patients presenting without persistent ST-segment elevation: Task Force for the Management of Acute Coronary Syndromes in Patients Presenting Without Persistent ST-Segment Elevation of the European Society of Cardiology (ESC). *Eur Heart J.* 2016;37(3):267–315.

10. Giugliano RP, Braunwald E. Non–ST elevation acute coronary syndromes. In: Zipes DP, Libby P, Bonow RO, Mann DL, Tomaselli GF, eds. *Braunwald's Heart Disease: A Textbook of Cardiovascular Medicine.* 11th ed. Philadelphia, PA: Elsevier/Saunders; 2019:1181–1202.

11. Thygesen K, Alpert JS, Jaffe AS, et al. Third universal definition of myocardial infarction. *Circulation.* 2012;126(16):2020–2035.

12. Segraves JM, Frishman WH. Highly sensitive cardiac troponin assays: a comprehensive review of their clinical utility. *Cardiol Rev.* 2015;23(6):282–289.

13. Moliterno DJ, Januzzi JL. Evaluation and management of non–ST-segment elevation myocardial infarction. In: Fuster F, Harrington RA, Narula J, Eapen JZ, eds. *Hurst's the Heart.* 14th ed. New York: McGraw-Hill; 2017:995–1016.

14. Mokhtari A, Borna C, Gilje P, et al. A 1-h combination algorithm allows fast rule-out and rule-in of major adverse cardiac events. *J Am Coll Cardiol.* 2016;67(13):1531–1540.

15. Sabatine MS, Morrow DA, de Lemos JA, et al. Multimarker approach to risk stratification in non-ST elevation acute coronary syndromes: simultaneous assessment of troponin I, C-reactive protein, and B-type natriuretic peptide. *Circulation.* 2002;105(15):1760–1763.

16. Amsterdam EA, Wenger NK, Brindis RG, et al. 2014 AHA/ACC guideline for the management of patients with non-ST-elevation acute coronary syndromes: a report of the American College of Cardiology/American Heart Association Task Force on Practice Guidelines. *J Am Coll Cardiol.* 2014;64:e139–e228.

17. Hulten E, Pickett C, Bittencourt MS, et al. Outcomes after coronary computed tomography angiography in the emergency department: a systematic review and meta-analysis of randomized, controlled trials. *J Am Coll Cardiol.* 2013;61(8):880–892.

18. Dewey M, Rief M, Martus P, et al. Evaluation of computed tomography in patients with atypical angina or chest pain clinically referred for invasive coronary angiography: randomised controlled trial. *BMJ.* 2016;355:i5441.

19. SCOT-HEART Investigators. CT coronary angiography in patients with suspected angina due to coronary heart disease (SCOT-HEART): an open-label, parallel-group, multicenter trial. *Lancet.* 2015;385(9985):2383–2391.

20. Rybicki FJ, Udelson JE, Peacock WF, et al. 2015 ACR/ACC/AHA/AATS/ACEP/ASNC/NASCI/SAEM/SCCT/SCMR/SCPC/SNMMI/STR/STS appropriate utilization of cardiovascular imaging n emergency department patients with chest pain: a joint document of the American College of Radiology Appropriateness Criteria Committee and the American College of Cardiology Appropriate Use Criteria Task Force. *J Am Coll Cardiol.* 2016;67(7):853–879.

21. Laimoud M, Faris F, Elghawaby H. Coronary atherosclerotic plaque vulnerability rather than stenosis predisposes to non-ST elevation acute coronary syndromes. *Cardiol Res Pract.* 2019;2019:2642740.

22. Antman EM, Cohen M, Bernink PJ, et al. The TIMI risk score for unstable angina/non–ST elevation MI: a method for prognostication and therapeutic decision making. *JAMA.* 2000;284(7):835–842.

23. Boersma E, Pieper KS, Steyerberg EW, et al. Predictors of outcome in patients with acute coronary syndromes without persistent ST-segment elevation. Results from an international trial of 9461 patients. The PURSUIT Investigators. *Circulation.* 2000;101(22):2557–2567.

24. Fox KA, Dabbous OH, Goldberg RJ, et al. Prediction of risk of death and myocardial infarction in the six months after presentation with acute coronary syndrome: prospective multinational observational study (GRACE). *BMJ.* 2006;333(7578):1091.

25. Perez MI, Musini VM, Wright JM. Effect of early treatment with anti-hypertensive drugs on short and long-term mortality in patients with an acute cardiovascular event. *Cochrane Database Syst Rev.* 2009;4, CD006743.

26. Kontos MC, Diercks DB, Ho PM, et al. Treatment and outcomes in patients with myocardial infarction treated with acute beta-blocker therapy: results from the American College of Cardiology's NCDRw. *Am Heart J.* 2011;161:864–870.

27. Chatterjee S, Biondi-Zoccai G, Abbate A, et al. Benefits of β blockers in patients with heart failure and reduced ejection fraction: network meta-analysis. *BMJ.* 2013;346:f55.

28. Packer M, O'Connor CM, Ghali JK, et al. Effect of amlodipine on morbidity and mortality in severe chronic heart failure. Prospective Randomized

Amlodipine Survival Evaluation Study Group. *N Engl J Med.* 1996;335:1107–1114.

29. Parodi G, Bellandi B, Xanthopoulou I, et al. Morphine is associated with a delayed activity of oral antiplatelet agents in patients with ST-elevation acute myocardial infarction undergoing primary percutaneous coronary intervention. *Circ Cardiovasc Interv.* 2015;8(1):e001593.
30. Grosser T, Fries S, Lawson JA, et al. Drug resistance and pseudoresistance: an unintended consequence of enteric coating aspirin. *Circulation.* 2013;127(3):377–385.
31. Mehta SR, Bassand JP, Chrolavicius S, et al. Dose comparisons of clopidogrel and aspirin in acute coronary syndromes. *N Engl J Med.* 2010;363(10):930–942.
32. Schomig A, Neumann FJ, Kastrati A, et al. A randomized comparison of antiplatelet and anticoagulant therapy after the placement of coronary-artery stents. *N Engl J Med.* 1996;334:1084–1089.
33. Valgimigli M, Bueno H, Byrne RA, et al. 2017 ESC focused update on dual antiplatelet therapy in coronary artery disease developed in collaboration with EACTS: The Task Force for dual antiplatelet therapy in coronary artery disease of the European Society of Cardiology (ESC) and of the European Association for Cardio-Thoracic Surgery (EACTS). *Eur Heart J.* 2018;39(3):213–260. https://doi.org/10.1093/eurheartj/ehx419.
34. Yusuf S, Zhao F, Mehta SR, et al. Effects of clopidogrel in addition to aspirin in patients with acute coronary syndromes without ST-segment elevation. *N Engl J Med.* 2001;345(7):494–502.
35. Levine GN, Bates ER, Bittl JA, et al. 2016 ACC/AHA guideline focused update on duration of dual antiplatelet therapy in patients with coronary artery disease: a report of the American College of Cardiology/American Heart Association Task Force on Clinical Practice Guidelines. *J Am Coll Cardiol.* 2016;68(10):1082–1115.
36. Wiviott SD, Braunwald E, McCabe CH, et al. Intensive oral antiplatelet therapy for reduction of ischaemic events including stent thrombosis in patients with acute coronary syndromes treated with percutaneous coronary intervention and stenting in the TRITON-TIMI 38 trial: a subanalysis of a randomised trial. *Lancet.* 2008;371 (9621):1353–1363.
37. Roe MT, Armstrong PW, Fox KA, et al. Prasugrel versus clopidogrel for acute coronary syndromes without revascularization. *N Engl J Med.* 2012;367(14):1297–1309.
38. Montalescot G, Bolognese L, Dudek D, et al. Pretreatment with prasugrel in non-ST-segment elevation acute coronary syndromes. *N Engl J Med.* 2013;369(11):999–1010.
39. Gurbel PA, Bliden KP, Butler K, et al. Randomized double-blind assessment of the ONSET and OFFSET of the antiplatelet effects of ticagrelor versus clopidogrel in patients with stable coronary artery disease: the ONSET/OFFSET study. *Circulation.* 2009;120(25):2577.
40. Wallentin L, Becker RC, Budaj A, et al. Ticagrelor versus clopidogrel in patients with acute coronary syndromes. *N Engl J Med.* 2009;361(11):1045–1057.

41. Mahaffey KW, Wojdyla DM, Carroll K, et al. Ticagrelor compared with clopidogrel by geographic region in the Platelet Inhibition and Patient Outcomes (PLATO) trial. *Circulation.* 2011;124(5):544–554.
42. Mehran R, Baber U, Sharma SK, et al. Ticagrelor with or without aspirin in high-risk patients after PCI. *N Engl J Med.* 2019;381(21):2032–2042.
43. Teng R. Ticagrelor: pharmacokinetic, pharmacodynamic and pharmacogenetic profile: an update. *Clin Pharmacokinet.* 2015;54:1125–1138.
44. Steg PG, Bhatt DL, Hamm CW, et al. Effect of cangrelor on periprocedural outcomes in percutaneous coronary interventions: a pooled analysis of patient-level data. *Lancet.* 2013;382(9909):1981–1992.
45. Giugliano RP, White JA, Bode C, et al. Early versus delayed, provisional eptifibatide in acute coronary syndromes. *N Engl J Med.* 2009;360(21):2176–2190.
46. Murphy SA, Gibson CM, Morrow DA, et al. Efficacy and safety of the low-molecular weight heparin enoxaparin compared with unfractionated heparin across the acute coronary syndrome spectrum: a meta-analysis. *Eur Heart J.* 2007;28:2077–2086.
47. Ferguson JJ, Califf RM, Antman EM, et al. Enoxaparin vs unfractionated heparin in high-risk patients with non-ST-segment elevation acute coronary syndromes managed with an intended early invasive strategy: primary results of the SYNERGY randomized trial. *JAMA.* 2004;292 (1):45–54.
48. Collet JP, Montalescot G, Lison L, et al. Percutaneous coronary intervention after subcutaneous enoxaparin pretreatment in patients with unstable angina pectoris. *Circulation.* 2001;103(5):658–663.
49. Lincoff AM, Bittl JA, Harrington RA, et al. Bivalirudin and provisional glycoprotein IIb/IIIa blockade compared with heparin and planned glycoprotein IIb/IIIa blockade during percutaneous coronary intervention: REPLACE-2 randomized trial. *JAMA.* 2003;289(7):853–863.
50. Stone GW, McLaurin BT, Cox DA, et al. Bivalirudin for patients with acute coronary syndromes. *N Engl J Med.* 2006;355(21):2203–2216.
51. Kastrati A, Neumann FJ, Mehilli J, et al. Bivalirudin versus unfractionated heparin during percutaneous coronary intervention. *N Engl J Med.* 2008;359:688–696.
52. Yusuf S, Mehta SR, Chrolavicius S, et al. Comparison of fondaparinux and enoxaparin in acute coronary syndromes. *N Engl J Med.* 2006;354:1464–1476.
53. Steg PG, Jolly SS, Mehta SR, et al. Low-dose vs standard-dose unfractionated heparin for percutaneous coronary intervention in acute coronary syndromes treated with fondaparinux: the FUTURA/OASIS-8 randomized trial. *JAMA.* 2010;304:1339–1349.
54. Giugliano RP, Wiviott SD, Blazing MA, et al. Long-term safety and efficacy of achieving very low levels of low-density lipoprotein cholesterol. *JAMA Cardiol.* 2017;2(5):547–555.
55. Hulten E, Jackson JL, Douglas K, et al. The effect of early, intensive statin therapy on acute coronary syndrome: a

meta-analysis of randomized controlled trials. *Arch Intern Med.* 2006;166(17):1814–1821.

56. Sun YY, Liu LY, Sun T, Wu MY, Ma FZ. Prophylactic atorvastatin prior to intra-arterial administration of iodinated contrast media for prevention of contrast-induced acute kidney injury: a meta-analysis of randomized trial data. *Clin Nephrol.* 2019;92(3):123–130.
57. Cannon CP, Blazing MA, Giugliano RP, et al. Ezetimibe added to statin therapy after acute coronary syndromes. *N Engl J Med.* 2015;372(25):2387–2397.
58. Grundy SM, Stone NJ, Bailey AL, et al. 2018 AHA/ACC/AACVPR/AAPA/ABC/ACPM/ADA/AGS/APhA/ASPC/NLA/PCNA guideline on the management of blood cholesterol: a report of the American College of Cardiology/American Heart Association Task Force on Clinical Practice Guidelines. *J Am Coll Cardiol.* 2019;73(24):e285–e350.
59. Mach F, Baigent C, Catapano AL, et al. 2019 ESC/EAS Guidelines for the management of dyslipidaemias: lipid modification to reduce cardiovascular risk. *Eur Heart J.* 2020;41(1):111–188.
60. Bavry AA, Kumbhani DJ, Rassi AN, Bhatt DL, Askari AT. Benefit of early invasive therapy in acute coronary syndromes: a meta-analysis of contemporary randomized clinical trials. *J Am Coll Cardiol.* 2006;48:1319–1325.
61. Neumann FJ, Sousa-Uva M, Ahlsson A, et al. 2018 ESC/EACTS guidelines on myocardial revascularization. *Eur Heart J.* 2019;40(2):87–165.
62. Mega JL, Braunwald E, Wiviott SD, et al. Rivaroxaban in patients with a recent acute coronary syndrome. *N Engl J Med.* 2012;366:9–19.
63. Damman P, Clayton T, Wallentin L, et al. Effects of age on long-term outcomes after a routine invasive or selective invasive strategy in patients presenting with non-ST segment elevation acute coronary syndromes: a collaborative analysis of individual data from the FRISC II–ICTUS–RITA-3 (FIR) trials. *Heart.* 2012;98(3):207–213.
64. Mccullough PA. Interface between renal disease and cardiovascular illness. In: Zipes DP, Libby P, Bonow RO, Mann DL, Tomaselli GF, eds. *Braunwald's Heart Disease: A Textbook of Cardiovascular Medicine.* 11th ed. Philadelphia, PA: Elsevier/Saunders; 2019:1910–1929.
65. Charytan DM, Wallentin L, Lagerqvist B, et al. Early angiography in patients with chronic kidney disease: a collaborative systematic review. *Clin J Am Soc Nephrol.* 2009;4(6):1032–1043.
66. Nakayama N, Kaikita K, Fukunaga T, et al. Clinical features and prognosis of patients with coronary spasm–induced non–ST-segment elevation acute coronary syndrome. *J Am Heart Assoc.* 2014;3(3):e000795.
67. Picard F, Sayah N, Spagnoli V, et al. Vasospastic angina: a literature review of current evidence. *Arch Cardiovasc Dis.* 2019;112(1):44–55.

# CHAPTER 24

# Stable Ischemic Heart Disease

MAJID KYAVAR • MOHAMMAD JAVAD ALEMZADEH-ANSARI
Cardiovascular Intervention Research Center, Rajaie Cardiovascular, Medical & Research Center, Iran
University of Medical Sciences, Tehran, Iran

---

**KEY POINTS**

- Myocardial oxygen supply–demand imbalance is a major mechanism of the development of angina in patients with stable ischemic heart disease (SIHD).
- Recognition about characteristics and types of angina pectoris as a most common presentation of SIHD is mandatory.
- Consideration of differential diagnosis of angina, especially gastrointestinal disorders, is necessary.
- The use of noninvasive and invasive modalities for diagnosis and estimating the prognosis of patients should be considered.
- Management (pharmacologic and nonpharmacologic) of patients with goals of an increase in survival and reliving symptoms should be considered.
- For patients who do not have a response to optimal medical therapy, coronary revascularization could be mentioned.
- For coronary revascularization decisions, both anatomy and functional evaluation must be considered.

---

## INTRODUCTION

Stable ischemic heart disease (SIHD) is most commonly caused by atherosclerotic plaque that formats over a number of years, and angina pectoris is the initial manifestation of ischemic heart disease (IHD) in approximately 50% of patients.[1] The lifetime risk of developing IHD after 40 years of age is 49% for men and 32% for women. IHD remains a major public health problem nationally and internationally. Although the age-adjusted mortality rate from IHD has steadily declined over the past several decades, the total number of cardiovascular deaths increased.[2,3] IHD is now the leading cause of death worldwide, and the prevalence of coronary artery disease (CAD) is expected to increase, especially in younger population with increasing cardiovascular risk factors such as increases in the worldwide prevalence of obesity, diabetes mellitus, metabolic syndrome, and physical inactivity.

## PATHOPHYSIOLOGY

Myocardial ischemia develops when myocardial oxygen supply (coronary blood flow) becomes inadequate to meet myocardial oxygen requirements. In the majority of cases, angina pectoris occurs in the setting of obstructive atherosclerotic plaque, which limits blood flow in the setting of increased myocardial demand. At the primary stages of atherosclerosis formation, plaque may extend eccentrically and outward without compromising the lumen (positive remodeling). In this stage, stress testing or angiography may not suggest the presence of CAD. However, imaging modalities such as cardiac computed tomography angiography (CCTA), intravascular ultrasonography (IVUS), or optical coherence tomography (OCT) can reveal the presence, extension, and even content of atherosclerotic plaque. By atherosclerosis progression and propagation, the plaque into the lumen can result in hemodynamic obstruction and angina.[4] Increased myocardial demand, such as exertion or emotional or mental stress, is directly related to increases in heart rate and blood pressure, and can induce myocardial ischemia. Although coronary vasospasm in the setting of Prinzmetal angina is a potential cause of flow reduction leading to myocardial ischemia, acute blood flow reduction after ulceration or erosion of the fibrous cap is a prominent feature of acute presentations of CAD such as myocardial infarction (MI). Prolonged ischemia can lead to electrocardiographic (ECG) and echocardiography changes. The progression of manifestations and laboratory findings of ischemia based on the severity of coronary artery narrowing best is illustrated in Fig. 24.1.

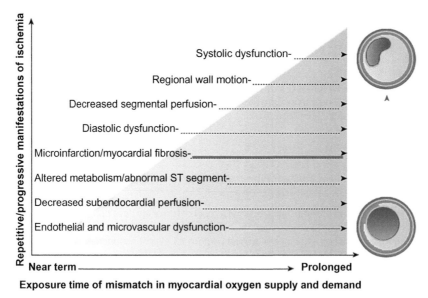

**FIG. 24.1** The progression of signs and symptoms of ischemia by narrowing the coronary artery over time. (From Shaw LJ, Bugiardini R, Merz CNB. Women and ischemic heart disease: evolving knowledge. *J Am Coll Cardiol.* 2009;54(17):1561–1575; with permission.)

The major factors that determine an increase in myocardial oxygen demand and a decrease in myocardial oxygen supply are listed in Table 24.1. The increase in oxygen demand can be observed in patients with hypertrophic cardiomyopathy, aortic stenosis, dilated cardiomyopathy, tachycardia, hyperthermia, hyperthyroidism, hypertension, anxiety, arteriovenous fistulae, and sympathomimetic toxicity (e.g., cocaine use). On the other hand, the decrease in oxygen supply can be observed patients with aortic stenosis, hypertrophic cardiomyopathy, anemia, hypoxemia, hyperviscosity (polycythemia, leukemia, thrombocytosis, hypergammaglobulinemia), and sickle cell disease.[5] Anemia is a common condition that could influence myocardial oxygen supply so that when hemoglobin level drops to lower than 9 g/dL, cardiac output rises, and when it drops to lower than 7 g/dL, ST-T-wave changes can occur.[5] Usage of cocaine increases myocardial oxygen demand, and coronary vasospasm can lead to infarction, especially in young individuals. Moreover, long-term cocaine usage can cause premature development of atherosclerosis.[6–8]

## CLINICAL MANIFESTATIONS

The majority of patients with SIHD present with typical angina pectoris as the primary clinical manifestation.[9] Typical angina pectoris presents as a retrosternal discomfort that patients may describe as pressure, heaviness, tightness, or constriction (Table 24.2). Typical characteristics of anginal pain are described in Table 24.3. Generally, typical angina pectoris is not described as sharp, knife like, stabbing, or needle like. Also, sharp or stabbing pain is a low-risk description of myocardial ischemia, especially when pain is pleuritic or positional and reproducible fully by palpation or movement.[10] Anginal discomfort may sensate at the epigastrium alone or be accompanied by chest pressure, but discomfort above the mandible or below the epigastrium is rare related to myocardial ischemia. Anginal equivalents, such as dyspnea, faintness, fatigue, diaphoresis, nausea and emesis, lightheadedness, and eructations, are common in women and older adults. In patients with SIHD, postprandial angina may be assigned as severe CAD, presumably caused by redistribution of coronary blood flow (steal phenomenon) after a meal.[11] If the duration of angina after rest or nitroglycerin was more than 5–10 min, this suggests that the pain may be secondary to other causes or severe ischemia, as with acute coronary syndrome (ACS). Response to nitroglycerin may be observed in the setting of esophageal pain and other syndromes.[12] First-effort or warm-up angina is described as angina that develops with exertion, but continue at the same or even greater level the exertion by a brief rest period, symptoms are significantly reduced or even relived. The main

**TABLE 24.1**
**Factors That Increase Myocardial Oxygen Demand and Decrease Myocardial Oxygen Supply**

| Myocardial Oxygen Demand | Myocardial Oxygen Supply |
|---|---|
| Increase in heart rate | Decrease in oxygen-carrying capacity of the blood (oxygen tension, hemoglobin concentration) |
| Increase in systolic blood pressure (afterload) | Decrease in coronary artery diameter |
| Increase in myocardial wall tension (the product of ventricular end-diastolic volume or preload and myocardial muscle mass) | Increase in coronary artery tone (resistance) |
| Increase in myocardial contractility | Diminished collateral blood flow |
| | Diminished perfusion pressure (pressure gradients from the aorta to the coronary arteries) |
| | Increase in heart rate (decrease in duration of diastole; coronary artery flow primarily occurs during diastole) |

**TABLE 24.2**
**Clinical Classification of Chest Pain**

| Typical (definite) angina | 1. Retrosternal discomfort with a characteristic quality and duration<br>2. Provoked by exertion or emotional stress<br>3. Relieved by rest or nitroglycerin |
|---|---|
| Atypical (probable) angina | Meets two of the above characteristics |
| Noncardiac chest pain | Meets one or none of the typical anginal characteristics |

**TABLE 24.3**
**Typical Characteristics of Chest Discomfort**

| Quality | Sense of strangling and anxiety Constricting, suffocating, crushing, heavy, and squeezing Other patients sensate more vague (mild pressure-like discomfort, tightness, an uncomfortable numbness, or a burning sensation) |
|---|---|
| Onset and offset | Intensity of the discomfort begins gradually over several minutes Relieved within several minutes by rest or the use of short-acting nitroglycerin (no more than 5–10 min) |
| Location | The site of the discomfort is usually retrosternal |
| Radiation | The radiation generally occurs toward the ulnar surface of the left arm but may also move toward the right arm and the outer surfaces of both arms |
| Timing | More common in the morning (secondary to a circadian variation in sympathetic tone) |
| Provoking factors | Physical activity, sexual activity, exposure to cold temperature, emotional or mental stress, meals, or cocaine use |

Some patients, especially the women, experience the typical anginal symptoms with objective evidence of myocardial ischemia despite normal coronary angiograms (angina without flow-limiting epicardial coronary stenosis, or syndrome X). These patients have ECG changes (ST-segment depression, T-wave inversions, or both) at rest or during the stress test, as well as evidence of reversible stress-induced myocardial perfusion defects on nuclear imaging. Although the benign long-term prognosis is generally emphasized for this syndrome, recently increased risk for adverse outcomes in certain subsets of these patients has been recognized.[14,15] Although the exact pathophysiologic mechanism of this syndrome is still unclear, potential explanations include endothelial and microvascular dysfunction and impaired coronary flow reserve. Other mechanisms include coronary vasospasm and myocardial metabolic abnormalities. However, chest discomfort without ischemia in some individuals may be caused by abnormal pain perception or sensitivity.[16]

The presence of objective evidence of ischemia in the absence of symptoms related to ischemia is considered as silent myocardial ischemia. These patients remain asymptomatic despite ischemic changes on resting or

mechanism of this phenomenon is ischemic preconditioning and collateral recruitment.[13] The classifications of the severity of angina pectoris based on the New York Heart Association, Canadian Cardiovascular Society, and Specific Activity Scale scores are listed in Table 24.4.

**TABLE 24.4**
**Grading the Severity of Angina Pectoris**

| Class | NYHA Functional Classification | CCS Functional Classification | Specific Activity Scale Classification |
|---|---|---|---|
| I | Patients with cardiac disease but without resulting limitations of physical activity<br>Ordinary physical activity does not cause undue fatigue, palpitation, dyspnea, or anginal pain | Ordinary physical activity, such as walking and climbing stairs, does not cause angina. Angina occurs with strenuous or rapid or prolonged exertion at work or recreation | Patients can perform to completion any activity requiring ≥7 METs |
| II | Patients with cardiac disease resulting in slight limitation of physical activity<br>They are comfortable at rest. Ordinary physical activity results in fatigue, palpitation, dyspnea, or angina pain | Slight limitation of ordinary activity Walking or climbing stairs rapidly, walking uphill, walking, or stair climbing after meals, in cold, in wind, or when under emotional stress, or only during the few hours after awakening<br>Walking more than two blocks on the level and climbing more than one flight of ordinary stairs at a normal pace and in normal conditions | Patients can perform to completion any activity requiring ≥5 METs but cannot and do not perform to completion activities requiring ≥7 METs |
| III | Patients with cardiac disease resulting in marked limitation of physical activity<br>They are comfortable at rest. Less than ordinary physical activity causes fatigue, palpitation, dyspnea, or anginal pain | Marked limitation of ordinary physical activity<br>Walking one to two blocks on the level and climbing more than one flight of ordinary stairs in normal conditions | Patients can perform to completion any activity requiring ≥2 METs but cannot and do not perform to completion any activities requiring ≥5 METs |
| IV | Patients with cardiac disease resulting in inability to carry on any physical activity without discomfort Symptoms of cardiac insufficiency or of the anginal syndrome may be present even at rest. If any physical activity is undertaken, discomfort is increased | Inability to carry on any physical activity without discomfort; anginal syndrome may be present at rest | Patients cannot or do not perform to completion activities requiring ≥2 METs. They cannot carry out activities listed for class III above |

*CCS*, Canadian Cardiovascular Society; *METs*, metabolic equivalents; *NYHA*, New York Heart Association.
Data from Goldman L, Hashimoto B, Cook E, et al. Comparative reproducibility and validity of systems for assessing cardiovascular functional class: advantages of a new specific activity scale. *Circulation.* 1981;64(6):1227–1234.

stress tests. During ambulatory ECG monitoring, transient ST-segment depression of 0.1 mV or greater that lasts longer than 30 s is a rare finding in normal subjects, but in these patients, this finding is accomplished with impaired regional myocardial perfusion and ischemia. The important cause of this condition is contributed to differences in both peripheral and central neural processing of pain. The prognosis of these patients is the same as for other patients with symptomatic IHD.[17,18] It is interesting that antianginal agents (e.g., nitrates,

beta-blockers, calcium channel blockers) can reduce or eliminate episodes of silent ischemia, as well as symptomatic ischemia. Also, other management, including preventive therapy, coronary angiography, and revascularization, should be similar.

## PHYSICAL EXAMINATION

Generally, the physical examination findings of patients with SIHD are normal. However, elevated blood pressure, xanthomas, and retinal exudates suggest the presence of CAD risk factors. It is also recommended that the body mass index is calculated, and a search done for the detection of peripheral vascular disease as well as comorbid conditions such as thyroid disease, renal disease, and diabetes. Examination during an episode of myocardial ischemia may reveal an increase in heart rate and blood pressure, new mitral regurgitation murmur caused by papillary muscle dysfunction or an increase in left ventricular (LV) filling pressure, pulmonary congestion findings (e.g., rales on auscultation) caused by decreased LV compliance, paradoxic S2 splitting caused by delayed relaxation of the LV myocardium and delayed closure of the aortic valve, S4 caused by a decrease in LV compliance, and S3 caused by LV systolic dysfunction. Relief of ischemia results in a cessation of symptoms and the signs that occurred during the episode.[19-21]

## DIFFERENTIAL DIAGNOSIS

Gastrointestinal disorders, especially gastroesophageal reflux, are common conditions that may simulate the coronary symptoms or coexist with IHD. Although nitroglycerin can reduce or relieve angina pectoris, in some cases, esophageal pain can be suppressed by this drug. However, the consumption of antacids, milk, foods, or warm liquids often relieves the esophageal pain.[22] The other differential diagnoses of angina pectoris are listed in Table 24.5.

## DIAGNOSIS

### Resting Electrocardiogram

A resting 12-lead ECG should be obtained for all patients with suspected CAD. Approximately half of the patients with SIHD have normal resting ECG findings, even in those with severe CAD, and this finding suggests the presence of normal resting LV function and good long-term prognosis. Patients with previous MI have specific ECG findings, including ST-T-wave changes or Q-wave formation. Other abnormalities such as conduction abnormalities, mainly left bundle branch block (LBBB) and impairment of atrioventricular conduction, may be present. However, the most common abnormal findings on ECGs in patients with SIHD are nonspecific ST-T-wave changes with or without abnormal Q waves.

Also, a resting ECG is recommended in all patients during or immediately after an episode of angina. About 50% of patients have new ECG changes during an episode of angina; the most common is ST-segment

**TABLE 24.5**
**Differential Diagnosis of Angina Pectoris**

| | |
|---|---|
| Nonischemic cardiovascular | Aortic dissection<br>Pericarditis<br>Myocarditis |
| Gastrointestinal | Esophageal reflux<br>Esophageal spasm<br>Esophagitis<br>Biliary colic<br>Cholecystitis<br>Choledocholithiasis<br>Cholangitis<br>Peptic ulcer<br>Pancreatitis |
| Pulmonary | Pulmonary embolism<br>Pulmonary infarction<br>Pneumothorax<br>Pneumonia<br>Pleuritis<br>Severe pulmonary hypertension |
| Chest wall | Costochondritis<br>Fibrositis<br>Rib fracture<br>Sternoclavicular arthritis<br>Herpes zoster (before the rash) |
| Psychiatric | Anxiety disorders<br>Hyperventilation<br>Panic disorder<br>Primary anxiety<br>Affective disorders (e.g., depression)<br>Somatiform disorders<br>Thought disorders (e.g., fixed delusions) |

Data from Fihn SD, Gardin JM, Abrams J, et al. 2012 ACCF/AHA/ACP/AATS/PCNA/SCAI/STS guideline for the diagnosis and management of patients with stable ischemic heart disease: a report of the American College of Cardiology Foundation/American Heart Association task force on practice guidelines, and the American College of Physicians, American Association for Thoracic Surgery, Preventive Cardiovascular Nurses Association, Society for Cardiovascular Angiography and Interventions, and Society of Thoracic Surgeons. *J Am Coll Cardiol.* 2012;60(24):e44–e164; and Mann DL, Zipes DP, Libby P, et al. *Braunwald's Heart Disease: A Textbook of Cardiovascular Medicine.* 10th ed. Philadelphia: Saunders; 2015.

depression. The presence of ST-T-wave changes, especially during an episode of angina, can correlate with the severity of the CAD and an adverse prognosis. The probability of IHD based on ECG changes and clinical status is illustrated in Table 24.6.[23] ST-segment depression during supraventricular tachyarrhythmias should not be used as evidence of obstructive CAD.[24]

**TABLE 24.6**
Probability of Ischemic Heart Disease Based on Clinical and Electrocardiogram Findings

| Probability of IHD | Clinical Findings | ECG Changes |
|---|---|---|
| High | Pain >20 min at rest; similar prior pain diagnosed as angina; and/or hypotension, diaphoresis, rales, transient mitral regurgitation | New ST-segment depression ≥0.5 mm, T-wave inversion ≥2 mm, recent left bundle branch block or life-threatening ventricular arrhythmia, and/or diagnostic elevations in biomarkers |
| Intermediate | Pain >20 min relieved by rest or nitroglycerin, male, age ≥70 years, coexistence of diabetes or extracardiac disease | Fixed Q waves and resting ST-segment depression ≤1 mm in multiple lead groups, LV hypertrophy, and/or traditional risk factors suggestive but not necessary for the diagnosis |
| Low | Absence of above; history of panic attacks, hyperventilation, or cocaine use; chest wall tenderness | ECG normal or unchanged, T-wave inversions in leads with dominant R waves, or T-wave flattening |

*ECG*, electrocardiogram; *IHD*, ischemic heart disease; *LV*, left ventricular.
From Kones R, Rumana U. Stable ischemic heart disease. *Heart Failure Clin.* 2016;12(1):11–29; with permission.

The presence of conduction disturbances, including left bundle branch block and left anterior fascicular block, is often associated with LV dysfunction, multivessel CAD, and a poor prognosis.[25–27] Arrhythmias, especially ventricular premature beats, have low sensitivity and specificity for detecting CAD. ECG findings in favor of LV hypertrophy correlate with systemic hypertension, aortic stenosis, hypertrophic cardiomyopathy, or previous MI with remodeling. Thus, in these patients, echocardiography for further evaluation is recommended.

Ambulatory ECG monitoring may reveal evidence of silent myocardial ischemia in patients with SIHD but rarely adds relevant diagnostic or prognostic information that cannot be derived from stress testing. ECG changes suggesting ischemia on ambulatory ECG monitoring are very frequent in women but do not correlate with findings during stress testing. Most importantly, therapeutic strategies targeting silent ischemia detected by ambulatory monitoring have not demonstrated clear survival benefits.[24]

## Biochemical Tests

Biochemical markers are used in patients with documented or suspected CAD to establish cardiovascular risk factors and associated conditions and to determine prognosis. Hemoglobin and thyroid hormone levels provide information related to possible causes of ischemia. Also, hemoglobin may add prognostic information.[28–30] The high-sensitivity C-reactive protein (hsCRP) has a prognostic value additive to traditional risk factors, including lipids; however, clinical value for the screening of CAD is debated.[31,32] Some professional society guidelines recommend the use of hsCRP in individuals at moderate global risk as a risk indicator to support statin therapy for primary prevention of CAD.[33] Detection of cardiac markers, especially sensitive troponin, in patients with SIHD is related to subsequent risk for cardiovascular mortality and heart failure[34–36]; however, the clinical use of troponin in patients without evidence of acute symptoms is currently not recommended.[37] Blood tests in the assessment of patients with known or suspected SIHD are listed in Table 24.7.[21]

## Echocardiography at Rest

According to the European Society of Cardiology (ESC) guidelines, resting transthoracic echocardiography is recommended in all patients for the exclusion of alternative causes of angina, regional wall motion abnormalities suggestive of CAD, measurement of LV ejection fraction for risk stratification purposes, and evaluation of diastolic function (class IB).[21] However, American College of Cardiology Foundation/American Heart Association (ACCF/AHA) guidelines do not recommend routine resting echocardiography for assessment of LV function in patients with a normal ECG, no history of MI, no symptoms or signs suggestive of heart failure, and no complex ventricular arrhythmias (class III). These guidelines recommended a resting Doppler echocardiography for assessment of LV systolic and diastolic function and evaluation for myocardium, heart valves, or pericardium in patients with known or suspected

**TABLE 24.7**
**Blood Tests in Assessment of Patients With Known or Suspected Stable Ischemic Heart Disease**

| Recommendations | Class | Level |
|---|---|---|
| If evaluation suggests clinical instability or ACS, repeated measurements of troponin, preferably using high-sensitivity or ultrasensitive assays, are recommended to rule out myocardial necrosis associated with ACS | I | A |
| Full blood count, including hemoglobin and WBC count, is recommended in all patients | I | B |
| It is recommended that screening for potential T2DM in patients with suspected and established SIHD is initiated with HbA1c and fasting plasma glucose and that an OGTT is added if HbA1c and fasting plasma glucose are inconclusive | I | B |
| Creatinine measurement and estimation of renal function (creatinine clearance) are recommended in all patients | I | B |
| A fasting lipid profile (including LDL) is recommended in all patients | I | C |
| If indicated by clinical suspicion of thyroid disorder, assessment of thyroid function is recommended | I | C |
| Liver function tests are recommended in patients early after beginning statin therapy | I | C |
| Creatine kinase measurements are recommended in patients taking statins and complaining of symptoms suggestive of myopathy | I | C |
| Annual control of lipids, glucose metabolism (fasting plasma glucose and HbA1c, if needed OGTT), and creatinine is recommended in all patients with known SIHD | I | C |
| BNP/NT-proBNP measurements should be considered in patients with suspected heart failure | IIa | C |

*ACS*, acute coronary syndrome; *BNP*, B-type natriuretic peptide; *HbA1c*, glycated hemoglobin; *LDL*, low-density lipoprotein; *NT-proBNP*, N-terminal pro-B-type natriuretic peptide; *OGTT*, oral glucose tolerance test; *SIHD*, stable ischemic heart disease; *T2DM*, type 2 diabetes mellitus; *WBC*, white blood cell.
From Montalescot G, Sechtem U, Achenbach S, et al. 2013 ESC guidelines on the management of stable coronary artery disease. *Eur Heart J.* 2013;34(38):2949–3003; with permission.

IHD and symptoms or signs of heart failure, a history of previous MI, pathologic Q waves on the ECG, complex ventricular arrhythmias, or an undiagnosed heart murmur (class I). Also, they mentioned that echocardiography may be considered for patients with hypertension or diabetes mellitus and abnormal findings on an ECG (class IIb). Routine reassessment (<1 year) of LV function is not recommended in SIHD patients with no change in clinical status and for whom no change in therapy is contemplated (class III).[5]

## Chest X-Ray

Although chest X-ray is frequently used in the assessment of patients with chest pain, it does not provide specific information for diagnosis or event risk stratification in patients with SIHD. The test may occasionally be helpful in assessing patients with suspected HF. Chest X-ray may also be useful in patients with pulmonary problems, which often accompany CAD, or to rule out another cause of chest pain in atypical presentations.[24]

## Probability Estimate of CAD

Estimation of the pretest probability of significant CAD based on clinical data is strongly recommended before a decision is made for standard stress testing (Table 24.8). When performing further testing in a patient with a probability of CAD less than 5%, the likelihood of a false-positive test result is actually higher than that of a true positive. On the other hand, with negative stress testing results in a patient with a very high pretest probability of CAD, the chance of falsely negative results in this patient is high, and more testing may be considered. Thus, further testing for patients with a pretest probability of CAD between 20% and 70% is most useful.[5] Additional factors, including ECG findings and cardiovascular risk factors, could help the physician in estimating the pretest probability of significant CAD (Table 24.9).[5,38]

Clinical models that included more information about risk factors for CVD, resting ECG changes, or coronary calcification have improved the identification of patients with obstructive CAD compared with age, sex,

**TABLE 24.8**

Pretest Likelihood of Significant Coronary Artery Disease in Patients According to Age, Sex, and TYPE of Angina

| | NONANGINAL CHEST PAIN | | ATYPICAL ANGINA | | TYPICAL ANGINA | |
|---|---|---|---|---|---|---|
| Age (years) | Men (%) | Women (%) | Men (%) | Women (%) | Men (%) | Women (%) |
| 30–39 | 4 | 2 | 34 | 12 | 76 | 26 |
| 40–49 | 13 | 3 | 51 | 22 | 87 | 55 |
| 50–59 | 20 | 7 | 65 | 31 | 93 | 73 |
| 60–69 | 27 | 14 | 72 | 51 | 94 | 86 |

**TABLE 24.9**

Pretest Likelihood of Significant Coronary Artery Disease in Low-Risk Symptomatic Patients Compared With High-Risk Symptomatic Patients Based on the Duke Database[a]

| | NONANGINAL CHEST PAIN | | ATYPICAL ANGINA | | TYPICAL ANGINA | |
|---|---|---|---|---|---|---|
| Age (Mid-decade), years | Men | Women | Men | Women | Men | Women |
| 35 | 3–35 | 1–19 | 8–59 | 2–39 | 30–88 | 10–78 |
| 45 | 9–47 | 2–22 | 21–70 | 5–43 | 51–92 | 20–79 |
| 55 | 23–59 | 4–21 | 45–79 | 10–47 | 80–95 | 38–82 |
| 65 | 49–69 | 9–29 | 71–86 | 20–51 | 93–97 | 56–84 |

[a]Each value represents a percentage, and in each box, the first number indicates the probability of coronary artery disease (CAD) in low-risk patients (without diabetes mellitus, smoking, or hyperlipidemia). The second numbers are for high-risk patients (with diabetes mellitus, smoking, and hyperlipidemia) in the same age bracket. If electrocardiogram changes, including ST-T-wave changes or Q waves, had been present, the likelihood of CAD would be higher in each box.
Data from Fihn SD, Gardin JM, Abrams J, et al. 2012 ACCF/AHA/ACP/AATS/PCNA/SCAI/STS guideline for the diagnosis and management of patients with stable ischemic heart disease: a report of the American College of Cardiology Foundation/American Heart Association task force on practice guidelines, and the American College of Physicians, American Association for Thoracic Surgery, Preventive Cardiovascular Nurses Association, Society for Cardiovascular Angiography and Interventions, and Society of Thoracic Surgeons. *J Am Coll Cardiol*. 2012;60(24): e44–e164; and Pryor DB, Shaw L, Harrell FE, et al. Estimating the likelihood of severe coronary artery disease. *Am J Med*. 1991;90(5):553–562.

and symptoms alone. Therefore, the presence of risk factors for CVD (such as the family history of CVD, dyslipidemia, diabetes, hypertension, smoking, and other lifestyle factors) that increase the probability of obstructive CAD can be used as modifiers of the pretest probability of significant CAD. If available, Q-wave, ST-segment, or T-wave changes on the ECG, LV dysfunction suggestive of ischemia, and findings on exercise ECG, as well as information on coronary calcium obtained by computed tomography, can be used to improve estimations of the pretest probability of obstructive CAD. In particular, the absence of coronary calcium (Agatston score = 0) is associated with a low prevalence of obstructive CAD (<5%), and a low risk of death or nonfatal MI (<1% annual risk). However, it should be noted that coronary calcium imaging does not exclude coronary stenosis caused by a noncalcified atherosclerotic lesion, and the presence of coronary calcium is a weak predictor of obstructive CAD.[24]

### Noninvasive Stress Testing

Noninvasive stress (functional) testing to detect inducible ischemia has been the gold standard technique to diagnose and estimate the severity of CAD in patients with suspected SIHD and to estimate prognosis in patients with known CAD.[39] These tests can provoke ischemia by using exercise or pharmacologic agents either to increase myocardial work (oxygen demand) or to induce vasodilation-elicited heterogeneity in induced coronary flow. It is important that coronary artery narrowing less than 70% is often undetected by stress testing. Noninvasive stress testing is most valuable when the pretest likelihood of CAD is intermediate. Also, it should be remembered that stress testing should be used only in patients in whom the further information delivered by testing can alter the planned management strategy.[40]

Although in previous exercise ECG was commonly used as an initial method to begin an evaluation in patients suspected to have CAD, recent evidence showed that exercise ECG has inferior diagnostic performance compared with diagnostic imaging tests and has limited power to rule-in or rule-out obstructive CAD.[41]

An exercise ECG alone may be considered as an alternative to diagnose obstructive CAD if imaging tests are not available, keeping in mind the risk of false-negative and false-positive test results.

Stress imaging is recommended in patients with uninterpretable ECGs (e.g., complete left bundle branch block, paced ventricular rhythm, and preexcitation syndrome), ECG changes (ST-segment depression at rest >1 mm, LV hypertrophy), or those taking digoxin. Also, the stress imaging for localizing ischemia is reasonable in patients with CAD who have undergone previous revascularization. In symptomatic women with a pretest likelihood of CAD more than intermediate, especially those with abnormal resting ECG, stress imaging or CCTA as an initial modality is recommended.[42] However, the noninvasive functional tests for ischemia typically have better rule-in power.

In asymptomatic individuals without known CAD, exercise testing usually is not recommended; however, in some conditions, this testing may be appropriate such as in asymptomatic individuals with diabetes who plan to begin a vigorous exercise or those with severe coronary calcifications on cardiac CT. Although using CCTA can effectively rule out obstructive CAD (especially in emergency departments), recent data showed that CCTA in patients with suspected angina caused by CAD helps to clarify the diagnosis and enables better-targeted interventions that might reduce the future risk of MI compared with standard care alone.[43] Also, the CONSERVE (Coronary Computed Tomographic Angiography for Selective Cardiac Catheterization) trial, presented at the ESC Congress 2016 in Rome, showed the computed tomography-guided strategy was associated with an 86% reduction in invasive coronary angiography compared with the direct invasive angiography approach.[44]

The risk stratification according to the noninvasive modalities, including exercise ECG, MPI, and stress echocardiography, is illustrated in Table 24.10. According to the guidelines, patients with high-risk noninvasive test results, regardless of the symptom severity, have a high likelihood of CAD; therefore, coronary arteriography should be done if they have no contraindications to revascularization.[45]

### Invasive Testing

Today, the gold standard modality for the detection of presence, extent, and the severity of CAD is coronary angiography (Table 24.11). Some patients had myocardial ischemia in the absence of epicardial coronary stenosis[14,15]; in about 15%–30% in some series, coronary

---

**TABLE 24.10**

**Risk Stratification According to Noninvasive Modalities in Patients With Stable Ischemic Heart Disease**

*High risk (>3% annual risk for death or MI)*

1. Severe resting left ventricular dysfunction (LVEF <35%) not readily explained by noncoronary causes
2. Resting perfusion abnormalities involving ≥10% of the myocardium without previous known MI
3. High-risk stress findings on the ECG, including
   - ≥2-mm ST-segment depression at low workload or persisting into recovery
   - Exercise-induced ST-segment elevation
   - Exercise-induced VT/VF
4. Severe stress-induced LV dysfunction (peak exercise LVEF <45% or drop in LVEF with stress ≥10%)
5. Stress-induced perfusion abnormalities encompassing ≥10% of the myocardium or stress segmental scores indicating multiple vascular territories with abnormalities
6. Stress-induced LV dilation
7. Inducible wall motion abnormality (involving >2 segments or 2 coronary beds)
8. Wall motion abnormality developing at a low dose of dobutamine (≤10 mg/kg/min) or at a low heart rate (<120 beats/min)
9. CAC score > 400 Agatston units
10. Multivessel obstructive CAD (≥70% stenosis) or left main stenosis (≥50% stenosis) on CCTA

*Continued*

---

**TABLE 24.10**

**Risk Stratification According to Noninvasive Modalities in Patients With Stable Ischemic Heart Disease—cont'd**

*Intermediate risk (1%–3% annual risk for death or MI)*

1. Mild-to-moderate resting LV dysfunction (LVEF of 35%–49%) not readily explained by noncoronary causes
2. Resting perfusion abnormalities involving 5%–9.9% of the myocardium in patients without a history or previous evidence of MI
3. ≥1-mm ST-segment depression occurring with exertional symptoms
4. Stress-induced perfusion abnormalities encompassing 5%–9.9% of the myocardium or stress segmental scores (in multiple segments) indicating one vascular territory with abnormalities but without LV dilation
5. Small wall motion abnormality involving one or two segments and only one coronary bed
6. CAC score of 100–399 Agatston units
7. One-vessel CAD with ≥70% stenosis or moderate CAD stenosis (50%–69% stenosis) in ≥2 arteries on CCTA

*Low risk (<1% annual risk for death or MI)*

1. Low-risk treadmill score (score ≥5) or no new ST-segment changes or exercise-induced chest pain symptoms when achieving maximal levels of exercise
2. Normal or small myocardial perfusion defect at rest or with stress encompassing ≥5% of the myocardium[a]
3. Normal stress or no change in limited resting wall motion abnormalities during stress
4. CAC score < 100 Agatston units
5. No coronary stenosis >50% on CCTA

*CAC*, coronary artery calcium; *CAD*, coronary artery disease; *CCTA*, coronary computed tomography angiography; *MI*, myocardial infarction; *VF*, ventricular fibrillation; *VT*, ventricular tachycardia.
[a]Although the published data are limited; patients with these findings will probably not be at low risk in the presence of either a high-risk treadmill score or severe resting left ventricular (LV) dysfunction (ventricular ejection fraction [LVEF] <35%).
Data from Fihn SD, Gardin JM, Abrams J, et al. 2012 ACCF/AHA/ACP/AATS/PCNA/SCAI/STS guideline for the diagnosis and management of patients with stable ischemic heart disease: a report of the American College of Cardiology Foundation/American Heart Association task force on practice guidelines, and the American College of Physicians, American Association for Thoracic Surgery, Preventive Cardiovascular Nurses Association, Society for Cardiovascular Angiography and Interventions, and Society of Thoracic Surgeons. *J Am Coll Cardiol*. 2012;60(24):e44–e164.

---

angiography showed no critical obstruction in these patients.[22] However, 5%–10% have significant left main coronary artery obstruction. The survival rate of patients with significant left main coronary stenosis or its equivalent [severe proximal left anterior descending coronary artery (LAD) and proximal left circumflex stenosis] is significantly reduced if they undergo medical treatment alone. Moreover, patients with left main coronary stenosis greater than 70%, especially if accomplished with reduced LV systolic function, have lower survival rates than patients with 50%–70% stenosis.

Measuring the extension of the severity of epicardial CAD for a better decision on the next therapeutic strategy could be done by scoring systems such as SYNTAX (synergy between percutaneous coronary intervention with TAXUS and cardiac surgery).[46] The presence of LV regional wall motion abnormalities during contrast ventriculography provides more characteristics of CAD. Elevated LV end-diastolic pressure may be predictive of the presence of reduced LV compliance or LV

systolic failure.[22] During catheterization, using advanced IVUS, OCT, angioscopy, or thermography provides further information about the detection and quantification of intracoronary lesions.[47–50] Also, fractional flow reserve (FFR) is an important modality for determining the functional significance of epicardial coronary stenosis.[51–53]

## TREATMENT

The main aims of treatment of patients with SIHD are to minimize the risk of death and maximize health and function. To reach these goals, five fundamental, complementary, and overlapping strategies should be used:

1. The patient is educated about the cause, clinical manifestations, and prognosis of CAD and who then participates in treatment decisions.
2. Identification of appropriate treatment for comorbid conditions
3. Modification of cardiovascular risk factors

**TABLE 24.11**

**Indications for Coronary Angiography in Patients With Stable Ischemic Heart Disease**

| Class I | Class IIa | Class IIb | Class III |
|---|---|---|---|
| • Patients with presumed SIHD who have unacceptable ischemic symptoms despite GDMT and who are amenable to and candidates for coronary revascularization. (Level of evidence: C) <br><br> • Patients with SIHD who have survived sudden cardiac death or potentially life-threatening ventricular arrhythmia should undergo coronary angiography to assess cardiac risk. (Level of evidence: B) <br><br> • Patients with SIHD who develop symptoms and signs of heart failure should be evaluated to determine whether coronary angiography should be performed for risk assessment. (Level of evidence: B) <br><br> • Patients with SIHD whose clinical characteristics and results of noninvasive testing indicate a high likelihood of severe IHD and when the benefits are deemed to exceed risk. (Level of evidence: C) | • To define the extent and severity of CAD in patients with suspected SIHD whose clinical characteristics and results of noninvasive testing (exclusive of stress testing) indicate a high likelihood of severe IHD and who are amenable to and candidates for coronary revascularization. (Level of Evidence: C) <br><br> • Patients with suspected symptomatic SIHD who cannot undergo diagnostic stress testing or have indeterminate or nondiagnostic stress tests when there is a high likelihood that the findings will result in important changes to therapy. (Level of Evidence: C) <br><br> • To further assess risk in patients with SIHD who have depressed LV function (EF <50%) and moderate risk criteria on noninvasive testing with demonstrable ischemia. (Level of evidence: C) <br><br> • To further assess risk in patients with SIHD and inconclusive prognostic information after noninvasive testing or in patients for whom noninvasive testing is contraindicated or inadequate. (Level of evidence: C) <br><br> • Risk assessment is reasonable for patients with SIHD who have unsatisfactory quality of life from angina, have preserved LV function (EF >50%), and have intermediate risk criteria on noninvasive testing. (Level of evidence: C) | • Patients with stress test results of acceptable quality that do not suggest the presence of CAD when clinical suspicion of CAD remains high and there is a high likelihood that the findings will result in important changes to therapy. (Level of Evidence: C) | • Risk assessment is not recommended in patients with SIHD who elect not to undergo revascularization or who are not candidates for revascularization because of comorbidities or individual preferences. (Level of evidence: B) <br><br> • Assess risk in patients with SIHD who have preserved LV function (EF >50%) and low-risk criteria on noninvasive testing. (Level of evidence: B) <br><br> • Assess risk in patients who are at low risk according to clinical criteria and who have not undergone noninvasive risk testing. (Level of evidence: C) <br><br> • Assess risk in asymptomatic patients with no evidence of ischemia on noninvasive testing. (Level of evidence: C) |

CAD, coronary artery disease; EF, ejection fraction; GDMT, guideline-directed medical therapy; IHD, ischemic heart disease; LV, left ventricular; SIHD, stable ischemic heart disease.

Data from Fihn SD, Gardin JM, Abrams J, et al. 2012 ACCF/AHA/ACP/AATS/PCNA/SCAI/STS guideline for the diagnosis and management of patients with stable ischemic heart disease: a report of the American College of Cardiology Foundation/American Heart Association task force on practice guidelines, and the American College of Physicians, American Association for Thoracic Surgery, Preventive Cardiovascular Nurses Association, Society for Cardiovascular Angiography and Interventions, and Society of Thoracic Surgeons. J Am Coll Cardiol. 2012;60(24):e44–e164; and Fihn SD, Blankenship JC, Alexander KP, et al. 2014 ACC/AHA/AATS/PCNA/SCAI/STS focused update of the guideline for the diagnosis and management of patients with stable ischemic heart disease: a report of the American College of Cardiology/American Heart Association Task Force on Practice Guidelines, and the American Association for Thoracic Surgery, Preventive Cardiovascular Nurses Association, Society for Cardiovascular Angiography and Interventions, and Society of Thoracic Surgeons. J Am Coll Cardiol. 2014;64(18):1929–1949.

4. Utilization of evidence-based medical treatment to maximize health, function, and survival of patients
5. Revascularization should be used in selected patients based on guideline recommendations

## Medical Management

In patients with SIHD, antianginal therapy is used to safely relieve symptoms and extend exercise duration. However, the standard treatment with long-acting nitrates, beta-blockers, or calcium channel blockers do not have a beneficial effect on disease progression, frequency of MI, and mortality. All standard antianginal agents act by predominantly affecting either the heart rate or vascular tone (physiologic effect). Some emerging therapies have a direct effect on myocardial metabolism; others have physiologic effects.[54] The major considerations in the prescription of antianginal agents are described in Table 24.12. A suggested approach for the use of different types of antianginal therapies based on clinical status is illustrated in Fig. 24.2.

On the other hand, some drugs benefit the effect on atherosclerotic plaque stabilizing and in cases, plaque regression, can lead to preventing cardiovascular events. Evidence has shown that in patients with SIHD and preserved LV function, using aspirin (or clopidogrel in case of aspirin intolerance), angiotensin-converting enzyme inhibition, and statins could prevent cardiovascular events and, therefore, reduce mortality and morbidity. In patients with SIHD and LV dysfunction or previous MI, addition of beta-blocking agents reduces both mortality and the risk for repeat MI. Guidelines recommend that optimal medical treatment includes at least one drug for angina relief plus drugs for event prevention for all patients with SIHD. Also, it is recommended that patients should be educated about CAD, risk factors, and treatment strategy, and the patient's response should be reviewed soon after starting therapy.[21]

Although the guidelines recommended achieving a goal blood pressure of less than 140/90 mmHg in hypertensive SIHD patients,[5] recent data showed that systolic blood pressure of less than 120 mmHg and diastolic blood pressure of less than 70 mmHg were each associated with adverse cardiovascular outcomes and mortality, probably because of inadequate myocardial perfusion (J-curve phenomenon for blood pressure in patients with CAD).[55]

Patients with diabetes are more prone to atherosclerotic plaque formation and cardiovascular events.[56–58] Although there is enough evidence about the control of blood glucose in the cardiovascular outcome of patients with diabetes, the results of intensive therapy in these patients are mixed. A favorable impact of intensive diabetes therapy in patients with type 1 diabetes on the risk of cardiovascular disease was shown at long-term follow-up[59]; however, this effect was not shown in patients with type 2 diabetes and was even associated with adverse outcomes in some cases.[60–62] The long-term follow-up of patients with diabetes showed that treatment with metformin compared with insulin or sulfonylurea had a lower incidence of MI and death.[63]

## Nonpharmacologic Treatment of Refractory Angina

Nonpharmacologic treatments, including enhanced external counterpulsation (EECP), transmyocardial laser revascularization (TMLR), and spinal cord stimulation, can be considered in patients with refractory ischemic symptoms after optimal medical treatment and coronary revascularization. ECCP, by increasing myocardial perfusion and oxygen supply, decreasing myocardial oxygen demand and improving endothelial function and vascular remodeling, could reduce the frequency of angina, increase cardiac output, and improve exercise tolerance and quality of life.[64–67] TMLR, by creating small channels from the epicardial to the endocardial surfaces and exposing the oxygenated blood directly from the LV to the myocardium, can improve refractory angina.[68] Compared with the surgical approach, percutaneous TMLR has lower procedural complication and mortality rates.[69] Spinal cord stimulation by neuromodulation of pain (based on the gate control theory of pain transmission) and prevention of transmission pain to the brain can reduce the frequency and severity of angina and improve quality of life. However, the efficacy of this method on angina improvement in different studies has been debated.[70–73]

## Coronary Artery Disease Revascularization

The main goals of revascularization for patients with CAD are improved survival and symptom relief. Based on the previous evidence, anatomically significant coronary stenosis is defined as 50% diameter narrowing for the left main and 70% for other coronary arteries. Also, FFR of 0.80 or less and instantaneous wave-free ratio (iwFR) of 0.89 or less can also be considered to be significant hemodynamic flow reduction. The Society of Thoracic Surgeons (STS) score and the SYNTAX score have been shown to predict adverse outcomes in patients undergoing coronary artery bypass grafting (CABG) and percutaneous coronary intervention (PCI), respectively, and are often useful in making revascularization decisions, especially for patients with an unprotected left main artery and complex CAD.[74–77]

**TABLE 24.12**

**Considerations for Prescription of Emerging Antianginal Drugs to Patients With Stable Ischemic Heart Disease**

| Agent | Common Side Effects | Contraindications | Potential Drug Interactions |
|---|---|---|---|
| *Agents that have a physiologic effect* | | | |
| Short- and long-acting nitrates | Headache, flushing, hypotension, syncope and postural hypotension, reflex tachycardia, methemoglobinemia | Hypertrophic obstructive cardiomyopathy | Phosphodiesterase type 5 inhibitors (sildenafil and similar agents), α-adrenergic blockers, CCBs |
| Beta-blockers | Fatigue, depression, bradycardia, heart block, bronchospasm, peripheral vasoconstriction, postural hypotension, impotence, masked signs of hypoglycemia | Low heart rate or heart conduction disorder, cardiogenic shock, asthma, severe peripheral vascular disease, decompensated heart failure, vasospastic angina; use with caution in patients with COPD (cardioselective beta-blockers may be used if patient receives adequate treatment with inhaled glucocorticoids and long-acting beta agonists) | Heart rate-lowering CCBs, sinus node or AV conduction depressors |
| *Calcium channel blockers* | | | |
| Nondihydropyridine (heart rate-lowering agents) | Bradycardia, heart conduction defect, low EF, constipation, gingival hyperplasia | Cardiogenic shock, severe aortic stenosis, obstructive cardiomyopathy | CYP3A4 substrates (digoxin, simvastatin, cyclosporine) |
| Dihydropyridine | Headache, ankle swelling, fatigue, flushing, reflex tachycardia | Low heart rate or heart rhythm disorder, sick sinus syndrome, CHF, low blood pressure | Agents with cardiodepressant effects (beta-blockers, flecainide), CYP3A4 substrates |
| Ivabradine | Visual disturbances, headache, dizziness, bradycardia, atrial fibrillation, AV block | Low heart rate or heart rhythm disorder, severe hepatic disease; not to be prescribed with verapamil and diltiazem; caution for use in patients with AF | QTc-extending drugs, macrolide antibiotics, anti-HIV drugs, antifungal drugs |
| Nicorandil | Headache, facial flushing, dizziness and weakness, nausea, hypotension; oral, anal, or gastrointestinal ulceration | Cardiogenic shock, heart failure, low blood pressure (<100 mmHg systolic) | Phosphodiesterase type 5 inhibitors (e.g., sildenafil or similar drugs) |
| Molsidomine | Headache, hypotension | None reported | None reported |
| *Agents that affect myocardial metabolism* | | | |
| Ranolazine | Dizziness, constipation, nausea, QT-interval prolongation | Liver cirrhosis, long QT | CYP3A4 substrates (digoxin, simvastatin, cyclosporine), drugs that prolong the corrected QT interval |
| Trimetazidine | Gastric discomfort, nausea, headache, movement disorders | Allergy, Parkinson disease, tremors, movement disorders, severe renal impairment | None reported |
| Perhexiline | Dizziness, nausea, vomiting, lethargy, tremors | Slow hydroxylators of cytochrome P450, abnormal liver function, neuropathy | Cytochrome P450 substrates |
| Allopurinol | Rash, gastric discomfort | Hypersensitivity, renal failure | Mercaptopurine, azathioprine |

*AF*, atrial fibrillation; *AV*, atrioventricular; *CCB*, calcium channel blocker; *CHF*, congestive heart failure; *COPD*, chronic obstructive pulmonary disease; *EF*, ejection fraction.
Data from Ohman EM. Chronic stable angina. *N Engl J Med.* 2016;2016(374):1167–1176; and Husted SE, Ohman EM. Pharmacological and emerging therapies in the treatment of chronic angina. *Lancet.* 2015;386(9994):691–701.

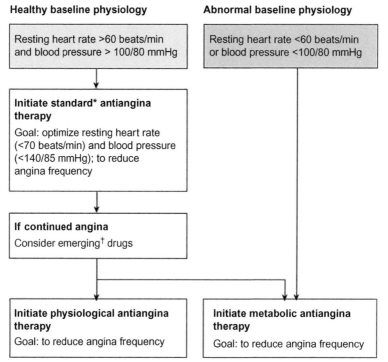

**FIG. 24.2** Approach to the use of antianginal therapy based on baseline physiologic findings. *Asterisk* indicates that standard antianginal agents (physiologic effect) include beta-blockers, calcium channel blockers, and long-acting nitrates. *Dagger* indicates that emerging antianginal agents with a physiologic effect include ivabradine (used only in patients with heart failure), nicorandil, and molsidomine. Emerging agents with myocardial metabolism affect include ranolazine, trimetazidine, perhexiline, and allopurinol. (From Husted SE, Ohman EM. Pharmacological and emerging therapies in the treatment of chronic angina. *Lancet.* 2015;386 (9994):691–701; with permission.)

In patients undergoing CABG, use of arterial conduits, especially the left internal mammary artery, has a major effect on long-term outcomes.[78] This benefit has been suggested to be associated with the higher patency of arterial conduits than saphenous vein grafts (90% vs 50% after 10 years). Moreover, the survival benefit will be higher if the surgeon uses the bilateral internal mammary artery. However, grafting of the bilateral internal mammary artery may increase the rate of sternal wound infections, especially in older patients or those with diabetes. Although the patency rate of radial artery conduits is lower than for the internal mammary artery, they have better long-term patency and clinical outcomes than saphenous vein grafts. Also, when the diameter stenosis of the target vessel is 90% or larger, the patency rate of the radial artery is excellent. An algorithm for selecting conduits for patients with SIHD undergoing elective CABG is illustrated in Fig. 24.3.[79]

## Revascularization (Coronary Artery Bypass Grafting or Percutaneous Coronary Intervention) vs Medical Therapy

Evidence shows that CABG offers survival advantage and relieves angina symptoms over medical therapy for patients with left main or three-vessel CAD.[80] Also, patients with multivessel CAD who were treated with CABG were found to be less likely to have a subsequent MI, need additional revascularization, or experience cardiac death compared with medical therapy on long-term follow-up.[81] By improving guideline-directed medical therapy (GDMT) during the past years, the relative benefits for survival and angina relief with CABG diminished compared with GDMT.[5] Thus, patients with more extensive and severe CAD, especially those with left main and three-vessel CAD, LV systolic dysfunction, and high-risk noninvasive testing, experience more benefit from CABG over medical therapy.

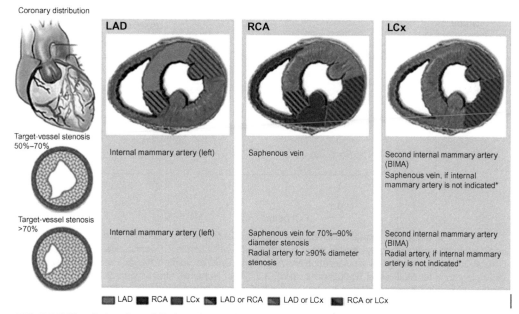

FIG. 24.3 The choice of conduits in patients with stable ischemic heart disease undergoing elective coronary artery bypass grafting. The *colored areas* represent the myocardium at risk. *Asterisk* indicates that the benefit–risk assessment should be considered by attention to a higher risk of sternal wound infection (especially in patients with diabetes and elderly patients). *BIMA*, bilateral internal mammary artery; *LAD*, left anterior descending artery; *LCx*, left circumflex coronary artery; *RCA*, right coronary artery. (From Piccolo R, Giustino G, Mehran R, et al. Stable coronary artery disease: revascularisation and invasive strategies. *Lancet.* 2015;386(9994): 702–713; with permission.)

Although PCI has a beneficial effect on the reduction of the incidence of angina, it did not reduce the risk of death or MI in patients without recent ACS in some studies.[82–84] A recent meta-analysis from three randomized trials [COURAGE (Clinical Outcomes Utilizing Revascularization and Aggressive Drug Evaluation), Nuclear Substudy 0, FAME-2 (Fractional Flow Reserve vs Angiography for Multivessel Evaluation-2), and SWISSI II (Silent Ischemia After Myocardial Infarction II)] suggests that mortality rates may be lower with PCI plus medical therapy vs medical therapy alone in patients with SIHD and significant ischemia based on noninvasive stress imaging or abnormal FFR ($\leq$0.80) (Fig. 24.4).[85]

A large network meta-analysis in 2014 demonstrated that CABG and new-generation drug-eluting stents (DESs) were associated with improved survival rates in patients with SIHD compared with a strategy of initial medical treatment. However, balloon angioplasty, bare-metal stents (BMS), or early-generation DESs did not have such an effect (Fig. 24.5).[86] Based on other evidence, today new-generation DESs are the standard of care for patients undergoing PCI.[87–90] Based on the

ESC 2019 guidelines, decisions for revascularization by PCI or CABG are based on clinical presentation and prior documentation of ischemia (ischemia >10% of the left ventricle). In the absence of prior documentation of ischemia, indications for revascularization depend on the invasive evaluation of stenosis severity or prognostic indications (diameter of stenosis >90%, FFR $\leq$0.80 or instantaneous wave-free ratio $\leq$0.89 in the major vessel, or LVEF $\leq$35% due to CAD).[24]

## Coronary Artery Bypass Grafting vs Percutaneous Coronary Intervention

Based on evidence, CABG comparing PCI is more effective in relieving angina and led to fewer repeated coronary revascularizations at long-term follow-up but had a higher risk for procedural stroke.[79,80] The superiority of CABG for lower risk of repeat revascularization may be due to more frequent revascularization of nonculprit lesions that do not intervene during the PCI.[79]

Results of the SYNTAX trial after 3 years showed that the major adverse cardiac events (MACEs), a composite of death, stroke, MI, or repeat revascularization, were

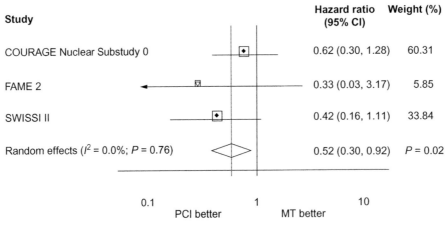

FIG. 24.4 The significant mortality benefit with percutaneous coronary intervention plus medical therapy compared with medical therapy alone in patients with significant ischemia. *CI*, confidence interval; *COURAGE*, Clinical Outcomes Utilizing Revascularization and Aggressive DruG Evaluation; *FAME*, Fractional Flow Reserve vs Angiography for Multivessel Evaluation-2; *SWISSI II*, Silent Ischemia After Myocardial Infarction II. (From Gada H, Kirtane AJ, Kereiakes DJ, et al. Meta-analysis of trials on mortality after percutaneous coronary intervention compared with medical therapy in patients with stable coronary heart disease and objective evidence of myocardial ischemia. *Am J Cardiol.* 2015;115(9):1194–1199; with permission.)

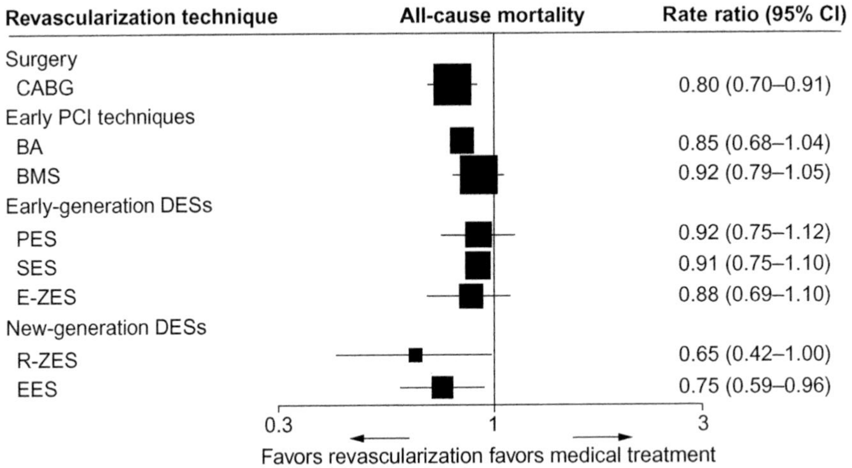

FIG. 24.5 The all-cause mortality based on different revascularization techniques compared with medical treatment in patients with SIHD. *BA*, balloon angioplasty; *BMS*, bare-metal stents; *CABG*, coronary artery bypass grafting; *CI*, confidence interval; *EES*, everolimus-eluting stent; *E-ZES*, endeavor zotarolimus-eluting stent; *PCI*, percutaneous coronary intervention; *PES*, paclitaxel-eluting stent; *SES*, sirolimus-eluting stent; *R-ZES*, resolute zotarolimus-eluting stent. (From Piccolo R, Giustino G, Mehran R, et al. Stable coronary artery disease: revascularisation and invasive strategies. *Lancet.* 2015;386(9994):702–713; with permission.)

significantly more often observed in PCI with the DES group compared with the CABG group.[74,75,91] The rates of death and stroke were similar; however, MI and repeat revascularization were more likely to occur with DES implantation.[91] The patients with higher SYNTAX scores have higher MACEs (Fig. 24.6).[91] The 5-year follow-up of the SYNTAX trial showed that although the rate of all-cause death was not significantly different between PCI and CABG, MI-related death significantly increased in the PCI group (Fig. 24.7), especially in

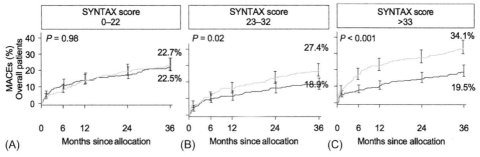

FIG. 24.6 The frequency of major adverse cardiac events (MACEs) based on SYNTAX (synergy between percutaneous coronary intervention with TAXUS and cardiac surgery) score in percutaneous coronary intervention and coronary artery bypass grafting groups after 3-year follow-up. (From Kappetein AP, Feldman TE, Mack MJ, et al. Comparison of coronary bypass surgery with drug-eluting stenting for the treatment of left main and/or three-vessel disease: 3-year follow-up of the SYNTAX trial. *Eur Heart J.* 2011;32(17):2125–2134; with permission.)

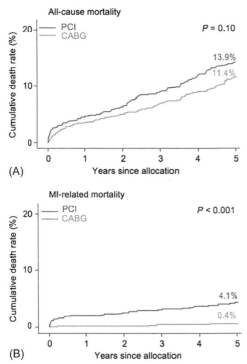

FIG. 24.7 (A and B) Five-year follow-up of the SYNTAX (synergy between percutaneous coronary intervention with TAXUS and cardiac surgery) trial. *CABG,* coronary artery bypass graft; *MI,* myocardial infarction; *PCI,* percutaneous coronary intervention. (From Milojevic M, Head SJ, Parasca CA, et al. Causes of death following PCI versus CABG in complex CAD: 5-year follow-up of SYNTAX. *J Am Coll Cardiol.* 2016;67(1):42–55; with permission.)

patients with diabetes, three-vessel CAD, or high SYNTAX scores.[92] Recently, a large registry study showed that PCI with everolimus-eluting stents (new-generation) compared with CABG is associated with a similar risk of death, a higher risk of MI (among patients with incomplete revascularization), and a higher risk of repeat revascularization but a lower risk of stroke.[93]

Although the gold standard treatment for unprotected left main CAD revascularization has been CABG, recently PCI has been considered as an alternative mode, especially in patients with left main ostium or trunk involvement, lower SYNTAX score, and higher STS score.[74,94,95] The decision between PCI or CABG for patients with multivessel and left main CAD based on a local heart team approach (incorporating input from interventional cardiologists and cardiothoracic surgeons) for careful evaluation of the possible benefits and risks inherent to both revascularization methods is recommended.[79] Today, routine angiographic follow-up after stenting for unprotected left main CAD is not recommended.[96] The choice of revascularization in patients with CAD and LV systolic dysfunction is made based on multiple variable considerations, including extension of CAD, the presence of diabetes mellitus, the presence of renal impairment, severity of LV systolic dysfunction, patient preferences, clinical judgment, and consultation between the interventional cardiologist and the cardiac surgeon.[5] An algorithm for revascularization based on anatomic and clinical status in patients with SIHD is illustrated in Fig. 24.8.

Repeat revascularization in symptomatic patients after CABG is most likely to improve survival in those

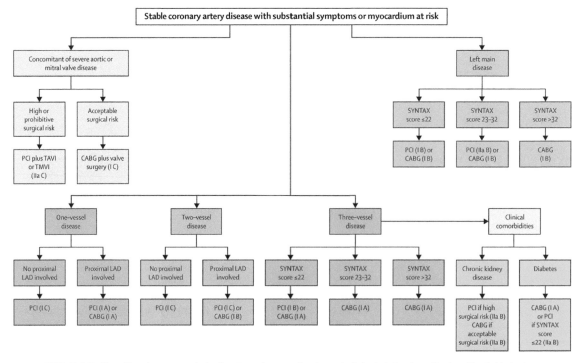

**FIG. 24.8** Algorithm for revascularization based on anatomic and clinical status in patients with stable ischemic heart disease based on 2014 European guidelines. *CABG*, coronary artery bypass graft; *LAD*, left anterior descending artery; *PCI*, percutaneous coronary intervention; *SYNTAX*, synergy between percutaneous coronary intervention with TAXUS and cardiac surgery; *TAVI*, transcatheter aortic valve implantation; *TMVI*, transcatheter mitral valve implantation. (Data from Piccolo R, Giustino G, Mehran R, Windecker S. Stable coronary artery disease: revascularisation and invasive strategies. *Lancet.* 2015;386(9994):702–713; and Windecker S, Kolh P, Alfonso F, et al. 2014 ESC/EACTS Guidelines on myocardial revascularization. *Eur Heart J.* 2014;35:2541–2619.)

with the highest risk (e.g., proximal LAD artery obstruction accomplished with extensive anterior ischemia).[97–99] However, in those with ischemia in other territories and those with a patent left internal mammary artery (LIMA) to the LAD artery, repeat revascularization is unlikely to increase the survival rate.[100] In patients with early graft failure after postoperative MI, PCI is a valuable option to revascularization; however, PCI in patients with degenerated saphenous vein grafts is often associated with poor angiographic and clinical outcomes.[101] Thus, the best option for repeat revascularization in patients with previous CABG multiple variables should be considered, such as the number of diseased bypass grafts, availability of the internal mammary artery for grafting, distal targets for bypass graft placement, areas of ischemia causing symptoms, a patent graft to the LAD artery, and comorbid conditions.

## SPECIAL GROUPS

### Women

Several large studies showed that women had worse outcomes after surgical or percutaneous coronary revascularization compared with men.[102–106] A recent study showed that despite young women having less severe angiographic CAD, they have an increased risk of the target vessel and target lesion failure at 5 years of follow-up after PCI.[106] In-hospital mortality and perioperative morbidity rates after CABG are higher in women than in men. This may be because the women referred for CABG are sicker (older age, comorbid conditions, more severe angina, and history of heart failure) than the men.[107,108] Some believe that after adjustment, the greater risk profile of women referred for CABG, short-term mortality rates, and long-term outcomes are similar to men, and female sex should not be a significant factor in decisions regarding whether to offer CABG.[22] Guidelines recommend that initial management with optimal medical therapy based on GDMT for women with SIHD must be considered. If symptoms of the patient are refractory or adverse effects of SIHD are present, angiography and revascularization could be performed.[5]

## Older Patients

The mortality and morbidity of older patients ($\geq$75 years of age) undergoing revascularization are higher compared with younger patients; this is because of a higher frequency of comorbid conditions such as peripheral vascular and cerebrovascular disease, advanced CAD, renal impairment, and LV dysfunction.[109–112] The results of revascularization compared with medical therapy based on previous studies are mixed, although some studies showed that long-term outcomes of older patients were better after revascularization.[113–118] By attention to the high risk of adverse effects after invasive treatments, it was recommended that decisions to recommend revascularization should be undertaken only after careful consideration of coronary anatomy, technical feasibility, risks of complication, patient preferences, functional capacity, quality of life, life expectancy, and end-of-life issues, as well as alternative therapies.[5] In those candidates for angiography and PCI, radial access is recommended whenever possible to reduce access-site complications. The use of DES, compared with bare-metal stents in this group, in combination with a short duration of DAPT is associated with significant safety and efficacy.[24]

## Diabetes Mellitus

Evidence shows that in patients with diabetes with multivessel CAD, and CABG has more benefit in long-term clinical outcomes (death and MI) compared with PCI.[119–122] A large analysis from 10 randomized trials showed a worse long-term survival rate in diabetic patients after PCI (balloon angioplasty or BMS implantation) than CABG.[123] The FREEDOM (Future REvascularization Evaluation in patients with Diabetes mellitus: Optimal management of Multivessel disease) trial compared the outcomes of CABG and PCI with DES in patients with diabetes with patients with multivessel CAD and found that all-cause mortality and the composite of death and MI was significantly reduced in the CABG group.[119] Although a recent meta-analysis showed that PCI with DES compared with CABG had a similar risk of MACEs in patients with diabetes with low and intermediate SYNTAX scores (0–32), MACEs were increased in the group with high SYNTAX scores

($>$32).[124] Recommendations for revascularization in patients with diabetes based on guidelines are illustrated in Fig. 24.7.

## Renal Insufficiency

Cardiovascular disease is the major cause of death in patients with end-stage renal disease. In these patients, risk factors, including diabetes, hypertension, LV systolic and diastolic dysfunction, abnormal lipid metabolism, anemia, and increased homocysteine levels, are associated with increased CAD and its complications. Also, surgical or percutaneous coronary revascularization is associated with higher complication rates.[125,126] Despite a higher early mortality rate in patients with the end-stage renal disease after CABG, these patients have lower late mortality, MI, and repeat revascularization at long-term follow-up compared with patients who undergo PCI.[125,127] Recommendations for revascularization in patients with diabetes based on guidelines are illustrated in Fig. 24.8.

## After Heart Transplantation

Transplant CAD is largely an immunological phenomenon and remains the most significant cause of morbidity and mortality after orthotopic heart transplantation.[128] Invasive coronary angiography is recommended for the assessment of transplant CAD and should be performed annually for 5 years after transplantation. If there are no significant abnormalities, angiograms can be performed biannually thereafter. Moreover, intravascular ultrasound (IVUS) may be useful for detecting and assessing cardiac allograft vasculopathy and plaque stability. Treatment options for CAD in these patients include pharmacotherapy and revascularization. PCI in the transplanted heart has become an established therapy.[24]

## Cancer

Advances in treatment have led to improved survival of patients with cancer but have also increased morbidity and mortality due to treatment side effects. Cardiovascular diseases (CVDs) are one of the most frequent of these side effects, and there is a growing concern that they may lead to premature morbidity and death among cancer survivors.[129] An increase in CAD in these patients may be due to a side effect of cancer therapy (i.e., radiotherapy to the thorax/mediastinum, cardiotoxic chemotherapy, or immunotherapies) or a result of extended cancer therapies in elderly individuals. The decision for CAD treatment should be based on life expectancy, additional comorbidities such as thrombocytopenia, increased thrombosis and bleeding propensity, and potential interactions between drugs used in SIHD management and antineoplastic drugs. In cancer patients with increased frailty, the least invasive revascularization procedures are recommended.[24]

## FOLLOW-UP OF PATIENTS WITH STABLE ISCHEMIC HEART DISEASE

Follow-up visits of patients with SIHD are recommended for monitoring symptoms and evaluation of progression or complications of CAD and patients' adherence to and effectiveness of therapy. The recommended intervals for visits based on guidelines are every 4–6 months during the first year of therapy and then every 6–12 months if the patient is stable and insightful about worsening symptoms and alarming signs. During each visit, a cardiovascular physical examination should be performed, and a resting 12-lead ECG is necessary when angina patterns change or there is evidence of arrhythmia or a conduction abnormality.[5] The presence of ECG changes (repolarization abnormalities) should be compared with previous ECGs to improve diagnostic accuracy and help the physician make decisions for the next step.[130–132] Appropriate noninvasive and invasive testing in the evaluation of new or worsening symptoms of patients with known SIHD should be considered if indicated. The diagnostic accuracy of noninvasive stress testing is similar in patients with and without known SIHD. Whenever possible, using the same noninvasive stress modalities in initial and follow-up testing should be performed. With this approach, the physician can make better decisions about the association between changes in clinical status and stress testing.[5]

## REFERENCES

1. Lloyd-Jones D, Adams RJ, Brown TM, et al. Heart disease and stroke statistics—2010 update. A report from the American Heart Association. *Circulation.* 2010;121(7): e46–e215.
2. Ford ES, Capewell S. Coronary heart disease mortality among young adults in the US from 1980 through 2002: concealed leveling of mortality rates. *J Am Coll Cardiol.* 2007;50(22):2128–2132.
3. Lozano R, Naghavi M, Foreman K, et al. Global and regional mortality from 235 causes of death for 20 age groups in 1990 and 2010: a systematic analysis for the Global Burden of Disease Study 2010. *Lancet.* 2013;380 (9859):2095–2128.
4. Abrams J. Chronic stable angina. *N Engl J Med.* 2005;352 (24):2524–2533.
5. Fihn SD, Gardin JM, Abrams J, et al. 2012 ACCF/AHA/ ACP/AATS/PCNA/SCAI/STS guideline for the diagnosis and management of patients with stable ischemic heart disease: a report of the American College of Cardiology Foundation/American Heart Association task force on practice guidelines, and the American College of Physicians, American Association for Thoracic Surgery, Preventive Cardiovascular Nurses Association, Society for Cardiovascular Angiography and Interventions, and Society of Thoracic Surgeons. *J Am Coll Cardiol.* 2012;60 (24):e44–e164.
6. Hollander JE. The management of cocaine-associated myocardial ischemia. *N Engl J Med.* 1995;333(19): 1267–1272.
7. McCord J, Jneid H, Hollander JE, et al. Management of cocaine-associated chest pain and myocardial infarction: a scientific statement from the American Heart Association Acute Cardiac Care Committee of the Council on Clinical Cardiology. *Circulation.* 2008;117 (14):1897–1907.
8. Stankowski RV, Kloner RA, Rezkalla SH. Cardiovascular consequences of cocaine use. *Trends Cardiovasc Med.* 2015;25(6):517–526.
9. Shaw LJ, Bugiardini R, Merz CNB. Women and ischemic heart disease: evolving knowledge. *J Am Coll Cardiol.* 2009;54(17):1561–1575.
10. Lee TH, Cook EF, Weisberg M, Sargent RK, Wilson C, Goldman L. Acute chest pain in the emergency room: identification and examination of low-risk patients. *Arch Intern Med.* 1985;145(1):65–69.
11. Chung W-Y, Sohn D-W, Kim Y-J, et al. Absence of postprandial surge in coronary blood flow distal to significant stenosis: a possible mechanism of postprandial angina. *J Am Coll Cardiol.* 2002;40(11):1976–1983.
12. Henrikson CA, Howell EE, Bush DE, et al. Chest pain relief by nitroglycerin does not predict active coronary artery disease. *Ann Intern Med.* 2003;139(12):979–986.
13. Tomai F. Warm up phenomenon and preconditioning in clinical practice. *Heart.* 2002;87(2):99–100.
14. Marzilli M, Merz CNB, Boden WE, et al. Obstructive coronary atherosclerosis and ischemic heart disease: an elusive link. *J Am Coll Cardiol.* 2012;60(11):951–956.
15. Pepine CJ, Douglas PS. Rethinking stable ischemic heart disease: is this the beginning of a new era? *J Am Coll Cardiol.* 2012;60(11):957–959.
16. Valeriani M, Sestito A, Le Pera D, et al. Abnormal cortical pain processing in patients with cardiac syndrome X. *Eur Heart J.* 2005;26(10):975–982.
17. Conti CR, Bavry AA, Petersen JW. Silent ischemia: clinical relevance. *J Am Coll Cardiol.* 2012;59(5):435–441.
18. Schoenenberger AW, Kobza R, Jamshidi P, et al. Sudden cardiac death in patients with silent myocardial ischemia after myocardial infarction (from the Swiss Interventional Study on Silent Ischemia Type II [SWISSI II]). *Am J Cardiol.* 2009;104(2):158–163.
19. Goldman L, Hashimoto B, Cook E, Loscalzo A. Comparative reproducibility and validity of systems for assessing cardiovascular functional class: advantages of a new specific activity scale. *Circulation.* 1981;64(6): 1227–1234.

20. Benjamin I, Griggs RC, Wing EJ, Fitz JG. *Andreoli and Carpenter's Cecil Essentials of Medicine*. Philadelphia: Elsevier Health Sciences; 2015.

21. Montalescot G, Sechtem U, Achenbach S, et al. 2013 ESC guidelines on the management of stable coronary artery disease. *Eur Heart J*. 2013;34(38):2949–3003.

22. Mann DL, Zipes DP, Libby P, Bonow RO. *Braunwald's Heart Disease: A Textbook of Cardiovascular Medicine*. Philadelphia: Elsevier Health Sciences; 2014.

23. Kones R, Rumana U. Stable ischemic heart disease. *Heart Fail Clin*. 2016;12(1):11–29.

24. Knuuti J, Wijns W, Saraste A, et al. 2019 ESC Guidelines for the diagnosis and management of chronic coronary syndromes. *Eur Heart J*. 2020;41:407–477.

25. Daly CA, De Stavola B, Sendon JLL, et al. Predicting prognosis in stable angina—results from the Euro heart survey of stable angina: prospective observational study. *BMJ*. 2006;332(7536):262–267.

26. Daly C, Norrie J, Murdoch D, Ford I, Dargie H, Fox K. The value of routine non-invasive tests to predict clinical outcome in stable angina. *Eur Heart J*. 2003;24(6): 532–540.

27. Hammermeister K, DeRouen T, Dodge H. Variables predictive of survival in patients with coronary disease. Selection by univariate and multivariate analyses from the clinical, electrocardiographic, exercise, arteriographic, and quantitative angiographic evaluations. *Circulation*. 1979;59(3):421–430.

28. Madjid M, Fatemi O. Components of the complete blood count as risk predictors for coronary heart disease. *Tex Heart Inst J*. 2013;40(1):17–29.

29. Hosseini SK, Alemzadeh-Ansar MJ, Tokaldany ML, Sharafi A, Kazazi EH, Poorhosseini H. Association between preprocedural hemoglobin level and 1-year outcome of elective percutaneous coronary intervention. *J Cardiovasc Med*. 2014;15(4):331–335.

30. Yaghoubi A, Golmohamadi Z, Alizadehasl A, Azarfarin R. Role of platelet parameters and haematological indices in myocardial infarction and unstable angina. *J Pak Med Assoc*. 2013;63(9):1133–1137.

31. Buckley DI, Fu R, Freeman M, Rogers K, Helfand M. C-reactive protein as a risk factor for coronary heart disease: a systematic review and meta-analyses for the US Preventive Services Task Force. *Ann Intern Med*. 2009;151(7):483–495.

32. Greenland P, Lloyd-Jones D. Defining a rational approach to screening for cardiovascular risk in asymptomatic patients. *J Am Coll Cardiol*. 2008;52(5):330–332.

33. Genest J, McPherson R, Frohlich J, et al. 2009 Canadian Cardiovascular Society/Canadian guidelines for the diagnosis and treatment of dyslipidemia and prevention of cardiovascular disease in the adult—2009 recommendations. *Can J Cardiol*. 2009;25(10):567–579.

34. Omland T, de Lemos JA, Sabatine MS, et al. A sensitive cardiac troponin T assay in stable coronary artery disease. *N Engl J Med*. 2009;361(26):2538–2547.

35. Ndrepepa G, Braun S, Mehilli J, et al. Prognostic value of sensitive troponin T in patients with stable and unstable angina and undetectable conventional troponin. *Am Heart J*. 2011;161(1):68–75.

36. Everett BM, Brooks MM, Vlachos HE, Chaitman BR, Frye RL, Bhatt DL. Troponin and cardiac events in stable ischemic heart disease and diabetes. *N Engl J Med*. 2015;373(7):610–620.

37. de Lemos JA, Morrow DA. Highly sensitive troponin assays and the cardiology community: a love/hate relationship? *Clin Chem*. 2011;57(6):826–829.

38. Pryor DB, Shaw L, Harrell FE, et al. Estimating the likelihood of severe coronary artery disease. *Am J Med*. 1991;90(5):553–562.

39. Morrow DA. Cardiovascular risk prediction in patients with stable and unstable coronary heart disease. *Circulation*. 2010;121(24):2681–2691.

40. Ohman EM. Chronic stable angina. *N Engl J Med*. 2016;2016(374):1167–1176.

41. Zacharias K, Ahmed A, Shah BN, et al. Relative clinical and economic impact of exercise echocardiography vs. exercise electrocardiography, as first line investigation in patients without known coronary artery disease and new stable angina: a randomized prospective study. *Eur Heart J Cardiovasc Imaging*. 2017;18:195–202.

42. Mieres JH, Gulati M, Merz NB, et al. Role of noninvasive testing in the clinical evaluation of women with suspected ischemic heart disease: a consensus statement from the American Heart Association. *Circulation*. 2014;130(4):350–379.

43. The SCOT-HEART Investigators. CT coronary angiography in patients with suspected angina due to coronary heart disease (SCOT-HEART): an open-label, parallel-group, multicentre trial. *Lancet*. 2015;385(9985):2383–2391.

44. ESC. *CONSERVE: Direct Catheterization vs. Selective Catheterization Guided by Coronary CT Angiography in Patients with Stable Suspected CAD*; 2016. Available from https://www.escardio.org/The-ESC/Press-Office/Press-releases/the-conserve-trial-non-invasive-imaging-can-guide-more-selective-invasive-corona.

45. Levine GN, Bates ER, Blankenship JC, et al. 2011 ACCF/AHA/SCAI guideline for percutaneous coronary intervention: a report of the American College of Cardiology Foundation/American Heart Association Task Force on Practice Guidelines and the Society for Cardiovascular Angiography and Interventions. *J Am Coll Cardiol*. 2011;58(24):e44–e122.

46. Serruys PW, Onuma Y, Garg S, et al. Assessment of the SYNTAX score in the Syntax study. *EuroIntervention*. 2009;5(1):50–56.

47. Falk E, Wilensky RL. Prediction of coronary events by intravascular imaging. *JACC Cardiovasc Imaging*. 2012;5 (3s1):S38–S41.

48. Claessen BE, Maehara A, Fahy M, Xu K, Stone GW, Mintz GS. Plaque composition by intravascular ultrasound and distal embolization after percutaneous coronary intervention. *JACC Cardiovasc Imaging*. 2012;5(3s1): S111–S118.

49. Chan PH, Alegria-Barrero E, Di Mario C. Tools & techniques: intravascular ultrasound and optical coherence tomography. *EuroIntervention*. 2012;7 (11):1343–1349.

50. Puri R, Worthley MI, Nicholls SJ. Intravascular imaging of vulnerable coronary plaque: current and future concepts. *Nat Rev Cardiol.* 2011;8(3):131–139.

51. De Bruyne B, Pijls NH, Kalesan B, et al. Fractional flow reserve-guided PCI versus medical therapy in stable coronary disease. *N Engl J Med.* 2012;367(11):991–1001.

52. Pijls NH, Sels J-WE. Functional measurement of coronary stenosis. *J Am Coll Cardiol.* 2012;59(12):1045–1057.

53. Fihn SD, Blankenship JC, Alexander KP, et al. 2014 ACC/AHA/AATS/PCNA/SCAI/STS focused update of the guideline for the diagnosis and management of patients with stable ischemic heart disease: a report of the American College of Cardiology/American Heart Association Task Force on Practice Guidelines, and the American Association for Thoracic Surgery, Preventive Cardiovascular Nurses Association, Society for Cardiovascular Angiography and Interventions, and Society of Thoracic Surgeons. *J Am Coll Cardiol.* 2014;64 (18):1929–1949.

54. Husted SE, Ohman EM. Pharmacological and emerging therapies in the treatment of chronic angina. *Lancet.* 2015;386(9994):691–701.

55. Vidal-Petiot E, Ford I, Greenlaw N, et al. Cardiovascular event rates and mortality according to achieved systolic and diastolic blood pressure in patients with stable coronary artery disease: an international cohort study. *Lancet.* 2016;388(10056):2142–2152.

56. Alderman EL, Corley SD, Fisher LD, et al. Five-year angiographic follow-up of factors associated with progression of coronary artery disease in the Coronary Artery Surgery Study (CASS). *J Am Coll Cardiol.* 1993;22 (4):1141–1154.

57. Haffner SM. Coronary heart disease in patients with diabetes. *N Engl J Med.* 2000;342(14):1040–1042.

58. Yaghoubi A, Safaie N, Azarfarin R, Alizadehasl A, Samad E-G. Evaluation of cardiovascular diseases and their risk factors in hospitalized patients in East Azerbaijan province, northwest Iran: a review of 18323 cases. *J Tehran Heart Cent.* 2015;8(2):101–105.

59. Nathan DM, Cleary PA, Backlund JY, et al. Intensive diabetes treatment and cardiovascular disease in patients with type 1 diabetes. *N Engl J Med.* 2005;2005 (353):2643–2653.

60. Group AS, Gerstein HC, Miller ME, et al. Long-term effects of intensive glucose lowering on cardiovascular outcomes. *N Engl J Med.* 2011;2011(364):818–828.

61. Duckworth W, Abraira C, Moritz T, et al. Glucose control and vascular complications in veterans with type 2 diabetes. *N Engl J Med.* 2009;360(2):129–139.

62. Patel A, MacMahon S, Chalmers J, et al. Intensive blood glucose control and vascular outcomes in patients with type 2 diabetes. *N Engl J Med.* 2008;2008(358):2560–2572.

63. Holman RR, Paul SK, Bethel MA, Matthews DR, Neil HAW. 10-Year follow-up of intensive glucose control in type 2 diabetes. *N Engl J Med.* 2008;359(15):1577–1589.

64. Braith RW, Casey DP, Beck DT. Enhanced external counterpulsation for ischemic heart disease: a look behind the curtain. *Exerc Sport Sci Rev.* 2012;40(3):145–152.

65. Casey DP, Beck DT, Nichols WW, et al. Effects of enhanced external counterpulsation on arterial stiffness and myocardial oxygen demand in patients with chronic angina pectoris. *Am J Cardiol.* 2011;107(10):1466–1472.

66. Ahlbom M, Hagerman I, Ståhlberg M, et al. Increases in cardiac output and oxygen consumption during enhanced external counterpulsation. *Heart Lung Circ.* 2016;25(11):1133–1136.

67. Shah SA, Shapiro RJ, Mehta R, Snyder JA. Impact of enhanced external counterpulsation on Canadian cardiovascular society angina class in patients with chronic stable angina: a meta-analysis. *Pharmacotherapy.* 2010;30(7):639–645.

68. Szatkowski A, Ndubuka-Irobunda C, Oesterle SN, Burkhoff D. Transmyocardial laser revascularization. *Am J Cardiovasc Drugs.* 2002;2(4):255–266.

69. Salem M, Rotevatn S, Stavnes S, Brekke M, Vollset SE, Nordrehaug JE. Usefulness and safety of percutaneous myocardial laser revascularization for refractory angina pectoris. *Am J Cardiol.* 2004;93(9):1086–1091.

70. Taylor RS, De Vries J, Buchser E, DeJongste MJ. Spinal cord stimulation in the treatment of refractory angina: systematic review and meta-analysis of randomised controlled trials. *BMC Cardiovasc Disord.* 2009;9(1):1.

71. Eldabe S, Thomson S, Duarte R, et al. The effectiveness and cost-effectiveness of spinal cord stimulation for refractory angina (RASCAL study): a pilot randomized controlled trial. *Neuromodulation.* 2016;19(1):60–70.

72. Tsigaridas N, Naka K, Tsapogas P, Pelechas E, Damigos D. Spinal cord stimulation in refractory angina. A systematic review of randomized controlled trials. *Acta Cardiol.* 2015;70(2):233–243.

73. Andrell P, Yu W, Gersbach P, et al. Long-term effects of spinal cord stimulation on angina symptoms and quality of life in patients with refractory angina pectoris—results from the European Angina Registry Link Study (EARL). *Heart.* 2010;96(14):1132–1136.

74. Morice M-C, Serruys PW, Kappetein AP, et al. Outcomes in patients with de novo left main disease treated with either percutaneous coronary intervention using paclitaxel-eluting stents or coronary artery bypass graft treatment in the Synergy Between Percutaneous Coronary Intervention with TAXUS and Cardiac Surgery (SYNTAX) trial. *Circulation.* 2010;121(24):2645–2653.

75. Serruys PW, Morice M-C, Kappetein AP, et al. Percutaneous coronary intervention versus coronary-artery bypass grafting for severe coronary artery disease. *N Engl J Med.* 2009;360(10):961–972.

76. Chakravarty T, Buch MH, Naik H, et al. Predictive accuracy of SYNTAX score for predicting long-term outcomes of unprotected left main coronary artery revascularization. *Am J Cardiol.* 2011;107(3):360–366.

77. Shahian DM, O'Brien SM, Normand S-LT, Peterson ED, Edwards FH. Association of hospital coronary artery bypass volume with processes of care, mortality, morbidity, and the Society of Thoracic Surgeons composite quality score. *J Thorac Cardiovasc Surg.* 2010;139(2):273–282.

78. Head SJ, Kieser TM, Falk V, Huysmans HA, Kappetein AP. Coronary artery bypass grafting: part 1—the evolution over the first 50 years. *Eur Heart J.* 2013;34(37):2862–2872.

79. Piccolo R, Giustino G, Mehran R, Windecker S. Stable coronary artery disease: revascularisation and invasive strategies. *Lancet.* 2015;386(9994):702–713.

80. Yusuf S, Zucker D, Passamani E, et al. Effect of coronary artery bypass graft surgery on survival: overview of 10-year results from randomised trials by the Coronary Artery Bypass Graft Surgery Trialists Collaboration. *Lancet.* 1994;344(8922):563–570.

81. Hueb W, Lopes N, Gersh BJ, et al. Ten-year follow-up survival of the Medicine, Angioplasty, or Surgery Study (MASS II): a randomized controlled clinical trial of 3 therapeutic strategies for multivessel coronary artery disease. *Circulation.* 2010;122(10):949–957.

82. Trikalinos TA, Siebert U, Lau J. Decision-analytic modeling to evaluate benefits and harms of medical tests: uses and limitations. *Med Decis Making.* 2009;29:E22–E29.

83. Boden WE, O'Rourke RA, Teo KK, et al. Optimal medical therapy with or without PCI for stable coronary disease. *N Engl J Med.* 2007;356(15):1503–1516.

84. Sedlis SP, Hartigan PM, Teo KK, et al. Effect of PCI on long-term survival in patients with stable ischemic heart disease. *N Engl J Med.* 2015;373(20):1937–1946.

85. Gada H, Kirtane AJ, Kereiakes DJ, et al. Meta-analysis of trials on mortality after percutaneous coronary intervention compared with medical therapy in patients with stable coronary heart disease and objective evidence of myocardial ischemia. *Am J Cardiol.* 2015;115 (9):1194–1199.

86. Windecker S, Stortecky S, Stefanini GG, et al. Revascularisation versus medical treatment in patients with stable coronary artery disease: network meta-analysis. *BMJ.* 2014;348:g3859.

87. Piccolo R, Stefanini GG, Franzone A, et al. Safety and efficacy of resolute zotarolimus-eluting stents compared with everolimus-eluting stents: a meta-analysis. *Circ Cardiovasc Interv.* 2015;8(4), e002223.

88. Kedhi E, Joesoef KS, McFadden E, et al. Second-generation everolimus-eluting and paclitaxel-eluting stents in real-life practice (COMPARE): a randomised trial. *Lancet.* 2010;375 (9710):201–209.

89. Stefanini GG, Baber U, Windecker S, et al. Safety and efficacy of drug-eluting stents in women: a patient-level pooled analysis of randomised trials. *Lancet.* 2013;382 (9908):1879–1888.

90. Windecker S, Kolh P, Alfonso F, et al. 2014 ESC/EACTS Guidelines on myocardial revascularization. *Eur Heart J.* 2014;35:2541–2619.

91. Kappetein AP, Feldman TE, Mack MJ, et al. Comparison of coronary bypass surgery with drug-eluting stenting for the treatment of left main and/or three-vessel disease: 3-year follow-up of the SYNTAX trial. *Eur Heart J.* 2011;32 (17):2125–2134.

92. Milojevic M, Head SJ, Parasca CA, et al. Causes of death following PCI versus CABG in complex CAD: 5-year follow-up of SYNTAX. *J Am Coll Cardiol.* 2016;67(1):42–55.

93. Bangalore S, Guo Y, Samadashvili Z, Blecker S, Xu J, Hannan EL. Everolimus-eluting stents or bypass surgery for multivessel coronary disease. *N Engl J Med.* 2015;372(13):1213–1222.

94. Chieffo A, Park SJ, Valgimigli M, et al. Favorable long-term outcome after drug-eluting stent implantation in nonbifurcation lesions that involve unprotected left main coronary artery a multicenter registry. *Circulation.* 2007;116(2):158–162.

95. Cavalcante R, Sotomi Y, Lee CW, et al. Outcomes after percutaneous coronary intervention or bypass surgery in patients with unprotected left main disease. *J Am Coll Cardiol.* 2016;68(10):999–1009.

96. Kushner FG, Hand M, Smith SC, et al. 2009 focused updates: ACC/AHA guidelines for the management of patients with ST-elevation myocardial infarction (updating the 2004 guideline and 2007 focused update) and ACC/AHA/SCAI guidelines on percutaneous coronary intervention (updating the 2005 guideline and 2007 focused update): a report of the American College of Cardiology Foundation/American Heart Association Task Force on Practice Guidelines. *J Am Coll Cardiol.* 2009;54(23):2205–2241.

97. Weintraub WS, Jones EL, Morris DC, King SB, Guyton RA, Craver JM. Outcome of reoperative coronary bypass surgery versus coronary angioplasty after previous bypass surgery. *Circulation.* 1997;95(4):868–877.

98. Brener SJ, Lytle BW, Casserly IP, Ellis SG, Topol EJ, Lauer MS. Predictors of revascularization method and long-term outcome of percutaneous coronary intervention or repeat coronary bypass surgery in patients with multivessel coronary disease and previous coronary bypass surgery. *Eur Heart J.* 2006;27(4):413–418.

99. Stephan WJ, O'Keefe JH, Piehler JM, et al. Coronary angioplasty versus repeat coronary artery bypass grafting for patients with previous bypass surgery. *J Am Coll Cardiol.* 1996;28(5):1140–1146.

100. Subramanian S, Sabik JF, Houghtaling PL, Nowicki ER, Blackstone EH, Lytle BW. Decision-making for patients with patent left internal thoracic artery grafts to left anterior descending. *Ann Thorac Surg.* 2009;87 (5):1392–1400.

101. Scarsini R, Zivelonghi C, Pesarini G, Vassanelli C, Ribichini FL. Repeat revascularization: percutaneous coronary intervention after coronary artery bypass graft surgery. *Cardiovasc Revasc Med.* 2016;17(4):272–278.

102. Swaminathan RV, Feldman DN, Pashun RA, et al. Gender differences in in-hospital outcomes after coronary artery bypass grafting. *Am J Cardiol.* 2016;118(3):362–368.

103. Jacobs AK, Johnston JM, Haviland A, et al. Improved outcomes for women undergoing contemporary percutaneous coronary intervention: a report from the National Heart, Lung, and Blood Institute Dynamic registry. *J Am Coll Cardiol.* 2002;39(10):1608–1614.

104. Holubkov R, Laskey WK, Haviland A, et al. Angina 1 year after percutaneous coronary intervention: a report from the NHLBI Dynamic Registry. *Am Heart J.* 2002;144 (5):826–833.

105. Vaccarino V, Abramson JL, Veledar E, Weintraub WS. Sex differences in hospital mortality after coronary artery bypass surgery evidence for a higher mortality in younger women. *Circulation.* 2002;105(10):1176–1181.

106. Epps KC, Holper EM, Selzer F, et al. Sex differences in outcomes following percutaneous coronary intervention according to age. *Circ Cardiovasc Qual Outcomes.* 2016;9(2 suppl 1):S16–S25.

107. Saxena A, Dinh D, Smith JA, Shardey G, Reid CM, Newcomb AE. Sex differences in outcomes following isolated coronary artery bypass graft surgery in Australian patients: analysis of the Australasian Society of Cardiac and Thoracic Surgeons cardiac surgery database. *Eur J Cardiothorac Surg.* 2012;41(4):755–762.

108. Hakim S, Alizadehasl A, Azarfarin R, Samadikhah J. The influence of gender on outcome in patients with first acute myocardial infarction. *Iran Heart J.* 2007;8(1):30–32.

109. Hillis LD, Smith PK, Anderson JL, et al. 2011 ACCF/AHA guideline for coronary artery bypass graft surgery: a report of the American College of Cardiology Foundation/American Heart Association task force on practice guidelines developed in collaboration with the American Association for Thoracic Surgery, Society of Cardiovascular Anesthesiologists, and Society of Thoracic Surgeons. *J Am Coll Cardiol.* 2011;58(24):e123–e210.

110. Kaneko H, Yajima J, Oikawa Y, et al. Impact of aging on the clinical outcomes of Japanese patients with coronary artery disease after percutaneous coronary intervention. *Heart Vessels.* 2014;29(2):156–164.

111. Afilalo J, Mottillo S, Eisenberg MJ, et al. Addition of frailty and disability to cardiac surgery risk scores identifies elderly patients at high risk of mortality or major morbidity. *Circ Cardiovasc Qual Outcomes.* 2012;5(2):222–228.

112. Dai X, Busby-Whitehead J, Forman DE, Alexander KP. Stable ischemic heart disease in the older adults. *J Geriatr Cardiol.* 2016;13(2):109–114.

113. Pfisterer M, Trial of Invasive versus Medical therapy in Elderly patients Investigators. Long-term outcome in elderly patients with chronic angina managed invasively versus by optimized medical therapy: four-year follow-up of the randomized Trial of Invasive versus Medical Therapy in Elderly patients (TIME). *Circulation.* 2004;110(10):1213–1218.

114. Maron DJ, Spertus JA, Mancini GJ, et al. Impact of an initial strategy of medical therapy without percutaneous coronary intervention in high-risk patients from the Clinical Outcomes Utilizing Revascularization and Aggressive DruG Evaluation (COURAGE) trial. *Am J Cardiol.* 2009;104(8):1055–1062.

115. Pfisterer M, Buser P, Osswald S, et al. Outcome of elderly patients with chronic symptomatic coronary artery disease with an invasive vs optimized medical treatment strategy: one-year results of the randomized TIME trial. *JAMA.* 2003;289(9):1117–1123.

116. Tao T, Wang H, Wang S-X, Guo Y-T, Zhu P, Wang Y-T. Long-term outcomes of high-risk elderly male patients with multivessel coronary disease: optimal medical therapy versus revascularization. *J Geriatr Cardiol.* 2016;13(2):152.

117. Lee SH, Yang JH, Choi S-H, et al. Long-term clinical outcomes of medical therapy for coronary chronic total occlusions in elderly patients (≥75 years). *Circ J.* 2015;79(8):1780–1786.

118. Wang TY, Gutierrez A, Peterson ED. Percutaneous coronary intervention in the elderly. *Nat Rev Cardiol.* 2011;8(2):79–90.

119. Farkouh ME, Domanski M, Sleeper LA, et al. Strategies for multivessel revascularization in patients with diabetes. *N Engl J Med.* 2012;367(25):2375–2384.

120. Verma S, Farkouh ME, Yanagawa B, et al. Comparison of coronary artery bypass surgery and percutaneous coronary intervention in patients with diabetes: a meta-analysis of randomised controlled trials. *Lancet Diabetes Endocrinol.* 2013;1(4):317–328.

121. Kurlansky P, Herbert M, Prince S, Mack MJ. Improved long-term survival for diabetic patients with surgical versus interventional revascularization. *Ann Thorac Surg.* 2015;99(4):1298–1305.

122. Roffi M, Angiolillo DJ, Kappetein AP. Current concepts on coronary revascularization in diabetic patients. *Eur Heart J.* 2011;32(22):2748–2757.

123. Hlatky MA, Boothroyd DB, Bravata DM, et al. Coronary artery bypass surgery compared with percutaneous coronary interventions for multivessel disease: a collaborative analysis of individual patient data from ten randomised trials. *Lancet.* 2009;373(9670):1190–1197.

124. Hakeem A, Garg N, Bhatti S, Rajpurohit N, Ahmed Z, Uretsky BF. Effectiveness of percutaneous coronary intervention with drug-eluting stents compared with bypass surgery in diabetics with multivessel coronary disease: comprehensive systematic review and meta-analysis of randomized clinical data. *J Am Heart Assoc.* 2013;2(4), e000354.

125. Zheng H, Xue S, Lian F, Huang R-T, Hu Z-L, Wang Y-Y. Meta-analysis of clinical studies comparing coronary artery bypass grafting with percutaneous coronary intervention in patients with end-stage renal disease. *Eur J Cardiothorac Surg.* 2013;43(3):459–467.

126. Boulton BJ, Kilgo P, Guyton RA, et al. Impact of preoperative renal dysfunction in patients undergoing off-pump versus on-pump coronary artery bypass. *Ann Thorac Surg.* 2011;92(2):595–602.

127. Möckel M, Searle J, Baberg HT, et al. Revascularisation of patients with end-stage renal disease on chronic haemodialysis: bypass surgery versus PCI—analysis of routine statutory health insurance data. *Open Heart.* 2016;3(2), e000464.

128. Zimmer RJ, Lee MS. Transplant coronary artery disease. *JACC Cardiovasc Interv.* 2010;3:367–377.

129. Zamorano JL, Lancellotti P, Rodriguez Munoz D, et al. 2016 ESC Position Paper on cancer treatments and cardiovascular toxicity developed under the auspices of the ESC Committee for Practice Guidelines: The Task Force for cancer treatments and cardiovascular toxicity of the European Society of Cardiology (ESC). *Eur Heart J.* 2016;37:2768–2801.

130. Lee TH, Cook EF, Weisberg MC, Rouan GW, Brand DA, Goldman L. Impact of the availability of a prior electrocardiogram on the triage of the patient with acute chest pain. *J Gen Intern Med.* 1990;5(5):381–388.

131. O'Donnell D, Mancera M, Savory E, Christopher S, Schaffer J, Roumpf S. The availability of prior ECGs improves paramedic accuracy in recognizing ST-segment elevation myocardial infarction. *J Electrocardiol.* 2015;48(1):93–98.

132. Fesmire F, Percy R, Wears R. Diagnostic and prognostic importance of comparing the initial to the previous electrocardiogram in patients admitted for suspected acute myocardial infarction. *South Med J.* 1991;84 (7):841–846.

## FURTHER READING

Sharma K, Kohli P, Gulati M. An update on exercise stress testing. *Curr Probl Cardiol.* 2012;37(5):177–202.

Mieres JH, Shaw LJ, Arai A, et al. Role of noninvasive testing in the clinical evaluation of women with suspected coronary artery disease consensus statement from the Cardiac Imaging Committee, Council on Clinical Cardiology, and the Cardiovascular Imaging and Intervention Committee, Council on Cardiovascular Radiology and Intervention, American Heart Association. *Circulation.* 2005;111 (5):682–696.

Shaw LJ, Mieres JH, Hendel RH, et al. Comparative effectiveness of exercise electrocardiography with or without myocardial perfusion single photon emission computed tomography in women with suspected coronary artery disease results from the What Is the Optimal Method for Ischemia Evaluation in Women (WOMEN) trial. *Circulation.* 2011;124(11):1239–1249.

# CHAPTER 25

# Percutaneous Coronary Intervention

ATA FIROUZI

Rajaie Cardiovascular, Medical & Research Center, Tehran, Iran

Coronary artery disease (CAD) is one of the most common causes of death worldwide.[1] Fortunately, percutaneous coronary intervention (PCI) has revolutionized the management of CAD and has opened a new field for treatment.

The first coronary intervention was performed by Andreas Gruentzig in 1977.[1] Ever since, major improvements have been made in techniques and instruments. Some devices, such as drug-eluting stents (DESs), were magic bullets for the treatment of CAD and decreased coronary restenosis after PCI. However, some important problems remain, such as stent thrombosis and the need for revascularization, with these devices.

This chapter summarizes PCI for general cardiologists. First, an explanation of some general topics in coronary intervention is provided.

## PLAIN OLD BALLOON ANGIOPLASTY

Plain old balloon angioplasty (POBA) is balloon angioplasty without stenting. Angiographically successful POBA is defined as less than 50% stenosis at the side of balloon angioplasty with Thrombolysis In Myocardial Infarction (TIMI) III flow.[2] The most important problem with this procedure is elastic recoil.[3] POBA has caused about a 40% restenosis rate, which is unacceptably high. In addition, in a high percentage of these patients, balloon-induced dissection is a big problem that can cause abrupt closure, which is a nightmare for interventionists.[3]

## BARE METAL STENTS

The first instrument that interventionists used for a perfect result after angioplasty with POBA was bare metal stents (BMSs). The device was initially used as walled off, for dissection flaps after POBA, and for elimination of elastic recoil afterward.

A successful result after BMS means less than 20% stenosis at the site of stent deployment, with TIMI III flow. However, the Achilles heel of this procedure is restenosis, which is as high as 20%–30%.[4] The main cause of restenosis is endothelial hyperplasia at the site of stenting.[3]

## DRUG-ELUTING STENTS

As stated earlier, endothelial hyperplasia was the main cause of restenosis after angioplasty with BMS.[3] For resolving this issue, another class of stents called DESs was invented in which cytotoxic or cytostatic drugs were added to BMSs for decreasing endothelial proliferation. As a result, stent restenosis was decreased to 10%–15%. DES has three components: the stent, polymer, and active drug.[4]

The most important problem associated with DESs is stent thrombosis. Active drug with cytotoxic or cytostatic effect causes delayed endothelialization of the stent. Instead of 1 month for BMS dual antiplatelet therapy, it should be expanded to 1 year (based on the guidelines).[4] Because of discontinuation of dual antiplatelets, incomplete endothelialization of the stent is the main cause of stent thrombosis.[5]

New devices such as bioabsorbable polymer stents and totally absorbable stents such as the bioresorbable vascular scaffold system are available to decrease the rate of stent thrombosis.

## STENT THROMBOSIS

When PCI was first used, restenosis was the most important problem. But with DES, there was a dramatic decrease in stent restenosis. However, the active drug component of DESs decreases the speed of stent endothelialization, which in turn creates thrombosis, which is a catastrophic complication of PCI.[4]

Several studies have shown that the incidence of stent thrombosis is about 0.5%–2%, but it is worth noting that the mortality rate of stent thrombosis is about 45%.[5] The incidence of stent thrombosis is not high, but unfortunately, if it occurs, it is catastrophic.

The most famous definition of stent thrombosis is offered by the Academic Research Consortium and includes:

- **Definite stent thrombosis:** acute coronary syndrome (ACS) and pathologic or angiographic evidence of thrombosis
- **Probable stent thrombosis:** death within 30 days after PCI or target vessel myocardial infarction (MI) without angiographic confirmation
- **Possible stent thrombosis:** unexplained death 30 days after PCI

The timing of stent thrombosis is important, and it can be defined as *acute* (in the first 24 h after PCI), *subacute* (within 24 h to 30 days of PCI), and *late* (30 days to 1 year). Additionally, very late stent thrombosis can happen 1 year after PCI.[6]

There are several risk factors for stent thrombosis, which are provided in Box 25.1.

---

### BOX 25.1
### Variables Associated With Stent Thrombosis

Clinical variables
- Acute myocardial infarction
- Clopidogrel noncompliance and discontinuation
- Clopidogrel bioavailability
- Diabetes
- Renal failure
- Congestive heart failure
- Previous brachytherapy
  Anatomic variables
- Long lesions
- Smaller vessels
- Multivessel disease
- Acute myocardial infarction
- Bifurcation lesions
  Procedural factors
- Stent underexpansion
- Incomplete wall apposition
- Residual inflow and outflow disease
- Margin dissections
- Crush technique
- Overlapping stent
- Polymer materials

From Mauri L, Bhatt DL. Percutaneous coronary intervention. In: Mann DL, Zipes DP, Libby P, et al., eds. *Braunwald's Heart Disease: A Textbook of Cardiovascular Medicine.* 10th ed. Philadelphia: Saunders; 2015:1258, with permission.

---

## CHRONIC STABLE ANGINA

There are important debates about coronary intervention in patients with chronic stable angina. As per guidelines, medical management and risk factor modification are the main goals of treatment.[7]

It is very important to have realistic expectations from any sort of treatment. Although PCI is widely used for patients with chronic stable angina, almost all of the studies available on intervention in chronic stable angina, such as the COURAGE trial, indicate that PCI is not superior to optimal medical treatment (OMT) in decreasing the rate of MI or death in these patients, but PCI improves functional class in patients with chronic stable angina.[8]

A few studies such as FAME11 have shown that fractional flow reserve (FFR)-guided PCI in chronic stable angina may be helpful for improving survival, but most studies such as the COURAGE trial proved that intervention in chronic stable angina should be done only in patients with functional classes poorer than class II despite OMT.[9]

The Ischemia Trial that compared invasive vs conservative strategy in patients with stable angina showed medical treatment and doing revascularization if medical treatment fails has the same clinical outcomes in comparison with doing PCI or CABG in these patients. However, the quality of life and angina relief will be better in the invasive group.[10]

## PERCUTANEOUS CORONARY INTERVENTION IN LEFT MAIN CORONARY ARTERY LESIONS

About 5%–7% of patients who underwent angiography have unprotected left main coronary artery (LMCA) lesions. When considering LMCA intervention, a good approach is to define LMCA involvement to the ostium, midportion, or distal part. If LMCA involvement is limited to the ostial or midportion of the LMCA without involvement of the distal part (left anterior descending coronary artery–left circumflex bifurcation), the PCI result will be excellent.[11] However, with involvement of the distal LMCA, PCI is more complex with a poorer long-term result. The most important studies that exist with respect to unprotected LMCA stenting are SYNTAX and PRECOMBAT, which compared coronary artery bypass graft (CABG) surgery with PCI. In PRECOMBAT, patients were followed up for at least 2 years, and the results showed that PCI and CABG are comparable with respect to death, MI, and stroke rates.[12] However, the revascularization rate was lower in the CABG arm. Furthermore, SYNTAX showed that in 3 years of follow-up, the MI and death rates in PCI were not lower than in CABG. However, the rate of revascularization was higher in the PCI group. Based on the SYNTAX and PRECOM-BAT trials, it is obvious that PCI in LMCA lesions can be a valid option, especially in patients with low-to-intermediate SYNTAX scores.[11–15]

## MULTIVESSEL DISEASE

In recent years, PCI for multivessel disease has increased dramatically, and the rate of CABG has decreased. Despite advances in PCI (techniques and instruments) until now, CABG has been the preferred treatment for patients with multivessel disease. One of the most prominent studies that we have about PCI or CABG in multivessel diseases is SYNTAX.

In a comparison between PCI and CABG for multives-sel disease, SYNTAX showed that the MI, death, and revas-cularization rates in CABG were lower than in PCI. However, in 3 years of follow-up in patients with low and intermediate SYNTAX scores, multivessel PCI and CABG outcomes were similar with regard to MI and death; however, the need for revascularization in PCI patients was higher. When we review large RCTs like SYNTAX BEST and FREEDOM trials, it seems that CABG remains the best revascularization method in patients with multivessel dis-eases specially in SYNTAX score >22.[11,16,17]

## PATIENTS WITH DIABETES MELLITUS

The prevalence of diabetes in patients with multivessel diseases is high. Subgroup analysis of patients with dia-betes in the SYNTAX study showed that PCI, regardless of MI and death, is comparable with CABG in 1 and 3 years of follow-up. However, the rate of revasculariza-tion was three times higher in the PCI group.[11]

Another important study that assessed PCI vs CABG in patients with diabetes was FREEDOM, in which patients were followed up for at least 2 years. The study showed that the outcome of CABG was better than PCI with regard to the MI and death rates, although the rate of stroke in the CABG group was higher.[18] Based on these studies, it can be concluded that PCI is a feasible way for treating patients with diabetes mellitus, but CABG is the preferred approach if there is a lower prob-ability of need for revascularization.[18–20]

## PERCUTANEOUS CORONARY INTERVENTION IN ACUTE CORONARY SYNDROME

About 29%–47% of patients admitted to hospitals with ACS have ST-segment elevation myocardial infarction

(STEMI). Based on different studies, if the door-to-balloon time is less than 90 min, primary PCI is the treatment of choice for reperfusion in STEMI. We know that if PCI is carried out with a delay of more than 120 min, the advantages of primary PCI will disappear. Thus, it is recommended that patients with STEMI be referred for primary PCI if delay will not be more than 120 min. It is important to know that the TRANSFER study showed that early PCI after fibrinolysis is helpful in decreasing MI and death without an increase in major bleeding at 1-year follow-up. American College of Cardiology/American Heart Association (ACC/AHA) guidelines recommend PCI within 3–24 h after fibrinolysis.[21,22]

In patients with ACS NSTEMI with a high-risk state, such as refractory angina, severe left ventricular systolic dysfunction, life-threatening arrhythmia, or unstable hemodynamics, urgent catheterization should be done in less than 2 h. For patients with GRACE (Global Reg-istry of Acute Coronary Events) scores greater than 140, an invasive strategy within 24 h is recommended. How-ever, for patients with GRACE scores less than 108 (low-risk patients), ACC/AHA guidelines recommend a delayed invasive (ischemia-guided) strategy.[23–25]

The COMPLETE trial showed that doing stage PCI on nonculprit significant lesion during 45 days after pri-mary PCI was superior than culprit only in reduction of cardiovascular death and MI.[26]

## INTRAVASCULAR ULTRASONOGRAPHY

Intravascular ultrasonography (IVUS) is a valuable instrument that can be helpful in conventional angiog-raphy for diagnosis and treatment. IVUS is a tomo-graphic assessment of the coronary lumen that can analyze lumen area, plaque size, and plaque character-istics. It is very helpful for qualification of lesions, espe-cially in LMCA, and is a preferred way for diagnosis of transplant vasculopathy.[27,28]

Obviously, atherosclerosis is a diffuse process, and for assessment of the stenosis rate, the true lumen size of normal coronary arteries should be clear. However, with diffuse involvement of coronary arteries, conven-tional angiography is not accurate in determining the true lumen size. In these situations, IVUS can help in accurately measuring the true lumen size[27,29,30] (Figs. 25.1–25.7).

Therefore, IVUS is helpful for ostial lesions, diffuse lesions, bifurcation lesions, and eccentric lesions and is diagnostic in hidden lesions because of overlapping and foreshortening in conventional angiography. Other new intravascular imaging devices, such as optical

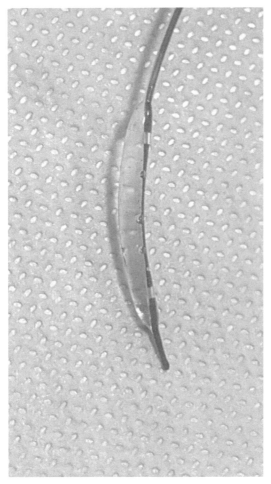

FIG. 25.1 Coronary balloon.

coherence tomography and Fourier-domain optical coherence tomography, can help in better evaluation of coronary arteries.[27]

## FRACTIONAL FLOW RESERVE

FFR is an instrument for measuring blood flow and pressure through a coronary artery. FFR is a guidewire-based device that can measure pressure drop along the coronary lesions after injection of adenosine. After adenosine injection, pressure distal to the coronary lesion is less than 75% or 80% when compared with guiding catheter pressure. It can be claimed that this lesion is significant, and scores above this threshold are not significant.[31,32]

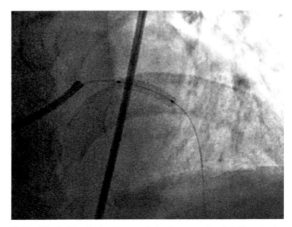

FIG. 25.3 Stent deployment in the proximal left anterior descending coronary artery.

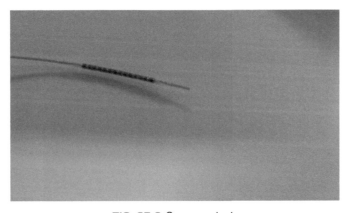

FIG. 25.2 Coronary stent.

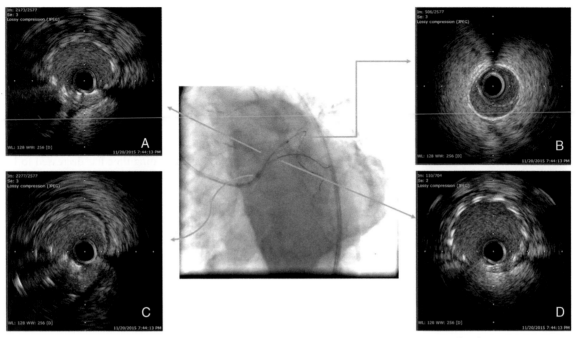

FIG. 25.4 Intravascular ultrasound image of the left anterior descending coronary artery (LAD) left main coronary artery (LMCA): (A) underdeployed stent, (B) LAD dissection, (C) unstented LMCA, and (D) stent lumen.

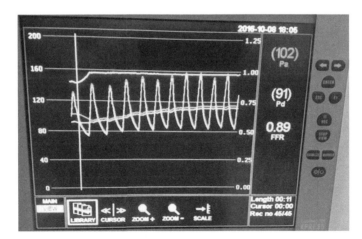

FIG. 25.5 Fractional flow reserve on the left anterior descending coronary artery.

## ROTABLATOR (ROTATIONAL ATHERECTOMY)

A rotablator is a diamond-tipped burr that is designed for ablation of plaque in coronary arteries and is always used for undilatable calcified lesions. It is important to know that this procedure is complex, and in patients who undergo this procedure, the risk of MI and other complications such as arrhythmia and distal coronary embolization is higher than with conventional angioplasty; thus, close observation and monitoring after the procedure are required.[32,33]

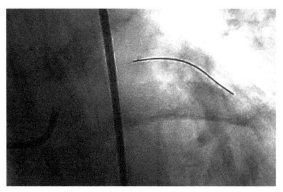

FIG. 25.6 Fractional flow reserve wire on the left anterior descending coronary artery.

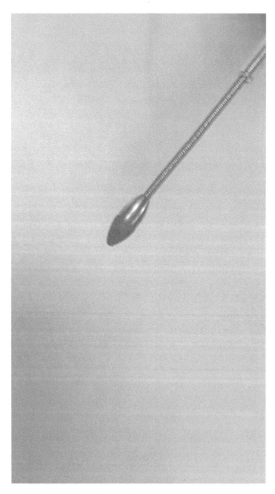

FIG. 25.7 Rotational atherectomy with a 1.75 burr.

## POSTINTERVENTION CARE

Coronary intervention is an invasive procedure on coronary arteries, and it is important to note that after PCI, patients are at risk for arrhythmia and infarction; thus, cardiac monitoring and bed rest are necessary. In addition, patients should be observed for chest pain, hemorrhage, and hematoma at the puncture site.

In the femoral approach, because high-dose anticoagulants are used, patients are transferred to the ward with side sheaths. These sheaths should be removed when the activating clotting time has decreased to less than 180. After sheath removal, patients should stay in bed for at least 1 h per sheath size.

In the radial approach, the operator removes the sheath in the catheterization laboratory, and local compression is mandatory for about 4 h.

## REFERENCES

1. Gruentzig AR. Transluminal dilatation of coronary artery stenosis. *Lancet.* 1978;1:263.
2. Serruys PW, de Jaegere P, Kiemeneij F, et al. A comparison of balloon-expandable-stent implantation with balloon angioplasty in patients with coronary artery disease. Benestent Study Group. *N Engl J Med.* 1994;331 (8):489–495.
3. Schwartz RS, Henry TD. Pathophysiology of coronary artery restenosis. *Rev Cardiovasc Med.* 2002;3(suppl. 5): S4–S9.
4. Malenka DJ, Kaplan AV, Lucas FL, Sharp SM, Skinner JS. Outcomes following coronary stenting in the era of bare-metal vs the era of drug eluting stents. *JAMA.* 2008;299:2868–2876.
5. Luscher TF, Steffel J, Eberli FR, et al. Drug-eluting stent and coronary thrombosis: biological mechanisms and clinical implications. *Circulation.* 2007;115(8):1051–1058.
6. Laskey WK, Yancy CW, Maisel WH. Thrombosis in coronary drug-eluting stents: report from the meeting of the Circulatory System Medical Devices Advisory Panel of the Food and Drug Administration Center for Devices and Radiologic Health, December 7–8, 2006. *Circulation.* 2007;115:2352–2357.
7. Gibbons RJ, Abrams J, Chatterjee K, et al. ACC/AHA 2002 guideline update for the management of patients with chronic stable angina—summary article: a report of the American College of Cardiology/American Heart Association Task Force on practice guidelines (Committee on the Management of Patients With Chronic Stable Angina). *J Am Coll Cardiol.* 2003;41: 159–168.
8. Teo KK, Sedlis SP, Boden WE, et al. Optimal medical therapy with or without percutaneous coronary intervention in older patients with stable coronary disease: a pre-specified subset analysis of the COURAGE

(Clinical Outcomes Utilizing Revascularization and Aggressive druG Evaluation) trial. *J Am Coll Cardiol.* 2009;54(14):1303–1308.

9. Pijls NH, Fearon WF, Tonino PA, et al. Fractional flow reserve versus angiography for guiding percutaneous coronary intervention in patients with multivessel coronary artery disease: 2-year follow-up of the FAME (Fractional Flow Reserve versus Angiography for Multivessel Evaluation) study. *J Am Coll Cardiol.* 2010;56:177–184.

10. Maron DJ, Hochman JS, O'Brien SM, et al. International Study of Comparative Health Effectiveness with Medical and Invasive Approaches (ISCHEMIA) trial: rationale and design. *Am Heart J.* 2018;201:124–135.

11. Sianos G, Morel MA, Kappetein AP, et al. The SYNTAX Score: an angiographic tool grading the complexity of coronary artery disease. *EuroIntervention.* 2005;1:219–227.

12. Ahn J-M, Roh J-H, Kim Y-H, et al. Randomized trial of stents versus bypass surgery for left main coronary artery disease 5-year outcomes of the PRECOMBAT study. *J Am Coll Cardiol.* 2015;65(20):2198–2206. (2015). https://doi.org/10.1016/j.jacc.2015.03.033.

13. Seung KB, Park DW, Kim YH, et al. Stents versus coronary-artery bypass grafting for left main coronary artery disease. *N Engl J Med.* 2008;358:1781–1792.

14. Meliga E, Garcia-Garcia HM, Valgimigli M, et al. Longest available clinical outcomes after drug-eluting stent implantation for unprotected left main coronary artery disease: the DELFT (Drug Eluting stent for LeFT main) Registry. *J Am Coll Cardiol.* 2008;51:2212–2219.

15. Park SJ, Kim YH, Park DW, et al. Randomized trial of stents versus bypass surgery for left main coronary artery disease. *N Engl J Med.* 2011;364:1718–1727.

16. Wijns W, Kolh P, Danchin N, et al. Guidelines on myocardial revascularization: the Task Force on Myocardial Revascularization of the European Society of Cardiology (ESC) and the European Association for Cardio-Thoracic Surgery (EACTS). *Eur Heart J.* 2010;31:2501–2555.

17. Mercado N, Wijns W, Serruys PW, et al. One-year outcomes of coronary artery bypass graft surgery versus percutaneous coronary intervention with multiple stenting for multisystem disease: a meta-analysis of individual patient data from randomized clinical trials. *J Thorac Cardiovasc Surg.* 2005;130:512–519.

18. Farkouh ME, Domanski M, Sleep LA, et al. Strategies for multivessel revascularization in patients with diabetes. *N Engl J Med.* 2012;367:2375–2384.

19. Hlatky MA. Compelling evidence for coronary-bypass surgery in patients with diabetes. *N Engl J Med.* 2012;367:2437–2478.

20. Farkouh ME, Dangas G, Leon MB, et al. Design of the Future REvascularization Evaluation in patients with Diabetes mellitus: optimal management of Multivessel disease (FREEDOM) Trial. *Am Heart J.* 2008;155:215–223.

21. O'Gara PT, Kushner FG, Ascheim DD, et al. 2013 ACCF/AHA guideline for the management of ST-elevation myocardial infarction: a report of the American College of Cardiology Foundation/American Heart Association Task Force on Practice Guidelines. *Circulation.* 2013;127(4):e362–e425.

22. Keeley EC, Boura JA, Grines CL. Primary angioplasty versus intravenous thrombolytic therapy for acute myocardial infarction: a quantitative review of 23 randomised trials. *Lancet.* 2003;361(9351):13–20.

23. Boden WE, O'Rourke RA, Crawford MH, et al. Outcomes in patients with acute non-Q-wave myocardial infarction randomly assigned to an invasive as compared with a conservative management strategy. Veterans Affairs Non-Q-Wave Infarction Strategies in Hospital (VANQWISH) Trial Investigators. *N Engl J Med.* 1998;338(25):1785–1789.

24. Mehta SR, Cannon CP, Fox KA, et al. Routine vs selective invasive strategies in patients with acute coronary syndromes: a collaborative meta-analysis of randomized trials. *JAMA.* 2005;293(23):2908–2917.

25. Mehta SR, Granger CB, Boden WE, et al. Early versus delayed invasive intervention in acute coronary syndromes. *N Engl J Med.* 2009;360(21):2165–2175.

26. Bainey KR, Mehta SR, Lai T, Welsh RC. Complete vs culprit-only revascularization for patients with multivessel disease undergoing primary percutaneous coronary intervention for ST-segment elevation myocardial infarction: a systematic review and meta-analysis. *Am Heart J.* 2014;167(1):1–14.

27. Gussenhoven EJ, Essed CE, Lancee CT, et al. Arterial wall characteristics determined by intravascular ultrasound imaging: an in vitro study. *J Am Coll Cardiol.* 1989;14:947–952.

28. Uretsky BF, Murali S, Reddy PS, et al. Development of coronary artery disease in cardiac transplant patients receiving immunosuppressive therapy with cyclosporine and prednisone. *Circulation.* 1987;76:827–834.

29. Hodgson JM, Graham SP, Savakus AD, et al. Clinical percutaneous imaging of coronary anatomy using an over-the-wire ultrasound catheter system. *Int J Card Imaging.* 1989;4:187–193.

30. Nissen SE, Grines CL, Gurley JC, et al. Application of a new phased-array ultrasound imaging catheter in the assessment of vascular dimensions: in vivo comparison to cineangiography. *Circulation.* 1990;81:660–666.

31. Fischer JJ, Samady H, McPherson JA, et al. Comparison between visual assessment and quantitative angiography versus fractional flow reserve for native coronary narrowings of moderate severity. *Am J Cardiol.* 2002;90(3):210–215.

32. Zimarino M, Corcos T, Favereau X, et al. Rotational coronary atherectomy with adjunctive balloon angioplasty for the treatment of ostial lesions. *Cathet Cardiovasc Diagn.* 1994;33(1):22–27.

33. Reifart N, Vandormael M, Krajcar M, et al. Randomized comparison of angioplasty of complex coronary lesions at a single center. Excimer Laser, Rotational Atherectomy, and Balloon Angioplasty Comparison (ERBAC) Study. *Circulation.* 1997;96(1):91–98.

# CHAPTER 26

# Transcatheter Therapies for Structural Heart Diseases

HAMIDREZA SANATI

Cardiovascular Intervention Research Center, Rajaei Cardiovascular Research and Medical Center, Iran University of Medical Sciences, Tehran, Iran

## KEY POINTS

- Percutaneous closure of patent foramen ovale might be a therapeutic option in some patients after transient ischemic attack or stroke if there is convincing evidence for its causal relationship after a thorough case study.
- Atrial and ventricular septal defects are amenable to percutaneous closure if they are hemodynamically significant and have suitable anatomy.
- Percutaneous closure of ventricular septal rupture following myocardial infarction (MI) might be tried, but the results are suboptimal in most patients, especially if performed in the early phase after MI.
- Left atrial appendage closure is an emerging technique for preventing stroke in patients with contraindications for anticoagulant therapy.
- Transcatheter closure of paravalvular leaks is a complex procedure requiring adequate preplanning using imaging modalities.
- Percutaneous balloon mitral valvuloplasty is a well-established treatment for rheumatic mitral stenosis with good early and long-term clinical results.
- Emerging techniques for mitral valve repair and replacement need future studies to be applied as a viable therapeutic option.
- Transcatheter aortic valve replacement is a class I recommendation in patients with severe aortic stenosis who are at high or prohibitive risk for surgery.

## INTERVENTION IN STRUCTURAL HEART DISORDERS

Although percutaneous interventions of structural heart diseases date back many years, the current advent of new procedures and devices has expanded this field. This chapter is a brief review on the structural heart lesions amenable to transcatheter therapy in adults.

## OCCLUSION OF CARDIAC DEFECTS

### Patent Foramen Ovale

The foramen ovale remains open in 15%–25% of individuals after birth and is traditionally not considered an important health problem. There is a paucity of data regarding the natural history of patent foramen ovale (PFO), but there are a few studies that have shown a reduced survival rate in some patients. PFO is not closed spontaneously with age; therefore, a possible explanation of this finding is the gradual elimination of individuals with PFO over time because of the related adverse events.[1] The prevalence of PFO is estimated to be 40%–60% in cryptogenic stroke (CS) patients younger than 55 years of age.[2] A weaker association is also evident in older patients.[3]

### Cryptogenic stroke

PFO might facilitate paradoxic embolism from the venous system and contribute to transient ischemic attack and stroke. Rarely, the defect itself is a source for thromboembolism, especially when associated with atrial septal aneurysm. Different regimens of medical therapies (antiplatelets and anticoagulants) have been investigated, but none of them was superior or even effective in the prevention of recurrent stroke in CS patients.[4]

### Patent foramen ovale closure

There are large quantities of data derived from nonrandomized single-center studies that have shown the superiority of transcatheter PFO closure over medical therapy in preventing recurrent events in patients with CS, but these studies have been criticized because of methodologic issues. Recently, new evidences from randomized controlled trials and meta-analyses have shown encouraging results that can change the older recommendations in the near future.[5,6] Until then, clinicians need to individualize the pros and cons of PFO closure based on the clinical scenario and anatomic considerations (Fig. 26.1). Apparently, PFO closure is much more likely to be efficient in certain subgroups of patients (Box 26.1). The Food and Drug Administration (FDA) has approved the Amplatzer PFO Occluder and the GORE CARDIOFORM Septal Occluder for PFO closure to reduce the risk of recurrent ischemic stroke in patients, predominantly between 18 and 60 years, who have had a CS due to a presumed paradoxical embolism.

### Other Possible Links

PFO might play a role in the pathophysiology of several other conditions. Of them, platypnea–orthodeoxia syndrome is highly associated with PFO, and PFO closure is its definitive therapy. Other conditions that might be related to PFO are decompression illness, migraine with aura, high-attitude pulmonary edema, and exacerbations of sleep apnea.

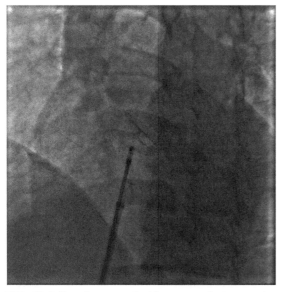

FIG. 26.1 Percutaneous patent foramen ovale closure using the Occlutech device.

---

BOX 26.1
**Cryptogenic Stroke Patients With a Higher Possibility of Therapeutic Yield After Patent Foramen Ovale Closure**

Recurrent events, especially if they occur despite medical therapy
   Recent (≤6 months) ischemic stroke
   Younger age (younger than 60 years of age)
   Large patent foramen ovale (≥2 mm)
   Large right-to-left shunt (>20 microbubbles)
   Unprovoked right-to-left shunt (resting bubble passage)
   The presence of aneurysmal or hypermobile interatrial septum
   Clinical or imaging evidence for deep vein thrombosis
   History of stroke after the activities associated with Valsalva maneuver or a period of immobility
   DW-MRI lesions compatible with cardioembolic events

*DW-MRI*, diffusion-weighted magnetic resonance imaging.

### Atrial Septal Defect

Percutaneous transcatheter atrial septal defect (ASD) closure is a reasonable alternative to surgical repair and is often preferred in patients with suitable anatomic characteristics (Fig. 26.2). When performed by an experienced operator, it is safe and effective with a high success rate and fewer complications compared with surgical closure.[7] A wide variety of devices have been introduced; three of them, the Amplatzer Septal Occluder, the GORE HELEX Septal Occluder (discontinued), and the GORE CARDIOFORM Septal Occluder, are currently FDA approved. Several other devices are currently in use with comparable procedural outcomes. The ostium secundum defect is particularly amenable to transcatheter closure when it is hemodynamically significant. Detection of the evidence of right ventricular volume overload might suffice, but in borderline cases, measurement of left-to-right shunt is useful. The defects with a pulmonary flow to systemic flow (Qp/Qs) ratio greater than 1.5:1.0 should be closed. Smaller defects might be considered for closure in patients with stroke to avoid paradoxic embolism.[8] In patients with pulmonary hypertension, closure might be still reasonable in case there is a net left-to-right shunt of at least 1.5:1.0 or if pulmonary vascular resistance does not exceed 8 Wood units on 100% oxygen.[8] For the procedure to be successful, the stretched diameter of the defect should not be more than 36 mm, and the rims toward the adjacent structures need to be sufficient (>5 mm) and firm. Nevertheless, a deficient or even absent aortic rim does

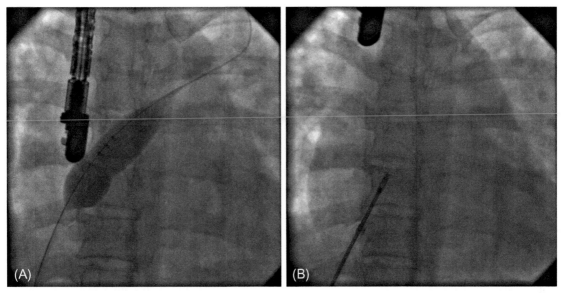

FIG. 26.2 Percutaneous atrial septal defect closure. (A) Balloon sizing for estimating the device size. (B) Device connected to the delivery cable before the releasing process.

not preclude a successful device deployment because the aorta provides a secure anchoring for the device. Primum or sinus venosus ASDs or those associated with abnormal drainage of pulmonary veins are traditionally being considered for surgery. Procedural complications are uncommon and include cardiac perforation, air embolism, device embolization, cardiac arrhythmias, device thrombosis, and late erosion. Late erosion is a rare but serious complication that happens mostly during the first year after device implantation and should be considered in every patient who presents with chest pain (often pleuritic) and pericardial or pleural effusion. It results from erosion of the aortic root or atrial roof by an oversized device, especially if the aortic rim is deficient. If it remains untreated, it causes cardiac perforation, hemothorax, and hemodynamic collapse. Upon diagnosis, the patient should be referred for emergent surgery.[9]

### Ventricular Septal Defect

A ventricular septal defect (VSD) that is indicated to be closed is not common in the adult period. Significant VSDs are often diagnosed in childhood and undergo surgical or percutaneous closure. The majority of cases that are appreciated in adults are very small and restrictive defects that do not need closure or very large nonrestrictive defects that have the Eisenmenger physiology.[10] Residual defects from previous surgical patch repair might be seen after childhood. Transcatheter closure is an alternative to surgery in high surgical risk patients and could be a good initial approach in

muscular VSDs. Perimembranous and residual defects might also be considered for transcatheter closure if the anatomy is suitable. The defect should be repaired in patients with symptoms or with the evidence of left ventricular volume overload. In those with pulmonary hypertension, closure is reasonable when there is a net left-to-right shunt (Qp/Qs) ratio >1.5 and pulmonary arterial pressure less than two-thirds of systemic pressure on baseline or after the vasodilator challenge.[8] Ventricular septal rupture (VSR) is a serious mechanical complication after myocardial infarction (MI) that needs particular attention. It should be closed urgently before the patient develops hemodynamic instability and biventricular failure. Transcatheter closure has been proposed for post-MI VSR, but the role is limited because of the high mortality rate and suboptimal results from the complex anatomy and frequently large size of the defects.

### Left Atrial Appendage Occlusion

Stroke is the third leading cause of death in developed countries and the number one reason for disability worldwide. A great proportion of cardioembolic strokes occur in patients with atrial fibrillation (AF), and AF-related strokes are associated with worse outcomes compared with non-AF-related strokes,[11] signifying the importance of effective preventive strategies. The left atrial appendage (LAA) is thought to be the source of thrombus and emboli in the majority of patients with AF who have a stroke.[12,13] The vitamin K antagonist, warfarin, is very effective and reduces the risk of stroke compared with aspirin and the combination of aspirin and clopidogrel and had long been considered the standard preventive regimen in these patients. Unfortunately, warfarin-related bleeding complications are common and sometimes serious, including intracranial hemorrhage. In addition, the lack of patient adherence is a common problem, and therapeutic levels cannot be appropriately maintained in many cases.

Non-vitamin K antagonist oral anticoagulants (NOACs [dabigatran, rivaroxaban, apixaban, and edoxaban]) have been recently proposed to overcome shortcomings of conventional anticoagulant therapy. They are currently considered the preferred anticoagulant agents in patients with nonvalvular AF who are at increased risk of embolic events because of their safety, efficacy, and ease of use. Nevertheless, there are still controversies about the risk of related major bleeding events (other than intracranial hemorrhage) compared with warfarin or antiplatelet agents.[14] Percutaneous LAA occlusion is now feasible and could be performed with a high success rate and a low rate of complications (Fig. 26.3). Mechanical occlusion of the LAA can theoretically reduce the risk of embolic events mitigating the adherent bleeding risks of oral anticoagulant agents. Several types of devices are now in use; of them, the Watchman device (Boston Scientific, Natick, MA) has been approved by the FDA. According to the latest guidelines, percutaneous LAA occlusion may be considered in patients with a high stroke risk and contraindications for long-term oral anticoagulation (class IIb).[15] Different categories of patients with nonvalvular AF in whom the candidacy for LAA occlusion might be evaluated are summarized in Box 26.2.[16] The role of LAA occlusion in the context of current safer NOAC therapy warrants further investigations in randomized trials and meta-analyses.

## Paravalvular Leak Closure

Paravalvular leak (PVL) results from incomplete sealing between the outer aspect of the prosthetic valve and native annular tissue which allows for regurgitation of blood, similar to valvular regurgitation. PVL occurs with both mechanical and biologic prostheses and is more common with prosthetic valves in the mitral than the aortic position. PVL occurs more frequently after transcatheter aortic valve replacement (TAVR) compared with surgical aortic valve replacement (SAVR). Fortunately, most PVLs are not significant after TAVR and do not need any specific intervention. Technical parameters, severe calcification of the annulus, native annular tissue friability, and infection are predisposing factors for the development of PVL.[4] The majority of PVLs are asymptomatic, but large defects can cause congestive heart failure, hemolysis, or both. Hemolysis may occur even with small PVLs because of the high-velocity jets through the defect, especially with mitral PVLs.[17]

Transcatheter intervention is a reasonable alternative to reoperation that is associated with high rates of

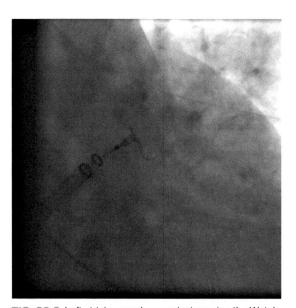

FIG. 26.3 Left atrial appendage occlusion using the Watchman device. The Watchman left atrial appendage occluder is delivered through a dedicated delivery system and sheath. Device sizing is the most crucial part in the procedure. The device is finally released after the confirmation of the appropriate position, stability, sealing, and size.

---

**BOX 26.2**
**Potential Candidates for Left Atrial Appendage Occlusion**

Nonvalvular AF patients at high risk for stroke (CHA2DS2-VASc $\geq$1 in men and $\geq$2 in women) if:

- Long-term contraindication to oral anticoagulants (history of significant bleeding without reversible cause)
- Bleeding risk is unexpectedly high (e.g., triple antiplatelet therapy, ESRD, labile INR)
- Recurrent embolic event despite adequate oral anticoagulation
- A patient wishes to discontinue an oral anticoagulant after AF ablation

*AF*, atrial fibrillation; *ESRD*, end-stage renal disease; *INR*, international ratio.

morbidity and mortality. It is less invasive and is associated with similar outcomes compared with surgical reoperation. With regard to recent advances, it is becoming the first-line approach in many centers. The indications for closure are congestive heart failure with a New York Heart Association functional class (NYHA FC) of II or greater despite optimal medical therapy and hemolytic anemia requiring multiple blood transfusions to maintain a hemoglobin level above 10 g/dL.[18] Percutaneous PVL intervention is a complex procedure and needs a high level of experience, adoption of different imaging modalities for preplanning and guiding the procedure, and availability of suitable devices. The American College of Cardiology/American Heart Association (ACC/AHA) guidelines for valvular heart disease give percutaneous PVL closure a level IIa recommendation when performed in experienced centers.

## MITRAL VALVE INTERVENTIONS
### Balloon Mitral Valvuloplasty
Mitral stenosis (MS) develops as a delayed sequela of rheumatic fever with adverse impact on the functional status and survival of the patients.[19] Balloon mitral valvuloplasty (BMV) improves symptoms and has a favorable impact on long-term survival of patients with MS.[20] Until now, different techniques and balloons have been introduced. Of them, retrograde balloon valvuloplasty via right femoral venous and transseptal access has

gained popularity. The Inoue balloon with its unique sequential distal to proximal dilation mode is well studied and is currently the most frequently used balloon (Fig. 26.4).[20] The balloon size is selected using a height-based formula or echocardiographic intercommissural diameter.[19,21] The procedure is relatively safe in experienced hands with final mitral valve areas (MVAs) comparable with surgical commissurotomy. Major complications are uncommon and include cardiac perforation, stroke, and severe mitral regurgitation (MR).

### Indications
Rheumatic MS with commissural fusion is the subject for BMV if it is severe (MVA $\leq 1.5$ cm$^2$) and symptomatic with favorable valve morphology in the absence of contraindications (class I).[22] BMV is reasonable in asymptomatic very severe MS with an MVA of 1 cm$^2$ or less (class IIa).[22] BMV in severe MS patients with new AF and in symptomatic patients with pulmonary hypertension and evidence of increased left atrial pressure but with an MVA of larger than 1.5 cm$^2$ is controversial (class IIb).[22] The morphologic characteristics of the mitral valve are best evaluated using echocardiographic Wilkins score, which predicts postprocedural results based on the degree of thickness, mobility, calcification, and subvalvular degeneration of the mitral valve.[23] BMV could have the best results when performed in patients with low Wilkins scores ($\leq 8$), without commissural

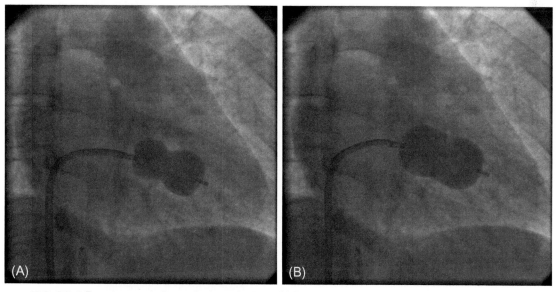

FIG. 26.4 Percutaneous balloon mitral valvuloplasty. (A) Sequential dilation of the distal and proximal parts of the balloon. (B) Final full balloon dilation.

calcification, and a history of previous commissurotomy. BMV is not successful in the absence of commissural fusion that is seen in the other causes of MS or in some patients with previous commissurotomy and is therefore generally prohibited. Left atrial and LAA thrombus, more than moderate mitral and aortic regurgitation, and fluoroscopic calcification of the mitral valve are contraindications for BMV.

## Percutaneous Mitral and Tricuspid Valve Repair and Replacement

There is a lot of experience with surgical mitral valve repair and replacement in patients with MR during recent decades. Despite low rates of morbidity and mortality with surgery, there is a subset of patients with high or prohibitive risk for surgery. Transcatheter mitral valve repair is an alternative treatment option in these patients, if they have symptomatic chronic significant MR (3 to 4+). Based on recent studies, selected patients with both primary (degenerative) and secondary (functional) MR can benefit from transcatheter mitral valve repair. Of the different and emerging transcatheter systems, the MitraClip and PASCAL system have been associated with acceptable results in the trials.[24,25] The latest European Society of Cardiology guidelines give percutaneous mitral valve repair (edge-to-edge procedure) a class IIb recommendation in some patients with chronic severe primary and secondary MR who remain symptomatic despite optimal medical therapy. Transcatheter mitral valve replacement is another emerging treatment option for selected patients. The development of percutaneous techniques for tricuspid regurgitation is still in the early phases, but there is growing evidence to support the application of these approaches, including edge-to-edge repair and annuloplasty.

The mitral and tricuspid valve-in-valve implantation is now feasible and seems to be a reasonable alternative in high-risk patients with degenerated bioprosthetic valves.[26]

## AORTA AND AORTIC VALVE INTERVENTIONS

### Balloon Aortic Valvuloplasty

After the advent of transcatheter aortic valve implantation (TAVI), the use of balloon aortic valvuloplasty (BAV) was again increased for predilation of severely stenotic aortic valves. Even recently, many TAVI cases are performed without predilation, and it is not a crucial part of the procedure in all cases. As a therapeutic procedure, its role is limited because of the suboptimal acute results, high rate of restenosis, and possible occurrence of life-threatening acute severe aortic regurgitation. BAV results in the fracture of calcific nodules of the aortic valve and opening

of fused commissures, which improves the valve area. However, restenosis is highly expected, and initial improvement often disappears after a 6-month period. As a result, its therapeutic use is limited to certain conditions in very high-risk or inoperable patients with severe calcific aortic stenosis (AS) (class IIb).[22] According to the results of BAV in noncalcific AS in children and adolescence, there may be a role for BAV in the treatment of young adult patients without significant valve calcification (Box 26.3).[27]

### Transcatheter Aortic Valve Implantation

AS is the most common degenerative heart valve disease in developed countries, affecting 2% of the population older than 65 years of age.[28] Congenital and rheumatic heart diseases are the other causes of AS. Symptomatic AS links with a poor prognosis and patients should be referred for SAVR. SAVR is now considered the preferred therapeutic strategy because it is associated with improved survival rates in patients who are not high risk for surgery. The management of patients with asymptomatic severe AS is more controversial, and the decision should be made based on careful interpretation of the results of echocardiography and exercise tolerance test. The younger patients with rheumatic and congenital AS, including bicuspid aortic valve, are traditionally being considered for SAVR, but a considerable percentage of older patients with senile AS ($\approx$30%) have significant comorbidities or contraindications for surgery and would not undergo SAVR.

TAVR was first introduced in 2002 as an alternative to SAVR.[29] It has gained rapidly rising popularity in recent years with ongoing advancements in techniques and devices. The Edwards Sapien (Edwards Lifesciences, Irvine, CA) and Medtronic CoreValve (Medtronic, Minneapolis, MN) valves are the dominant devices in the

---

**BOX 26.3**
**Possible Indications for Balloon Aortic Valvuloplasty in Patients With Symptomatic Severe Aortic Valve Stenosis**

Cardiogenic shock
Bridge to AVR or TAVI
Emergent high-risk noncardiac surgery
Poor candidates for AVR and TAVI
Predilation, sizing, and postdilation during the TAVI procedure
Congenital aortic stenosis (if symptomatic or the peak pressure gradient >50 mmHg)

*AVR*, aortic valve replacement; *TAVI*, transcatheter aortic valve implantation.

market, and their new generations (Sapien 3, CoreValve Evolut R and Evolut PRO) have become currently available (Fig. 26.5). Several new transcatheter aortic valves are currently in early clinical evaluation, including the DirectFlow, Boston Lotus, and St Jude Portico devices.[30] It is widely accepted that TAVR is superior over medical therapy in inoperable patients and is comparable to SAVR in high-risk patients. According to the ACC/AHA guidelines, TAVR is a class I recommendation in patients with severe symptomatic AS (stage D) who are at high or prohibitive surgical risk. Recent studies on intermediate-risk patients have shown promising results.[31]

In 2016 and 2017, the FDA approved an expanded indication for the Sapien XT, Sapien 3, and CoreValve series of TAVR systems for patients at intermediate risk for death and complications associated with SAVR. At present, TAVR is a class IIa recommendation in these patients. Apparently, further recommendations of TAVR for low-risk patients depend on the future availability of devices that abolish important concerns such as post-procedural conduction abnormalities and PVLs. Valve-in-valve procedure has gained popularity as a quite acceptable alternative in patients with failed aortic bioprosthetic valves. Surgical risk scores, including the Society of Thoracic Surgeons (STS) score, the Euroscore II, and the Logistic Euroscore, are used to stratify the patients who are candidates for SAVR. It should be noted that these risk prediction models might underestimate the surgical risk in high-risk patients, and they do not include some surgical risk factors such as frailty, poor mobility, obesity, severe liver disease, and history of chest wall radiation.[26] As a result, a heart team approach is highly recommended by the guidelines for patient selection based on the risk prediction models and individual basis.[32] A multidisciplinary imaging approach is needed for selecting anatomically appropriate patients and for preplanning and guiding the procedure. Currently, the retrograde transfemoral approach is the most popular method. Other approaches (transapical, transaortic, or subclavian) are usually reserved for patients with poor peripheral access.[33–35] The type of valve system (self-expanding and balloon expandable) probably does not have any impact on the mortality rate of the procedure, but the rate of some specific procedural complications may vary.[36]

Conduction disturbances caused by compression of the conduction system are more common with the CoreValve than with the Sapien (24%–33% vs 5%–12%).[37,38] Accordingly, the need for permanent pacing is more common with the CoreValve. PVLs are common and result from incomplete sealing between the device and the annulus caused by severe or asymmetrical calcification of the annulus, undersizing of the device, and the presence of a bicuspid aortic valve.[39] PVLs are mostly mild in severity and well tolerated (70%) and do not need any intervention. More severe PVLs are associated

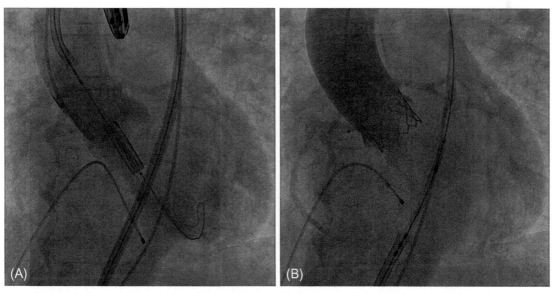

FIG. 26.5 Transcatheter aortic valve implantation. (A) Aortography for adjusting the Sapien 3 balloon-expandable valve on the annulus. (B) Implanted valve without significant paravalvular leak and patent coronary arteries.

with increased mortality rates and should be approached according to the cause.[40] Other complications include vascular injury, bleeding, valve thrombosis, and stroke.

### Coarctation of the Aorta

Coarctation of the aorta is seen in 0.04% of the population and accounts for 5% of all congenital heart defects.[41] It could be associated with a bicuspid aortic valve or even cerebral aneurysm in some patients. Therefore, meticulous attention should be paid to detecting the possible complications of these associated conditions beyond early childhood.[42] Adult patients with isolated discrete coarctation of the aorta often present with systemic hypertension. In addition, some patients have recurrent coarctation after the initial surgical or interventional treatment early in childhood. Coarctation of the aorta should be repaired in patients with a greater than 20-mmHg peak-to-peak gradient or in patients with a less than 20-mmHg peak-to-peak gradient but with significant angiographic evidence of a narrowing, especially when systemic hypertension is present. Primary stenting is the preferred therapeutic strategy in adult patients and is associated with good short- and medium-term outcomes even when it is performed in recurrent coarctation (Fig. 26.6). Balloon angioplasty and surgical repair are often reserved for small children and infants.

## PULMONARY VALVE INTERVENTION
### Pulmonary Valvuloplasty

The typical form of congenital pulmonary valve stenosis (PS) is usually sporadic and is characterized by a dome-shaped tricuspid pulmonary valve with commissural fusion, but the leaflets are not thickened and the arterial wall is normal. The so-called dysplastic PS is associated with a severely thickened valve tissue and is typically seen in the context of Noonan syndrome and some other genetic disorders. The management of neonates with PS and those with nonvalvular pulmonic obstruction is beyond the scope of this chapter. Patients with isolated PS might first be diagnosed beyond adolescence. Adult patients who have mild PS often do not experience significant change in the severity of the stenosis and rarely need therapeutic intervention in the future. A subset of PS patients with moderate severity would progress with time and require intervention. Severe PS needs to be treated with balloon valvuloplasty or surgical valvotomy. Balloon valvuloplasty, which is very safe and effective, has been accepted as the preferred therapeutic intervention in patients with isolated PS (Fig. 26.7). Balloon valvuloplasty is recommended when the transvalvular gradient is greater than 50 mmHg or when the patient is symptomatic.[8] In case of timely and successful balloon valvuloplasty, most patients do well, but 25% might need further intervention many years later.[43] A trial of balloon valvuloplasty

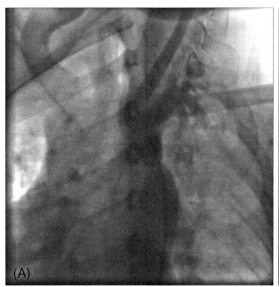
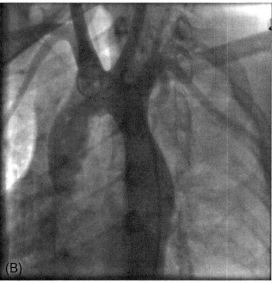

FIG. 26.6 Coarctoplasty using a self-expanding stent. (A) Discrete postductal coarctation of the aorta with a 60-mmHg peak-to-peak gradient. (B) Final result after deployment of a self-expanding stent followed by balloon postdilation.

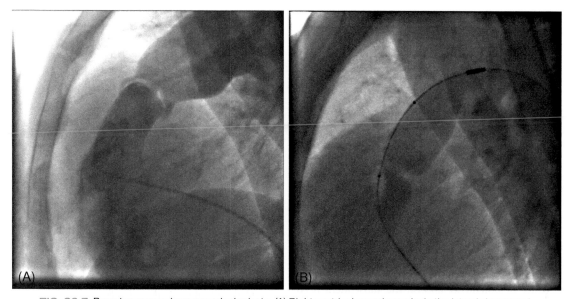

FIG. 26.7 Percutaneous pulmonary valvuloplasty. (A) Right ventricular angiography in the lateral view revealing a dome-shaped pulmonary valve with a central stenotic orifice and poststenotic dilation of the pulmonary artery. (B) Balloon inflation across the pulmonary valve with a waist appeared on the surface of the balloon caused by fused commissures. The balloon will be further dilated until the waist disappears.

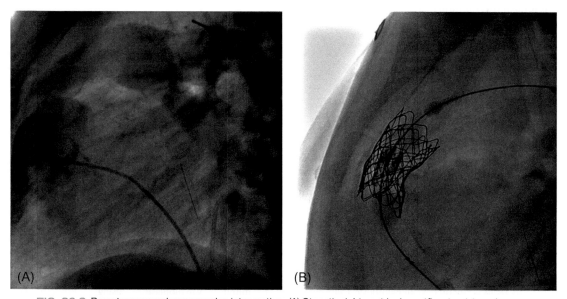

FIG. 26.8 Percutaneous pulmonary valve intervention. (A) Stenotic right ventricular outflow tract-to-pulmonary artery conduit in a patient after the Rastelli operation. (B) Prestenting of the stenotic conduits followed by implantation of a Sapien XT valve.

should be attempted in patients with dysplastic PS, but it might be ineffective because of the thickened leaflets and the absence of commissural fusion. Surgical valvotomy is reserved for patients who do not respond to percutaneous treatment.

## Percutaneous Pulmonary Valve Implantation

Right ventricular outflow tract pulmonary artery dysfunction, as pulmonary regurgitation or stenosis, is a frequent complication that happens years after surgical correction of congenital heart diseases. Right ventricular-to-pulmonary artery conduits are especially prone to late dysfunction, which needs subsequent surgical valve replacement. Although safe, surgery is limited by its long-term efficacy and need for reoperation in a significant number of patients in the next years.[44] Percutaneous pulmonary valve implantation (PPVI) has been introduced as a safe and minimally invasive procedure to reduce or potentially abolish the subsequent need for surgery (Fig. 26.8). Both stenotic and regurgitant pulmonary valves or right ventricular-to-pulmonary artery conduits are amenable to transcatheter therapy. Currently, two valve systems, the Melody transcatheter pulmonary valve and the Edwards Sapien valve, have received most of the experience in this field. Data regarding the long-term function of the valves and need for reintervention (surgery or second PPVI) are lacking. Medium-term follow-up studies have shown that restenosis is the most common reason for reintervention, but pulmonary regurgitation rarely occurs that is predominantly after infective endocarditis.[45]

## REFERENCES

1. Hagen PT, Scholz DG, Edwards WD. Incidence and size of patent foramen ovale during the first 10 decades of life: an autopsy study of 965 normal hearts. In: Mayo Clinic Proceedings, Elsevier; 1984.
2. Thaler DE, Di Angelantonio E, Di Tullio MR, et al. The Risk of Paradoxical Embolism (RoPE) Study: initial description of the completed database. *Int J Stroke.* 2013;8(8): 612–619.
3. Hijazi ZM, Feldman T, Al-Qbandi MHA, et al. *Transcatheter Closure of ASDs and PFOs: A Comprehensive Assessment.* Cardiotext Publishing; 2010.
4. Homma S, Sacco RL, Di Tullio MR, et al. Atrial anatomy in non-cardioembolic stroke patients: effect of medical therapy. *J Am Coll Cardiol.* 2003;42(6):1066–1072.
5. Mars JL, Derex L, Guerin P, et al. Reprint of: Transcatheter closure of patent foramen ovale to prevent stroke recurrence in patients with otherwise unexplained ischaemic stroke: expert consensus of the French Neurovascular Society and the French Society of Cardiology. *Rev Neurol (Paris).* 2020;176(1–2):53–61. https://doi.org/10.1016/j.neurol.2019.10.002.
6. Søndergaard L, Kasner SE, Rhodes JF, et al. Patent foramen ovale closure or antiplatelet therapy for cryptogenic stroke [published correction appears in N Engl J Med. 2020 Mar 5;382(10):978]. *N Engl J Med.* 2017;377(11): 1033–1042. https://doi.org/10.1056/NEJMoa1707404.
7. Abdi S, Kiani R, Momtahen M, et al. Percutaneous device closure for secundum-type atrial septal defect: short and intermediate-term results. *Arch Iran Med.* 2012;15(11):693.
8. Baumgartner H, Bonhoeffer P, De Groot NM, et al. Task Force on the Management of Grown-up Congenital Heart Disease of the European Society of Cardiology (ESC); Association for European Paediatric Cardiology (AEPC); ESC Committee for Practice Guidelines (CPG). ESC Guidelines for the management of grown-up congenital heart disease (new version 2010). *Eur Heart J.* 2010;ehq249.
9. Crawford GB, Brindis RG, Krucoff MW, et al. Percutaneous atrial septal occluder devices and cardiac erosion: a review of the literature. *Catheter Cardiovasc Interv.* 2012;80(2): 157–167.
10. Perloff JK, Child JS, Aboulhosn J. *Congenital Heart Disease in Adults.* Elsevier Health Sciences; 2009.
11. Lin HJ, Wolf PA, Kelly-Hayes M, et al. Stroke severity in atrial fibrillation. The Framingham Study. *Stroke.* 1996; 27(10):1760–1764.
12. Blackshear JL, Odell JA. Appendage obliteration to reduce stroke in cardiac surgical patients with atrial fibrillation. *Ann Thorac Surg.* 1996;61(2):755–759.
13. Tamura H, Watanabe T, Nishiyama S, et al. Prognostic value of low left atrial appendage wall velocity in patients with ischemic stroke and atrial fibrillation. *J Am Soc Echocardiogr.* 2012;25(5):576–583.
14. Gu ZC, Wei AH, Zhang C, et al. Risk of major gastrointestinal bleeding with new vs conventional oral anticoagulants: a systematic review and meta-analysis. *Clin Gastroenterol Hepatol.* 2020;18(4)https://doi.org/10.1016/j.cgh.2019.05.056 792–799.e61.
15. Kirchhof P, Benussi S, Kotecha D, et al. 2016 ESC Guidelines for the management of atrial fibrillation developed in collaboration with EACTS. *Europace.* 2016; euw295.
16. Meier B, Blaauw Y, Khattab AA, et al. EHRA/EAPCI expert consensus statement on catheter-based left atrial appendage occlusion. *Europace.* 2014;euu174.
17. Braunwald E, Bonow RO. *Braunwald's Heart Disease.* Elsevier Saunders; 2012.
18. Eeckhout E, Serruys PW, Wijins W, et al. *PCR–EAPCI Textbook of Percutaneous Interventional Cardiovascular Medicine.* London: Europa Publications; 2012.
19. Sanati HR, Zahedmehr A, Shakerian F, et al. Percutaneous mitral valvuloplasty using echocardiographic intercommissural diameter as reference for balloon sizing: a randomized controlled trial. *Clin Cardiol.* 2012; 35(12):749–754.

20. Rahimtoola SH, Durairaj A, Mehra A, Nuno I. Current evaluation and management of patients with mitral stenosis. *Circulation.* 2002;106(10):1183–1188.

21. Sanati HR, Kiavar M, Salehi N, et al. Percutaneous mitral valvuloplasty—a new method for balloon sizing based on maximal commissural diameter to improve procedural results. *Am Heart Hosp J.* 2010;8:29–32.

22. Nishimura RA, Otto CM, Bonow RO, et al. American College of Cardiology/American Heart Association Task Force on Practice Guidelines. 2014 AHA/ACC guideline for the management of patients with valvular heart disease: executive summary: a report of the American College of Cardiology/American Heart Association Task Force on Practice Guidelines. *J Am Coll Cardiol.* 2014; 63(22):2438–2488.

23. Wilkins GT, Weyman AE, Abascal VM, et al. Percutaneous balloon dilatation of the mitral valve: an analysis of echocardiographic variables related to outcome and the mechanism of dilatation. *Br Heart J.* 1988;60(4):299–308.

24. Whitlow PL, Feldman T, Pedersen WR, et al. Acute and 12-month results with catheter-based mitral valve leaflet repair: the EVEREST II (Endovascular Valve Edge-to-Edge Repair) High Risk Study. *J Am Coll Cardiol.* 2012;59(2): 130–139.

25. O'Gara PT, Calhoon JH, Moon MR, Tommaso CL. American College of Cardiology; American Association for Thoracic Surgery; Society for Cardiovascular Angiography and Interventions; Society of Thoracic Surgeons. Transcatheter therapies for mitral regurgitation: a professional society overview from the American College of Cardiology, the American Association for Thoracic Surgery, Society for Cardiovascular Angiography and Interventions Foundation, and the Society of Thoracic Surgeons. *J Am Coll Cardiol.* 2014;63(8):840–852.

26. Kappetein AP, Head SJ, Généreux P, et al. Updated standardized endpoint definitions for transcatheter aortic valve implantation: the Valve Academic Research Consortium-2 consensus document. *J Am Coll Cardiol.* 2012;60(15):1438–1454.

27. Czarny MJ, Resar JR. Diagnosis and management of valvular aortic stenosis. Clinical Medicine Insights. *Cardiology.* 2014;15 suppl. 1.

28. Stewart BF, Siscovick D, Lind BK, et al. Clinical factors associated with calcific aortic valve disease. Cardiovascular Health Study. *J Am Coll Cardiol.* 1997;29(3):630–634.

29. Cribier A, Eltchaninoff H, Bash A, et al. Percutaneous transcatheter implantation of an aortic valve prosthesis for calcific aortic stenosis first human case description. *Circulation.* 2002;106(24):3006–3008.

30. Bourantas CV, Farooq V, Onuma Y, et al. Transcatheter aortic valve implantation: new developments and upcoming clinical trials. *EuroIntervention.* 2012;8(5): 617–627.

31. Leon MB, Smith CR, Mack MJ, et al. Transcatheter or surgical aortic-valve replacement in intermediate-risk patients. *N Engl J Med.* 2016;374(17):1609–1620.

32. Webb JG, Wood DA. Current status of transcatheter aortic valve replacement. *J Am Coll Cardiol.* 2012;60(6): 483–492.

33. Lichtenstein SV, Cheung A, Ye J, et al. Transapical transcatheter aortic valve implantation in humans initial clinical experience. *Circulation.* 2006;114(6):591–596.

34. Ruge H, Lange R, Bleiziffer S, et al. First successful aortic valve implantation with the CoreValve ReValving System via right subclavian artery access: a case report. *Heart Surg Forum.* 2008;11(5):E323–E324.

35. Bapat VV, Attia R. Transaortic transcatheter aortic valve implantation using Edwards Sapien valve. *Catheter Cardiovasc Interv.* 2012;79(5):733–740.

36. Moretti C, D'Ascenzo F, Mennuni M, et al. Meta-analysis of comparison between self-expandable and balloon-expandable valves for patients having transcatheter aortic valve implantation. *Am J Cardiol.* 2015;115(12): 1720–1725.

37. Salizzoni S, Anselmino M, Fornengo C, et al. One-year follow-up of conduction disturbances following transcatheter aortic valve implantation. *J Cardiovasc Med.* 2015;16(4):296–302.

38. Hamm CW, Arsalan M, Mack MJ. The future of transcatheter aortic valve implantation. *Eur Heart J.* 2015; ehv574.

39. Krishnaswamy A, Tuzcu EM, Kapadia SR. Update on transcatheter aortic valve implantation. *Curr Cardiol Rep.* 2010;12(5):393–403.

40. Tarantini G, Gasparetto V, Napodano M, et al. Valvular leak after transcatheter aortic valve implantation: a clinician update on epidemiology, pathophysiology and clinical implications. *Am J Cardiovasc Dis.* 2011;1(3): 312–320.

41. Hoffman JI, Kaplan S. The incidence of congenital heart disease. *J Am Coll Cardiol.* 2002;39(12):1890–1900.

42. Connolly HM, Huston 3rd J, Brown Jr. RD, et al. Intracranial aneurysms in patients with coarctation of the aorta: a prospective magnetic resonance angiographic study of 100 patients. In: *Mayo Clinic Proceedings.* Elsevier; 2003.

43. Chen CR, Cheng TO, Huang T, et al. Percutaneous balloon valvuloplasty for pulmonic stenosis in adolescents and adults. *N Engl J Med.* 1996;335(1):21–25.

44. Tweddell JS, Pelech AN, Frommelt PC, et al. Factors affecting longevity of homograft valves used in right ventricular outflow tract reconstruction for congenital heart disease. *Circulation.* 2000;102(suppl. 3) Iii-130–Iii-135.

45. Lurz P, Coats L, Khambadkone S, et al. Percutaneous pulmonary valve implantation impact of evolving technology and learning curve on clinical outcome. *Circulation.* 2008;117(15):1964–1972.

# CHAPTER 27

# Aortic Disorders and Their Management

OMID SHAFE

Cardiovascular Interventional Research Center, Rajaie Cardiovascular, Medical & Research Center,
Iran University of Medical Sciences, Tehran, Iran

## KEY POINTS

- Aorta is the largest vessel in the body. Its histologic structure varies from origin to distal. Therefore, different pathologies and pathophysiologic processes are responsible for its disorders.
- Ascending aorta and arch are mostly involved in patients with heredity connective tissue disorders such as Marfan syndrome and Loeys-Dietz syndrome.
- Uncomplicated Type B aortic dissection treatment other than medical treatment is debated due to emerging new less invasive approaches, i.e., TEVAR.
- Ruptured AAA is a potentially lethal situation and its treatment needs especial facilities. AAA is relatively asymptomatic until becomes impending to rupture. Given its high mortality rate after becoming rupture there should be a screening algorithm to find AAA patients and risk stratify them.

## AORTIC DISEASES

Atherosclerosis is a diffuse disorder that involves every vascular bed, including the aorta. Similar to other vascular territories, atherosclerotic involvement of the aorta may be evident from significant stenosis to severe dilatation (i.e., aneurysm formation). Apart from atherosclerosis, some other specific types of disorders (e.g., aortic dissection) have their own unique pathophysiology and epidemiology. In this chapter, these various pathologies are discussed, along with the best diagnostic and therapeutic approach for each.

### Epidemiology and Screening Strategies of Aortic Aneurysms

Aneurysm dilatation of the aorta may be discovered at any site through the aortic length. Because there are different histologic properties within the aortic length, the epidemiologic and pathologic features of each are also different (Fig. 27.1).

### Abdominal Aortic Aneurysms

The abdominal aorta is more prone to atherosclerotic formation than other parts of the aorta. This predisposition explains why aneurysm formation is more common in this part of the aorta. The prevalence of abdominal aortic aneurysm (AAA) is estimated to be more than 6% in selected patients.[1] It is most common in men who are smokers and have hypertension and who are between 65 and 75 years of age (Table 27.1). AAA has a silent course, and most patients are asymptomatic until the AAA becomes ruptured or discovered during routine physical examination. If ruptured, AAA is highly lethal, and the mortality rate is more than 80% and even 100% if left untreated.[2-4] Even with open surgery or endovascular aortic repair (EVAR), the mortality rate is as high as 50% (25%–40% in the IMPROVE trial).[5] The most important risk factor for rupture is the size of the aneurysm (Table 27.2). Considering its silent course in the shadow of its lethal consequences, screening strategies are helpful to discover a clinically quiet AAA. The use of radiologic modalities as well as physical examination during routine ambulatory visits are recommended in selected higher risk patients. The most accessible radiologic modality is sonography, which has a high sensitivity and specificity for detection of AAA. Computed tomography angiography (CTA) and magnetic resonance angiography (MRA) are reserved for detecting AAAs, which are more accurate in determining size measurements and anatomic properties that are needed to help treatment planning (Fig. 27.2). Population-based screening plans reduce the risk of AAA death among men by 50%, but there is no benefit of such plans among women (Fig. 27.3 and Table 27.3).

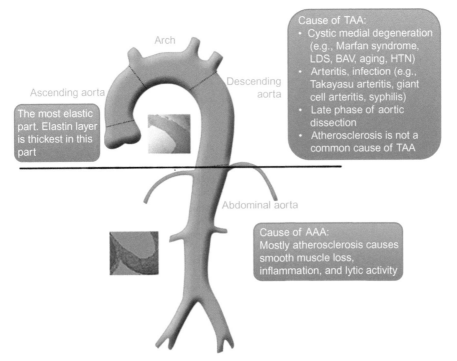

Arch

Ascending aorta

Descending aorta

The most elastic part. Elastin layer is thickest in this part

Cause of TAA:
- Cystic medial degeneration (e.g., Marfan syndrome, LDS, BAV, aging, HTN)
- Arteritis, infection (e.g., Takayasu arteritis, giant cell arteritis, syphilis)
- Late phase of aortic dissection
- Atherosclerosis is not a common cause of TAA

Abdominal aorta

Cause of AAA:
Mostly atherosclerosis causes smooth muscle loss, inflammation, and lytic activity

**FIG. 27.1** Anatomy of aorta and histologic specification of each part. The causes of the aortic aneurysms are mentioned at each level. Note that at ascending part there are thicker elastin layer than at abdominal part. *AAA*, abdominal aortic aneurysm; *BAV*, bicuspid aortic valve; *HTN*, hypertension; *LDS*, Loeys–Dietz syndrome; *TAA*, thoracic aortic aneurysm.

## Thoracic Aortic Aneurysms

Anatomically, the thoracic aorta is divided into the ascending aorta, arch, and descending aorta (see Fig. 27.1). The thoracic part of the aorta, especially at the ascending part, is more elastic than the abdominal part. This is because at the proximal parts, elastic media are thicker than at the distal parts. Considering this histologic difference, the pathophysiologic and pathologic pathways that may lead to thoracic aortic aneurysm (TAA) are different from those that lead to AAA. Although AAAs are a consequence of atherosclerotic degeneration of the aortic wall, this is not true for more proximal thoracic parts. From an epidemiologic point of view, it is difficult to estimate the true incidence and prevalence of TAAs because of the lack of an approved screening algorithm. However, there are subsets of patients who have substantial susceptibility to TAA. Marfan syndrome, a fibrillin-1 gene mutation, and other heredity connective tissue disorders are some examples. Also, probands of families with a previous history of any aneurysm have a substantial lifelong risk of aneurysm formation.[10,11] These patients are categorized as having familial thoracic aortic aneurysm syndrome (FTAAS).

Interestingly, it has been shown that there is a relationship between the aneurysm site in patients with TAA and their family members who had had a previous aneurysm.[12] There are recognized genes that are related to this pathology. Using genetic assays on a blood sample may determine the presence of an aneurysm at the thoracic aorta with more than 80% accuracy.[13] Despite these encouraging results, no routine genetic assay is recommended for screening purposes in clinical practice. Therefore, imaging modalities may be considered for screening of supposedly more susceptible patients (see Table 27.1); of course, there is no algorithm for screening of TAAs.

## PATHOLOGY AND PATHOPHYSIOLOGY OF AORTIC ANEURYSMS

### Abdominal Aortic Aneurysm (Fig. 27.4)

It has been shown that AAA has an association, in terms of epidemiologic and genetic perspectives, with other major vessel aneurysms, such as popliteal artery aneurysms.[14] Also, major vessels distant from an AAA have different biomechanics in patients with AAA. These

**TABLE 27.1**
**Risk Factors That Contribute in Aneurysm Formation Within the Thoracic and Abdominal Aorta**

| Abdominal Aortic Aneurysm | Thoracic Aortic Aneurysm |
|---|---|
| **Age >60 years** | **Cystic medial fibrosis (CMF)** |
| The prevalence is 1% between 55 and 64 years and increases by 2%–4% each decade | *HTN:* Aging and HTN lead to degenerative changes within elastic media |
| **Male sex** | *Connective tissue disorders:* Marfan syndrome, EDS, Turner |
| More than six times more prevalent in men than women | syndrome. Marfan syndrome is the fibrillin-1 gene mutation, with annuloaortic ectasia. BAV is also a congenital condition |
| **Smoking** | that is associated with CMF. Annuloaortic ectasia may |
| Its association is independent of atherosclerosis and relates to increase activity of oxidation and proteolysis within the aortic wall[2] | accompany this disorder |
| | *FTAAS:* It has been shown that many other gene mutations |
| The association is decreased after smoke cessation, although the risk of AAA formation persists for 10 years after cessation. The duration of smoking is more important than the number of cigarettes[3] | may be involved in TAA formation, apart from Marfan syndrome and other known syndromes. They seem sporadic, but more investigation is needed to clarify their familial origin |
| **More common in patients with CAD HTN** | **Arteritis** |
| It may have effects on AAA formation in rats but has not been approved in humans yet[4] | *Infective arteritis:* Such as syphilis, may be the etiology of TAA. Syphilis as a cause of TAA has faded because of aggressive antibiotic therapy. Also, infective endocarditis hampers the |
| **HLP** | risk of TAA |
| There are controversial results on the relationship between both higher cholesterol levels and statin therapy and risk of AAA | *Vasculitis:* Large-artery vasculitis, Takayasu arteritis, and giant cell arteritis are the most important causes. Although ESR rises in giant cell arteritis, it is not a determinant marker in |
| **Positive family history of AAA** | Takayasu arteritis |
| Its existence doubles the risk of AAA; it is independent of atherosclerosis and sex | **Chronic aortic dissection** |
| | Imaging surveillance is mandated in uncomplicated type B |
| **Obesity** | aortic dissection to recognize the progressive dilation of the |
| Waist-to-hip ratio and waist circumference are independently associated with AAA[5] | aorta |
| | **Atherosclerosis** |
| **Diabetes** | It is not a common cause of TAA. Descending aorta |
| Has a protective effect against AAA development | aneurysms have more association with atherosclerosis than ascending and arch aneurysms |

*AAA,* abdominal aortic aneurysm; *BAV,* bicuspid aortic valve; *CAD,* coronary artery disease; *EDS,* Ehlers–Danlos syndrome; *ESR,* erythrocyte sedimentation rate; *FTAS,* familial thoracic aortic aneurysm syndrome; *HLP,* hyperlipidemia; *HTN,* hypertension; *TAA,* thoracic aortic aneurysm.

**TABLE 27.2**
**Factors Associated With Risk of Aneurysm Rupture**

Aneurysm size: annual risk of rupture
- <4.0 cm in diameter: 0%
- 4.0–4.9 cm in diameter 0.5%–5%
- 5.0–5.9 cm in diameter: 3%–15%
- 6.0–6.9 cm in diameter: 10%–20%
- 7.0–7.9 cm in diameter: 20%–40%
- ≥8.0 cm in diameter: 30%–50%

Female gender
Elevated inflammatory biomarkers
- Fibrinogen
- Alpha 1-antitrypsin

Aneurysm expansion (growth)
- >1 cm per year shows rapid expansion

observations signify the generalized features of AAA rather than a focal destructive state of the aortic wall, which may accompany atherosclerosis alone. In fact, atherosclerosis, systemic hypertension, and smoking are factors that have both focal and generalized effects on AAA formation. Smoking leads to generalized inflammation throughout the arterial vascular system. Inflammatory cell infiltration within vessel walls is accompanied by proteolysis, which may lead to elastin and collagen degradation. These inflammatory responses, which are followed by many traditional atherosclerotic risk factors, along with background susceptibility (e.g., lack of elastogenesis during the embryonic period) and mechanical stress caused by systemic hypertension and increased pulse pressure at the abdominal aorta can lead to AAA formation.

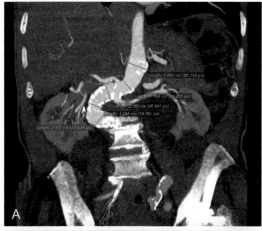

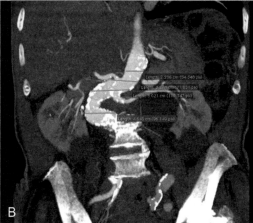

FIG. 27.2 Avoiding off-axis diameter measurement is crucial to avoid mistakes. It is very critical in a tortuous anatomy. (A) Correct diameter measurement according to centerline axis of the aorta in this tortuous segment. (B) Incorrect off-axis diameter measurement causes a significant error in tortuous segments.

## Thoracic Aortic Aneurysm (Fig. 27.5)

Age-related degeneration of elastic media is a part of the natural history of the aorta. However, this elastic degeneration is prompted in certain genetic disorders. As the proximal part of the aortic wall contains more elastin fibers, a TAA is the resultant of such genetic disorders. Some of these genetic disorders can manifest with a specific phenotype and syndromic appearance, but others have no specific phenotype or clinical feature until a dissection occurs or an aneurysm becomes symptomatic.

### Marfan syndrome

Patients with Marfan syndrome have a special appearance; they are taller and more elongated than the general population and have elongated faces, lens dislocation, and arachnodactyly. As a genetically inherent disorder, this syndrome is relatively common worldwide. This syndrome is a result of the fibrillin-1 gene (FBN1) mutation. Fibrillin-1 is an element of the connective tissue all over the body, so its lack has devastating consequences on connective tissue. Disordered transforming growth factor-β signaling also contributes to the abnormal and disordered incorporation of fibrillin-1 into the connective tissue.[15] In this respect, there is an overlap in terms of structural disorders within connective tissue between Marfan syndrome and Loeys–Dietz syndrome (LDS), as a syndrome with a specific appearance (craniosynostosis, scoliosis, hypertelorism, bifid uvula, and cleft palate) (Fig. 27.6).

### Ehlers–danlos syndrome

This syndrome is divided into three types: classic, hypermobile, and vascular. In contrast to Marfan syndrome and LDS in which the abnormality is limited to elastin processing, patients with vascular-type Ehlers–Danlos syndrome have abnormal collagen type III. Clinical manifestations include easy bruising, arterial and intestinal fragility, gastrointestinal perforation, and vascular dissection or perforation. Because elastin disorder is not present in these patients, aneurysm formation as well as acute aortic events occurs more frequently at the distal parts of the thoracic aorta and at the abdominal aorta.

### Bicuspid aortic valve

Fusion of two aortic valve leaflets creates a bicuspid aortic valve (BAV). It has familial clustering and is associated with some other congenital malformations such as coarctation of the aorta and patent ductus arteriosus (PDA). It has been shown that fibrillin-1 protein has a role in aneurysm formation in patients with BAV. Apart from fibrillin-1 itself, transcriptional elements that control fibrillin-1 production may be defective.[16] Annuloaortic ectasia, which refers to a combination of dilation of the aortic valve annulus, dilated aortic root and ascending aorta, and significant aortic valve regurgitation, is a morphologic finding that can be seen in relatively all patients with BAV and ascending aortic aneurysm and many patients with Marfan syndrome or LDS and ascending aortic aneurysm as well. However, there are subsets of patients with annuloaortic ectasia

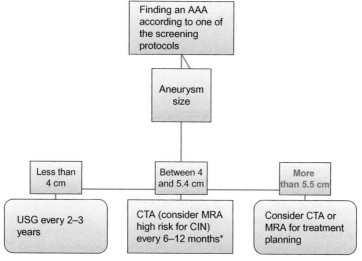

FIG. 27.3 Screening algorithm for abdominal aortic aneurysm (AAA). Asterisk indicates that if CTA is not available, ultrasonography (US) should be considered. *CIN*, contrast-induced nephropathy; *CTA*, computed tomography angiography; *MRA*, magnetic resonance angiography.

## TABLE 27.3
## Guidelines on Screening for Abdominal Aortic Aneurysm

**USPSTF**
- Men ages 65–75 years who have ever smoked should be screened once for AAA by US. There is no benefit to repeat screening in men who have negative US results and who are older than 75 years of age
- Men ages 65–75 years who have never smoked: There is benefit for routine US screening in these patients, but the physician can selectively offer screening for AAA to this age group of men
- Women ages 65–75 years who have ever smoked: The current evidence is insufficient to assess the balance of benefits and harms of screening for AAA in women ages 65–75 years who have ever smoked
- Women who have never smoked: The USPSTF is against routine screening for AAA in women who have never smoked

**ACC/AHA**
- Men ages 65–75 years who have ever smoked should undergo a physical examination and one-time US
- Men older than 60 years who are siblings or offspring of patients with AAA should undergo a physical examination and one-time US

**CSVS**
- Men ages 65–75 years who are potential candidates for surgery should undergo US
- Women older than 65 years with multiple risk factors (smoking, family history, and CVD) should selectively undergo US
- Women older than 65 years should not undergo US routinely

or aneurysm at the other parts of the thoracic aorta (even the abdominal aorta) who have no specified morphologic appearance. A detailed family history inspection may reveal a sort of family clustering of aneurysm formation. This subset of patients has familial thoracic aortic aneurysm and dissection (FTAAD).

Because this seems to be a hereditary disorder, genetic evaluation may reveal a genetic disorder; in many of these patients, none of the known genetic disorders can be found. ACTA2 gene mutation is associated with FTAAD and premature coronary or cerebrovascular obstruction.

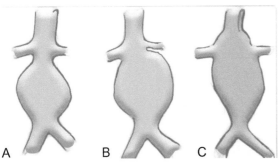

FIG. 27.4 Abdominal aortic aneurysms (AAAs) classification according to the distance from renal arteries and involvement of visceral arteries. From left to right, infrarenal, juxtarenal, pararenal, and suprarenal AAAs. Proximal neck of an AAA is defined as the distance between the lowest renal artery separation and aneurysm initiation. If there is a normal segment of aorta (at least 1–2 cm) within the proximal neck, the aneurysm is categorized as infrarenal AAA (as in A). If the proximal neck length is lesser than 1 cm, then the aneurysm is categorized as juxta- or pararenal AAA (as in B). If there is no neck and the aneurysm is initiated above the renal arteries, the aneurysm is categorized as suprarenal AAA (as in C).

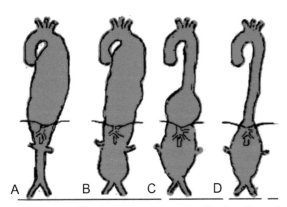

FIG. 27.5 Thoracic aortic aneurysm classification. (Type A) Aneurysmal Involvement of the descending thoracic aorta after the left subclavian artery (LSA) up to the suprarenal segment. (Type B) Aneurysmal involvement of the whole aorta from the LSA to the aortic bifurcation. (Type C) Aneurysmal involvement of the aorta from the supradiaphragmatic part of the descending aorta to the aortic bifurcation. (Type D) Aneurysmal involvement of the distal descending aorta to the aortic bifurcation

Other factors that may damage the aortic wall, such as vasculitis or infective endocarditis or endarteritis, are the causes of TAA. TAA is also common after surgical Dacron patch aortoplasty in patients with coarctation of the aorta (Fig. 27.7).

## MANAGEMENT (FIG. 27.8)
### Medical Therapy
#### Thoracic aortic aneurysms
To date, no valid medical therapy has been introduced for treatment for TAA. Blood pressure control may have some benefits in reducing expansion of aneurysms or the probability of acute aortic events.

#### Abdominal aortic aneurysm
Because these aneurysms are associated with widespread atherosclerosis, blood pressure control, smoking cessation, and dyslipidemia control may have some benefits to at least reduce the overall risk of cardiovascular mortality. Indeed, there are some recommendations that beta-blockers may reduce aneurysm expansion.[18] It has been shown that continued smoking raises the rate of aneurysm expansion up to 25%.[19]

### Open Surgery or Endovascular Therapy
For proximal parts of the thoracic aorta (ascending and arch and some descending aorta aneurysms), the treatment of choice is surgery. According to the severity of involvement of the aortic valve, the surgical technique is different (Fig. 27.9).

With the emergence of custom-made devices that are appropriate for individual patients as well as newer endovascular techniques, some centers perform endovascular endograft placement in the ascending aorta instead of open repair among selected patients.

Either open surgery or thoracic endovascular aortic repair (TEVAR) is the treatment strategy for descending aorta aneurysms. If the anatomy is feasible, TEVAR has a lower procedural risk of mortality and morbidity. The most notable complication in this region is spinal cord injury, which may occur after both open surgery and TEVAR; however, its rate is higher after open surgery than TEVAR. Spinal cord injury presents with paraparesis or paraplegia after the procedure. It is the result of damage or occlusion of vessels directing blood toward the spinal cord.

Either open surgery or EVAR can be considered in patients with AAAs with diameters larger than 5.5 cm (Fig. 27.10). EVAR has a lower procedural mortality and morbidity than open surgery. However, this benefit does not last over long-term follow-up (Table 27.4).

## ACUTE AORTIC SYNDROMES
### Aortic Dissection and Its Variants
#### Aortic dissection (Figs. 27.11 and 27.12)
Aortic dissection is one of the most catastrophic events with a high mortality rate. During the early hours after

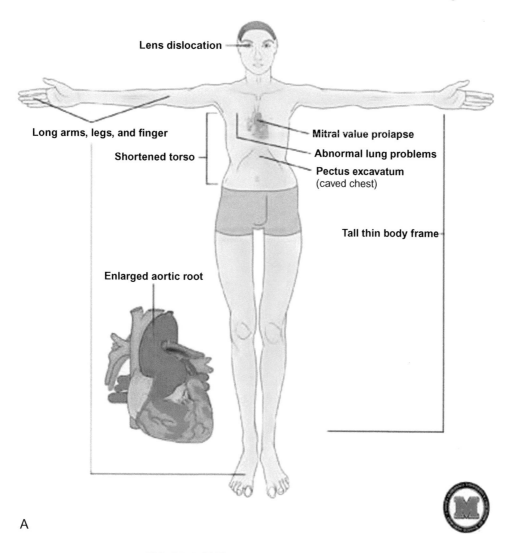

**Lens dislocation**

**Long arms, legs, and finger**

**Shortened torso**

**Mitral value prolapse**

**Abnormal lung problems**

**Pectus excavatum**
(caved chest)

**Tall thin body frame**

**Enlarged aortic root**

A

FIG. 27.6 (A) Phenotype of Marfan syndrome.

*Continued*

type A aortic dissection, the mortality risk increases about 1% per hour.[21] As time passes, the mortality rate increase slows down but is still high. The in-hospital mortality rate is about 59% among medically treated patients with type A aortic dissection.[22] Also, the in-hospital mortality rate is about 13% among patients with type B aortic dissections.[23] The incidence of aortic dissection has been rising, partly because of the improvement in and availability of diagnostic methods.

Aging increases its incidence as degenerative aortic wall changes and the rate of systemic hypertension increase. Thoracic aneurysms and diameter of the aorta, especially in patients with genetic disorders, are two of the most important risk factors of aortic dissection; however, only 16% of patients with thoracic aortic dissection have known aneurysms. It is noteworthy that thoracic aortic dissection is a common cause of TAAs (see Table 27.1).[24]

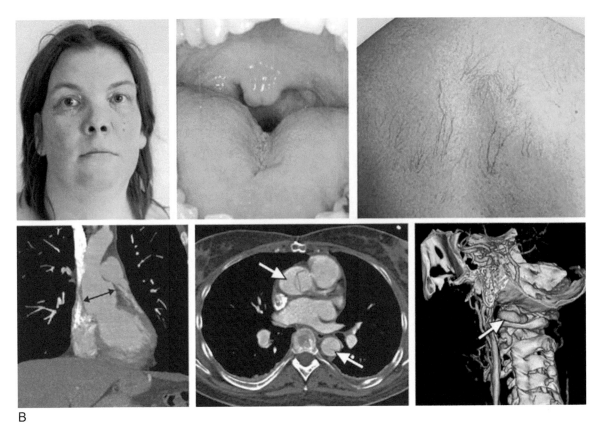

B

FIG. 27.6, Cont'd (B) Phenotype of Loeys–Dietz syndrome, including hypertelorism and uvula bifida. Part B: From left to right, annuloaortic ectasia, ascending aorta dissection and aneurysm formation, highly tortuous vertebral artery. (Panel (B): From van de Laar IMBH, Oldenburg RA, Pals G, et al. Mutations in SMAD3 cause a syndromic form of aortic aneurysms and dissections with early-onset osteoarthritis. *Nat Genet*. 2011;43(2): 121–128, with permission.)

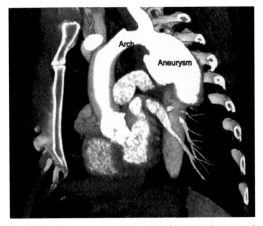

FIG. 27.7 An aneurysm at the site of the previous surgical Dacron patch aortoplasty for coarctation of the aorta. The treatment threshold for this aneurysm is lower than for regular, fusiform aneurysms.

### Pathophysiology

An intimal tear is known as the initiating event. Uncontrolled systemic hypertension and degenerated media of the aorta, either genetic or depending on age, are the precipitating factors. After the intimal tear occurs, the hemodynamic load exerts over the medial layer in a longitudinal manner and causes tearing of media and separation of the aortic wall layers through its length, most commonly within the media (Fig. 27.13).

There are also some other proposed mechanisms that may lead to aortic dissection. Ruptured vasa vasorum is considered an initiating event by some authors. As mentioned before, in patients with aortic wall degenerative disorders (e.g., Marfan syndrome, LDS, BAV) and even age-related media degeneration, dissection may occur without an aneurysm or dilatation (Table 27.5). Type A aortic dissection may be

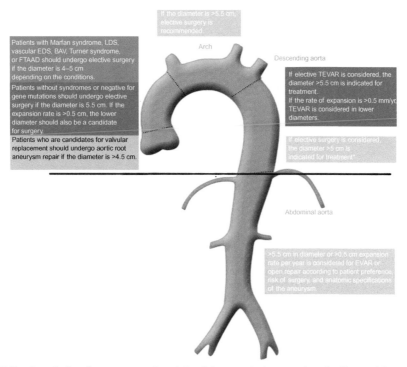

FIG. 27.8 Treatment of aortic aneurysm at each level. In some instances when the figure of the aneurysm is not fusiform and is bizarre or saccular, the lower diameter of the aneurysm should be considered for treatment.[17] *BAV*, bicuspid aortic valve; *EDS*, Ehlers–Danlos syndrome; *EVAR*, endovascular aortic repair; *FTAAD*, familial thoracic aortic aneurysm and dissection; *LDS*, Loeys–Dietz syndrome; *TEVAR*, thoracic endovascular aortic repair. (Data from Grabenwoger M, Alfonso F, Bachet J, et al. Thoracic endovascular aortic repair (TEVAR) for the treatment of aortic diseases: a position statement from the European Association for Cardio-Thoracic Surgery (EACTS) and the European Society of Cardiology (ESC), in collaboration with the European Association of Percutaneous Cardiovascular Interventions (EAPCI). *Eur Heart J.* 2014; and Rooke TW, Hirsch AT, Misra S, et al. 2011 ACCF/AHA focused update of the guideline for the management of patients with peripheral artery disease (updating the 2005 guideline). A report of the American College of Cardiology Foundation/American Heart Association Task Force on Practice Guidelines. *Circulation*. 2011;124:2020–2045.)

accompanied by aortic valve regurgitation, tamponade, and [AU17] obstruction of arch vessels, as well as coronary artery and aortic rupture. Aortic rupture in this setting is the leading mechanism of death. Because type B aortic dissection happens more distant from heart structures and arch branches, its lethality is lower, but it still exists. Aortic rupture and occlusion of branch vessels (i.e., mesenteric artery, celiac artery, or renal arteries) are the causes of death in type B aortic dissection. However, if type B aortic dissection has an uncomplicated acute course, a good survival rate is anticipated even with medical therapy alone.

### Clinical manifestations

Sudden, severe tearing pain, which is in its maximum intensity at first and radiates to the back or lower extremities, is the typical pain associated with aortic dissection. However, many individuals have different presentations. These may include syncope, sudden cardiac death, ischemic-like pain, abdominal pain, limb pain caused by ischemia, hypoperfusion syndrome and shock caused by severe aortic regurgitation or tamponade, cerebrovascular accidents, and hypertensive crisis caused by obstruction of the renal arteries. Pain accompanies these symptoms, but because it may resolve early, the presenting symptom might obscure the initial pain. Migratory pain may be present because the dissection may extend to more distal parts of the aorta and hampers a higher risk of complications. To diagnose aortic dissection, the physician should estimate the likelihood of aortic dissection as the cause of chest pain as well as other symptoms that

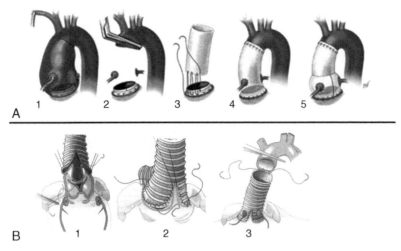

FIG. 27.9 (A) Ascending aorta aneurysm repair using a modified Bentall procedure. (B) Valve-sparing root replacement. A1 and 2: Removing the aneurysmal part of the ascending aorta after valve replacement; A3–5: reimplantation of coronaries and suturing proximal and distal parts of the prosthetic graft. B1–3: Removing the aneurysmal part with graft placement with coronary reimplantation without valve replacement. (Panel (A): From Malekan R, Spielvogel D, Saunders P, et al. The completion Bentall procedure. *Ann Thorac Surg.* 2011;92 (1):362–363, with permission. Panel (B): From Sin YK, Pillai RG. Valve-sparing aortic root replacement. *J Card Surg.* 2000;15:424–427, with permission.)

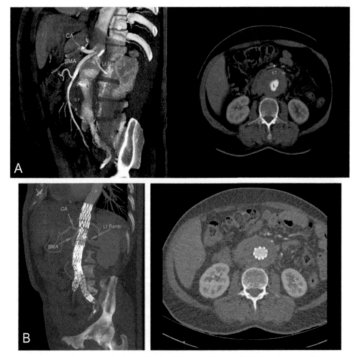

FIG. 27.10 Endovascular aortic repair for a patient with an infrarenal abdominal aortic aneurysm. Pre- (A) and postprocedure (B) computed tomography angiography. *CA,* celiac artery; *Lt,* left; *SMA,* superior mesenteric artery.

**TABLE 27.4**
**Guidelines on Treatment of Abdominal Aortic Aneurysm[20]**

| | |
|---|---|
| • Open surgery or EVAR of infrarenal AAAs and/or common iliac aneurysms is indicated in patients who are good surgical candidates[a] | I(A) |
| • Periodic long-term surveillance imaging should be performed to monitor endoleak, confirm graft position, and document shrinkage or stability of the excluded aneurysm sac | I(A) |
| • Open aneurysm repair is reasonable to perform in patients who are good candidates but who cannot comply with periodic long-term surveillance required after endovascular repair | IIA (C) |
| • Endovascular repair of infrarenal aortic aneurysms in patients who are at high surgical or anesthetic risk as determined by the presence of coexisting severe cardiac, pulmonary, or renal disease is of uncertain effectiveness | IIB (B) |

[a]Patients with AAA larger than 5-5.5 cm in diameter who are likely to live > 2 years and are good surgical risk candidates.

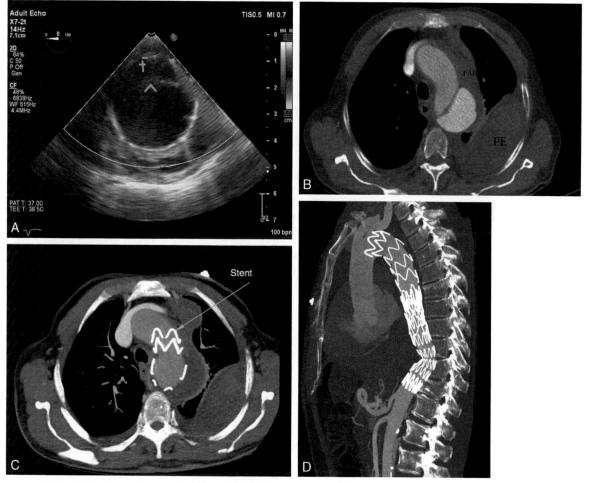

FIG. 27.11 Type B aortic dissection (TBAD) before thoracic endovascular aortic repair (TEVAR) shown on transesophageal echocardiography (A) and computed tomography angiography (B) images. (C, D) Post-TEVAR imaging. This is an example of a complicated TBAD. There is a rupture with resultant periaortic hematoma (PAH) and pleural effusion (PE). *F*, false lumen.

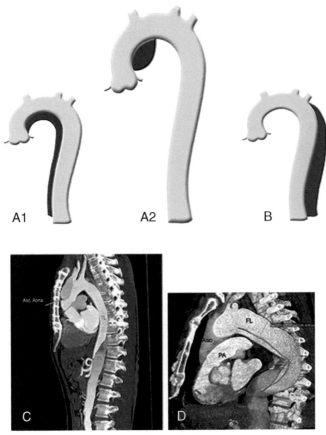

FIG. 27.12 Aortic dissection classification. A1, Type A1 with involvement of the ascending aorta (Asc aorta). Computed tomography angiography (CTA) shows a typical type A1 dissection. Note the true lumen (TL) and false lumen (FL). A2, Type A2 with involvement of the ascending aorta only. B, Type B with involvement of the descending aorta and further. Typically, the entry tear is just after the left SCA, and the TL is almost always smaller than the FL. C, D, CTA shows a type B aortic dissection (TBAD) in the chronic phase; note how dilated the aorta is (i.e., aneurysm formation). The diameter is larger than 5 cm, and the aorta is severely tortuous, making any intervention difficult.

are related to dissection (Fig. 27.14). Certain clinical presentations put the patient in a higher risk category. These include syncope, sudden cardiac death, hypotension, symptoms related to branch vessel involvement (i.e., ischemic-type chest pain that may relate to myocardial infarction [MI]), neurologic deficits, abdominal pain that may relate to intestinal ischemia, severe uncontrolled hypertension despite appropriate drug therapy that may relate to renal artery involvement, acute limb ischemia, and paraplegia. Paraplegia occurs after occlusion of spinal cord ischemia as a dissection flap obstructs vessels supplying blood to the spinal cord.

## Approach to Patients With Suspicious Aortic Dissection (Fig. 27.14)

Because chest pain has several important differential diagnoses, when encountered in an emergency department (ED), it is reasonable to direct workups in a way that the more likely and more dangerous causes have more probability to be discovered. Routinely, more attention and force are paid to find coronary-related chest pain because it is highly lethal and more common and, of course, is treatable. But other differential diagnoses, including aortic dissection and pulmonary thromboembolism, also must be considered. This perspective makes many experts use a diagnostic algorithm,

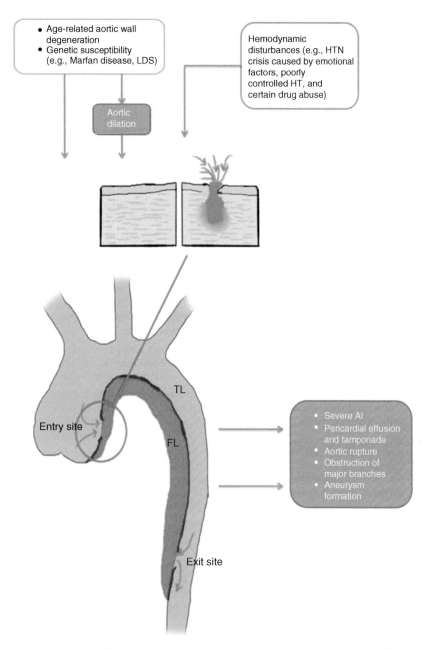

FIG. 27.13 An illustration of the conditions that lead to dissection initiation and propagation. Consequent events that lead to mortality or morbidity. *AI*, aortic insufficiency; *FL*, false lumen; *HTN*, hypertension; *LDS*, Loeys–Dietz syndrome; *TL*, true lumen.

which can help to diagnose these lethal conditions in an ED. These approaches are based on the patient's risk and probability of having these highly lethal conditions. However, a practitioner should always be cautious because these algorithms reach the diagnosis in many cases, but not all of them. There might be some situations in which even the existence of a clearly diagnosed differential diagnosis does not rule out other differential diagnoses. Let us clear it up by supplying an example. There are some type A aortic dissections which present

**TABLE 27.5**
**Association of Different Factors With Aortic Dissection**

| Factor | Comments |
|---|---|
| Sex | Dissection is more common among men |
| Age | Has bimodal distribution; genetically susceptible patients are younger. The average age of onset of TAAD is lower than TBAD (61 years vs 66 years) |
| Aortic diameter | A more dilated aorta confers a higher risk of dissection. Of course, there are specific diameter points at which the risk of dissection jumps (i.e., hinge points, from 3% to 30% if the diameter reaches to 6 cm for the ascending aorta and 7 cm for the descending aorta). However, it should be kept in mind that the height and weight of the patient affect the diameter in which the probability of the occurrence of the dissection becomes considerable[24] |
| Atherosclerosis | There is not a direct relationship between atherosclerosis and typical aortic dissection; however, PAU, a dissection variant, is more common in higher atherosclerotic burden |
| Hypertension | Hypertension is an independent risk factor of dissection, even in aortic diameters smaller than 5.5 cm |
| Diabetes | The prevalence of diabetes is low among patients with dissection. The protective effect of diabetes over the aortic dilation may in part explain this observation |
| Aortitis | Large vessel arteritis, Takayasu arteritis, or giant cell arteritis can lead to dissection |
| Pregnancy | It is not clear that pregnancy has an independent relationship with dissection. However, among pregnant patients with genetic disorders of the connective tissue (e.g., Marfan syndrome), the risk of dissection is much higher than in nonpregnant genetically affected patients |
| Trauma | Dissection caused by blunt trauma is rare. However, iatrogenic dissection after CABG or cardiac catheterization is well recognized. About 90% of iatrogenic TBADs result from cardiac catheterization, and more than 65% of iatrogenic TAADs result from CABG at the aortic cannulation site |
| Drugs | Both cocaine and amphetamine raise the risk of dissection in a temporal manner. However, the risk estimation attributed to amphetamine is higher than for cocaine. There are a few case reports on about the association of sildenafil administration and the risk of aortic dissection |
| Genetic factors | With cardiovascular defects<br>BAV is associated with aortic dissection<br>Coarctation of the aorta: Dissection may occur during interventional coarctoplasty; most are local and do not need any further treatment or can be treated by covered stents during coarctoplasty. Spontaneous dissection is not frequent among patients with coarctation<br><br>With syndromic features<br>Marfan syndrome, LDS, EDS, Turner syndrome (see text)<br><br>Without syndromic features<br>FTAAD (see text) |

*BAV*, bicuspid aortic valve; *CABG*, coronary artery bypass graft; *EDS*, Ehlers–Danlos syndrome; *FTAAD*, familial thoracic aortic aneurysm and dissection; *LDS*, Loeys–Dietz syndrome; *PAU*, penetrating atherosclerotic ulcer; *TAAD*, type A aortic dissection; *TBAD*, type B aortic dissection.
Data from LeMaire SA, Russell L. Epidemiology of thoracic aortic dissection. *Nat Rev Cardiol.* 2011;8(2):103–113.

with acute inferior ST-segment elevation MI. This is because the frequency of involvement of the right coronary artery is more than that of other coronary artery ostia while a type A dissection occurs. In such patients, thrombolytic therapy is contraindicated because the thrombosed flap may extend farther antegradely or retrogradely, worsening the patient's conditions. So it is recommended to fully evaluate the patients with chest pain to discover these atypical presentations that are potentially dangerous.

### Treatment (Fig. 27.15)

After the diagnosis is confirmed, medical treatment should be conducted without wasting time. Blood pressure should be controlled with respect to the patient's baseline levels. A normal blood pressure is considered

Diagnostic pathway

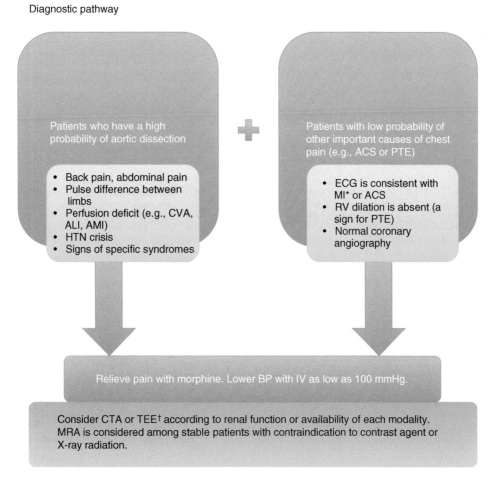

**FIG. 27.14** Diagnostic approach to a patient suspected of having aortic dissection. (*ACS*, acute coronary syndrome; *ALI*, acute limb injury; *AMI*, acute myocardial infarction; *BP*, blood pressure; *CVA*, cerebrovascular accident; *ECG*, electrocardiogram; *HTN*, hypertension; *IV*, intravenous; *MI*, myocardial infarction; *MRA*, magnetic resonance angiography; *PE*, pleural effusion; *RV*, right ventricular; *TEE*, transesophageal echocardiography.)

a hypotension state for a patient with a history of poorly uncontrolled hypertension. It is crucial to treat hypotensive patients with fluid replacement and even blood injection because hypotension is an important sign of aortic rupture as well as tamponade or cardiogenic shock caused by acute severe aortic regurgitation. However, there are some situations when a dissection flap may obstruct arch vessels, so the resultant hypotension is false. CTA findings help to find this subset of patients.

Traditionally, it is recommended to reduce the blood pressure to prevent dissection extension or aortic rupture. This approach is the most important part of medical treatment in all dissection types. As described earlier, consideration of the baseline blood pressure is essential. Drugs that are used to achieve a blood pressure level less than 100–120 mmHg are parenteral and usually include labetalol, esmolol, propranolol, and metoprolol. In patients with contraindications to beta-

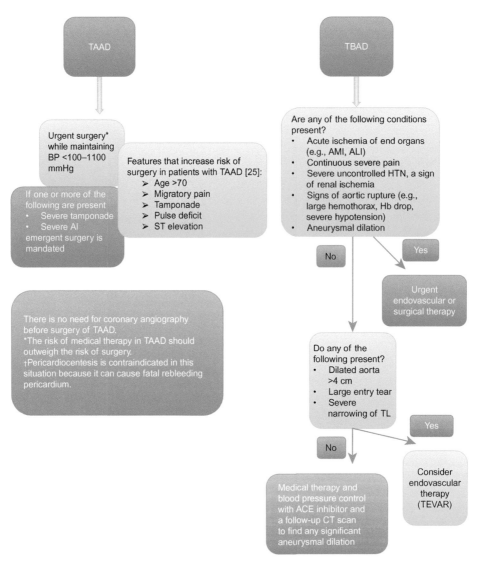

FIG. 27.15 Therapeutic pathway in patients with dissection of the aorta, thoracic aortic aneurysm and dissection (TAAD), and type B aortic dissection (TBAD).[25] *ACE*, angiotensin-converting enzyme; *AI*, aortic insufficiency; *ALI*, acute limb injury; *AMI*, acute myocardial infarction; *BP*, blood pressure; *Hb*, hemoglobin; *HTN*, hypertension; *TEVAR*, thoracic endovascular aortic repair; *TL*, true lumen.

blockers, calcium channel blockers are the best option (e.g., verapamil and diltiazem). Nitroprusside and nitroglycerine should not be used alone because they cause increased dP/dt (i.e., peak cardiac effect and LV contractility force) and extend dissection. Patients with type A aortic dissection and complicated type B aortic dissection always need surgical or endovascular therapy. A surgical approach is the method of choice for the treatment of nearly all TAAs. Today, TEVAR is the method of choice for the treatment of complicated type B aortic dissections (see Fig. 27.10).

## Aortic Dissection Variants

Aortic dissection variants include intramural hematoma (IMH) and penetrating atherosclerotic ulcer (PAU). IMH is less common than typical dissection.

IMH and PAU are quite similar in terms of clinical manifestations, indications of treatment, and even diagnostic imaging (Fig. 27.16).

Penetrating atherosclerotic ulcer is different from typical dissection. In this pathology, an atherosclerotic plaque penetrates the aortic wall and causes a painful ulcer within the wall. Although infrequent, it can cause

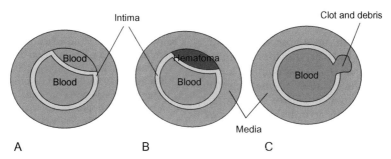

FIG. 27.16 Aortic dissection variants. (A) Presence of blood in true lumen and false lumen. (B) Hematoma within the aortic wall. Note that if the false lumen of a true dissection is thrombosed during aortic remodeling, radiologic differentiation of a thrombosed FL from IMH as the primary pathology is very difficult. (C) Penetrating atherosclerotic ulcer.

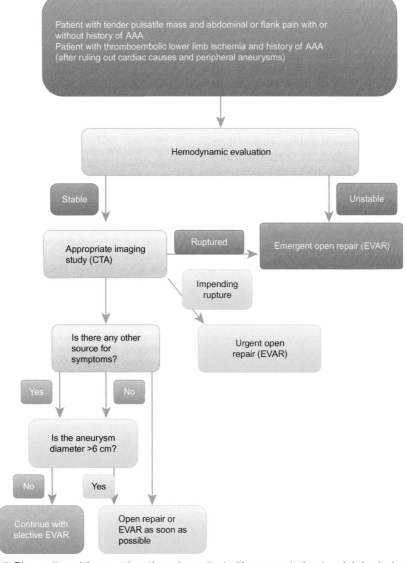

FIG. 27.17 Diagnostic and therapeutic pathway in a patient with a suspected ruptured abdominal aortic aneurysm (AA). *CTA*, computed tomography angiography; *EVAR*, endovascular aortic repair.

a local dissection. It also can create a pseudoaneurysm at the site of ulceration, which has a risk for rupture. Its location is usually at the level of the abdominal aorta, where the atherosclerotic plaques can be detected much more frequently than in other parts of the aorta. The therapeutic strategies vary according to the site of PAU and the pathology that is created by the complicated plaque. If the ulcer was localized and the dissection was localized as well and the pain is to be relieved, then medical therapy is the choice, but if there is a pseudoaneurysm, especially within an acceptable distance from branches of the abdominal aorta, endovascular therapy is the best option. Usually, surgery is reserved for situations when endovascular therapy is impossible.

### Ruptured abdominal aortic aneurysm

Symptoms of abdominal or flank pain and acute limb ischemia caused by embolization in a patient with known AAA should be considered complicated AAA (i.e., ruptured or impending to rupture AAA). The mortality rate of ruptured AAA is very high. It has been shown that up to 50% of patients with ruptured AAA die before hospital admission, and about 40% of them die before treatment at a hospital. The operative mortality rate is also high but is lower with EVAR. Nearly all of the patients with AAA who have symptoms related to AAA should be treated, but the timing varies in different clinical scenarios (Fig. 27.17).

## REFERENCES

1. McFarlane MJ. The epidemiologic necropsy for abdominal aortic aneurysm. *JAMA.* 1991;265:2085–2088.
2. Verhoeven EL, Kapma MR, Groen H, et al. Mortality of ruptured abdominal aortic aneurysm treated with open or endovascular repair. *J Vasc Surg.* 2008;48:1396–1400.
3. Basnyat PS, Biffin AH, Moseley LG, Hedges AR, Lewis MH. Mortality from ruptured abdominal aortic aneurysm in Wales. *Br J Surg.* 1999;86:765–770.
4. Karthikesalingam A, Holt PJ, Vidal-Diez A, et al. Mortality from ruptured abdominal aortic aneurysm: clinical lessons from a comparison of outcomes in England and the USA. *Lancet.* 2014;383:963–969.
5. Powell JT, Hinchliff RJ, Thompson MM, et al. Endovascular or open repair strategy for ruptured abdominal aortic aneurysm: 30 day outcomes from IMPROVE randomised trial. *BMJ.* 2014;348:f7661.
6. Knuutinen A, et al. Smoking affects collagen synthesis and extracellular matrix turnover in human skin. *Br J Dermatol.* 2002;146:588–594.
7. Forsdahl SH, Singh K, Solberg S, et al. Risk factors for abdominal aortic aneurysms: a 7-year prospective study: the Trosmo study, 1994-2001. *Circulation.* 2009;119: 2202–2208.
8. Wanhainen A, et al. Risk factors associated with abdominal aortic aneurysm: a population-based study with historical and current data. *J Vasc Surg.* 2005;41:390–396.
9. Long A, et al. Prevalence of abdominal aortic aneurysm and large infrarenal aorta in patients with acute coronary syndrome and proven coronary stenosis: a prospective monocenter study. *Ann Vasc Surg.* 2010;24:602–608.
10. Dawson J, Choke E, Sayed S, et al. Pharmacotherapy of abdominal aortic aneurysms. *Curr Vasc Pharmacol.* 2006;4:129–149.
11. Coady MA, Davies RR, Roberts M, et al. Familial patterns of thoracic aneurysms. *Arch Surg.* 1999;134:361–367.
12. Lorelli DR, Jean-Cloude JM, Fox CJ, et al. response of plasma matrix metalloproteinase-9 to conventional abdominal aortic aneurysm and repair or endovascular exclusion: implications for endoleak. *J Vasc Surg.* 2002 may;35(5):916–922.
13. Hasham SN, Willing MC, Guo DC, et al. Mapping a locus for familial thoracic aneurysms and dissections (TAAD2) to 3p2425. *Circulation.* 2003;107:3184–3190.
14. Abdul-Hussien H, Hanemaaijer R, Kleemann R, et al. The pathophysiology of abdominal aortic aneurysm growth: corresponding and discordant inflammatory and proteolytic processes in abdominal aortic and popliteal artery aneurysms. *J Vasc Surg.* 2010;51:6.
15. Loeys CJ, Neptune ER, et al. A syndrome of altered cardiovascular, craniofacial, neurocognitive and skeletal development caused by mutations in TGFBR1 or TGFBR2. *Nat Genet.* 2005;37(3):275–281.
16. Epstein JA, Buck CA. Transcriptional regulation of cardiac development: implications for congenital heart disease and DiGeorge syndrome. *Pediatr Res.* 2000;48:717–724.
17. Grabenwöger M, Alfonso F, Bachet J, et al. Thoracic Endovascular Aortic Repair (TEVAR) for the treatment of aortic diseases: a position statement from the European Association for Cardio-Thoracic Surgery (EACTS) and the European Society of Cardiology (ESC), in collaboration with the European Association of Percutaneous Cardiovascular Interventions (EAPCI). *Eur Heart J.* 2012;33(13):1558–1563.
18. Gadowski GR, Pilcher DB, Ricci MA. Abdominal aortic aneurysm expansion rate: effect of size and beta-adrenergic blockade. *J Vasc Surg.* 1994;19:727–731.
19. Powell JT, Greenhalgh RM. Clinical practice. Small abdominal aortic aneurysms. *N Engl J Med.* 2003;348:1895–1901.
20. Rooke TW, Hirsch AT, Misra S, et al. 2011 ACCF/AHA focused update of the guideline for the management of patients with peripheral artery disease (updating the 2005 guideline). A report of the American College of Cardiology Foundation/American Heart Association Task Force on Practice Guidelines. *Circulation.* 2011;124:2020–2045.
21. Mészáros I, Mórocz J, Szlávi J, et al. Epidemiology and clinicopathology of aortic dissection. *Chest.* 2000;117:1271–1278.
22. Trimarchi S, Eagle KA, Nienaber CA, et al. Role of age in acute type A aortic dissection outcome: report from the

International Registry of Acute Aortic Dissection (iRAD). *J Thorac Cardiovasc Surg.* 2010;140:784–789.

23. Tsai TT, Fattori R, Trimarchi S, et al. Long-term survival in patients presenting with type B acute aortic dissection: insights from the International Registry of Acute Aortic Dissection. *Circulation.* 2006;114:2226–2231.

24. LeMaire SA, Russell L. Epidemiology of thoracic aortic dissection. *Nat Rev Cardiol.* 2011;8(2):103–113.

25. Eleftriades JA. Natural history of thoracic aortic aneurysms: indications for surgery, and surgical versus nonsurgical risks. *Ann Thorac Surg.* 2002;74:S1877–S1880.

26. Rampoldi V, Trimarchi S, Eagle KA, et al. Simple risk models to predict surgical mortality in acute type A aortic dissection: the International Registry of Acute Aortic Dissection score. *Ann Thorac Surg.* 2007;83(1): 55–61.

# CHAPTER 28

# Peripheral Artery Disease

JAMAL MOOSAVI, MD
Cardiovascular Intervention Research Center, Rajaie Cardiovascular, Medical & Research Center, Iran University of Medical Sciences, Tehran, Iran

---

### KEY POINTS

- In the presence of peripheral artery disease (PAD), the risk of cardiovascular events increases three- to fourfold, even in asymptomatic patients.
- Smoking and diabetes are the most predominant risk factors of PAD.
- The ankle-brachial index (ABI) is the method of choice to screen and establish the PAD diagnosis and has more than 90% sensitivity and specificity.
- Various imaging modalities have different indications for diagnosis of PAD and treatment planning.
- For the classification of PAD severity, Rutherford or Fontaine (clinical) and Trans-Atlantic Inter-Society Consensus II (TASC II) (anatomic) are commonly used.
- PAD screening programs with the main goal of cardiovascular event reduction are recommended to resolve the main concerns with PAD: underdiagnosis and undertreatment.
- Smoking cessation, antiplatelet therapy, statins, supervised exercise training, and cilostazol are the mainstays of non-invasive management of patients with PAD.
- If first-line therapies fail to improve patient symptoms, an endovascular-first approach is the preferred revascularization technique.
- In the setting of diabetic foot or critical limb ischemia (CLI), early diagnosis, proper management, and consistent follow-up in the context of a multidisciplinary approach remain the only solution to prevent amputation.

---

## EPIDEMIOLOGY

The prevalence of peripheral artery disease (PAD) as a reflection of systemic atherosclerosis is dramatically increasing with aging of the population. According to abnormal preliminary diagnostic tests such as the ankle-brachial index (ABI), the overall 3%–10% prevalence of PAD increases to 15%–20% in ages older than 70 years.[1]

The inflammatory nature and atherosclerotic basis of PAD pathology make this entity a mirror of increased risk of myocardial infarction (MI) and stroke in addition to impaired quality of life (QoL). The least important consequence of PAD underdiagnosis and undertreatment is the potential of developing critical limb ischemia (CLI). The risk of cardiovascular events, even in asymptomatic patients, increases three- to fourfold.[2]

The prevalence of PAD is similar between older men and postmenopausal women, but the classic symptoms of disease are more common among men, especially at a younger age.[3] A higher incidence of symptomatic PAD in men mirrors their greater disease severity.[4]

Among common risk factors of PAD with other atherosclerotic diseases, smoking and diabetes are predominant and independent, but hypertension and dyslipidemia contribute less risk.[5] It is worth pointing out that the leg amputation rate in diabetic patients is an indicator of health systems performance.[6]

## CLINICAL MANIFESTATIONS

Intermittent claudication (IC), as a typical and classic symptom of PAD, was originally described by Dr. Rose for the purposes of epidemiologic study. Nearly 50% of patients with PAD are asymptomatic, and only 10%–30% complain of IC. The remaining patients may have atypical leg pain on exertion or at rest or other symptoms such as reduced leg strength, impaired balance, slow walking speed, ischemic peripheral neuropathy, and functional decline.[7,8] These symptoms are in differential diagnosis with other causes of limb pain, including spinal stenosis, statin-induced myalgia, and orthopedic disorders.[9] Patients with atypical symptoms, compared with patients with classical IC, have poorer nerve sensation and a higher prevalence of diabetes and spinal stenosis with more comorbid conditions.[7] It is important to know that the greater functional decline means more advanced disease and increased cardiovascular events.

IC is defined by exercise-provoked muscular discomfort, primarily in the calf, which is relieved at rest. In PAD, progressive atherosclerosis leads to chronic occlusion of lower extremity arteries, and in contrast with coronary circulation, plaque rupture does not have any role in manifestations.[10]

CLI is the most severe clinical manifestation of PAD and presents as ischemic rest pain or a lesion with risk of tissue loss. CLI has a chronic nature and presents for a period of more than 2 weeks. Although only 1%–2% of patients with PAD develop CLI, the prognosis is very poor, with a 30% amputation rate and a 25% mortality during just 1 year after index presentation.[11]

Signs of PAD may include weak pulses, arterial bruits caused by turbulent flow, impaired capillary refill, pallor on elevation (or dependent rubor caused by impaired autoregulation in dermal arterioles), trophic changes, and skin discoloration as a consequence of chronic vasodilation, all of them present in advanced stages of the disease. Arterial ulcerations have a characteristic well-demarcated, "punched-out" appearance (Fig. 28.1).[12,13] Ulceration or gangrene of the toes occurs in the CLI group of patients[14] (Fig. 28.2).

Acute limb ischemia (ALI) is a vascular emergency caused by the sudden disruption of an extremity blood flow. The causes of ALI are acute thrombosis and, less commonly, embolic events from a central or proximal source such as cardiac structures. The "six Ps"—pain, pallor, pulselessness, paresthesia, paralysis, and poikilothermia—are the classical presentation of patients with ALI.

## DIAGNOSIS

ABI is the method of choice to screen and establish the diagnosis of a lower extremity PAD. ABI is an inexpensive and reproducible physiologic test that measures the ratio of the highest ankle systolic pressure in each leg, at the level of dorsalis pedis and posterior tibialis arteries using a handheld CW Doppler probe, to the highest brachial artery pressure.

$$ABI = \frac{\text{Highest ankle systolic pressure in each leg(mmHg)}}{\text{Highest brachial artery pressure in either arm}}$$

Patients with PAD typically have an ABI less than 0.90 at rest (90% sensitivity and 95% specificity), and this

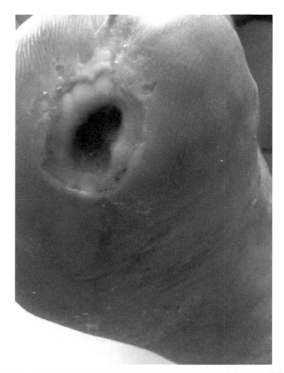

FIG. 28.1 Lower extremity ulceration induced by arterial insufficiency. The wound is located in an area of repetitive trauma and is characterized by a "punched-out" appearance. (From Foley TR, Armstrong EJ, Waldo SW. Contemporary evaluation and management of lower extremity peripheral artery disease. *Heart.* 2016;102:1436–1441, with permission.)

finding is associated with a higher than twice the mortality that is associated with an ABI of 1.1–1.4.[3] (Table 28.1).

An ABI of more than 1.40 indicates arterial calcification and noncompressibility of the tibial arteries, mostly caused by advanced age, diabetes, and chronic kidney disease (CKD). The toe-brachial index (TBI) is used in this situation. A TBI of less than 0.70 is considered diagnostic for lower extremity PAD.

In healthy adults, the dynamic system of rest-to-exercise transition increases limb blood flow 10-fold at low levels of exercise and 40-fold at high levels.[15] In patients with PAD, this system is markedly blunted, which is the result of fixed stenosis becoming flow limiting (critical arterial stenosis). In addition, significant abnormality of endothelium-dependent vasodilation of peripheral circulation contributes to the exercise impairment in PAD.[16]

Postexercise ABI enables the detection of patients who have normal or borderline ABI at rest but with a high clinical suspicion of PAD. Using a treadmill test for this purpose also helps to differentiate vascular

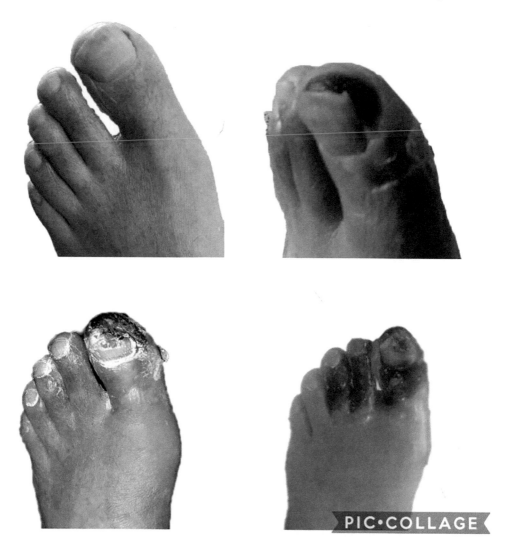

FIG. 28.2 Rapid progression of critical limb ischemia in an unlucky diabetic patient who did not seek proper care.

claudication from pseudoclaudication (leg pressure remains stable or even increases).[17] The exercise treadmill test with or without ABI is recommended as the most objective evidence of patients' functional limitation and to document the response to therapy.[18] A postexercise ABI of 0.90 or less or 20% or a greater drop in ABI after exercise is considered abnormal.

## Imaging

Duplex ultrasonography as an accurate imaging for assessment of lower extremity PAD location and severity is also useful to follow the patients after endovascular or surgical procedures, including femoral popliteal bypass with a venous conduit. The ultrasound criteria for diagnosis of a stenosis greater than 50% include[19]:

- Peak systolic velocity (PSV) greater than 200 cm/s
- PSV ratio (between the site of stenosis and adjacent normal vessel) more than 2.0
- Aliasing with color Doppler

Digital subtraction angiography (DSA) is the gold standard for diagnosis of PAD, but it will be gradually replaced by noninvasive imaging, including magnetic resonance angiography (MRA) and computed tomography angiography (CTA).

According to the American College of Cardiology/ American Heart Association (ACC/AHA) and European Society of Cardiology (ESC) guidelines, use of CTA or

**TABLE 28.1**
**Normal and Abnormal Values of Ankle-Brachial Index (ABI)**

| ABI | |
|---|---|
| 1–1.40 | Normal |
| 0.91–0.99 | Borderline |
| ≤0.90 | Abnormal |
| >1.40 | Noncompressible |
| **ABNORMAL ABI** | |
| 0.70–0.90 | Mild ischemia |
| 0.40–0.69 | Moderate ischemia |
| <0.40 | Critical ischemia |

MRA is supported for the diagnosis of anatomic location and degree of PAD stenosis, especially for patients who are candidates for surgical or endovascular intervention. The sensitivity and specificity of CTA or MR in this field reach up to 95% and more, especially in aortoiliac and femoral levels, compared with tibial arteries.[17,18]

Although duplex ultrasonography, CTA, and MRA all can be used to evaluate venous graft patency, duplex ultrasonography is not suitable for patency follow-up of synthetic conduits. Generally, CTA is superior to MRA for evaluation of stents (metallic or grafted) and is the diagnostic modality of choice.[20]

Visualization of calcification, stents, and bypasses is the great advantage of CTA, although in direct comparison, MRA has the ability to replace DSA to assist therapeutic decision-making, especially in the case of major allergies.[17] Overall, heavy calcification is a major limitation for noninvasive diagnostic purposes, but MRA is considered the modality of choice in this setting, which is common among patients with diabetes and CKD. In the presence of renal insufficiency, duplex ultrasonography and noncontrast MRA can be safely used.[20] As a nonradiation modality, MRA is technically more challenging than CTA and has some limitations, including an inability to use it in patients who have certain metallic or electronic implants and risk of nephrogenic systemic fibrosis caused by gadolinium in patients with CKD.[3]

Contrast angiography and DSA give detailed information about anatomy and are recommended when revascularization is planned for patients with lower extremity PAD.

Assessment of the affected arterial territory, including arterial inflow and outflow, is the main indication of contrast angiography. When the significance of an obstructive lesion is ambiguous, taking more angiographic views with different angulations and obtaining transstenotic gradients are indicated.

## Disease Severity Classification

Two most commonly used classifications for PAD symptoms are the Fontaine and Rutherford-Becker classifications (Table 28.2). Another classification system for PAD is the Trans-Atlantic Inter-Society Consensus (TASC II), which defines anatomic distribution of PAD at aortoiliac (Fig. 28.3) or femoropopliteal levels.

Typical IC characteristically manifests in the calves during walking, which quickly disappears at rest. In more proximal PAD (aortoiliac level), pain extends into the thighs and buttocks. Rest pain in the supine position (Rutherford category IV, Fontaine stage III) often is localized in the foot accompanied by a permanent cold sensation in the feet. Arterial ulcers are often painful and begin mostly at the level of toes or limb distal portions. These ulcers can be secondary to local trauma, mostly minor, and their healing process is often complicated by infection.[17] Limb ulcers caused by peripheral neuropathy are more common and in the absence of pain should be considered.

## Screening

Its asymptomatic nature, poor prognosis, and known treatment for PAD have led many guidelines to recommend screening programs for PAD in selected groups of

**TABLE 28.2**
**Peripheral Artery Disease Symptom Classification**

| | RUTHERFORD | | Fontaine |
|---|---|---|---|
| | Category | Grade | Stage |
| Asymptomatic | 0 | 0 | I |
| Mild claudication | 1 | I | IIa |
| Moderate claudication | 2 | | IIb |
| Severe claudication | 3 | | |
| Ischemic rest pain | 4 | II | III |
| Minor tissue loss | 5 | III | IV |
| Major tissue loss | 6 | | |

Mild claudication: for distances >200 m. Moderate claudication: for distances <200 m.

| | |
|---|---|
| **TASC A lesions**<br>• Unilateral or bilateral CIA stenoses<br>• Unilateral or bilateral single short (3 cm) EIA stenosis | 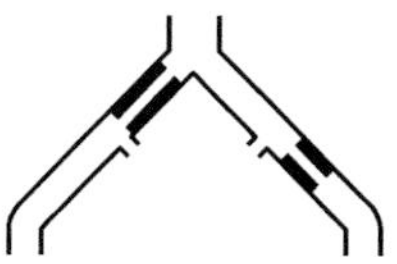 |
| **TASC B lesions**<br>• Short (3 cm) stenosis of the infrarenal aorta<br>• Unilateral CIA occlusion<br>• Single or multiple stenosis totaling 3–10 cm involving the EIA not extending into the CFA<br>• Unilateral EIA occlusion not involving the origins of the internal iliac or CFA | 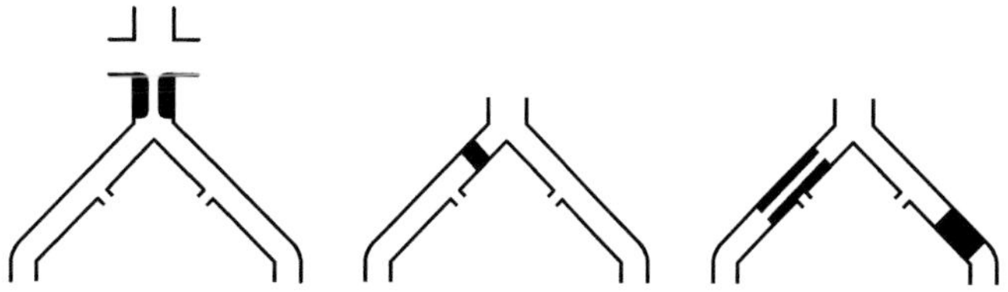 |
| **TASC C lesions**<br>• Bilateral CIA occlusions<br>• Bilateral EIA stenoses 3–10 cm long not extending into the CFA<br>• Unilateral EIA stenosis extending into the CFA<br>• Unilateral EIA occlusion involving the origins of the internal iliac and/or CFA<br>• Heavily calcified unilateral EIA occlusion with or without involvement of the origins of the internal iliac and/or CFA | 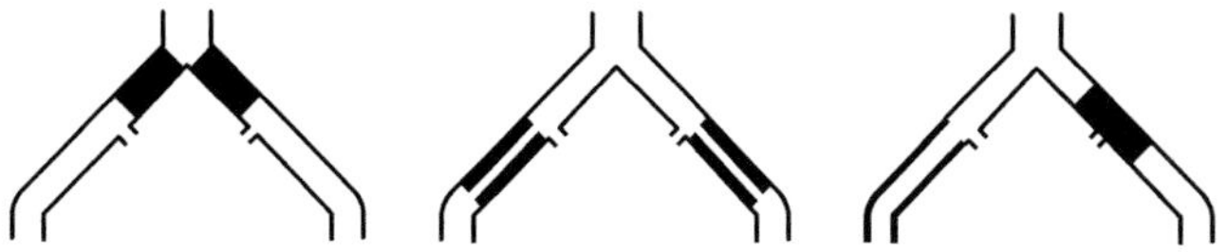 |
| **TASC D lesions**<br>• Infrarenal aortoiliac occlusion<br>• Diffuse disease involving the aorta and both iliac arteries<br>• Diffuse multiple stenoses involving the unilateral CIA, EIA, and CFA<br>• Unilateral occlusions of both CIA and EIA<br>• Bilateral EIA occlusions<br>• Iliac stenoses in patients with AAA not amenable to endograft placement | 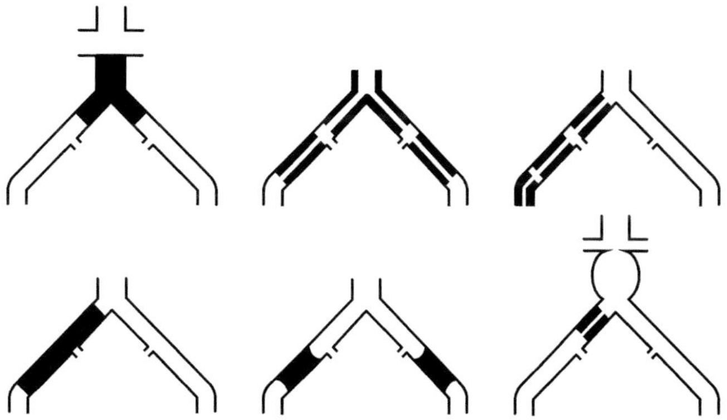 |

FIG. 28.3 Intersociety consensus for the management of peripheral arterial disease (Trans-Atlantic Inter-Society Consensus [TASC]) classification of aortoiliac lesions. *AAA*, abdominal aortic aneurysm; *CFA*, common femoral artery; *CIA*, common iliac artery; *EIA*, external iliac artery. (From the TASC Steering Committee. An update on methods for revascularization and expansion of the TASC lesion classification to include below-the-knee arteries: a supplement to the Inter-Society Consensus for the Management of Peripheral Arterial Disease (TASC II). *Ann Vasc Dis.* 2015;8(4):343–357, with permission.)

patients. The main goal of screening is to identify these patients to reduce their increased cardiovascular events. Progressive and nonhealing wounds and disabling amputations are other major concerns among these patients.

The ACC/AHA recommendation is to consider diagnostic ABI for the following conditions[18,21]:
• Age 65 years old or older
• Abnormal findings in history or examination suggestive of PAD

- Age 50–64 years with risk factors for atherosclerosis, including diabetes mellitus, smoking, hyperlipidemia, hypertension, or family history of PAD
- Age younger than 50 years with diabetes and one additional atherosclerosis risk factor
- Atherosclerotic involvement of another vascular bed including a coronary, carotid, subclavian, renal, mesenteric or abdominal aortic aneurysm

## TREATMENT

Current treatment of PAD is focused on four strategies:
1. Cardiovascular risk modification
2. Supervised exercise training
3. Medical therapy
4. Endovascular or surgical interventions

The goals of these therapies are to improve cardiovascular outcome and functional capacity in addition to preserving limb viability.[3]

### Antiplatelet and Anticoagulant Therapy

According to the updated recommendation of the ACC/AHA guidelines, antiplatelet therapy—typically aspirin in daily doses of 75–325 mg—in patients with PAD has a different level of indication as follows[18]:

a. Individuals with symptomatic atherosclerotic lower extremity PAD, including those with IC or CLI, have a class I indication to reduce the risk of MI, stroke, and vascular death. Clopidogrel (75 mg/day) is a safe alternative with the same indication.

b. Asymptomatic patients with ABIs of 0.90 or less have a class IIa indication.

c. For asymptomatic individuals who have borderline ABIs (0.91–0.99), antiplatelet therapy usefulness is not well established (class IIb).

Dual antiplatelet therapy (DAPT), including low-dose aspirin and clopidogrel, can be considered in patients with symptomatic PAD who do not have an increased risk of bleeding (class IIb).[18,22] The main use of DAPT is a 1–3-month prescription after endovascular intervention. Addition of warfarin to daily antiplatelet therapy in the absence of proven indications has no benefit (class III).

Vorapaxar as a novel antagonist of thrombin receptors has been studied in a randomized controlled trial (TRA2P-TIMI 50), which resulted in no reduction of cardiovascular death, MI, or stroke among patients with PAD, but vorapaxar significantly reduced the rate of ALI and peripheral revascularization despite an increased risk of bleeding.[23]

In the Cardiovascular Outcomes for People using Anticoagulant Strategies (COMPASS) trial on 27,395 patients with stable CAD/PAD, the rate of the primary outcomes, including of a composite of cardiovascular death, stroke, or MI, reduced by 24% with rivaroxaban 2.5 mg twice daily plus aspirin than with aspirin alone. Importantly, major bleeding was higher by 70% in the rivaroxaban group. The rate of ALI, major adverse limb event (MALE), and all vascular amputation (including major amputation) was significantly lower in the rivaroxaban arm of the PAD subgroup.[24–26]

The COMPASS trial has not included patients in the early period after surgical or endovascular revascularization. In the Vascular Outcomes studY of ASA alonG with rivaroxaban in Endovascular or surgical limb Revascularization for Peripheral Artery Disease (VOYAGER PAD) trial, rivaroxaban 2.5 mg twice daily plus aspirin, compared to aspirin alone, decreased the rate of ALI, major amputation, MI, and ischemic stroke from 19.9% to 17.3% although bleeding concerns still persist.[27]

### Statins

In all patients with PAD, guidelines support treatment with a high-intensity statin to achieve a low-density lipoprotein (LDL) level of less than 70 mg/dL or decreased by at least 50% if the initial LDL level is between 70 and 135 mg/dL.[17]

Otherwise, the REACH (Reduction of Atherothrombosis for Continued Health) registry showed strain therapy impact on limb prognosis in symptomatic patients with PAD. Adverse limb outcomes, including amputation, with statin therapy reduced significantly ($\approx$18%), in addition to a decrease in cardiovascular events.[28,29]

### Glycemic Control

The prognosis of PAD in patients with diabetes is poorer, with a risk of amputation five times more than in patients without diabetes.[30] The severity and duration of diabetes influence the incidence and the extent of PAD, particularly in active smokers and men with hypertension.[30,31] However, tight glycemic control does not reduce macrovascular complications in patients with PAD, in contrast with microvascular diseases.

However, current guidelines recommend an $HbA_1C$ of less than 7% by glucose control therapies to improve both microvascular and probably cardiovascular outcomes in patients with PAD (class IIa).[32] On the other hand, proper foot care with urgent treatment of skin lesions is of the utmost importance.

### Smoking Cessation

Most studies have shown that smoking is the strongest and most modifiable independent risk factor for PAD development. PAD incidence among smokers increases about fourfold, even more than the risk of atherosclerosis in the other arterial territories.[33] Smoking cessation decreases the rate of cardiovascular events, CLI, and amputations; thus, patients with PAD should be helped to quit smoking using behavioral and pharmacologic strategies. All modalities that help patients to stop smoking, including varenicline, bupropion, and nicotine replacement, have a class I recommendation in the guidelines.[18]

### Antihypertensive Therapy

Hypertension treatment in PAD patients has a class I recommendation to reduce the risk of stroke and cardiovascular events. Angiotensin-converting enzyme (ACE) inhibitors, especially ramipril, are the most well-known class of antihypertensives studied in patients with PAD. To reduce the risk of cardiovascular events, ACE inhibitors are recommended in the guidelines for symptomatic patients with PAD as a class IIa recommendation and for asymptomatic patients with PAD as a class IIb recommendation,[18] irrespective of hypertension.

Otherwise, among patients with PAD, the target level of blood pressure should be less than 140/90 mmHg for patients without diabetes and less than 130/80 mmHg for patients with diabetes or CKD (class I). In a randomized trial, targeting a systolic blood pressure of less than 120 mmHg among a high-risk group of patients resulted in lower rates of cardiovascular events and death.[34]

For the treatment of hypertension in patients with PAD, even beta-adrenergic blockers are effective and are not contraindicated, although ACE inhibitors are the preferred class of antihypertensives for them.

### Supervised Exercise Training

Among patients with PAD, peak exercise performance has a claudication-limited peak that is improved by exercise training.[35] The main goal of supervised exercise training is an improvement in the QoL and patient function.[8] To achieve the best result, a minimum of 12 weeks of exercise at least three sessions per week for 30–45 min is recommended as an initial therapy of IC (class I recommendation).[18] Another benefit of exercise training in patients with PAD is reduction of all-cause and cardiovascular mortality.[36]

ERASE (Endovascular Revascularization and Supervised Exercise for Peripheral Artery Disease) is a randomized controlled trial among patients complaining of IC, which showed a combination therapy, including endovascular revascularization followed by supervised exercise training, has the greatest improvement in QoL among patients with PAD.[37]

Even a structured community or home-based exercise program with the guidance of healthcare providers is reasonable (class IIa) and can be beneficial to improve walking ability.

### Specific Drugs for Treatment of Claudication

Dedicated drugs for treatment or improvement of PAD symptoms (namely IC) in current practice are limited. Traditional vasoactive drugs, including cilostazol and pentoxifylline, in addition to other vasoactive agents such as naftidrofuryl and inositol nicotinate, are prescribed by vascular specialists for symptom relief of these patients.

#### Cilostazol

This drug is an oral phosphodiesterase-3 inhibitor with both a vasodilatory effect and platelet aggregation inhibitory mechanism. Cilostazol improves maximum walking distance by more than 50%.[38] Some data suggest that cilostazol may decrease intimal hyperplasia growth after endovascular therapy and reduce the rate of restenosis.[39]

Cilostazol (100 mg twice daily) is a class I recommendation of guidelines to improve symptoms in the absence of heart failure and should be considered for a primary therapeutic trial in all patients with lifestyle-limiting claudication. Maximum benefits of cilostazol take 4 months to occur. The most known adverse effects of cilostazol include tachycardia, diarrhea, headache, dizziness, and increased bleeding tendency. Mechanistic similarity to other type III phosphodiesterase inhibitors such as milrinone is the main reason for contraindication of cilostazol in heart failure patients. About 20% of patients may discontinue this drug during 3 months of treatment.

#### Pentoxifylline

In today's practice, this drug is rarely prescribed to improve claudication because functional benefit compared with placebo is marginal. Alteration in the hemorheologic profile of red blood cells and blood viscosity reduction are the main mechanisms of action of pentoxifylline. Current guidelines believe pentoxifylline is not effective for treatment of claudication and no longer is recommended (class III).

#### Other Treatments

As a serotonin 5-Hz receptor blocker, naftidrofuryl has vasoactive and hemorheologic properties with favorable effects on oxidative metabolism and peripheral transcutaneous oxygen pressure.[40] Naftidrofuryl has been available in Europe for more than 3 decades and increases pain-free walking distance significantly ($\approx$26% compared with placebo). This drug is more cost-effective than cilostazol.[41]

Chelation therapy and homocysteine level lowering have no benefit for treatment of IC and reducing cardiovascular events in PAD patients (class III).

Annual influenza vaccination is strongly recommended in PAD patients (class I).

## Endovascular or Surgical Intervention

If the patient's symptoms and lifestyle fail to improve favorably after first-line treatments, including risk factor modification in addition to exercise and medical therapy, invasive strategies are indicated. An endovascular-first approach is the preferred revascularization technique mostly because of the shorter length of hospitalization and lower procedural morbidity and mortality rates with comparable results.

The TASC category of lesion length does not predict restenosis, so even most complex lesions can be addressed by endovascular strategy if operator expertise and institutional capabilities are appropriate.[8] Three levels of obstruction—aortoiliac, femoropopliteal, and tibioperoneal—will be discussed here.

### Aortoiliac Disease

For the treatment of aortoiliac occlusive disease, the most recommended points include:

- Endovascular-first approach
- The primary patency rate during 24 months is more than 85%.
- In borderline lesions, the translesional pressure gradient should be obtained.
- Stenting is effective primary therapy, especially for nonfocal common iliac occlusions.
- Stenting of the common femoral artery is generally avoided because of stent fracture risk caused by hip movements.
- A covered stent is an option, preferably for long total occlusions with probably a lower restenosis rate compared with noncovered stents (COBEST [Covered versus Balloon Expandable Stent Trial]) in addition to minimizing the fatal bleeding risk.

### Femoropopliteal Disease

The superficial femoral artery (SFA), as the longest artery with the fewest side branches, is subjected to external mechanical stresses, including flexion, compression, and torsion, which significantly affect clinical outcomes and the patency results of this region after endovascular revascularization. Restenosis, stent fracture, and thrombosis are the major concerns after SFA intervention.[42] Practical points for endovascular intervention in this territory are as follows:

- Endovascular-first approach
- Primary stenting efficacy is not well established, and there is controversy in the guidelines. Currently, intermediate to long SFA lesions (more complex occlusions) are treated by primary stenting.[8]
- Other adjunctive therapies such as atherectomy devices or cutting balloons may be used.

- If stenting is planned, nitinol self-expanding stents should be deployed because of external pressure in this region, which distorts the stents.
- Drug-coated balloons offer some advantages for intervention of femoropopliteal lesions, including a superior patency rate compared with percutaneous transluminal angioplasty alone or bare metal stents and avoiding stent complications such as stent fracture.
- Other technologies such as dedicated covered or drug-coated stents have shown very promising results in treatment of femoropopliteal lesions.
- Prophylactic endovascular intervention in asymptomatic patients with lower extremity PAD has no indication.

### Tibioperoneal Disease

For patients with below-the-knee disease, revascularization is indicated just for limb salvage in the CLI stage, and claudication rarely mandates invasive strategy. Practical pearls for the intervention in the context of CLI include:

- Endovascular-first strategy
- In patients with CLI with both inflow and outflow occlusions, the inflow level should be treated first.
- In current practice and guidelines, balloon angioplasty alone is the standard of therapy. Bare metal stents are used just in bailout situations such as flow-limiting flap of dissection.
- The concept of endovascular intervention in CLI patients is to establish at least a straight-line flow from the hip to the foot ulcer.[8]
- Intervention according to the feeding vascular territory of the foot ulcer is a relatively new strategy (angiosome concept) that improves the prognosis of the disease.
- Ongoing trials about the use of dedicated drug-coated stents or balloons may change the future guidelines.

## REFERENCES

1. Dua A, Lee CJ. Epidemiology of peripheral arterial disease and critical limb ischemia. *Tech Vasc Interv Radiol.* 2016; 19 (2):91–95. (2016). https://doi.org/10.1053/j.tvir.2016.04.001 Epub 2016 Apr 22.
2. Leng GC, Fowkes FG, Lee AJ, Dunbar J, Housley E, Ruckley CV. Use of ankle brachial pressure index to predict cardiovascular events and death: a cohort study. *BMJ.* 1996; 313:1440–1444.
3. Kullo IJ, Rooke TW. Peripheral artery disease. *N Engl J Med.* 2016; 374:861–871. (2016). https://doi.org/10.1056/NEJMcp1507631 March 3, 2016.

4. Collins TC, Suarez-Almazor M, Bush RL, et al. Gender and peripheral arterial disease. *J Am Board Fam Med.* 2006; 19:132–140.

5. Joosten MM, Pai JK, Bertoia ML, et al. Associations between conventional cardiovascular risk factors and risk of peripheral artery disease in men. *JAMA.* 2012; 308: 1660–1667.

6. Carinci F, Massi Benedetti M, Klazinga NS, Uccioli L. Lower extremity amputation rates in people with diabetes as an indicator of health systems performance. A critical appraisal of the data collection 2000-2011 by the Organization for Economic Cooperation and Development (OECD). *Acta Diabetol.* 2016; 53(5): 825–832. https://doi.org/10.1007/s00592-016-0879-4.

7. McDermott MM, Greenland P, Liu K, et al. Leg symptoms in peripheral arterial disease: associated clinical characteristics and functional impairment. *JAMA.* 2001; 286:1599–1606.

8. Olin JW, White CJ, Armstrong EJ, Kadian-Dodov D, Hiatt WR. Peripheral artery disease: evolving role of exercise, medical therapy, and endovascular options. *J Am Coll Cardiol.* 2016; 67(11):1338–1357. (2016). https://doi.org/10.1016/j.jacc.2015.12.049 Review.

9. Hiatt WR, Armstrong EJ, Larson CJ, Brass EP. Pathogenesis of the limb manifestations and exercise limitations in peripheral artery disease. *Circ Res.* 2015; 116(9): 1527–1539. (2015). https://doi.org/10.1161/CIRCRESAHA. 116.303566.

10. Goldschmidt-Clermont PJ, Creager MA, Losordo DW, et al. Atherosclerosis 2005: recent discoveries and novel hypotheses. *Circulation.* 2005; 112:3348–3353. (2005). https://doi.org/10.1161/CIRCULATIONAHA.105.577460.

11. Norgren L, Hiatt WR, Dormandy JA, et al. Inter-society consensus for the management of peripheral arterial disease (TASC II). *J Vasc Surg.* 2007; 45(suppl. S):S5–S67.

12. Foley TR, Armstrong EJ, Waldo SW. Contemporary evaluation and management of lower extremity peripheral artery disease. *Heart.* 2016; 102(18):1436–1441. (2016). https://doi.org/10.1136/heartjnl-2015-309076 Epub 2016 Jun 1.

13. Wennberg PW. Approach to the patient with peripheral arterial disease. *Circulation.* 2013; 128:2241–2250.

14. Shafe O, et al. Multidisciplinary therapeutic and active follow-up protocols to reduce the rate of amputations and cardiovascular morbidities in patients with critical limb ischemia: IRANCLI study design and rationale—a prospective single-center registry in Iran. *Res Cardiovasc Med.* 2019; 8(2):46–53. https://doi.org/10.4103/rcm.rcm_22_19.

15. Hiatt WR, Marsh RC, Brammell HL, Fee C, Horwitz LD. Effect of aerobic conditioning on the peripheral circulation during chronic beta-adrenergic blockade. *J Am Coll Cardiol.* 1984; 4:958–963.

16. Bragadeesh T, Sari I, Pascotto M, Micari A, Kaul S, Lindner JR. Detection of peripheral vascular stenosis by assessing skeletal muscle flow reserve. *J Am Coll Cardiol.* 2005; 45:780–785. (2005). https://doi.org/10.1016/j. jacc.2004.11.045.

17. Aboyans V, et al. 2017 ESC Guidelines on the Diagnosis and Treatment of Peripheral Arterial Diseases, in collaboration with the European Society for Vascular Surgery (ESVS). *Eur J Vasc Endovasc Surg.* 2018; 55(3):305–368. (2018). https://doi.org/10.1016/j.ejvs.2017.07.018.

18. Gerhard-Herman MD, et al. 2016 AHA/ACC guideline on the management of patients with lower extremity peripheral artery disease. *Vasc Med.* 2017; 22(3): NP1–NP43. (2017). https://doi.org/10.1177/1358863X 17701592.

19. Rooke TW, Hirsch AT, Misra S, et al. Management of patients with peripheral artery disease (compilation of 2005 and 2011 ACCF/AHA guideline recommendations): a report of the American College of Cardiology Foundation/American Heart Association Task Force on Practice Guidelines. *J Am Coll Cardiol.* 2013; 61:1555–1570.

20. Pollak AW, Norton PT, Kramer CM. Multimodality imaging of lower extremity peripheral arterial disease: current role and future directions. *Circ Cardiovasc Imaging.* 2012; 5(6):797–807. Review. No abstract available. PMID 23169982 (web archive link)(2012). https://doi.org/10.1161/CIRCIMAGING.111.970814.

21. Sorensen J, Wilks SA, Jacob AD, Huynh TT. Screening for peripheral artery disease. *Semin Roentgenol.* 2015; 50(2): 139–147. (2015). https://doi.org/10.1053/j.ro.2014.10. 011 Epub 2014 Oct 18.

22. Cacoub PP, Bhatt DL, Steg PG, Topol EJ, Creager MA. Patients with peripheral arterial disease in the CHARISMA trial. *Eur Heart J.* 2009; 30:192–201.

23. Bonaca MP, Scirica BM, Creager MA, et al. Vorapaxar in patients with peripheral artery disease: results from TRA2° P-TIMI 50. *Circulation.* 2013; 127(14):1522–1529. 1529e1–1529e6(2013). https://doi.org/10.1161/CIRCUL ATIONAHA.112.000679.

24. Eikelboom JW, Connolly SJ, Bosch J, et al. Rivaroxaban with or without aspirin in stable cardiovascular disease. *N Engl J Med.* 2017; 377(14):1319–1330.

25. Anand SS, Bosch J, Eikelboom JW, et al. Rivaroxaban with or without aspirin in patients with stable peripheral or carotid artery disease: an international, randomized, double-blind, placebo-controlled trial. *Lancet.* 2018; 391 (10117):219–229.

26. Anand SS, Caron F, Eikelboom JW, et al. Major adverse limb events and mortality in patients with peripheral artery disease: the COMPASS Trial. *J Am Coll Cardiol.* 2018; 71(20):2306–2315.

27. Bonaca MP, Bauersachs RM, Anand SS, et al. Rivaroxaban in peripheral artery disease after revascularization. *N Engl J Med.* 2020; 382(21):1994–2004.

28. Kumbhani DJ, Steg PG, Cannon CP, et al. Statin therapy and long-term adverse limb outcomes in patients with peripheral artery disease: insights from the REACH registry. *Eur Heart J.* 2014; 35:2864–2872.

29. Piepoli MF, Hoes AW, Agewall S, et al. 2016 European Guidelines on cardiovascular disease prevention in clinical practice: the Sixth Joint Task Force of the European Society of Cardiology and Other Societies on Cardiovascular

Disease Prevention in Clinical Practice (constituted by representatives of 10 societies and by invited experts). Developed with the special contribution of the European Association for Cardiovascular Prevention & Rehabilitation (EACPR). *Eur Heart J.* 2016; 37:2315e81.

30. Jude EB, Oyibo SO, Chalmers N, Boulton AJ. Peripheral arterial disease in diabetic and nondiabetic patients: a comparison of severity and outcome. *Diabetes Care.* 2001; 24(8):1433–1437.

31. Marso SP, Hiatt WR. Peripheral arterial disease in patients with diabetes. *J Am Coll Cardiol.* 2006; 47:921–929. PMID 16516072 (web archive link)(2006). https://doi.org/10.1016/j.jacc.2005.09.065.

32. Foley TR, Waldo SW, Armstrong EJ. Medical therapy in peripheral artery disease and critical limb ischemia. *Curr Treat Options Cardiovasc Med.* 2016; 18(7):42. Review. PMID 27181397 (web archive link)(2016). https://doi.org/10.1007/s11936-016-0464-8.

33. Criqui MH, Aboyans V. Epidemiology of peripheral artery disease. *Circ Res.* 2015; 116(9):1509–1526. Review. Erratum in: *Circ Res.* 2015;117(1):e12. PMID 25908725 (web archive link)(2015). https://doi.org/10.1161/CIRCRESAHA.116.303849.

34. Wright JT, Williamson JD, Whelton PK, et al. A randomized trial of intensive versus standard blood-pressure control. *N Engl J Med.* 2015; 373:2103–2116.

35. Hiatt WR, Regensteiner JG, Wolfel EE, Carry MR, Brass EP. Effect of exercise training on skeletal muscle histology and metabolism in peripheral arterial disease. *J Appl Physiol.* 1985; 1996(81):780–788.

36. Sakamoto S, Yokoyama N, Tamori Y, Akutsu K, Hashimoto H, Takeshita S. Patients with peripheral artery disease who complete 12-week supervised exercise training program show reduce cardiovascular mortality and morbidity. *Circ J.* 2009; 73:167–173.

37. Fakhry F, Spronk S, van der Laan L, et al. Endovascular revascularization and supervised exercise for peripheral artery disease and intermittent claudication: a randomized clinical trial. *JAMA.* 2015; 314:1936–1944.

38. Thompson PD, Zimet R, Forbes WP, et al. Meta-analysis of results from eight randomized, placebo-controlled trials on the effect of cilostazol on patients with intermittent claudication. *Am J Cardiol.* 2002; 90:1314–1319.

39. Benjo AM, Garcia DC, Jenkins JS, et al. Cilostazol increases patency and reduces adverse outcomes in percutaneous femoropopliteal revascularisation: a meta-analysis of randomised controlled trials. *Open Heart.* 2014; 1: e000154.

40. Barradell LB, Brogden RN. Oral naftidrofuryl. A review of its pharmacology and therapeutic use in the management of peripheral occlusive arterial disease. *Drugs Aging.* 1996; 8(4):299–322.

41. Lehert P, Comte S, Gamand S, Brown TM. Naftidrofuryl in intermittent claudication: a retrospective analysis. *J Cardiovasc Pharmacol.* 1994; 23(suppl. 3):S48–S52.

42. Thukkani AK, Kinlay S. Endovascular intervention for peripheral artery disease. *Circ Res.* 2015; 116 (9):1599–1613. Review. PMID 25908731 (web archive link)(2015). https://doi.org/10.1161/CIRCRESAHA.116.303503.

# CHAPTER 29

# Cardiomyopathies and Myocarditis

NASIM NADERI

Rajaie Cardiovascular, Medical & Research Center, Iran University of Medical Sciences, Tehran, Iran

## BACKGROUND

Cardiomyopathy is a cardiac disorder leading to cardiac muscle dysfunction. Mechanical or electrical abnormalities of cardiac muscle cells causing impaired myocardial performance may lead to heart failure, arrhythmias, or both.

Cardiomyopathies are complex disorders of multifactorial pathogenesis and have a high mortality and morbidity. The pathogenesis of each subtype is unique, and diagnosis of the type of cardiomyopathy is essential for prognostication and care management options. In the past decades, there have been many definitions of cardiomyopathies and revisions of classification systems due to new results of investigations.

The MOGE(S) classification system for cardiomyopathies was proposed by Arbustini et al. in 2013. It is a phenotype–genotype-based classification system based on five attributes, including morpho-functional characteristics (M), organ involvement (O), genetic or familial inheritance pattern (G), etiological annotation (E), and optional information about the heart failure functional status (S), the functional status (S) using the heart failure A–D stages and/or NYHA functional classes I–IV (Table 29.1).

The morphological and functional subtype provides the basis of this classification system and the major clinical decisions are still based on morphofunctional characteristics.

The genetic information is also important for the diagnostic assessments, treatment decisions, and follow-up plans. The consideration of genotype in the description of the cardiomyopathies is increasingly becoming a routine, as it has been shown that mutations in the same gene may lead to different phenotypes, whereas different gene mutations can lead to indistinguishable phenotypes.[1,2]

## DILATED CARDIOMYOPATHY[1–12]

Dilated cardiomyopathy is characterized by increased cardiac chamber size (most commonly the left ventricle [LV]). The ventricular wall thickness may be normal or decreased. DCM is a common cause of heart transplantation and is classified into several subtypes. The mainstay of treatment in all forms of DCM is to appropriately address the underlying cause accompanied by implementation of guideline-directed heart failure therapies. Table 29.2 presents the subtypes of DCM.

### Key Points About Peripartum Cardiomyopathy[8,11–13]

The exact cause of peripartum cardiomyopathy (PPCM) is not known, but nutritional deficiency, salt overload, myocarditis, and autoimmune processes and genetic causes have been suggested.

The first step in diagnosis is to exclude the usual causes of LV systolic dysfunction.

Preeclampsia has been proposed as a risk factor.

Echocardiography should be performed as soon as possible in all women suspected with PPCM. Normal echocardiography suggests noncardiogenic pulmonary edema or lung disorders.

Severe diastolic dysfunction in the setting of preeclampsia makes patients prone to the development of pulmonary edema.

Patients with heart failure with reduced ejection fraction (HFrEF) during pregnancy are treated the same as nonpregnant women.

Loop diuretics, hydralazine and nitrates, beta-blockers, and digoxin can be used in pregnancy.

Angiotensin-converting enzyme (ACE) inhibitors and angiotensin receptor blockers (ARBs) are contraindicated and should be avoided because of the risk of fetal renal dysgenesis and death.

Anticoagulation with heparin should also be instituted because of the risk of thromboembolism in PPCM. Warfarin can be used safely in the third trimester and then switched to heparin before delivery.

Close monitoring in an intensive care unit is recommended in this setting, and it is better for both the mother and the fetus if the patients are transferred to a tertiary care center.

## TABLE 29.1
### Attributes of the MOGE(S) Classification

| Morphofunctional | Organ/System Involvement | Genetic | Etiology | | Stage | |
|---|---|---|---|---|---|---|
| D—dilated | H—heart | N—family history negative | G—genetic etiology | G-OC—obligate carrier | ACC-AHA | A |
| | | | | G-ONC—obligate noncarrier | | B |
| | | | | G-DN—de novo | | C |
| | | | | G-Neg—genetic test negative | | D |
| | | | | G-N—genetic test not identified | | NU—not used |
| | | | | G-A—genetic amyloidosis | | NA—not applicable |
| H—hypertrophic | M—muscle/skeletal | U—family history unknown | 0—no genetic test | | NYHA | I |
| | | | | | | II |
| | | | | | | II |
| | | | | | | IV |
| H(Obs)—hypertrophic obstructive | N—nervous | AD—autosomal dominant | M—myocarditis | | | |
| H(noObs)—hypertrophic non obstructive | C—cutaneous | AR—autosomal recessive | V—viral infection | | | |
| R—restrictive | E—eye | XLR—X-linked recessive | AI—autoimmune/immune-mediated | | | |
| A—ARVC | A—auditory | XLD—X-linked dominant | AI-S—autoimmune immune-mediated suspected | | | |
| NC—LVNC | K—kidney | XL—X-linked | AI-P—autoimmune immune-mediated proven | | | |
| NS—nonspecific phenotype | G—gastrointestinal | M—matrilinear | A—amyloidosis | | | |
| NA—information not available | S—skeletal | 0 | I—infectious, nonviral | | | |
| E(D)—early diagnosis of dilated | Lu—lung | Under—inheritance still undetermined | T—toxicity | | | |
| E(H)—early diagnosis of hypertrophic | Li—liver | S—phenotypically sporadic | Eo—hypereosinophilic heart disease | | | |
| 0—unaffected | 0—absence of organ/system involvement | | A-K amyloidosis type K | | | |
| E(R)—early diagnosis of restrictive | | | A-L—amyloidosis type L | | | |
| E(A)—early diagnosis of ARVC | | | A-SAA—amyloidosis type SAA | | | |
| R EMF—endomyocardial fibrosis | | | Other | | | |

Attributes of cardiomyopathies available in the MOGE(S) classification.

From Westphal JG, Rigopoulos AG, Bakogiannis C, et al. The MOGE(S) classification for cardiomyopathies: current status and future outlook. *Heart Fail Rev.* 2017;22(6):743–752.

**TABLE 29.2**
**Subtypes of Dilated Cardiomyopathies**

| Subtype | Description |
|---|---|
| Ischemic (most common cause of DCM) | The cause of cardiac dysfunction is ischemic heart disease. |
| Idiopathic | The cause of cardiac dysfunction remains unexplained in many cases of DCM. However, it may be caused by failure to identify known causes (e.g., myocarditis, toxin). |
| Familial | The presence of idiopathic DCM in two (or more) first- or second-degree relatives of an individual with idiopathic DCM. Genetic testing is indicated in patients with these criteria. Inheritance is generally autosomal dominant; however, autosomal recessive and X-linked cases have also been reported. Family screening is recommended for all patients with idiopathic DCM. |
| Alcoholic | Long-term and heavy alcohol consumption can be an etiology for DCM. These patients have history of excessive alcohol intake and physical signs of alcohol abuse (mental status change, telangiectasia and spider angiomata, cirrhosis, and parotid disorder). The mainstay of therapy for alcoholic cardiomyopathy is complete and everlasting abstinence from alcohol consumption. Alcohol abstinence is more efficacious in the early stages of disease. Conventional heart failure therapies should also be initiated for these patients. |
| Peripartum (PPCM) | An idiopathic cardiomyopathy presents at the last month of pregnancy or in up to 6 months after delivery. PPCM manifests clinically by heart failure signs and symptoms. It is more common in multiparous women. The patients develop severe left ventricular systolic dysfunction with pulmonary and systemic congestion, which may be complicated by ventricular arrhythmias and thromboembolism. However, PPCM has the best prognosis among all forms of DCM. |
| Chemotherapy induced | Anthracyclines, widely used antineoplastic agents, have a high degree of cardiotoxicity. The development of heart failure with these agents is dose dependent and may present both early acute (from the onset of exposure to several weeks after drug infusion) and chronic forms of cardiotoxicity. Other chemotherapy agents with cardiotoxic effects include cyclophosphamide, trastuzumab, and other monoclonal antibody-based tyrosine kinase inhibitors. See also Chapter 41 for more details |
| AIDS induced | Development of DCM in patients with AIDS. The mechanism of cardiomyopathy is poorly understood. The potential causes of AIDS CMP are inflammatory reactions, cytokine effects, HIV-1, various opportunistic infections, and cardiotoxicity of prescribed antiretrovirals or illicit drugs. |
| Tachycardia induced | In this type of cardiomyopathy, LV function becomes normal after successful and on-time treatment of tachycardia. The LV dysfunction may be irreversible if the arrhythmia is left untreated. Thus, a high level of suspicion is needed for early detection and treatment. Common causes include chronic atrial fibrillation with rapid ventricular response and frequent premature ventricular contractions (more than thousands daily). |
| Associated with collagen vascular disease | Development of DCM in patients with any type of connective tissue disease, including SLE, systemic sclerosis, or Takayasu arteritis. |

*CMP*, cardiomyopathy; *DCM*, dilated cardiomyopathy; *LV*, left ventricular; *SLE*, systemic lupus erythematosus.

Vaginal delivery is the preferred method for delivery. Stable patients should be managed medically until spontaneous vaginal delivery.

For women with unstable hemodynamics and progressive cardiac dysfunction despite medical therapies, intra-aortic balloon pump (IABP), mechanical circulatory support (MCS), or heart transplantation may be considered.

Inotropic agents can be used in the setting of cardiogenic shock.

After delivery, standard heart failure therapies should be continued, and the combination of hydralazine and nitrate can be replaced by an ACE inhibitor or ARB. There is some evidence that postpartum use of bromocriptine and pentoxifylline could be useful in improving LV systolic function and outcomes in PPCM.

## ARRHYTHMOGENIC RIGHT VENTRICULAR CARDIOMYOPATHY[14-17]

In ARVC, the myocardium of the right ventricle (RV) is replaced by fibrofatty tissue, leading to an increased risk of arrhythmia and sudden cardiac death. The disease is inherited as autosomal dominant, and the LV can also be involved in some cases. The RV and right ventricular outflow tract (RVOT) are dilated.

- Cardiac magnetic resonance (CMR) imaging is very useful in the diagnosis of ARVC (see also Chapter 8).
- The mainstays of treatment are prevention and suppression of ventricular arrhythmias.
- An implantable cardioverter defibrillator (ICD) is recommended in patients with syncope, aborted sudden cardiac death, and LV systolic dysfunction.
- Catheter ablation of ventricular tachycardia is recommended in some patients.
- Treatment of the sign and symptoms of RV failure has been discussed in more detail in Chapter 12.

## RESTRICTIVE CARDIOMYOPATHY[1,18-34]
### Background

Restrictive cardiomyopathy is a rare condition in which the cardiac chambers are stiff and sometimes thick. The stiff myocardium cannot be relaxed in diastole (diastolic stiffness or reduced compliance), leading to elevation of ventricular filling pressures. The systolic function is usually normal or near normal, except in the late stage of the disease. An inability of optimal ventricular filling leads to failure in augmentation of stroke volume during exercise and development of heart failure symptoms.

Restrictive cardiomyopathy is grouped into four categories: idiopathic, infiltrative, malignancy, and treatment induced.

### Key Points About Restrictive Cardiomyopathy

RCM is the least common type of cardiomyopathy and may have a genetic cause. However, only a few mutations have been found in this regard.

The most important differential diagnosis of RCM is constrictive pericarditis.

RCM is asymptomatic in the early stages, so establishment of the diagnosis is very difficult early in the clinical course, and many cases are diagnosed very late. Therefore, the prognosis is usually poor in this condition.

### Idiopathic Primary Restrictive Cardiomyopathy[19,24,27]

Patients with idiopathic RCM have heart failure symptoms and restrictive hemodynamics without significant ventricular hypertrophy and endocardial fibrosis or thickening. Male and female patients are equally affected. The disease is more aggressive in children, and LV dysfunction is frequently seen in pediatric RCM. A familial pattern is seen in some cases.

The presenting symptoms are left- and right-sided heart failure, and as many as one-third of patients may present with thromboembolic events such as deep vein thrombosis, pulmonary emboli, or systemic emboli. Atrial fibrillation is common in idiopathic RCM. These patients are at very high risk for systemic embolic events.

### Infiltrative Restrictive Cardiomyopathy[18,21,22,26,29,30,32,33,35,36]

The site of infiltration in infiltrative RCM may be the myocardium or endocardium and may be caused by the following:

- Eosinophilic cardiomyopathy and endomyocardial fibrosis
- Amyloidosis
- Hemochromatosis
- Sarcoidosis
- Carcinoid syndrome
- Glycogen storage diseases (Fabry disease)
- Metastatic malignancy
- Radiation-induced cardiomyopathy

### Key Points About Eosinophilic Cardiomyopathy (Loeffler Endocarditis) and Endomyocardial Fibrosis[32,33,37]

Severe prolonged eosinophilia from any reason (idiopathic, allergic, leukemic, autoimmune, or parasitic) may lead to eosinophilic infiltration.

This type of RCM is associated with dense fibrosis of the endomyocardium and intracavitary thrombus formation, which may lead to obliteration of the LV cavity in late stages.

Echocardiography may be helpful for diagnosis. The apex of both ventricles is obliterated by the thrombus in the absence of regional wall motion abnormality. The mitral valve is thickened with significant mitral regurgitation.

Due to its ability to better characterize endomyocardial tissue involvement, the CMR is a valuable tool for accurate diagnosing, monitoring the Loeffler endocarditis at any stage of the disease.

The prognosis is poor, and there is no specific therapy. Corticosteroids interferon, hydroxyurea, and other immunosuppressant or cytotoxic medications as well as endocardiectomy have been recommended.

## Amyloidosis[20,23,25,34–36,38–40]

Its characteristic is intracellular accumulation of amyloid protein. Amyloidosis has four types with different clinical manifestations and prognoses:

- Light chain amyloidosis (AL). The source of amyloid protein is light chains produced by plasma cells in the bone marrow.
- Hereditary transthyretin amyloidosis (ATTRm), caused by a genetic mutation of transthyretin (TTR) protein. The source of amyloid protein is an unstable mutant transthyretin produced in the liver
- Nonhereditary TTR or senile amyloidosis or wild-type ATTR (ATTRwt)
- Secondary amyloidosis (secondary to chronic diseases)

### Key points about amyloidosis

Cardiac amyloidosis should be considered in all patients with unexplained heart failure.

About 50% of patients with AL amyloidosis have cardiac involvement. AL cardiac amyloidosis manifests with rapidly progressive heart failure in which the right-sided heart failure signs are more prominent.

In AL amyloidosis, monoclonal gammopathy can be detected in the blood and urine by immune electrophoresis and light chain assay methods. In bone marrow biopsy, plasma cells are increased.

ATTRm amyloidosis is an autosomal dominant disease. It is caused by a point mutation of transthyretin (TTR) protein.

In younger patients, the ATTRm manifests as sinus node dysfunction and mild cardiac infiltration as well as neuropathy. If it occurs in middle age, cardiomyopathy is more prominent.

ATTRwt, also known as systemic senile amyloidosis, is caused by deposition of normal TTR protein. It is emerging as one of the major specific causes of HFpEF. It occurs predominantly in men at the end of the seventh decade of life and can progress to severe biventricular failure.

Median survival in patients with untreated ATTRm and ATTRwt is about 2.5 and 3.6 years, respectively:

Secondary amyloidosis is secondary to an inflammatory process, and the heart is rarely involved.

For the diagnosis of cardiac amyloidosis, clinical manifestations, imaging features, and blood and tissue analysis should be considered (Fig. 29.1).

The sparkling appearance on echocardiography may be present and is typical of cardiac amyloidosis, but it is not diagnostic.

CMR imaging has diagnostic value in diagnosis of amyloidosis (Figs. 29.2 and 29.3).

Endomyocardial biopsy should be performed to confirm the diagnosis (Fig. 29.4).

The mainstay of treatment is management of heart failure, particularly RV failure.

### Treatment of cardiac amyloidosis

Cardiologic aspects:

Diuretics are the cornerstone therapy for the treatment of fluid overload in cardiac amyloidosis (see Chapter 12 for more detail)

Calcium channel blockers, beta-blockers, and digoxin should be avoided in these patients

Be aware of hypotension with ACE-I/ARBs

Pacemaker therapy is frequently needed; however, the role of ICDs and CRT is unclear

Heart transplantation may be an option in highly selected patients

MCS currently plays a minor role in cardiac amyloid

Specific therapies:

Chemotherapy with a combination of multiple classes of antineoplastic drugs is recommended for AL amyloidosis secondary to plasma cell dyscrasia.

Due to marked improvement in chemotherapy plans in recent decades, the circulating light chains reduce or even normalize in most patients.

Autologous stem cell transplantation is another treatment option in selected cases.

Chemotherapy has no role in ATTR amyloidosis. Multiple agents have been introduced as disease modifying medications for ATTR amyloidosis including: tafamidis, dilunisal, and ribonucleic acid (RNA) interference approaches.

Recently, the phase 3 study for investigating the utility of tafamidis in ATTR cardiomyopathy has been finished and this drug in now approved for both ATTRwt and ATTRm.

ATTRm can be treated with liver or combined liver and heart transplantation.

## Hemochromatosis[22,26,31]

In hemochromatosis, iron is accumulated and deposited in many organs, including the heart and endocrine tissues, leading to toxicity and organ dysfunction.

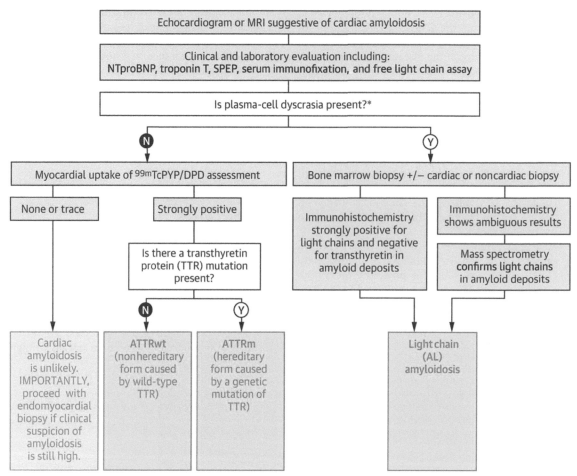

FIG. 29.1 Diagnosing and typing cardiac amyloidosis in a patient with unexplained heart failure. *The finding of evidence of a plasma cell dyscrasia does not necessarily confirm light chain (AL) amyloidosis because monoclonal gammopathy of unknown significance (MGUS) might coexist with transthyretin (TTR) amyloidosis. Thus, if the clinical picture suggests TTR amyloidosis (e.g., isolated cardiac amyloidosis in an elderly man with a history of carpal tunnel syndrome and no proteinuria or neuropathy), further workup is required to exclude transthyretin amyloidosis (ATTR). A classical appearance on imaging for amyloidosis, with a strong 99mtechnetium pyrophosphate (Tc99mPYP) (or 2,3-dicarboxypropane-1,1-diphosphonate [DPD] in Europe) cardiac uptake, and no evidence of a plasma cell dyscrasia appears to be diagnostic of TTR amyloidosis, without the need for a biopsy. *ATTRm* = mutant transthyretin amyloidosis; *ATTRwt* = wild-type transthyretin amyloidosis; *MRI* = magnetic resonance imaging; *NT-proBNP* = N-terminal pro-B-type natriuretic peptide; *SPEP* = serum protein electrophoresis. (From Falk RH, Alexander KM, Liao R, Dorbala S. AL (light-chain) cardiac amyloidosis: a review of diagnosis and therapy. *J Am Coll Cardiol.* 2016;68(12):1323–1341.)

Cardiomyopathy secondary to hemochromatosis is an RCM that presents at early stages with diastolic dysfunction and progresses to dilated cardiomyopathy. RCM secondary to iron overload is the most important determinant of survival in patients with major beta-thalassemia.

Hemochromatosis has two main types, primary (hereditary, idiopathic) hemochromatosis and secondary hemochromatosis.

Primary hemochromatosis has four types. In type 1, which is the classical type and an autosomal recessive disorder, there is mutation in the *HFE* gene.

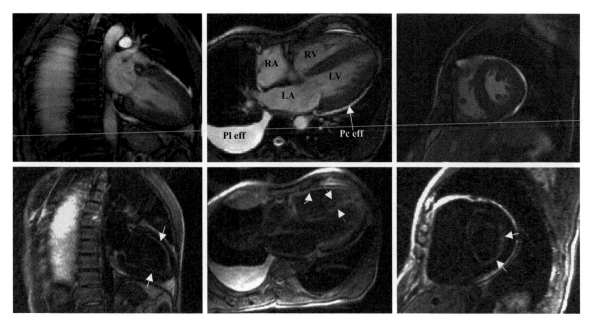

FIG. 29.2 Cardiac magnetic resonance (CMR) imaging in a patient with systemic amyloid light chain (AL) amyloidosis. *Top row* shows diastolic frames from cines (vertical long axis, horizontal long axis, and short axis, respectively) showing a thickened LV and pleural effusions (Pl eff) and pericardial effusions (Pc eff) associated with heart failure. *Bottom row* shows late gadolinium enhancement images in the same planes. The CMR sequence forces the myocardium remote from the pathology to be nulled (*black*) such that the abnormal region is enhanced. In cardiac amyloidosis, however, the region of greatest abnormality is enhanced as the entire myocardium is affected by amyloid infiltration, and the result is diffuse global subendocardial enhancement (*straight arrows*). The endocardium of the right ventricle (RV) is also heavily loaded with amyloid, and therefore the septum in the horizontal long-axis view shows biventricular subendocardial enhancement with a dark midwall (zebra appearance; *dotted arrows*). The RV free wall is also enhanced (*curved arrow*). Note that the blood pool is dark, which does not occur in other reported conditions, indicating abnormal gadolinium handling in these patients. *LA*, left atrium; *RA*, right atrium. (From Maceira AM, Joshi J, Prasad SK, et al. Cardiovascular magnetic resonance in cardiac amyloidosis. *Circulation.* 2005;111(2):188; with permission.)

Secondary hemochromatosis is a secondary iron overload that occurs primarily in patients with hemoglobinopathies (thalassemias and sickle cell anemia) who have repeated blood transfusions and increased gastrointestinal iron absorption because of ineffective erythropoiesis.

Complications of iron overload include:
- Cardiomyopathy and heart failure
- Liver dysfunction and cirrhosis
- Diabetes
- Arteritis
- Hypogonadism, impotence, and amenorrhea
- Osteoporosis

Cardiovascular abnormalities include:
- Diastolic and systolic dysfunction
- Sinoatrial node and atrioventricular node disease, various arrhythmias, and sudden cardiac death
- Increased risk of myocardial ischemia and infarction
- Pulmonary hypertension and RV dysfunction (in patients with hemoglobinopathies)
- Chronic thromboembolic diseases

### Diagnosis

Most patients with primary hemochromatosis are asymptomatic and are diagnosed when increased serum iron levels are noted on routine biochemistry tests or when screening is performed in a patient with a family history of hemochromatosis.

Iron profile in patients with primary hemochromatosis:
- Serum transferrin saturation greater than 45%
- Serum ferritin level 300 mg/L or greater in men and postmenopausal women and 200 mg/L or greater in premenopausal women

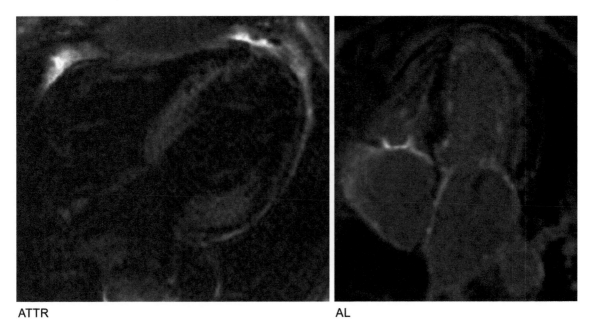

ATTR                                                    AL

**FIG. 29.3** Two different types of cardiac amyloidosis. *Left*: A horizontal long-axis late gadolinium enhancement (LGE) image from a patient with familial amyloidosis (ATTR) amyloidosis, highlighting the base–apex gradient. *Right*: A horizontal long-axis image from a patient with cardiac amyloid light chain (AL) amyloidosis with global subendocardial LGE. (From Dungu JN, Valencia O, Pinney JH, et al. CMR-based differentiation of AL and ATTR cardiac amyloidosis. *JACC Cardiovasc Imaging.* 2014;7(2):138; with permission.)

Note: The serum ferritin level may be elevated in the setting of infection, inflammation, cancer, or infection.

Imaging techniques such as echocardiography and CMR have diagnostic and prognostic significance in hemochromatosis.

### Key points about hemochromatosis

Conventional echocardiographic measures of systolic and diastolic parameters are insensitive for detecting iron overload of the heart in the early stages.

Strain rate imaging is a more sensitive measure in detecting the effects of iron overload on cardiac function and allows early detection of systolic and diastolic dysfunction in these patients.

The evaluation of the T2 relaxation time by CMR is a useful noninvasive technique for estimating the myocardial iron deposition as well as the response to iron chelation therapy.

Given the inherent risks of endomyocardial biopsy, it is not routinely used for the diagnosis of hemochromatosis.

The mainstay therapy for iron overload in patients with primary hemochromatosis is phlebotomy.

The aims of phlebotomy are to keep the serum ferritin level to less than 50 ng/mL and to prevent reaccumulation of iron.

Iron chelation therapy is the main therapy in patients with a secondary iron overload.

It is recommended that parenteral (deferoxamine) and oral (deferiprone) chelators be used together.

Standard heart failure as well as RV therapies should be implemented in these patients.

Some investigators recommend the use of a calcium channel blocker and antioxidant to prevent the effects of iron-induced oxidative stress.

### Cardiac Sarcoidosis[21,27,29]

Cardiac sarcoidosis is an idiopathic inflammatory granulomatous disease with multiorgan involvement, including the lung, heart, eyes, skin, and kidneys.

### Key points about cardiac sarcoidosis

Heart block, ventricular tachycardia, and sudden cardiac death may occur.

Prophylactic ICD should be considered in patients with cardiac sarcoidosis.

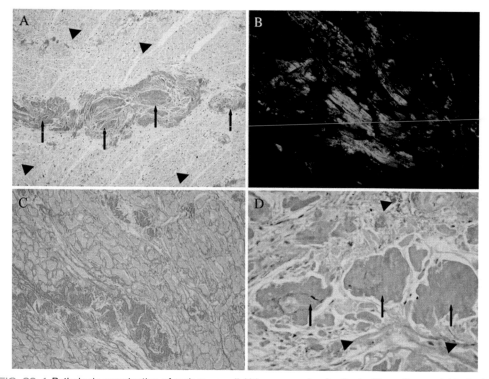

FIG. 29.4 Pathologic examination of endomyocardial biopsy sample of patient with cardiac amyloidosis. (A) Congo red staining of section from postmortem heart. Substantial amyloid deposition is seen as red nodules (*straight arrows*), and there is fine interstitial infiltration around individual myocytes (*arrowheads*), confirmed by green birefringence under polarized light (B). (C) Sirius red stains both amyloid and collagen, with myocytes staining yellow. Confirmation that the dominant component is amyloid comes from the elastin van Gieson stain (D), with amyloid showing as yellow (*straight arrows*) and collagen as dark pink (*arrowheads*). Note that there is only a small component of fibrosis. (From Maceira AM, Joshi J, Prasad SK, et al. Cardiovascular magnetic resonance in cardiac amyloidosis. *Circulation.* 2005;111(2):191; with permission.)

Bundle branch blocks and fragmented QRS are seen in ECG; patients with such ECG changes should have further workup for cardiac involvement.

CMR is useful in the diagnosis of cardiac sarcoidosis. Natriuretic peptides are also elevated in these patients. Corticosteroids should be administered for treatment of cardiac involvement.

## Constrictive vs Restrictive Physiology[41–43]

Abnormal ventricular filling and diastolic heart failure are characteristic of both constrictive pericarditis (CP) and restrictive cardiomyopathy (RCM) (Fig. 29.5). However, differentiating between these two conditions is necessary because of the different treatment strategies.

Practical points in catheterization of CP:
- Equalization and elevation of diastolic filling pressures is required for the diagnosis of CP.

- In the early stages of disease or in patients with low intravascular volume, diastolic equalization may not be present.
- In CP patients with low intravascular volume, cardiac output is decreased, so the presence of normal filling pressures accompanied by a normal cardiac output precludes the diagnosis of CP.

Practical points for differentiating RCM and CP:
- The equalization is more pronounced in CP than in RCM. This means that the difference between the end-diastolic LV and RV pressures is 5 mmHg or less in CP but more than 5 mmHg in RCM.
- RV end-diastolic pressure is more than one-third of RV systolic pressure in CP but not in RCM.
- The respiratory variation in the right atrial pressure waveform is absent in CP but present in RCM.

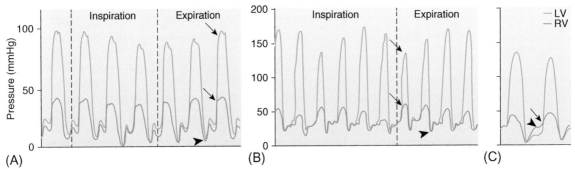

FIG. 29.5 Cardiac catheterization in constrictive pericarditis to differentiate between restrictive cardiomyopathy and constrictive pericarditis. (A) Simultaneous left (LV) and right ventricular (RV) pressure tracings in restrictive cardiomyopathy. (B) Simultaneous LV and RV pressure tracings in constrictive pericarditis. In both panels, ventricular pressures rise and equalize with a dip–plateau waveform (*arrowhead*) indicating restrictive ventricular filling. During inspiration and expiration, LV and RV pressure changes are concordant in restrictive cardiomyopathy and discordant in constrictive pericarditis, identified by peak LV and RV pressures (*arrows*) and areas under the respective pressure tracing. (C) In tricuspid regurgitation, RV pressure rises sharply during diastole (*arrowhead*) to reach a higher level (*arrow*) than LV pressure. (From Syed FF, Schaff HV, Oh JK. Constrictive pericarditis: a curable diastolic heart failure. *Nat Rev Cardiol*. 2014;11(9):530–544; with permission.)

- The respiratory gradient of pulmonary capillary wedge pressure and LV is 5 mmHg or more in CP and less than 5 mmHg in RCM.
- The pulmonary artery pressure (PAP) is not elevated in CP (usually <50 mmHg), but in RCM, the PAP is usually more than 50 mmHg.
  Similarities between CP and RCM:
- The dip and plateau (square root sign) of ventricular pressure during diastole is seen in both CP and RCM.
- In the right atrial waveform, a prominent "y" descent is seen in both CP and RCM.

## HYPERTROPHIC CARDIOMYOPATHY[44–47]
### Background
Hypertrophic cardiomyopathy is the most common genetic disorder of the heart. It is also the most common cause of sudden cardiac death among athletes and affects men and women equally. The hallmark of HCM is left ventricular hypertrophy (LVH), which cannot be explained by abnormal loading conditions. HCM is caused by mutations in cardiac sarcomere protein genes. The inheritance is commonly autosomal dominant with variable penetrance and expression.

### Key Points About Hypertrophic Cardiomyopathy
The hypertrophy can be in any region of the LV and is usually asymmetric.

The majority of cases are caused by mutations in the genes encoding beta-myosin heavy chain and myosin-binding protein C.

Other affected genes are cardiac troponin I and T, tropomyosin alpha-1 chain, and myosin light chain 3.

The prevalence of a family history of HCM and sudden cardiac death is higher in patients with mutations in sarcomeric proteins.

Several other genetic and nongenetic disorders mimic HCM, including metabolic disorders (Anderson–Fabry disease), mitochondrial cardiomyopathies, neuromuscular disease (Friedreich ataxia), malformation syndromes, infiltrative disorders (amyloidosis), and endocrine disorders (neonates born from mothers with diabetes).

### Diagnostic Criteria
A wall thickness in one or more segments of the LV 15 mm or greater measured by any imaging modality that cannot be explained by an abnormal loading condition is necessary for diagnosis of the HCM in adults.

In the presence of lesser wall thickness (13–14 mm), other genetic and nongenetic disorders may be present, and other features are required to be considered for the differential diagnosis, including family history, extracardiac signs and symptoms, ECG abnormalities, and cardiac imaging findings.

The diagnosis of HCM in children requires an increase in LV wall thickness more than two standard deviations of the predicted mean.

Common challenging issues in the diagnosis of HCM include:

- Athlete's heart
- Infiltrative cardiomyopathies including amyloidosis or glycogen/lysosmal storage diseases (such as Fabry's or Danon disease)
- Presence of coexisting pathologies such as hypertension and valvular heart disease
- Burned-out HCM (late phase of disease presenting with thin and dilated LV)
- Isolated basal septum hypertrophy in older adults

The first-degree relatives of patients with definite HCM should be evaluated for HCM by any imaging modality (echocardiography, CMR, and computed tomography [CT]). The presence of unexplained increased LV wall thickness of 13 mm or more in one or more LV segments is considered to be HCM.

### Key Points About Hypertrophic Cardiomyopathy

Clinical presentation includes dyspnea, presyncope, syncope, palpitation, angina, dizziness, heart failure symptoms, and sudden cardiac death.

The most common symptom is dyspnea, which is caused by severe LV diastolic dysfunction, decreased LV compliance, and elevated LV filling pressures.

48-h ECG Holter monitoring is recommended for all patients with HCM to detect ventricular and atrial arrhythmias.

Assessment of left ventricular outflow (LVOT) obstruction by echocardiography (at rest, during Valsalva maneuver, and during standing or exercise echocardiography) should be performed in all patients with HCM.

The presence and extent of myocardial fibrosis and hypertrophy should be evaluated by CMR in all patients with hypertrophic cardiomyopathy. CMR can be helpful for differentiation of etiology of left ventricular hypertrophy.

Genetic counseling is recommended for all patients with definite HCM.

Coronary angiography or CT angiography is recommended in survivors of sudden cardiac death (SCD), patients with ventricular arrhythmia, patients

with anginal chest pain, and patients who are candidates for septal reduction therapies.

Treatment may be medical or surgical. The aim of treatment is to increase ventricular compliance and LVOT dimension and reduce ventricular contractility and the pressure gradient across LVOT in patients with obstructive HCM (HOCM).

The value of medical treatment in asymptomatic patients with HCM is not clear.

For patients who are at high risk for sudden cardiac death, ICD should be implanted. These high-risk patients include:

- A positive family history of premature sudden cardiac death caused by HCM
- Presence of nonsustained ventricular tachycardia in Holter monitoring
- Abnormal blood pressure response during exercise defined as less than a 20-mmHg increase in systolic blood pressure from baseline value, progressive decrease in systolic blood pressure, or a decrease more than 20 mmHg after a rise in systolic blood pressure during exercise.
- Syncope at rest or during exercise
- Late gadolinium enhancement (LGE) 15% or greater of LV mass in CMR

### Treatment of Obstructive Hypertrophic Cardiomyopathy

- Dehydration and alcohol should be avoided, so diuretics should be used with caution.
- Vasodilators such as nitrates and phosphodiesterase 3 inhibitors are contraindicated.
- Atrial fibrillation rhythm should be managed by restoration of the sinus rhythm or by controlling the ventricular response.
- Digoxin should not be used in patients with LVOT obstruction.
- The initial treatment in patients with HOCM is a nonvasodilating beta-blocker; it should be titrated to the maximal tolerated dose.
- If beta-blocker therapy fails, disopyramide (maximum dose, 400–600 mg/day) can be used.
- Verapamil can be used when beta-blockers are contraindicated.
- Verapamil should be used with caution in patients with a severe LVOT gradient (>100 mmHg) or pulmonary hypertension because it may provoke pulmonary edema.
- The dosage of verapamil is 40 mg three times daily to a maximum of 48 mg/day.

- Diltiazem can also be used in patients who cannot tolerate beta-blockers or verapamil.
- Amlodipine and nifedipine should not be used.
- Vasodilators and inotropes are contraindicated in patients with HCM with severe provocable LVOT obstruction who have developed hypotension and pulmonary edema.
- The recognition of this condition is very important, and the treatment consists of intravenous vasoconstrictors (phenylephrine, metaraminol, and norepinephrine) and a beta-blocker.
- In patients who are highly symptomatic with an LVOT gradient greater than 50 mmHg or who have recurrent syncope despite maximally tolerated drug therapy, invasive therapy with surgery or septal alcohol ablation is recommended.
- Septal alcohol ablation should be performed only in experienced centers.
- In selected patients who are refractory to drug therapy and have a contraindication for invasive therapy, sequential AV pacing with an optimal AV interval to reduce the LVOT gradient or to facilitate drug therapy is recommended.
- Drug therapy in symptomatic patients with nonobstructive HCM includes beta-blockers, verapamil, diltiazem, and diuretics to improve heart failure symptoms.

- Patients with HCM who have reduced LV ejection fraction (<50%) should be medically treated as recommended for HFrEF.

### Hemodynamic Study of Hypertrophic Cardiomyopathy[45,46]

Cardiac catheterization is not necessary for the evaluation of HOCM. During HOCM catheterization, the pressures are measured in a hyperdynamic LV with small cavity, so specific considerations are needed.

The best method for precise measurement of LV pressure gradients is a transseptal approach. In the retrograde approach, the catheter may be entrapped in the cardiac muscles, resulting in incorrect measurement.

The pressure gradient in typical forms of HOCM is between the LV apex and outflow tract. The most important differential diagnosis of HOCM is valvular aortic stenosis.

The Brockenbrough–Braunwald sign is helpful to differentiate HOCM from valvular aortic stenosis. In the Brockenbrough–Braunwald response after premature ventricular contraction, the pulse pressure is decreased, and the pressure gradient is increased. Increased dynamic obstruction secondary to postextrasystole potentiation results in a reduction in stroke volume and pulse pressure and elevation in the LVOT pressure gradient (Fig. 29.6).

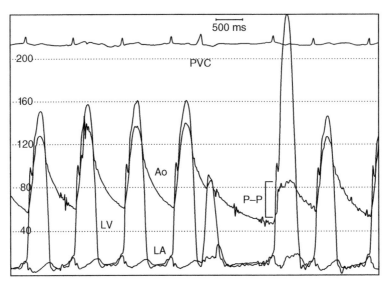

FIG. 29.6 Brockenbrough–Braunwald response after premature ventricular contraction in patient with obstructive hypertrophic cardiomyopathy. *Ao,* Aorta; *LA,* left atrium; *LV,* left ventricle; *PVC,* premature ventricular contraction. (From Nishimura RA, Carabello BA. Hemodynamics in the cardiac catheterization laboratory of the 21st century. *Circulation.* 2012;125(17):2144; with permission.)

## Myocarditis[48–54]

### Background

One of the most important causes of DCM is myocarditis. It is an inflammation of the heart muscle secondary to the infectious and noninfectious triggers. Myocarditis can be precipitated by various causes including infections, autoimmune disorder such as collagen vascular diseases, and drugs such as immune checkpoint inhibitors. Myocarditis is diagnosed by histologic, immunologic, and immunohistochemical criteria. The prognosis of myocarditis depends on the cause, disease stage, and clinical presentation.

### Key points

The most common causes of myocarditis are viral infections and postviral immune-mediated responses.

Myocarditis may be seen in all ages, but it is more frequent in younger individuals.

There are local and temporal differences concerning the distribution of virus species, which should be considered in diagnostic approaches and care management of patients with myocarditis.

Viral myocarditis has three phases (Fig. 29.7):

1. Acute phase: This takes a few days. A specific receptor mediates virus entry into the myocyte, and virus replication leads to acute myocardial injury; exposure of the intracellular antigens to the host's immune system; and invasion of natural killer cells, macrophages, and T lymphocytes.

2. Subacute phase: This takes a few weeks to several months. Activated virus-specific T lymphocytes invade myocardial cells and cause cardiac cell damage and contractile dysfunction. Antibodies to viral and cardiac proteins and cytokine activation aggravate myocardial damage.

3. Chronic phase: Although LV function recovers as immune response declines with virus elimination in most patients, in some patients, autoimmune processes persist and lead to myocardial remodeling and development of DCM.

- The diagnosis of acute myocarditis based on clinical manifestations is not usually simple. There is a spectrum of manifestations from asymptomatic illness to cardiogenic shock. The following features support the clinical suspicion of myocarditis:
- Previously suspected or definite myocarditis
- Fever of 38°C or above at presentation or within the preceding month with or without evidence of respiratory or gastrointestinal infection
- Peripartum period
- Personal or family history of any type of allergic disorder, including allergic asthma, extracardiac autoimmune disorder, or exposure to toxic agents
- Family history of myocarditis or DCM

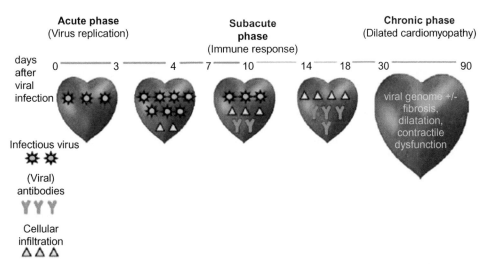

FIG. 29.7 Phases of myocarditis. *DCM*, dilated cardiomyopathy. (From Kindermann I, Barth C, Mahfoud F, et al. Update on myocarditis. *J Am Coll Cardiol.* 2012;59(9):781; with permission.)

**TABLE 29.3**
Diagnostic Criteria for Myocarditis

**CLINICAL MANIFESTATIONS**

1. Acute atypical nonangina or pericarditic chest pain
2. New onset (<3 months) or worsening of dyspnea (at rest or on exertion) and/or fatigue with or without heart failure signs
3. Subacute or chronic (>3 months) or worsening of dyspnea (at rest or on exertion) and/or fatigue with or without heart failure signs
4. Palpitations and/or unexplained arrhythmias and/or syncope and/or aborted sudden cardiac death

**DIAGNOSTIC CRITERIA**

1. ECG, Holter, stress test: presence of new abnormalities include:
   AV block (I–III degree)
   Sinus arrest
   Widening QRS (BBBs, intraventricular conduction delay)
   ST-T changes (ST-segment elevation, depression, T inversion)
   QRS: poor R progression low voltage, abnormal Q wave
   Frequent premature beats, AF rhythm, VT or VF
2. Cardiac biomarkers: elevated troponin T and I levels
3. Structural and functional abnormalities on cardiac imaging (echocardiography, CMR, or angiography):
   New and unexplained LV or RV function and structure abnormality (may be an incidental finding in an asymptomatic patient)
   Systolic and diastolic dysfunction or regional wall motion abnormality with or without ventricular dilatation, increased wall thickness pericardial effusion, or thrombus in cardiac chambers
4. Lake Louise criteria in CMR:
   Edema
   LGE of classical myocarditic pattern

*AF*, atrial fibrillation; *AV*, atrioventricular; *BBB*, bundle branch block; *CMR*, cardiac magnetic resonance imaging; *LGE*, late gadolinium enhancement; *LV*, left ventricular; *RV*, right ventricular; *VF*, ventricular fibrillation; *VT*, ventricular tachycardia.

Diagnostic criteria for myocarditis are shown in Table 29.3. Myocarditis should be suspected if there are one or more clinical manifestations and one or more diagnostic criteria from different categories in the absence of:
- A significant coronary artery disease (≥50% stenosis) in coronary angiography
- Known preexisting cardiovascular disorders (e.g., valvular disorder, congenital heart disease) or extracardiac etiologies that could explain the syndrome (e.g., hyperthyroidism)

***Key points about myocarditis***
A higher number of criteria increases the suspicion level. In asymptomatic patients, two or more diagnostic criteria should be met.

Recommendations for clinical assessment of myocarditis:
- A 12-lead ECG should be performed in all patients with suspected myocarditis.
- Erythrocyte sedimentation rate (ESR) and C-reactive protein (CRP) may be elevated and should be measured in all patients with suspected myocarditis.
- Cardiac troponins and NPs are sensitive to myocardial injury and should be measured in all patients with suspected myocarditis.
- Chronic skeletal diseases may be associated with mild increases in cardiac troponins.
- Heterophil antibodies may interfere with troponin T assay (falsely elevated troponin T level). The troponin I level should be measured to clarify the cardiac origin of the biomarker.

- ESR, CRP, and cardiac biomarkers are nonspecific, and normal values do not rule out myocarditis.
- Transthoracic echocardiography (TTE) should be performed in all patients with suspected myocarditis. TTE should be repeated during hospital admission if there is any worsening in hemodynamic conditions.
- Nuclear imaging may only be useful in patients suspected of having cardiac sarcoidosis and is not recommended in all patients with suspected myocarditis.
- Cardiovascular magnetic resonance findings should be consistent with myocarditis (Lake Louise criteria) (Fig. 29.8).
- CMR can be considered before endomyocardial biopsy (EMB) in stable patients. EMB should not be replaced by CMR in critically ill patients.
- Recently, fluorodeoxyglucose (FDG)-labeled positron emission tomography (PET) along with CMR (PET/CMR) or computed tomography (PET/CT) has increased the ability to detect the metabolic activity of myocardial inflammation.
- Routine viral serology measurement is not recommended.
- Serum levels of cardiac auto antibodies should be assessed if possible depending on center expertise.
- All patients suspected of having myocarditis should undergo coronary angiography and EMB.

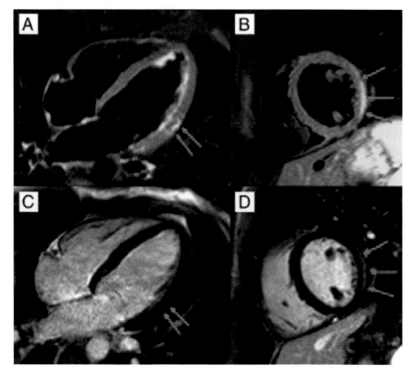

FIG. 29.8 Cardiac magnetic resonance images of a young patient presenting with acute chest pain syndrome caused by acute myocarditis. Long-axis (A) and short-axis (B) T2-weighted edema images demonstrating focal myocardial edema in the subepicardium of the left midventricular lateral wall (*red arrows*). Corresponding long-axis (C) and short-axis (D) T1-weighted late gadolinium enhancement images demonstrate the presence of typical late gadolinium enhancement in the subepicardium of the left midventricular lateral wall and the basal septum (*red arrows*). (From Kindermann I, Barth C, Mahfoud F, et al. Update on myocarditis. *J Am Coll Cardiol.* 2012;59(9):783; with permission.)

- Viral polymerase chain reaction (PCR) should be performed on myocardial tissue obtained from EMB as well as blood sample.
- The myocardial tissues obtained from EMB should also be analyzed using histology and immunohistochemistry.
- EMB may be repeated to monitor response to the treatments or if a sampling error is suspected.

### Treatment of myocarditis

- Patients with critical conditions should be transferred to an expert center for cardiac catheterization, EMB, and hemodynamic monitoring.
- Management of patients with heart failure should be initiated according to the current heart failure guidelines.
- In patients with hemodynamic instability, mechanical circulatory support may be needed as a bridge to recovery or as a bridge to transplantation.
- Because recovery may occur, the patient can referred for heart transplantation in the acute phase unless she or he cannot be hemodynamically stabilized by pharmacologic support and MCS, particularly in those with giant cell myocarditis.
- Treatment of arrhythmias should be based on guideline recommendations, and ICD implantation should be deferred in the acute phase because recovery may occur.
- In the acute phase and for at least 6 months (the time for complete recovery), physical activity should be restricted in athletes and nonathletes. After 6 months, clinical reassessment should be performed before resumption of competitive sports.
- Before starting specific antiviral therapies, an infectious disease specialist should be involved in decision-making.
- There is still no approved antiviral therapy for acute myocarditis. The efficacy of antiviral therapies for specific viruses is unproven (e.g., interferon beta for enterovirus and adenovirus or acyclovir, valganciclovir, or ganciclovir for herpesvirus).
- There is some supportive evidence for intravenous immunoglobulin (IVIG) therapy in acute myocarditis. Recent studies show that IVIG can accelerate the recovery of LV function, result in lower hospital mortality, and increase the survival in acute myocarditis.

- The use of immunoadsorption is still not recommended due to lack of evidence.
- The immunosuppressive regimens currently used in myocarditis are steroids alone; azathioprine and steroids; or steroids, cyclosporine A, and azathioprine.
- Active infection should be ruled out by PCR on EMB samples before starting immunosuppressive therapy.
- Immunosuppression is recommended in patients with infection-negative autoimmune myocarditis with no contraindication of immunosuppressive therapy, including cardiac sarcoidosis, giant cell myocarditis and myocarditis secondary to known systemic autoimmune disorders, and lymphocytic myocarditis refractory to standard therapies.
- Combined immunosuppressive therapy (steroid and cyclosporine with or without azathioprine) may improve the poor prognosis in giant cell myocarditis.
- Patients with cardiac sarcoidosis should be treated with steroids in the presence of heart failure or arrhythmias.
- Steroids are also indicated in some forms of toxic myocarditis or infection-negative eosinophilic myocarditis in the presence of arrhythmias or ventricular dysfunction.
- To guide the intensity and duration of immunosuppressive therapies, follow-up EMB is recommended.
- Patients with myocarditis can be discharged from the hospital when their cardiac enzymes come to the normal range and ventricular function is preserved.
- Patients with myocarditis can partially or fully recover.
- Some patients may relapse several years later, which should be managed similarly to the first episode.
- All patients with myocarditis should have long-term cardiologist follow-up with clinical assessment, cardiac biomarkers, ECG, echocardiography, or CMR.
- Patients with progression of left or RV dysfunction or persistent elevated cardiac markers should be readmitted for EMB.

An algorithmic approach to myocarditis is shown in Fig. 29.9. Figs. 29.10–29.12 show pathologic examination of myocarditis.

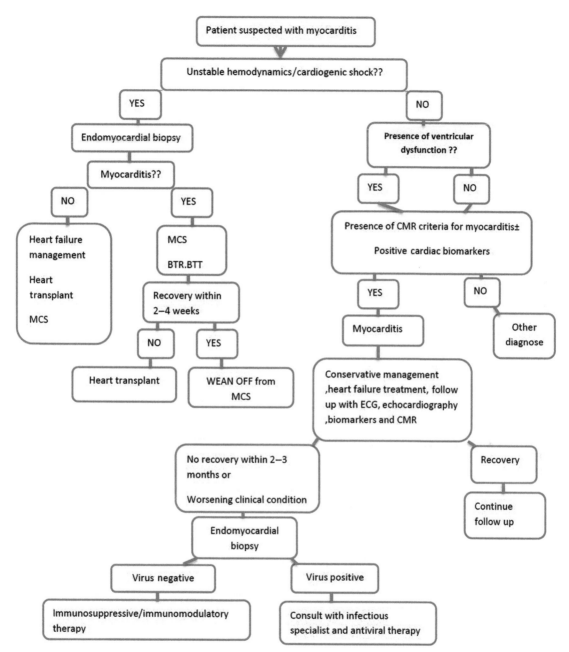

FIG. 29.9 Algorithmic approach to myocarditis. *BTR*, bridge to recovery; *BTT*, bridge to transplantation; *CMR*, cardiac magnetic resonance imaging; *ECG*, electrocardiography; *MCS*, mechanical circulatory support.

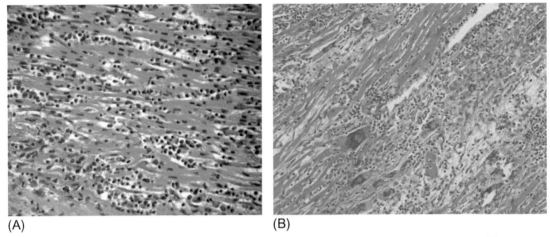

FIG. 29.10 Pathologic examination of endomyocardial biopsy sample of a patient with myocarditis. (A) Lymphocytic myocarditis. (B) Giant cell myocarditis. (From Tavora FR. Myocarditis pathology. 2015. http://emedicine.medscape.com/article/1612533-overview#a1%20%20, Multimedia.)

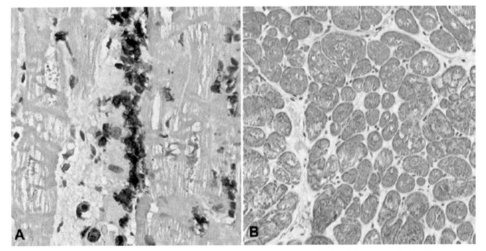

FIG. 29.11 Pathologic examination of endomyocardial biopsy sample obtained from a patient with myocarditis who has improved after therapy. LV endomyocardial biopsy of a 19-year-old young man before and after 6 months of immunosuppressive therapy. Marked reduction of left ventricular volumes and increase in LVEF (from 24% to 50%) were associated with disappearance of CD45RO-positive activated T lymphocytes and myocyte necrosis present at baseline (A, immunoperoxidase, ×200), both replaced by fibrosis in control biopsy (B, Masson trichrome, ×100). (From Frustaci A, Russo MA, Chimenti C. Randomized study on the efficacy of immunosuppressive therapy in patients with virus-negative inflammatory cardiomyopathy: the TIMIC study. *Eur Heart J.* 2009;30(16):1995–2002; with permission.)

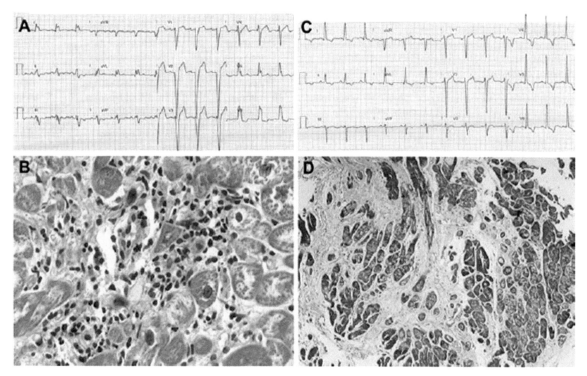

FIG. 29.12 Electrocardiography and pathologic examination of a patient with myocarditis who has improved after therapy. A 12-lead ECG (A and C) and endomyocardial biopsy (B and D) from a 54-year-old man before (A and B) and after (C and D) 6 months of immunosuppression. Severely dilated (left ventricular end diastolic diameter = 90 mm) and hypokinetic (ejection fraction = 18%) left ventricle recovered significantly after treatment (end-diastolic diameter = 73 mm, ejection fraction = 38%), and left ventricle improvement was associated with disappearance of left bundle branch block (A and C), while an active lymphocytic myocarditis (B) progressed to a healed phase (D). (From Frustaci A, Russo MA, Chimenti C. Randomized study on the efficacy of immunosuppressive therapy in patients with virus-negative inflammatory cardiomyopathy: the TIMIC study. *Eur Heart J.* 2009;30(16):1995–2002; with permission.)

## REFERENCES

1. Elliott P, Andersson B, Arbustini E, et al. Classification of the cardiomyopathies: a position statement from the European Society of Cardiology Working Group on Myocardial and Pericardial Diseases. *Eur Heart J.* 2007;29:270–276.
2. Westphal JG, Rigopoulos AG, Bakogiannis C, et al. The MOGE(S) classification for cardiomyopathies: current status and future outlook. *Heart Fail Rev.* 2017;22(6):743–752.
3. Fuster V, Gersh BJ, Giuliani ER, Tajik AJ, Brandenburg RO, Frye RL. The natural history of idiopathic dilated cardiomyopathy. *Am J Cardiol.* 1981;47(3):525–531.
4. Lewis W. AIDS cardiomyopathy. *Ann N Y Acad Sci.* 2001;946(1):46–56.
5. Piano MR. Alcoholic cardiomyopathy: incidence, clinical characteristics, and pathophysiology. *Chest.* 2002;121(5):1638–1650.
6. Nakatani BT, Minicucci MF, Okoshi K, Okoshi MP. Tachycardia-induced cardiomyopathy. *BMJ Case Rep.* 2012;2012:bcr2012006587.
7. Florescu M, Cinteza M, Vinereanu D. Chemotherapy-induced cardiotoxicity. *Maedica (Buchar).* 2013;8(1):59–67.
8. Haghikia A, Podewski E, Libhaber E, et al. Phenotyping and outcome on contemporary management in a German cohort of patients with peripartum cardiomyopathy. *Basic Res Cardiol.* 2013;108(4):1–13.
9. Hershberger RE, Hedges DJ, Morales A. Dilated cardiomyopathy: the complexity of a diverse genetic architecture. *Nat Rev Cardiol.* 2013;10(9):531–547.
10. Ahmadi A, Zolfi-Gol A, Arasteh M. Tachycardia-induced cardiomyopathy. *ARYA Atheroscler.* 2014;10(3):175.
11. Hilfiker-Kleiner D, Sliwa K. Pathophysiology and epidemiology of peripartum cardiomyopathy. *Nat Rev Cardiol.* 2014;11(6):364–370.
12. Sliwa K, Hilfiker-Kleiner D, Mebazaa A, et al. EURObservational Research Programme: a worldwide

registry on peripartum cardiomyopathy (PPCM) in conjunction with the Heart Failure Association of the European Society of Cardiology Working Group on PPCM. *Eur J Heart Fail.* 2014;16(5):583–591.

13. Sliwa K, Blauwet L, Tibazarwa K, et al. Evaluation of bromocriptine in the treatment of acute severe peripartum cardiomyopathy: a proof-of-concept pilot study. *Circulation.* 2010;121(13):1465–1473.

14. McKenna WJ, Thiene G, Nava A, et al. Diagnosis of arrhythmogenic right ventricular dysplasia/cardiomyopathy. Task Force of the Working Group Myocardial and Pericardial Disease of the European Society of Cardiology and of the Scientific Council on Cardiomyopathies of the International Society and Federation of Cardiology. *Br Heart J.* 1994;71(3):215.

15. Basso C, Corrado D, Bauce B, Thiene G. Arrhythmogenic right ventricular cardiomyopathy. *Circ Arrhythm Electrophysiol.* 2012;5(6):1233–1246.

16. Marra MP, Rizzo S, Bauce B, et al. Arrhythmogenic right ventricular cardiomyopathy. *Herz.* 2015;40(4):600–606.

17. Howlett JG, McKelvie RS, Arnold JMO, et al. Canadian Cardiovascular Society Consensus Conference guidelines on heart failure, update 2009: diagnosis and management of right-sided heart failure, myocarditis, device therapy and recent important clinical trials. *Can J Cardiol.* 2009;25(2):85–105.

18. Kushwaha SS, Fallon JT, Fuster V. Restrictive cardiomyopathy. *N Engl J Med.* 1997;336(4):267–276.

19. Mogensen J, Kubo T, Duque M, et al. Idiopathic restrictive cardiomyopathy is part of the clinical expression of cardiac troponin I mutations. *J Clin Invest.* 2003;111(2):209–216.

20. Maceira AM, Joshi J, Prasad SK, et al. Cardiovascular magnetic resonance in cardiac amyloidosis. *Circulation.* 2005;111(2):186–193.

21. Doughan AR, Williams BR. Cardiac sarcoidosis. *Heart.* 2006;92(2):282–288.

22. Gujja P, Rosing DR, Tripodi DJ, Shizukuda Y. Iron overload cardiomyopathy better understanding of an increasing disorder. *J Am Coll Cardiol.* 2010;56(13):1001–1012.

23. Rapezzi C, Quarta CC, Obici L, et al. Disease profile and differential diagnosis of hereditary transthyretin-related amyloidosis with exclusively cardiac phenotype: an Italian perspective. *Eur Heart J.* 2013;34(7):520–528.

24. Ammash N, Tajik A. *Idiopathic Restrictive Cardiomyopathy.* Waltham, MA: UpToDate; 2014 Up to Date.

25. Dungu JN, Valencia O, Pinney JH, et al. CMR-based differentiation of AL and ATTR cardiac amyloidosis. *JACC Cardiovasc Imaging.* 2014;7(2):133–142.

26. Gulati V, Harikrishnan P, Palaniswamy C, Aronow WS, Jain D, Frishman WH. Cardiac involvement in hemochromatosis. *Cardiol Rev.* 2014;22(2):56–68.

27. Merlo M, Abate E, Pinamonti B, et al. Restrictive cardiomyopathy: clinical assessment and imaging in diagnosis and patient management. In: Pinamonti B, Sinagra G, eds. *Clinical Echocardiography and Other Imaging Techniques in Cardiomyopathies.* Cham: Springer; 2014:185–206.

28. Quarta CC, Solomon SD, Uraizee I, et al. Left ventricular structure and function in transthyretin-related versus light-chain cardiac amyloidosis. *Circulation.* 2014;129 (18):1840–1849.

29. Kusano KF, Satomi K. Diagnosis and treatment of cardiac sarcoidosis. *Heart.* 2016;102(3):184–190.

30. Latona J, Jayasinghe R, Niranjan S. Restrictive cardiomyopathy as a result of endomyocardial fibrosis from hypereosinophilia. *Intern Med J.* 2015;45(1):115–117.

31. Oudit GY, Backx PH. Amlodipine therapy for iron-overload cardiomyopathy: the enduring value of translational research. *Can J Cardiol.* 2016;32(8):938–940.

32. Freers J, Masembe V, Schmauz R, Kidaaga F, Mayanja-Kizza H. Endomyocardial fibrosis: is it a systemic disease? *South Sudan Med J.* 2016;9(3):52–55.

33. Grimaldi A, Mocumbi AO, Freers J, et al. Tropical endomyocardial fibrosis natural history, challenges, and perspectives. *Circulation.* 2016;133(24):2503–2515.

34. Muchtar E, Blauwet LA, Gertz MA. Restrictive cardiomyopathy: genetics, pathogenesis, clinical manifestations, diagnosis, and therapy. *Circ Res.* 2017;121(7):819–837.

35. Falk RH, Alexander KM, Liao R, Dorbala SAL. (Light-chain) cardiac amyloidosis: a review of diagnosis and therapy. *J Am Coll Cardiol.* 2016;68(12):1323–1341.

36. Dorbala S, Cuddy S, Falk RH. How to image cardiac amyloidosis: a practical approach. *JACC Cardiovasc Imaging.* 2020;13(6):1368–1383.

37. Alam A, Thampi S, Saba SG, Jermyn R. Loeffler endocarditis: a unique presentation of right-sided heart failure due to eosinophil-induced endomyocardial fibrosis. *Clin Med Insights Case Rep.* 2017;10:1179547617723643.

38. Kyriakou P, Mouselimis D, Tsarouchas A, et al. Diagnosis of cardiac amyloidosis: a systematic review on the role of imaging and biomarkers. *BMC Cardiovasc Disord.* 2018;18(1):221.

39. Amin HZ, Mori S, Sasaki N, Hirata K. Diagnostic approach to cardiac amyloidosis. *Kobe J Med Sci.* 2014;60(1):E5–e11.

40. Maurer MS, Schwartz JH, Gundapaneni B, et al. Tafamidis treatment for patients with transthyretin amyloid cardiomyopathy. *N Engl J Med.* 2018;379(11):1007–1016.

41. Talreja DR, Nishimura RA, Oh JK, Holmes DR. Constrictive pericarditis in the modern era: novel criteria for diagnosis in the cardiac catheterization laboratory. *J Am Coll Cardiol.* 2008;51(3):315–319.

42. Garcia MJ. Constrictive pericarditis versus restrictive cardiomyopathy? *J Am Coll Cardiol.* 2016;67 (17):2061–2076.

43. Syed FF, Schaff HV, Oh JK. Constrictive pericarditis—a curable diastolic heart failure. *Nat Rev Cardiol.* 2014;11 (9):530–544.

44. Gersh BJ, Maron BJ, Bonow RO, et al. 2011 ACCF/AHA guideline for the diagnosis and treatment of hypertrophic cardiomyopathy: executive summary: a report of the American College of Cardiology Foundation/American Heart Association Task Force on

Practice Guidelines developed in collaboration with the American Association for Thoracic Surgery, American Society of Echocardiography, American Society of Nuclear Cardiology, Heart Failure Society of America, Heart Rhythm Society, Society for Cardiovascular Angiography and Interventions, and Society of Thoracic Surgeons. *J Am Coll Cardiol.* 2011;58(25):2703–2738.

45. Elliott PM, Anastasakis A, Borger MA, et al. 2014 ESC Guidelines on diagnosis and management of hypertrophic cardiomyopathy: the Task Force for the Diagnosis and Management of Hypertrophic Cardiomyopathy of the European Society of Cardiology (ESC). *Eur Heart J.* 2014;35(39):2733–2779 ehu284.

46. Brockenbrough E. The Brockenbrough-Braunwald-Morrow sign. *N Engl J Med.* 1994;1994(331):1589–1590.

47. Rowin EJ, Maron MS. The role of cardiac MRI in the diagnosis and risk stratification of hypertrophic cardiomyopathy. *Arrhythm Electrophysiol Rev.* 2016;5(3):197–202.

48. Caforio AL, Pankuweit S, Arbustini E, et al. Current state of knowledge on aetiology, diagnosis, management, and therapy of myocarditis: a position statement of the European Society of Cardiology Working Group on Myocardial and Pericardial Diseases. *Eur Heart J.* 2013;34 (33):2636–2648.

49. Biesbroek PS, Beek AM, Germans T, Niessen HW, van Rossum AC. Diagnosis of myocarditis: current state and future perspectives. *Int J Cardiol.* 2015;191:211–219.

50. Kafil TS, Tzemos N. Myocarditis in 2020. *Adv Imaging Clin Manag.* 2020;2(2):178–179.

51. Frustaci A, Russo MA, Chimenti C. Randomized study on the efficacy of immunosuppressive therapy in patients with virus-negative inflammatory cardiomyopathy: the TIMIC study. *Eur Heart J.* 2009;30(16):1995–2002.

52. Kindermann I, Barth C, Mahfoud F, et al. Update on myocarditis. *J Am Coll Cardiol.* 2012;59(9):779–792.

53. Li Y, Yu Y, Chen S, Liao Y, Du J. Corticosteroids and intravenous immunoglobulin in pediatric myocarditis: a meta-analysis. *Front Pediatr.* 2019;7:342.

54. Huang X, Sun Y, Su G, Li Y, Shuai X. Intravenous immunoglobulin therapy for acute myocarditis in children and adults. *Int Heart J.* 2019;60(2):359–365.

# CHAPTER 30

# Valvular Heart Disease

FERIDOUN NOOHI[a] • ANITA SADEGHPOUR[b,c] • AZIN ALIZADEHASL[d]

[a]Rajaie Cardiovascular, Medical & Research Center, Iran University of Medical Sciences, Tehran, Iran, [b]Rajaie Cardiovascular, Medical & Research Center, Tehran, Iran, [c]Visiting Research Scholar in Duke Cardiovascular MR Center, Durham, NC, United States, [d]Cardio-Oncology Research Center, Rajaie Cardiovascular, Medical & Research Center, Iran University of Medical Sciences, Tehran, Iran

## AORTIC VALVE

### Aortic Stenosis

#### Epidemiology

Among all the diseases of the heart valves, aortic valve (AV) stenosis is the most common valve disease, and aortic valve replacement (AVR) accounts for about two-thirds of all heart valve surgeries in developed countries. Aortic stenosis (AS) is a progressive disease, and its prevalence increases with aging, reaching 9.8% in octogenarians.[1,2]

#### Causes and pathology

Obstruction to the left ventricular outflow tract (LVOT) can occur at three levels: the AV, above the valve (supravalvular stenosis), and below the valve (as in discrete subvalvular stenosis or as dynamic obstruction in hypertrophic obstructive cardiomyopathy).[3]

The most common type of LVOT obstruction occurs at AV level because of:

1. Degenerative senile calcification of a tricuspid AV
2. Degenerative calcification of a congenital bicuspid AV (BAV)
3. Rheumatic involvement of the AV (Fig. 30.1)

Calcific AV disease, formerly termed "degenerative or senile AS," is the most common type of AV stenosis and affects a normal tricuspid AV or a congenital BAV.

Aortic valve sclerosis is defined as an irregular thickening of the AV leaflets without significant stenosis and is seen in 29% of individuals 65 years of age or older. However, significant AS occurs in 2% of these individuals.

Aortic sclerosis, which is diagnosed by echocardiography or cardiac computed tomography (CT), is the early stage of calcified AV disease and suggests a 50% increased risk of myocardial infarction (MI) or cardiovascular death at about 5 years' follow-up. It has common risk factors with mitral annular calcification (MAC) and shares many of the pathophysiologic features of atherosclerosis.[1–4]

The typical features of rheumatic AS are as follows:

- Adhesions and fusions of the cusps and commissures
- Retraction of the margins of the cusps
- Reduced orifice of the valve, giving it a round or triangular shape and resulting in stenosis as well as regurgitation
- Frequent involvement of the mitral valve (MV)

#### Pathophysiology

Previously, calcified AS was considered the simple result of the wearing and tearing of the valve tissue in a passive mechanism. However, this idea was changed by studies showing that the mechanism of calcified AS is more complex with the involvement of the active inflammatory process and genetic factors.[1,3]

In adults with AV disease, a significant burden of leaflet involvement is present before the development of the outflow obstruction. Consequently, when mild obstruction occurs, hemodynamic progression happens in almost all patients. Natural history studies on AS have shown a long latent period of progressive AS followed by symptomatic AS. Table 30.1 demonstrates the clinical stages of valvular AS.

The AV area has to be reduced to about half of the normal value until a measurable gradient occurs. When a pressure gradient develops between the aorta and the left ventricle (LV), LV pressure rises to maintain aortic pressure within the normal range. Indeed, the LV responds to AS by left ventricular hypertrophy (LVH). LVH may induce LV diastolic dysfunction. Systolic heart failure (HF) occurs at the end stage of the disease. Fig. 30.1 depicts that pathophysiology of myocardial ischemia in severe AS.

Interestingly, more women have "excessive" LVH compared with men despite similar degrees of AS severity with "supernormal" left ventricular ejection fraction (LVEF)—associated with a small, thick-walled LV and lower end-systolic wall stress.[5,6]

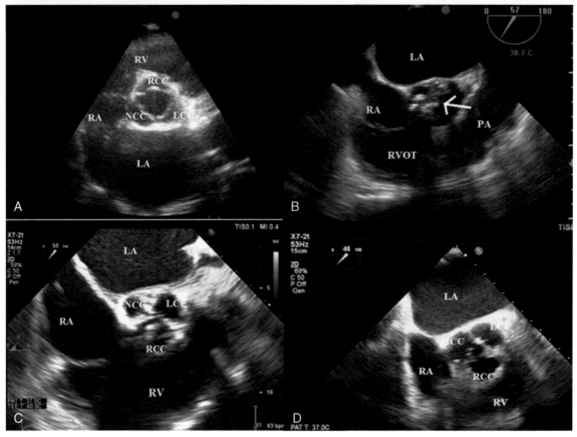

FIG. 30.1 (A) Normal tricuspid aortic valve (AV). (B) Thickened and calcified bicuspid AV. (C) Tricuspid, degenerative, calcified AV. (D) Rheumatic AV with thickened cusps and fusions of the commissures. *LA*, left atrium; *LCC*, left coronary cusp; *NCC*, noncoronary cusp; *PA*, pulmonary artery; *RA*, right atrium; *RCC*, right coronary cusp; *RV*, right ventricle; *RVOT*, right ventricular outflow tract.

**TABLE 30.1**
**Clinical Stages of Valvular Aortic Stenosis**

| Stage | Definition | Valve Anatomy | Valve Hemodynamics | Hemodynamic Consequences | Symptoms |
|-------|-----------|---------------|--------------------|-----------------------|----------|
| A | At risk of AS | • Bicuspid aortic valve (or other congenital valve anomaly)<br>• Aortic valve sclerosis | • Aortic $V_{max}$ <2 m/s | None | None |
| B | Progressive AS | • Mild-to-moderate leaflet calcification of a bicuspid or trileaflet valve with some reduction in systolic motion or rheumatic valve changes with commissural fusion | • Mild AS: aortic $V_{max}$ 2.0–2.9 m/s or mean $\Delta P$ <20 mmHg<br>• Moderate AS: aortic $V_{max}$ 3.0–3.9 m/s or mean $\Delta P$ 20–39 mmHg | • Early LV diastolic dysfunction may be present<br>• Normal LVEF | None |
| C: Asymptomatic severe AS | | | | | |
| C1 | Asymptomatic severe AS | • Severe leaflet calcification or congenital stenosis | • Aortic $V_{max}$ ≤4 m/s or mean $\Delta P$ ≤40 mmHg | • LV diastolic dysfunction | None; exercise testing is reasonable to |

*Continued*

**TABLE 30.1**
Clinical Stages of Valvular Aortic Stenosis—cont'd

| Stage | Definition | Valve Anatomy | Valve Hemodynamics | Hemodynamic Consequences | Symptoms |
|---|---|---|---|---|---|
| | | with severely reduced leaflet opening | • AVA typically is $\leq 1.0$ cm$^2$ (or AVAi $\leq 0.6$ cm$^2$/m$^2$)<br>• Very severe AS is an aortic $V_{max} \leq 5$ m/s or mean $\Delta P$ $\leq 60$ mmHg | • Mild LV hypertrophy<br>• Normal LVEF | confirm symptom status |
| C2 | Asymptomatic severe AS with LV dysfunction | • Severe leaflet calcification or congenital stenosis with severely reduced leaflet opening | • Aortic $V_{max} \leq 4$ m/s or mean $\Delta P$ $\leq 40$ mmHg<br>• AVA typically $\leq 1.0$ cm$^2$ (or AVAi $\leq 0.6$ cm$^2$/m$^2$) | • LVEF <50% | None |
| **D: Symptomatic severe AS** | | | | | |
| D1 | Symptomatic severe high-gradient AS | • Severe leaflet calcification or congenital stenosis with severely reduced leaflet opening | • Aortic $V_{max} \leq 4$ m/s or mean $\Delta P$ $\leq 40$ mmHg<br>• AVA typically $\leq 1.0$ cm$^2$ (or AVAi $\leq 0.6$ cm$^2$/m$^2$) but may be larger with mixed AS/AR | • LV diastolic dysfunction<br>• LV hypertrophy<br>• Pulmonary hypertension may be present | • Exertional dyspnea or decreased exercise tolerance<br>• Exertional angina<br>• Exertional syncope or presyncope |
| D2 | Symptomatic severe low-flow, low-gradient AS with reduced LVEF | • Severe leaflet calcification with severely reduced leaflet motion | • AVA $\leq 1.0$ cm$^2$ with resting aortic $V_{max}$ <4 m/s or mean $\Delta P$ <40 mmHg<br>• Dobutamine stress echocardiography shows AVA $\leq 1.0$ cm$^2$ with $V_{max} \leq 4$ m/s at any flow rate | • LV diastolic dysfunction<br>• LV hypertrophy<br>• LVEF <50% | • HF<br>• Angina<br>• Syncope or presyncope |
| D3 | Symptomatic severe low-gradient AS with normal LVEF or paradoxical low-flow severe AS | • Severe leaflet calcification with severely reduced leaflet motion | • AVA $\leq 1.0$ cm$^2$ with aortic $V_{max}$ <4 m/s or mean $\Delta P$ <40 mmHg<br>• Indexed AVA $\leq 0.6$ cm$^2$/m$^2$ and<br>• Stroke volume index <35 mL/m$^2$<br>• Measured when patient is normotensive (systolic BP <140 mmHg) | • Increased LV relative wall thickness<br>• Small LV chamber with low stroke volume<br>• Restrictive diastolic filling<br>• LVEF $\geq 50$% | • HF<br>• Angina<br>• Syncope or presyncope |

*AR*, aortic regurgitation; *AS*, aortic stenosis; *AVA*, aortic valve area; *AVAi*, aortic valve area indexed to body surface area; *BP*, blood pressure; *HF*, heart failure; *LV*, left ventricular; *LVEF*, left ventricular ejection fraction; *ΔP*, pressure gradient; *V$_{max}$*, maximum aortic velocity.

From Nishimura RA, Otto CM, Bonow RO, et al. 2014 AHA/ACC guideline for the management of patients with valvular heart disease: a report of the American College of Cardiology/American Heart Association Task Force on Practice Guidelines. *J Am Coll Cardiol.* 2014;63(22):e57–e185; with permission.

Severe AS has been defined based on the natural history of unoperated patients with AS, showing a poor prognosis when peak AV velocity becomes greater than 4 m/s or AV mean gradient reaches more than 40 mmHg.[4,7,8]

The risk of sudden death is less than 1% in asymptomatic patients with severe AS; clinical decision making is therefore based on the patient's symptoms and LV function as well as the hemodynamic severity of the valve. Indeed, the onset of symptoms such as dyspnea, angina, and syncope in patients with severe AS shows the subsequent clinical events.

### Clinical findings

The cardinal symptoms of AS are dyspnea on exertion, angina, syncope, HF, and death in the end stages.[9] When symptoms occur, it means that the lifespan of the patient is becoming short without therapeutic interventional treatment. The typical symptoms of AS in patients with BAV begin at age 50–70 years and in calcified tricuspid AV begins at age 70 years or older. Even 40% of patients with AS who are 70 years or older have congenital BAV.[10] The most common symptom in patients with AS is a gradual decrease in exercise capacity, which may be due to a high LV end-diastolic pressure in LV diastolic dysfunction or limited ability in increasing the cardiac output after exercise. Angina is seen in about two-thirds of patients with severe AS, with about 50% of the patients having associated significant coronary artery disease (CAD). In patients without CAD, angina is a consequence of the combination of increased

---

myocardial demands and reduced oxygen supply, resulting in myocardial ischemia (Fig. 30.2).

Syncope occurs in severe AS most commonly during exertion because of cerebral hypoperfusion. Box 30.1 presents some other causes of severe AS.

Gastrointestinal bleeding in patients with severe AS is often associated with angiodysplasia (mostly of the right colon) and is corrected by AV repair.

### Physical examination

The physical findings of patients with AS depend on the severity of valvular stenosis, LV function, and stroke volume.

The most important features of severe AS are as follows[4,7]:

1. *Parvus et tardus arterial pulse*, which means a slow-rising, low-amplitude, and late-peaking carotid pulse, is specific for severe AS; however, associated

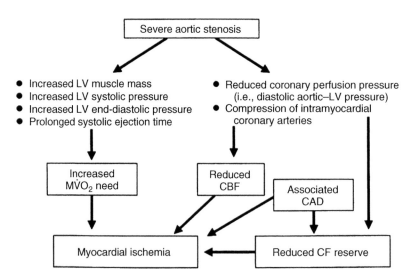

FIG. 30.2 Pathophysiology of myocardial ischemia in severe aortic stenosis. *CAD,* coronary artery disease; *CBF,* cerebral blood flow; *CF,* coronary flow; *MVO$_2$,* myocardial oxygen consumption; *LV,* left ventricular. (From Fuster V, O'Rourke RA, Walsh RA, et al. *Hurst's the Heart.* 12th ed. New York: McGraw-Hill; 2007; with permission.)

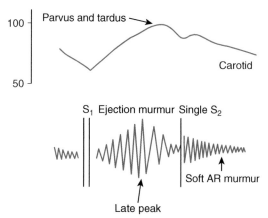

FIG. 30.3 Slow-rising, low-amplitude, and late-peaking aortic pressure waveform of the carotid pulse with a late-peaking crescendo–decrescendo systolic murmur in severe aortic stenosis. *AR*, aortic regurgitation. (From Otto CM, Bonow RO. Valvular heart disease. In: Mann DL, Zipes DP, Libby P, et al., eds. *Braunwald's Heart Disease: A Textbook of Cardiovascular Medicine.* 10th ed. Philadelphia: Saunders; 2015; with permission.)

systemic hypertension or aortic regurgitation (AR) can affect the arterial pulse (Fig. 30.3).

2. *Late-peaking systolic ejection murmur (SEM)* is best heard at the base of the heart in the aortic region (upper right sternal border) and can be a musical or seagull sound.
3. Radiation of the high-frequency components of SEM to the apex is termed "Gallavardin phenomenon" and can be mistaken with the murmur of mitral regurgitation (MR).
4. Change in the intensity of the murmur by the Valsalva and standing maneuver is in favor of AS.
5. *Carotid shudder or palpable systolic thrill* is a specific, albeit not sensitive, the sign of severe AS.
6. *Single $S_2$ or paradoxical $S_2$* happens because of late $A_2$.
7. $S_4$ gallop sound.
8. In young patients with BAV, $A_2$ can be heard normally or accentuated in association with aortic ejection sound, showing a flexible and noncalcified valve.

### Diagnostic testing
#### Electrocardiography
- The main finding of AS is LVH, which is seen in about 85% of patients with severe AS. Consequently, the absence of LVH cannot rule out the presence of severe AS.
- The presence of LV strain associated with ST-segment depressions is suggestive of severe LVH.
- Left atrial (LA) enlargement is found in more than 80% of patients with isolated severe AS.

- Atrial fibrillation (AF) may occur in 10%–15% of patients with AS.[4,7]
- Loss of atrial contraction may cause serious hypotension, and AF rhythm should be reversed immediately, usually with cardioversion.

**Chest radiography.** A normal-sized heart and a dilated ascending aorta (poststenotic dilation) constitute the usual findings in a patient with AS. The calcification of the AV is present in almost all adult patients with significant AS and is visible by fluoroscopy and CT but rarely is seen in chest radiography. However, a calcified AV does not constitute severe AS.[3,6]

**Echocardiography.** Transthoracic echocardiography (TTE) is the gold-standard imaging modality for the initial evaluation and follow-up of patients with AS.[1,4] Box 30.2 lists the data that can be provided by two-dimensional (2D) TTE can confer.

The hemodynamic severity of AS is evaluated via Doppler echocardiography by measuring blood flow velocity and pressure gradient from the Bernoulli equation.

The Bernoulli equation, which was initially simplified to $\Delta P = 4 \ (V2^2 - V1^2)$, was subsequently simplified further to $\Delta P = 4 \ V2^2$ if LVOT velocity is less than 1 m/s:

$V2$ = Transaortic velocity measured by continuous-wave Doppler study

$V1$ = LVOT velocity measured by pulsed-wave Doppler study

The accuracy of Doppler-derived pressure gradients has been confirmed by simultaneous cardiac catheterization data.[11,12]

Because the most variables are derived from aortic peak velocity, a careful evaluation of maximal aortic velocity from different views and windows (apical

---

**BOX 30.2**

**Information Provided by Transthoracic Echocardiography in Patients With Aortic Stenosis**

Cause of aortic valve stenosis

Aortic valve morphology and severity of calcification

Severity of aortic stenosis (aortic valve peak velocity, mean pressure gradient, and aortic valve area)

Concomitant aortic regurgitation and other valve diseases

Left ventricular hypertrophy and left ventricular function

Size of the aortic root and the ascending aorta

Systolic pulmonary artery pressure

five- and three-chamber views and suprasternal and right parasternal windows) is mandatory. Interestingly, the highest velocities are commonly found in the right parasternal window.[2,3]

The severity of AS has been classified based on echocardiography-derived hemodynamic data as follows: aortic $V_{max}$, mean $\Delta P$, aortic valve area (AVA) by continuity evaluation, and LVOT-to-AV velocity time integral (TVI) ratio = (LVOT/AVTI).

The typical findings in severe AS are as follows:
- Aortic peak V of 4 m/s or greater
- Mean pressure gradient 40 mmHg or greater
- AVA 1 cm² or less or AVA index 0.6 cm²/m² or less by continuity evaluation
- LVOT-to-AV TVI ratio = (LVOT/AVTI) 0.25 or less[4] (Fig. 30.4)

**Transesophageal echocardiography.** Transesophageal echocardiography (TEE) is not recommended for the routine evaluation of AS, but when TTE is inconclusive and difficult to perform or there is serial stenosis or AS is associated with dynamic LVOT obstruction, TEE can be used to clearly show the valve morphology and the number of AV cusps and to measure AV area by direct planimetry. TEE helps evaluate the severity of associated MR.[3]

**Cardiac imaging.** Cardiac CT is a useful method for the evaluation of the aortic root and ascending aorta dilatation in patients who are candidates for AV surgery because it can determine the type of surgery.

Cardiac CT can measure AV calcification with the Agatston method, and AV calcification greater than 1651 Agatston Units (AU) provides the sensitivity of 80% and specificity of 87% for severe AS, which is useful even in patients with a reduced LVEF.[13]

Cardiac magnetic resonance (CMR) is a valuable method for evaluating LV volume and function, especially when echocardiography is not conclusive.

**Cardiac catheterization and angiography.** In most patients, echocardiography can provide sufficient hemodynamic data for patient management. Cardiac catheterization is reserved for patients who need coronary angiography before surgery or when there is a discrepancy between noninvasive data and clinical findings.[14,15]

**Exercise stress testing.** The use of the exercise test in patients with severe asymptomatic AS is reasonable (class IIa) in that it can both evaluate exercise capacity, ST-segment abnormalities, and blood pressure response and determine whether the patient is asymptomatic.

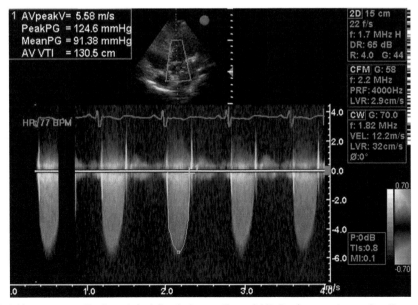

FIG. 30.4 Very severe aortic stenosis is defined when aortic peak V is 5 m/s or greater or when the mean pressure gradient is 60 mmHg or greater.

Exercise testing is not recommended (class III) in patients with severe AS who are symptomatic.[4]

**Hemodynamic progression.** The progression rate is very variable. Older age, more calcification of the AV, hypertension, hyperlipidemia, and smoking have been proposed as risk factors for rapid progression. The average rate of the annual decrease in AV area is about 0.12 $cm^2$/year.[3] When symptoms occur, the survival rate will be poor unless the LVOT obstruction is relieved.

### Low-flow, low-gradient aortic stenosis

In patients with LV systolic dysfunction, aortic velocity and pressure gradient can be reduced even if the calculated AV area is less than 1 $cm^2$. In this situation, one must differentiate between true anatomically severe AS and pseudofunctional AS. In true anatomically severe AS, LV systolic dysfunction and low transaortic flow occur because of afterload mismatch. In primary LV myocardial dysfunction, the AV opening is reduced because of a low transaortic flow rate. It can even occur in moderate AS.

Low-dose dobutamine stress echocardiography (DSE) is a class IIa indication in patients with stage D2 AS and is recommended in patients with the following:
a. Calcified AV with calculated AV area 1 $cm^2$ or less
b. LVEF less than 50%
c. Aortic velocity less than 4.0 m/s
d. Mean pressure gradient less than 40 mmHg

True anatomically severe AS is defined whenever the following data are obtained during DSE:
- Maximum AV velocity 4.0 m/s or greater with AV area 1.0 $cm^2$ or less

DSE is useful in identifying the presence of myocardial contractile reserve, which means a 20% or greater increase in stroke volume in DSE.
- Patients without contractile reserve have a poor prognosis even with surgical therapy. However, there is evidence that survival improves because afterload is reduced after AV repair.[4,16,17]
- In patients without myocardial contractile reserve, AV repair can increase survival if AV means pressure gradient is greater than 20 mmHg.

### Low-flow, low-gradient aortic stenosis with normal left ventricular systolic function

It has been suggested that 5%–25% of patients with severe AS have low-flow, low-gradient AS with preserved systolic function. The typical finding is a small hypertrophied LV with a preserved ejection fraction EF in hypertensive older adult patients. A low transaortic flow rate (<35 mL/$m^2$) is mainly due to a small LV cavity. It is very important to distinguish moderate AS from true anatomically severe AS because many of these patients have a small body size with only moderate AS, and others have severe true AS and as such need AV repair. The management of these patients is very challenging and needs reevaluation of the symptoms after controlling hypertension (normotensive patients with systolic blood pressure < 140 mmHg) and calculating indexed AV area, which should be 10.6 $cm^2$/$m^2$ or less.[18,19]

### Management

Principles in the management of patients with AS are as follows:
- Patients should be informed to report their symptoms when they become symptomatic.
- Patients with severe AS should avoid vigorous physical activities and sports.
- Conventional CAD risk factors should be treated based on the guidelines.
- Large randomized controlled trials have not shown the beneficial effects of lipid-lowering therapy (statins) in patients with AS in terms of hemodynamic progression.
- Management of patients with severe AS is shown in Fig. 30.5.

Recommendations for the timing of therapeutic intervention (either surgical AV repair or transcatheter AV repair) for AS are summarized in Table 30.2 based on the guidelines.

Transcatheter AV repair (TAVR) or transcatheter aortic valve implantation, which uses bioprostheses, is an alternate approach for patients who need AV repair.

TAVR is a class I recommendation for patients who are candidates for AV repair with excessive risk for surgery and a predicted survival rate longer than 12 months after TAVR.

The choice of intervention, which means surgical versus TAVR, relies on multiple parameters such as comorbidity, risk of surgery, and the patient's frailty. The decision should be made by a heart-valve team.[4]

### Bicuspid Aortic Valve
#### Epidemiology
Bicuspid aortic valve is a common congenital disease and is seen in 1%–2% of the general population with a male predominance. Familial clustering with an autosomal dominant pattern has been reported.[10]

#### Pathophysiology
The most common type of BAV, seen in 70%–80% of patients, is the fusion of the left and right coronary cusps and results in the left-right systolic opening. In

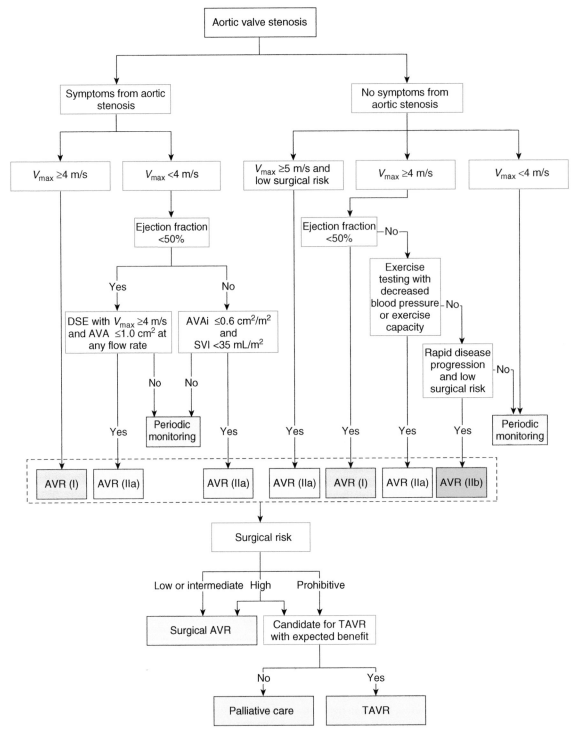

FIG. 30.5 Algorithm management of patients with severe aortic stenosis (AS). *AVAi*, aortic valve area indexed to body surface area; *AVR*, aortic valve replacement; *DSE*, dobutamine stress echocardiography; *SVI*, stroke volume index; *TAVR*, transcatheter aortic valve repair.

## TABLE 30.2
### Recommendation for Timing of Intervention in Severe Aortic Stenosis

| Recommendation | COR | LOE |
| --- | --- | --- |
| AVR is recommended with severe high-gradient AS who have symptoms by history or on exercise testing (stage D1) | I | B |
| AVR is recommended for asymptomatic patients with severe AS (stage C2) and LVEF <50% | I | B |
| AVR is recommended for patients with severe AS (stage C or D) when undergoing other cardiac surgery | I | B |
| AVR is reasonable for asymptomatic patients with very severe AS (stage C1, aortic velocity ≤5 m/s) and low surgical risk | II$_a$ | B |
| AVR is reasonable for asymptomatic patients (stage C) with severe AS and decreased exercise tolerance or an exercise fall in BP | II$_a$ | B |
| AVR is reasonable in symptomatic patients with low-flow, low-gradient severe AS with reduced LVEF (stage D2) with a low-dose dobutamine stress study that shows an aortic velocity 24.0 m/s (or mean pressure gradient ≥49 mmHg) with a valve area ≥1.0 cm² at any dobutamine dose | II$_a$ | B |
| AVR is reasonable in symptomatic patients who have low-flow/low-gradient severe AS (stage D3) who are normotensive and have and LVEF ≥50% if clinical, hemodynamic and anatomic data support valve obstruction as the most likely cause of symptoms | II$_a$ | C |
| AVR is reasonable for patients with moderate AS (stage B) (aortic velocity, 3.0–3.9 m/s) who are undergoing other cardiac surgery | II$_b$ | C |
| AVR may be considered for asymptomatic patients with severe AS (stage C1) and rapid disease progression and low surgical risk | II$_b$ | C |

*AS*, aortic stenosis; *AVR*, aortic valve replacement by either surgical or trans catheter approach; *BP*, blood pressure; *COR*, Class of Recommendation; *LOE*, level of evidence; *LVEF*, left ventricular ejection fraction; *N/A*, not applicable.
From Nishimura RA, Otto CM, Bonow RO, et al. 2014 AHA/ACC guideline for the management of patients with valvular heart disease: a report of the American College of Cardiology/American Heart Association Task Force on Practice Guidelines. *J Am Coll Cardiol.* 2014;63(22):e57–e185; with permission.

20%–30% of the patients, the fusion of the right and noncoronary cusps occurs and results in anterior–posterior orientation.

The echocardiographic diagnosis of BAV is based on the oval-shaped systolic opening of the AV. Evaluating BAV in diastole can be misleading, and the raphe—which is the prominent tissue ridge—mimics a tricuspid AV. BAV is associated with aortopathy and dilation of the ascending aorta. The severity of the aortopathy does not seem to be related to the severity of AS. BAV patients have a five- to ninefold higher risk of aortic dissection[20-23] (Fig. 30.6).

### Clinical presentation and disease course
Although most BAVs have an acceptable function until late in life, these patients are at risk of the following:
- Significant AR (≈ 20% of the patients need AV repair) at age 10–40 years
- Increased risk of infective endocarditis (IE)
- Aortopathy, aortic dilatation, and increased risk of aortic dissection (five to nine times higher risk)
- Severe AS (after the age of 50, most of the patients have severe calcified AS)

### Management
Currently, there is no proven medication for the prevention of BAV deterioration. Patients should be followed for valve dysfunction besides aortopathy of the ascending aorta.

In patients who are candidates for AV replacement, aortic root or ascending aorta replacement should be considered if the maximum end-diastolic diameter of the aorta exceeds 4.5 cm.

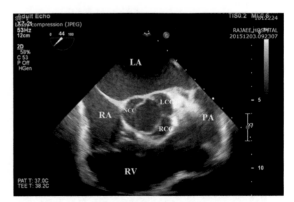

FIG. 30.6 Oval-shaped systolic opening of the aortic valve with the fusion of the left and right coronary cusps. *LA*, left atrium; *LCC*, left coronary cusp; *NCC*, noncoronary cusp; *PA*, pulmonary artery; *RA*, right atrium; *RCC*, right coronary cusp; *RV*, right ventricle.

In patients with acceptable functioning of the BAV, aortic replacement is indicated if the maximum end-diastolic diameter of the aorta reaches 5.5 cm or when it reaches 5 cm and there is a rapid progression of aortic dilatation (≥0.5 cm/year) or malignant positive family history.[24,25]

## Aortic Regurgitation

### Epidemiology and pathology

Similar to all other valve diseases, AR is divided into primary AR, secondary AR, or complex AR (meaning both). Primary AR is caused by primary involvement of the AV as in IE, and secondary AR can result from the aortic root abnormality such as aortic root disease in Marfan syndrome (Fig. 30.7 and Box 30.3).

It has been suggested that the rate of secondary AR is increasing and accounts for more than 50% of the patients who need AV replacement. Congenital involvement of the AV (BAV) account for the second most cause of AR.[3,14,26]

The overall prevalence of AR has been suggested to be about 10% as shown in the Strong Heart Study, although most of the participants had mild AR. The aortic root diameter and age were the independent predictors of AR.[27]

### Pathophysiology

By definition, AR is a diastolic reversal of the flow from the aorta to the LV, which occurs because of aortic cusp disease or malcoaptation of the cusps.

Aortic regurgitation differs from MR; in MR, the regurgitant fraction empties to the LA, which is a low-pressure

---

**BOX 30.3**
**Primary and Secondary Cause of Aortic Regurgitation (AR)**

**PRIMARY AR (AV DISEASE)**

Degenerative or calcified AV results AS and in most patients some degree of AR

Infective endocarditis results perforation and destruction of the AV

Trauma

Congenital BAV causing prolapse or incomplete closure of the valves

Rheumatic heart disease is common cause of primary AR

AR in patients with congenital heart disease such as in large VSD or in patients with subaortic stenosis

Myxomatous change of the AV

In unicommissural and quadricuspid aortic valves

**SECONDARY AR (CAUSED BY MARKED DILATION OF THE AORTIC ROOT OR ASCENDING AORTA)**

Degenerative aortic dilation (age related)

Cystic medial necrosis as isolated or seen in Marfan syndrome

Aortopathy associated with bicuspid valves

Chronic systemic hypertension

Aortic dissection

Systemic disease such as ankylosing spondylitis, Behçet syndrome, or syphilitic aortitis

*AS*, aortic stenosis; *BAV*, bicuspid aortic valve; *VSD*, ventricular septal defect.

---

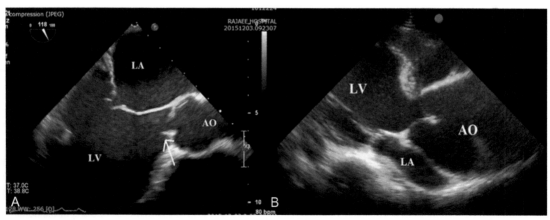

FIG. 30.7 (A) Primary involvement of the aortic valve caused by infective endocarditis. (B) Secondary aortic regurgitation in a patient with Marfan syndrome. The surgical approach differs in these two patients. *AO*, aorta; *LA*, left atrium; *LV*, left ventricle.

chamber, but in AR, the whole left ventricle stroke volume ejects to the aorta, which is a high-pressure chamber.

Indeed, severe chronic AR imposes a severe volume and pressure overload on the LV. The volume overload results from added regurgitant volume to the forward stroke volume, and pressure overload results from increased total stroke volume, which ejects to the aorta in systole and results systolic hypertension.[3,6,26]

## MYOCARDIAL ISCHEMIA

Myocardial ischemia occurs in both acute and chronic AR. In acute AR, wall tension increases result in increased myocardial oxygen requirements. In severe chronic AR, as the LV mass increases, total myocardial oxygen demands also increases. On the other hand, coronary flow reserve is reduced because of the decreased diastolic pressure of the aorta and coronary perfusion pressure.

Consequently, the combination of the increased myocardial oxygen demands and reduced supply develop myocardial ischemia, particularly during exercise.

### Chronic Aortic Insufficiency

In the early phase of severe AR, LV compensation occurs by eccentric hypertrophy, which maintains LV filling pressure and LVEF in the normal range. Indeed, in chronic AR, both preload and afterload increase, and systolic function is preserved through LV dilation and hypertrophy.

Severe chronic AR results in the largest LV end-diastolic volume between all forms of heart diseases, which is called *cor bovinum heart*.

Over time, the LV progressively dilates and wall stress increases because of systolic hypertension, which results in latent myocardial dysfunction and preserved LVEF and in the cost of the increased preload.

Ultimately, LVEF reduces filling pressures increases, and LV systolic dysfunction and HF symptoms occur.[3,6,26]

### Acute Aortic Insufficiency

Usually acute AR is severe and causes the LV to enface a large volume of regurgitant blood during diastole. In this acute situation, there is no enough time for compensatory LV enlargement except for a mild increase in LV end-diastolic volume, which would be less than 20%–30%. Consequently, compensatory tachycardia, low forward stroke volume, hypotension, and pulmonary congestion occur, which are contrary to systolic hypertension that occurs in severe chronic AR.[3,4,6,26]

### Clinical findings

Usually, patients with mild or moderate AR are asymptomatic. Even severe chronic AR is well tolerated, and patients remain asymptomatic until considerable cardiac enlargement and dysfunction occur. In severe chronic AR, the LV gradually enlarges and results in the ejection of a large volume of the blood in the systole; consequently, patients feel palpitations and pounding of the head, especially during emotional stress and tachycardia. These symptoms may occur many years before overt LV systolic dysfunction.

Symptoms occur late in the course and mainly result from increased pulmonary venous pressure (dyspnea on exertion, paroxysmal nocturnal dyspnea, and orthopnea). Angina may occur in the late course of the disease as a result of the low arterial diastolic pressure and low heart rate at night (nocturnal angina).

### Physical examination

Many clinical signs in severe chronic AR have been suggested, mostly caused by increased stroke volume and systolic hypertension, although not all of them are very useful in clinical practice (Box 30.4).

---

**BOX 30.4**

**Physical Examination of Patients With Severe Chronic Aortic Regurgitation (AR) (Note: Some are seen in moderate AR.)**

Prominent arterial pulse (best examination is palpation of the radial artery when the arm is elevated)

Hyperdynamic impulse

De Musset sign (head bobbing with each heartbeat)

Water hammer pulses

Corrigan pulse (abrupt distention and quick collapse)

Quincke pulse (capillary pulsations)

Bisferiens pulse (double impulse during systole) may be appreciated in the femoral and brachial arteries

Traube sign (pistol shot sounds), which means booming of the systolic and diastolic sounds over the femoral artery

Wide pulse pressure (elevated systolic arterial pressure and low diastolic pressure)

Korotkoff sounds often persist to zero even though the intra-arterial pressure rarely falls below 30 mmHg

Diffuse and hyperdynamic apical impulse, which is inferiorly and laterally displaced

The systolic arterial pressure is increased (in severe AR, it averages 145–160 mmHg), and the diastolic pressure is reduced (in severe AR, it averages 45–60 mmHg)

Persistent Korotkoff sounds (down to 0 mmHg), although intra-arterial pressure usually remains above 30 mmHg

In patients with LV systolic dysfunction, systolic blood pressure may fall and diastolic pressure rise because of the peripheral vasoconstriction and should not be mistaken for improvement in the severity of AR.

### Auscultation
- High-frequency decrescendo blowing diastolic murmur (over the third or fourth left intercostal space) is the typical finding for chronic AR and may be associated with diastolic thrill.
- Single $S_2$ caused by incomplete closure of the AV.
- Mid and late diastolic rumble in the apex (Austin-Flint murmur) caused by the struck of the mitral leaflet with the AR jet.
- Systolic ejection murmur in severe AR demonstrates the increased ejection volume.

### Diagnostic testing
**Electrocardiography.** The electrocardiogram (ECG) may show:
- Left axis deviation.
- LV strain pattern, which correlates with LV dilatation and hypertrophy.
- Normal sinus rhythm is the usual pattern; in the case of AF, HF, or the presence of the mitral disease should be considered.

**Chest radiography.** In the presence of the significant AR and LV enlargement, the cardiothoracic ratio increases, and the apex displaces downward and to the left side of the thorax.

The ascending aorta and aortic knob may be dilated (Fig. 30.8).[3,4,6,25]

**Echocardiography.** Echocardiography plays a key role in the initial evaluation and follow-up of patients with AR[4,25] (Box 30.5 and Table 30.3).

**Cardiac imaging.** Multidetector CT (MDCT) and CMR are useful methods for evaluating the entire thoracic aorta and more importantly, for the distal part of the ascending aorta in patients who are candidates for surgery because of the ascending aortic dilatation or in patients with echocardiographic suboptimal imaging quality.[14]

**Cardiac magnetic resonance imaging.** CMR imaging accurately assess LV volume and function and is a valuable method for AR severity quantification whenever the echocardiography image quality is suboptimal or there is the controversy between clinical data and echocardiography findings.[3,4,25,26] CMR is a useful method for accurate measurement of the LV volume and function in asymptomatic patients with severe AR.[25]

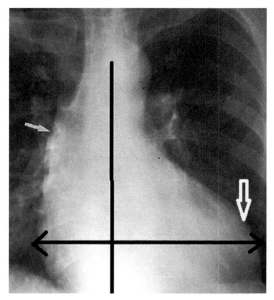

FIG. 30.8 Typical chest radiograph of a patient with severe chronic aortic regurgitation. *Arrows* indicate increased cardiothoracic ratio (cardiomegaly).

---

**BOX 30.5**
**Valuable Information Provided by Transthoracic Echocardiography in Patients With Aortic Regurgitation (AR)**

Presence and etiology of AR

Assessment of the AV morphology, aortic root, and ascending aorta size and anatomy

Severity of the AR (aortic valve peak velocity, mean pressure gradient, AV area).

Concomitant valve disease or congenital heart disease

LV volume and function

Systolic PA pressure

---

*AV*, aortic valve; *LV*, left ventricular; *PA*, pulmonary artery.

**Cardiac catheterization.** Cardiac catheterization is helpful whenever there is a discrepancy between clinical data and imaging modalities regarding the AR severity or hemodynamic studies. However, angiographic evaluation of AR, which usually a visual assessment, requires the correct amount of contrast media injection, more importantly in dilated ventricles with a rapid injection rate of about 25–35 mL/s.[3,4,28]

Although TTE is a valuable imaging modality for assessing LV size and function and AR severity, cardiac catheterization and coronary angiography may be

**TABLE 30.3**
**Echocardiographic Evaluation of Aortic Regurgitation Severity Circulation and Guideline**

| Mild AR | Moderate AR | Severe AR |
|---|---|---|
| • Jet width <25% of LVOT | • Jet width 25%–64% of LVOT | • Jet width ≤65% of LVOT |
| • Vena contracta <0.3 cm | • Vena contracta 0.3–0.6 cm | • Vena contracta >0.6 cm |
| • RVol <30 mL/beat | • RVol 30–59 mL/beat | • Holodiastolic flow reversal in the proximal abdominal aorta |
| • RF <30% | • RF 30%–49% | |
| • ERO <0.10 cm$^2$ | • ERO 0.10–0.29 cm$^2$ | • RVol ≥60 mL/beat |
| • Pressure half time (PHT) more than 500 ms | • Normal LV size or mild LV enlargement | • RF ≥50% |
| • Normal LV size | | • Evidence of LV enlargement |
| | | • PHT <200 ms |

*AR*, aortic regurgitation; *ERO*, effective regurgitant orifice; *LV*, left ventricular; *LVOT*, left ventricular outflow tract; *RV*, right ventricular; *RVol*, regurgitant volume.
Data from Nishimura RA, Otto CM, Bonow RO, et al. 2014 AHA/ACC guideline for the management of patients with valvular heart disease: a report of the American College of Cardiology/American Heart Association Task Force on Practice Guidelines. *J Am Coll Cardiol.* 2014;63(22):e57–e185.

required in patients who are candidates for surgery and need coronary artery evaluation, including men aged 35 years or older, premenopausal women aged 35 years or older with CAD risk factors, and postmenopausal women.[26]

### Hemodynamic and natural history

Significant chronic AR often is tolerated well provided that the patient remains asymptomatic with preserved systolic function.

In a study that involved relatively young asymptomatic patients with severe chronic AR and normal LV function, there was a low mortality rate of about 1%. However, similar to severe AS, when the patient develops symptoms, the prognosis becomes worse.

In asymptomatic patients, LV systolic volume and function remain the greatest predictors of clinical outcomes in severe AR.

The stages of AR have been categorized based on the valve anatomy, hemodynamic consequence, LV enlargement, and systolic function and symptoms (Table 30.4).

### Management

Patients with chronic AR who have systolic hypertension (blood pressure >140 mmHg) or diastolic hypertension should receive medical treatment, preferably vasodilators such as angiotensin-converting enzyme (ACE) inhibitors or nifedipines to decrease the regurgitant volume. Beta-blocking agents must be used with caution.[3]

The routine use of vasodilators in asymptomatic patients with severe chronic AR who have normal LV function is not recommended.[4]

However, medical treatment is useful in patients who have symptomatic severe AR with or without LV dysfunction and are not candidates for AV replacement because of comorbidities.

**Surgical.** Aortic valve replacement is the only definite treatment for symptomatic patients. Fig. 30.9 shows the optimal timing of AVR in patients with chronic AR based on the latest American College of Cardiology (ACC) guideline.

Patients with severe chronic AR need surgical treatment:
1. If symptoms develop, regardless of the LV size and function.
2. Asymptomatic or symptomatic patients with LVEF less than 50%.
3. Severe LV enlargement defined as an end-systolic diameter more than 50 mm.[3,4]

Comments:
- Patients with very severe LV systolic dysfunction (LVEF <25%) are considered as high risk for surgery, but their prognosis is very poor too if they are treated medically alone. So these patients should be managed individually.
- In patients with severe asymptomatic AR and LV dysfunction or LV enlargement, the decision for AVR should be based on the several serial measurements in 2- to 4-month intervals to overcome the possible measurement variability that may be found in echocardiography.
- All patients who are candidates for AVR should undergo concomitant aortic root surgery or ascending aorta replacement if aortic dilation exceeds 45 mm.[4,29]
- The mortality rate of surgical AVR is about 3%–8% based on the patient general condition, LV systolic function, and expertise of the surgical team.
- Surgical treatment of the AR may need concomitant replacement of the aortic root and ascending aorta. In these patients, the AV may be saved (valve-sparing procedure) if the AR is caused by root dilatation. Aneurysmal dilation of the ascending aorta requires excision, replacement with a graft that contains a

**TABLE 30.4**
**Stages of Chronic Aortic Regurgitation**

| Stage | Definition | Valve Anatomy | Valve Hemodynamics | Hemodynamic Consequences | Symptoms |
|-------|-----------|---------------|--------------------|-----------------------|----------|
| A | At risk of AR | • Bicuspid aortic valve (or other congenital valve anomaly)<br>• Aortic valve sclerosis<br>• Diseases of the aortic sinuses or ascending aorta<br>• History of rheumatic fever or known rheumatic heart disease<br>• IE | • AR severity: none or trace | None | None |
| B | Progressive AR | • Mild-to-moderate calcification of a trileaflet valve bicuspid aortic valve (or other congenital valve anomaly)<br>• Dilated aortic sinuses<br>• Rheumatic valve changes<br>• Previous IE | • Mild AR:<br> o Jet width <25% of LVOT<br> o Vena contracta <0.3 cm<br> o RVol <30 mL/beat<br> o RF <30%<br> o ERO <0.10 cm$^2$<br> o Angiography grade 1+<br>moderate AR<br> o Jet width 25%–64% of LVOT<br> o Vena contracta 0.3–0.6 cm<br> o RVol 30–59 mL/beat<br> o RF 30%–49%<br> o ERO 0.10–0.29 cm$^2$<br> o Angiography grade 2+ | • Normal LV systolic function<br>• Normal LV volume or mild LV dilation | None |
| C | Asymptomatic severe AR | • Calcific aortic valve disease<br>• Bicuspid valve (or other congenital abnormality)<br>• Dilated aortic sinuses or ascending aorta<br>• Rheumatic valve changes | • Severe AR:<br> o Jet width ≤65% of LVOT<br> o Vena contracta >0.6 cm<br> o Holodiastolic flow reversal in the proximal abdominal aorta<br> o RVol ≥60 mL/beat | • C1: Normal LVEF (≥50%) and mild-to-moderate LV dilation (LVESD ≤50 mm)<br>• C2: abnormal LV systolic function with depressed LVEF (<50%) or severe LV dilatation (LVESD >50 mm or | • None; exercise testing is reasonable to confirm symptom status |

*Continued*

**TABLE 30.4**
**Stages of Chronic Aortic Regurgitation—cont'd**

| Stage | Definition | Valve Anatomy | Valve Hemodynamics | Hemodynamic Consequences | Symptoms |
|-------|-----------|---------------|-------------------|--------------------------|----------|
| | | • IE with abnormal leaflet closure or perforation | ○ RF $\geq$50%<br>○ ERO $\geq$0.3 cm$^2$<br>○ Angiography grade 3+ to 4+<br>○ In addition, diagnosis of chronic severe AR requires evidence of LV dilation | indexed LVESD >25 mm/m$^2$) | |
| D | Symptomatic severe AR | • Calcific valve disease<br>• Bicuspid valve (or other congenital abnormality)<br>• Dilated aortic sinuses or ascending aorta<br>• Rheumatic valve changes<br>• Previous IE with abnormal leaflet closure or perforation | • Severe AR:<br>○ Doppler jet width $\geq$ 65% of LVOT<br>○ Vena contracta >0.6 cm<br>○ Holodiastolic flow reversal in the proximal abdominal aorta,<br>○ RVol $\geq$60 mL/beat<br>○ RF $\geq$50%<br>○ ERO $\geq$0.3 cm$^2$<br>○ Angiography grade 3+ to 4+<br>○ In addition, diagnosis of chronic severe AR requires evidence of LV dilation | • Symptomatic severe AR may occur with normal systolic function (LVEF $\geq$50%), mild-to-moderate LV dysfunction (LVEF 40%–50%), or severe LV dysfunction (LVEF <40%)<br>• Moderate-to-severe LV dilation is present | • Exertional dyspnea or angina or more severe HF symptoms |

*AR*, aortic regurgitation; *ERO*, effective regurgitant orifice; *HF*, heart failure; *IE*, infective endocarditis; *LV*, left ventricular; *LVEF*, left ventricular ejection fraction; *LVESD*, left ventricular end-systolic dimension; *LVOT*, left ventricular outflow tract; *RF*, regurgitant fraction; *RVol*, regurgitant volume.
From Nishimura RA, Otto CM, Bonow RO, et al. 2014 AHA/ACC guideline for the management of patients with valvular heart disease: a report of the American College of Cardiology/American Heart Association Task Force on Practice Guidelines. *J Am Coll Cardiol.* 2014;63(22):e57–e185; with permission.

prosthetic valve, and reimplantation of the coronary arteries. In some patients with aortic root disease, the native valve can be spared when the aortic root is replaced or repaired.

## Acute Aortic Regurgitation

Acute AR is a life-threatening disease with the three most common causes being aortic dissection, IE, and trauma.

As the LV is acutely faced with a large regurgitant volume, tachycardia occurs as a compensatory mechanism,

and LV diastolic pressure rises above the LA pressure and causes premature closure of the MV. Both together reduce the diastolic filling time and cause pulmonary congestion as well as severe hypotension because of the reduced cardiac output.

### Clinical findings

The diagnosis of acute AR, which usually is severe, is not easy, and requires knowledge and a high index of suspicion.

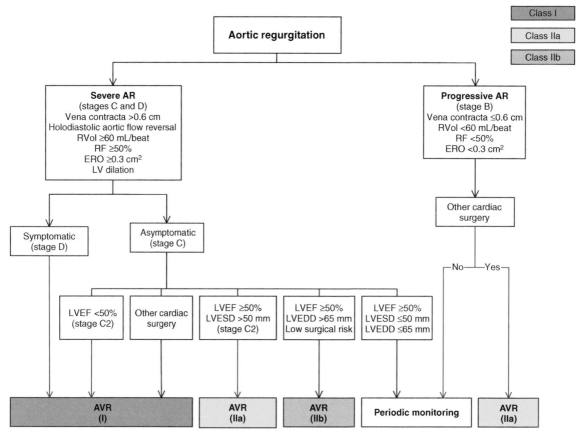

FIG. 30.9 Surgical management of patients with severe chronic aortic regurgitation (AR). *AVR*, aortic valve replacement (valve repair may be appropriate in selected patients); *ERO*, effective regurgitant orifice; *LV*, left ventricular; *LVEDD*, left ventricular end-diastolic dimension; *LVEF*, left ventricular ejection fraction; *LVESD*, left ventricular end-systolic dimension; *RF*, regurgitant fraction; *RVol*, regurgitant volume. (From Nishimura RA, Otto CM, Bonow RO, et al. 2014 AHA/ACC guideline for the management of patients with valvular heart disease: a report of the American College of Cardiology/American Heart Association Task Force on Practice Guidelines. *J Am Coll Cardiol*. 2014;63(22):e57–e185; with permission.)

Most clinical signs of chronic AR are caused by increased stroke volume and systolic hypertension, which are both absent in acute AR. The wide pulse pressure is absent because of the peripheral vasoconstriction. The murmur of acute AR is an early low-pitched diastolic murmur with shorter duration that is not impressive and dramatic as severe chronic AR.

### Echocardiography
Echocardiography is a valuable method to identify the cause of the acute AR; evaluate the AV morphology, aortic root, and ascending aorta anatomy; and assess the AR

severity, LV size and function, and premature closure of the MV besides the pulmonary pressure.

### Management
Acute AR requires a rapid diagnosis and early surgery because frequently LV failure occurs, even in patients with normal LV function. Diastolic closure of the MV is an alarm sign.

Patients should be managed by intravenous agents such as positive inotrope agents (dobutamine or dopamine) or even vasodilator agents such as nitroprusside based on the patient's arterial pressure. In the setting of acute AR, one should be aware that an intra-aortic balloon pump and beta blockers are contraindicated,

In patients with active IE who hemodynamically are stable, the surgery may be postponed for 5–7 days to allow the patient to receive intense antibiotic therapy. AV replacement with or without root replacement is the treatment of choice.

## MITRAL VALVE DISEASE
### Mitral Stenosis
#### Pathology
The main cause of mitral stenosis (MS) is rheumatic fever, with rheumatic changes present in 99% of stenotic MVs removed at the time of MV surgery. Rheumatic fever creates characteristic changes in the MV, including fusion of the commissures, thickening at the leaflet edges, and chordal fusion and shortening.[30,31]

#### Pathophysiology
The most beneficial descriptor and definition of the severity of MV stenosis is the degree of diastolic valve opening or, in other words, the MV orifice area. This obstruction and stenosis result in the creation and development of a pressure gradient through the valve in diastole and causes a rise in LA and pulmonary venous pressures.

High LA pressures lead to LA enlargement, predisposing the patient with MS to AF and systemic thromboembolism. Also, elevated pulmonary venous pressures create pulmonary edema and congestion. Finally, in advanced stages, patients with MS develop pulmonary artery hypertension (PAH) and even significant right-sided HF.[3,31–34]

#### Clinical findings
Patients with MS can present with exertional dyspnea, palpitation, fatigue, atrial arrhythmias, hemoptysis, embolic events, angina-like chest pain, and finally right-sided HF. Previously stable and asymptomatic patients might decompensate acutely during emotional stress, exercise, infection, or pregnancy or when they have uncontrolled AF.[3,33,34]

**Atrial fibrillation.** Atrial fibrillation is the most common complication of MS. The prevalence of AF in patients with MS is related to the degree of valve obstruction and the patient's age. Of course, when MS is severe, the prevalence of AF is related to age. AF is frequently episodic at first; however, it subsequently becomes more persistent. AF per se creates significant diffuse atrophy of atrial muscle, atrial enlargement, and further inhomogeneity of conduction and refractoriness. These changes result in irreversible AF.[3,33–35]

**Pulmonary artery hypertension.** In patients with mild and sometimes moderate MS without increased pulmonary vascular resistance, pulmonary arterial pressure (PAP) might be normal or only slightly elevated at rest; however, this pressure increases during exercise. In individuals with severe MS and those in whom pulmonary vascular resistance is considerably increased, resting PAP is high. Infrequently, in patients with enormously elevated pulmonary vascular resistance, even PAP can exceed systemic arterial pressure. More elevations of LA and pulmonary vascular pressures happen during tachycardia and exercise.

*Causes of pulmonary hypertension in patients with mitral stenosis*
- Passive backward transmission of high LA pressures.
- Pulmonary arteriolar narrowing and constriction, which apparently are triggered by LA and pulmonary venous hypertension or reactive PAH.
- Anatomic obliterated changes in the pulmonary vascular bed, which can be considered an important complication of long-lasting and severe MS.

With moderately high PAPs, the right ventricular (RV) function is frequently maintained. Nevertheless, severe PAH usually results in right-sided HF, dilation of the RV and its annulus, secondary tricuspid regurgitation (TR), and sometimes pulmonary valve regurgitation.[3,31,35]

#### Physical examination
The typical findings of MS on auscultation are a highlighted first heart sound ($S_1$), an opening snap, and mid-diastolic rumble. Of course, $S_1$ may be weakened in intensity if the MV is heavily calcified, with reduced and limited mobility. Interestingly, if the patient is in sinus rhythm, there is the presystolic accentuation of the diastolic murmur during the atrial contraction phase (Fig. 30.10).

With a further gradual increase in the severity of stenosis, the duration of the murmur rises, the opening snap happens earlier during diastole because of a higher LA pressure, and there is the accentuation of $P_2$ when PAH is present. If the crossing flow of the MV is diminished because of HF, PAH, or AS, the murmur of MS can be reduced in intensity or even may be inaudible.[3,32–34]

#### Hemodynamics
In patients with MS and sinus rhythm, the mean LA pressure is high, and the LA pressure curve displays a prominent atrial contraction (a wave), with a gradual pressure reduction after MV opening (y descent) (Fig. 30.11).

#### Diagnostic testing
**Electrocardiography.** The ECG may show evidence of LA enlargement (P-wave duration in lead II $\geq$0.12 s or a

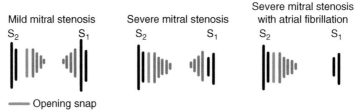

FIG. 30.10 The murmur of mitral stenosis in different degrees of severity.

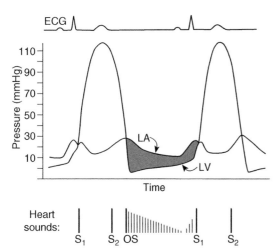

FIG. 30.11 Schematic illustration of left ventricular (LV) and left atrial (OV) pressures in patients with mitral stenosis. Classic auscultatory signs of mitral stenosis are shown at the *bottom* of the diagram. *ECG,* electrocardiogram.

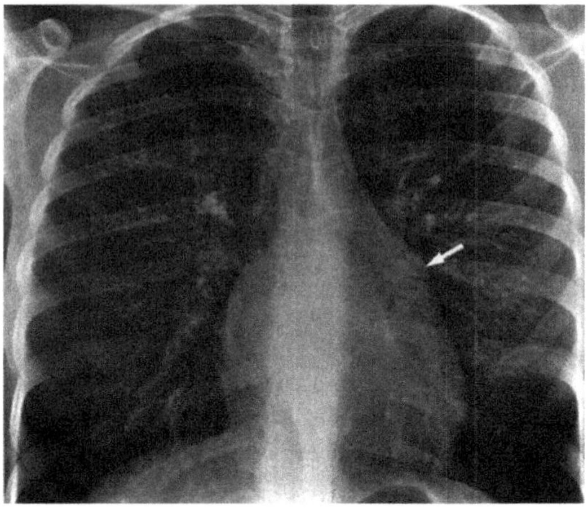

FIG. 30.12 Chest radiography of a patient with isolated mitral stenosis, demonstrating a prominent left atrial appendage (*white arrow*) as a classic sign of left atrial enlargement.

P-wave axis between +45 and −30 degrees). When the disease is more severe, AF or RV hypertrophy caused by PAH may be present.[3,34]

**Chest radiography.** On chest radiography, the typical findings of MS are LA enlargement without cardiomegaly, enlargement of the main pulmonary arteries, and sometimes pulmonary congestion. The enlargement of the right atrium, RV, and pulmonary artery also happens in patients with severe MS and pulmonary hypertension[3,30–32] (Fig. 30.12).

**Echocardiography.** Transthoracic echocardiography is indicated for all patients with suspected MS to confirm the diagnosis, to determine hemodynamic severity (mean pressure gradient across the valve, MV area, and PAP), to identify concomitant valvular lesions, and to study valve morphology with a view to defining suitability for balloon mitral commissurotomy and even as a guide for selecting the sizing balloon. The main findings of MS contain valve thickening, anterior leaflet doming, restricted valve opening, and fusion of the leaflets at the commissures (Fig. 30.13).

In patients with MS, the mean pressure gradient across the MV on Doppler echocardiography is at least 5 mmHg, and it is frequently greater than 10 mmHg in severe stenosis. Importantly, because the transvalvular gradient is flow dependent, the severity of MS is more precisely defined by the MV area [by tracing the MV opening area in cross-section by 2D or three-dimensional (3D) echocardiography] (Fig. 30.14).

Also, the MV area is measured using the pressure half time (PHT) (pressure × ½t), which is the amount of time it takes for the transmitral pressure to fall to half its initial value (MV area = 220/[$P \times \frac{1}{2}t$]) (Fig. 30.15).

Transesophageal echocardiography must be performed in patients considered for percutaneous mitral balloon commissurotomy (PBMC) to evaluate the absence or

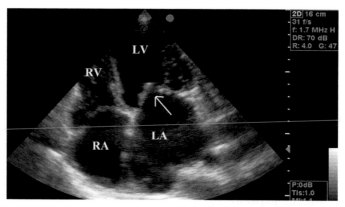

FIG. 30.13 Apical four-chamber view, showing valve thickening associated with anterior leaflet doming and restricted motion of the valve opening. *LA*, left atrium; *LV*, left ventricle; *RA*, right atrium; *RV*, right ventricle.

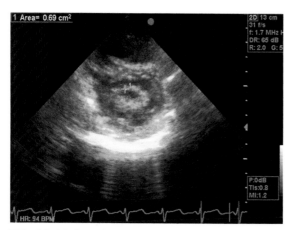

FIG. 30.14 Commissural fusion and valve stenosis of a patient with severe mitral stenosis. Mitral valve area is measured by tracing the valve opening in the parasternal short-axis view.

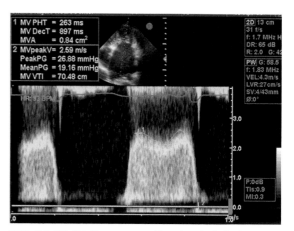

FIG. 30.15 Continuous-wave Doppler study in the transthoracic apical four-chamber view, showing severely increased mean pressure gradient and pressure half time (PHT) across the mitral valve.

presence of LA thrombi and to precisely study the MV and the severity of MR. Exercise testing or invasive hemodynamic study is suggested to assess the response of the mean MV gradient and PAP in patients with MS when there is a discrepancy between baseline resting echocardiographic findings and clinical symptoms.[3,36]

**Exercise testing.** Exercise testing using either a treadmill or a supine bicycle is beneficial to define symptoms and functional capacity, mostly if it is difficult to confirm the presence of symptoms by history. Indeed, Doppler echocardiography, joined with exercise, makes available additional essential hemodynamic data regarding the amount of the MV gradient and PAP during exercise because symptoms are frequently most prominent at upper heart rates.[3,36,37]

**Catheterization.** Catheter-based study of LA and LV pressures reveals the expected hemodynamics and permits the measurement of the mean transmitral pressure gradient, transmitral volume flow rate, and MV area using Gorlin formula. Rarely, diagnostic cardiac catheterization is needed when echocardiography is nondiagnostic or the results have discrepancy with the clinical symptoms. Of course, these studies are recorded for monitoring before, during, and after PBMC. Accordingly, routine diagnostic cardiac catheterization is not suggested for the assessment of MS.[3,34,38]

## Management

**Medical.** In patients with MS, medical management has no role in changing the natural history or even delaying the need for surgery (Fig. 30.16). Medical treatment includes diuretics for alleviating the pulmonary congestion, treating AF, and anticoagulating patients who are at increased risk of systemic embolic events.

Tachycardia is poorly tolerated in patients with MS and can lead to acute worsening and deterioration; consequently, diastolic filling time might be short and inadequate. Mainly, heart rate control can be beneficial in patients with MS and AF and rapid ventricular response. Nonetheless, heart rate control might also be considered for patients in normal sinus rhythm and with symptoms associated with exercise.

Beta-blockers, calcium channel blockers, digoxin, and recently ivabradine have been used to control the ventricular rate.

An effort to restore the sinus rhythm with direct current cardioversion or antiarrhythmic drugs might be considered.

Anticoagulation is indicated to prevent thromboembolic events in the following[33]:
- AF rhythm (permanent, persistent, or paroxysmal)
- Previous history of thromboembolism
- LA or LA appendix thrombus

Also, anticoagulation might be considered if the LA is noticeably dilated ($\geq 5.0$ cm) or if there is spontaneous contrast on TEE.

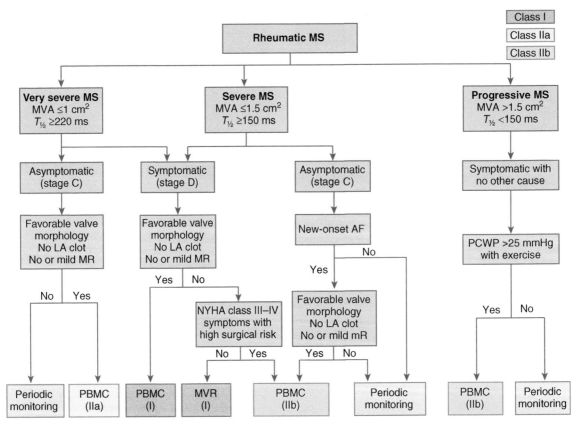

FIG. 30.16 Indications for intervention for rheumatic MS. *AF*, atrial fibrillation; *LA*, left atrial; *MR*, mitral regurgitation; *MVA*, mitral valve area; *MVR*, mitral valve surgery (repair or replacement); *NYHA*, New York Heart Association; *PBMC*, percutaneous balloon mitral commissurotomy; *PCWP*, pulmonary capillary wedge pressure; $T_{1/2}$, pressure half time. (From Otto CM, Bonow RO. Valvular heart disease. In: Mann DL, Zipes DP, Libby P, et al., eds. *Braunwald's Heart Disease: A Textbook of Cardiovascular Medicine.* 10th ed. Philadelphia: Saunders; 2015; with permission.)

Long-term secondary prophylaxis, favorably with penicillin, is suggested for all patients with a history of rheumatic fever, rheumatic carditis, or rheumatic valve disease. The duration of prophylaxis depends on the number of factors, including time from the last attack, the age of the patient, the extent of cardiac involvement, and the patient's risk of exposure to streptococcal infections. Nevertheless, routine antibiotic prophylaxis for endocarditis is no longer recommended for patients with MS.[3,11,30–32]

### Percutaneous mitral balloon commissurotomy.

PMBC is a catheter-based procedure in which a balloon is inflated across the obstructed and stenotic valve to split the fused commissures and increase the valve area. Hemodynamic and clinical improvements may be immediately seen. Interestingly, the results are even typically comparable with those reached with open MV commissurotomy.

Mitral valve morphology, especially calcification, is an important predictor of successful PMBC. Severe valve calcification or significant thickening or specially calcification of the subvalvular apparatus on echocardiography before PMBC is related to a higher rate of complications and a greater risk of relapse.

PMBC must be considered for those with symptomatic severe MS without LA thrombi or more than moderate MR because the degree of MR frequently increases after the procedure.

PMBC is also indicated for symptomatic patients with less valve stenosis (area > 1.5 cm$^2$) if there is evidence of hemodynamically significant MS during stress and exercise—for example, if pulmonary capillary wedge pressure is greater than 25 mmHg (Fig. 30.17).

If the valve anatomy is suboptimal, PMBC may also be considered only for patients with severe MS who have more progressive symptoms (New York Heart Association [NYHA] class III–IV) and are not candidates for surgery or are at higher risk for surgery. PMBC is indicated in even asymptomatic patients if they have either very severe MS (area ≤1 cm$^2$) or severe MS with new-onset AF. In a large study by Noohi et al. consisting of 2531 patients who underwent 3138 PMBCs, they showed high immediate success results and successful long-term outcomes (success rate, 72.9% after 8 years). The complications of PMBC are severe MR (in 3%), systemic thromboembolism (in 3%), and residual atrial septal defect (ASD), of course, with significant shunting (<5%). Importantly, the mortality rate with this procedure in experienced hands is less than 1%.[3,35,39–42]

### Surgical intervention

*Closed and open mitral valvotomy.* Surgical mitral commissurotomy was performed for the first time in

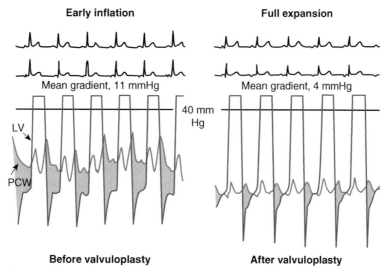

**Early inflation**  **Full expansion**

Mean gradient, 11 mmHg    Mean gradient, 4 mmHg

40 mm Hg

LV

PCW

**Before valvuloplasty**    **After valvuloplasty**

FIG. 30.17 Successful percutaneous balloon mitral valvotomy results in a significant increase in the mitral valve area, as reflected by a reduction in the diastolic pressure gradient between the left ventricle (*magenta*) and the pulmonary capillary wedge (*blue*) pressure, as indicated by the *shaded area*. *LV*, left ventricle; *PCW*, pulmonary capillary wedge pressure. (From Otto CM, Bonow RO. Valvular heart disease. In: Mann DL, Zipes DP, Libby P, et al., eds. *Braunwald's Heart Disease: A Textbook of Cardiovascular Medicine*. 10th ed. Philadelphia: Saunders; 2015; with permission.)

1925 as a closed method (which does not require using full cardiopulmonary bypass and is done through an incision in the LA appendage). This modality is still widely used in some developing countries. Open surgical mitral commissurotomy involves the full use of cardiopulmonary bypass pump and the repair of a diseased MV by direct access and visualization. It can be considered in patients with MS, but the valve anatomy is unsuitable for PMBC (including the presence of LA thrombi and surgery necessitated by other associated valvular diseases or coronary artery disease). Surgical MV commissurotomy (open or closed) may be carried out through either a median sternotomy or a left thoracotomy opening incision.[3,30,33–35]

*Mitral valve replacement.* PMBC and surgical MV commissurotomy are palliative techniques, and in many patients, more intervention such as MV replacement is required. MV replacement may be considered as a first-line procedure in patients with either a heavily calcified MV or significant MR. Needless to say, both mechanical and biological prostheses are used for MV replacement; the choice of the valve often depends on other factors such as age, necessity of associated anticoagulation, and LV size. MV replacement surgery is indicated in severely symptomatic patients (NYHA class III/IV) who are not at high risk for surgery and who are not candidates for (or failed previous) PMBC.

Associated MV surgery is designated for patients with severe or even moderate MS undergoing other cardiac surgery. MV surgery with the excision of the LA appendage might also be considered for patients with severe MS who have had recurrent systemic embolic events while receiving sufficient and sufficient anticoagulation.[3,30,33–35]

### Follow-Up

Patients with MS must be followed up with yearly history taking and physical examinations. Repeat echocardiography must be considered every 3–5 years for those with progressive but not severe MS (MV area >1.5 cm$^2$). For asymptomatic patients with severe MS, serial echocardiography is advised every 1–2 years for those with MV areas of 1.0–1.5 cm$^2$ and every year for those with MV areas less than 1.0 cm$^2$.[3,5,32–35]

### Pregnancy

Pregnancy creates increased plasma volume, reduced afterload, and higher heart rate. These features tend to increase the transmitral pressure gradient (sometimes even to double that of the baseline), leading to increased LA pressures and raised pulmonary venous pressures, which may result in pulmonary congestion and edema. Moreover, increased LA pressures can lead to atrial

arrhythmias (e.g., AF), which are not well tolerated by pregnant patients and patients with MS and as such result in clinical failure and decompensation. Indeed, patients with asymptomatic moderate to severe MS can decompensate during phases of higher physiologic stress, such as pregnancy.

Before pregnancy, all individuals with severe MS must undergo prepregnancy counseling with the relevant expertise comprising a discussion of the benefits and risks of the operative interventions, including mechanical prostheses, bioprostheses, and valve repair. Indeed, valve intervention is recommended before pregnancy for symptomatic patients with severe MS and for asymptomatic patients with severe MS who have valve morphology favorable for PMBC. Pregnant patients with severe MS must be checked in a tertiary care center with a dedicated heart valve team featuring cardiologists, surgeons, anesthesiologists, and also obstetricians with expertise in the management of high-risk cardiac patients during pregnancy.

PMBC is reasonable for pregnant patients with severe MS with valve morphology favorable for PMBC who are symptomatic with NYHA class III–IV HF symptoms despite full medical therapy. Valve surgery is reasonable for pregnant patients with severe MS and valve morphology not favorable for PMBC only if there are refractory NYHA class IV HF symptoms.

In asymptomatic patients with severe MS whose valve morphology is not favorable for PMBC, it can be reasonable to proceed with moderate risk elective noncardiac surgery combined with proper intraoperative and postoperative hemodynamic monitoring.

During pregnancy, women with MS must receive appropriate medical therapy, containing beta-blockers and—in certain patients—diuretics but never ACE inhibitors or angiotensin II receptor blockers because of their teratogenic potential. Importantly, those at risk for thromboembolization must be anticoagulated. In general, this is accomplished with warfarin during the second and third trimesters, with a change to unfractionated heparin before labor and delivery.[30–35]

## MITRAL REGURGITATION
### Etiology and Pathology

Mitral regurgitation may result from the disease of the valve leaflets themselves or any the adjacent structures, consisting of the MV apparatus. The leading reason for MR is rheumatic heart disease in developing countries and degenerative diseases of the MV (myxomatous disease with fibroelastic deficiency) in the United States and other developing areas. Less common disorders contain MAC and congenital anomalies such as clefts in the MV. Other infrequent causes of MR are endomyocardial fibrosis, carcinoid disease, radiation therapy, ergotamine toxicity, systemic lupus erythematosus (SLE), and diet or drug toxicity.

In developed countries, the second leading cause of MR is functional, which results from the dilatation of the MV annulus or from myocardial ischemia and infarction. Specially, infarctions involving the papillary muscles (inferolateral and posteromedial) create tethering of the leaflets, preventing normal coaptation and as such leading to functional MR, although the valve leaflets themselves are structurally normal.[43]

### Pathophysiology

As a rule, MR is slowly progressive, and the LV can develop compensatory changes. Thus, symptoms are either absent or slowly progressive over many years. The adaptive changes consist of LV dilatation and eccentric hypertrophy. The LA being the chamber of lesser pressure, it also enlarges because the regurgitant volume ejects into it.[44] Although patients with compensated and chronic MR can remain asymptomatic for many years, decompensation may finally develop if the MR is adequately severe. LVEF in chronic MR can be greater than normal because of an increase in preload and also afterload, which decreases the effect of ejection into the low-impedance LA. Accordingly, LVEF may be confusing as a measure of real contractile function in this disease. Indeed, advanced myocardial dysfunction may happen while LVEF is still good and normal. Therefore, the outcome after MV surgery is poorer in patients with a preoperative LVEF less than 60%.[45,46]

### Physical examination

The physical examination of a patient with severe chronic MR varies based on the degree of the decompensation of the patient. The carotid upstroke is sharp in patients with compensated MR; however, the volume of the carotid pulse is considerably reduced in the presence of advanced failure.[43] Usually, the apical impulse is brisk and hyperdynamic. In patients with severe MR, it can be enlarged and displaced laterally. $S_1$ is typically soft, and a wide splitting of $S_2$ is common. $S_3$ and a diastolic rumble may be present and not essentially indicate LV failure.[44] Commonly, the systolic murmur of MR differs according to the etiology of the MR. This murmur is typically heard best at the apex in the left lateral decubitus position. Early systolic murmurs are characteristic of acute MR. Late systolic murmurs are representative of MV prolapse and papillary muscle dysfunction. The signs of PAH such as a loud $P_2$ are

generally threatening and represent an advanced form of the disease[45,46] (Fig. 30.18).

### Diagnostic testing

**Chest radiography.** Cardiomegaly caused by LV and LA enlargement is common in patients with chronic severe MR. In patients with PAH, right-sided chamber enlargement is also a common finding. Kerley B lines and interstitial edema might be seen in patients with acute severe MR or progressive LV dysfunction (Fig. 30.19).

**Electrocardiography.** Left atrial enlargement and AF are the most common ECG findings in patients with MR. LV enlargement is noted in about one-third of the patients, and RV hypertrophy is observed in 15%.

**Echocardiography.** Echocardiography is the most generally used instrument to study patients with supposed MR. It provides information about the cause, mechanism, and severity of MR, as well as the function and size of the LV and RV, the size of the LA, the grade of

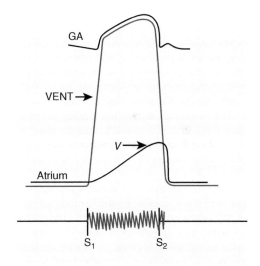

FIG. 30.18 Illustration of great arterial (GA), ventricular (VENT), and atrial pressure pulses with phonocardiogram, displaying the physiological mechanism of a holosystolic murmur in mitral regurgitation. Ventricular pressure exceeds atrial pressure at the very onset of systole, so the regurgitant flow and murmur begins with the first heart sound ($S_1$). The murmur persists up to or faintly beyond the second heart sound ($S_2$) because the regurgitation persists until the end of systole (ventricular pressure still exceeds atrial pressure). *V*, atrial v wave. (From Mann DL, Zipes DP, Libby P, et al., eds. *Braunwald's Heart Disease: A Textbook of Cardiovascular Medicine.* 10th ed. Philadelphia: Saunders; 2015; with permission.)

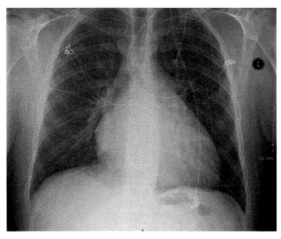

FIG. 30.19 Chest radiography showing Kerley B lines and interstitial edema.

PAH, and the presence of other related valve lesions.[35] Also, the Doppler study provides quantitative measurements of the severity of MR, which have been revealed to be the main predictors of prognosis and outcome.[45,46]

**Exercise testing.** Exercise testing is valuable in determining functional capacity, mainly when the symptoms are unclear. The measurement of the severity of MR and PAP before and after exercise testing via Doppler echocardiography can provide additional beneficial information, particularly if surgical intervention is being anticipated.[44] This method is especially useful in symptomatic patients in whom there is inconsistency between the symptoms and the resting measurements of LV function and PAP.

**Cardiac catheterization.** Cardiac catheterization is usually performed to evaluate the hemodynamic severity of MR when noninvasive testing is indecisive and questionable or a disagreement exists between clinical and also noninvasive findings. Coronary angiography is indicated for patients who are scheduled to undergo surgery and are at risk of CAD.

**Hemodynamics.** Forward cardiac output typically is low in severely symptomatic patients with MR, but total LV output (the summation of forward and also regurgitant flow) typically is high until the late course of the disease. The atrial contraction "a" wave in LA pressure pulse frequently is not as noticeable in patients with MR as that in patients with MS; however, the "v" wave is typically much taller because it is inscribed during ventricular systole when the LA is being filled with blood from the pulmonary veins and from the LV.

Rarely, the backward transmission of the tall "v" wave into the pulmonary arterial bed might result in an early diastolic pulmonary arterial "v" wave. In patients with isolated MR, the "y" descent in the pulmonary capillary pressure pulse is chiefly rapid because the distended LA empties quickly during early diastole[45–47] (Fig. 30.20).

### Treatment: Medical, surgical, and percutaneous techniques

Patients with severe chronic MR may remain asymptomatic for years. Patients with mild MR and overall normal hearts can be followed up with yearly clinical studies, undertaking echocardiography only if their clinical situation changes (e.g., the intensity of the murmur). In patients with moderate to severe MR, clinical examination and echocardiography must be done annually or even sooner if symptoms develop.

Recently, LV systolic dysfunction in severe MR has been defined as an LVEF of 60% or less or an end-systolic dimension 40 mm or greater, and these situations must have immediate surgical referral. Likewise, asymptomatic patients with severe MR must be considered for surgically correction, particularly if the valve could be repaired. If these patients decline surgery, they must be followed up with clinical evaluations and echocardiography each 6–12 months and must be referred for surgery immediately if they develop symptoms, AF, PAH, or LV systolic dysfunction.[44,47]

The timing of surgery is partly associated with whether the patient is a candidate for MV repair or replacement. It is thus critical that patients with severe type of MR who might need surgery be referred to high-volume experienced MV surgical centers, with a high likelihood of a successful repair.[44,48] Usually, nonrheumatic posterior MV prolapse (MVP) or degenerative MV disease and ruptured chordae tendineae may be repaired. The involvement of the anterior MV leaflet or both leaflets needs more experience, which decreases the likelihood of a successful for repair because it needs some convoying interventions such as chordal transfers or chordal shortening[44] (Fig. 30.21).

For patients with asymptomatic degenerative MR, no accepted medical therapy has been revealed to delay the necessity for surgical intervention. Furthermore, in asymptomatic patients with severe MR and normal LV function, the repair might prevent sequelae of chronic severe MR. Of course, this must be considered only when the probability of a successful valve repair is more than 90% in a skilled and experienced center.[44]

In patients with functional MR related with LV dysfunction, beta-blockers, ACE inhibitors, and biventricular pacing have been revealed to yield useful reverse

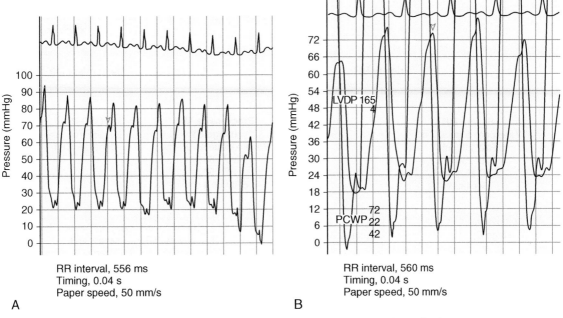

FIG. 30.20 (A) A pulmonary artery tracing in mitral regurgitation revealing an elevated pulmonary artery pressure, with a peak early systolic pressure of approximately 70 mmHg (*red arrowhead*) followed by a V wave, which further elevates the pulmonary-artery pressure. (B) The pulmonary capillary wedge pressure (PCWP) tracing is characterized by a V wave (*red arrowhead*), which ranges from 64 to 78 mmHg. The left ventricular diastolic pressure (LVDP) curve shows that the pressure in the LV is normal from the onset of diastole to the beginning of the A wave (*upper black arrow*). With atrial contraction, however, there is a marked increase in pressure of 24 mmHg (the area between the two *black arrows*). (From Otto CM, Bonow RO. Valvular heart disease. In: Mann DL, Zipes DP, Libby P, et al., eds. *Braunwald's Heart Disease: A Textbook of Cardiovascular Medicine.* 10th ed. Philadelphia: Saunders; 2015; with permission.)

remodeling, and a decrease in LV end-diastolic and end-systolic volumes with these treatments is allied to the reduced severity of MR.[49–52]

Percutaneous methods for MV repair are under improvement, and several of them are currently undergoing clinical trials.[44,49] Of course, these methods will probably not be as effective as surgical repair done in experienced centers. Be that as it may, because percutaneous methods to MV repair probably pose less risk to patients than open-heart surgery, they can be effective enough to be used in particular higher-risk people such as older patients with multiple comorbid situations or patients with severe LV failure.[50,51]

## Acute Mitral Regurgitation

Significant causes of acute MR are the chordae tendineae rupture, IE with the disruption of the MV leaflets or chordal rupture, ischemic dysfunction, or rarely the rupture of a papillary muscle, as well as malfunction of a prosthetic valve.

Acute severe MR causes a marked reduction in the forward stroke volume, minor reduction in the end-systolic volume, and a rise in the end-diastolic volume. One main hemodynamic difference between acute and chronic MR originates from the differences in LA compliance. Patients who develop acute severe MR typically have a normal-sized LA, with normal or reduced LA compliance. The LA pressure increases suddenly, which frequently leads to pulmonary edema, a marked rise in pulmonary vascular resistance, and eventually right-sided HF. In addition, in severe MR secondary to acute myocardial infarction (AMI), pulmonary edema, hypotension, and frank cardiogenic shock can develop.

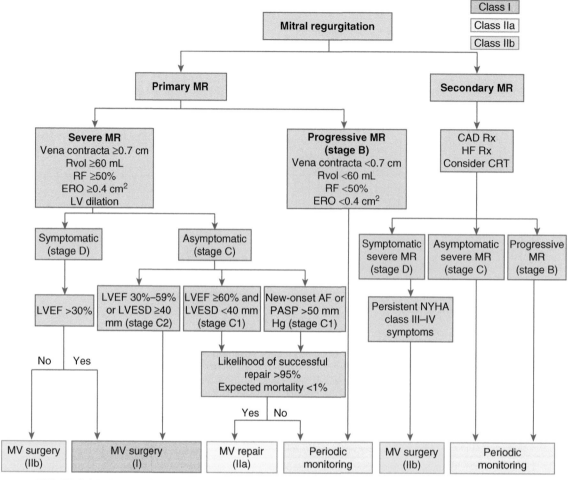

FIG. 30.21 Indications for mitral valve (MV) surgery for chronic severe MR. *Asterisk* indicates that MV repair is preferred over MV replacement when possible. *AF,* atrial fibrillation; *CAD,* coronary artery disease; *CRT,* cardiac resynchronization therapy; *ERO,* effective regurgitant orifice; *HF,* heart failure; *LVEF,* left ventricular ejection fraction; *LVESD,* left ventricular end-systolic dimension; *PASP,* pulmonary artery systolic pressure; *RF,* regurgitant fraction; *RVol,* regurgitant volume; *Rx,* therapy. (From Otto CM, Bonow RO. Valvular heart disease. In: Mann DL, Zipes DP, Libby P, et al., eds. *Braunwald's Heart Disease: A Textbook of Cardiovascular Medicine.* 10th ed. Philadelphia: Saunders; 2015; with permission.)

Because the "v" wave is significantly elevated in these patients, the reverse pressure gradient between the LV and LA drops at the end of systole, and the murmur can be decrescendo rather than holosystolic, ending well before the $A_2$. It is typically lower pitched and softer than the murmur of chronic MR. A left-sided $S_4$ commonly is found. Common PAH might increase the intensity of $P_2$, and the murmurs of PI and TR also may be heard together with a right-sided $S_4$. In patients with severe acute MR, a late systolic pressure rise (a v wave) may rarely cause the premature closure of the pulmonary valve, an early $P_2$, and the paradoxical splitting of $S_2$.

Acute MR, even if severe, frequently does not rise the whole cardiac size, as is seen on chest radiography, and might produce only mild LA enlargement despite a marked raise in LA pressure.

Echocardiography may display little increase in the internal diameter of the LA or LV, but the augmented systolic motion of the LV is noticeable. The main findings on Doppler echocardiography are the severe jet of MR and the increase in the pulmonary artery pressure.[51-55]

## Management

Afterload lessening is chiefly important in treating patients with acute severe MR. Intravenous nitroprusside may be lifesaving in patients with acute severe MR caused by the rupture of the head of a papillary muscle, complicating an AMI. It can stabilize clinical status, thereby permitting coronary arteriography and surgery to be performed with the patient in an ideal situation. In patients with acute severe MR who are hypotensive, an inotropic agent such as dobutamine must be administered with nitroprusside. Intra-aortic balloon counterpulsation may be necessary to stabilize the patient while preparations for surgery are made.

Emergency surgical management may be essential for patients with acute LV failure caused by acute severe MR. Emergency surgery is correlated with higher mortality rates than those for elective surgery for chronic MR. Nonetheless, unless patients with acute severe MR and HF are treated aggressively, a fatal outcome is nearly certain.

Acute papillary muscle rupture needs emergency surgery with MV repair or replacement. However, in patients with papillary muscle dysfunction, early treatment must contain hemodynamic stabilization, generally with the aid of intra-aortic balloon counterpulsation, and surgery must be considered for patients who do not experience improvement with aggressive medical therapy. If patients with MR can be stabilized by medical management, it is advisable to defer surgery until 4–6 weeks after the MI if possible. Vasodilator treatment can be beneficial during this period, but medical management must not be prolonged if multisystem (especially renal and pulmonary) failure develops.

Surgical mortality rates also are greater in patients with severe acute MR and refractory HF (NYHA functional class IV), those with prosthetic valve dysfunction, and those with active IE (of a native or prosthetic valve). Despite the higher surgical risks, the efficacy of early surgery has been established in patients with IE complicated by medically uncontrollable congestive HF and recurrent emboli.

## MITRAL VALVE PROLAPSE

Mitral valve prolapse is one of the most prevalent cardiac valvular disorders. Using valid echocardiographic diagnostic criteria, previous community-based studies have revealed that the MVP syndrome happens in 2.4% of the population. MVP is twofold as frequent in women as in men, but serious MR happens more often in older men (especially older than 50 years of age) with MVP than in younger women with this disorder.[56–58]

The clinical and echocardiographic criteria for the diagnosis of MVP have been well proven. The typical systolic click and the mid-to-late systolic murmur are the main diagnostic criteria. Echocardiographically, MVP is well defined as the superior displacement of the leaflet tissue into the LA past the MV annular plane. In the early era of diagnostic echocardiography, even a mild billowing of the anterior leaflet in the systole MV annular plane was considered as MVP and these observations were taken to recommend that the diagnosis of MVP could just be made in the long-axis view. Nonetheless, in the modern era of TTE- and TEE-based diagnosis of MVP, the shape of the annulus has a slight significance. The term "billowing MV" must be limited to describing the superior motion of the body of the leaflet. Of course, the longer anterior leaflet typically shows mild billowing during ventricular systole. The billowing at the base of the leaflet can be considered abnormal when it goes beyond 2 mm above the annular plane in a long-axis view about 130 degrees in the mid-esophageal plane by TEE and 5 mm in the four-chamber view (0 degrees in the mid-esophageal plane). In addition, localized prolapse might involve P1, P2, or P3 scallops and A1, A2, and A3 scallops as isolated abnormalities[57–61] (Fig. 30.22).

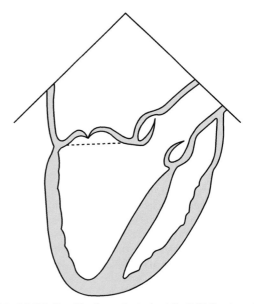

FIG. 30.22 Graphic views displaying bileaflet billowing with mitral valve prolapse in which both leaflets prolapse above the annular plane.

Several causes of MVP have been recognized:

1. *Degenerative or myxomatous MVP* can also be defined as primary or idiopathic. This is the most common cause of MVP, and although it is seen in youth or young adulthood, it is more frequently present in older adults. In its characteristic form as defined by Barlow, it is correlated with the global involvement of redundant leaflets, excess tissue, enlarged chords, and dilated annuli. Interestingly, some patients might present with focal myxomatous change. MV regurgitation becomes progressive, with the enlargement of the chambers and progress to heart failure.

2. *Fibroelastic deficiency* is a less common entity and can be seen in older patients past age 70 years. The valve involvement is more focal, and whole leaflets are not redundant or thickened. The valves are thin and friable. Rarely, the same valve may exhibit fibroelastic deficiency as well as focal myxomatous change in different parts.

3. *Acute rheumatic MV disease:* Typical MVP has been explained with acute rheumatic valvulitis in countries where rheumatic fever is prevalent. Nevertheless, chronic rheumatic valve disease is not allied to MVP.

4. *Marfan syndrome* is a common manifestation of global valve degeneration, with dilated annulus mimicking Barlow's valve. The characteristic aortic root and aorta involvement and other systemic abnormalities help discriminate it from idiopathic degenerative MVP.

5. *Bacterial IE:* Acute and subacute bacterial endocarditis can result in ruptured chordae and flail MVP. This is frequently correlated with vegetation, perforation of the leaflets, and annular abscess. Clinical data and positive blood cultures can help differentiate this disorder.

6. *Papillary muscle rupture:* AMI may be associated with the rupture of a main papillary muscle, resulting in massive MR and acute pulmonary edema. Nonetheless, the rupture of one head of the papillary muscles can present as the flail valve syndrome with severe MR. Typically, TEE shows a ruptured papillary muscle head, flail chords, and severe MR.

7. *AMI and acute ischemia* involving a papillary muscle can result in MVP. This mechanism was experimentally confirmed by Tei et al. The mechanisms of chronic ischemic MR are associated with leaflet tethering rather than MVP.[60–64]

## Management
### Medical
Although symptoms related to MVP are frequently improved with beta-blockers, there is no medication to inhibit the progression of MVP. Antibiotic prophylaxis against bacterial endocarditis is no longer suggested unless the patient has had prior endocarditis or has undergone MV replacement.

### Surgical
**Mitral valve repair.** The commonly used surgical methods contain leaflet resection, plication, artificial chords, and leaflet reduction such as sliding plasty for the posterior leaflet and annuloplasty rings or bands. The success of surgery and the late outcome is determined by the use of the correct surgical way and approach for a given pathology. The prolapse of the P2 scallop is detected in more than 60% of patients undergoing surgery. Patients with Barlow valve display diffuse bileaflet prolapse, although the severity of MVP as well as the origin of MR jets may vary. It is widely documented that a careful valuation of valve pathology using TEE before the establishment of cardiopulmonary bypass pump is a prerequisite to a successful outcome.[63–66]

**Intraoperative transesophageal echocardiography.** All patients considered for MV repair undergo intraoperative TEE to permit careful planning of surgery as well as discussion on the feasibility of repair and appropriateness for slightly invasive surgical approaches.

Appropriate measurements using 2D TEE for the measurements of the anterior and posterior leaflet heights and the annular diameter are best made in the long-axis view ($\approx 135$ degrees). These are essential in defining the suitable size of the mitral annular ring or band to avoid postrepair systolic anterior motion of the MV (SAM).[64–66]

**Postrepair assessment.** It is essential to assess the anatomic as well as functional aspects of the repaired valve. Structurally, the tip coaptation must be subannular and must have a surface coaptation near the free edge of about 5–10 mm.

Functionally, the absence of any regurgitation is a favorite outcome. Of course, it is not rare to see trivial or mild MR after a successful repair. This valuation must be made with a sufficiently filled ventricle and with the systolic blood pressure of 110–140 mmHg. If the MR is moderate or greater, a careful echocardiographic assessment of its localization can be useful in the revision of the repair on a second pump run. Usually, the second pump run might be needed in about 10% of patients and usually results in a successful repair in 75% of these patients. Multiple echocardiographic views must be imaged to look for paravalvular MR. Low-velocity small jets are frequently correlated to "stitch" regurgitation, and these are eliminated after the administration of protamine. However, a turbulent paravalvular jet, albeit small, must not be ignored because it could show a progression or may be related to clinical hemolysis. Postrepair SAM has been known to happen in 5%–10% of patients with myxomatous degenerative MVP. When SAM occurs, it is vitally important to establish good ventricular filling, slower heart rates, and normal blood pressures. If SAM is persistent and is related to MR, corrective action should be accepted. This may entail lessening the amount of leaflet tissues or implanting a larger annuloplasty band or ring.[62–66]

**Mitral valve replacement.** After MV replacement, it is important to define the presence and severity of paravalvular regurgitation and to study transvalvular gradients. TEE identifies SAM and LVOT and provides a guarantee of not only normal prosthetic valve function, the normal opening of bileaflet discs, and normal flow and hemodynamics but also the absence of the central regurgitation of bioprosthetic valves.[65,66]

## TRICUSPID VALVE DISEASE

### Normal Anatomy

Of the cardiac valves, the tricuspid valve (TV) is the most caudal and the largest valve. Classically, the TV has three unequal-sized leaflets: septal (smallest), posterior, and anterior (the largest).[67–69] The septal TV leaflet normally has a unique attachment to the interventricular septum as opposed to the MV.

### Pathology

**Tricuspid valve diseases:** These diseases are divided into pure TR, pure tricuspid stenosis (TS), and mixed TR and TS.

**Tricuspid regurgitation:** Mild-degree TR can be seen in about 70% of the normal population. TR is divided into primary (organic) and secondary (functional) TR.

In the setting of pathologic TR, the secondary or functional TR is the most common cause of TR in that it often occurs in the setting of the left-heart valve disease.[70]

**Primary or organic TR:** This kind of TR occurs in the setting of a structurally abnormal TV apparatus. It can be congenital such as Ebstein anomaly and involvement in an atrioventricular septal defect or can be acquired such as carcinoid syndrome, rheumatic heart disease (which usually involves the MV as well), trauma, IE, and a floppy or prolaptic TV.

**Secondary or functional TR:** This kind of TR occurs in a structurally normal TV but with the abnormal geometry of the TV apparatus such as RV and TV annulus dilation. RV failure—as is the case in RV MI, cardiomyopathies, pulmonary hypertension (usually RV systolic pressure > 55 mmHg) in MV disease, and Eisenmenger syndrome—causes secondary TR.[3,33–35,70–72]

### Clinical Findings

Patients with significant TR can stay asymptomatic even in the late stage. However, TR in the presence of pulmonary hypertension is less tolerated. The common symptoms that may occur are as follows:

- Fatigue caused by low cardiac output
- Cachexia and weight loss
- Painful liver congestion, liver enlargement, and liver systolic pulsation may disappear in chronic TR because cirrhosis may occur.
- Ascites and leg edema caused by fluid retention

In secondary TR, the symptoms of the primary disease such as MV disease are predominant; however, when the severity of TR increases, the symptoms of pulmonary congestion decrease and are replaced with fatigue and weakness caused by low cardiac output.

### Physical Examination
#### Cardiac auscultation

High-pitched holosystolic murmurs with an accentuated $P_2$ in the fourth intercostal space at the left sternal border are heard in secondary TR associated with pulmonary hypertension.

Low-intensity early systolic murmurs occur in primary low-pressure TR. Characteristically, the TR murmur is augmented with inspiration (Carvallo sign).

#### Diagnostic testing

**Jugular venous waveform examination.** Jugular vein distension occurs in severe TR. The V wave and C wave will merge (as the antegrade right atrial filling occurs with the retrograde TR flow) and make ventricularization with an absent "x" descent and a prominent "y" descent[3,35] (Fig. 30.23).

**Electrocardiography.** The ECG can be nonspecific, although it may offer some clues such as incomplete right bundle branch block, prominent P wave with RA enlargement, and AF rhythm.

**Chest radiography.** In significant TR, cardiomegaly caused by RA enlargement and prominent right-sided borders may be seen (Fig. 30.24).

**Catheterization.** Nowadays, cardiac catheterization is not recommended only for the diagnosis or quantitation

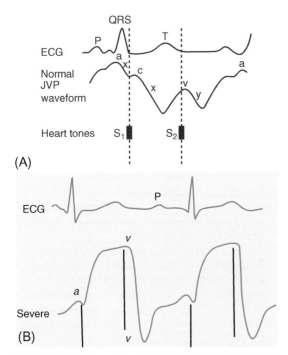

(A)

(B)

FIG. 30.23 (A) Normal jugular venous waveform in concomitant with ECG and normal heart sounds and (B) severe tricuspid regurgitation. *ECG*, electrocardiogram; *JVP*, jugular venous pressure. (From Mann DL, Zipes DP, Libby P, et al., eds. *Braunwald's Heart Disease: A Textbook of Cardiovascular Medicine.* 10th ed. Philadelphia: Saunders; 2015; with permission.)

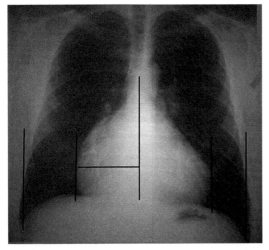

FIG. 30.24 Ebstein anomaly with severe right atrial enlargement and cardiomegaly and normal or reduced pulmonary vascularity; an increased cardiothoracic ratio is notable.

of TR severity. However, hemodynamic evaluation can be helpful in differentiating primary TR (PAP or RV systolic pressure < 40 mmHg) from secondary TR (PAP or RV systolic pressure > 55 mmHg). In significant TR, RA, and RV end-diastolic pressures are often elevated.[3,33,34]

**Echocardiography.** Echocardiography is the technique of choice for the evaluation of TR. Most often, TTE is sufficient; however, TEE may be used in patients where the image quality is poor with TTE.[3,33–35,73]

The following data should be obtained by echocardiography:

1. Presence of TR using color-flow imaging (as trivial TR is a frequent finding in normal subjects)
2. Presence of pathologic TR and differentiating between primary TR (structurally abnormal TV) and secondary TR (2D echocardiography assists in determining the TR etiology, e.g., vegetations in endocarditis, prolaptic TV in myxomatous changes, and retracted and thickened valves in rheumatic heart disease vs structurally normal leaflets in functional TR)
3. TR severity (Table 30.5)
4. TV annulus diameter and leaflet tethering in functional TR (It is measured in diastole and is defined as significant when the diameter is ≥40 mm or ≤21 mm/m$^2$ in the apical four-chamber view in TTE.)
5. TR peak velocity and peak pressure gradient for the estimation of RV systolic and pulmonary artery pressures and the differentiation between primary TR and secondary TR[34]
6. RV size and function based on the latest guidelines[74,75]
7. Involvement of the other valves and associated lesions (Figs. 30.25–30.27)

## Medical and Surgical Treatment of Severe Tricuspid Regurgitation

The medical management for severe TR is limited. Loop diuretics decrease systemic congestion (ascites and peripheral edema), resulting in the low-flow syndrome. Aldosterone antagonists can be added and should be considered in hepatic congestion. Also, the primary cause of functional TR should be corrected. There are limited data regarding the natural history of severe TR; they, however, suggest that even if TR has been well-tolerated for years, the prognosis is poor.[33,34,76,77] Patients can be candidates for surgical treatment based on Fig. 30.28.

## Tricuspid Stenosis
### Pathology
Rheumatic heart disease is the most common cause of TS and generally is associated with MV disease and AV

**TABLE 30.5**
**Echocardiographic Evaluation of Tricuspid Regurgitation Severity**

| Tricuspid Regurgitation Severity | Mild | Moderate | Severe |
| --- | --- | --- | --- |
| Jet area by CFI (cm$^2$) | <5 | 5–10 | >10 |
| Vena contracta width | Not defined | 0.7 cm | >0.7 cm |
| Jet contour and density | Soft and parabolic jet | Variable contour | Dense, triangular, and early peaking |
| Hepatic vein flow study | Dominant systolic flow | Blunted systolic flow | Systolic flow reversal in the hepatic vein |
| RA and RV size | Normal RA and RV size | No or mild RA enlargement; normal RV size | RA and RV enlargement |
| PISA radius with Nyquist's limit 28 cm/s (mm) | <6 | 6–9 | >9 |

*CFI*, color-flow imaging; *RA*, right atrium; *RV*, right ventricle; *PISA*, proximal isovelocity surface area.

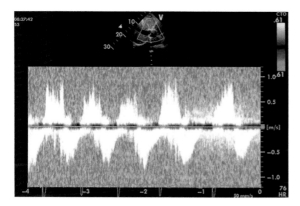

FIG. 30.25 Systolic flow reversal in the hepatic vein.

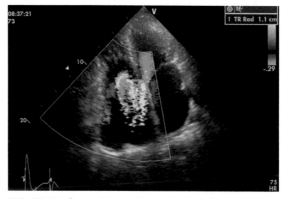

FIG. 30.27 Severe tricuspid regurgitation with proximal iso-velocity surface area radius larger than 9 mm.

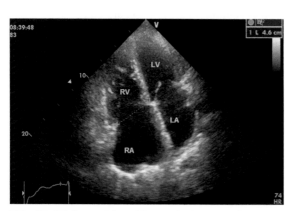

FIG. 30.26 Severe tricuspid regurgitation, resulting in right atrial (RA) and right ventricular (RV) enlargement and annuls dilatation. *LA*, left atrium; *LV*, right ventricle.

involvement. However, TS is not a frequent finding in patients with rheumatic involvement of the MV (only 3%–5% of patients).[3,33]

The typical changes of TS are similar to those in MS, which include commissural fusion, valve thickening, chordal shortening, and rarely valve calcification.

### Pathophysiology

Rheumatic changes of the TV result in a central fix opening, which is usually stenotic and regurgitant and causes pressure gradient between the RA and RV in diastole, associated with RA enlargement and passive congestion of the liver and spleen.

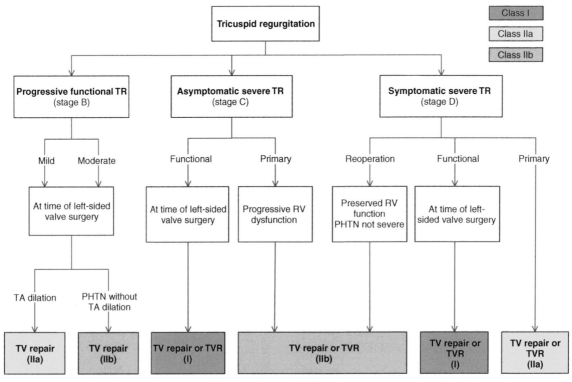

FIG. 30.28 Indications for surgery. *LV*, left ventricular; *PHTN*, pulmonary hypertension; *RV*, right ventricular; *TA*, tricuspid annular; *TR*, tricuspid regurgitation; *TTE*, transthoracic echocardiogram; *TV*, tricuspid valve; *TVR*, tricuspid valve replacement. (From Nishimura RA, Otto CM, Bonow RO, et al. 2014 AHA/ACC guideline for the management of patients with valvular heart disease: a report of the American College of Cardiology/American Heart Association Task Force on Practice Guidelines. *J Am Coll Cardiol.* 2014;63(22):e57–e185; with permission.)

### Clinical findings
Symptoms may be masked by the concomitant MV disease. TS generally causes symptoms of:
- Low cardiac output such as fatigue
- Systemic venous congestion such as hepatomegaly, peripheral edema, and ascites

### Physical examination
The venous pressure is elevated with a prominent a wave and slow y descent. An opening snap followed by a diastolic rumbling murmur at the right sternal border that varies with respiration is characteristic. As with TR, physical examination findings may be subtle and the murmur often inaudible.

### Hemodynamic
The diagnosis of TS is based on the morphologic changes of TV associated with a diastolic mean pressure gradient of 2 mmHg. The pressure gradient is flow

dependent and increases with deep inspiration, exercise, and fluid administration and decreases with the restriction of sodium intake or using diuretics.

### Electrocardiography
In patients with sinus rhythm, the P wave is tall and more than 0.25 mV in lead II is suggestive of RA enlargement.

### Chest radiography
Chest radiography may show cardiomegaly caused by the prominent right-sided heart.

### Echocardiography
Transthoracic echocardiography provides an accurate diagnosis of the TS besides evaluating the severity of TS and associated TR. Echocardiographic evaluation of severe TS consists of:
- Thickened TV leaflets with TV mean pressure gradient greater than 5 mmHg,

- PHT of 190 ms or greater
- TV area 1.0 cm$^2$ or less by the continuity equation
- RA and inferior vena cava dilatation

### Catheterization

Cardiac catheterization for hemodynamic evaluation of TS is rarely needed.

### Management

In patients with hepatic and systemic congestion, loop diuretics can be used to relieve the symptoms. However, the isolated TV surgery is a class I recommendation for patients with severe symptomatic TS and in patients with severe TS who are candidates for left-sided valve surgery.

Percutaneous balloon commissurotomy of the TV is a class IIb recommendation in patients with severe symptomatic TS and no TR.[3,33,35]

## PULMONARY VALVE STENOSIS

Pulmonary valve stenosis (PS) repeatedly presents with an asymptomatic systolic murmur but rarely with exercise intolerance. Mild PS is seldom progressive; nonetheless, moderate PS might progress to considerable stenosis and secondary hypertrophy in the subpulmonic and infundibulum. Of course, this lesion exists as a range, from isolated mild valvular PS to the complete atresia of the whole pulmonary outflow tract. The shape of the pulmonary valve (PV) in patients with valvular PS varies from a trileaflet valve with different degrees of commissural fusion to even an imperforate membrane.[78–80]

### Clinical Findings

Whereas patients with isolated mild-to-moderate PS typically are asymptomatic, patients with severe PS may present with dyspnea, exercise intolerance, light-headedness, and sometimes chest pain (RV angina caused by RV pressure overload). Physical examination may reveal a prominent jugular A wave, an RV heave, and a thrill on the left sternal border. Auscultation shows a normal $S_1$, a single or split $S_2$ with a weakened $P_2$, and a systolic ejection murmur that is best heard on the second intercostal space at the left sternal border. Interestingly, if the PV is flexible and thin, a systolic ejection click can be heard, which decreases with inspiration. Importantly, as the severity of PS increases, the interval between $S_1$ and the systolic ejection click develops to be shorter, $S_2$ becomes widely split, $P_2$ weakens or even disappears, and the systolic ejection murmur prolongs and peaks later—frequently until beyond $A_2$. Cyanosis might be present when a patent foramen ovale or an atrial septal defect allows

right-to-left shunting. Atrial arrhythmias resulting from RV pressure overload and TR can happen.[80–82]

### Diagnostic Testing

#### Electrocardiography

In adults, ECG findings depend on the severity of PS. In milder PS, ECG must be normal. As the stenosis progresses, ECG evidence of RV hypertrophy appears. Severe stenosis is seen in the form of a tall R wave in lead $V_4R$ or $V_1$ with a deep S wave in lead $V_6$. The existence of an RV strain pattern reflects severe PS. If an rSR pattern is detected in lead $V_1$, typically, RV pressures are lower than in patients with a pure R wave even with equal amplitude. RA overload is correlated to moderate to severe PS.[80–83]

#### Chest radiography

In patients with mild or moderate PS, chest radiography frequently reveals a normal-sized heart and normal pulmonary vascularity. Poststenotic dilatation of the main and left pulmonary arteries is repeatedly seen. RA and RV enlargement is detected in patients with severe obstruction and secondary RV failure. Pulmonary vascularity is generally normal without a right-to-LA shunt; however, it might be reduced in patients with severe PS and RV failure.[82–84]

#### Echocardiography

Combined 2D echocardiographic and continuous-wave (CW) Doppler studies characterize the anatomy of the PV and the severity of PS. Basically, echocardiography has obviated the need for diagnostic cardiac catheterization. The PS severity has been graded as mild, moderate, or severe based on the echocardiographically measured peak velocity and peak pressure gradient (Table 30.6).

Although maximum instantaneous gradients have typically been used in choosing patients for balloon valvuloplasty, recent data recommend that mean Doppler gradients (which associate better with catheter-derived peak-to peak gradients) with a value of 50 mmHg be the cutoff point for commencing intervention.[78,85–87] During the intervention, RV size, pulmonary artery pressure, TV morphology and function, and the status of the interatrial septum may be addressed by echocardiography.[86–88]

| TABLE 30.6 Grading of the Pulmonary Stenosis | | | |
|---|---|---|---|
| | **Mild** | **Moderate** | **Severe** |
| Peak velocity (m/s) | <3 | 3–4 | >4 |
| Peak gradient (mmHg) | <36 | 36–64 | >64 |

## Management and Follow-up

Balloon valvuloplasty is recommended when the gradient through the PV is greater than 50 mmHg at rest and when the patient is symptomatic. Some patients undergo surgery and have excellent survival rates (survival rate after surgical valvotomy, 95.7%). Be that as it may, after a mean follow-up period of 33 years after surgery, 53% of patients needed further intervention, mostly because of severe pulmonary regurgitation, and 38% of them had either ventricular or atrial arrhythmias.[86–89]

## PULMONIC REGURGITATION

### Pathology

Pulmonic regurgitation (PR) in low grades is the most common valvular disease and may result from the dilation of the pulmonary artery or from the dilation of the valve annulus caused by pulmonary hypertension. Rarely, IE can involve the pulmonic valve and result in PR. Because there are more patients with congenital heart disease, there is an increasing number of young adults with residual PR after the surgical treatment of tetralogy of Fallot (ToF) or surgical or transcatheter treatment of congenital pulmonic stenosis such as absent, malformed, and fenestrated leaflets. These abnormalities may happen as isolated lesions but more often are associated with other congenital heart diseases.

Rare reasons for PR contain carcinoid syndrome, rheumatic involvement, injury created by a pulmonary artery flow-directed catheter, syphilis, and chest trauma.[80,90]

### Clinical Presentation

Similar to TR, isolated PR leads to RV volume overload and may be tolerated for many years without trouble—unless complicated by pulmonary hypertension. In this case, PR frequently exacerbates RV failure. Patients with PR caused by IE who develop septic pulmonary emboli and pulmonary hypertension frequently show severe RV failure. In most situations, the clinical appearances of the primary disease are severe and usually overshadow the PR, which is frequently found only in the incidental examination and auscultatory findings.

### Physical Examination

The RV is hyperdynamic and yields palpable systolic pulsation in the left parasternal border. There is an enlarged pulmonary artery, frequently producing another systolic pulsation in the second left intercostal space. Occasionally, systolic and diastolic thrills are felt, too. Pulmonary valve closure typically is palpable in patients with pulmonary hypertension and secondary PR.[80,90,91]

### Auscultation

$P_2$ is inaudible in patients with the congenital absence of the pulmonary valve, but this sound is emphasized in patients with PR secondary to pulmonary hypertension. The wide splitting of $S_2$ is produced by the prolongation of RV ejection caused by high RV stroke volume. The abrupt expansion of the pulmonary artery by the augmented RV stroke volume produces a systolic ejection click, which is followed by a midsystolic ejection murmur in the left second intercostal space. $S_3$ and $S_4$ originating from the RV are often audible.

In the absence of pulmonary hypertension, the diastolic murmur of PR is low pitched and typically is heard best at the third and fourth left intercostal spaces nearby the sternum. The murmur becomes louder during inspiration. When systolic pulmonary artery pressure goes above 55 mmHg, the dilation of the pulmonic annulus results in a high-velocity regurgitant jet and leads to an audible murmur of PR (or Graham Steell murmur). Occasionally, a low-frequency presystolic murmur is present, originating from the augmented diastolic flow across the TV.[90–92]

### Diagnostic Testing
#### Electrocardiography

Without pulmonary hypertension, PR frequently results in an ECG that reflects RV diastolic overload—an rSr (or rsR) shape in the right precordial leads. PR secondary to pulmonary hypertension is typically associated with the ECG sign of RV pressure overload and hypertrophy.[80]

#### Chest radiography

Both the pulmonary artery and RV are typically enlarged; however, these signs are nonspecific. Fluoroscopy can demonstrate marked pulsation of the main pulmonary artery. PR may be diagnosed by observing the opacification of the RV after the injection of the contrast material into the main pulmonary artery; nonetheless, this diagnosis is made in nearly all patients with echocardiography or CMR.[80]

#### Echocardiography

Two-dimensional echocardiography shows RV dilation and in patients with pulmonary hypertension and RV hypertrophy as well. RV function can be assessed. The abnormal motion of the septum, typical of the volume overload of the RV in diastole, and sometimes septal flutter can be obvious. The systolic notching of the posterior leaflet of the pulmonary valve suggests pulmonary hypertension, and a large a wave denotes pulmonary stenosis. Doppler and color-flow imaging is very precise in detecting PR and in helping with the assessment of its severity. When the flow velocity drops during diastole, the pulmonary artery pressure is commonly normal, and the regurgitation is caused by an abnormality of the valve itself.[91,93]

Severe PR is characterized with:

- Deformed or absent PV leaflets; annular dilation
- Color-flow fills the RV outflow tract
- Dense jet of PR detected by CW Doppler
- Steep deceleration and short PHT
- Abnormal septal motion compatible with volume overload
- RV enlargement

### Cardiac magnetic resonance imaging

CMR imaging plays a central role in evaluating pulmonary artery dilation, imaging the regurgitant jet, and calculating PR severity. CMR also is valuable in assessing RV dilation and its systolic function.[80,93]

### Treatment

Except for patients with a previous surgery of ToF, PR alone is rarely severe enough to need specific treatment. The management of the primary condition such as IE or the reason for pulmonary hypertension such as MV disorders significantly improves PR. The timing of surgery for severe PR after the correction of ToF is contentious, with current recommendations based on the degree of RV dilation and evidence of RV systolic dysfunction. In these patients, valve replacement can be carried out, if possible with a pulmonary allograft. There is increasing experience with catheter-based approaches to pulmonary valve replacement in native pulmonary valve disease and in PR after the surgical correction of congenital heart diseases.[80,92–94]

### Prosthetic Heart Valves

Despite the noticeable improvements in prosthetic heart valve (PHV) design and surgical techniques over the past years, PHV replacement does not provide an absolute cure for valvular heart disease. Native VHD is just changed to "prosthetic valve disease," and the outcome of patients undergoing valve replacement surgery is affected by prosthetic valve durability, hemodynamics, and thrombogenicity.[95,96]

There are two major types of prosthetic valves: mechanical prostheses and bioprostheses. Excellent durability for mechanical valves has been suggested, although there is a risk of thrombosis with all mechanical valves with greater risk in the mitral position compared with the aortic position.

### Mechanical Valves

Three basic types of mechanical PHV exist: monoleaflet, bileaflet, and caged ball (Table 30.7).

The most essential factors that necessity to be considered are the age of patient, life expectancy, preference, indications, and contraindications for warfarin therapy, and comorbidities. In the recent ACC/American Heart Association and European guidelines, the weight for patient age has been decreased, but much greater significance is now agreed to the patient's preference. The major criteria in favor of using a mechanical PHV contain the following: (1) an informed patient who wants

| **TABLE 30.7** Factors Used for Shared Decision Making About Type of Valve Prosthesis | |
|---|---|
| **Favor Mechanical Prosthesis** | **Favor Bioprosthesis** |
| Age <50 years | Age >70 years |
| Increased incidence of structural deterioration with bioprosthesis (15-year risk: 30% for age 40 years, 50% for age 20 years) | Low incidence of structural deterioration (15-year risk: <10% for age >70 years) |
| Lower risk of anticoagulation complications | Higher risk of anticoagulation complications |
| Patient preference (avoid risk of reintervention of valve sounds) | Patient preference (avoid risk and inconvenience of anticoagulation and absence) |
| Low risk of long-term anticoagulation | High risk of long-term anticoagulation |
| Compliant patient with either home monitoring or close access to INR monitoring | Limited access to medical care or inability to regulate VKA |
| Other indication for long-term anticoagulation (e.g., AF) | Access to surgical centers with low reoperation mortality rate |
| High-risk reintervention (e.g., porcelain aorta, prior radiation therapy) | |
| Small aortic root size for AVR (may preclude valve-in-valve procedure in future). | |

*AF*, atrial fibrillation; *AVR*, aortic valve replacement; *INR*, international normalized ratio; *VKA*, vitamin K antagonist.

**TABLE 30.8**
Grading of the Prosthesis–Patient Mismatch (PPM)[a]

| THRESHOLD VALUES OF INDEXED PROSTHETIC VALVE EOA FOR THE IDENTIFICATION AND QUANTIFICATION OF PPM | | |
| --- | --- | --- |
| | Mild or Not Clinically Significant ($cm^2/m^2$) | Moderate ($cm^2/m^2$) | Severe ($cm^2/m^2$) |
| Aortic Position | >0.85 (0.8–0.9) | ≤0.85 (0.8–0.9) | ≤0.65 (0.6–0.7) |
| Mitral Position | >1.2 (1.2–1.3) | ≤1.2 (1.2–1.3) | ≤0.9 (0.9) |

*EOA*, effective orifice area.
[a]Numbers in parentheses represent the range of threshold values that have been used in the literature.

a mechanical PHV and has no contraindication for lasting anticoagulation, (2) the patient is previously on anticoagulation (another mechanical PHV or at high risk for thromboembolism), (3) the patient is at risk of speeded bioprosthesis structural degeneration (younger age, renal insufficiency, and hyperparathyroidism), and (4) the patients is younger than 65 years of age and has a lengthy life expectancy. Also, a bioprosthesis might be preferred in the following conditions: (1) an informed patient who desires a bioprosthesis, (2) contraindication or high risk for anticoagulation, (3) the patient is 65 years of age or older or has a restricted life expectancy, and (4) a woman of childbearing age because bioprostheses degenerate more quickly in younger patients and in pregnancy. Therefore, a woman who has complete her family must most likely be recommended to have a mechanical PHV.[95–97]

The baseline postoperative echocardiography study should be performed in about 6 weeks to 3 months after the valve surgery and be repeated in case of new symptoms or signs.

In bioprosthetic valves after 10 years of implantation, annual TTE is recommended even in the absence of new symptoms.[33]

There is distinctive auscultation for different prosthetic valves Figs. 30.29 and 30.30).

## Measurable Parameters

### Transprosthetic velocity and gradient

The fluid dynamics characteristics of mechanical PHVs may differ noticeably from those of native valves. The regurgitant flow is eccentric in monoleaflet and combined with three discrete jets in the bileaflet valves. Because the direction of the tran-prosthetic jet might be eccentric, all windows must be studied cautiously to notice the highest velocity signal in the prosthetic AV. Infrequently, an abnormally high jet gradient corresponding to a local high-velocity might be recorded by CW Doppler examination through the smaller central orifice of bileaflet mechanical prostheses in the AV or MV position. This issue might lead to an overestimation of gradient and a false doubt of prosthesis dysfunction.[97]

A normally functioning mitral prostheses is confirmed by normal bileaflet motion or monoleaflet disc excursion of the prostheses associated with the following Doppler parameters: mitral valve peak E velocity less than 1.9 (m/s), mean gradient less than 6 mmHg, and PHT less than 100–130 ms (Figs. 30.31 and 30.32).

### Effective orifice area

The effective orifice area (EOA) is measured by the "continuity equation," similar to the native AV area. When the EOA of a prosthetic valve is measured, a few particular cautions must be taken into consideration. The replacement of the LVOT diameter by the labeled prosthesis size in the continuity equation is not a valid way to define the EOA of aortic prostheses. For MV prostheses, the EOA is measured by the "continuity equation" using the stroke volume calculated in the LVOT. It is important to give emphasis to that the PHT is not valid for estimation the valve EOA of MV prostheses.[96,97]

### Doppler velocity index

The Doppler velocity index (DVI) is a dimension-less ratio of the proximal velocity (or VTI) in the LVOT to that of flow velocity (or VTI) through the prosthesis: DVI = V of LVOT/V of PV. This parameter can be used to monitor for valve obstruction, mainly when the cross-sectional area of the LVOT cannot be achieved.[95–97]

### Prosthesis–patient mismatch

The term valve *prosthesis–patient mismatch* (PPM) was first suggested in 1978 by Rahimtoola. PPM happens

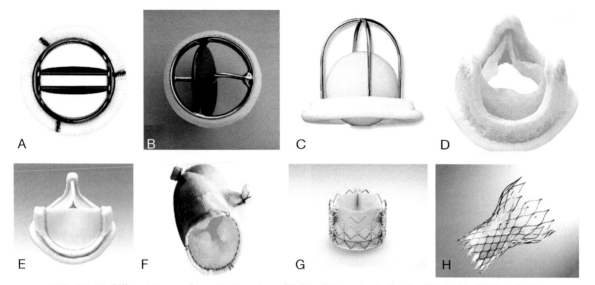

FIG. 30.29 Different types of prosthetic valves. (A) Bileaflet mechanical valve (St. Jude). (B) Monoleaflet mechanical valve (Medtronic Hall). (C) Caged ball valve (Starr-Edwards). (D) Stented porcine bioprosthesis (Medtronic Mosaic). (E) Stented pericardial bioprosthesis (Carpentier-Edwards Magna). (F) Stentless porcine bioprosthesis (Medtronic Freestyle). (G) Percutaneous bioprosthesis expanded over a balloon (Edwards Sapien). (H) Self-expandable percutaneous bioprosthesis (CoreValve). (From Pibarot P, Dumesnil JG. Prosthetic heart valves, selection of the optimal prosthesis, and long-term management. *Circulation*. 2009;119:1034–1048; with permission.)

| Type of Valve | Aortic Prosthesis | | Mitral Prosthesis | |
|---|---|---|---|---|
| | Normal Findings | Abnormal Findings | Normal Findings | Abnormal Findings |
| Caged ball (Starr-Edwards) | OC S₁ ·····CC P₂ SEM | Aortic diastolic murmur Decreased intensity of opening or CC | CC OC S₂ SEM | Low-frequency apical diastolic murmur High-frequency holosystolic murmur |
| Single-tilting-disc (Björk-Shiley or Medtronic-Hall) | OC CC S₁ P₂ SEM DM | Decreased intensity of CC | CC OC S₂ DM | High-frequency holosystolic murmur Decreased intensity of CC |
| Bileaflet-tilting-disc (St. Jude Medical) | OC CC S₁ P₂ SEM | Aortic diastolic murmur Decreased intensity of CC | CC OC S₂ DM | High-frequency holosystolic murmur Decreased intensity of CC |
| Heterograft bioprosthesis (Hancock or Carpentier-Edwards) | AC S₁ P₂ SEM | Aortic diastolic murmur | MC S₂ MO SEM DM | High-frequency holosystolic murmur |

FIG. 30.30 Auscultatory characteristics of various prosthetic valves in the aortic and mitral positions, with schematic diagrams of normal findings and descriptions. of abnormal findings. *AC*, aortic closure; *CC*, closing click; *DM*, diastolic murmur; *MC*, mitral valve closure; *MO*, mitral opening; *OC*, opening click; *SEM*, systolic ejection murmur. (From Vongpatanasin W, Hillis LD, Lange RA. Prosthetic heart valves. *N Engl J Med*. 1996;335:407; with permission.)

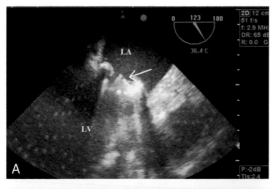

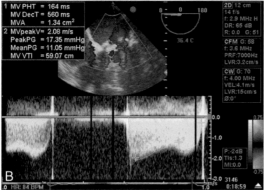

FIG. 30.31 (A) Transesophageal echocardiography shows a stuck anterior leaflet of the bileaflet mitral prostheses (*arrow*). (B) Doppler study showing increased mean pressure gradient, pressure half time (PHT), and peak E velocity suggestive of significant stenosis. *LA*, left atrium; *LV*, left ventricle.

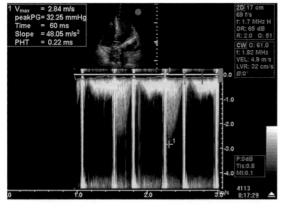

FIG. 30.32 Normal Doppler study in aortic prostheses. Peak velocity is less than 3 m/s, mean gradient is less than 20 mmHg, and acceleration time (AT) is less than 80 ms.

when the EOA of a normally functioning prosthesis is too small in relation to the patient's body size, resulting in abnormally high postoperation gradients. The most widely accepted and validated parameter for recognizing PPM is the indexed EOA [EAO/body surface area (BSA)]. Moderate PPM might be common in both the AV (20%–70%) and MV (30%–70%) positions, but the occurrence of severe PPM varieties from 2% to 10% in both valve positions (Tables 30.7 and 30.8).

The impact of AV PPM is most important in patients with reduced LV function with regard to HF and mortality after AVR. These definitions reflect the fact that an increased gradient is less well accepted by a poorly functioning LV than by a normal one. Also, the influence of PPM is more prominent in younger patients, which might be related to higher cardiac output requirements. Mitral PPM is independently associated with persisting PAH, augmented incidence of congestive HF, and reduced survival rates after MVR[95–99] (Fig. 30.33).

### Assessment and elucidation of prosthetic valve regurgitation

The approach to identifying prosthesis regurgitation is similar to that for native valves and contains an assessment of several Doppler echocardiographic indexes. But care is needed to distinct physiological from pathological regurgitation. Mechanical prostheses have a normal regurgitant flow recognized as leakage backflow to prevent blood stasis and clot formation by a washing effect. The normal leakage backflow jets are considered by being narrow, short duration, and symmetrical.

In prosthetic AV regurgitation, TEE may provide important fundamental information such as flail bioprosthetic cusp, the existence of pannus or thrombus interacting with leaflet closure, prosthesis dehiscence, and the site and size of paravalvular jets.

However, about the prosthetic MV regurgitation, the presence of "occult" regurgitation must be supposed when the following signs are present: flow convergence downstream of the prosthesis during systole, increased MV peak E-wave velocity (>2 m/s) or mean gradient (>5–7 mmHg), DVI less than 0.45, or inexplicable or new worsening of PAH. A decision tree analysis such as that suggested by Fernandes et al.[99] using multiple parameters can also be beneficial. TEE must be done systematically when a clinical or TTE doubt of pathological MV prosthesis regurgitation is present (Fig. 30.34).

Significant paravalvular leakage classically is caused by infection, suture dehiscence, or fibrosis and calcification of the native annulus, leading to insufficient contact between the sewing ring and annulus. Small

High transprosthetic gradients

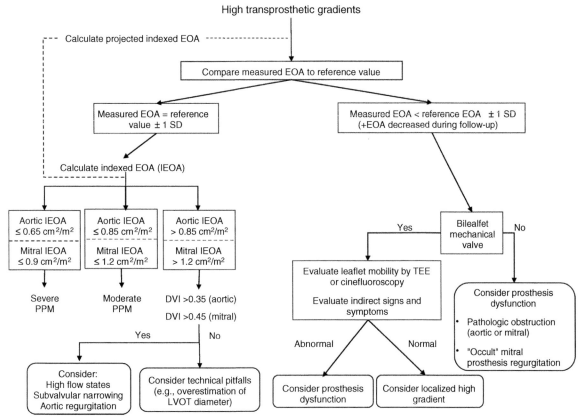

FIG. 30.33 Algorithm for the interpretation of high transprosthetic gradient. *DVI*, Doppler velocity index; *EOA*, effective orifice area; *IEOA*, indexed effective orifice area; *LOVT*, left ventricular outflow tract; *PPM*, prosthesis–patient mismatch; *SD*, standard deviation, *TEE*, transesophageal echocardiography. (From Pibarot P, Dumesnil JG. Prosthetic heart valves, selection of the optimal prosthesis, and long-term management. *Circulation*. 2009;119:1034–1048; with permission.)

paravalvular regurgitant jets are often (10%–25%) seen on intraoperative TEE before cardiopulmonary bypass weaning and may meaningfully decrease after the injection of protamine or in the days, weeks, or months after the operation as the healing process evolves. Moderate or severe paravalvular leakage is rare (1%–2%) and requires returning to cardiopulmonary bypass for speedy correction. Dehiscence of the prosthesis in the late postoperative period may be related to operative technical factors but is most often caused by endocarditis, in which case emergency surgical treatment is usually required.

The paravalvular leakages can be repaired without valve replacement in about 50% of patients. In patients with severe paravalvular MR refractory to aggressive medical therapy who are not candidates for surgical intervention, percutaneous implantation of an Amplatzer septal occluder device offers an alternative therapeutic option.[95–98]

### Prosthesis dysfunction

The function and size of the LV and the atrial chambers and the level of systolic PAP can be used to confirm prosthesis dysfunction severity. These measurements may be compared with previous quantities and frequently are the first sign to alert attention when the regurgitation is hard to imagine.[95,96]

### Prosthetic valve thrombosis

Obstruction of PHV might be caused by thrombus, pannus, or a combination of both. Pannus may present as a gradually progressive obstruction in both bioprosthesis and mechanical valves.

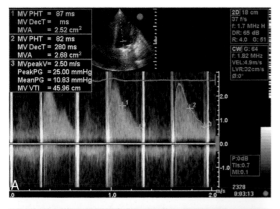

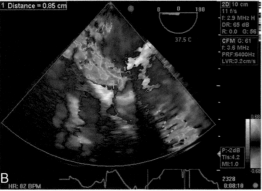

FIG. 30.34 (A) Increased peak E velocity and mean pressure gradient with reduced pressure half time (PHT) are suggestive of a typical Doppler study of a patient with significant paravalvular leakage of the mitral prostheses. (B) Transesophageal echocardiography confirms the significant paravalvular leakage from the medial side of the mitral prostheses.

Prosthetic valve thrombosis (PVT) is most frequently encountered in patients with mechanical valves and insufficient antithrombotic therapy. Thrombosis also might be seen in bioprosthetic valves, where it most repeatedly happens in the early postoperative time. Pannus and thrombosis might be present alone or together and cause acute or subacute obstruction. The incidence of PVT differs between 0.3% and 1.3% per patient-year in patients with mechanical valves.

PVT must be suspected in any patient with any type of prosthetic valves who presents with a new increase in dyspnea or fatigue because PVT can develop slowly over several days or weeks with a period of interrupted or subtherapeutic anticoagulation. In such patients, echocardiography must be done quickly and must contain TEE, principally if the prosthesis is in the MV position.

In nonobstructive left-sided PVT established by TTE or TEE, management consists of a short course of intravenous heparin with close echocardiographic follow-up plus modification of warfarin therapy and addition of aspirin (100 mg). But if the medical treatment is unsuccessful, surgery must be considered in patients with large (>5–10 mm as defined by TEE) or mobile thrombi; thrombolysis with urokinase, streptokinase, or recombinant tissue plasminogen activator is suggested in other patients. Highly mobile, filamentous masses smaller than 1 mm in thickness (named *fibrin strands*) can be found in prosthetic valves during TEE. An association between fibrin strands and cerebral ischemic events has been suggested[95–97,100–102] (Table 30.9).

### Valve degeneration

Mechanical prostheses have outstanding durability, and valve degeneration is very rare with new valves, although mechanical failure (strut fracture, leaflet seepage, occluder dysfunction by lipid and calcium adsorption) has happened with some models in the past. The rate of valve degeneration in bioprosthetic valves rises over time, principally after the initial 7–8 years after insertion. Risk factors until that time found to be related to bioprosthetic valve degeneration include young age, MV position, renal insufficiency, and hyperparathyroidism. Hypertension, LVH, poor LV function, and prosthesis size also have

**TABLE 30.9**
**Fibrinolysis Versus Surgery for Prosthetic Valve Thrombosis**

| Favor Surgery | Favor Fibrinolysis |
| --- | --- |
| Readily available surgical expertise | No surgical expertise available |
| Low surgical risk | High surgical risk |
| Contraindication to fibrinolysis | No contraindication to fibrinolysis |
| Recurrent valve thrombosis | First-time episode of valve thrombosis |
| NYHA class IV | NYHA class I–III |
| Large clot (>0.8 cm$^2$) | Small clot (≤0.8 cm$^2$) |
| Left atrial thrombus | No left atrial thrombus |
| Concomitant CAD in need of revascularization | No or mild CAD |
| Other valve disease | No other valve disease |
| Possible pannus | Thrombus visualized |
| Patient choice | Patient choice |

*CAD*, coronary artery disease; *NYHA*, New York Heart Association.

been reported as predictors of valve degeneration in bioprostheses inserted in the AV position.[95,96,99,103]

In the pulmonary position, most valves are replaced with an allograft or xenograft, and mechanical valves are less favorable regarding the theory of the higher risk of thrombosis in the right-sided valves. However, the mechanical valves are also less likely to require reoperation and can be considered as an alternative to bioprostheses (which are at risk of denegation) in patients with another mechanical valve or patients with severe RV dysfunction who are at high risk for reoperation.[100–108]

### Infective endocarditis

The incidence of prosthetic valve IE is about 0.5% per patient-year, even with suitable antibiotic prophylaxis. Prosthetic valve IE is an extremely serious condition with high mortality rates (30%–50%). The diagnosis relies mainly on the combination of positive blood cultures and echocardiographic evidence of prosthetic infection, containing vegetations, paraprosthetic abscesses, or a new paravalvular regurgitation. TEE is crucial because of its greater sensitivity in detecting these abnormalities. Despite immediate and appropriate antibiotic treatment, many patients with prosthetic valve IE will eventually require surgery. Medical treatment alone is more likely to succeed in late prosthetic valve IE (occurring >6 months after surgery) and in nonstaphylococcal infections. Surgery must be considered in the following situations: failure of medical treatment; hemodynamically significant prosthesis regurgitation, especially if related with the deterioration of LV function; large vegetations; and development of intracardiac fistulas.[96,98,107,108]

## PERCUTANEOUS VALVE REPLACEMENT

The field of percutaneous valve replacement and repair is currently developing at a rapid pace: percutaneous treatment of valvular heart disease is now one of the fastest developing areas of cardiology. Transcatheter aortic and pulmonary valve replacement and a variety of mitral and tricuspid valves therapy approaches have been successfully performed in hundreds of patients.

Actually, efforts to develop and refine percutaneous catheter-based approaches to cardiac valve repair and replacement have advanced rapidly over the past several years. Such clinical strategies were initiated as early as the 1950s with the introduction of simple catheter devices for treating pulmonic stenosis.

Treatment of stenotic lesions matured in the early 1980s with the advent of balloon valvuloplasty, which has become the predominant therapy for primary pulmonic and mitral stenosis lesions. Percutaneous aortic balloon valvuloplasty, however, has yielded largely unfavorable results and is now seldom performed because of its substantial risks and short-lived benefits, but percutaneous aortic valves have been developed and experience is accumulating in humans.

Importantly, with incremental use of percutaneous valve replacements, it is imperative that all physicians involved in all aspects of device development and clinical use insist on properly conducted clinical trials to assure the safety and efficacy of percutaneous techniques against current clinical standards of care to produce the best outcome of this promising clinical area.[106–108]

## CONCLUSIONS

Rapid recognition of valve malfunction and dysfunction permits immediate treatment, frequently with repeat surgical intervention. Some recent developments, including the rapidly evolving field of percutaneous valve implantation, lifestyle, and pharmacologic interventions for the prevention of bioprosthetic valve degeneration, and patient self-management of oral anticoagulation, might change the face of the current practice for the surgical management of valve disease in the future.

## REFERENCES

1. Otto C, Prendergast B. Aortic-valve Stenosis—from patients at risk to severe valve obstruction. *N Engl J Med.* 2014;371:744–756.
2. Saikrishnan N, Kumar G, Sawaya FJ, Lerakis S, Yoganathan AP. Accurate assessment of aortic stenosis: a review of diagnostic modalities and hemodynamics. *Circulation.* 2014;129:244–253.
3. Zipes D, Libby P, Bonow R. *Braunwald's Heart Disease: A Textbook of Cardiovascular Medicine.* 10th ed. Saunders: Elsevier Inc; 2018.
4. Nishimura R, Otto C, Bonow R, et al. 2017 AHA/ACC focused update of the 2014 AHA/ACC guideline for the management of patients with valvular heart disease. A report of the American College of Cardiology/American Heart Association Task Force on Clinical Practice Guidelines. *Circulation.* 2017;135:e1159–e1195. https://doi.org/10.1161/CIR.0000000000000503.
5. Tobin Jr JR, Rahimtoola SH, Blundell PE, et al. Percentage of left ventricular stroke work loss: a simple hemodynamic concept for estimation of severity in valvular aortic stenosis. *Circulation.* 1967;35:868–879. 6021776.
6. Fuster V, Walsh RA, O'Rourke RA, Poole-Wilson P. *Hurst's the Heart.* 12th ed. McGrow-Hill; 2007.
7. Otto CM, Burwash IG, Legget ME, et al. Prospective study of asymptomatic valvular aortic stenosis. Clinical, echocardiographic, and exercise predictors of outcome. *Circulation.* 1997;95:2262–2270.
8. Rosenhek R, Zilberszac R, Schemper M, et al. Natural history of very severe aortic stenosis. *Circulation.* 2010;121:151–156.

9. Carabello BA, Paulus WJ. Aortic stenosis. *Lancet.* 2009;373:956.

10. Braverman AC. The bicuspid aortic valve. In: Otto CM, Bonow RO, eds. *Valvular Heart Disease: A Companion to Braunwald's Heart Disease.* 4th ed. Philadelphia: Saunders; 2013:179–198.

11. Currie PJ, Seward JB, Reeder GS, et al. Continuous-wave Doppler echocardiographic assessment of severity of calcific aortic stenosis: a simultaneous Doppler-catheter correlative study in 100 adult patients. *Circulation.* 1985;71:1162–1169.

12. Ilegrenaes I, Hatle L. Aortic stenosis in adults: non-invasive estimation of pressure differences by continuous wave Doppler echocardiography. *Br Heart J.* 1985;54:396–404.

13. Cueff C, Serfaty JM, Cimadevilla C, et al. Measurement of aortic valve calcification using multislice computed tomography: correlation with haemodynamic severity of aortic stenosis and clinical implication for patients with low ejection fraction. *Heart.* 2011;97:721–726.

14. Vahanian A, Alfieri O, Andreotti F, et al. Guidelines on the management of valvular heart disease (version 2012). Joint Task Force on the Management of Valvular Heart Disease of the European Society of Cardiology and the European Association for Cardio-Thoracic Surgery. *Eur Heart J.* 2012;33:2451.

15. Shavelle DM. Evaluation of valvular heart disease by cardiac catheterization and angiography. In: Otto CM, Bonow RO, eds. *Valvular Heart Disease: A Companion to Braunwald's Heart Disease.* 4th ed. Philadelphia: Saunders; 2013:91–106.

16. Clavel MA, Dumesnil JG, Capoulade R, et al. Outcome of patients with aortic stenosis, small valve area, and low-flow, low-gradient despite preserved left ventricular ejection fraction. *J Am Coll Cardiol.* 2012;60:1259.

17. Fougeres E, Tribouilloy C, Monchi M, et al. Outcomes of pseudo-severe aortic stenosis under conservative treatment. *Eur Heart J.* 2012;33:2426.

18. Jander N, Minners J, Holme I, et al. Outcome of patients with low-gradient "severe" aortic stenosis and preserved ejection fraction. *Circulation.* 2011;123:887.

19. Herrmann HC, Pibarot P, Hueter I, et al. Predictors of mortality and outcomes of therapy in low-flow severe aortic stenosis: a placement of aortic transcatheter valves (PARTNER) trial analysis. *Circulation.* 2013;127:2316.

20. Schaefer BM, Lewin MB, Stout KK, et al. Usefulness of bicuspid aortic valve phenotype to predict elastic properties of the ascending aorta. *Am J Cardiol.* 2007;99:686.

21. Fernandez B, Duran AC, Fernandez-Gallego T, et al. Bicuspid aortic valves with different special orientations of the leaflets are distinct etiological entities. *J Am Coll Cardiol.* 2009;54:2312.

22. Kang JW, Song HG, Yang DH, et al. Association between bicuspid aortic valve phenotype and patterns of valvular dysfunction and bicuspid aortopathy. *J Am Coll Cardiol Img.* 2013;6:150.

23. Bonow RO. Bicuspid aortic valves and dilated aortas: a critical review of the critical review of the ACC/AHA guidelines recommendations. *Am J Cardiol.* 2008; 102:111.

24. Leong DP, Joseph MX, Selvanayagam JB. The evolving role of multimodality imaging in valvular heart disease. *Heart.* 2014;100:336.

25. Charitos EI, Stierle U, Petersen M, et al. The fate of the bicuspid valve aortopathy after aortic valve replacement. *Eur J Cardiothorac Surg.* 2014;45:e128.

26. Bekeredjian R, Grayburn PA. Valvular heart disease aortic regurgitation. *Circulation.* 2005;112:125–134.

27. Lebowitz NE, Bella JN, Roman MJ, et al. Prevalence and correlates of aortic regurgitation in American Indians: the Strong Heart Study. *J Am Coll Cardiol.* 2000;36:461–467.

28. Croft CH, Lipscomb K, Mathis K, et al. Limitations of qualitative angiographic grading in aortic or mitral regurgitation. *Am J Cardiol.* 1984;53:1593–1598.

29. Hiratzka FD, Bakris GL, Beckman JA, et al. 2010 ACCF/AHA/AATS/ACR/ASA/SCA/SCAI/SIR/STS/SVM guidelines for the diagnosis and management of patients with thoracic aortic disease: executive summary. A report of the American College of Cardiology Foundation/American Heart Association Task Force on Practice Guidelines, American Association for Thoracic Surgery, American College of Radiology, American Stroke Association, Society of Cardiovascular Anesthesiologists, Society for Cardiovascular Angiography and Interventions, Society of Interventional Radiology, Society of Thoracic Surgeons, and Society for Vascular Medicine. *Circulation.* 2010;121:1544.

30. Essop MR, Nkomo VT. Rheumatic and nonrheumatic valvular heart disease: epidemiology, management, and prevention in Africa. *Circulation.* 2005;112:3584.

31. Tsang W, Freed BH, Lang RM. Three-dimensional anatomy of the aortic and mitral valves. In: Otto CM, Bonow RO, eds. *Valvular Heart Disease: A Companion to Braunwald's Heart Disease.* 4th ed. Philadelphia: Saunders; 2013:14–29.

32. Iung B, Vahanian A. Rheumatic mitral valve disease. In: Otto CM, Bonow RO, eds. *Valvular Heart Disease: A Companion to Braunwald's Heart Disease.* 4th ed. Philadelphia: Saunders; 2013:255–277. 5.

33. Nishimura R, Otto C, Bonow R, et al. AHA/ACC guideline for the management of patients with valvular heart disease. *Circulation.* 2014;2014:129.

34. Vahanian A, Alfieri O, Andreotti F, et al. Guidelines on the management of valvular heart disease (version 2012). *Eur Heart J.* 2012;33:2451–2496. https://dx.doi.org/10.1093/eurheartj/ehs109.

35. Fuster V, Walsh R, O'Rourke R, Poole-Wilson Ph. Hurst's the Heart, 12th ed., (n.d.) McGraw Hill;1235–1256.

36. Min SY, Song JM, Kim YJ, et al. Discrepancy between mitral valve areas measured by two-dimensional planimetry and three-dimensional transoesophageal echocardiography in patients with mitral stenosis. *Heart.* 2013;99:253.

37. Wunderlich NC, Beigel R, Siegel RJ. Management of mitral stenosis using 2D and 3D echo-Doppler imaging. *J Am Coll Cardiol Img*. 2013;6:1191.

38. Shavelle DM. Evaluation of valvular heart disease by cardiac catheterization and angiography. In: Otto CM, Bonow RO, eds. *Valvular Heart Disease: A Companion to Braunwald's Heart Disease*. 4th ed. Philadelphia: Saunders; 2009:85–100.

39. Kaya MG, Akpek M, Elcik D, et al. Relation of left atrial spontaneous echocardiographic contrast in patients with mitral stenosis to inflammatory markers. *Am J Cardiol*. 2012;109:851.

40. Tuzcu EM, Kapadia SR. Long-term efficacy of percutaneous mitral commissurotomy for recurrent mitral stenosis. *Heart*. 2013;99:1307.

41. Song JK, Song JM, Kang DH, et al. Restenosis and adverse clinical events after successful percutaneous mitral valvuloplasty: immediate post-procedural mitral valve area as an important prognosticator. *Eur Heart J*. 2009;30:1254.

42. Jneid H, Cruz-Gonzalez I, Sanchez-Ledesma M, et al. Impact of pre- and postprocedural mitral regurgitation on outcomes after percutaneous mitral valvuloplasty for mitral stenosis. *Am J Cardiol*. 2009;104:1122.

43. Levine RA, Schwammenthal E. Ischemic mitral regurgitation on the threshold of a solution: from paradoxes to unifying concepts. *Circulation*. 2005; 112:745–758.

44. Borer JS, Bonow RO. Contemporary approach to aortic and mitral regurgitation. *Circulation*. 2003;108:2432–2438.

45. Enriquez-Sarano M, Avierinos JF, Messika-Zeitoun D, et al. Quantitative determinants of the outcome of asymptomatic mitral regurgitation. *N Engl J Med*. 2005; 352(9):875–883.

46. Zoghbi WA, Enriquez-Sarano M, Foster E, et al. Recommendations for evaluation of the severity of native valvular regurgitation with two-dimensional and Doppler echocardiography. *J Am Soc Echocardiogr*. 2003;16:777.

47. Rosenhek R, Rader F, Klaar U, et al. Outcome of watchful waiting in asymptomatic severe mitral regurgitation. *Circulation*. 2006;113(18):2238–2244.

48. Enriquez-Sarano M, Schaff HV, Orszulak TA, Tajik AJ, Bailey KR, Frye RL. Valve repair improves the outcome of surgery for mitral regurgitation: a multivariate analysis. *Circulation*. 1995;91:1022–1028.

49. Capomolla S, Febo O, Gnemmi M, et al. Beta blockade in chronic HF: diastolic function and mitral regurgitation improvement by carvedilol. *Am Heart J*. 2000; 139:596–608.

50. Stout KK, Verrier ED. Acute valvular regurgitation. *Circulation*. 2009;119:3232.

51. Roes SD, Hammer S, van der Geest RJ, et al. Flow assessment through four heart valves simultaneously using 3-dimensional 3-directional velocity-encoded magnetic resonance imaging with retrospective valve tracking in healthy volunteers and patients with valvular regurgitation. *Invest Radiol*. 2009;44(10): 669–675.

52. Dujardin KS, Enriquez-Sarano M, Schaff HV, et al. Mortality and morbidity of aortic regurgitation in clinical practice: a long-term follow-up study. *Circulation*. 1999;99:1851–1857.

53. Greenberg BH, DeMots H, Murphy E, et al. Beneficial effects of hydralazine on rest and exercise hemodynamics in patients with chronic severe aortic insufficiency. *Circulation*. 1980;62:49–55.

54. Shen WF, Roubin GS, Hirasawa K, et al. Noninvasive assessment of acute effects of nifedipine on rest and exercise hemodynamics and cardiac function in patients with aortic regurgitation. *J Am Coll Cardiol*. 1984;4:902–907.

55. Lin M, Chiang HT, Lin SL, et al. Vasodilator therapy in chronic asymptomatic aortic regurgitation: enalapril versus hydralazine therapy. *J Am Coll Cardiol*. 1994;24: 1046–1053.

56. Omran AS, Woo A, David TE, Feindel CM, Rakoswki H, Siu SC. Intraoperative transesophageal echocardiography accurately predicts mitral valve anatomy and suitability for repair. *J Am Soc Echocardiogr*. 2002;15:950–957.

57. Shah PM, Raney AA. Echocardiographic roadmap of the mitral valve. *J Heart Valve Dis*. 2003;12:551–552.

58. Omoto R, Kyo S, Matsumura M, et al. Bi-plane color transesophageal Doppler echocardiography (color TEE): its advantages and limitations. *Int J Card Imaging*. 1989;4:57–58.

59. Kyo S, Takamoto S, Matsumura M, et al. Immediate and early postoperative evaluation of results of cardiac surgery by transesophageal two-dimensional Doppler echocardiography. *Circulation*. 1987;76(suppl. V):V113–V121.

60. Sugeng L, Lang RM. Current status of three-dimensional color flow Doppler. *Cardiol Clin*. 2007;25:297–303.

61. Ahmed S, Nanda NC, Miller AP, et al. Usefulness of transesophageal three-dimensional echocardiography in the identification of individual segment/scallop prolapse of the mitral valve. *Echocardiography*. 2003;20: 203–209.

62. Shiota T. 3D echocardiography: the present and the future. *J Cardiol*. 2008;52:169–185.

63. Otsuji Y, Levine RA, Takeuchi M, Sakata R, Teo C. Mechanism of ischemic mitral regurgitation. *J Cardiol*. 2008;51:145–156.

64. Yamada R, Watanabe N, Kume T, et al. Quantitative measurement of mitral valve coaptation in functional mitral regurgitation: in vivo experimental study by real-time three-dimensional echocardiography. *J Cardiol*. 2009;53:94–101.

65. Shah PM, Raney AA. Echocardiographic correlates of left ventricular outflow obstruction and systolic anterior motion following mitral valve repair. *J Heart Valve Dis*. 2001;10:302–306.

66. McCarthy PM, McGee EC, Rigolin VH, et al. Initial clinical experience with Myxo-ETlogix mitral valve ring. *J Thorac Cardiovasc Surg.* 2008;136:73–81.

67. Muraru DMD, Surkova E, Badano L. Revisit of functional tricuspid regurgitation; current trends in the diagnosis and management. *Korean Circ J.* 2016;46(4):443–455.

68. Sadeghpour A, Kyavar M, Alizadehasl A. *Comprehensive Approach to Adult Congenital Heart Disease.* London: Springer-Verlag; 2014. https://dx.doi.org/10.1007/978-1-4471-6383-1_2.

69. Tornos Mas P, Rodríguez-Palomares JF, Antunes MJ. Secondary tricuspid valve regurgitation: a forgotten entity. *Heart.* 2015;101:1840–1848.

70. Bruce CJ, Connolly HM. Right-sided valve disease deserves a little more respect. *Circulation.* 2009;119:2726.

71. Rogers JH, Bolling SF. The tricuspid valve: current perspective and evolving management of tricuspid regurgitation. *Circulation.* 2009;119:2718.

72. Dreyfus GD, Corbi PJ, Chan KM, Bahrami T. Secondary tricuspid regurgitation or dilatation: which should be the criteria for surgical repair? *Ann Thorac Surg.* 2005;79:127–132. TV annulus 4 am.

73. Van de Veire NR, Braun J, Delgado V, et al. Tricuspid annuloplasty prevents right ventricular dilatation and progression of tricuspid regurgitation in patients with tricuspid annular dilatation undergoing mitral valve repair. *J Thorac Cardiovasc Surg.* 2011;141:1431–1439.

74. Lang RM, Badano LP, Mor-Avi V, et al. Recommendations for cardiac chamber quantification by echocardiography in adults: an update from the American Society of Echocardiography and the European Association of Cardiovascular Imaging. *J Am Soc Echocardiogr.* 2015;28:1–39.

75. Rudski LG, Lai WW, Afilalo J, Hua L, Handschumacher MD, Chandrasekaran K. Guidelines for the echocardiographic assessment of the right heart in adults: a report from the American Society of Echocardiography. *J Am Soc Echocardiogr.* 2010;23:685–713.

76. Sadeghpour A, Hassanzadeh M, Kyavar M, et al. Impact of severe tricuspid regurgitation on long term survival. *Res Cardiovasc Med.* 2013;2(3):121.

77. Nath J, Foster E, Heidenreich PA. Impact of tricuspid regurgitation on long-term survival. *J Am Coll Cardiol.* 2004;43:405–409 [TR prognosis].

78. Guidelines and Standards. Echocardiographic Assessment of Valve Stenosis: EAE/ASE Recommendations for Clinical Practice. Helmut Baumgartner, Judy Hung, Javier Bermejo, John B. Chambers, Arturo Evangelista, Brian P. Griffin, Bernard Iung, Catherine M. Otto, MD, Patricia A. Pellikka, and Miguel Quiñones.

79. Anita S, Majid K, Azin A. *Comprehensive Approach to Adult Congenital Heart Disease.* Springer London Heidelberg New York Dordrecht; 2014.

80. Warnes CA, Williams RG, Bashore TM, et al. ACC/AHA 2008 guidelines for the management of adults with congenital heart disease. *J Am Coll Cardiol.* 2008;52: e1–e121.

81. Broadbent JC, Wood EH, Burchell HB. Left-to-right intra-cardiac shunts in the presence of pulmonary stenosis. *Proc Staff Meet Mayo Clin.* 1953;28:101.

82. Callahan JA, Brandenburg RO, Swan HJC. Pulmonary stenosis and ventricular septal defect with arteriovenous shunts: a clinical and hemodynamic study of eleven patients. *Circulation.* 1955;12:994.

83. Blount Jr SG, McCord MC, Moller H, Swan H. Isolated valvular pulmonic stenosis: clinical and physiologic response to open valvuloplasty. *Circulation.* 1954;10:161.

84. Campbell M. Simple pulmonary stenosis; pulmonary valvular stenosis with a closed ventricular septum. *Br Heart J.* 1954;16(3):273–300.

85. Silvilairat S, Cabalka AK, Cetta F, et al. Echocardiographic assessment of isolated pulmonary valve stenosis: which outpatient Doppler gradient has the most clinical validity? *J Am Soc Echocardiogr.* 2005;18:1137.

86. Bonow RO, Carabello BA, Chatterjee K, et al. ACC/AHA 2006 guideline for the management of patients with valvular heart disease. *J Am Coll Cardiol.* 2006;48(3): e1–148.

87. Vahanian A, Baumgartner H, Bax J, et al. Guidelines on the management of valvular heart disease: the task force on the Management of Valvular Heart Disease of the European Society of Cardiology. *Eur Heart J.* 2007;28 (2):230–268.

88. Karagoz T, Asoh K, Hickey E, et al. Balloon dilation of pulmonary valve stenosis in infants less than 3 kg: a 20-year experience. *Catheter Cardiovasc Interv.* 2009;74:753.

89. Earing MG, Connolly HM, Dearani JA, et al. Long-term follow-up of patients after surgical treatment for isolated pulmonary valve stenosis. *Mayo Clin Proc.* 2005;80:871.

90. Huehnergarth KV, Gurvitz M, Stout KK, Otto CM. Repaired ToF in the adult: monitoring and management. *Heart.* 2008;94:1663.

91. Sommer RJ, Hijazi ZM, Rhodes JF. Pathophysiology of congenital heart disease in the adult: part III: complex congenital heart disease. *Circulation.* 2008;117:1340.

92. McElhinney DB, Hellenbrand WE, Zahn EM, et al. Short- and medium-term outcomes after transcatheter pulmonary valve placement in the expanded multicenter US melody valve trial. *Circulation.* 2010;122:507.

93. Am Li W, Davlouros PA, Kilner PJ, et al. Doppler-echocardiographic assessment of pulmonary regurgitation in adults with repaired tetralogy of Fallot: comparison with cardiovascular magnetic resonance imaging. *Heart J.* 2004;147:165–172.

94. Silversides CK, Veldtman GR, Crossin J, et al. Pressure half-time predicts hemodynamically significant pulmonary regurgitation in adult patients with repaired tetralogy of fallot. *J Am Soc Echocardiogr.* 2003;16:1057–1062.

95. Nishimura Rick A, Otto Catherine M, Bonow Robert O, et al. 2014 AHA/ACC guideline for the management of patients with valvular heart disease. A report of the

American College of Cardiology/American Heart Association Task Force on Practice Guidelines. *Circulation.* 2014;129:e521–e643.

96. Zoghbi WA, Chambers JB, Dumesnil JG, et al. Recommendations for evaluation of prosthetic valves with echocardiography and Doppler ultrasound. *JASE.* 2009;22(9):975–1014.

97. Pibarot P, Dumesnil JG. Prosthetic heart valves, selection of the optimal prosthesis and long-term management. *Circulation.* 2009;119:1034–1048.

98. Bonow RO, Carabello BA, Kanu C, et al. ACC/AHA 2006 guidelines for the management of patients with valvular heart disease: a report of the American College of Cardiology/American Heart Association Task Force on Practice Guidelines. *Circulation.* 2006;114:e84–e231.

99. Fernandes V, Olmos L, Nagueh SF, Quinones MA, Zoghbi WA. Peak early diastolic velocity rather than pressure half-time is the best index of mechanical prosthetic mitral valve function. *Am J Cardiol.* 2002;89:704–710.

100. Lancellotti P, Pibarot P, Chambers J, et al. Recommendations for the imaging assessment of prosthetic heart valves: a report from the European Association of Cardiovascular Imaging endorsed by the Chinese Society of Echocardiography, the Inter-American Society of Echocardiography, and the Brazilian Department of Cardiovascular Imaging. *Eur Heart J Cardiovasc Imaging.* 2016;17:589–590.

101. Merie C, Kober L, Skov Olsen P, et al. Association of warfarin therapy duration after bioprosthetic aortic valve replacement with risk of mortality, thromboembolic complications, and bleeding. *JAMA.* 2012;308:2118–2125.

102. Kiavar M, Sadeghpour A, Bakhshandeh H, et al. Are prosthetic valve fibrin strands negligible? The associations and significance. *J Am SocEchocardiogr.* 2009;22:890–894.

103. Botzenhardt F, Eichinger WB, Bleiziffer S, et al. Hemodynamic comparison of bioprostheses for complete supra-annular position in patients with small aortic annulus. *J Am Coll Cardiol.* 2005;45:2054–2060.

104. Zakkar M, Amirak E, Chan KM, Punjabi PP. Rheumatic mitral valve disease: current surgical status. *Prog Cardiovasc Dis.* 2009;51:478.

105. Sadeghpour A, Kyavar M, Javani B, et al. Mid-term outcome of mechanical pulmonary valve prostheses: the importance of anticoagulation. *J Cardiovasc Thorac Res.* 2014;6(3):163–168.

106. Sadeghpour A, Javani B, Peighambari M, Kyavar M, Khajali Z. Mid-term follow-up of pulmonary valve bioprostheses in adults with congenital heart disease. *Anadolu Kardiyol Derg.* 2012;12:434–436.

107. Piper C, Körfer R, Horstkotte D. Prosthetic valve endocarditis. *Heart.* 2001;85:590–593.

108. Nishimura RA, Otto CM, Bonow, et al. 2017 AHA/ACC focused update of the 2014 AHA/ACC guideline for the management of patients with valvular heart disease: a report of the American College of Cardiology/American Heart Association Task Force on clinical practice guidelines. *Circulation.* 2017;135:e1159–e1195. https://doi.org/10.1161/CIR.0000000000000503.

# CHAPTER 31

# Infective Endocarditis

AZIN ALIZADEHASL[a] • ANITA SADEGHPOUR[b,c]
[a]Cardio-Oncology Research Center, Rajaie Cardiovascular, Medical & Research Center, Iran University of Medical Sciences, Tehran, Iran, [b]Rajaie Cardiovascular, Medical & Research Center, Tehran, Iran, [c]Visiting Research Scholar in Duke Cardiovascular MR Center, Durham, NC, United States

Infective endocarditis (IE) is a worldwide, potentially fatal disease, which is caused by infection of the endocardial surface of the heart, native or prosthetic heart valves, or indwelling cardiac leads and devices. The causes and epidemiology of the disease have evolved in the recent decades with a doubling of the average patient age and an increased incidence in patients with indwelling cardiac devices. The microbiology of the disease has also altered, and staphylococci, most frequently related to health-care contact and invasive procedures, have overtaken streptococci as the most common reason of the disease. IE is a heterogeneous disease with different epidemiology in the developed and developing countries. Interestingly, there are regional differences even in the developing countries, regarding the clinical manifestation, underlying heart disease and microorganism.[1–5]

## EPIDEMIOLOGY

Infective endocarditis is an uncommon infectious disease with high morbidity and mortality in the world. The annual incidence of IE range from 3 to 7 per 100,000 person-years, and IE is known the third or fourth most common life-threatening infection syndrome, after sepsis, pneumonia, and intraabdominal abscess.

Several global surveys have confirmed that the epidemiologic profile of IE has changed substantially. Although the overall IE incidence has remained stable, the incidence of IE caused by *Staphylococcus aureus* has increased, especially in the industrialized world.

Features of IE cases have also shifted toward higher mean of patient age, a higher amount of prosthetic valves and other new cardiac devices, and a reducing proportion of rheumatic heart disease (RHD). Furthermore, the fraction of IE patients undergoing surgery has augmented over the time to reach about 50%.

In addition to these temporal epidemiologic changes, major new diagnostic, prognostic, and therapeutic methods such as the rapid detection of pathogens

from valve tissue of patients undergoing surgery for IE by polymerase chain reaction (PCR), new imaging techniques such as three-dimensional (3D) echocardiography, multislice computed tomography (MSCT), $^{18}$F-fluorodeoxyglucose (FDG) positron emission tomography (PET)/computed tomography (CT), and cardiac magnetic resonance imaging (MRI) have been helpful in studies for diagnosis and management of IE complications.

Despite notable advances in diagnostic technology and improvements in antimicrobial selection, as well as presentation of new guidelines to proper management of disease, the morbidity and mortality remain high.[1–7]

Patients with the highest risk of IE are shown in Table 31.1.

Although the recent studies have shown that bicuspid aortic valve and degenerative heart diseases including flail mitral valves and mitral valve prolapse can be considered as high-risk group for IE and may benefit from IE prophylaxis.[4,8]

## MICROBIOLOGY

### Blood Culture-Positive Infective Endocarditis

- Positive blood cultures are the most important basis of diagnosis and are used for identification and susceptibility testing.
- At least three 30-min intervals set, each containing 10 mL of blood from a peripheral vein and using a meticulous sterile technique, are virtually always sufficient to identify the usual causative microorganisms.
- A single positive blood culture must be regarded cautiously for establishing the diagnosis of IE. When a microorganism has been identified, blood cultures must be repeated after 48–72 h to check the effectiveness of treatment.
- Presumptive identification is done based on Gram staining to adapt presumptive antibiotic therapy by clinicians. Complete identification is routinely

**TABLE 31.1**
**Cardiac Conditions at Highest Risk of Infective Endocarditis**

| Recommendations | Class of Recommendation | Level of Evidence |
|---|---|---|
| Antibiotic prophylaxis should be considered for patients at highest risk for IE:<br>1. Patients with any prosthetic valve, including a transcatheter valve, or those in whom any prosthetic material was used for cardiac valve repair<br>2. Patients with a previous episode of IE<br>3. Patients with CHD:<br>  a. Any type of cyanotic CHD<br>  b. Any type of CHD repaired with a prosthetic material, whether placed surgically or by percutaneous techniques, up to 6 months after the procedure or lifelong if residual shunt or valvular regurgitation remains | IIa | C |
| Antibiotic prophylaxis is not recommended in other forms of valvular or CHD | III | C |

CHD, congenital heart disease; IE, infective endocarditis.
From Habib G, Lancellotti P, Antunes MJ, et al. 2015 ESC Guidelines for the management of infective endocarditis. *Eur Heart J.* 2015;36(44): 3075–3128, with permission.

achieved within 2 days, however, might require longer for fastidious or atypical organisms.

- In many cases, because the results of blood cultures are taken for hours to days until a pathogen is identified, the empirical therapy of IE is started with the expectation that the regimen will be revised after a pathogen is defined and susceptibility results are obtained. The selection of an optimal empiric regimen depends on patient characteristics, prior antimicrobial exposures, microbiologic findings, and epidemiologic features.
- It is rational to acquire two sets of blood cultures every 24–48 h until the bloodstream is cleared of infection. However, if a patient have undergone valve surgery and the resected tissue is culture-positive or there was a perivalvular abscess in surgery, then an entire period of antimicrobial therapy is rational after valve surgery.
- Some studies suggest 2 weeks of antibiotic therapy for patients who undergo valve surgery and have negative valve tissue cultures, particularly in patients with IE caused by *Viridans* group streptococci or *Streptococcus gallolyticus* (*bovis*).[1,2,6,7]

**Blood Culture-Negative Infective Endocarditis** (Table 31.2)
- Blood culture-negative IE (BCNIE), which means no causative microorganism is found when the usual blood culture methods are used, can be seen in about 30% of all cases of IE, creating a significant dilemma in diagnostic and therapeutic managements.
- BCNIE most commonly is caused by previous antibiotic therapy; consequently, antibiotics should be held, and blood cultures should be repeated.

- BCNIE can be caused by fungi or fastidious bacteria, notably obligatory intracellular bacteria, which requires culturing them on specialized media, and their growth is relatively slow.
- According to the local epidemiology, systematic serologic testing for *Coxiella burnetii*, *Bartonella* spp., *Aspergillus* spp., *Mycoplasma pneumoniae*, *Brucella* spp., and *Legionella pneumophila* must be proposed followed by specific PCR assays for *Tropheryma whipplei*, *Bartonella* spp., and fungi (*Candida* spp. and *Aspergillus* spp.).
- In some countries, there is a higher prevalence of Q fever IE, in patients with culture-negative IE (30%) and checking for *C. burnetii* infections is highly recommended.[9]
- Blood PCR for the diagnosis of BCNIE has highlighted the importance of *S. gallolyticus* and *Streptococcus mitis*, enterococci, *S. aureus*, *Escherichia coli*, and fastidious bacteria.
- When all microbiologic assays are negative, the diagnosis of noninfectious endocarditis must be performed by antinuclear antibodies as well as antiphospholipid syndrome {anticardiolipin antibodies [immunoglobulin (Ig) G] and anti-b2-glycoprotein 1 antibodies [IgG and IgM]}. In a patient with a porcine bioprosthesis and negative blood culture with markers of allergic response, anti-pork antibodies must be sought.[5,6,10,11]

**Histologic Features of Infective Endocarditis**
Pathological examination of resected valvular tissue or embolic fragments remains the gold standard for the diagnosis of IE. For this purpose, all tissue samples that are obtained from surgical removal of cardiac valves

**TABLE 31.2**

Epidemiological and Etiological Clues in Culture-Negative Endocarditis

| Epidemiologic Feature | Common Microorganism |
| --- | --- |
| IDU | *Staphylococcus aureus*, including community-acquired oxacillin-resistant strains<br>Coagulase-negative staphylococci<br>β-Hemolytic streptococci<br>Fungi<br>Aerobic Gram-negative bacilli, including *Pseudomonas aeruginosa*<br>Polymicrobial |
| Indwelling cardiovascular medical devices | *S. aureus*<br>Coagulase-negative staphylococci<br>Fungi<br>Aerobic Gram-negative bacilli<br>*Corynebacterium* spp. |
| Genitourinary disorders, infection, and manipulation, including pregnancy, delivery, and abortion | *Enterococcus* spp.<br>Group B streptococci (*Streptococcus agalactiae*)<br>*Listeria monocytogenes*<br>Aerobic Gram-negative bacilli<br>*Neisseria gonorrhoeae* |
| Chronic skin disorders, including recurrent infections | *S. aureus*<br>β-Hemolytic streptococci |
| Poor dental health, dental procedures | VGS<br>Nutritionally variant streptococci<br>*Abiotrophia defectiva*<br>*Granulicatella* spp.<br>*Gemella* spp.<br>HACEK organisms |
| Alcoholism, cirrhosis | *Bartonella* spp.<br>*Aeromonas* spp.<br>*Listeria* spp.<br>*Streptococcus pneumoniae*<br>β-Hemolytic streptococci |
| Burn | *S. aureus*<br>Aerobic Gram-negative bacilli, including *P. aeruginosa*<br>Fungi |
| Diabetes mellitus | *S. aureus*<br>β-Hemolytic streptococci<br>*S. pneumoniae* |
| Early (≤1 year) prosthetic valve placement | Coagulase-negative staphylococci<br>*S. aureus*<br>Aerobic gram-negative bacilli<br>Fungi<br>*Corynebacterium* spp.<br>*Legionella* spp. |
| Late (≥1 year) prosthetic valve placement | Coagulase-negative staphylococci<br>*S. aureus*<br>VGS<br>*Enterococcus* spp.<br>Fungi<br>*Corynebacterium* spp. |

*Continued*

**TABLE 31.2**
Epidemiological and Etiological Clues in Culture-Negative Endocarditis—cont'd

| Epidemiologic Feature | Common Microorganism |
|---|---|
| Dog or cat exposure | *Bartonella* spp.<br>*Pasteurella* spp.<br>*Capnocytophaga* spp. |
| Contact with contaminated milk or infected farm animals | *Brucella* spp.<br>*Coxiella burnetii*<br>*Erysipelothrix* spp. |
| Homeless, body lice | *Brucella* spp. |
| AIDS | *Salmonella* spp.<br>*S. aureus*<br>*S. pneumoniae* |
| Pneumonia, meningitis | *S. pneumoniae* |
| Solid organ transplantation | *S. aureus*<br>*Aspergillus fumigatus*<br>*Enterococcus* spp.<br>*Candida* spp. |
| Gastrointestinal lesions | *Streptococcus gallolyticus* (*bovis*)<br>*Enterococcus* spp.<br>*Clostridium septicum* |

*HACEK, Haemophilus* spp., *Aggregatibacter* spp., *Cardiobacterium hominis, Eikenella corrodens*, and *Kingella* spp.; *IDU*, injection drug use; *VGS, Viridans* group streptococci.
From Baddour LM, Wilson WR, Bayer AS, et al. Infective endocarditis in adults: diagnosis, antimicrobial therapy, and management of complications a scientific statement for healthcare professionals from the American Heart Association. *Circulation.* 2015;132(15):1435–1486, with permission.

must be collected in a sterile container without fixative or culture medium and sent to a diagnostic microbiology laboratory for optimal recovery and identification of microorganisms.[1,2,6,12]

A proposed strategy for a microbiological diagnostic algorithm in suspected IE is depicted in Fig. 31.1.

## DIAGNOSIS
### Clinical Presentation
Infective endocarditis is known with a variety of very different clinical situations from an acute, rapidly progressive infection to a subacute or chronic disease with low-grade fever and nonspecific symptoms. This highly variable clinical presentation is according to the causative microorganism, the presence or the absence of preexisting cardiac disease, the presence or the absence of prosthetic valves or cardiac devices, and the mode of presentation.

In the International Collaboration on Endocarditis (ICE-PCS) study of the patients with definite IE, native valve IE was the most common (72%), which was followed by prosthetic valve IE (21%) and implantable cardioverter defibrillator or pacemaker IE (7%).

They also found that vegetations were most commonly found on the mitral valve (41%) followed by the aortic valve (38%), tricuspid (12%), and pulmonary (1%) valves.

- The most common symptoms are fever (>38°C in up to 90% of the patients), often associated with systemic symptoms of chills, poor appetite, weight loss, and heart murmurs.
- Up to 25% of IE patients have experienced embolic complications at the time of diagnosis, which makes IE a possible diagnosis in any patient presenting with fever and embolic phenomena.
- Vascular and immunologic phenomena such as splinter hemorrhages, Roth spots, and glomerulonephritis are other signs that became uncommon because of the advances in diagnosis and treatment.
- Petechiae, occurring on the conjunctivae oral mucosa or extremities[1,6,13,14] (Figs. 31.2–31.4).
- Emboli to the brain, lung, or spleen occur in 30% of cases. In a febrile patient, diagnostic suspicion might be strengthened by laboratory signs of infection, such as elevated C-reactive protein (CRP) or erythrocyte sedimentation rate (ESR), leukocytosis, anemia,

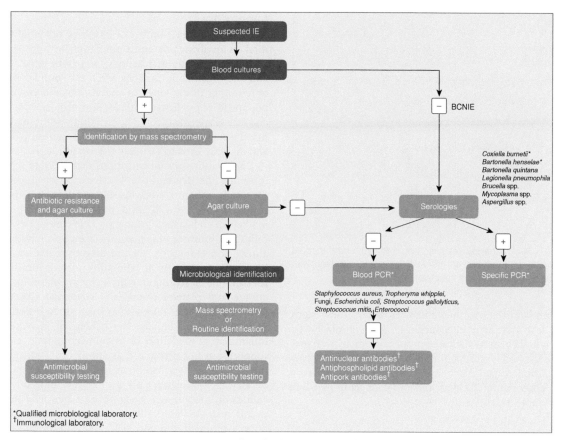

FIG. 31.1  Blood cultures and tests for IE.

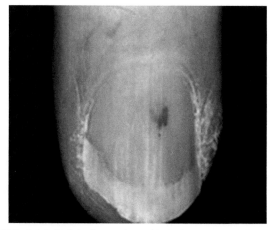

FIG. 31.2  Splinter hemorrhage. Embolic subungual hemorrhages in the midportion of the nail bed.

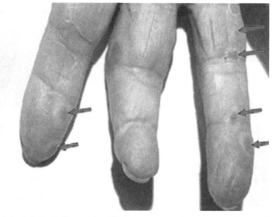

FIG. 31.3  Osler nodes. Violaceous, tender nodules (*arrows*) on volar fingers associated with minute infective emboli or immune complex deposition.

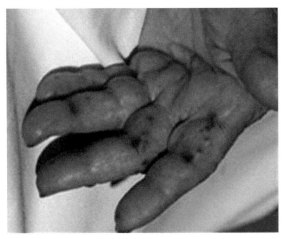

FIG. 31.4 Janeway lesions. Hemorrhagic and infarcted macules and papules on the volar fingers in a patient with *Staphylococcus aureus* infective endocarditis.

and microscopic hematuria. However, these signs have not been integrated into current diagnostic criteria because they are not specific. An atypical presentation is more common in older or immunocompromised patients than in younger patients. Fever is less common in elderly older in younger individuals (Table 31.3).[4,6–17]

**TABLE 31.3**
**Physical Findings in Infective Endocarditis**

| Sign | Patients Affected (%) |
|---|---|
| Fever | 80–90 |
| Heart murmur | 75–85 |
| New murmur | 10–50 |
| Changing murmur | 5–20 |
| Central neurologic abnormality | 20–40 |
| Splenomegaly | 10–40 |
| Petechial or conjunctival hemorrhage | 10–40 |
| Splinter hemorrhages | 5–15 |
| Janeway lesions | 5–10 |
| Osler nodes | 3–10 |
| Retinal lesion or Roth spot | 2–10 |

From Mann DL, Zipes DP, Libby P, et al, eds. *Braunwald's Heart Disease: A Textbook of Cardiovascular Medicine.* 10th ed. Philadelphia: Saunders; 2015:1528, with permission.

## Laboratory Findings

Although the large number of proposed potential biomarkers involving pro- and antiinflammatory processes, humoral and cellular reactions, and both circulatory and end-organ abnormalities reflect the complex pathophysiology of the sepsis or endocarditis process, their poor positive predictive value for the diagnosis of sepsis and lack of specificity for endocarditis, these biomarkers have been excluded from being major diagnostic criteria and are only used to facilitate risk stratification.

Some laboratory investigations that indicate sepsis, including the degree of leukocytosis or leucopoenia, the number of immature white blood cell (WBC) forms, concentrations of CRP and procalcitonin, ESR and markers of end-organ dysfunction (lactatemia, elevated bilirubin, thrombocytopenia, and changes in serum creatinine concentration), are not diagnostic markers for IE. Furthermore, certain laboratory investigations are used in surgical scoring systems including bilirubin, creatinine and platelet count, and creatinine clearance (EuroSCORE) are relevant to risk stratification in patients with IE. Finally, the pattern of increase in inflammatory mediators or immune complexes might support, but not prove, the diagnosis of IE, including the finding of hypocomplementemia in the presence of elevated antineutrophil cytoplasmic antibody in endocarditis-associated vasculitis or, when lead infection is suspected clinically, the laboratory finding of a normal procalcitonin and WBC count in the presence of significantly elevated CRP or ESR.[6,17–19]

## Imaging Techniques

Imaging, particularly echocardiography, plays a key role in the diagnosis, management, prognostic assessment, and decision-making in IE. Echocardiography is particularly useful for initial assessment of the embolic risk. TEE plays a major role both before and during surgery (intraoperative echocardiography).

### Echocardiography

Echocardiography [transthoracic echocardiography (TTE) or TEE] is the technique of choice for the diagnosis, management, and monitoring of patients with IE. TEE must be performed in case of negative TTE when there is a high index of suspicion for IE and in patients with positive TTE to rule out local complications. In patients with *S. aureus* bacteremia, TTE or TEE must be considered based on individual patient risk factors and the mode of acquirement of *S. aureus* bacteremia.

Three echocardiographic feathers are major criteria in the diagnosis of IE: vegetation, abscess or pseudoaneurysm, and new dehiscence of a prosthetic valve. However, identification of vegetations might be difficult in the presence of preexisting valvular lesions (mitral valve prolapse, degenerative calcified lesions), prosthetic valves, small vegetations (2–3 mm), and recent embolization and in nonvegetant IE. Identification of small abscesses might be difficult, too, particularly in the earliest stage of the disease or in the presence of a prosthetic valve. False diagnosis of IE might occur, and in some instances, it might be difficult to differentiate vegetations from thrombi, Lambl's excrescences, cusp prolapse, chordal rupture, valve fibroelastoma, degenerative or myxomatous valve disease, strands, systemic lupus (Libman–Sacks) lesions, primary antiphospholipid syndrome, rheumatoid lesions, or marantic vegetations. Therefore, the results of the echocardiographic study must be interpreted with caution, taking into account the patient's clinical presentation and the likelihood of IE.[2,14–16]

In patients with an initially negative examination, repeat TTE or TEE must be performed 5–7 days later if the clinical level of suspicion is still high or even earlier in the case of *S. aureus* infection.

Finally, follow-up echocardiography to monitor complications and response to treatment must be done. For this purpose, real-time 3D TEE is used because it is a feasible technique for the analysis of vegetation morphology and size that might overcome the shortcomings of conventional TEE, leading to a better prediction of the embolic risk in IE, and it is particularly useful in the assessment of perivalvular extension of the infection, prosthetic valve dehiscence, and valve perforation (Figs. 31.5 and 31.6).[1,3,6,10–22]

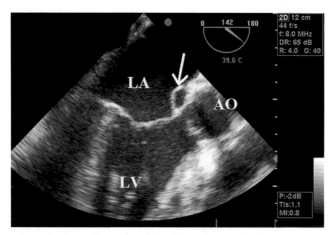

FIG. 31.5 Transesophageal echocardiography of the midesophagus showing a pseudoaneurysm of the intervalvular fibrosa (IVF), *arrow*. *AO*, aorta; *LA*, left atrium; *LV*, left ventricle.

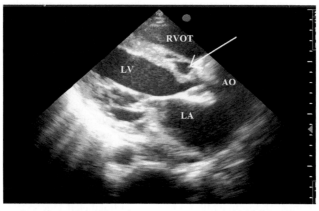

FIG. 31.6 Transthoracic echocardiography of a myocardial abscess in infective endocarditis (*arrow*). *AO*, aorta; *LA*, left atrium; *LV*, left ventricle; *RVOT*, right ventricular outflow tract.

### Multislice computed tomography

MSCT can be used for coronary angiography and to identify abscesses and pseudoaneurysms with a diagnostic accuracy similar to TEE and is probably superior in the providing of data regarding the extent and concerns of any perivalvular extension, containing the anatomy of abscesses, pseudoaneurysms, and fistulae. In aortic IE, CT might in addition be beneficial to define the size and anatomy of the aortic valve, aortic root, and ascending aorta, which might be used to inform the surgical planning. In pulmonary or right-sided IE, CT might reveal associated pulmonary disease containing abscesses and infarcts. MSCT might be equivalent or superior to echocardiography for the demonstration of prostheses-related vegetations, abscesses, pseudoaneurysms, and dehiscence in the evaluation of prosthetic valve dysfunction.

In critically ill patients, CT might be more feasible and practical and is an acceptable alternative when MRI is not available despite the higher sensitivity of MRI compared with CT for the detection of cerebral lesions.

Because of the higher sensitivity of MSCT angiography compared with conventional digital subtraction angiography and because it carries a lower contrast burden, it is useful for visualization of the intracranial vascular tree. When subarachnoid or intraparenchymal hemorrhage is detected, other vascular imaging (i.e., angiography) is required to diagnose or exclude a mycotic aneurysm if not detected on CT.[1,2,6,21,23]

### Magnetic resonance imaging

MRI is one of the best methods to detect the cerebral consequences of IE. Regardless of neurologic signs and symptoms, most pathologies are ischemic lesions (in 50%–80% of patients), with more common small ischemic lesions than larger infarcts. Other lesions are found in 10% of patients and are parenchymal or subarachnoid hemorrhages, abscesses, and mycotic aneurysms.

Cerebral MRI has an influence on the diagnosis of IE as one minor Duke criterion in patients who have cerebral MRI lesions and no neurologic symptoms.

Cerebral microbleeds are detected only when using gradient echo T2-weighted sequences and are found in 50%–60% of patients. Although IE and the presence of microbleeds are powerfully linked, microbleeds must not be considered as a minor criterion in the Duke classification.

Systematic abdominal MRI discovers lesions in one-third of patients assessed, most frequently affecting the spleen. Ischemic lesions are most common followed by abscesses or hemorrhagic lesions. Abdominal MRI findings have no incremental impact on the diagnosis of IE

when taking into account the findings of cerebral MRI. To summarize, cerebral MRI permits better lesion characterization in patients with IE and neurologic symptoms, but its impact on IE diagnosis is noticeable in patients with noncertain IE and without neurologic symptoms.[1–3,21–27]

### Nuclear imaging

With the introduction of hybrid equipment for both conventional nuclear medicine [e.g., single-photon emission CT (SPECT) and PET (e.g., PET/CT)], nuclear molecular methods are evolving as an important supplementary technique for patients with suspected IE and diagnostic problems. SPECT and CT imaging rely on the use of autologous radiolabeled leucocytes ($^{111}$In-oxine or $^{99m}$Tc-hexamethylpropyleneamine oxime) that collect in a time-dependent fashion in late images vs former images. PET/CT is usually performed using a single acquisition time point (generally at 1 h) after administration of $^{18}$F-FDG, which is actively incorporated in vivo by activated leucocytes, monocyte–macrophages, and CD4$^+$ T-lymphocytes collecting at the sites of infection.

Also, an additional promising role of $^{18}$F-FDG PET/CT might be seen in patients with recognized IE, in whom it could be used to monitor response to antimicrobial treatment (Table 31.4). However, sufficient data are not available at this time to make a general recommendation.[1,23–27]

### Diagnostic Criteria

The modified Duke criteria were recommended for diagnostic classification. These criteria are based on clinical, echocardiographic, and biologic findings, as well as the results of blood cultures and serologies (Tables 31.5–31.7). However, a lower diagnostic accuracy of modified Duke criteria for early diagnosis in clinical practice, especially in the case of prosthetic valve endocarditis (PVE) and pacemaker or defibrillator lead IE, and on the other, the recent advances in imaging modalities such as cardiac or whole-body CT scan, cerebral MRI, $^{18}$F-FDG PET/CT, and radiolabeled leucocyte SPECT/CT caused to be added three further points in the diagnostic criteria:

1. The identification of paravalvular lesions by cardiac CT must be considered as a major criterion.
2. In the setting of the suspicion of endocarditis on a prosthetic valve, abnormal activity around the site of implantation detected by $^{18}$F-FDG PET/CT (only if the prosthesis was implanted for 3 months) or radiolabeled leucocyte SPECT/CT must be considered as a major criterion.

## TABLE 31.4
### Care During and After Completion of Antimicrobial Treatment

**INITIATION BEFORE OR AT COMPLETION OF THERAPY**

- Echocardiography to establish new baseline
- Drug rehabilitation referral for patients who use illicit injection drugs
- Education on the signs of endocarditis and need for antibiotic prophylaxis for certain dental, surgical, and invasive procedures
- Thorough dental evaluation and treatment if not performed earlier in evaluation
- Prompt removal of intravenous catheter at completion of antimicrobial therapy

**SHORT-TERM FOLLOW-UP**

- At least three sets of blood cultures from separate sites for any febrile illness and before initiation of antibiotic therapy
- Physical examination for evidence of heart failure
- Evaluation for toxicity resulting from current or previous antimicrobial therapy

**LONG-TERM FOLLOW-UP**

- At least three sets of blood cultures from separate sites for any febrile illness and before initiation of antibiotic therapy
- Evaluation of valvular and ventricular function (echocardiography)
- Scrupulous oral hygiene and frequent dental professional office visits

From Habib G, Lancellotti P, Antunes MJ, et al. 2015 ESC Guidelines for the management of infective endocarditis. *Eur Heart J.* 2015;36(44): 3075–3128, with permission.

## TABLE 31.5
### Modified Duke Criteria for the Diagnosis of Infectious Endocarditis

**MAJOR CRITERIA**

Blood culture positive for IE
- Typical microorganisms consistent with IE from two separate blood cultures:
- *Viridans* streptococcus, *Streptococcus bovis*, HACEK group, *Staphylococcus aureus*, or community-acquired enterococci in the absence of primary focus
- Microorganisms consistent with IE from two persistently positive blood cultures:
  - At least two positive blood cultures of blood samples drawn >12 h apart or all of three or a majority of four or more separate cultures of blood with first and last sample drawn at least 1 h apart
  - Single positive blood culture for *Coxiella burnetii* or phase I IgG antibody titer >1:800

Evidence of endocardial involvement
- Echocardiogram positive for IE (vegetation, abscess, new partial dehiscence of prosthetic valve)
- New valvular regurgitation

**MINOR CRITERIA**

- Predisposition: predisposing heart condition, IDU
- Fever temperature >38°C
- Vascular phenomena: major arterial emboli, septic pulmonary infarcts, mycotic aneurysms
- Intracranial hemorrhages, conjunctival hemorrhages, Janeway lesions
- Immunologic phenomena: glomerulonephritis Osler node, Roth spot, rheumatoid factor
- Microbiological evidence: positive blood culture but does not meet a major criterion or serologic evidence of active infection with organism consistent with IE

*HACEK, Haemophilus* spp., *Aggregatibacter* spp., *Cardiobacterium hominis*, *Eikenella corrodens*, and *Kingella* spp.; *IDU*, injection drug use; *IE*, infective endocarditis.
Adapted from Li JS, Sexton DJ, Mick N, et al. Proposed modifications to the Duke criteria for the diagnosis of infective endocarditis. *Clin Infect Dis.* 2000;30:633, with permission.

**TABLE 31.6**
**Diagnosis of Infective Endocarditis**

| Diagnosis Is *Definite* in the Presence of | Diagnosis of *Possible* in the Presence of |
|---|---|
| Two major criteria or One major and three minor criteria or Five minor criteria | One major and one minor criteria or Three minor criteria |

3. The identification of the recent embolic events or infectious aneurysms by imaging only (silent events) must be considered as a minor criterion.

The diagnosis of IE is still based on the Duke criteria, with a major role of echocardiography and blood cultures. When the diagnosis remains only "possible" or even "rejected," however, with a persisting high level of clinical suspicion, echocardiography and blood culture must be repeated, and other imaging techniques must be used, either for diagnosis of cardiac involvement (cardiac CT, [18]F-FDG PET/CT, or radiolabeled leucocyte SPECT/CT) or for imaging embolic events (cerebral MRI, whole-body CT, and/or PET/CT).[1,2,6,12]

In summary, echocardiography (TTE and TEE), positive blood cultures, and clinical features remain the cornerstones of IE diagnosis. When blood culture results are negative, further microbiological studies are needed. The sensitivity of the Duke criteria can be improved by new imaging modalities (MRI, CT, and PET/CT) that allow the diagnosis of embolic events and cardiac involvement when TTE/TEE findings are negative or doubtful. These criteria are useful, but they do not replace the clinical judgment of the endocarditis team.[6,12]

## TREATMENT

### Antimicrobial Therapy (Tables 31.8–31.11)

Successful treatment of IE relies on antimicrobial therapy. Aminoglycosides synergize with cell-wall inhibitors (e.g., beta-lactams and glycopeptides) for bactericidal activity and are beneficial for shortening the duration of treatment (e.g., oral streptococci) and eliminating problematic organisms (e.g., *Enterococcus* spp.). One major limitation to drug-induced killing is antibiotic tolerance for bacteria. Actually, tolerant microbes are not resistant (still they are vulnerable to growth inhibition via the drug) but escape drug-induced killing and might resume growth even after treatment discontinuation. Slow-growing and latent microbes show

**TABLE 31.7**
**The Clinical Terminology of IE**

| | Surgery or Necropsy | Echocardiography |
|---|---|---|
| Vegetation | Infected mass attached to an endocardial structure or an implanted intracardiac material | Oscillating or nonoscillating intracardiac mass or other endocardial structures or nonimplanted intracardiac material |
| Abscess | Perivalvular cavity with necrosis and purulent material not communicating with the cardiovascular lumen | Thickened nonhomogeneous perivalvular area with echo-dense or echo-lucent appearance |
| Pseudoaneurysm | Perivalvular cavity communicating with the cardiovascular lumen | Pulsatile perivalvular echo-free space with color-flow Doppler detected |
| Perforation | Interruption of endocardial tissue continuity | Interruption of endocardial tissue continuity traversed by color-flow Doppler |
| Fistula | Communication between two neighboring cavities through as perforation | Color-flow Doppler communication between two neighboring cavities through a perforation |
| Valve aneurysm | Saccular outpouching of valvular tissue | Saccular bulging of valvular tissue |
| Dehiscence of a prosthetic valve | Dehiscence of prosthesis | Paravalvular regurgitation identified by TEE or TTE with or without a rocking motion of the prosthesis |

*TEE*, transesophageal echocardiography; *TTE*, transthoracic echocardiography.
From Habib G, Hoen B, Tornos P, et al. Guidelines on the prevention, diagnosis, and treatment of infective endocarditis (new version 2009). *Eur Heart J*. 2009;30(19):2369–2413, with permission.

**TABLE 31.8**

**Antibiotic Treatment of Infective Endocarditis Caused by Oral Streptococci and Streptococcus Bovis Group**

| Antibiotic | Dosage and Route | Duration (Weeks) | Class b |
|---|---|---|---|
| Strains penicillin-susceptible (MIC ≥0.125 mg/L) oral and digestive streptococci Standard treatment: 4-week duration | | | |
| Penicillin G or | 12–18 million U/day IV either in 4–6 doses or continuously | 4 | I |
| Amoxicillin or | 100–200 mg/kg/day IV in 4–6 doses | 4 | I |
| Ceftriaxone | 2 g/day IV or IM in 1 dose | 4 | I |
| **PEDIATRIC DOSAGES:** Penicillin G 200,000 U/kg/day IV in 4–6 divided doses Amoxicillin 300 mg/kg/day IV in 4–6 equally divided doses Ceftriaxone 100 mg/kg/day IV or IM in 1 dose | | | |
| Standard treatment: 2-week duration | | | |
| Penicillin G or Netilmicin | 12–18 million U/day IV either in 4–6 doses or continuously | 2 | I |
| Amoxicillin or | 100–200 mg/kg/day IV in 4–6 doses | 2 | I |
| Ceftriaxone combined with | 2 g/day IV or IM in 1 dose | 2 | I |
| Gentamicin or | 3 mg/kg/day IV or IM in 1 dose | 2 | I |
| Netilmicin | 4–5 mg/kg/day IV or IM in 1 dose | 2 | I |
| Pediatric dosages: penicillin G, amoxicillin, and ceftriaxone as above Gentamicin 3 mg/kg/day IV or IM in 1 dose or 3 equally divided doses | | | |
| **IN BETA-LACTAM ALLERGIC PATIENTS** | | | |
| Vancomycin | 30 mg/kg/day IV in 2 doses | 4 | I |
| Strains relatively resistant to penicillin (MIC 0.250–2 mg/L) | | | |
| **STANDARD TREATMENT** | | | |
| Penicillin G or | 24 million U/day IV either in 4–6 doses or continuously | 4 | I |
| Amoxicillin or | 200 mg/kg/day IV in 4–6 doses | 4 | I |
| Ceftriaxone combined with | 2 g/day IV or IM in 1 dose | 4 | I |
| Gentamicin | 3 mg/kg/day IV or IM in 1 dose | 2 | I |
| **IN BETA-LACTAM ALLERGIC PATIENTS** | | | |
| Vancomycin with | 30 mg/kg/day IV in 2 doses | 4 | 1 |
| Gentamicin | 3 mg/kg/day IV or IM in 1 dose | 2 | 1 |
| Pediatric doses: as above | | | |

*IM*, intramuscular; *IV*, intravenous; *MIC*, minimum inhibitory concentration; *U*, unit.

**TABLE 31.9**
Antibiotic Treatment of Infective Endocarditis Caused by *Staphylococcus* spp.

| Antibiotic | Dosage and Route | Duration (Weeks) | Class |
|---|---|---|---|
| | **NATIVE VALVES** | | |
| | **METHICILLIN-SUSCEPTIBLE STAPHYLOCOCCI** | | |
| (Flu) cloxacillin or oxacillin | 12 g/day IV in 4–6 doses | 4–6 | I |
| **PEDIATRIC DOSAGES: 200–300 MG/KG/DAY IV IN 4–6 EQUALLY DIVIDED DOSES** | | | |
| Alternative therapy Cotrimoxazole with | Sulfamethoxazole 4800 mg/day and Trimethoprim 960 mg/day (IV in 4–6 doses) | 1 IV + 5 oral intake | IIb |
| Clindamycin | 1800 mg/day IV in 3 doses | 1 | IIb |
| **PEDIATRIC DOSAGES:** Sulfamethoxazole 60 mg/kg/day and trimethoprim 12 mg/kg/day (IV in 2 doses) Clindamycin 40 mg/kg/day (IV in 3 doses) | | | |
| | **PENICILLIN-ALLERGIC PATIENTS OR METHICILLIN-RESISTANT STAPHYLOCOCCI** | | |
| Vancomycin | 30–60 mg/kg/day IV in 2–3 doses | 4–6 | I |
| **PEDIATRIC DOSAGES: 40 MG/KG/DAY IV IN 2–3 EQUALLY DIVIDED DOSES** | | | |
| Alternative therapy: Daptomycin | 10 mg/kg/day IV once daily | 4–6 | IIa |
| **PEDIATRIC DOSAGES: 10 MG/KG/DAY IV ONCE DAILY** | | | |
| Alternative therapy* Cotrimoxazole with | Sulfamethoxazole 4800 mg/day and Trimethoprim 960 mg/day (IV in 4–6 doses) | 1 IV + 5 oral intake | IIb |
| Clindamycin | 1800 mg/day IV in 3 doses | 1 | IIb |
| | **PROSTHETIC VALVES** | | |
| | **METHICILLIN-SUSCEPTIBLE STAPHYLOCOCCI** | | |
| (Flu) cloxacillin or oxacillin with | 200 mg/kg/day IV in 4–6 doses | ≥6 | 1 |
| Rifampin and | 900–1200 mg IV or PO in 2 or 3 divided doses | ≥6 | 1 |
| Gentamicin | 3 mg/kg/day IV or IM in 1 or 2 doses | 2 | 1 |
| Pediatric dosages: Oxacillin and (flu) cloxacillin as above Rifampin 20 mg/kg/day IV or PO in 3 equally divided doses | | | |
| | **PENICILLIN-ALLERGIC PATIENTS AND METHICILLIN-RESISTANT STAPHYLOCOCCI** | | |
| Vancomycin with | 30–60 mg/kg/day IV in 2–3 doses | ≥6 | 1 |
| Rifampin | 900–1200 mg IV or PO in 2 or 3 divided doses | ≥6 | 1 |
| Gentamicin | 3 mg/kg/day IV or IM in 1 or 2 doses | ≥6 | |
| Pediatric dosages: as above | | | |

*IM*, intramuscular; *IV*, intravenous; *PO*, oral.

**TABLE 31.10**
Antibiotic Treatment of Infective Endocarditis Caused by to *Enterococcus* spp.

| Antibiotic | Dosage and Route | Duration (Weeks) | Class |
|---|---|---|---|
| | **BETA-LACTAM AND GENTAMICIN-SUSCEPTIBLE STRAINS** | | |
| Amoxicillin with | 200 mg/kg/day IV in 4–6 doses | 4–6 | I |
| Gentamicin | 3 mg/kg/day IV or IM in 1 dose | 2–6 | I |
| **PEDIATRIC DOSAGES:** Ampicillin 300 mg/kg/day IV in 4–6 equally divided doses Gentamicin 3 mg/kg/day IV or IM in 3 equally divided doses | | | |
| Ampicillin with | 200 mg/kg/day IV in 4–6 doses | 6 | I |
| Ceftriaxone | 4 g/day IV or IM in 2 doses | 6 | I |
| Pediatric dosages: Amoxicillin as above Ceftriaxone 100 mg/kg/12 h IV or IM | | | |
| Vancomycin with | 30 mg/kg/day IV in 2 doses | 6 | I |
| Gentamicin | 3 mg/kg/day IV or IM in 1 dose | 6 | 1 |
| **PEDIATRIC DOSAGES:** Vancomycin 40 mg/kg/day IV in 2–3 equally divided doses. Gentamicin as above | | | |

*IM*, intramuscular; *IV*, intravenous.

**TABLE 31.11**
Antibiotic Treatment of Blood Culture-Negative Infective Endocarditis

| Pathogens | Proposed Therapy | Treatment Outcome |
|---|---|---|
| *Brucella* spp. | Doxycycline (200 mg/24 h) plus cotrimoxazole (960 mg/12 h) plus rifampin (300–600/24 h) for ≥3–6 months PO | Treatment success defined as an antibody titer <1:60 Some authors recommend adding gentamicin for the first 3 weeks |
| *Coxiella burnetii* (agent of Q fever) | Doxycycline (200 mg/24 h) plus hydroxychloroquine (200–600 mg/24 h) PO (>18 months of treatment) | Treatment success defined as antiphase I IgG titer <1:200, and IgA and IgM titers <1:50 |
| *Bartonella* spp. | Doxycycline 100 mg/12 h PO for 4 weeks plus gentamicin (3 mg/24 h) IV for 2 weeks | Treatment success expected in ≥90% |
| *Legionella* spp. | Levofloxacin (500 mg/12 h) IV or PO for >6 weeks or clarithromycin (500 mg/12 h) IV for 2 weeks, then PO for 4 weeks plus rifampin (300–1200 mg/24 h) | Optimal treatment unknown |
| Mycoplasma spp. | Levofloxacin (500 mg/12 h) IV or PO for ≥6 months | Optimal treatment unknown |
| *Tropheryma whipplei* (agent of Whipple disease) | Doxycycline (200 mg/24 h) plus hydroxychloroquine (200–600 mg/24 h) PO for >18 months | Long-term treatment, optimal duration unknown |

*IM*, intramuscular; *IV*, intravenous; *PO*, oral; *q*, every.

phenotypic tolerance toward most antibiotics (excluding rifampin to some extent). They are existing in vegetations (e.g., in PVE) and justify the need for lengthy therapy (6 weeks) to fully sterilize infected heart valves. Drug management of PVE must last longer (at least 6 weeks) than that of native valve endocarditis (NVE, 2–6 weeks) but is otherwise similar, except for staphylococcal PVE, wherever the regimen must contain rifampin whenever the strain is vulnerable. In NVE requiring valve replacement by a prosthesis during antibiotic therapy, the postoperative antibiotic regimen must be that suggested for NVE, not for PVE. In both PVE and NVE, the duration of management is based on the first day of effective antibiotic therapy (negative blood culture in the case of primary positive blood culture), not on the day of surgery. A new complete course of management must only start if valve cultures are positive, with the choice of antibiotic being based on the susceptibility of the latest recovered bacterial isolate.

In conclusion, there are six central considerations in the current recommendations: (1) the indications and outline of use of aminoglycosides have altered. They are no longer recommended in staphylococcal NVE because their significant clinical benefits have not been established; however, they may increase renal toxicity. When they are specified in other situations, aminoglycosides must be given in a single daily dose to decrease nephrotoxicity. (2) Rifampin must be used only in foreign body infections such as PVE after 3–5 days of effective antibiotic therapy after the bacteremia has been cleared. (3) Daptomycin and fosfomycin have been suggested for treating staphylococcal endocarditis and netilmicin for treating penicillin-susceptible streptococci. When daptomycin is indicated, it must be given at high doses (≥10 mg/kg once daily) and combined with a second antibiotic to increase activity and avoid the development of resistance. (4) Only published antibiotic efficacy data from clinical trials and cohort studies in patients with endocarditis (or bacteremia if there are no endocarditis data) have been considered in these guidelines. Data from experimental endocarditis models have not been taken into account in most cases. (5) We are still using the Clinical and Laboratory Standards Institute minimum inhibitory concentration (MIC) breakpoints instead of the European Committee on Antimicrobial Susceptibility Testing ones because most endocarditis data are derived from studies using the former breakpoints. (6) Although a consensus was obtained for the majority of antibiotic treatments, the optimal management of staphylococcal IE and the empirical treatment are still questioned.[1,15–18,23,28]

## Indications and Timing of Surgery

There is a prevailing opinion that valve surgery is crucial for optimal therapy in selected patients with complicated IE. Studies showed the proportion of IE patients undergoing valve surgery increased 7% per decade between 1969 and 2000. In population-based surveys, about 50% of both NVE and PVE patients undergo valve surgery during the active phase of IE (during initial hospitalization before completion of a full therapeutic course of antibiotics).

Although valve replacement surgery has served as an important option in the management of individual IE patients, firm conclusions from studies cannot be drawn on the effect of early surgery on mortality. Despite the availability of new studies, the indications for surgery have not changed appreciably over time.

Decisions on surgical intervention are complex and must be determined by a multispecialty team with expertise in cardiology, imaging, cardiothoracic surgery, and infectious diseases. These decisions depend on many clinical and prognostic factors, including infecting organism, vegetation size, the presence of perivalvular infection, the presence of embolism or heart failure, age, noncardiac comorbidities, and available surgical expertise.

Indeed, developing IE team has potential to enhance patient management and even reduce the cardiac and extracardiac burden of the IE.

Early surgery in patients with recurrent emboli and persistent vegetations has generally been enacted after clinical events. Whether recurrent, asymptomatic emboli detected on advanced imaging studies must be considered on an individual basis (Table 31.12).[23–27,29]

## Outpatient Management and Follow-Up Evaluation

After inhospital treatment, the main complications include recurrence of infection, heart failure, need for valve surgery, and death.

The actual risk of recurrence of IE is between 2% and 6% among survivors. Two main types of recurrence are distinguishable: relapse (a repeat episode of IE caused by the same microorganism) and reinfection (an infection caused by a different microorganism). In cases of same species during a subsequent episode of IE, molecular methods including strain typing techniques must be used, and when these techniques or the identity of both isolates is unavailable, the timing of the second episode of IE might be used to distinguish relapse from reinfection. Generally speaking, a recurrence caused by the same species within 6 months after the initial infection represents relapse, but later events suggest reinfection.

**TABLE 31.12**
Surgery in Infective Endocarditis

| Early Valve Surgery in Left-Sided NVE | Class and Level of Evidence |
|---|---|
| 1 Early surgery (during initial hospitalization and before completion of a full course of antibiotics) is indicated in patients with IE who present with valve dysfunction resulting in symptoms or signs of heart failure | Class I; level of evidence: B |
| 2 Early surgery must be considered, particularly in patients with IE caused by fungi or highly resistant organisms (e.g., vancomycin-resistant *Enterococcus*; multidrug-resistant, Gram-negative bacilli) | Class I; level of evidence: B |
| 3 Early surgery is indicated in patients with IE complicated by heart block, annular or aortic abscess, or destructive penetrating lesions | Class I; level of evidence: B |
| 4 Early surgery is indicated for evidence of persistent infection (manifested by persistent bacteremia or fever lasting >5–7 days and provided that other sites of infection and fever have been excluded) after the start of appropriate antimicrobial therapy | Class I; level of evidence: B |
| 5 Early surgery is reasonable in patients who present with recurrent emboli and persistent or enlarging vegetations despite appropriate antibiotic therapy | Class IIa; level of evidence: B |
| 6 Early surgery is reasonable in patients with severe valve regurgitation and mobile vegetations >10 mm | Class IIa; level of evidence: B |
| 7 Early surgery might be considered in patients with mobile vegetations >10 mm, particularly when involving the anterior leaflet of the MV and associated with other relative indications for surgery | Class IIb; level of evidence: C |
| **EARLY VALVE SURGERY IN PVE** | |
| 1 Early surgery is indicated in patients with symptoms or signs of heart failure resulting from valve dehiscence, intracardiac fistula, or severe prosthetic valve dysfunction | Class I; level of evidence: B |
| 2 Early surgery must be done in patients who have persistent bacteremia despite appropriate antibiotic therapy for 5–7 days in whom other sites of infection have been excluded | Class I; level of evidence: B |
| 3 Early surgery is indicated when IE is complicated by heart block, annular or aortic abscess, or destructive penetrating lesions | Class I; level of evidence: B |
| 4 Early surgery is indicated in patients with PVE caused by fungi or highly resistant organisms | Class I; level of evidence: B |
| 5 Early surgery is reasonable for patients with PVE who have recurrent emboli despite appropriate antibiotic treatment | Class IIa; level of evidence: B |
| 6 Early surgery is reasonable for patients with relapsing PVE | Class IIa; level of evidence: C |
| 7 Early surgery might be considered in patients with mobile vegetations >10 mm | Class IIb; level of evidence: C |
| **VALVE SURGERY IN CASES WITH RIGHT-SIDED IE** | |
| 1 Surgical intervention is reasonable for patients with certain complications | Class IIa; level of evidence: C |
| 2 Valve repair rather than replacement must be performed when feasible | Class I; level of evidence: C |
| 3 If valve replacement is performed, then an individualized choice of prosthesis by the surgeon is reasonable | Class IIa; level of evidence: C |
| 4 It is reasonable to avoid surgery when possible in patients who with IDU | Class IIa; level of evidence: C |
| **VALVE SURGERY IN CASES WITH PRIOR EMBOLI/HEMORRHAGE/STROKE** | |
| 1 Valve surgery might be considered in IE patients with stroke or subclinical cerebral emboli and residual vegetation without delay if intracranial hemorrhage has been excluded by imaging studies and neurologic damage is not severe (i.e., coma) | Class IIb; level of evidence: B |
| 2 In patients with major ischemic stroke or intracranial hemorrhage, it is reasonable to delay valve surgery for at least 4 weeks | Class IIa; level of evidence: B |

*IE*, infective endocarditis; *MV*, mitral valve; *NVE*, native valve endocarditis; *PVE*, prosthetic valve endocarditis.

**TABLE 31.13**
**Factors Associated With an Increased Rate of Relapse**

- Inadequate antibiotic treatment (agent, dose, duration)
- Resistant microorganism: *Brucella* spp., *Legionella* spp., *Chlamydia* spp., *Mycoplasma* spp., *Mycobacterium* spp., *Bartonella* spp., *Coxiella burnetii*, fungi
- Polymicrobial infection in an IVDA
- Empirical antimicrobial therapy for BCNIE
- Periannular extension
- Prosthetic valve IE
- Persistent metastatic foci of infection (abscesses)
- Resistance to conventional antibiotic regimens
- Positive valve culture
- Persistence of fever at the seventh postoperative day
- Chronic dialysis

*BCNIE*, blood culture-negative infective endocarditis; *IE*, infective endocarditis; *IVDA*, intravenous drug abuser.
From Habib G, Lancellotti P, Antunes MJ, et al. 2015 ESC Guidelines for the management of infective endocarditis. *Eur Heart J.* 2015;36 (44):3075–3128, with permission.

Factors associated with an increased rate of relapse are listed in Table 31.13. Relapses are most often caused by insufficient duration of original treatment, suboptimal choice of initial antibiotics, or a persistent focus of infection. Relapse must be treated for a further 4–6 weeks depending on the causative microorganism and its antibiotic susceptibility (remembering that resistance might develop in the meantime).

Patients with previous IE are at risk of reinfection, and prophylactic measures must be very strict. These patients are at higher risk of death and need for valve replacement. Reinfection is more frequent in IVDAs (especially in the year after the initial episode), in PVE, in patients undergoing chronic dialysis, and in those with multiple risk factors for IE.[1,2,30–33]

### Short-Term Follow-Up

A first episode of IE must not be considered as an ending after the patient has been discharged. Residual severe valve regurgitation might decompensate left ventricular function, or valve deterioration might progress despite bacteriological cure, usually presenting with acute HF.

Recurrences are rare after IE and might be associated with inadequate initial antibiotic therapy, resistant microorganisms, persistent focus of infection, IV drug abuse, or chronic dialysis. Patients must be aware that recurrence signs and symptoms of IE, including new onset of fever, chills, or other signs of infection, which mandates immediate evaluation, including procurement of blood cultures before empirical use of antibiotics. To monitor the development of secondary HF, an initial clinical evaluation and baseline TTE must be performed at the completion of antimicrobial therapy and repeated serially, particularly during the first year of follow-up. Regular clinical and echocardiographic follow-up, laboratory examination (e.g., WBC and CRP), and blood cultures must be performed during the first year after the completion of treatment.

### Long-Term Prognosis

The crude long-term survival rates after the completion of treatment of IE were estimated to be 80%–90% at 1 year, 70%–80% at 2 years, and 60%–70% at 5 years. The main predictors of long-term mortality are older age, comorbidities, recurrences, and heart failure, especially when cardiac surgery cannot be performed.

Late complications such as heart failure, higher risk of recurrences, and higher patient vulnerability are caused by excess mortality, especially within the first few years after hospital discharge.[1–3,32,33]

### REFERENCES

1. Habib G, Lancellotti P, Antunes MJ, et al. ESC Guidelines for the management of infective endocarditis. *Eur Heart J.* 2015;36(44):3075–3128. https://doi.org/10.1093/eurheartj/ehv319.
2. Cahill TJ, Prendergast BD. Infective endocarditis. *Lancet.* 2016;387(10021):882–893.
3. Habib G, Erba PA, Iung B, et al. Clinical presentation, aetiology and outcome of infective endocarditis. Results of the ESC-EORP EURO-ENDO (European infective endocarditis) registry: a prospective cohort study. *Eur Heart J.* 2019;40(39):3222–3232.
4. Sadeghpour A, Maleki M, Movassaghi M, et al. Iranian Registry of Infective Endocarditis (IRIE): time to relook at the guideline, regarding to regional differences. *Int J Cardiol Heart Vasc.* 2020;26:100433. https://doi.org/10.1016/j.ijcha.2019.100433.
5. Gouriet F, Chaudet H, Gautret P, et al. Endocarditis in the mediterranean basin. *New Microbes New Infect.* 2018;26:S43–S51.
6. Baddour LM, Walter R, et al. Infective endocarditis in adults: diagnosis, antimicrobial therapy, and management of complications: a scientific statement for healthcare professionals from the American Heart Association. *Circulation.* 2015;132.
7. De Sa DD, Tleyjeh IM, Anavekar NS, et al. Epidemiological trends of infective endocarditis: a population-based study

in Olmsted County, Minnesota. *Mayo Clin Proc.* 2010;85:422.

8. Zegri-Reiriz I, de Alarcon A, Munoz P, et al. Infective endocarditis in patients with bicuspid aortic valve or mitral valve prolapse. *J Am Coll Cardiol.* 2018;71(24):2731–2740.

9. Moradnejad P, Esmaeili S, Maleki M, et al. Q fever endocarditis in Iran. *Sci Rep.* 2019;9(1):1–7.

10. Fedeli U, Schievano E, Buonfrate D, et al. Increasing incidence and mortality of infective endocarditis: a population-based study through a record-linkage system. *BMC Infect Dis.* 2011;11:48.

11. Siegman-Ingra Y, Keifman B, Porat R, Giladi M. Healthcare associated infective endocarditis: a distinct entity. *Scand J Infect Dis.* 2008;40:474.

12. Li JS, Sexton DJ, Mick N, et al. Proposed modifications to the Duke criteria for the diagnosis of infective endocarditis. *Clin Infect Dis.* 2000;30:633.

13. Murdoch DR, Corey GR, Hoen B, et al. Clinical presentation, etiology, and outcome of infective endocarditis in the 21st century: the International Collaboration on Endocarditis-Prospective Cohort Study. *Arch Intern Med.* 2009;169:463.

14. Bonow RO, Mann DL, Zipes DP, Lippy P, eds. *Braunwald's Heart Disease: A Text Book of Cardiovascular Medicine.* 10th ed. Philadelphia: Saunders Elsevier; 2015:1528. Infective endocarditis chapter.

15. Jain V, Kovacicova-Lezcano G, Juhle LS, et al. Infective endocarditis in an urban medical center: association of individual drugs with valvular involvement. *J Infect.* 2008;57:132.

16. Nadji G, Rusinaru D, Remadi JP, et al. Heart failure in left-sided native valve infective endocarditis: characteristics, prognosis, and results of surgical treatment. *Eur J Heart Fail.* 2009;11:668.

17. Thuny F, Disalvo G, Belliard O, et al. Risk of embolism and death in infective endocarditis: prognostic value of echocardiography. A prospective multicenter study. *Circulation.* 2005;112:69.

18. Tornos P, Gonzalez-Alujas T, Thuny F, Habib G. Infective endocarditis: the European viewpoint. *Curr Probl Cardiol.* 2011;36:175.

19. Casella F, Rana B, Casazza G, et al. The potential impact of contemporary transthoracic echocardiography on the management of patients with native valve endocarditis: a comparison with transesophageal echocardiography. *Echocardiography.* 2009;26:900.

20. Habib G, Badano L, Tribouilloy C, et al. Recommendations for the practice of echocardiography in infective endocarditis. *Eur J Echocardiogr.* 2010;11:202.

21. Hansalia S, Biswas M, Dutta R, et al. The value of live/real time three-dimensional transesophageal echocardiography in the assessment of valvular vegetations. *Echocardiography.* 2009;26:1264.

22. Banchs J, Yusuf SW. Echocardiographic evaluation of cardiac infections. *Expert Rev Cardiovasc Ther.* 2012;10:1.

23. Nishimura RA, Otto CM, Bonow RO, et al. AHA/ACCF guideline for the management of patients with valvular heart disease. A report of the American College of Cardiology Foundation/American Heart Association Task Force on Practice Guidelines. *Circulation.* 2014;129:2440–2492.

24. Bannay A, Hoen B, Duval X, et al. AEPEI Study Group: the impact of valve surgery on shortand long-term mortality in left-sided infective endocarditis: do differences in methodological approaches explain previous conflicting results? *Eur Heart J.* 2011;2003:32.

25. Di Salvo G, Habib G, Pergola V, et al. Echocardiography predicts embolic events in infective endocarditis. *J Am Coll Cardiol.* 2001;37:1069.

26. Thuny F, Beurtheret S, Mancini J, et al. The timing of surgery influences mortality and morbidity in adults with severe complicated infective endocarditis: a propensity analysis. *Eur Heart J.* 2011;32:2027.

27. Iung B, Klein I, Mourvillier B, et al. Respective effects of early cerebral and abdominal magnetic resonance imaging on clinical decisions in infective endocarditis. *Eur Heart J Cardiovasc Imaging.* 2012;13:703.

28. Sadeghpour A, Boudagh S, Ghadrdoost B, et al. Acute kidney injury after nephrotoxic antibiotic therapy in patients with infective endocarditis. *Arch Clin Infect Dis.* 2019;14(5):e87617. https://doi.org/10.5812/archcid.87617.

29. Sadeghpour A, Maleki M, Boodagh S, et al. Impact of the Iranian Registry of Infective Endocarditis (IRIE) and multidisciplinary team approach on patient management. *Acta Cardiol.* 2020. https://doi.org/10.1080/00015385.2020.1781423.

30. Rossi M, Gallo A, De Silva RJ, Sayeed R. What is the optimal timing for surgery in infective endocarditis with cerebrovascular complications? *Interact Cardiovasc Thorac Surg.* 2012;14:72.

31. Ruttmann E, Legit C, Poelzl G, et al. Mitral valve repair provides improved outcome over replacement in active infective endocarditis. *J Thorac Cardiovasc Surg.* 2005;130:765.

32. Thuny F, Beurtheret S, Gariboldi V, et al. Outcome after surgical treatment performed within the first week of antimicrobial therapy during infective endocarditis: a prospective study. *Arch Cardiovasc Dis.* 2008;101:687.

33. Gaca JG, Sheng S, Daneshmand MA, et al. Outcomes for endocarditis surgery in North America: a simplified risk scoring system. *J Thorac Cardiovasc Surg.* 2011;141:98.

# CHAPTER 32

# Pericardial Disease

ANITA SADEGHPOUR[a,b] • AZIN ALIZADEHASL[c]

[a]Rajaie Cardiovascular, Medical & Research Center, Tehran, Iran, [b]Visiting Research Scholar in Duke Cardiovascular MR Center, Durham, NC, United States, [c]Cardio-Oncology Research Center, Rajaie Cardiovascular, Medical & Research Center, Iran University of Medical Sciences, Tehran, Iran

## NORMAL PERICARDIUM, ANATOMY, AND FUNCTION

The pericardium is a flask-like two-layered (visceral and parietal) sac that surrounds the heart. The outer layer (parietal layer) is mostly acellular and contains collagen and elastin fibers and normally has a 2-mm thickness. The visceral layer is a monolayer of mesothelial cells, collagen, and elastin fibers that cover the heart.

The pericardium covers most of the heart and proximal part of the great vessels. The pericardial space is between two layers and normally contains less than 50 mL of serous fluid. The visceral layer is continuous with the parietal layer and forms pericardial sinuses. Reflection of the serosal layer posterior to the ascending aorta forms the transverse sinus, and reflection behind the left atrium forms the oblique sinus. The parietal pericardium has some attachment to adjacent structures via ligaments such as the diaphragm and sternum.

There is some amount of adipose tissue under the visceral layer that is called the epicardial fat and is largely along the atrioventricular and interventricular grooves and around the right ventricle (RV) and contains coronary arteries, veins, and nerves. The pericardium has sympathetic and parasympathetic innervation. Arteries that supply the pericardium are derived from the descending thoracic aorta and internal thoracic artery.

Although congenital absence of the pericardium or surgical pericardectomy is not incompatible with life and humans can live without the pericardium, the pericardium has several functions such as:

- Fixation of the heart and preventing excessive heart motion
- Mechanical barrier against infection
- Lubricating function between the heart layers and surrounding structures
- Contains mechanoreceptors and chemoreceptors that have an autocrine–paracrine role and secrete prostaglandin and prostacyclin
- Limits cardiac distention by restraining effect

The pericardium can be involved as an isolated disease (viral pericarditis) after myocardial involvement [pericarditis after acute myocardial infarction (MI)] or may be part of a sign of systemic diseases such as pericardial effusion in collagen vascular disease (lupus) or hypothyroidism.[1–3]

## CAUSES, EPIDEMIOLOGY, AND PATHOPHYSIOLOGY OF ACUTE PERICARDITIS

Acute pericarditis is inflammation of the pericardium and is characterized by pleuritic chest pain of less than 2 weeks in duration.[3] Many causes, including viral and bacterial infections, have been suggested as the etiology of pericarditis, but it is deemed idiopathic because of the low yield of the routine diagnostic tests; therefore, the cause cannot be found (Table 32.1).

### Epidemiology

It is difficult to determine the precise incidence of pericarditis because of different clinical presentations and specific criteria for its diagnosis. Nonetheless, the incidence has been reported to be about 1% in autopsy. Nearly 5% of nonischemic chest pain in the emergency department is caused by pericarditis. Demography influences the prevalence of etiology, with infectious causes being more common in the developing countries.[4,5]

The signs and symptoms are caused by pericardial inflammation. Most cases are uncomplicated. Complicated cases are those that have large pericardial effusions (PEs) or left ventricular (LV) dysfunction, which are identified with increased troponin levels.

**TABLE 32.1**
**Pericardial Disease and Selected Specific Causes**

Idiopathic[a]

Infectious

Viral (echovirus, coxsackievirus, adenovirus, cytomegalovirus, hepatitis B, infectious mononucleosis, HIV/AIDS)

Bacterial (*Pneumococcus, Staphylococcus, Streptococcus, Mycoplasma* spp., others)

Mycobacteria (*Mycobacterium tuberculosis, Mycobacterium avium-intracellulare*)

HIV associated

Fungal (histoplasmosis, coccidioidomycosis)

Protozoal

Inflammatory

Connective tissue disease[a] (SLE, RA, scleroderma, dermatomyositis, Sjögren syndrome, mixed)

Drug-induced[a] (procainamide, hydralazine, isoniazid, cyclosporine)
Arteritis (polyarteritis nodosa, temporal arteritis)

Inflammatory bowel disease

After cardiotomy or thoracotomy,[a] after cardiac injury[a]

Miscellaneous: sarcoidosis, Erdheim–Chester disease, Churg–Strauss disease

After myocardial infarction

Early

Late (Dressler syndrome)[a]

Cancer

Primary: mesothelioma, fibrosarcoma, lipoma, and so on

Secondary[a]: breast and lung carcinoma, lymphomas, Kaposi sarcoma

Radiation induced[a]

Early after cardiac surgery and orthotopic heart transplantation

Hemopericardium

Trauma

Post-MI free wall rupture

Device and procedure related: percutaneous coronary procedures

Implantable defibrillators, pacemakers, after ablation of arrhythmia

After closure of an ASD, after valve repair or replacement

Dissecting aortic aneurysm

Congenital

Cysts, congenital absence pericardium

Miscellaneous

Stress cardiomyopathy

Cholesterol ("gold paint" pericarditis)

*Continued*

**TABLE 32.1**
**Pericardial Disease and Selected Specific Causes—cont'd**

Chronic renal failure, dialysis associated[a]

Hypothyroidism and hyperthyroidism

Amyloidosis

Pneumopericardium

*ASD*, atrial septal defect; *RA*, rheumatoid arthritis; *SLE*, systemic lupus erythematosus.
[a]Causes that can be manifested as the syndrome of acute pericarditis.
From LeWinter MM, Hopkins WE. Pericardial diseases. In: Mann DL, Zipes DP, Libby P, et al., eds. *Braunwald's Heart Disease: A Textbook of Cardiovascular Medicine*. 10th ed. Philadelphia: Saunders; 2015; with permission.

## Clinical Presentation, History, and Physical Examination

Pleuritic chest pain, which is the typical symptom of acute pericarditis, is characterized by the following:

- Sharp retrosternal pain with radiation to the trapezius muscle
- Exacerbation with inspiration and lying down and released by sitting up

It can be indistinguishable from pleurisy or even MI; nevertheless, age, quality of pain, and exacerbation with inspiration and lying down help to differentiate pericarditis from other diseases. Friction rub is the hallmark of pericarditis and resembles walking on snow owing to its superficial and scratchy character. It has three phases: systole, early diastole, and atrial contraction. Also, because friction may be dynamic, it can be heard before it then disappears after a period. This dynamic characterization necessitates frequent examinations for friction rub if pericarditis is suspected but not heard in the initial examination. Friction is independent of the respiratory cycle and can be heard during systole and diastole. It can be mistaken for heart murmur, especially if heard louder during systole or diastole. It may be heard all over the heart, but the best auscultation zone is the lower sternal border and the apex when the patient is lying leftward.

## Diagnosis

The diagnosis is based on the presence of at least two of the following four typical findings:

1. Typical pleuritic chest pain
2. Pericardial friction rub
3. Typical electrocardiography (ECG) changes consistent with pericarditis
4. New or worsening PE

Aside from these criteria, the diagnosis can be supported by some laboratory data such as acute phase reactants, including increased serum high-sensitivity C-reactive protein (hs-CRP) or erythrocyte sedimentation rate (ESR) (Table 32.2).[6,7]

**TABLE 32.2**
**Definitions and Diagnostic Criteria for Pericarditis**

| Pericarditis | Definition and Diagnostic Criteria |
|---|---|
| Acute | Inflammatory pericardial syndrome to be diagnosed with at least two of the four following criteria: |
| | (1) Pericarditic chest pain |
| | (2) Pericardial rubs |
| | (3) New widespread ST-elevation or PR depression on ECG |
| | (4) Pericardial effusion (new or worsening) |
| | Additional supporting findings: |
| | – Elevation of markers of inflammation (i.e., C-reactive protein, erythrocyte sedimentation rate, and white blood cell count); |
| | – Evidence of pericardial inflammation by an imaging technique (CT, CMR) |
| Incessant | Pericarditis lasting for >4–6 weeks but <3 months without remission |
| Recurrent | Recurrence of pericarditis after a documented first episode of acute pericarditis and a symptom-free interval of 4–6 weeks or longer[a] |
| Chronic | Pericarditis lasting for >3 months |

*CMR*, cardiac magnetic resonance; *CT*, computed tomography; *ECG*, electrocardiogram.
[a]Usually within 18–24 months but a precise upper limit of time has not been established.

### Electrocardiography

In acute pericarditis, ECG has been suggested as the most important test with a typical finding of diffuse ST-segment elevation. ECG changes have four phases, but only half of patients show all of the following four stages:

1. *First stage*: There is a diffuse ST-segment elevation in most leads except aVR and $V_1$ and can be associated with PR depression. It occurs within a few hours of the onset of chest pain and lasts hours to days.
2. *Second stage*: The ST segments return to an isoelectric line.
3. *Third stage*: T-wave inversion occurs. These ECG changes can last weeks to months or even indeterminately in tuberculosis (TB) and uremia.[1]
4. *Fourth stage*: ECG may show normalization.

Electrocardiographic findings can be mistaken for other diseases such as MI and early repolarization. History and physical examination help to distinguish.

### Laboratory findings
Nonspecific serum markers like increased white blood cell (WBC) count and ESR can be detected. In about 75% of patients, hs-CRP is elevated. In about 1 week in most patients, hs-CRP returns to the normal value. However, in some cases, it may take longer ($\approx 4$ weeks). Serial measurements of hs-CRP may be used for disease monitoring.

The myocardium may be involved in 15% of patients, and troponin is elevated in those with coexisting myocarditis.

In one study, half of the patients exhibited elevated troponin, and in half of these patients, troponin was in the range of MI diagnosis; nonetheless, none of these patients with high levels of troponin had coronary artery disease on angiography.[1] Still, MI should be taken into consideration if the troponin level is high.[8]

### Imaging: Echocardiography, computed tomography, and magnetic resonance imaging
Transthoracic echocardiography (TTE) is the first-line imaging modality and should be done in all patients with acute pericarditis. Most patients have normal echocardiography results, and the absence of PE may be seen in up to 60% of patients, but the presence of effusion (usually small) can confirm the diagnosis.[4,9]

Rarely, PE is large and even progresses to tamponade physiology (especially in nonidiopathic effusions). TTE can not only detect PE but also help distinguish other diseases and underlying pathologies such as MI. Even though about 5% of patients with acute pericarditis have wall motion abnormality on TTE, this finding is important as it can be an indication for ischemic evaluation.[4]

Cardiac imaging modalities such as computed tomography (CT) and cardiac magnetic resonance imaging (CMR) are rarely indicated in uncomplicated cases (Table 32.3). However, CT shows loculated PE and thickened pericardium and distinguishes exudative, transudative, and hemorrhagic fluids by the density of

**TABLE 32.3**

Recommendations for Cardiovascular Imaging in Noncomplicated Pericarditis From the European Association of Cardiovascular Imaging, 2014

| | |
|---|---|
| TTE to confirm the diagnosis of noncomplicated acute pericarditis with small or no pericardial effusion | Recommended |
| CT or CMR to confirm the associated myocarditis in case of clinically suspected myocarditis | Recommended |
| CT, CMR, or TEE in case of inconclusive TTE | Not recommended |

*CMR*, cardiac magnetic resonance imaging; *CT*, computed tomography; *TEE*, transesophageal echocardiography; *TTE*, transthoracic echocardiography.
Data from Cosyns B, Plein S, Nihoyanopoulos P, et al. European Association of Cardiovascular Imaging (EACVI) position paper: multimodality imaging in pericardial disease. *Eur Heart J Cardiovasc Imaging*. 2014;16(1):12–31.

the fluid based on the Hounsfield unit (HU). An HU less than 10 suggests transudative effusion, and an HU of 20–60 denotes exudative effusion.[2]

Magnetic resonance imaging (MRI) detects localized PE and similar to CT can differentiate transudative fluids from exudative fluids by signal characteristics. It also can demonstrate myocarditis by edema and wall motion abnormality.

### Natural History and Management
Acute pericarditis is usually self-limited with uncomplicated course in 70%–90% of patients. Patients with small PE scan be treated on an outpatient basis.[5,10]

*Admission should be considered in the following situations:*
1. Moderate- to large-sized effusion
2. Not responding to the initial treatment
3. Nonidiopathic causes
4. Elevated temperature (temperature $>38°C$)
5. Immunosuppression
6. Anticoagulation
7. Myopericarditis
8. Trauma[7,11–13]

In cases of idiopathic pericarditis, nonsteroidal antiinflammatory drugs (NSAIDs) are the first line of treatment.

Colchicine is recommended for initial therapy in conjunction with NSAIDs or monotherapy. When colchicine is used as initial therapy with NSAIDs, it reduces the recurrence of the episodes. Its dosages are 0.5 mg/day for patients weighing less than 70 kg and 0.5 mg every

12 h for patients weighing more than 70 kg for 3 months.[1] Corticosteroids can be used in patients who poorly respond to NSAIDs. Prednisone (0.2–0.5 mg/kg/day) is initiated and may be tapered every 2–4 weeks.

Colchicine in conjunction with prednisone is recommended. However, given the increased risk of gastrointestinal disorder, NSAIDs should be discontinued[14,15] (Table 32.4).

## Relapsing and Recurrent Pericarditis

About 15%–30% of patients experience relapses, which can even occur many years after the initial pericarditis.[3,12] Those in whom the initial treatment has failed and women are at an increased risk of relapse.[3] It is, therefore, advisable that follow-up evaluation be undertaken. Pericardial biopsy without PE is not appropriate because the specific agent is rarely obtained and will seldom affect the management.[3] The management includes NSAIDs, to which patients often respond. CRP can be used for guiding the therapy.[3] Colchicine for 6–12 months is effective for treatment and prophylaxis. Patients with difficult cases who do not respond to NSAIDs and colchicine may respond to a short duration of high-dose corticosteroids. Azathioprine and cyclophosphamide are used, although no systemic evidence exists. Pericardiectomy is only for those who do not respond to medical treatment, and quality of life in those subjected to it is not satisfactory (Table 32.5).

## PERICARDIAL EFFUSION

Any inflammation (e.g., idiopathic, viral or bacterial, neoplastic, autoimmune, and postsurgical) that involves the pericardium can induce PE. Effusion can be transudate, exudate, hemopericardium, or pyo-pericardium. Effusion without inflammation is seen in uremia or idiopathic pericarditis. After orthotopic heart transplantation, effusion is common, but tamponade is rare and is usually resolved within a few weeks or

### TABLE 32.4
Commonly Prescribed Antiinflammatory Therapy for Acute Pericarditis

| Drug | Usual Dosing | Tx Duration | Tapering[a] |
|---|---|---|---|
| Aspirin | 750–1000 mg every 8 h | 1–2 weeks | Decrease doses by 250–500 mg every week for 2–3 weeks, then discontinue |
| Ibuprofen | 600 mg every 8 h | 1–2 weeks | Decrease doses by 200–400 mg every week for 2–3 weeks, then discontinue |
| Colchicine | 0.5 mg once (<70 kg) or 0.5 mg b.i.d. (≥70 kg) | 3 months | Not mandatory, alternatively 0.5 mg every other day (<70 kg) or 0.5 mg once (≥70 kg) in the last weeks |

[a]Therapy duration is mainly individualized and conducted by symptoms and hs-CRP. Maintain initial dose and taper only if patient is asymptomatic and hs-CRP is normalized.
Modified from Zipes DP, Libby P, Bonow RO, Mann DL, Tomaselli GF. Braunwald's Heart Disease; A Textbook of Cardiovascular Medicine Internet. 11th ed. Elsevier Health Sciences; 2018:1666 [chapter 83].

### TABLE 32.5
Commonly Prescribed Antiinflammatory Therapies for Recurrent Pericarditis

| Tx Duraion | Usual Dosing | Tx Duration | Tapering |
|---|---|---|---|
| Aspirin | 500–100 mg every 6–8 h (range 1.5–4 g/day) | Weeks–months | Decrease doses by 250–500 mg every 1–2 weeks |
| Ibuprofen | 600 mg every 8 h (range 1200–2400 mg) | Weeks–months | Decrease doses by 200–400 mg every 1–2 weeks |
| Indomethacin | 25–50 mg every 8 h start at lower end of dosing range and titrate upward to avoid headache and dizziness | Weeks–months | Decrease doses by 25 mg every 1–2 weeks |
| Colchicine | 0.5 mg twice or 0.5 mg daily for patients <70 kg or intolerant to higher doses | At least 6 months | Not necessary, alternatively 0.5 mg every other day (<70 kg)or 0.5 mg once (≥70 kg) in the last weeks |

months. Hemopericardium is seen after MI and free-wall rupture or aortic dissection. PE can be seen in some systemic diseases such as end-stage renal disease, hypothyroidism, and neoplasm.

## TAMPONADE

Tamponade is a life-threatening condition in which the pericardial pressure is elevated and equals the atrial pressure, inhibiting normal atrial filling and compressing the chambers.

### Pathophysiology and Hemodynamics

The critical point in effusion is the restriction of the cardiac volume and the filling of the chambers and, eventually, the cardiac output. The amount of effusion has a weak correlation with the hemodynamic effect and depends on the volume and speed of accumulation.

The pericardium has a low reserve volume, and the speed of accumulation is important because a rapid accumulation of even 150–200 mL of fluid can increase the pericardial pressure and exert a significant hemodynamic effect. In contrast, a slow accumulation of large effusion can be an incidental finding without symptoms caused by chronic change and the stretching of the pericardium.

Indeed, the pericardium responds to acute stretch in a manner different from gradual stretch. The gradual accumulation of PE within several weeks or months increases the pericardium compliance and shifts the pressure–volume curve to the right, which is contrary to the rapid accumulation of PE, which causes increased pericardial compliance and shifts the pressure–volume curve to the right.[16]

As fluid accumulation increases in the pericardium, LV and RV diastolic pressures and atrial pressures rise (20–25 mmHg) and equalize to the pressure of the pericardial sac. In response to the increased intrapericardial pressure, the venous pressures should increase to maintain normal cardiac filling. Consequently, the transmural pressure, which is intracavitary diastolic pressure minus intrapericardial pressure, will be close to zero or even become negative. Finally, the reduced preload with exhausted compensatory mechanisms results in a low cardiac output and hypotension. In severe tamponade with restricted cardiac volume and low transmural pressure, cardiac filling can occur only during systole while the heart is emptying. Consequently, the Y wave disappears because, during diastole, there is no space for blood emptying into the heart.

Paradoxical pulse is the characteristic finding of tamponade and is defined as greater than 10-mmHg decrease in systolic blood pressure during inspiration.[3] Paradoxical pulse can be seen in constrictive pericarditis, pulmonary embolism, and pulmonary disease. The paradoxical pulse occurs as the normal increase in systemic venous return sustains during inspiration and causing an increased filling of the right-sided cardiac chambers and consequently shifting the interventricular septum to the left and reducing the left-sided stroke volume. All of these changes happen mostly because total cardiac volume is fixed. In its severe form, there may be no peripheral pulse during inspiration.[3]

In response to the low cardiac output, adrenergic response increases, and parasympathetic withdrawal occurs. Compensatory tachycardia and increased contractility will maintain the output, and when the compensatory mechanism fails, hypotension occurs.

### Specific Types of Tamponade

- In some cases, paradoxical pulse may be absent because of a preexisting high diastolic pressure or volume such as in atrial septal defects, aortic regurgitation, and chronic LV dysfunction.
- Loculated effusion, which compresses selected chambers, results in tamponade without the typical hemodynamic or echocardiographic findings of tamponade. This form usually occurs after cardiac surgery.[3]
- Low-pressure tamponade occurs in the setting of a low intrapericardial and intracardiac diastolic pressure and is defined when the intrapericardial pressure is less than 7–10 mmHg and the right atrial (RA) pressure or the intracardiac diastolic pressure becomes less than 4 mmHg. Low-pressure tamponade is seen mostly in hemodialysis, traumatic hemorrhage, and diuretic usage.[17]

### Clinical Features

Large PE may be asymptomatic and found incidentally by cardiomegaly on chest radiography or on echocardiography when it is done for other reasons.

Patients with tamponade may complain of dyspnea, shortness of breath when lying down, and chest pain.

The Beck's triad, consisting of hypotension (and pulsus paradoxus), jugular vein distention, and muffled heart sounds (impalpable cardiac pulsation), may be seen in severe tamponade. Other findings include tachycardia, diaphoresis, and peripheral coldness or cyanosis. Bradycardia may be the last phase of tamponade.

Paradoxical pulse is measured as a decrease in systolic blood pressure during inspiration. When severe, paradoxical pulse can be detected by missing of the peripheral pulse in palpation during inspiration.

The differential diagnosis is every disorder that results in jugular vein distention and hypotension such as RV MI, pulmonary embolism, and right-heart failure.

## Diagnostic Testing

### Electrocardiography

The ECG shows tachycardia, low voltage, and electrical alternans caused by swinging heart.

**Chest radiography.** Moderate or more PE on chest radiography may be detected by flask-like cardiomegaly (Fig. 32.1).

### Echocardiography

Echocardiography is the first-choice imaging modality for the diagnosis of PE. The accuracy of TTE to detect PE is approximately 100%. On two-dimensional (2D) echocardiography, circumferential or localized PE (echo-free space between the visceral and parietal layers) can be seen (Fig. 32.2). When PE is detected only in systole, its amount is less than 50 mL, and it is seen in normal situations or suggests nonsignificant trivial PE.[6]

Small PE is initially seen in the basal posterior of the LV. The epicardial fat is often mistaken with it, but whereas PE is motionless and echolucent, the epicardial fat is brighter than the myocardium and moves with the heart.

Pericardial effusion is categorized semiquantitatively by measuring its size at end-diastole as follows:

Small: <1 cm
Moderate: 1–2 cm
Large: >2 cm
Very large: >2.5 cm

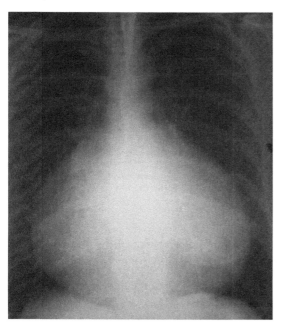

FIG. 32.1 Diffusely enlarged heart with obscured hilar shadows and no congestion in the lung parenchyma, which helps to differentiate it from the cardiomegaly in heart failure.

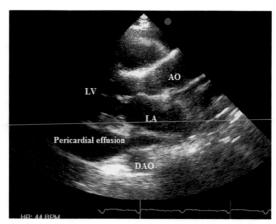

FIG. 32.2 Parasternal long-axis view showing pericardial effusion that extends to the descending thoracic aorta (AO) and posterior of the left atrium (LA). *DAO, LV,* left ventricle.

Echocardiographic findings in tamponade are as follows:

- The presence of PE.
- Inferior vena cava and hepatic vein dilatation (inferior vena cava >2.1 cm and <50% respiratory collapse).
- Chamber collapse (RA and RV diastolic collapse).
- Significant respiratory variation in the size of the RV and LV.
- Plethora of the inferior vena cava is seen in more than 90% of the cases except in low-pressure tamponade.[4]
- Right-heart chamber collapse occurs earlier because the right-heart chambers have low pressure compared with the left-heart chambers.
- RV early diastolic collapse and RA late diastolic collapse that lasts more than one-third of the cardiac cycle are sensitive and specific signs for the diagnosis of tamponade (Fig. 32.3). However, they appear relatively early, and the absence of chamber collapse is a very useful sign to *exclude* hemodynamically significant tamponade.[18,19]
- Conditions that are associated with late collapse are RV hypertrophy, pulmonary hypertension, and severe LV dysfunction.
- LV and LA collapse may be seen in posterior effusion after cardiac surgery and pulmonary arterial hypertension.
- Doppler flow study confirms respiratory ventricular interdependency as a 30% inspiratory reduction in mitral peak E-wave velocity and a 60% inspiratory increase in tricuspid E-wave velocity is diagnostic.

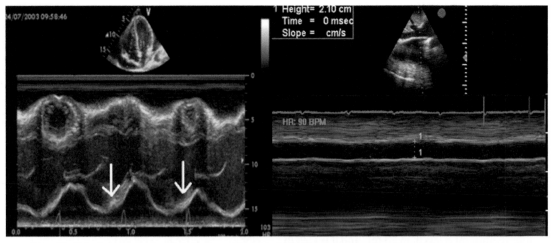

FIG. 32.3 *Left*: Large pericardial effusion with right atrial late diastolic and early systolic collapse (*arrows*). *Right*: Plethora of the inferior vena cava as a very sensitive sign of tamponade.

The greatest change is seen on the first beat of inspiration; nevertheless, Doppler flow study should not be a stand-alone criterion for tamponade.
- Transesophageal echocardiography may be helpful postoperatively for loculated effusion.

### Computed tomography and magnetic resonance imaging

Usually, CT and MRI are not requested. However, they are used in loculated effusion to distinguish transudate from exudative fluid and in unusual conditions.

### Management

In the presence of hemodynamically significant tamponade or threatened tamponade, urgent or emergency action comprising pericardiocentesis or careful hemodynamic monitoring with trial medical treatment is appropriate. However, in bacterial and TB pericarditis and in hemopericardium and nonchronic moderate to large PE, urgent diagnostic and therapeutic pericardiocentesis should be considered (Table 32.6).

In the absence of life-threatening tamponade, more diagnostic tests based on the patient's history and examination can be requested such as laboratory tests for neoplasm, hypothyroidism, and autoimmune disorders.

Usually, diagnostic pericardiocentesis in nonthreatening effusion is not needed.[3]

A course of NSAIDs or colchicine in large asymptomatic effusion may be helpful. Corticosteroids may have the same effect. Patients with mild tamponade who are chosen for conservative treatment should be under close hemodynamic monitoring. Pericardiocentesis in patients with hemopericardium can prove challenging because it

| **TABLE 32.6**<br>Approach to patients with pericardial effusion. |
| --- |
| 1. Determine the presence of tamponade or threatened tamponade based on the patient's history, physical examination, and echocardiography |
| 2. In the absence of tamponade or threatened tamponade: If the cause of pericardial effusion is not apparent, consider diagnostic tests as for acute pericarditis.<br>If the effusion is large, consider a course of an NSAID plus colchicine or a corticosteroid, and if the patient does not respond to it, consider closed pericardiocentesis |
| 3. If there is significant tamponade or threatened tamponade:<br>Urgent or emergency pericardiocentesis or careful hemodynamic monitoring with a trial of medication may be considered |

*NSAID*, nonsteroidal antiinflammatory drug.
Data from Mann DL, Zipes DP, Libby P, et al., eds. *Braunwald's Heart Disease: A Textbook of Cardiovascular Medicine*. 10th ed. Philadelphia: Saunders; 2015.

may exacerbate bleeding to the pericardial space. Pericardiocentesis is contraindicated in hemopericardium caused by trauma or LV free-wall rupture after MI and type A dissection.

Echocardiography should be repeated after pericardiocentesis.

### Analysis of the pericardial fluid

The pericardial fluid is similar to plasma with dominant lymphocytes. Although fluid analysis has a low diagnostic yield, the fluid should be analyzed for microorganisms and malignant cells. Pericardial biopsy may be helpful in some cases.

## CONSTRICTIVE PERICARDITIS

Constrictive pericarditis (CP) can be the final stage of any inflammatory disease with pericardial involvement because any inflammation of the pericardium can result in fibrosis, calcification, and adhesion of visceral and parietal layers.

In developed countries, the most common causes are idiopathic, postsurgical, and radiation; in developing countries, TB is another important cause (Table 32.7).

Sometimes CP is reversible using antiinflammatory drugs such as after cardiac surgery.

### Pathophysiology

Scarred pericardium restricts cardiac filling, which results in elevation and equalization of pressures in all cardiac chambers and pulmonary and systemic veins. Rapid cardiac filling occurs in early diastole because of high LA pressure, but in mid to late diastole, filling ceases because there is no more volume regarding the stiff pericardium.

The main hemodynamic mechanism in CP is based on the:

1. Intrathoracic and intracardiac pressure disassociation: During inspiration, pulmonary pressure decreases, but stiff pericardium interferes with falling of the left-heart pressure, so the gradient between the pulmonary vein and LA reduces (during inspiration), and left-heart filling decreases.
2. Exaggerated interventricular interdependence: Because the pericardium has a fixed volume in CP, role of the ventricular interdependence becomes more prominent. During inspiration, the LV filling decreases and allows the septum to shift to the left, increasing the RV filling. This interdependence becomes more obvious when the filling pressure is high.

### TABLE 32.7
### Most Prevalent Causes of Constrictive Pericarditis

| Idiopathic | Irradiation |
|---|---|
| Related to surgery | Infectious |
| Neoplastic | Autoimmune (connective tissue) disorders |
| Uremia | Posttrauma |

### Clinical Findings

Most symptoms are consequence of low cardiac output and systemic venous congestion with manifestation of right-sided heart failure signs and symptoms, including peripheral edema and abdominal complaints, which progress to ascites, anasarca, and cardiac cirrhosis; finally, low cardiac output results in fatigue and cachexia. Cough, dyspnea, and orthopnea appear later as a result of left-heart failure.

### Physical Examination

- The jugular vein is distended, and W- or M-shaped venous pressure waves are found because of a rapid Y descent and normal X descent. The Kussmaul sign is a usual finding, although not specific, and is defined as failing of decrease in venous pressure during inspiration. One-third of patients may have paradoxical pulse, especially in effusive CP.
- Pericardial knock is the most notable finding, which is an early diastolic sound heard after S2 at the left sternal border or the apex. This sound is the result of the abrupt cessation of the LV filling caused by the scarred pericardium.[3]

Palmar erythema and spider angioedema and jaundice are signs of cardiac cirrhosis.

### Diagnostic Findings
#### Electrocardiography

Electrocardiography findings are nonspecific and include ST-T change, low voltage, and LA abnormality. Atrial fibrillation rhythm is a common finding.

#### Chest radiography

Pericardial calcification and PE may be seen on chest radiography; however, pericardial calcification is neither diagnostic for CP nor a common finding but should raise the possibility of TB pericarditis.

#### Echocardiographic features of constrictive pericarditis
##### 2D findings

- Thickened pericardium (an absence of thickened pericardium does not exclude CP because 20% of patients have been reported as having normal thickness)
- Abnormal ventricular septal motion in early diastole (septal bounce)
- Respiratory variation in ventricular size
- Dilated hepatic vein and inferior vena cava
- Biatrial enlargement

## M-mode findings

- Flattened LV posterior wall in diastole
- Abrupt posterior displacement of the septum in early diastole (septal bounce or shudder)
- Competitive filling of the ventricles (respiratory variation in ventricular size by M-mode study)
- The propagation velocity of early diastolic mitral inflow usually exceeds 100 cm/s (Figs. 32.4 and 32.5)[10]

## Doppler findings

- Significant respiratory variation in mitral (25%–40%) and tricuspid valve (40%–60%) by pulsed-wave Doppler study as consensus for the calculation of the respiratory variation percentage in CP is the same for tamponade: for both the mitral and

tricuspid valves, inflow is (expiration – - inspiration)/expiration; the result is negative in a tricuspid inflow velocity study (Fig. 32.6).
- Mitral valve deceleration time is less than 160 ms (not in all patients).
- Hepatic vein flow Doppler study shows expiratory increased diastolic flow reversal.
- Significant variation can be found in the pulmonary venous Doppler study.
- A typical finding in patients with CP is expiratory increase 25% or more in mitral peak E velocity and expiratory increase in diastolic flow reversal of hepatic vein study.

However, about 20% of patients with CP do not have typical respiratory variation, mostly because of elevated left atrial pressure or mixed constrictive and restrictive myocardial involvement.

## Tissue Doppler imaging

- Annulus reversus: Prominent early diastolic velocity ($e'$) of medial annulus and decrease in lateral annulus caused by restricted motion of the lateral wall by a stiff pericardium (Fig. 32.7).
- Tissue Doppler is useful to discriminate CP from restrictive cardiomyopathy (RCM) that shows reduced $e'$.[1,3,18]

### Cardiac imaging

Normal pericardium thickness on CT is up to 2 mm. CT can reveal pericardial thickening and calcification. Pericardial thickness on MRI is 3–4 mm in normal population, and MRI can show active inflammation that is

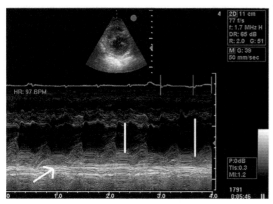

FIG. 32.4 Thickened pericardium, flattened left ventricular posterior wall, diastolic septal bounce, and competitive filling of the ventricles in short-axis view in favor of constrictive pericarditis.

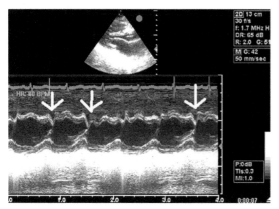

FIG. 32.5 Abrupt posterior displacement of the septum in early diastole (septal bounce or septal shudder, *arrows*).

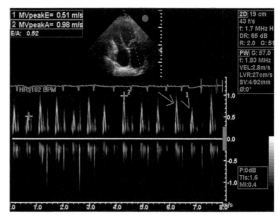

FIG. 32.6 Pulsed-wave Doppler study of the mitral inflow in a patient with constrictive pericarditis (noticeable respiratory variation) (*arrows*).

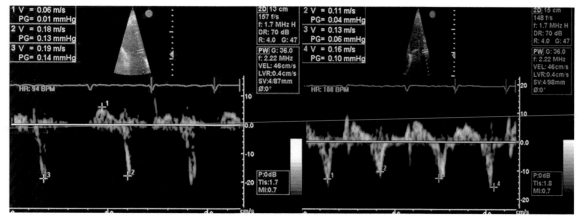

FIG. 32.7 Tissue Doppler imaging study in constrictive pericarditis shows annulus reversus associated with significant respiratory variation.

useful to predict patients who respond to antiinflammation therapy; CP is reversible.[11]

In the setting of clinical findings of CP, the presence of a thickened pericardium is diagnostic for CP, which can be associated with:

- Interventricular septum motion in early diastole (septal "bounce")
- Distorted ventricular contours
- Pericardial thickening that is absent in about 18% of hemodynamically proven CP

### Cardiac catheterization

Cardiac catheterization can provide precise hemodynamic evaluation, which is helpful in differentiation between CP and restrictive pericarditis. Coronary angiography should be done in patients who are candidates for pericardiectomy.

Hemodynamic findings in favor of CP:

- Elevated and equalization of RA, RV, and LV diastolic pressures and pulmonary capillary wedge pressure about 20 mmHg with less than 3–5 mmHg differences between them
- "Dip and plateau" or "square root" sign in ventricular pressure study
- Exaggerated ventricular interdependence
- Modestly elevated pulmonary artery pressure and RV systolic pressure, usually around 35–45 mmHg

### Differentiating Constrictive Pericarditis From Restrictive Cardiomyopathy

Differentiation of CP from RCM is challenging and important. Both have elevated diastolic pressure in left and right chambers, but in RCM, LV pressure is mildly higher than RV ($\approx$3–5 mmHg) (Table 32.8). Significant pulmonary hypertension is not present in typical CP.

Exaggerated respiratory variation in mitral inflow velocity, interventricular dependence, annulus reversus in tissue Doppler imaging study, and exaggerated diastolic flow reversal in hepatic vein study are detected during inspiration in RCM and in expiration in CP.

### Differentiating Constrictive Pericarditis From COPD

Sometimes differentiation of CP from COPD is challenging and difficult. Superior vena cava Doppler from a patient with CP shows little respiratory changes in systolic forward flow velocity from inspiration to expiration, in contrast to marked phasic inspiratory augmentation of forward flow velocity in chronic obstructive pulmonary disease (COPD); and this point is so important. Other echocardiographic and Doppler parameters are not significantly different (Figs. 32.8 and 32.9).

### Management

- Diuretic and salt restriction are used for decreasing edema, but definite therapy is surgical pericardiectomy. Pericardiectomy in patients with radiation-induced constriction should be avoided.
- Tachycardia is a compensatory mechanism, so beta-blockers and calcium channel blockers should not be used.

**TABLE 32.8**
**Constrictive Pericarditis vs Restrictive Cardiomyopathy A Brief Overview of Features for the Differential Diagnosis**

| Diagnostic Evaluation | Constrictive Pericarditic | Restrictive Cardiomyopathy |
|---|---|---|
| Physical findings | Kussmaul sign, pericardial knock | Regurgitant murmur, Kussmaul sign may be present, S3 (advanced) |
| ECG | Low voltages, nonspecfic ST/T changes, atrial fibrillation | Low voltages, pseudoinfarction, possible widening of QRS, left-axis deviation, atrial fibrillation |
| Chest X-ray | Pericardial calcifications (1/3 of cases) | No pericardial calcifications |
| Echocardiography | • Sepal bounce<br>• Pericardial thickening and calcifications<br>• Respiratory variation of the mitral peak $E$ velocity of >25% and variation in the pulmonary venous peak D flow velocity of >20%<br>• Color M-mode flow propagation velocity ($V_p$) >45 cm/s<br>• Tissue Doppler; peak $e'$ >8.0 cm/s | • Small left ventricle with large atria, possible increased wall thickness<br>• $E/A$ ratio >2 short DT<br>• Significant respiratory variations of mitral inflow are absent<br>• Color M-mode flow propagation velocity ($V_p$) <45 cm/s<br>• Tissue Doppler: peak $e'$ <80 cm/s |
| Cardiac catheterization | "Dip and plateau" or "square root" sign, right ventricular diastolic, and left ventricular diastolic pressures usually equal, ventricular interdependence (i.e., assessed by the systolic area index >1.1)[a] | Marked right ventricular systolic hypertension (>50 mmHg) and left ventricular diastole pressure exceeds right ventricular diastole pressure (LVEDP > RVEDP) at rest or during exercise by S mmHg or more (RVEDP <1/3 RVSP) |
| CT/CMR | Pericardial thickness >3–4 mm, pericardial calcifications (CT), ventricular interdependence (real-time cine CMR) | Normal pericardial thickness (<3.0 mm), myocardial involvement by morphology and functional study (CMR) |

[a]Hypovolemia (e.g., due to diuretic therapy) can mask hemodynamic findings. Rapid infusion of 1 L of normal saline over 6–8 min may reveal typical features.

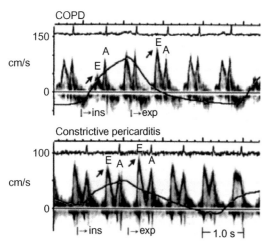

FIG. 32.8 Mitral inflow Doppler from patients with chronic obstructive pulmonary disease (COPD) *(top)* or constrictive pericarditis *(bottom)* showing respiratory variation in mitral *E* velocity *(arrows)*. *exp*, expiration; *ins*, inspiration.

• Digoxin is useful in patients with rapid ventricular response atrial fibrillation to maintain the heart rate to about 80–90 beats/min.

Hemodynamics and symptoms improve immediately after surgery or within weeks or months.

Long-term prognosis is worse in patients with history of radiation, low LV ejection fraction, low levels of sodium, renal failure, old age, and moderate to severe tricuspid regurgitation.[20,21]

Transient constriction may be seen after cardiac surgery, and effusion is present in two-thirds of these patients. Late gadolinium enhancement on MRI is associated with inflammation and fibrosis. Studies have demonstrated that this finding in MRI is correlated with responding to antiinflammatory drugs and reversibility. High CRP and ESR are useful to identify patients who may respond to antiinflammatory medication.[22]

Patients with CP, especially postsurgically, with late gadolinium enhancement on MRI and high CRP and

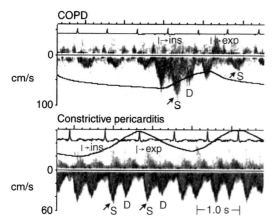

FIG. 32.9 Superior vena cava Doppler from a patient with constrictive pericarditis shows little respiratory changes in systolic forward flow velocity (*bottom*) from inspiration to expiration (*arrows*), in contrast to marked phasic inspiratory increase of forward flow velocity in chronic obstructive pulmonary disease (COPD) (*top*). *D*, diastolic forward flow; *exp*, expiration; *ins*, inspiration; *S*, systolic forward flow. (Boonyaratavej S, Oh JK, Tajik AJ, et al. Comparison of mitral inflow and superior vena cava Doppler velocities in chronic obstructive pulmonary disease and constrictive pericarditis. *J Am Coll Cardiol.* 1998;32:2043–2048.)

ESR may benefit from a 2- to 3-month course of antiinflammatory drugs.

In one study, NSAIDs, corticosteroids, and colchicine were not preferred to each other. A combination of a corticosteroid and colchicine has been recommended.[1]

## EFFUSIVE–CONSTRICTIVE PERICARDITIS

These patients have combination of inflammatory effusion in the early stage and constriction in the late phase. Its course is usually subacute but can present chronically up to 1 year. These patients are characterized with failure of hemodynamic return to normal after pericardiocentesis. Its definition is failing of decrease in RA pressure at least 50% or to a level less than 10 mmHg after pericardiocentesis and no residual PE.[3] The most common causes are idiopathic, malignancy, radiation, pericardiectomy, TB, and connective tissue disorders.

Physical and hemodynamic findings are a combination of symptoms of patients with effusion and constriction. Biopsy may be required for diagnosis. No agreement exists on preferred treatment. Management is based on the specific cause, and in cases of idiopathic effusive–constrictive physiology, antiinflammatory drugs, including colchicine and corticosteroids as an initial treatment, are recommended. Ultimately, pericardiectomy is needed in many patients.[23]

## SPECIFIC CAUSES OF PERICARDIAL DISEASE

### Infectious Disease

Viral pericarditis is the most common form of infectious pericarditis. Echovirus and coxsackievirus are most frequent.

In bacterial pericarditis, staphylococci, pneumococci, and streptococci are the most common agents. Pericardium can be infected because of direct extension of pneumonia or empyema and hematogenous, contiguous, and traumatic causes.

Bacterial pericarditis presents as fever, chills, dyspnea, and chest pain. It may progress to tamponade. Pericardial fluid has leukocytosis, low glucose, and high protein.

Treatment of bacterial pericarditis is immediate pericardiocentesis or surgical drainage with or without window. Pericardiectomy may be needed in cases of adhesive pericarditis for drainage and preventing constriction. Bacterial pericarditis has poor prognosis (Table 32.6).

### Pericardial Disease in Human Immunodeficiency Virus: Causes and Pathology

The most common cardiac presentation of HIV is pericardial disease, and PE is the most frequent form. Most patients are asymptomatic and have small effusions. Larger effusions are often observed in the advanced stage and are caused by malignancy or infection.

Most of them are idiopathic, and other causes include congestive heart failure, TB, and Kaposi sarcoma. Their presentation includes chest pain and dyspnea.

### Tuberculosis

Nearly 2% of patients with TB have pericardial abnormalities, which may lead to tamponade, constriction, or both. Pericardial involvement is usually caused by hematogenous spread from the primary site, retrograde from a lymph node, or contiguous from a lesion in the lung.

The clinical course is usually subacute or chronic and includes fever, night sweats, cough, and weight loss. Effusive constriction may be seen and can progress to CP in the late stage.

Definitive diagnosis is based on microorganisms in fluid or biopsy. Other diagnostic tests included a positive skin test result, ADA, and polymerase chain reaction of fluid, with a low threshold for pericardiocentesis.

Management consists of a 6-month course of the standard antimycobacterial therapy and likely pericardiocentesis or window.

There is controversy regarding the beneficial effects of corticosteroids. However, high doses of corticosteroids with tapering over 6–8 weeks have been suggested in some studies.[9,24,25]

### Pericarditis in Patients With Renal Disease

Widespread and available dialysis nearly abolished classic uremic pericarditis. It has a correlation with serum blood urea nitrogen (BUN) level. The pathophysiology includes toxic metabolites, hypercalcemia, autoimmune, viral, and hemorrhagic causes. It can progress to a thick and adhesive pericardium and constriction.

Dialysis-associated disease is more common today and is identified as pericardial disease despite chronic dialysis with normal or mildly elevated BUN and creatinine level.

Small effusion is often asymptomatic. In case of hypotension during or after dialysis, low-pressure tamponade should be kept in mind.

Management of classic uremic pericarditis is regular hemodialysis. Drainage in tamponade and window in recurrent effusion are effective management.[5,9]

### Dressler Syndrome and Postmyocardial Infarction Pericarditis

Early post-MI pericarditis occurs within the first week after transmural MI because of the inflamed visceral pericardium in transmural necrosis. It has a correlation with infarct size. Early reperfusion reduces this form of pericarditis.

Dressler syndrome is late-onset pericarditis, which usually occurs 1–8 weeks after MI. Reperfusion has decreased its incidence significantly. The mechanism of Dressler syndrome is autoimmune.

Early post-MI pericarditis may be asymptomatic or present with chest pain or friction rub. Usually PE is not large. In case of tamponade physiology, myocardial rupture should be ruled out. Because this form of pericarditis is localized inflammation of the pericardium, ST-segment elevation on ECG may be limited to initial involved leads.

Dressler syndrome presents with fever, chest pain, PE, friction rub, and ST-segment elevation.

Management of early post-MI pericarditis includes increased dose of usual ASA (650 mg 3 or 4 times a day) or acetaminophen. NSAIDs and corticosteroids should be avoided because they prevent scar formation of infarcted segments and predispose to rupture. Hemopericardium is rare early after MI, and there is no need to adjust the dose of anticoagulation.

Dressler syndrome is self-limited, and treatment consists of NSAIDs, colchicine, and rarely corticosteroids in a limited course.[3,5,9]

### Pericardial Disease in Cancer

The main cause of pericardial involvement in malignancy is implantation of the primary tumor into the pericardium. Malignancy accounts for the most important cause of tamponade in the developed countries. The most common tumors are lung carcinoma (40%) followed by breast cancer and lymphoma. About 18% of patients with symptomatic large effusion account for their first presentations of malignancy.

Management is based on survival and the severity of pericardial disease. Invasion of the primary tumor should be excluded by pericardial fluid analysis and pericardial biopsy if needed. In patients with end-stage malignancy, palliative drainage is reasonable. Single pericardiocentesis may be efficient for a long time, so as a first step, closed pericardiocentesis is recommended in most patients. Recurrence of effusion in malignancy is high, and intrapericardial installation of drugs such as tetracycline, bleomycin, and cisplatin is indicated. Pericardial window and pericardiectomy are performed in patients who are unresponsive to other treatment.[3,26–28]

#### Primary pericardial tumor

Primary pericardial neoplasms are rare and include mesothelioma, lymphangiomas, fibrosarcoma, hemangiomas, lipomas, and teratomas. They can be localized and present with chamber collapse or incidental abnormal silhouette on chest radiography. CT and MRI are useful to identifying tumor structure.

#### Pericarditis after radiation

The heart may be involved after radiation, which is the standard treatment of thoracic cancer. Factors that affect pericardial injury are age, dose, extent of cardiac exposure, radiation source, and duration of therapy. Left-sided breast tumors are more likely to be associated with pericardial disease.

Pericarditis after radiation has two forms. The acute form presents with chest pain and fever, and the delayed form may occur up to 20 years later. Small self-limited effusion is common, and tamponade is not a frequent finding. Effusion can progress to constriction. PE after radiation may be difficult to differentiate from malignant effusions.

Medical treatment is not usually effective, and surgical pericardiectomy is the choice treatment of constriction.[1]

## Postcardiac Surgery Pericarditis

Cardiac surgery, thoracotomy, chest trauma, and pacemaker insertion can cause pericarditis after days to months. About 15% of patients develop pericarditis after cardiac surgery. The pathology is related to the systemic inflammatory response to injured myocardium. Pleuritic chest pain, fever, and leukocytosis are common findings. TTE usually shows small- to moderate-sized PE, although tamponade is rare.

First-line treatment is NSAIDs with adding the colchicine and finally corticosteroid in severe, refractory cases.[29-33]

## Pericardial Effusion in Infective Endocarditis

Pericardial effusion in the setting of IE is a relatively common finding, however, most cases have mild effusion. It has been suggested that the presence of IE is not an independent predictor of in hospital mortality.[34,35]

## Stress Cardiomyopathy

The incidence of stress-induced cardiomyopathy (takotsubo) is increasing, and one study reported that 70% of patients with stress-induced cardiomyopathy had PE.[32]

## Hemopericardium

Hemopericardium can occur after MI following free-wall rupture, dissection type A, mitral valvuloplasty, device closure of an atrial septal defect (ASD), insertion of a Watchman device for LA appendage, transcutaneous aortic valve implantation, percutaneous coronary intervention, atrial fibrillation ablation, endomyocardial biopsy, and rarely as a complication of laparoscopic gastroesophageal surgery.

## CONCLUSION

Pericardial disease is so crucial, however, not so common in clinic. The most important one is "constrictive pericarditis"; it is the result of increased pericardial fluid or tissue or both. Increased fluid is treated by drainage; but increased tissue is treated by excision. In most patients with chronic constrictive pericarditis, the etiology is not apparent even after histologic examination of pericardium.

Despite a large amount of new data and many clinical trials that allow clinical management to be on the road to evidence-based medicine, there are several issues that require additional research and clarification about pericardium and pericardial disease.

Ongoing basic and clinical research is necessary and needed to address all these issues and provide additional diagnostic and therapeutic tools for individualized management of each patient and to improve the prognosis.[13,36,37]

## REFERENCES

1. Spodick DH. *Infectious pericarditis. The Pericardium: A Comprehensive Textbook.* New York: Marcel Dekker; 1997;260–290.
2. Tanaka T, Hasegawa K, Fujita M, et al. Marked elevation of brain natriuretic peptide levels in pericardial fluid is closely associated with left ventricular dysfunction. *J Am Coll Cardiol.* 1998;31(2):399–403. (1998). 9462585.
3. Bonow RO, Mann DL, Zipes DP, Lippy P, eds. *Braunwald's Heart Disease: A Text Book of Cardiovascular Medicine.* 10th ed. Philadelphia: Saunders Elsevier; 2015.
4. Dudzinski DM, Mak GS, Hung JW. Pericardial diseases. *Curr Probl Cardiol.* 2012;37:75.
5. Seferović PM, Ristić AD, Maksimović R, et al. Pericardial syndromes: an update after the ESC guidelines 2004. *Heart Fail Rev.* 2013;18:255.
6. Klein A, Abbara S, Agler D, et al. American Society of Echocardiography clinical recommendations for multimodality cardiovascular imaging of patients with pericardial disease. *J Am Soc Echocardiogr.* 2013; 26:965–1012.
7. Khandaker MH, Espinosa RE, Nishimura RA, et al. Pericardial disease: diagnosis and management. *Mayo Clin Proc.* 2010;85(6):572–593. https://doi.org/10.4065/mcp.2010.0046.
8. Imazio M, Brucato A, Maestroni S, et al. Prevalence of C-reactive protein elevation and time course of normalization in acute pericarditis: implications for the diagnosis, therapy, and prognosis of pericarditis. *Circulation.* 2011;123:1092.
9. Maisch B, Seferovic PM, Ristic AD, et al. Guidelines on the diagnosis and management of pericardial diseases executive summary; the task force on the diagnosis and management of pericardial diseases of the European Society of Cardiology. *Eur Heart J.* 2004;25:587.
10. Imazio M, Bobbio M, Cecchi E, et al. Colchicine as first-choice therapy for recurrent pericarditis: results of the CORE (COlchicine for REcurrent pericarditis) trial. *Arch Intern Med.* 2005;1987:165.
11. Cosyns B, Plein S, Nihoyanopoulos P. European Association of Cardiovascular Imaging (EACVI) position paper: multimodality imaging in pericardial disease. *Eur Heart J Cardiovasc Imaging.* 2015;16(1):12–31. https://doi.org/10.1093/ehjci/jeu128. PMID:25248336.
12. Lang RM, Goldstein SA, Kronzon I. *ASE's Comprehensive Echocardiography.* 2nd ed. Philadelphia: Saunders Elsevier; 2016.
13. Massimo I, Enrico C, Brunella D, et al. Indicators of poor prognosis of acute pericarditis. *Circulation.* 2007;115:2739–2744. https://doi.org/10.1161/CIRCULATIONAHA.106.662114.

14. Imazio M, Brucato A, Cumetti D, et al. Corticosteroids for recurrent pericarditis: high versus low doses: a nonrandomized observation. *Circulation*. 2008;118:667.

15. Lotrionte M, Biondi-Zoccai G, Imazio M, et al. International collaborative systematic review of controlled clinical trials on pharmacologic treatments for acute pericarditis and its recurrences. *Am Heart J*. 2010;160:662.

16. Ariyarajah V, Spodick D. Cardiac tamponade revisited. *Tex Heart Inst J*. 2007;34(3):347–351.

17. Jaume S-S, Juan A, Antonia S, Joan A, Gaietà P-M, Soler-Soler J. Low-pressure cardiac tamponade. *Circulation*. 2006;114:945–995.

18. Oh JK, Seward JB, Tajik AJ. *The Echo Manual*. 3rd ed. Philadelphia: Lippincott, Williams & Wilkins; 2006.

19. Veress G, Feng D, Oh JK. Echocardiography in pericardial diseases: new developments. *Heart Fail Rev*. 2013;18:267.

20. Ling LH, Oh JK, Schaff HV, et al. Constrictive pericarditis in the modern era: evolving clinical spectrum and impact on outcome after pericardiectomy. *Circulation*. 1999;100:1380.

21. Bertog SC, Thambidorai SK, Parakh K, et al. Constrictive pericarditis: etiology and cause specific survival after pericardiectomy. *J Am Coll Cardiol*. 2004;43:1445.

22. Haley JH, Tajik AJ, Danielson GK, et al. Transient constrictive pericarditis: causes and natural history. *J Am Coll Cardiol*. 2004;43:271.

23. Syed FF, Ntsekhe M, Mayosi BM, Oh JK. Effusive-constrictive pericarditis. *Heart Fail Rev*. 2013;18:277 And Braunwald (1).

24. Tuon FF, Litvoc MN, Lopes MI. Adenosine deaminase and tuberculous pericarditis—a systematic review with meta-analysis. *Acta Trop*. 2006;99:67.

25. Zamirian M, Mokhtarian M, Motazedian MH, et al. Constrictive pericarditis: detection of *Mycobacterium tuberculosis* in paraffin-embedded pericardial tissues by polymerase chain reaction. *Clin Biochem*. 2007;40:355.

26. Maisch B, Ristic A, Pankuweit S. Evaluation and management of pericardial effusion in patients with neoplastic disease. *Prog Cardiovasc Dis*. 2010;53:157.

27. Ben-Horin S, Bank I, Guetta V, Livneh A. Large symptomatic pericardial effusion as the presentation of unrecognized cancer: a study in 173 consecutive patients undergoing pericardiocentesis. *Medicine (Baltimore)*. 2006;85:49.

28. Imazio M. Pericardial involvement in systemic inflammatory diseases. *Heart*. 2011;97:1882.

29. Rosenbaum E, Krebs E, Cohen M, et al. The spectrum of clinical manifestations, outcome and treatment of pericardial tamponade in patients with systemic lupus erythematosus: a retrospective study and literature review. *Lupus*. 2009;18:608.

30. Erlich JF, Paz Z. Postpericardial injury syndrome: an autoimmune phenomenon. *Clin Rev Allergy Immunol*. 2010;38:156.

31. Cevik C, Wilborn T, Corona R, et al. Post-cardiac injury syndrome following transvenous pacemaker insertion: a case report and review of the literature. *Heart Lung Circ*. 2009;18:379.

32. Eitel I, Lucke C, Grothoff M, et al. Inflammation in takotsubo cardiomyopathy: insights from cardiovascular magnetic resonance imaging. *Eur Radiol*. 2010;20:422.

33. Imazio M, Brucato R, Rampello S, et al. Management of pericardial diseases during pregnancy. *J Cardiovasc Med*. 2010;11:557.

34. Youssef GS, Mashaal MS, El Remisy DR, Sorour KA, Rizk HH. Pericardial effusion in prosthetic and native valve infective endocarditis. *Indian Heart J*. 2019; 71:80–84. https://doi.org/10.1016/j.ihj.2018.12.002.

35. Firouzi A, Ahmadi R, Abbaszade Marzbali N, et al. Prevalence and prognostic significance of pericardial effusion in native valve endocarditis based on data from the Iranian registry of infective endocarditis (IRIE). *Iran Heart J*. 2018;19(2):36–43.

36. Smonporn B, Oh JK, Tajik AJ, Appleton CP, Seward JB. Comparison of mitral inflow and superior vena cava Doppler velocities in chronic obstructive pulmonary disease and constrictive pericarditis. *J Am Coll Cardiol*. 1998;32:2043–2048.

37. Adler Y, Charron P, Imazio M, et al. 2015 ESC guidelines for the diagnosis and management of pericardial diseases. The Task Force for the Diagnosis and Management of Pericardial Diseases of the European Society of Cardiology. *Eur Heart J*. 2015;36:2921–2964. https://doi.org/10.1093/eurheartj/ehv318.

## FURTHER READING

Edwards MH, Leak AM. Pericardial effusions on anti-TNF therapy for rheumatoid arthritis—a drug side effect or uncontrolled systemic disease? *Rheumatology (Oxford)*. 2009;48:316.

# CHAPTER 33

# Congenital Heart Disease

ZAHRA KHAJALI[a] • SEDIGHEH SAEDI[b]
[a]Rajaei Cardiovascular, Medical & Research Center, Iran University of Medical Sciences, Tehran, Iran,
[b]Rajaie Cardiovascular, Medical & Research Center, Tehran, Iran

## KEY POINTS

- During the past few years, considerable progress has been made in the management of patients with congenital heart disease, and now many of these patients have reached adulthood. Comprehensive and thorough knowledge about approach, evaluation, interventional options, and follow-up of these patients is necessary for all cardiologists in clinical practice with adult patients.
- Cardiologists without related training and expertise in the field of adult congenital heart disease (ACHD) should learn to manage and follow adults with congenital heart disease in cooperation with ACHD specialists.

## BASIC NOMENCLATURE AND SEGMENTAL APPROACH TO CONGENITAL HEART DISEASE

### Sidedness (Situs)

The term *sidedness* is used to describe the location of organs or structures that are not symmetric pairs in the body. Examples are abdominal or visceral situs (liver, spleen, and bronchus), great vessels situs (aorta and inferior vena cava), and atrial situs. Possible arrangements are solitus (normal), inversus (mirror image or reversed normal anatomy), and ambiguus (none of the previous forms).

- Situs solitus: The inferior vena cava (IVC), liver, and cecum are on the right side of the abdomen, and the spleen, stomach, and aorta are on the left side. The left atrium (LA) is located posterior to and to the left side of the right atrium (RA).
- Situs inversus: The IVC, liver, and cecum are on the left side of the abdomen, and the spleen, stomach, and aorta are located on the right side. The LA is posterior to, and to the right side of the RA.
- Situs ambiguus: Locations of the organs are not any of the above mentioned and include the cases of left isomerism and right isomerism. Examples are cases with both the aorta and IVC located in the left side, bilateral liver with no normal spleen, and two morphologic left atria with no morphologic RA (Fig. 33.1).
- Atrial situs: This generally follows abdominal situs in solitus and inversus types.

### Cardiac Orientation

Cardiac orientation is defined based on the orientation of the cardiac base to the apex axis.

- Levocardia: The cardiac apex is oriented toward the left side in the mediastinum.
- Dextrocardia: The cardiac apex is pointed toward the right side (Fig. 33.2).
- Mesocardia: The cardiac apex is located mostly midline (superior–inferior axis).

Cardiac position in the mediastinum could be levo-, dextro-, or mesoposition. The term *dextroposition* is used when most of the cardiac mass is in the right hemithorax. A patient with levocardia could have cardiac dextroposition caused by the shifting effect of a hypoplastic right lung.

### Atrioventricular Connections

- Concordant: The connection of the RA to the right ventricle (RV) and the LA to the left ventricle (LV) is normal.
- Discordant: The RA is connected to the LV and the LA to the RV (e.g., congenitally corrected transposition of the great arteries [ccTGA]) (Fig. 33.3).
- Univentricular connection: Both atria are mainly received by one ventricle (e.g., double-inlet RV [DORV]).

### Ventriculoarterial Connections

- Concordant: The pulmonary artery (PA) originates from the RV and the aorta from the LV.
- Discordant: The PA originates from the LV and the aorta from the RV (e.g., ccTGA).

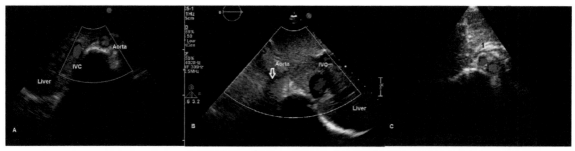

FIG. 33.1 Abdominal situs. (A) Situs solitus with aorta to the left of spine and IVC to the right. (B) Situs inversus. (C) Interrupted IVC and azygos continuity with aorta (1) and the left sided azygos (2) located on the left side.

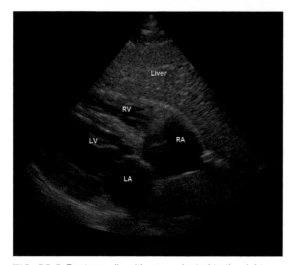

FIG. 33.2 Dextrocardia with apex oriented to the right.

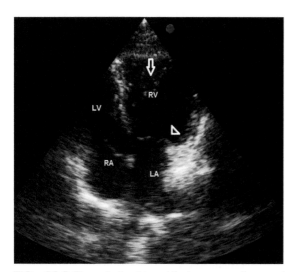

FIG. 33.3 Discordant atrioventricular connection and l-looped ventricles with RV located on the left side of LV. *Arrow*: moderator band; *arrow head*: tricuspid valve.

- Double outlet: Both great arteries mainly (more than 50% of both great arteries) originate from one ventricle (e.g., DORV).
- Single outlet: Both ventricles empty through a single great artery (e.g., truncus arteriosus).

The term *transposition* of the great arteries is used when the great arteries have changed places across the septum; the term *malposition* is used to describe any abnormal arrangement of the great arteries and includes the following:

- Normally related: The aorta is posterior, inferior, and to the right side of the PA.
- D-malposition: The aorta is located side by side or superior and to the right side of the PA.
- L-malposition: The aorta is located side by side or superior and to the left side of the PA (Fig. 33.4).
- Anterior aorta: The aorta is located completely anterior to the PA.

The cardiac chambers may be distinguished as described in the following:

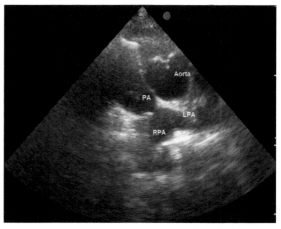

FIG. 33.4 L-malposition of great arteries. *LPA*, left branch of PA; *PA*, pulmonary artery; *RPA*, right branch of PA.

- RA: Usually receives systemic veins (superior vena cava [SVC] and IVC); has the limbus of fossa ovalis and a wide-based and triangular appendage along with prominent pectinate muscles
- LA: Narrow orifice and finger-like appendage
- Morphologic RV: Extensive trabeculations, moderator band, septal attachment of atrioventricular valve with chordal attachment to the interventricular septum (IVS), more apical position of the tricuspid valve
- Morphologic LV: Fine trabeculations and lack of septal attachments of the mitral valve (MV)
- Aorta: Origin of coronary arteries, arching and giving rise to innominate, carotid, and subclavian arteries
- PA: Branching into left and right PA branches
- Tricuspid valve: Always with the RV, and the MV with the LV
- If the morphologic RV is on the right side of the morphologic LV, the ventricles are said to have D (dextro) looping, and if the morphologic RV is on the left side of the morphologic LV, the ventricles are L (levo) looped[1-3] (Fig. 33.3).

## CLINICAL ISSUES IN CONGENITAL HEART DISEASE

### Cyanosis

Cyanosis is a manifestation of arterial oxygen desaturation caused by mixing or shunting of venous flow into the systemic arterial blood flow. When there is an obstruction in the way of pulmonary blood flow (PBF), such as severe pulmonary stenosis (PS) (low flow to lungs) or pulmonary hypertension (high flow to lungs), the blood circulates via a less obstructed route (i.e., through an atrial septal defect [ASD] or ventricular septal defect [VSD]) toward the systemic circulation, resulting in arterial desaturation and cyanosis. Cyanosis may also result from anatomic defects such as an unroofed coronary sinus emptying into the LA and pulmonary AV fistulas or right-sided heart failure (e.g., Ebstein's anomaly).

### Pathologic consequences

Hypoxemia stimulates the increased production of erythropoietin by the kidneys with resultant secondary erythrocytosis and elevated hematocrit. Hyperviscosity symptoms appear as fatigue, dizziness, lightheadedness, faintness, headaches, blurred vision, tinnitus, myalgia, and paresthesia. Iron deficiency may manifest by similar symptoms and is generally caused by frequent phlebotomies or bleeding.

Iron deficiency is a predictor of cerebrovascular events in this population and should be routinely investigated and addressed. Mean corpuscular volume (MCV) less than 80 fL warrants the need for iron replacement.

Hematologic abnormalities and bleeding tendency are common in cyanotic patients. There are decreased numbers and functions of platelets, prolonged prothrombin time, and partial thromboplastin time, lower levels of hemostatic factors (II, V, VII, VIII, IX, and X), and abnormally increased fibrinolysis. These abnormalities may cause life-threatening bleeding. During bleeding episodes, fresh-frozen plasma, vitamin K, cryoprecipitate, and platelet transfusion may be used. However, these patients are at risk for thrombosis as well, and the bleeding tendency does not neutralize the thrombotic events. Aspirin, warfarin, and heparin should not be administered unless the risk of thromboembolic events is higher than that of bleeding.

Increased breakdown of red blood cells and abnormal renal filtration of uric acid could lead to hyperuricemia, nephrolithiasis, and gout. Gouty arthritis can be treated with colchicine, probenecid, or allopurinol. Asymptomatic hyperuricemia does not require treatment.

Gallstones are common because of high red blood cell turnover. However, surgery should not be performed until the patient becomes symptomatic.

Other systemic disorders include renal dysfunction and proteinuria, clubbing, hypertrophic osteoarthropathy with bone pain, arthralgia and arthritis, and the risk of paradoxical emboli.

Phlebotomy is indicated for the alleviation of symptoms and sometimes before elective operations to ameliorate coagulation abnormalities but should not be performed in asymptomatic patients. Phlebotomy should be performed when there is no dehydration or iron depletion and the hematocrit is above 65%. During this procedure, 250–500 mL of blood is removed over a 30- to 45-min interval with concurrent intravascular volume replacement (750–1000 mL of isotonic saline or dextrose) and could be repeated 24–48 h later.

Routine laboratory workup, including complete blood count, MCV, serum iron, ferritin, and transferrin levels and saturation, serum uric acid, creatinine, coagulation, and evaluation of folic acid and vitamin $B_{12}$ status, should be performed in follow-up clinic visits.

## PULMONARY ARTERIAL HYPERTENSION AND EISENMENGER SYNDROME

Pulmonary hypertension is a common finding in patients with CHD. Eisenmenger syndrome is defined as severe PA hypertension (PAH) leading to bidirectional or reversed shunt through a large and unrestricted connection between pulmonary and systemic circulations and resultant cyanosis. The affected individuals usually become symptomatic and cyanotic in the second or third decade of life and develop heart failure after the age of 40 years. They also commonly present with hemoptysis and arrhythmias. Physical examination reveals central and nail bed cyanosis and clubbing. Treatment options include phosphodiesterase-5 inhibitors (e.g., sildenafil and tadalafil), endothelin receptor antagonists (e.g., bosentan and macitentan), and prostacyclins or heart–lung transplantation in end-stage patients.[1–4]

## HEART FAILURE

Patients with congenital heart disease are at increased risk of right, left, or biventricular failure due to anatomical defects resulting in chronic volume or pressure overload or myocardial injury related to previous surgeries. Management follows the guidelines on treatment systolic and diastolic heart failure and includes medical therapy with renin–angiotensin–aldosterone system (RAAS) blockers, β-blockers, diuretics, and mineralocorticoid receptor antagonists.

### Clinical Evaluation of Congenital Heart Disease
#### Physical Examination
The general examination should include a search for characteristic physical findings of syndromes, previous surgical scars, and cyanosis. Pulse oximetry should also be performed in patients with CHD. All areas of the anterior and posterior chest wall must be auscultated with special attention to murmurs of collaterals, shunts, or peripheral PS.

### Electrocardiography
Electrocardiogram (ECG) changes are discussed separately under the related CHD sections.

### Chest radiography
Chest radiography is particularly useful in patients with CHD for evaluation of PBF and vascularity, cardiac orientation, position, situs, and aortic arch sidedness. Increased pulmonary flow occurs with significant left-to-right shunts (shunt vascularity). Criteria for shunt vascularity include the following:
- Vascular markings are uniformly increased in the lung field. (Vascular markings are more prominent in the lower lobe in normal individuals.)
- Cross section and end of PA branches are larger than the accompanying bronchus.

- The diameter of the right descending PA is greater than 17 mm (or greater than 16 mm in men and greater than 14 mm in women).

Shunt vascularity becomes evident when there is a shunt with a pulmonary flow-to-systemic flow ratio ($Q_p/Q_s$) of at least 1.5:1. A shunt of more than 2.5:1 usually causes cardiomegaly.

Decreased pulmonary flow is seen in severe PS and tetralogy of Fallot.

### Echocardiography, Magnetic Resonance Imaging, and Computed Tomography
These tests in CHD are discussed in related chapters.

### Cardiac Catheterization and Hemodynamic Study
With the advent of multiple imaging modalities, cardiac catheterization is now performed mainly when imaging findings are inadequate or for the purpose of measuring pulmonary and systemic pressures and resistance, systolic and end-diastolic ventricular and atrial pressures, and pulmonary to systemic shunt quantification. It is also used to assess reversibility and vasoreactivity in patients with severe pulmonary hypertension and determine those who might benefit from surgical repair. Therapeutic catheterization is increasingly being performed for repair of lesions amenable to percutaneous interventions (e.g., ASD closure).

#### Evaluation of circulatory shunts
In healthy individuals, PBF is equal to systemic blood flow (SBF). Oximetry is the most common method for evaluating the amount of blood entering from systemic circulation to pulmonary circulation (left-to-right shunt) or from pulmonary to systemic flow (right-to-left shunt) or moving in both directions (bidirectional shunt). In this method, blood samples are obtained from different intracardiac and great arterial locations and analyzed for oxygen saturation. Sudden and significant (greater than 5%–7%) elevation in oxygen saturation from one location to the next in the right heart system, the so-called $O_2$ step-up, indicates a left-to-right shunt to that chamber. A significant (3%) decrease in oxygen saturation from one location in the left system to the next, the $O_2$ step-down, is an indicator of a right-to-left shunt in that chamber.

There are two methods for oximetric evaluation. First is a screening method when suspicion of significant shunts is low, during which blood samples are withdrawn from the SVC and PA. If the patient has equal or more than 8% step-up in oxygen saturation from the SVC to the PA, then a complete oximetric evaluation is undertaken. In a full oximetric study, blood sampling is done from high and low IVC; high and low SVC; high, middle, and low RA; RV inflow, RV apex, or midcavity and RV outflow; main PA and left or right PA branches for determination of left-to-right shunts (step-up); and pulmonary veins, the LA if possible [through an ASD or patent foramen ovale (PFO)], the LV and descending aorta for localization of right-to-left shunts (step-down).

To quantify the intracardiac shunt level, PBF or $Q_p$, SBF or $Q_s$, and effective blood flow (EBF), which is the amount of venous flow entering the lungs without mixing with the shunted blood, have to be determined and are calculated based on the Fick method for cardiac output estimation.

$$\text{Fick cardiac output}(L/\min) = \frac{\text{Oxygen consumption}(mL/\min)}{A - VO_2 \times 1.36 \times Hgb \times 10}$$

Oxygen consumption is assumed as 125 mL/m$^2$ in many laboratories. $A - VO_2$ is the arterial–venous oxygen saturation difference, and 1.36 is the constant for the oxygen-carrying capacity of hemoglobin (expressed in mL $O_2$/g Hgb). Hgb is the hemoglobin concentration (mg/dL). Multiplication by 10 is to convert deciliters to liters when the hemoglobin is measured as g/dL:

$$PBF = \frac{\text{Oxygen consumption}\left(\dfrac{mL}{\min}\right)}{(\text{Pulmonary venous } O_2 \text{ sat} - \text{Pulmonary arterial } O_2 \text{ sat}) \times 1.36 \times Hgb \times 10}$$

$$SBF = \text{Oxygen consumption}\left(\dfrac{mL}{\min}\right)(\text{Systemic arterial } O_2 \text{ sat} - \text{Mixed venous } O_2 \text{ sat}) \times 1.36 \times Hgb \times 10$$

$$EBF = \text{Oxygen consumption}\left(\dfrac{mL}{\min}\right)(\text{Pulmonary venous } O_2 \text{ sat} - \text{Mixed venous } O_2 \text{ sat}) \times 1.36 \times Hgb \times 10$$

If the saturation is 95%, use 0.95 in the formula, not 95.

Mixed venous oxygen saturation is calculated by averaging oxygen saturation of the chamber proximal to the location of the shunt. For example, in ASDs, mixed venous saturation/oxygen content (MVO$_2$) is the average of SVC and IVC oxygen saturation/content and is calculated as

$$MVO_2 = \frac{3(\text{SVCO}_2 \text{ sat}) + 1(\text{IVCO}_2 \text{ sat})}{4}$$

When pulmonary venous saturation is not available, systemic arterial oxygen saturation may be substituted.

If systemic arterial saturation is less than 93% because of a right-to-left shunt, pulmonary venous oxygen saturation is calculated as 98%. If arterial desaturation is secondary to pulmonary disease, hypoventilation, or a cause other than a right-to-left shunt, systemic arterial oxygen saturation is used. Systemic desaturation related to secondary causes is often improved if the patient takes deep breaths or 100% oxygen is administered.

A PBF-to-SBF ratio or $Q_p/Q_s$ less than 1.5:1 indicates a small left-to-right shunt. A ratio greater than 1.5:1 is considered significant and 1.5 to 2:1 is an indicator of a moderate shunt. $Q_p/Q_s$ of 2:1 or higher suggests a large left-to-right shunt. A ratio of less than 1 implies a net right-to-left shunt:

$$\begin{aligned} PBF/SBF &= \frac{Q_p}{Q_s} \\ &= \frac{\text{Systemic arterial } O_2 \text{ sat} - \text{Mixed venous } O_2 \text{ sat}}{\text{Pulmonary venous } O_2 \text{ sat} - \text{Pulmonary arterial } O_2 \text{ sat}} \end{aligned}$$

The amount of left-to-right shunt in liters is calculated as

$$\text{Left-to-right shunt} = PBF - SBF$$

In bidirectional shunts:

The estimated amount of left-to-right shunt $= PBF - EBF$

And the estimated amount of right-to-left shunt $= SBF - EBF$

### Vascular resistance

Cardiac catheterization is used to assess pulmonary (PVR) and systemic (SVR) vascular resistance for determination of operability and treatment options of patients with CHD. Calculation of these indices is also important before cavopulmonary anastomoses (Glenn or Fontan surgery) and cardiac transplantation because surgical risks are increased with a high PVR. The units for resistance are mm Hg/L/min or Wood units:

$$PVR = \frac{\text{Mean PAP} + \text{mean LAP}}{Q_p}$$

$$SVR = \frac{\text{Mean AoP} + \text{mean RAP}}{Q_s}$$

where PAP is pulmonary arterial pressure, LAP is left atrial pressure, RAP is right atrial pressure, and AoP is aortic pressure.

Multiplying the numerator of the fraction by constant 80 is used to convert units from Wood units to the absolute resistance units (dyn s cm$^{-5}$)—that is, PVR = 80 (mean PAP – mean LAP)/$Q_p$. Normal values are 700–1600 dyn s cm$^{-5}$ for SVR and 20–130 dyn s cm$^{-5}$ for PVR.

### Pulmonary vasoreactivity testing

In patients with severe PAH, pulmonary vasoreactivity tests are performed to assess whether pulmonary hypertension and increased PVR are fixed or reactive and the possibility of defect closure or responsiveness to medical treatment. The patients are given vasodilator agents (generally 100% inhaled oxygen or nitric oxide) in the catheterization laboratory. Those who show significant decreases in PVR, a reduction in mean PAP (mPAP) of at least 10 mmHg, a decrease in mPAP to lower than 40 mmHg in the presence of a constant or increased cardiac output, and a significant increase in left-to-right shunt (if existent) are considered to have reactive PAH.[3,5]

## SPECIFIC CONGENITAL CARDIAC DEFECTS

### Shunt Defects

#### Atrial septal defect

ASD is an abnormally persistent connection between the RA and LA. It is a common congenital heart defect, and there are four main types listed below in order of frequency (Fig. 33.5):

1. Ostium secundum defects (most common) are located in the fossa ovalis region.
2. Ostium primum defects are located near the cardiac crux and AV valves.
3. Sinus venosus defects are located around the SVC or the IVC entrance site to the heart. (The SVC type is almost always associated with an anomalous right pulmonary venous connection.)
4. Coronary sinus defects consist of defects in the roof of the coronary sinus that results in abnormal communications with the LA (Fig. 33.6).

ASDs cause a left-to-right and RV volume overload. The most frequent symptoms are exercise intolerance, dyspnea, and palpitation. Development of atrial arrhythmias, including atrial fibrillation, atrial flutter, or sick sinus syndrome, and PAH are common with long-standing RA and RV volume and pressure overload. Paradoxic embolism is also a possibility.

### Investigations

*Clinical examination.* Findings include equalization of *a* and *v* waves in the jugular venous pulse, wide and fixed splitting of S₂, systolic pulmonary ejection murmur, a diastolic rumble from overflow through the tricuspid valve, and a sometimes parasternal lift.

*Electrocardiography.* Incomplete right bundle branch block (RBBB), T wave inversion in V1–V3, "crochetage" sign or notching of the QRS complexes in the inferior leads in secundum ASDs, RV conduction delay with superior axis deviation in primum-type ASDs, and low atrial rhythm with negative P waves in the inferior leads in SVC-type sinus venosus defects may be found. Tall R in $V_1$ and right axis deviation is seen with pulmonary hypertension.

*Chest radiography.* The RA and RV are enlarged, and there is evidence of pulmonary overflow or shunt vascularity. Aortic knob might be small due to remarkable left-to-right shunting of blood at atrial level.

*Echocardiography.* The interatrial septal defect may be visualized by transthoracic echocardiography (TTE) in subcostal, apical four-chamber, and left parasternal short-axis views by two-dimensional (2D) and color Doppler study. Contrast echocardiography with intravenous agitated saline may also help in the diagnosis.

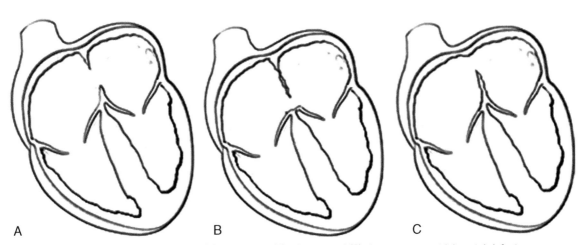

A          B          C

FIG. 33.5 Schematic views of (A) secundum, (B) primum, and (C) sinus venosus atrial septal defects.

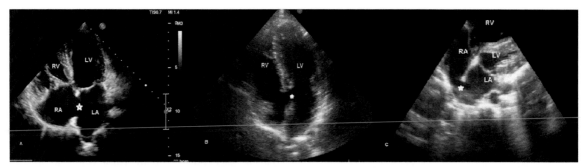

FIG. 33.6 Echocardiographic views of (A) secundum, (B) primum, and (C) sinus venosus ASDs (stars).

There is associated right-sided chamber enlargement and volume overload with paradoxical ventricular septal motion. The IVS becomes D shaped in the parasternal short-axis view during diastole (diastolic flattening) as a result of RV volume overload or in both systole and diastole with pressure overload and pulmonary hypertension. Attention should be paid to evidence of unroofed coronary sinus and blood shunting to the LA.

Transesophageal echocardiography (TEE) is generally performed for precise determination of size, location, and suitability of rims for percutaneous device closure, and to evaluate for any abnormal pulmonary vein connections or associated anomalies.

*Cardiac catheterization.* Catheterization is performed when other imaging modalities are inadequate or for evaluation of coronary arteries or pulmonary vascular resistance and reactivity in those with significant pulmonary hypertension and for the purpose of percutaneous device closure.

**Closure of atrial septal defect.** The following are indications for ASD closure:
- $Q_p/Q_s$ greater than 1.5:1 with RV volume overload
- RV and RA enlargement with or without symptoms
  Small ASDs (<5 mm) with no RV enlargement and $Q_p/Q_s$ less than 1.5 are closed only for prevention of paradoxical emboli after a stroke or documented orthodeoxia–platypnea. ASDs should not be closed in the presence of irreversible severe PAH without a significant left-to-right shunt.

Closure is achieved via surgery or device. Device closure is generally possible only for secundum-type ASDs with suitable rims as measured by TEE and in the absence of anomalous pulmonary venous drainage. All the rims except the anterosuperior rim should be at least 5 mm in length. Patients should receive antiplatelet therapy for at least 6 months after the procedure (Fig. 33.7).

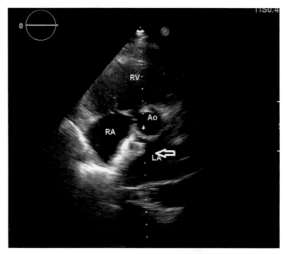

FIG. 33.7 Echocardiographic view of a secundum type ASD occluded with device (*arrow*).

ASDs larger than 38 mm are usually considered unsuitable for device closure.

It should be kept in mind that patients with unexplained RV enlargement and volume overload in TTE should be further evaluated by TEE for the presence of ASD.[1–6]

### Patent foramen ovale

Patent foramen ovale is a tunnel-like route between the overlap region of the septum primum and secundum that directs blood flow from the RA to LA during fetal life and closes in 75% of the population after birth.

Patent foramen ovale has been implicated as a potential cause of cryptogenic stroke, especially in the younger population and in those with aneurysmal interatrial septum by either paradoxic embolization or in situ thrombus formation in the tunnel of the PFO.[3]

### Ventricular septal defect

Various classification systems are used to describe a VSD's location, but it can generally be classified into four types:

- Perimembranous: In this most common type, the defect is in the membranous part of the septum and close to the septal leaflet of the tricuspid valve in the RV side and aorta in the LV side. It is best seen in TTE five-chamber view and parasternal short-axis view at the level of the aortic valve.
- Inlet: The defect is immediately under the mitral and tricuspid valves, best imaged in the TTE four-chamber view.
- Outlet (subarterial): The VSD is located directly under the semilunar valves and best imaged in the parasternal short-axis view of the TTE.
- Muscular: The defect is in the muscular part of the septum (Fig. 33.8).

VSDs are also classified based on their size and hemodynamic effects (i.e., increased volume load of LV and PBF):

- Restrictive or small
  - Small left-to-right shunt ($Q_p/Q_s \geq 1.4$:1)
  - Size less than one-third of the aortic root size
  - Pulmonary-to-aortic systolic pressure ratio of less than 0.3
  - A considerable pressure gradient between the LV and RV
  - Low chance of development of pulmonary hypertension
- Moderate
  - $Q_p/Q_s$ of 1.4:1 to 2.2:1
  - One-third to two-thirds of aortic root size
  - Pulmonary-to-aortic pressure ratio less than 0.66
- Nonrestrictive or large
  - $Q_p/Q_s$ greater than 2.2:1

- More than two-thirds of aortic root size
- Pulmonary-to-aortic systolic pressure ratio more than 0.66
- None or small-pressure gradient between the LV and RV
- Eisenmenger VSD
  - Net right-to-left shunt, $Q_p/Q_s$ less than 1:1, and suprasystemic pulmonary arterial pressure

### Investigations

*Clinical examination.* Small VSDs result in a high-pitched 3–4/6 pansystolic murmur in the left sternal border. In larger VSDs, the murmur intensity decreases and the cardiac apex is displaced to the left. With the development of pulmonary hypertension, there is a loud $P_2$ and RV heave. Patients with Eisenmenger VSDs have clubbing and cyanosis.

*Electrocardiography.* Changes reflect the hemodynamics of VSD. The ECG is normal in small VSDs. As the size increases, there is evidence of LA and LV enlargement and volume overload (tall R and T waves plus deep Q waves in $V_5$ and $V_6$). Right-axis deviation and evidence of RV pressure overload appear as pulmonary pressure increases.

*Chest radiography.* Left ventricular enlargement plus shunt vascularity is noted.

*Echocardiography.* Helps determine the location, type, and hemodynamics of the VSDs (Fig. 33.9).

**Closure of the ventricular septal defect.** Indications for closure include the following:

- $Q_p/Q_s$ ratio greater than 1.5:1
- LV and LA enlargement with or without symptoms
- Possibility of damage to the aortic valve and progressive or more than mild aortic regurgitation in perimembranous VSDs

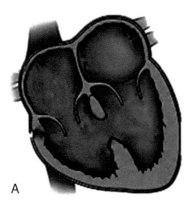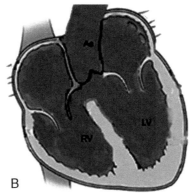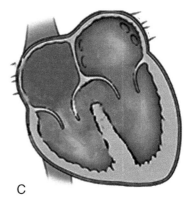

FIG. 33.8 (A) Muscular, (B) perimembranous, and (C) inlet ventricular septal defects.

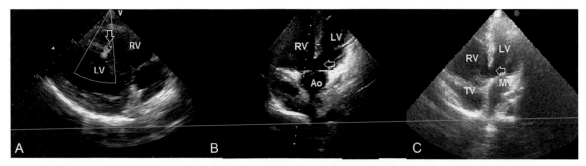

FIG. 33.9 Echocardiographic views of (A) midmuscular, (B) subaortic, and (C) inlet type VSDs (*arrow*).

- Recurrent endocarditis

Closure is achieved either percutaneously by device or through surgical repair.[1,4,5]

### Patent ductus arteriosus

Prenatally, the blood of a fetus does not go to the lungs to become oxygenated. The ductus arteriosus is patent and lets the unoxygenated blood move from the RV and PA to the descending aorta and the placenta, where the blood is oxygenated. Functional closure of the duct happens shortly after a term birth, but full anatomic closure takes several weeks. Patent ductus arteriosus (PDA) is an abnormally persistent connection between the aorta and the PA.

Patent ductus arteriosus is classified based on the size and degree of left-to-right shunting:

- Silent: very small duct, no murmur, usually detected only during echocardiography
- Small: continuous murmur; $Q_p/Q_s$ less than 1.5:1
- Moderate: continuous murmur; $Q_p/Q_s$ of 1.5–2.2
- Large: continuous murmur; $Q_p/Q_s$ greater than 2.2:1
- Eisenmenger: Significant pulmonary hypertension with differential hypoxemia and cyanosis (cyanosis in toes and not fingers); murmur is generally only systolic or not heard

### Investigations

*Clinical examination.* A continuous murmur is best heard in the first and second left intercostal space. Oxygen saturation of both upper and lower extremities should be measured.

*Electrocardiography.* Findings depend on the size and degree of shunting. The ECG is usually normal in a small PDA. In larger defects, there is evidence of LA and ventricular volume overload, including notched P waves with deep Q and tall R and T waves mainly in $V_5$ and $V_6$. PDAs with Eisenmenger physiology show evidence of right-axis deviation and RV hypertrophy on ECG.

*Chest radiography.* If there is a significant amount of left-to-right shunting, chest radiography shows LV enlargement and evidence of shunt vascularity or pulmonary hypertension.

*Echocardiography.* Patent ductus arteriosus is assessed in suprasternal and short-axis TTE views, where the descending aorta and LPA communication with its pertinent flow are visualized. The size and hemodynamic effects of the PDA can be defined with TTE (Fig. 33.10).

**Indications for intervention.** Patent ductus arteriosus with murmur and significant left-to-right shunting should be closed at any age before the establishment of irreversible pulmonary hypertension. Transcatheter device closure of PDA is now the procedure of choice, and surgery is performed only if the percutaneous method is unsuccessful.[3,5]

### Aortopulmonary window

In aortopulmonary window, an abnormal communication exists between the ascending aorta and PA. There are various classifications based on the size of the defect. Pulmonary hypertension and Eisenmenger syndrome develop early because of generally large and persistent left-to-right shunting. Physical examination, ECG, and chest radiography mimic those of large PDAs.[5]

### Atrioventricular septal defects

Endocardial cushion defect, or AV septal defect (AVSD), has some anatomic hallmarks independent of the type or the presence of ASD and VSD. All types of this anomaly have an absence of AV valve offsetting, elongated LVOT, and a cleft on the anterior leaflet of the MV.

There are four types of AVSDs: partial, transitional, intermediate, and complete forms. In the partial type, the patient has primum-type ASD and a cleft on the anterior MV leaflet. In transitional AVSD the physiology is similar to the partial form; in addition to ASD and cleft, small inlet-type VSD exists. Intermediate and

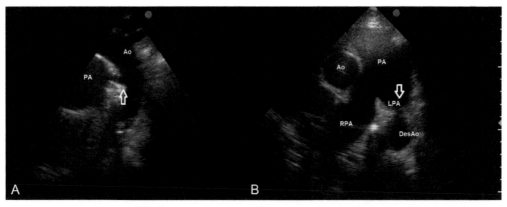

FIG. 33.10 Echocardiographic views of a patent ductus arteriosus from (A) suprasternal and (B) short axis windows (*arrow*).The defect is between left branch of pulmonary artery (LPA) and descending aorta (DesAo).

complete forms have similar physiologies with large inlet-type VSD.

This pathologic condition is the result of an endocardial cushion defect in the AV canal and an anomalous connection between the interatrial septum and interventricular septum, so the patients have low ASD, inlet-type VSD, and AV valve structure abnormalities. Because of the AV valve's annulus defect, the aortic valve, which is normally wedged between the tricuspid and mitral valves, is unwedged and displaced to an anterior position, and an elongated or gooseneck deformity develops.

In the complete form, a common AV valve junction and common AV valve are seen. This common AV valve has five leaflets: superior and inferior bridging leaflets and mural left, right anterior, and right posterior leaflets.

In the partial and transitional forms, the ventricular septum is connected to the valve and divided into two AV valves—the left with three and the right with four leaflets.

Between the superior and the inferior bridging leaflets in systole is a space called the cleft; from this, a cleft regurgitation is seen.

**Epidemiology.** The prevalence of AVSD is 3% among persons with CHD, and the anomaly is slightly more common in females. The complete form is more prevalent and is seen in 35% of patients with Down syndrome.

**Pathophysiology.** As pointed out previously, patients with the partial and transitional forms have pathophysiology similar to patients with ASD, but in patients with intermediate and complete forms, the clinical features are more similar to a large VSD.

**Clinical features.** Patients with partial AVSD, similar to those with ASD, have symptoms of dyspnea on exercise and palpitation during the third or fourth decade of life. They may have symptoms of mitral regurgitation (MR) simultaneously. The complete form of AVSD presents earlier in life with symptoms, similar to those of VSD, beginning in the early years of life, and pulmonary vascular resistance increases and stabilizes by 2 years of age, in patients with Down syndrome. Eisenmenger syndrome earlier.

**Investigations**

*Physical examination.* In partial AVSD, wide fixed S2 splitting and a systolic murmur in the upper left sternal border are heard. The apical murmur of MR is also audible. In the complete form, during the early years, the systolic murmur of the VSD is heard, but with increased PVR the murmur disappears, and a loud P2 and systolic murmur of common valve regurgitation become audible.

*Electrocardiography.* In the partial form, incomplete RBBB is seen, but unlike in secundum ASD, the QRS axis deviates to the left. This deviation is caused by left anterior fascicle hypoplasia. In the complete form, RV hypertrophy pattern and the left anterior descending coronary artery (LAD) are seen.

*Chest radiography.* In the partial form, RV enlargement and evidence of shunt vascularity are seen. In the complete form, cardiomegaly, dilation of PA branches, and pruning of the pulmonary branch are observed.

*Echocardiography.* Echocardiography is the best tool for the exact denotation of this disease. The four-chamber view is specified for primum ASD and inlet-type VSD. The best view for seeing the valve leaflets is subcostal. The cleft is also seen in the subcostal and short-axis view. MR grading can be determined, and LV outflow tract obstruction (LVOT) should also be checked.

*Cardiac catheterization.* For patients with the partial form, there is no need for catheterization. However, if patients have PAH, a hemodynamic workup is necessary for exact evaluation of PVR and pulmonary vascular response. In the complete form, for patients in whom Eisenmenger syndrome has developed, follow-up echocardiography is sufficient.

*Management.* Surgery is the main treatment for these patients. In every patient with the partial form, repair of ASD, mitral cleft, MR, and tricuspid regurgitation (TR) should be performed. The complete form should be corrected before 6 months of age because of the risk of pulmonary vascular disease. Before surgery in infants with heart failure symptoms, medical treatment is recommended. Surgery includes single- or double-patch repair.

*Surgical outcome.* The mortality rate for patients undergoing surgery is about 3%, and the 10-year survival rate is 90%, but the risk that reoperation will be required is 10%–20%. The top reason for reoperation is the progression of MR. After that, LVOT obstruction, valvular stenosis, and residual defects are reasons to redo surgery. Two possible complications during surgery are AV node damage and risk of complete heart block.

*Follow-up.* Patients with AVSD, whether repaired or nonrepaired, should have lifelong follow-up by a cardiologist with special training in CHD. Patients should be monitored for AV valve regurgitation, atrial arrhythmia, LVOT obstruction, and ventricular function.

*Pregnancy.* In repaired patients with no residual significant defect, pregnancy has no prohibition. In the partial nonrepaired form, pregnancy may also be tolerated. In patients with Eisenmenger syndrome, however, pregnancy is contraindicated.[2–4]

### Anomalous pulmonary venous connection

In anomalous pulmonary venous connection, all or some of the pulmonary veins (PVs) do not connect to the LA; therefore all or part of the pulmonary venous flow is returned to the right side of the heart, creating a left-to-right shunt.

**Total anomalous pulmonary venous connection.** Total anomalous pulmonary venous connection (TAPVC) might be supracardiac (more common) in which all the PVs connect to a vertical vein, which connects to the innominate vein, the SVC, and then the RA, or infracardiac in which the anomalous trunk connects to the portal vein or other abdominal veins that ultimately empty to the RA. Other anatomic variants are intracardiac (connection to coronary sinus) and mixed type.

*Physical examination.* There is a fixed and wide splitting of $S_2$ with accentuated $P_2$.

*Electrocardiography.* Right-axis deviation and right-sided enlargement are seen.

*Chest radiography.* The vertical vein, innominate vein, and SVC are dilated; enlarged right heart chambers are enlarged.

*Echocardiography.* The left vertical vein is visualized from the suprasternal view as a vessel parallel to the descending aorta with the flow being in the opposite direction of the descending aorta.

**Partial anomalous pulmonary venous connection.** Partial anomalous pulmonary venous connection (PAPVC) has various anatomic subtypes, all resulting in left-to-right shunt:

- Right-sided PVs connect to the SVC (most common).
- Right-sided PVs connect directly to the RA.
- Right-sided PVs connect to the IVC (scimitar syndrome).
- Left-sided PVs connect to a vertical vein with flow toward the innominate vein and then the SVC and RA.
- Rarely, PVs connect to the coronary sinus, and their blood reaches the RA.

*Physical examination, electrocardiography, and chest radiography.* Findings are similar to those of secundum-type ASDs. TEE, computed tomography (CT), and cardiac magnetic resonance imaging (CMR) are commonly used for diagnosis in adults.

*Cardiac catheterization.* Catheterization is used to measure pulmonary arterial pressure and calculate $Q_p/Q_s$. During catheterization, PA injection is performed, and PAPVCs are visualized in levophase. Right-sided PAPVCs might be directly entered. In the case of the significant left-to-right shunt, corrective surgery is indicated.[3,5,7]

### Cyanotic Heart Defects
#### Tetralogy of Fallot

Tetralogy of Fallot (ToF) is one of the most prevalent cyanotic CHD types. This condition consists of a tetrad that includes large subaortic VSD, overriding of the aorta, subvalvular pulmonary stenosis, and RV hypertrophy. All of these defects have an embryologic cause: anterocephalad deviation of the conal septum, which is misaligned with the rest of the septal part.

The pulmonary valve may have no anomaly, but in most cases, the valve is stenotic and thickened and may be bicuspid. For a better explanation, we divide patients with ToF into three groups: unrepaired patients, palliated patients, and totally corrected patients.

In large part, neonates with ToF are born with cyanosis, the degree of which depends on RV outflow tract (RVOT) obstruction. In a small subset of patients the clinical cyanosis is less, the so-called pink TOF patients. This group has less RVOT obstruction than in other cyanotic ToF. Infants with cyanotic ToF have cyanotic spells, which occur during crying or other activities that increase catecholamines, resulting in severe RVOT obstruction, restricted flow to the pulmonary arteries, and increased right-to-left shunt via VSD. For relief of this situation, the maneuvers and drugs for increasing systemic vascular resistance and decreasing pulmonary vascular resistance are helpful. These include squatting, oxygen, morphine, intravenous propranolol, and phenylephrine.

### Investigations

*Physical examination.* Patients with ToF have RV heave, single $S_2$, and, in auscultation, a harsh systolic murmur in the left sternal border, an aortic ejection sound in the aortic area because of an overridden aorta, and aortic overflow. A continuous murmur of collateral arteries is also heard on the chest or back. The intensity of the systolic murmur is inversely dependent on the degree of RVOT obstruction, while in isolated pulmonary stenosis the intensity of murmur has a direct relation with the severity of obstruction. In patients with absent pulmonary valve syndrome (a rare variant of ToF), to-and-fro murmur of PS and pulmonary regurgitation is auscultated. In the case of ToF with pulmonary atresia, systolic murmur of the PV is absent, and only a single $S_2$ and continuous murmur of collaterals are heard. In palliated patients with systemic shunt, in addition to this murmur, continuous soufflé of the shunt is heard.

In patients who have undergone repair, the sounds and murmur of a residual defect may be auscultated. A systolic murmur of residual VSD or residual PS is heard; in patients with pulmonary regurgitation, a soft short diastolic murmur is heard in upper LSB. If a harsh diastolic murmur is heard in these patients, it is caused by aortic regurgitation, which occurs in patients with nonrepaired or repaired ToF because of a dilated aorta and aortopathy.

*Electrocardiography.* In patients with native ToF, right ventricular hypertrophy (RVH) criteria are present. The QRS axis is right-sided, and RA enlargement (pulmonic P wave) is seen, but the strain pattern of RVH is seen mostly in $V_1$ to $V_3$, not in all the precordial leads as in isolated PS. Tall R in V1 with a sudden transition to RS in $V_2$ usually is seen. These changes are also seen in palliated patients. In totally repaired patients, RBBB is almost always seen because of right bundle branch injury during RVOT shaving in surgery. The QRS duration is related to RV enlargement, and widening of the S wave occurs in $V_5$ to $V_6$ through dilation of the RV and pulmonary regurgitation over the years.

*Chest radiography.* In patients with nonrepaired ToF, the boot-shaped sign, or *coeur en sabot*, is seen because of RVH, pulmonary vascular marking is decreased, and a concave left upper pulmonary border is seen. In palliated patients, one lung with a systemic shunt may have increased vascularity. In totally corrected patients, radiographs may be normal, or RV dilation and aneurysmal RVOT caused by pulmonary regurgitation may be seen (Fig. 33.11).

*Echocardiography.* In native ToF, in the four-chamber view, two developed ventricles are seen with significant hypertrophied RV. In the five-chamber view, a large subaortic VSD with an overridden aorta is seen; VSD flow is laminar and bidirectional. Findings are similar in the parasternal long-axis view. On the parasternal short-axis view, the VSD shows subvalvular and valvular PS. In palliated patients, the flow of shunt may be observed in suprasternal views; also, in this view, flow of collaterals is seen. In totally repaired patients, sequelae and surgery complications should be sought. Residual VSD is seen in five-chamber and parasternal short- and long-axis views. Residual PS is found in the parasternal short-axis view. The most prevalent abnormal finding is pulmonary regurgitation, which is

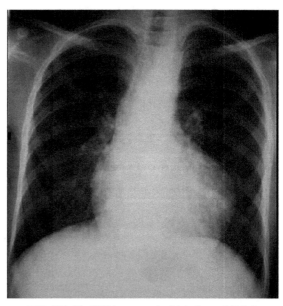

FIG. 33.11 CXR in unrepaired tetralogy of Fallot.

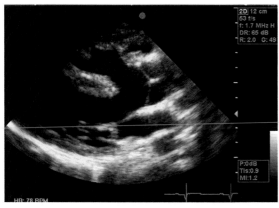

FIG. 33.12 Parasternal echocardiographic long axis view echo in unrepaired tetralogy of Fallot.

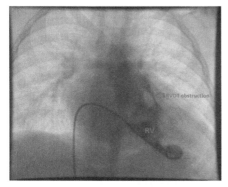

FIG. 33.13 Right ventricle angiogram in tetralogy of Fallot.

diagnosed by color-flow, pulsed wave, and continuous wave Doppler. Other findings that should be noted are TR, RV dilation and dysfunction, aortic regurgitation, aortic root dilation, and peripheral PS (Fig. 33.12).

*Cardiac catheterization.* Although CT angiography could answer most questions about the size of PA branches and collaterals and the coronary artery course in patients with native ToF who are candidates for surgery, catheterization should be done in pulmonary atresia for exact evaluation of collaterals and PA pressure in segments that are supplied by collaterals. In adult patients, coronary artery disease and PA pressure should be evaluated before surgery (Fig. 33.13).

*Cardiac computed tomography angiography.* This imaging is performed to evaluate PA branch size, course of the coronary artery and PA arborization, and size and location of collateral arteries.

*Cardiac magnetic resonance imaging.* The gold standard for imaging in patients with corrected ToF,

CMR is very useful for evaluating RV size, volume, and function for the timing of surgery for pulmonary regurgitation.

*Management.* For patients with native ToF, total correction in cyanotic patients of every age is recommended. The obstacles to this surgery include prematurity, low body weight, and small size of PA branches. Surgery is recommended even for older adults if they have appropriate ventricles and PA branches.

In palliated ToF, with passing years the shunt is not enough for oxygenation, and patients became more cyanotic. For this group, total corrective surgery and take down the shunt is recommended.

Survival of patients with corrected ToF is excellent, but about 10%–15% have complications, especially pulmonary regurgitation after 20 years. Surgery is indicated for these patients if residual VSD is seen in a left-to-right shunt with a $Q_s/Q_p$ greater than 1.5, or in patients with residual PS if RV to LV pressure is more than 60%. Surgery is indicated for pulmonary regurgitation if RV volume is more than 150 cc/m$^2$ or right ventricular ejection fraction (RVEF) less than 45%, the patient has exercise intolerance, or resistant arrhythmia, or progressive TR is seen in follow-up echocardiography. Left ventricular dysfunction and QRS widening greater than 180 ms are recommendations for pulmonary valve replacement.

Aortic regurgitation surgery is indicated if the patient meets the aortic insufficiency criteria for aortic valve replacement. Aortic root dilation greater than 55 mm is an indication for root surgery.

*Surgery.* In the past, surgery for patients with native ToF included VSD closure by patch and RVOT shaving to alleviate stenosis. One obstacle for RVOT shaving is an abnormal course of the LAD from the right coronary artery and passing anterior to the RVOT. In this situation, as in pulmonary atresia, a valve conduit is inserted between the RVOT and MPA. In patients with a hypoplastic annulus, a transannular patch has sometimes been a substrate for existing pulmonary insufficiency. Currently a transatrial and transpulmonary approach for surgery is used, with the belief that leaving some degree of stenosis is well tolerated and that this approach is better than a transannular patch that might cause pulmonary insufficiency in the future.

**Pulmonary valve replacement.** There are still questions in choosing the type of valve in the pulmonary position. High chance of thrombosis in mechanical valves vs biologic valve degeneration challenges valve type selection.[8]

*Percutaneous pulmonary valve replacement.* This is a new approach for valve replacement in pulmonary position, especially in conduits. For this approach, the size of the PV annulus and its relation to the coronary artery should be appropriate.

*Arrhythmia.* Atrial and ventricular arrhythmia in patients with ToF is common, especially after total correction. Atrial flutter is one of the most common atrial arrhythmias. Premature ventricular contractions and episodes of nonsustained ventricular tachycardia (VT) are also seen, but VT and sudden cardiac death are uncommon. An implantable cardiac defibrillator (ICD) is recommended for patients with documented VT or sudden death, but there is no clear indication for ICD implantation as primary prevention.

*Pregnancy.* In nonrepaired and palliated cyanotic patients, the risk associated with pregnancy is moderate, and the chance of prematurity of the neonate is high. For patients with total correction, if no sequelae have occurred, the risk associated with pregnancy is low. However, patients with significant pulmonary insufficiency may become decompensated during pregnancy.

*Follow-up.* Cyanotic nonrepaired and palliated patients should be under observation by a professional cardiologist experienced in CHD. Corrected patients should also have regular follow-up because of the risk of sequelae happening years later. Endocarditis prophylaxis is needed for all nonrepaired and palliated patients and patients with corrected but residual anomaly.[2-4,9]

### Transposition of the great arteries

In the transposition of the great arteries (TGA) pathologic complex, the aorta arises from the RV and the PA from the LV. Atrioventricular connections may be concordant or discordant. If the atrioventricular connection is concordant, the patient has two parallel circulations, but in a discordant atrioventricular connection the circulations are in series, which actually means that circulation physiology is corrected.

**Complete transposition.** In complete, TGA (DTGA), the atrioventricular connection is concordant, but the ventriculoarterial connection is discordant (Fig. 33.14). This abnormality is incompatible with life unless a shunt exists between these two circulations. All patients have ASD, two-thirds have PDA, and one-third have VSD. The fetus has normal growth and newborns usually weigh more than normal, but problems begin immediately after birth.

DTGA may occur as an isolated disorder or a part of a complex disease. The most prevalent associated anomalies in complex disease are VSD and PS.

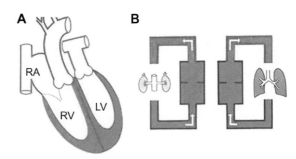

**FIG. 33.14** Schematic diagram showing complete TGA with parallel circulation.

*Clinical presentation.* Newborns have cyanosis or congestive failure symptoms, depending on the size of the shunt between two circulatory systems. If the shunt is limited, such as a small ASD without PDA and VSD, the neonate will have severe cyanosis.

*Management.* For newborns with DTGA, intervention should take place immediately after birth. First, a prostaglandin infusion is started for ductal patency and greater mixing at the atrial level. The next intervention is atrial septostomy or surgical septectomy to increase mixing and patient oxygen saturation. Today, the arterial switch operation is recommended in the first week of life.

Surgical interventions for these patients are atrial switch, arterial switch, and the Rastelli procedure. Atrial switch, or the Senning procedure, is now considered a historical method, and arterial switch is currently performed for most patients with complete TGA.

In the atrial switch procedure, the systemic venous drainage is deviated to the MV and LV, and the pulmonary venous drainage is left to conduct to the tricuspid valve and RV. To create this bypass an atrial septum baffle is used (Senning procedure) or a pericardial or synthetic patch is applied (Mustard procedure). Thus, in this procedure, the RV becomes the systemic ventricle (Fig. 33.15).

During the arterial switch, or Jatene procedure the aorta and PA are transected above the coronary artery, the PA is brought to an anterior position (Lecompte maneuver) and grafted to the proximal part of the previous aorta, the aorta is sewn to the previous PA so that the proximal part and root of the neoaorta are the previous main PA, and the coronary artery is reimplanted to the neoaorta.

The Rastelli procedure is performed for patients with complete TGA who have subaortic VSD and LVOT obstruction. For these patients, an arterial shunt may first be placed to improve oxygenation. In the procedure the

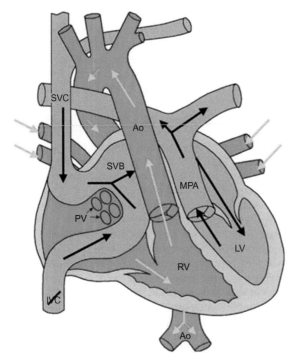
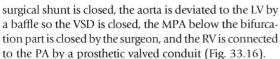

FIG. 33.15 Senning procedure.

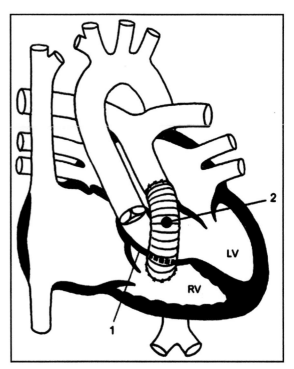

FIG. 33.16 Rastelli procedure.

surgical shunt is closed, the aorta is deviated to the LV by a baffle so the VSD is closed, the MPA below the bifurcation part is closed by the surgeon, and the RV is connected to the PA by a prosthetic valved conduit (Fig. 33.16).

*Postoperative considerations.* Patients after the atrial switch procedure have limited exercise capacity (functional class 1 or 2), most probably because of limited atrial baffle compliance and diastolic dysfunction. After a few years, systolic dysfunction symptoms may appear; 2%–15% have symptoms of congestive heart failure. Progressive TR subsequent to RV dilation and dysfunction is seen. Atrial arrhythmia, most commonly atrial flutter, is reported in 40%, and sinus node dysfunction after surgery is common. Pulmonary artery hypertension is seen in patients who had residual shunt or underwent surgery at an older age. In summary, patients undergoing the Senning procedure had 70%–80% survival after 20–30 years.

Cardiac examination of these patients shows RV heave, a normal $S_1$, but a single S2 heard because of the posterior location of the pulmonary valve. Right ventricular $S_4$ is also audible, and murmur of TR, which is not increased by respiration, is heard in the left sternal border.

On an electrocardiogram, a P wave may not be observed. Junctional rhythm or another atrial arrhythmia and signs of right-axis deviation and RVH may be seen.

In chest radiography the "egg on a string" sign is seen, caused by a narrow mediastinum (anterior posterior position of aorta and PA) on an enlarged heart.

Echocardiography is an important modality for evaluation of patients after the Senning procedure. The hallmark sign is the parallel position of the great arteries, with the aorta anterior and to the right side of the pulmonary valve. The atrial baffle should be checked for patency and leakage (Fig. 33.17). Velocity is less than 1 m/s, and flow is laminar. Pulmonary atrial baffle flow should be less than 2 m/s, SVC and IVC baffle flow is biphasic, and pulmonary atrial baffle flow is triphasic. The function of systemic RV and TR severity should be evaluated. The MR gradient is used for the measurement of PA pressure.

CMR is necessary for an exact evaluation of systemic RV function.

In the Rastelli procedure the LV becomes the systemic ventricle, so patients do not have symptoms of systemic ventricle failure as Senning procedure patients may. With passing time and growth of the child, however, the conduit becomes stenotic, and surgery for conduit replacement is necessary.

Cardiac examination of these patients shows normal $S_1$ and $S_2$, but blood flow passing through the conduit causes systolic murmur.

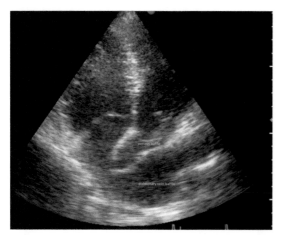

FIG. 33.17 Echocardiogram of a patient after senning procedure.

Most patients have RBBB on the electrocardiogram after surgery because of trauma to the right bundle branch.

Chest radiography findings are normal after surgery, but in time calcification of the conduit is observed.

In echocardiography the conduit may be seen with difficulty. Stenosis at the conduit should be noted; it may occur at the proximal or distal site of anastomosis or in the valve insertion area. Right ventricular function, TR severity, and TR gradient should be evaluated. Residual VSD and subaortic stenosis should be checked.

Cardiac catheterization and angiography are performed when conduit stenosis cannot be evaluated precisely by noninvasive imaging (Fig. 33.18).

In the arterial switch procedure, the LV becomes the systemic ventricle. If there was no complication of surgery, cardiac examination findings are completely normal.

Results of electrocardiography and chest radiography, despite the Lecompte maneuver, are normal.

In echocardiography, any complication should be evaluated. Regional wall motion abnormality, supravalvular stenosis of the PA, aortic root dilation, and aortic regurgitation should be noted.

*Reintervention.* As mentioned previously, patients who have had the Senning procedure have multiple complications, so a high percentage of them require reintervention. One common complication is TR in which tricuspid valve replacement should be performed if RVEF is more than 45%. If the RV has failed, the patient should be scheduled for cardiac transplantation or a double-switch procedure. Before the double-switch procedure the LV should be trained by PA banding until the LV is hypertrophied, at which time the PA is debanded, atrial baffles are removed, and the arterial switch is performed. In patients with atrial baffle obstruction, catheterization or surgical intervention is performed. Both the SVC and the IVC may be obstructed, but SVC obstruction is more common and benign because SVC drainage takes place via the azygos vein. Pulmonary venous baffle obstruction, with

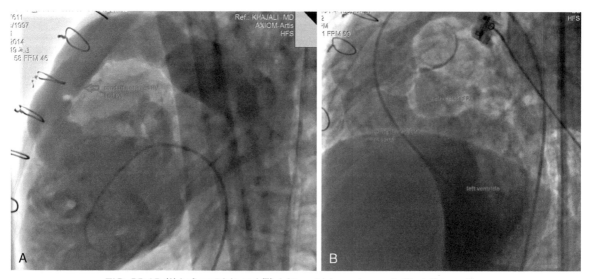

FIG. 33.18 (A) Left ventricle and (B) right ventricle angiogram in Rastelli operation.

symptoms of pulmonary venous congestion and pulmonary edema, is also alleviated by balloon and stenting or a surgical approach. A baffle leak with a right-to-left shunt should be closed, and if a left-to-right shunt ratio is more than 1.5:1, the baffle should be repaired. In junctional bradycardia or complete heart block, a cardiac pacemaker should be implanted, an atrial lead inserted into the baffle, and a ventricular lead implanted in the LV by active fixation.

After surgery with the Rastelli technique, the conduit becomes calcified and incompetent as the patient grows. The conduit should be replaced if the mean gradient is greater than 50 mmHg measured by echocardiography or the peak-to-peak gradient is greater than 50 mmHg in cardiac catheterization. Percutaneous pulmonary valve replacement could be performed successfully for these patients. Other indications for surgery are residual VSD with a left-to-right shunt ratio greater than 1.5:1 and subaortic stenosis with a gradient greater than 50 mmHg.

Patients who have undergone the arterial switch procedure stay asymptomatic for a long time. One complication that needs reintervention is coronary artery ostial stenosis, for which a bypass graft with an arterial conduit should be performed. Supravalvular stenosis with a mean gradient greater than 50 mmHg is another indication for redo surgery, as is aortic root dilation and aortic regurgitation in which the root size is more than 55 mm. Treatment of aortic insufficiency is the same as for other patients if symptoms occur or LV dilation or LV dysfunction should be repaired.

*Medical treatment.* Medical treatment may be indicated in patients with systemic RV dysfunction who have had the Senning procedure, but the efficacy of ACE inhibitors and beta-blockers in these patients with heart failure is debatable.

*Pregnancy.* Patients who have undergone the arterial switch or Rastelli procedure with no complications tolerate pregnancy well. Those who have had the Senning procedure should be discouraged from pregnancy if they have RV dysfunction (ejection fraction less than 45%). In patients with a history of Senning procedure who became pregnant RV failure may be worsened during pregnancy and this worsening persists after delivery.

*Follow-up.* Patients who have had an arterial switch and Rastelli procedures could be followed by periodic echocardiography, but patients after Senning procedures need periodic Holter monitoring and CMR in addition to echocardiography.

**Congenitally corrected transposition of great arteries.** In patients with ccTGA, atrioventricular connections such as the ventriculoarterial connection are discordant, so circulation is physiologically correct; that is, systemic venous drainage is to the pulmonary circulation, and pulmonary venous drainage is connected to the LA and then the RV and aorta (Fig. 33.19). However,

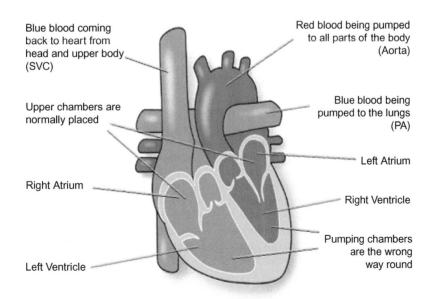

FIG. 33.19 AV and VA discordance in CCTGA.

in this anomaly, the RV stays as the systemic ventricle and with the passage of time becomes dysfunctional.

Although ccTGA or levo-transposition of the great arteries may occur in isolation without other anomalies, it is commonly associated with other heart defects. The most prevalent associated anomalies are VSD and PS. More than 75% of patients have an abnormal tricuspid valve, which often is an Ebstein-like deformity. The risk of complete heart block accompanying ccTGA is 5% at birth and increases by 2% each year after that.

*Pathophysiology.* Patients with isolated ccTGA who have no associated anomaly may have a long life expectancy, to the seventh or eighth decade. Patients may be asymptomatic to 30 years of age, but symptoms of systemic RV dysfunction and RV failure appear after the fourth decade. Palpitation and atrial arrhythmia begin from the fifth decade. The patients with associated anomalies have usually undergone a surgical procedure such as an arterial shunt or VSD and PS repair. Some patients with VSD and PS have a balanced physiology in which cyanosis is not severe or bothersome, and these patients remain asymptomatic for many years.

### Investigations

*Clinical examination.* Patients with isolated ccTGA remain asymptomatic to late adulthood. In auscultation $S_1$ is normal, but $S_2$ is single and $A_2$ is palpable. The murmur of TR may be audible in the left sternal border and is not intensified by respiration. In patients with an associated anomaly, the murmur of VSD or PS is heard. The murmur of PS radiates to the right sternal border because of the location of the pulmonary valve and PA.

*Electrocardiography.* Because of the inverse position of the ventricles in ccTGA, septal depolarization is inverse, so septal Q in $V_5$–$V_6$ and initial r wave are not seen, the QRS axis is deviated to the left, and the Q wave is visible in inferior leads. As noted before, 5% of those with ccTGA are born with complete heart block, and the rate of block increases significantly after surgery. In addition, 50% have first-degree AV block.

*Chest radiography.* The side-by-side orientation of the ventricles causes a hump shape appearance at the left border of the heart. The PA border is not seen because of the posterior location of the PA, and the entire upper left border is formed by the aorta. The waterfall sign in which the right PA has a more apparent course than in a normal heart is characteristic for ccTGA. Dextrocardia, commonly associated with situs solitus, occurs in 20%, and this is a radiographic clue for a ccTGA diagnosis.

*Echocardiography.* TTE is one of the first modalities for diagnosis of ccTGA, and an easy and important one. First, the atrial situs should be checked from a subcostal view. In this anomaly the atrioventricular connection is discordant, so the presentation is a normal atrial situs and a morphologic LV positioned at the right side of a morphologic RV. The RV has a triangular shape with a moderator band and is guarded by a tricuspid valve that is inserted more apically so that offsetting AV valves are reversed. The aorta is located anterior to and to the left of the PA. The function of the systemic RV, morphology of the tricuspid valve, and TR severity should be evaluated.

*Cardiac magnetic resonance imaging.* Because of limitations of TTE for exact evaluation of the systemic RV, periodic CMR for evaluation of RV function is necessary. For patients with a permanent pacemaker or claustrophobia, high-resolution nuclear imaging or perspective CT is recommended.

### Management

*Surgical treatment.* Tricuspid valve repair or replacement in cases of moderate to severe regurgitation is performed if the RVEF is more than 45%; for an RVEF less than 45% or RV failure the double-switch procedure is recommended. Before the double-switch procedure, LV training by PA banding is necessary. If the RV has failed severely, cardiac transplantation should be performed. If patients have previously undergone VSD and PS repair, reintervention is recommended if they have residual VSD with a left-to-right shunt ratio greater than 1.5:1 or residual PS, although some degree of PS in these patients is protective against RV dysfunction and TR progression. The Ilbawi procedure (atrial switch and Rastelli procedure) is recommended for patients with VSD and PS.

*Medical management.* Some studies have shown the efficacy of valsartan and carvedilol in RV failure of patients with ccTGA.

*Pregnancy.* If the RV has failed or RVFE is less than 45%, patients should be discouraged from becoming pregnant.

*Follow-up.* Lifelong periodic follow-up is recommended for all patients who have isolated ccTGA without a history of surgery or all of the patients with ccTGA who have had a surgical procedure performed.[2–4,9]

### Double-outlet right ventricle

In double-outlet right ventricle (DORV), both the aorta and the PA entirely or predominantly arise from the RV. Although anomalies such as ccTGA or univentricular heart may be associated with DORV, this section focuses on hearts with atrioventricular concordance and two ventricles of acceptable size.

**Pathophysiology.** A simple and understandable classification for DORV, especially from the standpoint of surgery, is based on the location of VSD in relation to the great arteries. The four categories are DORV with subaortic VSD, DORV with subpulmonic VSD, DORV with doubly committed VSD, and DORV with remote or noncommitted VSD.

- DORV with subaortic VSD: This variant is most common. Pathophysiologic features of this anomaly depend on the presence and degree of PS. In patients with PS, the pathophysiology resembles that of tetralogy of Fallot (ToF type). In the absence of PS the PBF is increased and the pathophysiology is like VSD (VSD type).
- DORV with subpulmonic VSD: In this variant of DORV the aorta arises completely from the RV, and streaming of blood flow from the LV is predominantly to the PA (TGA type). One anomaly in this variant group is Taussig–Bing anomaly in which the aorta is lateral and to the right of the PA and patients have severe PAH.
- DORV with doubly committed VSD: In this anomaly, the VSD is beneath both great arteries, and the interarterial septum is deficient. Management of this variant depends on association with PS and PBF.
- DORV with noncommitted VSD: In this variant both great arteries arise completely from the RV. Another name for this anomaly is DORV 200% (Figs. 33.20 and 33.21).

## Investigations

*Clinical examination.* Presentation depends on the type of DORV and associated anomalies and may include cyanosis or heart failure symptoms. Findings on cardiac auscultation also depend on association with PS.

*Electrocardiography.* Results depend on the DORV type, but most patients have evidence of RVH.

*Chest radiography.* Cardiomegaly and increased pulmonary vascular marking are seen in patients with a large VSD and without PS. In patients with PS, pulmonary vascular marking is reduced.

*Echocardiography.* This is an easy and important modality for the evaluation of patients. Size of the VSD and its relation to the great arteries should be evaluated.

## Management

*Surgical management.* Surgery for DORV is challenging, and the technique depends on the type. For the VSD type, the VSD is closed by a patch. In the ToF type, RVOT shaving, PV commissurotomy, and VSD closure are used. In the TGA type and Taussig–Bing anomaly, arterial switch and closing of the VSD are performed. The most demanding procedure is for patients with remote VSD because deviating the aorta to the LV is difficult and requires enlarging the VSD. Many surgeons use a univentricular approach and the Fontan procedure for these patients.

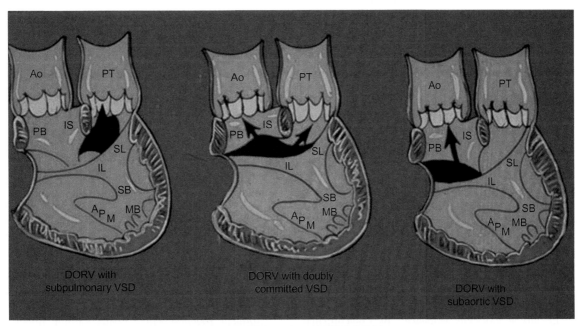

FIG. 33.20 Location of VSD in DORV.

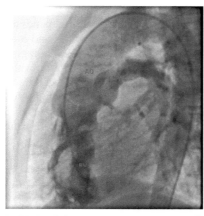

FIG. 33.21 RV angiogram in patient with DORV.

*Follow-up.* Lifelong follow-up is needed for all patients in whom surgery is performed and for patients with no surgical treatment recommended.[1–4]

### Truncus arteriosus

Truncus arteriosus is a cyanotic CHD in which a common arterial trunk arises from the heart and forms the aorta and the PA. There is a single outflow valve (truncal valve) that might be tricuspid or quadricuspid. A large interventricular communication is almost always present, and the common trunk seems to override it. A right aortic arch could also be present. Classifications vary, but a commonly used clinical classification is based on the anatomy of the PA and branches:

- Type I: The main PA arises from the common trunk (commonly the left posterolateral aspect) and then branches into the LPA and RPA.
- Type II: The PA branches originate directly from the posterior aspect of the trunk.
- Type III: The PA branches originate directly from the lateral aspect of the trunk.
- Type IV: One of the PA branches might be absent and the respective lung receives the blood through collaterals.

Severe pulmonary hypertension and Eisenmenger syndrome appear early and are usually established beyond the first year of age. Truncal valve regurgitation is prevalent and causes biventricular failure.

### Investigations

*Physical examination.* Adults' findings usually include pulmonary hypertension, cyanosis, and Eisenmenger physiology.

*Electrocardiography.* Evidence of biventricular hypertrophy and pulmonary hypertension is seen.

*Chest radiography.* Findings include cardiomegaly, increased pulmonary arterial flow, and pulmonary hypertension.

*Echocardiography.* VSD and overriding of the aorta, RVH, a large common trunk with possible regurgitation (tricuspid or quadricuspid), and a right-sided aortic arch are seen frequently. The PA anatomy might be difficult to visualize in adults.

*Cardiac catheterization.* Catheterization is not generally necessary because the diagnosis is readily made based on other imaging modalities, and the condition is irreversible when there is arterial desaturation as determined by noninvasive pulse oximetry.

*Surgical management.* Corrective surgery should be carried out in infancy before the development of the significant pulmonary arterial obstructive disease. It involves the separation of the PA from the trunk, reconstruction of RV outflow by a valved conduit, and VSD closure. Adults after surgery should be monitored for conduit valve stenosis and regurgitation, truncal valve regurgitation, and pulmonary hypertension if surgery was relatively late in life.[3–5]

### Tricuspid atresia

In the cyanotic anomaly tricuspid atresia, the right-sided AV valve, or tricuspid valve (TV), is absent or atretic with no antegrade flow and the RV is hypoplastic. The venous blood enters the LV via an ASD that is always present. The hypoplastic RV is usually connected to the LV by a VSD. Tricuspid atresia is classified based on the relation of the great arteries:

- Type I: Normally related
- Type II: D-transposed
- Type III: Forms of malposition other than D-transposition
- Type IV: Persistent truncus arteriosus

### Investigations

*Electrocardiography.* There is evidence of LV hypertrophy (because of the dominance of LV forces), left-axis deviation, and RA enlargement.

*Chest radiography.* This is not generally diagnostic.

*Echocardiography.* The atretic and fibrotic TV, ASD, VSD, size of the RV, and the relation of the great arteries (VA discordance might be present) should be evaluated.

*Cardiac catheterization.* Catheterization is not necessary for diagnosis. It is usually performed to measure PA pressure if the patient is a candidate for palliative or univentricular repair surgery.

*Surgical management.* Patients cannot undergo biventricular corrective surgery, and surgical options are palliative shunts or univentricular repair (Fontan and total cavopulmonary connection operations).[3–5]

### Hypoplastic left heart syndrome

Hypoplastic left heart syndrome (HLHS) consists of an anatomic spectrum of left-sided hypoplastic lesions, including varying degrees of mitral stenosis (from mild stenosis to atresia), LV hypoplasia, varying degrees of aortic valve stenosis, ascending and aortic arch hypoplasia, and coarctation. Systemic circulation is duct dependent, and patients become highly symptomatic as the duct starts to constrict. Prostaglandins should be started after birth, and the patient is scheduled for staged palliative surgery. The ECG shows right-axis deviation in HLHS.[3]

### Double-inlet ventricles

In the anomaly double-inlet ventricles, one ventricle is functionally dominant, and drainage through one AV valve plus more than 50% through the other AV valve is received by the dominant ventricle. Electrocardiographic forces depend on the dominant ventricle morphology. The dominant ventricle is generally connected to the rudimentary ventricle by a VSD. Surgical interventions include insertion of palliative shunts and the Fontan operation.[3]

### Isomerism

Isomerism consists of either bilateral right-sidedness or bilateral left-sidedness.

In bilateral right-sidedness (asplenia syndrome), both atria have the RA morphology, both lungs are trilobed, the liver is located midline, and the spleen is small or does not exist. The aorta and IVC are both located to the right of the spine.

In bilateral left-sidedness, both atria have the LA morphology and both lungs have the anatomy of the left lung. The patient has polysplenia and a frequently interrupted IVC with hemiazygos continuation. The sinus node is commonly absent, and P waves are generated from various atrial sites.

Atrioventricular septal defect is a common cardiac anomaly in both isomerism types, but the unbalanced type (RV dominant) and accompanying DORV are more often seen in right isomerism.[2–5]

### Outflow Tract Lesions

#### Left ventricular outflow tract lesions

Left ventricular outflow tract lesions include valvular, subvalvular, and supravalvular aortic stenosis and aortic coarctation.

**Congenital aortic valve stenosis.** This lesion is generally due to cusp fusion and thickening, resulting in bicuspid or monocuspid valves. The presence of associated anomalies should be considered. The ECG shows increased QRS voltage and LV hypertrophy. Interventional options are balloon valvuloplasty in earlier ages and surgical valve replacement. Mean Doppler aortic gradient or peak-to-peak gradients at catheterization greater than 50 mmHg in symptomatic patients and 60 mmHg in asymptomatic individuals are usually considered indications for intervention.

**Subaortic stenosis.** Subaortic stenosis is usually seen in the form of a discrete fibrous or fibromuscular ridge or ring that obstructs the LV outflow tract below the aortic valve (Fig. 33.22). Physical examination may reveal an ejection-type systolic murmur in the left sternal border without an ejection click. The ECG shows evidence of LVH. For echocardiography, the parasternal long-axis view best shows the anatomic type of subvalvular stenosis.

Subaortic stenosis is generally progressive. Surgery is indicated when there is a mean Doppler gradient of 30 mmHg, peak instantaneous gradient of greater than 50 mmHg, or progressive aortic regurgitation with considerable dilation of LV and an ejection fraction less than 55%. Because of the possibility of recurrence of stenosis after resection or the development of aortic regurgitation, patients should have a lifelong follow-up.

**Supravalvular aortic stenosis.** The fixed stenosis starts above the sinus of Valsalva and can extend distally to various lengths. The origin of the coronary arteries, which is proximal to obstruction, is subject to high

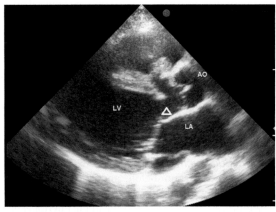

FIG. 33.22  Subaortic web with resultant obstruction in LVOT.

intra-LV pressure and thus prone to atherosclerotic or obstructive lesions, ectasia, or aneurysm formation. Supravalvular aortic stenosis is common in patients with Williams syndrome.

On physical examination, systolic pressure may be higher in the right arm than the left (Coanda effect) because of preferential blood flow to the brachiocephalic artery. Another finding is systolic thrill extending to the carotid arteries in the suprasternal notch. An ejection click is absent. The ECG shows LV hypertrophy and secondary ST-T changes. The presence of ischemic changes should be kept in mind. Narrowing in the supraaortic region can be seen by 2D echocardiography, but in long-segment stenosis, the precise pressure gradient measurement might be difficult.

Cardiac catheterization could be performed for precise gradient measurement. Delineation of coronary arteries should be done cautiously and preferably after evaluation of the coronary arteries by CT or CMR because of the possibility of ostial obstructive lesions. In patients with Williams syndrome, imaging of the entire aorta and pulmonary arteries is necessary because stenosis in the aortic branch (including renal arteries) and the peripheral pulmonary branch is common in this group.

When the patient is symptomatic or echocardiography shows a mean gradient greater than 50 mmHg and peak gradient greater than 70 mmHg, surgery is indicated.

**Aortic coarctation.** Aortic coarctation is a focal narrowing in the descending aorta caused by a shelf in the posterior aortic wall, usually after the left subclavian artery in the region of the ductus arteriosus. A bicuspid aortic valve is seen commonly. Presenting complaints may be hypertension, exertional headaches, or leg fatigue.

Physical examination reveals a delayed femoral pulse compared with the brachial pulse, and distal pulses might be weak. On auscultation a bruit might be detected in the left interscapular space, which is due to either well-developed collateral arteries or the coarctation. Other findings depend on the presence of a bicuspid aortic valve with stenosis or regurgitation. Aneurysm of the intracranial arteries might accompany coarctation.

*Electrocardiography.* Evidence of LV hypertrophy is seen on the ECG.

*Chest radiography.* The proximal descending aorta might show dilation before and after stenosis and together with the indentation at the coarctation site resembles a "3 sign." Rib notching in the inferior aspect of the third to ninth posterior ribs is due to collaterals.

*Echocardiography.* Narrowing and an increased gradient with a diastolic tail at the coarctation site are seen in the suprasternal view. The flow of the abdominal aorta has a slow and decreased upstroke.

*Computed tomography and chest magnetic resonance imaging.* These are helpful in delineating the anatomy and planning for intervention.

*Cardiac catheterization.* Catheterization is performed for measurement of gradients across the coarctation site and coarctation balloon dilation and stenting.

*Interventional options.* Significant coarctation is defined as a gradient equal to or greater than 20 mmHg across the coarctation site. Sometimes no significant gradient is detected because of an abundance of collaterals, and intervention is performed if there is systemic hypertension plus imaging or angiographic anatomic evidence of considerable narrowing in the aorta and significant flow through collateral arteries.

First-line therapy is percutaneous stenting, especially in focal coarctation. The long segment, tortuous, interruption and hypoplasia, and other anatomies not amenable to catheter interventions are referred for surgery. Lifelong follow-up should be performed for hypertension, restenosis, and interval imaging after surgical repair for aneurysm formation or restenosis. Guidelines recommend CT or magnetic resonance imaging in 5-year intervals or less after coarctation repair based on preoperative and postoperative anatomic findings.[2–5,9,10]

### Right ventricular outflow tract lesions

Congenital obstruction of the RVOT may be subvalvular, valvular, or supravalvular. Subvalvular stenosis is either infundibular (as commonly seen in ToF) or subinfundibular (with greater distance from the pulmonic valve).

In subinfundibular stenosis or double-chambered right ventricle (DCRV), aberrant anomalous muscle bundles divide the RV into two proximal (high-pressure) and distal (low-pressure) chambers. VSDs (usually small and perimembranous type) are seen commonly. In DCRV obstruction may be progressive.

### Investigations

*Physical examination.* An ejection systolic murmur might be audible in the upper left sternal border or covered by the systolic murmur of VSD. Right ventricular heave may be present.

*Electrocardiography.* The ECG commonly shows RV hypertrophy.

*Echocardiography.* The anomalous muscle bundle and turbulence in the RVOT are seen, especially in the precordial short-axis view. VSDs should be sought.

Superimposition of VSD flow might result in overestimate of the measured gradients.

*Cardiac catheterization.* Catheterization is performed for precise measurement of RVOT gradients.

**Indications for intervention.** These include RV systolic pressure in the proximal chamber greater than 60% of systemic blood pressure, mean Doppler gradient of greater than 40 mmHg and peak gradient greater than 60 mmHg by echocardiography across the obstruction site in asymptomatic patients and mean greater than 30 mmHg and peak greater than 50 mmHg in symptomatic patients, or VSD with a significant left-to-right shunt. The DCRV is repaired surgically by resection of aberrant muscle bundles and VSD closure.

## Valvular Pulmonary Stenosis

Valvular PS has three types:
- Nondysplastic valvular PS: The pulmonary valve is thick and domed with mobile leaflets and poststenotic dilation.
- Dysplastic pulmonary valve: The leaflets are myxomatous, thick, and dysplastic with little mobility and no commissural fusion. The annulus is small, and there is no poststenotic dilation. This type of PS is common in Noonan syndrome.
- Bicuspid or unicuspid pulmonary valve: This type is more common in ToF.

The PS is mild when the gradient across the valve is less than 30 mmHg, moderate when it is 30–50 mmHg, and severe when it is greater than 50 mmHg.

### Investigations

*Physical examination.* The patient may be asymptomatic or complain of dyspnea or exercise intolerance. In severe PS a loud systolic ejection murmur can be heard. Right ventricular lift and elevated jugular venous pressure may be present.

*Electrocardiography.* In severe stenosis, right-axis deviation and RV hypertrophy are seen.

*Chest radiography.* In nondysplastic valvular PS (first type mentioned above), the main PA is dilated and PBF is normal to reduced.

*Echocardiography.* This modality is useful in determining the gradients and type of stenosis and planning interventional procedures.

*Management.* The initial intervention of choice in nondysplastic valvular PS is balloon valvotomy. In asymptomatic patients mean Doppler gradients greater than 40 mmHg and peak Doppler gradients greater than 60 mmHg are indications for intervention, whereas in symptomatic patients mean gradients greater than 30 mmHg and peak gradients greater than 50 mmHg are considered significant. If balloon valvotomy is planned, pulmonary regurgitation should be less than moderate. For most dysplastic pulmonary valves, subvalvular and supravalvular stenosis, hypoplastic annulus, and the presence of associated cardiac lesions, surgery is preferred.

In peripheral (branch) pulmonary stenosis, percutaneous intervention is indicated when there is a greater than 50% diameter reduction or RV systolic pressure is greater than 50 mmHg. Percutaneous intervention is the first choice for focal stenosis.[2–5,7,9]

## Other Valvular and Miscellaneous Lesions
### Ebstein's anomaly

The main features in Ebstein's anomaly are apical displacement of the septal (and commonly posterior) tricuspid valve leaflets and tethering and redundancy of the anterior, resulting in TR of varying degrees and atrialization of the parts of the RV. The functional RV may be very small, and the RA is enlarged (Fig. 33.23). In about 50% of patients, ASD or PFO is seen with right-to-left shunt when RA pressure becomes higher than LA pressure. Right-sided accessory pathways are also frequently encountered.

Patients generally complain of exercise intolerance, cyanosis (caused by right-to-left shunting), palpitation, or right-sided heart failure symptoms. Paradoxic embolism is also a possibility.

### Investigations

*Physical examination.* Despite the presence of severe TR, the jugular venous pressure is usually normal

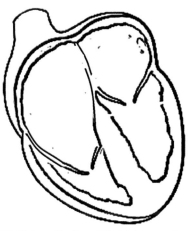

FIG. 33.23 Schematic view of Ebstein's anomaly of the right ventricle.

because of the compliant and enlarged RA. Central or peripheral cyanosis may be present. On auscultation a loud (T2 component), wildly split first heart sound (sail sound) and a holosystolic murmur of TR that increases with inspiration are heard.

*Electrocardiography.* Tall and peaked P waves (Himalayan P waves) and a prolonged PR interval are seen (unless there is PR shortening caused by preexcitation). The ECG may be low voltage with an RBBB pattern and QRS prolongation.

*Chest radiography.* Cardiomegaly with a globular heart and reduced pulmonary flow is observed. The great arteries (aortic arch and PA trunk) appear small.

*Echocardiography.* Apical displacement of the TV septal leaflet (more than $0.8 \text{ mm/m}^2$ distance between MV and TV), tethering, fenestration, and redundancy of the anterior TV leaflet are seen. The presence of ASD or PFO, TR severity, and RV function should be considered. Measurement of functional to anatomic RV ratio is important for surgical decision-making (Fig. 33.24).

*Cardiac catheterization.* Catheterization is performed if the measurement of pulmonary arterial pressure or shunt quantification is needed.

**Timing of intervention.** Intervention is indicated when the patient is symptomatic with deterioration in functional capacity (which could be assessed by an exercise test); if there is a progressive increase in RV size and dysfunction; if cyanosis ($SO_2$ less than 90%) or

paradoxic embolism occurs; or if an increased cardiothoracic ratio (greater than 60%) is seen on chest radiography or progressive cardiomegaly is found.

During surgery, the TV is repaired or replaced and interatrial communications are closed. If the functional RV is small (less than 35% of anatomic RV), the addition of a bidirectional Glenn shunt or a Fontan-type operation might be indicated.[3,5]

### Congenital mitral valve stenosis and regurgitation

Conditions include parachute MV, MV arcade, accessory MV tissue, supravalvular ring, and double-orifice MV. Congenital MV regurgitation is due mainly to a cleft or dysplastic MV.

### Cortriatriatum

In cortriatriatum, an abnormal fibromuscular diaphragm divides the LA into two chambers. The proximal chamber receives the PV and is connected to the rest of LA through an orifice, thus mimicking mitral stenosis (Fig. 33.25).

### Pulmonary arteriovenous fistulas

Pulmonary arteriovenous fistulas are abnormal communications between PA branches and PVs so that capillaries are bypassed. Many patients are asymptomatic, but cyanosis, dyspnea, and paradoxical emboli may occur. Treatment options in symptomatic patients include interventional embolization or surgery.

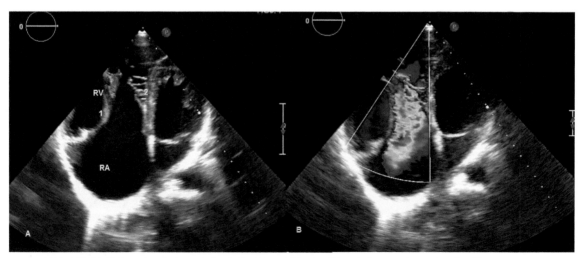

FIG. 33.24 Tethered and elongated anterior tricuspid leaflet (1) and displaced septal leaflet (2) with severe tricuspid regurgitation in Ebstein's anomaly.

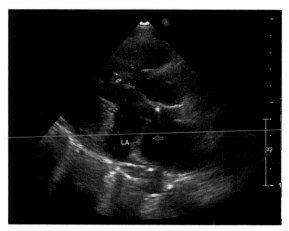

FIG. 33.25 Obstructive web in the left atrium or cortriatriatum.

### Vascular rings

In the vascular ring group of congenital defects, relations of the aortic arch or PA branches may be abnormal, or the vessels may produce a pressure effect on the esophagus or trachea. These abnormalities include right aortic arch with a left ductus, double aortic arch, retroesophageal descending aorta, abnormal origin of the right subclavian artery, and PA sling.

### Coronary-arteriovenous fistulas

An abnormal connection is present between coronary arteries and the PA (coronary-pulmonary fistulas), veins (coronary-arteriovenous fistulas), or cardiac chambers (coronary-cameral fistulas).

### Coronary abnormalities

Congenital anomalies occur in the origin, anatomy, course, and termination of coronary arteries. These anomalies could be isolated, but a variety of coronary abnormalities also accompany congenital heart defects, and these need to be evaluated and managed according to the underlying congenital anomaly.[3,5]

### Fontan Operation

In CHD there are two approaches for surgery: biventricular and univentricular repair. If patients do not have two ventricles with an acceptable size or have a large VSD resembling single-ventricle physiology, the Fontan procedure is chosen. These anomalies include tricuspid atresia, double-inlet ventricle, hypoplastic heart syndrome, and isomerism syndromes. Fontan is not a special procedure but rather a concept in which systemic veins are deviated to pulmonary arteries and systemic circulation is separated from the pulmonary circulation. This means that the RV is bypassed from circulation. Thus, in this procedure, there is no pump in the pulmonary circulation, and flow is completely streamlined. The mechanism for extending flow to the pulmonary arteries is pull and push, which means push by elevated pressure in the Fontan circuit and pull by systemic ventricle contraction, LA relaxation, and inspiration.

Fontan first performed the procedure in 1971 in a case of tricuspid atresia. The SVC was anastomosed to the RPA as a classic Glenn shunt, the RA appendage was anastomosed to the rest of the PA, the ASD was closed, and a homograft valve was inserted at the RA to PA anastomotic site and also in the IVC. These valves increased the risk of thrombosis. Two years later Kreutzer performed a procedure creating an atriopulmonary connection in which the RA appendage was anastomosed to PA branches.

In the classic Fontan procedure, the RA became dilated and a site for thrombosis and arrhythmic focus, so in the 1990s a modified procedure, the lateral tunnel technique, was developed in which a baffle and part of the RA wall were applied to direct blood from the IVC to the PA. In another modified procedure, the extracardiac Fontan or total cavopulmonary connection (TCPC), a Gore-Tex tube was used to connect the IVC to the RPA, and a bidirectional Glenn shunt was used for SVC flow to the RPA (Fig. 33.26).

### Investigations

**Physical examination.** In the patient after Fontan surgery, a quiet heart is expected. No murmur should be heard, and $S_1$ and $S_2$ are single. If a murmur is heard in these patients, it means a complication has happened.

**Electrocardiography.** Findings depend on the underlying anomaly. For example, in tricuspid atresia, left-axis deviation and signs of LV enlargement are seen.

**Chest radiography.** Again, findings depend on the primary pathologic condition, but overall, in these patients pulmonary vascular marking is decreased. In patients with an atriopulmonary connection, the right heart border bulges because of RA enlargement.

**Echocardiography.** This method is easy and the best modality for exact evaluation of patients after surgery (Fig. 33.27). Postsurgical complications should be evaluated by a combination of echocardiography and cardiac function. The Fontan circuit should be searched for

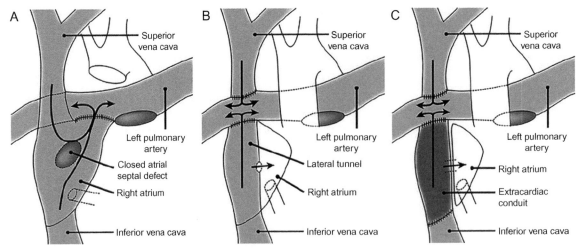

FIG. 33.26 Different types of the Fontan procedure.

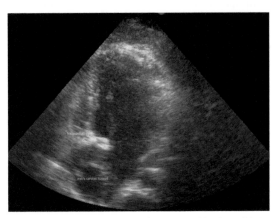

FIG. 33.27 Echocardiogram of a patient with tricuspid atresia who had undergone an extracardiac Fontan operation.

thrombosis, obstruction in the anastomotic site (IVC to conduit and PA) should be noted, and patency of the Glenn shunt should be checked. Flow in the IVC, SVC, and PA is biphasic and changes with respiration. In an atriopulmonary connection, flow is triphasic and retrograde flow by RA relaxation is seen. Detection of a gradient greater than 2 mmHg between IVC, and—conduit or conduit and—PA is important and a sign of stenosis. Flow should be laminar, and turbulent flow is a sign of obstruction. Systolic and diastolic function of the systemic ventricle should be evaluated closely. Normal diastolic function is important for optimal function of this circuit. Another parameter that is notable for assessment is systemic AV valve regurgitation. In the Fontan procedure surgeons

commonly create a fenestration in the conduit, which is a pop-off mechanism for the right-sided system and also increases preload, but may result in cyanosis. The fenestration should be found with echocardiography and the transpulmonary gradient measured; an acceptable range of the gradient is 5–8 mmHg.

**Computed tomography and chest magnetic resonance imaging.** CT and CMR are helpful in cases of suspected obstruction or thrombosis.

**Cardiac catheterization.** Catheterization is the gold standard for exact evaluation of pulmonary vascular resistance and pressure in the right-side circulation. It is performed when such interventions as stenting or closure of fenestration are planned.

### Fontan complications
*Arrhythmia.* Arrhythmias, especially atrial flutter and fibrillation, are one of the most common complications after Fontan surgery. The arrhythmia may be the consequence of abnormal hemodynamics, and also, they are deteriorated hemodynamic situation. Arrhythmias in Fontan patients are usually resistant to medical treatment. Treatment options are antiarrhythmic drugs, especially amiodarone and sotalol; direct-current shock; radiofrequency ablation; and Fontan conversion with a maze procedure. Ablation therapy is challenging, and the risk of recurrences for all treatment is high.

*Thrombosis and embolization.* Because of streamlined flow and the absence of pump function, the risk of thrombosis formation in Fontan circuit is increased, and fenestration raises the risk of paradoxical emboli. Pulmonary emboli may also occur. Anticoagulant drugs are used for prevention of and therapy for thrombosis and stroke. Warfarin therapy is recommended for post-Fontan patients with fenestration, thrombosis, and atrial tachyarrhythmia. Some recent studies showed that new oral anticoagulation could be used instead of warfarin in Fontan patients.

*Cyanosis.* One cause of cyanosis is right-to-left shunt via fenestration. Others are collateral formation, including venovenous collaterals, and pulmonary arteriovenous fistula.

*Fontan obstruction.* In most cases obstruction is due to thrombosis formation, but stenosis at the anastomotic site could be the result of Fontan circuit obstruction.

*Pulmonary vein compression and stenosis.* A dilated RA has a compressive effect on the pulmonary veins. This is seen most commonly in the right pulmonary veins and the atriopulmonary connection.

*Protein-losing enteropathy.* This devastating complication is the result of elevated pressure in the right circuit and enteric lymphangiectasia. In this situation, proteins and lymphocytes cannot be reabsorbed in the intestine and are excreted in the stool. Alpha$_1$-antitrypsin levels are elevated in stool, and the patient has lymphopenia and hypoproteinemia. Protein-losing enteropathy is resistant to medical treatment. Recommended drug therapy includes inotropes, medium-change triglycerides, albumin, diuretic therapy, octreotide, and corticosteroid therapy. Fontan conversion is a surgical approach, and the final step is cardiac transplantation.[2–4]

*Hepatic dysfunction.* Elevated central venous and portal vein pressure may cause some degree of liver fibrosis and hepatic function derangement.

*Plastic bronchitis.* This is an extremely rare but fatal complication after a Fontan operation.

## REFERENCES

1. Eidem BW, Cetta F, O'Leary PW, eds. *Echocardiography in Pediatric and Adult Congenital Heart Disease.* 1st ed. Philadelphia: Lippincott Williams & Wilkins; 2010.
2. Allen HD, Driscoll DJ, Shaddy RE, Moss Feltes TF. *Heart Adams' Disease in Infants, Children, and Adolescents: Including the Fetus and Young Adult.* 8th ed. Philadelphia: Lippincott Williams & Wilkins; 2013.
3. Mann DL, Zipes DP, Libby P, Bonow RO. *Braunwald's Heart Disease: A Textbook of Cardiovascular Medicine.* 9th ed. Philadelphia: Elsevier Health Sciences; 2014.
4. Warnes CA, Williams RG, Bashore TM, et al. ACC/AHA 2008 guidelines for the management of adults with congenital heart disease: a report of the American College of Cardiology/American Heart Association Task Force on Practice Guidelines (Writing Committee to Develop Guidelines for the Management of Adults With Congenital Heart Disease). *J Am Coll Cardiol.* 2008;52: e143–e263.
5. Vijayalakshmi IB, Syamasundar Rao P, Chugh RA. *A Comprehensive Approach to Congenital Heart Diseases.* 1st ed. New Delhi: Jaypee Brothers Medical Publishers; 2013.
6. Saedi S, Aliramezany M, Khajali Z, Sanati HR. Transcatheter closure of large atrial septal defects: a single-center experience. *Res Cardiovasc Med.* 2018;7(3):148.
7. Wong CP, Miller-Hance WC. *Transesophageal Echocardiography for Congenital Heart Disease.* 1st ed. London: Springer; 2014.
8. Khajali Z, Mohammadzadeh S, Maleki M, et al. Fibrinolytic therapy for mechanical pulmonary valve thrombosis. *Pediatr Cardiol.* 2015;36(1):171–176.
9. Baumgartner H, Bonhoeffer P, De Groot NM, et al. ESC guidelines for the management of grown-up congenital heart disease (new version 2010). *Eur Heart J.* 2010;31: 2915–2957. ehq249.
10. Saedi S, Aliramezany M, Moosavi J, Saedi T. Successful thoracic endovascular aortic repair for post-coarctoplasty aneurysm. *Egypt Heart J.* 2020;72(1):1–5.

# CHAPTER 34

# Venous Thromboembolism

FARSHAD SHAKERIAN[a] • PARHAM SADEGHIPOUR[b] •
AZITA HAJ HOSSEIN TALASAZ[c]
[a]Cardiovascular Intervention Research Center, Rajaie Cardiovascular, Medical & Research Center, Iran University of Medical Sciences, Tehran, Iran, [b]Rajaie Cardiovascular, Medical & Research Center, Iran University of Medical Sciences, Tehran, Iran, [c]Tehran Heart Center, Tehran University of Medical Sciences, Tehran, Iran

## KEY POINTS

- Venous thromboembolism (VTE)—consisting of pulmonary embolism (PE) and deep venous thrombosis (DVT)—is a common cardiovascular disease and step behind myocardial infarction and stroke and is among major public health concern.
- VTE is reported to be the second most common cardiovascular complication, might affect the hospitalization course of various medical and surgical illness, and is considered the second cause of a prolonged hospital stay.
- Major surgery and trauma, active cancer, immobility, hospitalization for acute medical illness, and pregnancy are among the most important clinical risk factors for VTE.
- Sign and symptoms of both PE and DVT might be too unspecific and the definite diagnosis demands the implication of accurate clinical risk stratification tools and diagnostic modalities.
- Although various novel therapies have been introduced for different situation in VTE, anticoagulation is still the cornerstone of the treatment.
- VTE is a preventable disease, and a prophylactic strategy has proven to reduce significantly the burden of the disease.

## INTRODUCTION

Deep venous thrombosis (DVT) of the upper and lower limbs and pulmonary embolism (PE) are among the most common and important thrombotic accidents of the venous circulation [i.e., venous thromboembolism (VTE)]. Today both conditions are among the major public health concerns: they have a considerable mortality rate, might affect the hospitalization course of various medical and surgical illness, causing significant "permanent work-related disability," and consequently have a great impact on the health economics. It should be added that prevention strategies showed very promising results on decreasing the mentioned impact.

In this chapter we review the different aspects of DVT and PE, emphasizing on the practical points of their management.

## EPIDEMIOLOGY

VTE is a common cardiovascular disease and a step behind myocardial infarction and stroke.[1] The annual incidence risk of VTE is estimated from 104 to 183 per 100,000 person-years in population with European origin and the estimated incidence of PE (with or without DVT) and DVT alone is between 29 and 78, and 45–117 per 100,000 person-years, respectively.[2] VTE occurrence increases with age[3] and interestingly, the contribution of PE on VTE incidence increases with age.[4] The prevalence in both sex varies by age: during childbearing years (16–44 years), the condition is more common in women, whereas it becomes more frequent in men during the following years.[2] VTE is reported to be the second most common cardiovascular complication[5]: a great proportion of hospitalized surgical and medical patients were complicated by VTE each year—4,000,000 and 8,000,000 patients, respectively.[6] Consequently, VTE significantly influences the clinical course of hospitalized patients and it is considered to be the second cause of the excess length of hospital stay (LOS), and the third one in excess mortality.[5]

## CLINICAL RISK FACTORS

VTE is a multifactorial disease, and various risk factors have been reported to impact its occurrence. A large population-based case–control study cited major surgery, active cancer (with or without concurrent chemotherapy), neurological disease with lower-limb paresis, hospitalization for acute medical illness, nursing-home residence, trauma or fracture, pregnancy or puerperium, oral contraception (OCP), and obesity as independent risk factors for VTE.[7] Other studies have also reported that age, varicose veins, central vein catheterization, or transvenous pacemaker placement, prior superficial vein thrombosis, urinary tract infection, increased baseline plasma fibrin D-dimer, family history of VTE and long haul (>4–6 h) air travel might potentially increase the risk of VTE.[3] Both hospitalization for medical illness and surgical hospitalization have almost similar proportion for VTE (22% vs 24%, respectively).[8] Age ≥65 years, surgical procedures like neurosurgery, major orthopedic surgery of the leg, renal transplantation, cardiovascular surgery, and thoracic, abdominal, or pelvic surgery for cancer, obesity and poor physical status are among risk factors increasing VTE in patients undergoing surgery.[2] Also for patients hospitalized with acute medical illness, several risk factors have been reported to increase the rate of VTE during their hospitalization: older age, obesity, previous VTE, thrombophilia, cancer, recent trauma or surgery, tachycardia, acute myocardial infarction or stroke, leg paresis, congestive heart failure, chronic obstructive pulmonary disease, prolonged immobilization (bed rest), acute infection or rheumatological disorder, hormone therapy, central venous catheter, admission to an intensive or coronary care unit, white blood cell count, and platelet count.[2] Several prediction models have been designed for predicting the occurrence of VTE in both surgical and medical population, but none of them reached acceptable generalizability and validity.[9] Patients with active cancer consist for approximately 20% of all VTE incident[10] and patients with cancers of the brain, pancreas, ovaries, colon, stomach, lungs, kidneys, or bones, are more susceptible to complications by VTE than other locations.[11] In addition, patients with metastasis and also those receiving chemotherapies are even at higher risk of venous thromboembolic complications.[11]

OCP, hormone therapy, pregnancy, and puerperium influence the incidence of VTE in women at childbearing age.[3] Regarding OCP, first-generation and third-generation oral contraceptives have higher risks than the second generation.[12] Hormone therapy increases two- to fourfold the risk of VTE.[13] Of note, intrauterine hormone-releasing devices and also progesterone-only OCPs do not result in a significant increase in VTE risk.[14] Pregnant women have a fourfold increased risk compared to a nonpregnant woman and the incidence of pregnancy-associated VTE is approximately 200 events per 100,000 women-years.[15] During the postpartum period, the risk of VTE is fivefold higher compared to pregnancy, which shows the importance of postpartum care.[15] Superficial vein thrombosis, history of varicose veins, urinary tract infection, preexisting diabetes mellitus, stillbirth, obesity, obstetric hemorrhage, preterm delivery, and delivery by cesarean section are among most important risk factors which increased the risk of VTE during pregnancy and the postpartum period.[16]

Among known clinical risk factors predisposing VTE, there are some anatomic variations also, which might increase the risk of VTE. May–Thurner's syndrome is the most famous one. Described firstly by May and Thurner in 1957, the syndrome is classically defined by a fibrotic and vascular thickening in the left common iliac vein which is the result of the compressive force of the right common iliac artery.[17] Other anatomic sites have also been recognized. Its incidence is reported between 18% and 49%; however, only 2%–3% of the affected population present with DVT.[18] The situation is more prevalent in women and commonly its acute presentation occurred in the third and fourth decade of life.[18] Venous stenting showed promising results in the treatment of VTE associated with May–Thurner syndrome.[19]

Among genetic cause of thrombophilia, factor V Leiden and the prothrombin mutation are the most common condition that increases the risk of VTE by 10- and 2-fold, respectively.[20] The antiphospholipid syndrome considered the most common form of acquired thrombophilia, might present with several episodes of VTE.[1] Of note, the potential risk of inherited thrombophilia increased remarkably by other risk factors like obesity, tobacco smoking, cancer, OCP, and pregnancy.[3]

Lastly, there is an important overlap between the clinical risk factors VTE and atherothrombosis (Fig. 34.1)[21]: a meta-analysis reviewing the data of over 60,000 patients with VTE has revealed that the relative risk for VTE was 2.3 for obesity, 1.5 for hypertension, 1.4 for diabetes mellitus, 1.2 for cigarette smoking, and 1.2 for hypercholesterolemia.[22] This overlap showed that with an integrated preventive approach, clinicians can considerably decrease the cardiovascular burden of their patients.[21] In a large randomized controlled trial (RCT), on healthy individuals with low-density lipoprotein (LDL) cholesterol levels below than 130 mg/dL and high-sensitivity C-reactive protein levels above 2.0 mg/L, rosuvastatin decrease significantly, the incidence of VTE.[23] In a prespecified analysis of the ODYSSEY trial, the addition of alirocumab in patients with the recent acute coronary syndrome has decreased the risk of VTE and peripheral vascular diseases events.[24]

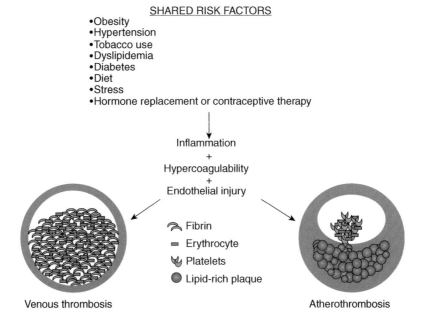

FIG. 34.1 Overlap between the clinical risk factors venous thromboembolism and atherothrombosis.[21]

Recent European Society of Cardiology (ESC) PE guideline categorized patients' risk factors into four groups based on their risk for VTE recurrence and preferred the mentioned classification compared to traditional "provoked" and "unprovoked" term: (1) patients with "a strong (major) transient or reversible risk factor," which can strongly be attributed to the current acute episode; (2) patients in whom the current acute episode might be partly attributed to "a weak (minor) transient or reversible risk factor," or the persistence of "nonmalignant risk factor for thrombosis"; (3) patients with no identifiable risk factors; (4) patients with a history of more than one episode of VTE, and also those "with a major persistent prothrombotic condition" like antiphospholipid antibody syndrome; and (5) patients with active cancer (Table 34.1).[27]

## PATHOPHYSIOLOGY OF VTE

VTE pathophysiology stands on three pillars of inflammation, endothelial injury, and hypercoagulability state ("Virchow's Triad"). In almost all patients at least one and, more often, more are in play (Fig. 34.2).[28]

In many instances of the so-called "unprovoked" VTE after careful study some abnormality can be found. The high recurrence rate of VTE in the absence of treatment together with the importance of inflammatory markers implies a systemic inflammatory disorder behind the scene.[27]

Obstruction of the affected veins (most often in legs) causes impaired drainage (edema) and inflammation in the area causes pain. Apart from pain edema and sometimes red discoloration of the limb, by far the most important consequence of VTE is PE.

Acute PE affects both the circulation system and gas exchange altogether. Right ventricular (RV) failure because of pressure overload is mainly the cause of mortality in massive PE.

Increase in PAP occurs only if more than about 50% of the cross-sectional area of the pulmonary artery circulation gets occluded by thromboemboli.[29] Release of mediators like thromboxane A2 and serotonin induces vasoconstriction and further increases the PAP. This part of PH can be decreased by vasodilators. So, a combination of anatomical obstruction and vascular constriction exists in patients with PE.[30]

The acute increase of pulmonary vascular resistance culminates in RV dilation, it alters the RV contractility by the Frank–Starling phenomenon. RV pressure and volume increase and leads to wall tension increase and stretching of the myocytes.

Activation of the neurohumoral pathways (mainly sympathetic) leads to an increase in cardiac contractility and heart rate. These mechanisms plus systemic

**TABLE 34.1**
**Clinical Risk Factors for Occurrence of Pulmonary Emboli**

| Estimated Risk for Long-Term Recurrence[a] | Risk Factor Category for Index PE | Examples[b] |
|---|---|---|
| Low (<3% per year) | Major transient or reversible factors associated with >10-fold increased risk for the index VTE event (compared to patients without the risk factor) | • Surgery with general anesthesia for >30 min<br>• Confined to bed in hospital (only bathroom privileges) for ≥3 days due to an acute illness, or acute exacerbation of a chronic illness<br>• Trauma with fractures |
| Intermediate (3%–8% per year) | Transient or reversible factors Associated with ≤10-fold increased risk for first (index) VTE | • Minor surgery (general anesthesia for <30 min)<br>• Admission to hospital for <3 days with an acute illness<br>• Estrogen therapy/contraception<br>• Pregnancy or puerperium<br>• Confined to bed out of hospital for ≥3 days with an acute illness<br>• Leg injury (without factor) associated with reduced mobility for ≥3 days<br>• Long-haul fight |
| | Nonmalignant persistent risk factors | • Inflammatory bowel disease<br>• Active autoimmune disease |
| | No identifiable risk factor | |
| High (>8% per year) | | • Active cancer<br>• One or more previous episodes of VTE in the absence of a major transient of reversible factor<br>• Antiphospholipid antibody syndrome |

PE, pulmonary embolism; VTE, venous thromboembolism.
[a]If anticoagulation is discontinued after the first 3 months.[25,26]
[b]The categorization of risk factors for the index VTE event is in line with that proposed by the International Society on Thrombosis and Hemostasis.[25]

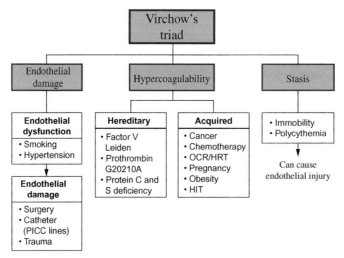

FIG. 34.2 Virchow's triad.

vasoconstriction induced by catecholamines, tries to compensate for the increase in pulmonary artery pressure and maintain systemic blood pressure (BP). Right ventricle is thin and unable to cope with high pulmonary pressures acutely so it tries to prolong its contraction time which forces the septum toward left and deteriorates left ventricular filling. Generally, it cannot produce pressures higher than 40 mmHg (mean) and if this pressure would not be enough, BP drops and cardiogenic shock happens (Fig. 34.3).[31] High RV pressures may lead to right bundle branch block (RBBB) that exacerbates ventricular dyssynchrony. The desynchronization of the ventricles may be exacerbated by the development of RBBB.

A massive neurohumoral response causes an increase in RV wall tension, increase in systemic vascular resistance, and in extreme cases even some sorts of apoptosis.[32]

Sometimes later deterioration (in terms of days) happens in the situation of patients which can be explained by the recurrence of PE or neurohumoral effect.[33]

In acute PE, the higher the levels of biomarkers of injury for cardiac myocytes (e.g., troponin) the higher is mortality. It further shows the role of RV myocardial injury as a pathophysiologic mechanism in this situation.[34] Fig. 34.3 shows the abovementioned in brief.

If respiratory failure happens in PE, is often secondary to circulatory collapse.[35]

Respiratory failure occurs secondary to circulatory compromise. Flow is reduced in obstructed vessels and increased in open capillary bed while ventilation is the same in both regions so ventilation–perfusion mismatch occurs. Decreased cardiac output also contributes to the desaturation of venous blood. All result in hypoxemia. Right to left shunting which occurs in one-third of patients via patent foramen ovale aggravates hypoxemia and can even cause paradoxical emboli and stroke.

In small, hemodynamically insignificant emboli alveolar hemorrhage occurs because of tiny pulmonary infarctions.

Its main significance is the point that it can be harbinger of a later coming larger or massive PE.

## APPROACH TO PATIENTS WITH ACUTE DVT
### History and Physical Examination (Table 34.2)

The most common symptoms of patients presented with acute DVT include swelling, pain, and discoloration of the affected extremity. There is no specific relation between the site of the symptoms and the location of thrombosis. The patient should be asked about the

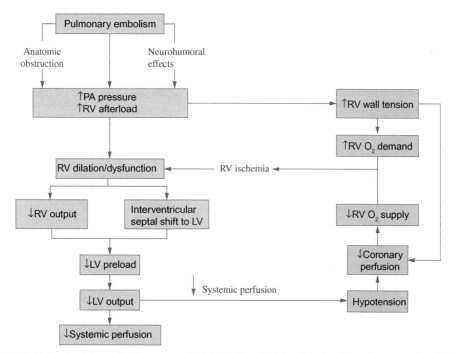

FIG. 34.3 Pathophysiology of pulmonary emboli. *LV,* left ventricle/ventricular; *PA,* pulmonary artery; *RV,* right ventricle/ventricular.

**TABLE 34.2**
**Most Common Symptoms and Signs of Pulmonary Embolism**

**SYMPTOMS**

Otherwise unexplained dyspnea

Chest pain, either pleuritic or atypical

Anxiety

Cough

**SIGNS**

Tachypnea

Tachycardia

Low-grade fever

Left parasternal lift

Jugular venous distension

Tricuspid regurgitant murmur

Accentuated $P_2$

Hemoptysis

Leg edema, erythema, tenderness

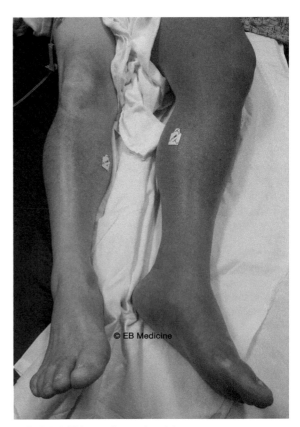

FIG. 34.4 Phlegmasia cerulea dolens.

potential clinical risk factors of VTE, emphasizing on a history of immobility, recent surgery, malignancies, and previous VTE. Also, symptoms duration and the intensity of the symptoms are important factors for potential invasive therapies.

In the physical examination unilateral swelling or edema, warmth, tenderness, and erythema might be prominent. Superficial veins dilation might be inspected in the whole affected limb and also in the pelvic and lower abdomen area in more proximal DVT. Calf swelling and the difference in the calf diameter have potential value for ruling out the diagnosis.[36] The thrombosis might be massive and possibly affect the visceral vein (e.g., hepatic vein thrombosis, i.e., Budd–Chiari syndrome, or renal vein thrombosis, i.e., nephrotic syndrome); therefore, a systemic physical examination is warranted. The famous Homans sign that was described by pain behind the knee during the dorsiflexion of the foot, have limited sensitivity and specificity.[37]

In the extreme cases of acute proximal DVT, the compressive effect of the dilated vein might compromise the arterial flow and result in critical limb ischemia and possible limb loss.[38] Phlegmasia alba dolens manifest by a swollen and white extremity present during the early stage of compromise arterial flow. The situation could aggravate by severe swelling, cyanosis, and blue discoloration (i.e., phlegmasia cerulea dolens) (Fig. 34.4). Both situations need prompt and immediate treatment and have significant morbidity (limb loss) and mortality.[38]

It should be noted that symptoms and sign of DVT are too unspecific and consequently additional testing is mandatory.

**Differential Diagnosis**

Muscle strain, tear, or twisting injury to the leg, leg swelling in paralyzed extremities, obstructive lymph diseases, chronic venous insufficiency diseases, Baker cyst, cellulitis, knee abnormalities are the most common situation which might mimic DVT and present with leg pain and/or swelling.[39] It is important to notice that only a small number of patients evaluated for acute DVT have actually the disease; therefore an integrated approach for an accurate diagnosis will prevent further unnecessary treatment, especially inappropriate anticoagulation.[40]

## Diagnostic Modalities

### Clinical prediction tools

Several scoring systems have been introduced for prediction of DVT.[41] Probably, the Wells score is the most commonly used one (Table 34.3). The Wells scoring will categorize the evaluated patients into one of the low (0 or less point), moderate (1 or 2 points), and high (3 or greater points) probability.[42] The median negative predictive value of Wells score in the low test probability category was 96% in a review of 15 studies, while its positive predicting value was estimated 75% in the high-risk group.[43] The main limitation of the Wells score is its subjectivity and the possible interaction of personal interpretation of each criterion. Therefore, the scoring will be complete by other diagnostic modalities.

**D-dimer.** D-dimer or "the degradation product of cross-linked fibrin" is the main laboratory test used in the diagnosis of DVT. An amount of greater than 500 ng/mL will be detected in nearly all the subjects with acute DVT.[44] Consequently, the negative predictive value of the test is considerable (94%) but the test lacks an acceptable positive predictive value.[45] Therefore, basically, the test helps to rule out the diagnosis. In addition, various clinical scenario such as myocardial infarction, stroke, limb ischemia, disseminated intravascular coagulation, congestive heart failure, sepsis, malignancy, pregnancy, old age, and recent surgery or trauma might increase the

### TABLE 34.3
### Wells Score for Acute DVT[42]

| Clinical Features | Score |
|---|---|
| Active cancer (treatment ongoing or within the previous 6 months or palliative) | 1 |
| Paralysis, paresis, or recent plaster immobilization of the lower extremities | 1 |
| Recently bedridden for more than 3 days or major surgery, within 4 weeks | 1 |
| Localized tenderness along the distribution of the deep venous system | 1 |
| Entire leg swollen | 1 |
| Calf swelling by more than 3 cm when compared to the asymptomatic leg (measured below the tibial tuberosity) | 1 |
| Pitting edema (greater in the symptomatic leg) | 1 |
| Collateral superficial veins (nonvaricose) | 1 |
| Alternative diagnosis as likely or more likely than that of deep venous thrombosis | −2 |

serum level of D-dimer.[44] It is important to notice that a negative D-dimer test in a high-risk population may be insufficient as a single test, and incomplete for ruling out the diagnosis in this category of the patients.[46]

The specificity of D-dimer test lessens with age. Recently, the age-adjusted cutoff (age × 10 mg/L, for patients above 50 years) has been validated[47] and recommended by the ESC PE guideline.[27]

**Ultrasonography.** Compression ultrasonography (CUS) has been considered the noninvasive approach of choice in patients with suspected acute DVT. Abnormality in the venous compressibility is the main finding during CUS. The test is highly sensitive (>95%) and specific (>95%) and could be easily performed in emergency department by portable devices.[48] Nevertheless, the test has some limitations. Iliac veins are usually difficult to be examined by ultrasound and therefore isolated thrombi in the iliac veins might possibly be missed. Consequently, some guidelines recommend complete venous ultrasonography in which color Doppler study is added.[49] Color Doppler US increases the sensitivity but decreases the specificity.[50] US is difficult to apply in patients with limb deformities and plaster, and finally, a small number of patients might have initial negative results and might need a serial imaging test in the following days.[51]

**Magnetic resonance venography (MRV).** MRV is among the most accurate diagnostic modalities for detecting DVT. With a high specificity (98%) and sensitivity (100%), the test might have comparable results to the invasive method. The imaging might especially be useful in various conditions in which ultrasonography is undetermined (e.g., iliac vein thrombosis) or difficult to be performed (patients with plaster and leg deformities). The test is considered a perfect substitute for contrast venography in patients allergic to the contrast agent. High cost and expertise for test interpretation are among the important limitations of the modality. Also, injection of gadolinium might be restricted in patients with renal failure.[52]

**Contrast venography.** Contrast venography is still considered the gold standard for the diagnosis of DVT. Substituted by noninvasive methods, the test is rarely performed today for diagnostic-only purposes and is reserved for the equivocal situation and high clinical suspicion. The invasiveness and the use of contrast materials are among the main drawbacks. It is important to notice that the test is mandatory when invasive therapy is planned.[53]

## Practical Approach for Patients With Suspected DVT

The American Guideline of Chest Physician gives detailed recommendations regarding the diagnosis of DVT.[54] The guideline emphasizes the importance of choosing the appropriate diagnostic modalities according to the patient's pretest probability test (e.g., Wells scoring system). The guideline recommendation can be simplified in the following way. In a patient with a low test probability, both negative D-dimer and compression ultrasound will rule out the diagnosis. In patients with a higher pretest probability (moderate and high risk), a negative D-dimer is better to be accompanied by a negative ultrasound to rule out DVT. In patients with a high pretest probability, a negative compression ultrasound must be completed by other imaging modalities (MRV or contrast venography) or the ultrasound exam must be repeated in the following days. In pregnant patients suspected having DVT, the guideline suggests that compression ultrasound should be the initial test; in case of a negative ultrasound, the guideline suggests to repeat the test in the following days.[54]

ESC guideline has also suggested assessing the clinical probability (two-level modified Wells score) of each patient: patients categorized as "unlikely," a D-dimer test is recommended. For patients with "likely" criteria, complete US (CUS along with color Doppler) is recommended.[49]

At last, it should be noted that some more sophisticated diagnostic modalities like or emerging imaging methods like CT venography were not explained here due to their less applicability.

## Approach to Patients With Acute PE

The vast array of different presentations for PE makes its diagnosis notoriously difficult. It can easily be misdiagnosed as an acute coronary syndrome, exacerbation of heart failure, or almost any other cardiovascular disease. Its concomitant occurrence and presence as a cause of any exacerbation in all preexisting heart and lung condition make it more important. The best approach is to have PE in mind as a probable diagnosis and careful use of well-tested likelihood diagrams together with careful use of diagnostic tests.[55,56]

### Clinical presentation (Table 34.2)

There are no specific sign or symptom of PE. High clinical suspicion together with the use of probability diagrams and algorithms is the key not to miss it.[56]

The most prevalent symptom is dyspnea. Tachypnea and tachycardia are the most prevalent signs.

| TABLE 34.4 Differential Diagnosis of Pulmonary Embolism |
| --- |
| Anxiety, pleurisy, costochondritis |
| Pneumonia, bronchitis |
| Acute coronary syndromes |
| Pericarditis |
| Congestive heart failure |
| Aortic dissection |
| Idiopathic pulmonary hypertension |

In the extreme cases of massive PE syncope, shock or sudden cardiac arrest can happen, most often not heralded by chest pain. Significant chest pain in the setting of PE usually is a sign of more peripheral, smaller, and less important PE. The cause is often plural irritation so the pain can be severe and pleuritic in nature.

In cases of large PE acute pulmonary hypertension happens and all manifestations can be attributed to it: prominent jugular veins, right-sided heave and S3, and in severe cases of hypotension and shock.

Absence of any of the above criteria does not rule out PE. As it is a disease of recurrence, failure to identify an even small unimportant PE can end up in a later devastating massive one.

### Differential diagnosis

Almost all acute cardiovascular or lung diseases from acute myocardial infarction to pneumonia are on the list of its differential diagnosis. Any exacerbation in the condition of a chronic problem like heart failure or chronic pulmonary disease, especially in hospitalized or critically ill patients should warn of the occurrence of PE (Table 34.4).

### Diagnostic Modalities

#### Clinical prediction tools

Wells rules (Table 34.5) and Geneva rules (Table 34.6) have both been validated and have simplified versions for predicting the PE occurrence.[42,57] When a "two-level classification" was implicated, the percentage of patients whom PE was confirmed is about 12% in the PE-unlikely population.[57]

**D-dimer.** See above.

**Electrocardiogram.** Signs of right ventricular strain like S1Q3T3, S1S2S3, inverted T wave in right precordial leads, new RBBB may be seen. It also helps in ruling out other diagnoses like myocardial infarction.[58]

<table>
<tr><td colspan="2">

**TABLE 34.5**
Well's Score for Acute Pulmonary Emboli

</td></tr>
</table>

| Criterion | Scoring[a] |
|---|---|
| DVT symptoms or signs | 3 |
| An alternative diagnosis is less likely than PE | 3 |
| Heart rate >100 bpm | 1.5 |
| Immobilization of surgery within 4 weeks | 1.5 |
| Previous DVT or PE | 1.5 |
| Hemoptysis | 1 |
| Cancer treated within 6 months or metastatic | 1 |

[a]>4 score points, high probability; ≤4 score points, nonhigh probability.

**TABLE 34.6**
Geneva Risk and Revised Geneva Risk Score for Predicting Pulmonary Emboli[57]

| Items | CLINICAL DECISION RULE POINTS | |
|---|---|---|
| | Original Version | Simplified Version |
| Previous PE or DVT | 3 | 1 |
| Heart rate | | |
|   75–94 bpm | 3 | 1 |
|   ≥95 bpm | 5 | 2 |
| Surgery or fracture within the past month | 2 | 1 |
| Active cancer | 2 | 1 |
| Unilateral lower-limb pain | 3 | 1 |
| Pain on lower-limb deep venous palpitation and unilateral edema | 4 | 1 |
| Age >65 years | 1 | 1 |
| Clinical probability | | |
|   Three-level score | | |
|     Low | 0–3 | 0–1 |
|     Intermediate | 4–10 | 2–4 |
|     High | ≥11 | ≥5 |
|   Two-level score | | |
|     PE-unlikely | 0–5 | |
|     PE-likely | ≥6 | ≥3 |

**Imaging methods.** *Echocardiography:* Depending on the severity of PE, from RV dilation and dysfunction together with pulmonary hypertension to near normal echocardiography in small PE all can be seen. McConnell's sign (RV dysfunction with apical hyperkinesis or normal motion) is most often seen in large PE. RV/LV ratio of >1.0 and TAPSE <16 mm are the best indicators in patients with high-risk PE.[27]

*Chest Radiography:* It is not conspicuous and many times normal. Like ECG, it helps exclude another diagnosis like pneumonia. Near normal chest radiograph in a patient with shock can be due to massive PE.

*Lung Scanning:* The use of perfusion lung scan with or without ventilation scan using radioactive-labeled particles has been abandoned because of widespread use of far better CT angiography. Its limited indications now are in patients intolerant of radiocontrast (because of nephropathy or sensitivity) and pregnancy (its radiation is much lower than CT).

*Chest Computed Tomography:* It is now the most reliable test for PE. With new ultrafast detectors almost all clinically important PE can be diagnosed except for very small peripheral emboli. It visualizes other chest structures so, it also is useful for ruling out other diagnoses like pulmonary conditions as well.[59]

*Magnetic Resonance Angiography:* It has less diagnostic accuracy than CT and it is more expensive and time consuming. So it should be reserved for patients with special concerns for CT (pregnancy, contrast sensitivity, etc.).[60]

*Pulmonary Angiography:* Its use is now confined to patients undergoing invasive treatment approaches [catheter-directed thrombolysis (CDT), etc.]. Thrombus if visible is in the form of filling defect.

### Practical approach to patients with PE

As the treatment of PE expanded and the option of thrombolytic and invasive therapy has been suggested for high-risk PE and also selective case of intermediate-risk PE, accurate risk stratification seems to be mandatory. Generally, PE has been categorized into high-risk (massive), intermediate-risk (submassive), and low-risk PE (Table 34.7).[27,61,62] Clinical appearance and vital sign, cardiac biomarker and RV function have been implicated in this categorization. Interestingly, the ESC guideline has introduced the PESI classification for risk stratification (Table 34.8).[27] Also, ESC guideline has divided the intermediate-risk category into two groups of intermediate-high and intermediate-low.[27] RV dysfunction means the presence of at least one of the following criteria[61]:
1. RV dilation: RV/LV diameter >0.9

**TABLE 34.7**
Pulmonary Emboli Risk Stratification[61–63]

| | | RISK PARAMETERS AND SCORES | | | |
|---|---|---|---|---|---|
| Risk | Incidence | Shock or Hypotension | PESI Class III–V or sPESI >1 | RV Function | Cardiac Biomarker |
| High | 5% | + | +[*] | + | +[*] |
| Intermediate | | | | | |
| Intermediate-high | 25%–30% | − | + | Both positive | |
| Intermediate-low | | − | + | Either one positive | |
| Low | 65%–70% | + | − | − | − |

**TABLE 34.8**
Pulmonary Embolism Severity Index (PESI) and
Simplified PESI: Predictors of Prognostic Risk

| Age >80 years | Age in years |
|---|---|
| **PESI CRITERIA**[a] | |
| Male sex | +10 |
| History of cancer | +30 |
| History of heart failure | +10 |
| History of chronic lung disease | +10 |
| Heart rate ≥110 bpm | +20 |
| Systolic blood pressure <100 mm/Hg | +30 |
| Respiratory rate ≥30 breaths/min | +20 |
| Temperature <36°C | +20 |
| Altered mental status | +60 |
| Arterial oxygen saturation <90% | +20 |
| **SIMPLIFIED PESI**[b] **CRITERIA** | |
| Age >80 years | +1 |
| History of cancer | +1 |
| History of heart failure or chronic lung disease | +1 |
| Heart rate >110 bpm | +1 |
| Systolic blood pressure <100 mm/Hg | +1 |
| Arterial oxygen saturation <90% | +1 |

[a]Class I = ≤65; Class II = 66–85; Class III = 86–105; Class
IV = 106–125; Class V ≥ 125. In the PESI score, Classes I and II are
considered low risk, and Classes III–V are considered high risk.
[b]Patients with a score of 0 are considered to be at low risk for PE;
those with scores ≥1 are considered at high risk.

2. RV dysfunction
3. BNP (>90 pg/mL) nt-BNP (>500 pg/mL)
4. ECG changes showing RV strain

In addition, positive cardiac biomarkers (myocardial necrosis) are defined as elevation of troponin I (>0.4 ng/mL) or troponin T (>0.1 ng/mL).[61]

It is very important to have PE in mind and use scientifically proven algorithms (Figs. 34.5 and 34.6) even in cases remotely suspicious. In patients with hemodynamic instability or after successful resuscitation, the routine diagnostic approach might be challenging. In this situation, ESC guideline suggests an RV function assessment as the primary step. If the RV function is normal, it is unlikely for PE to be the cause of hemodynamic deterioration. However, in patients with RV dysfunction, pulmonary CTA should be proceeded if the patient's general condition allows us. If pulmonary CTA is not feasible, high-risk PE treatment (e.g., thrombolytic therapy) can be applied, due to its potential impact on patient's survival.

### PE and pregnancy

PE diagnosis during pregnancy and postpartum is difficult because symptoms overlap with normal pregnancy. D-dimer also goes above threshold in about 25% of normal pregnant women, which made the diagnosis of PE very challenging.[64] Although no clinical probability prediction rule has been validated specifically for PE in pregnancy, recently it has been shown that a low-risk prediction rule along with normal D-dimer has acceptable accuracy for ruling out PE in pregnancy.[65] However, a considerable number of patients will have a positive D-dimer test which necessitates further evaluation.[65,66] Imaging should be saved for suspicious cases with a priority of more safe modalities: in patients with stable

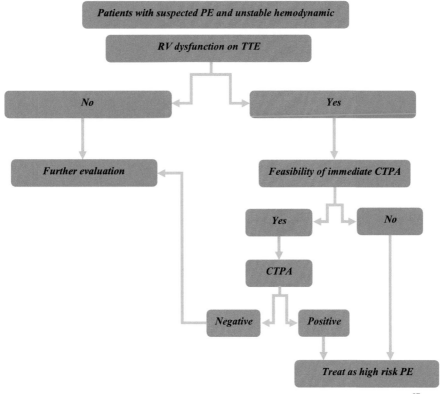

FIG. 34.5 Approach to the patient with hemodynamic instability pulmonary emboli.[27]

hemodynamic a positive venous US for acute DVT, omit further workup and necessitates treatment.[27] Otherwise, in patients with the normal US, pulmonary CTA or perfusion lung scan should proceed according to the availability and expertise (Fig. 34.7).[61]

High-risk PE should be treated like nonpregnant patients but thrombolytic therapy should not be used in peripartum period if alternatives are available.

## ADDITIONAL TEST FOR PATIENTS WITH ESTABLISHED VTE

### Screening for Hypercoagulable State

Since the beginning of modern management of VTE, the cost-effectiveness and true applicability of the identification of various inherited or acquired hypercoagulable state were debated. Studies have shown that the identification of an inheritable defect would not change the therapeutic or prophylactic treatment. In addition VTE

is multifactorial disease and mostly an acquired risk factor (e.g., surgery, immobility, pregnancy, etc.) plays a crucial role in the presentation of thrombotic events in patients with inherited hypercoagulability. Consequently, routine testing for hypercoagulable state is not warranted in patients with established VTE.[67] Some experts believe that the test might be useful in special groups of patients (Table 34.9). Common factors tested for inheritable coagulopathy are as follows: factor V Leiden (APC resistance), prothrombin gene mutation, protein C and S, and antithrombin. For antiphospholipid syndrome antiphospholipid antibodies (anticardiolipin and beta2-glycoprotein I antibodies) and lupus anticoagulant is commonly tested. It is important to notice that acute thrombotic state and the anticoagulation therapies affect the measurements of most of these factors, and it is usually advised to test for hypercoagulable state after a period of anticoagulation discontinuation of at least 2 weeks.[67]

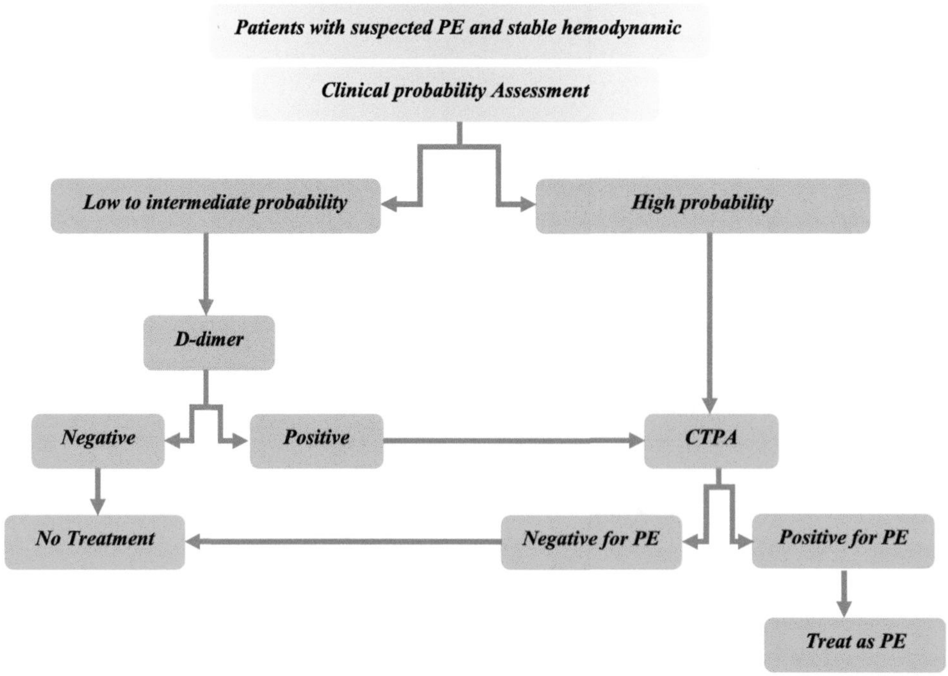

FIG. 34.6 Approach to the patient without hemodynamic instability pulmonary emboli.[27]

Finally, a common misconception is to order a hypercoagulable state screening for patients with the first episode of unprovoked VTE; the test is not routinely recommended unless a plausible explanation exists (Table 34.9).[69]

### Screening for Malignancies

Studies have reported an incidence of 2%–25% for the diagnosis of malignancies in patients presenting with VTE. The highest risk for cancer occurrence is during the first 6 months of initial diagnosis of VTE and cancer of ovaries, pancreas, liver, kidneys, and lungs are among the most common ones.[70] There is no specific recommendation regarding screening for cancer in VTE patients, but routine screening is not necessary.

## CLINICAL COURSE

We have reviewed the common short-term outcome of both DVT and PE: RV failure and limb ischemia are important and potentially devastating short-term

complications in PE and DVT, respectively. Apart from that, VTE has also important mid- and long-term consequences which have made DVT as one of the leading cause of rehospitalization and also disability.[2] Some of the more important consequences are explained here.

### Recurrent VTE

VTE has a substantial recurrence rate of 30%[71] and patients with symptomatic PE have a greater proportion of recurrency than their counterpart with only an episode of DVT.[72] It should be noted that the recurrence is more prevalent in men compared to women and also happens more frequently in patients with spontaneous VTE episode (i.e., unprovoked).[73] Also, some other risk factors might have a greater impact on VTE recurrence which active cancer, increasing body mass index (BMI), and neurological diseases with leg paresis are the most reported.[2] Importantly, an index VTE following pregnancy, fracture, and surgery, or trauma have no prognostic implication on VTE recurrence.[2] As explained before, the debate still continues on the true

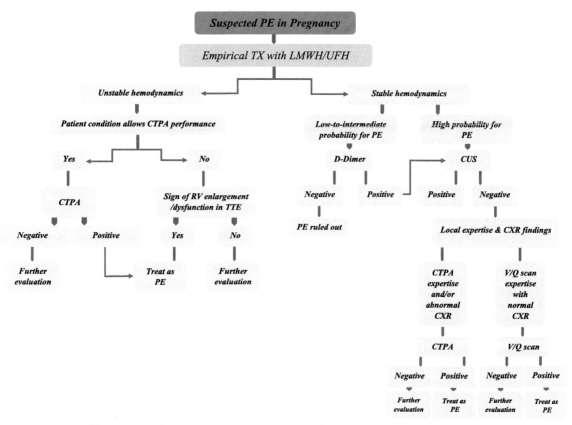

FIG. 34.7 Management of pulmonary emboli in pregnancy. *CTPA*, computed tomography pulmonary angiography; *CUS*, complete ultrasound; *CXR*, chest X-ray; *LMWH*, low-molecular-weight heparin; *PE*, pulmonary embolism; *RV*, right ventricle; *TTE*, transthoracic echocardiography; *TX*, treatment; *UFH*, unfractionated heparin; *V/Q* scan, ventilation perfusion scan.

## TABLE 34.9
### List of Patients Who Might Benefit From Hypercoagulable State Screening Test[68]

Patients with strong family history of VTE (first degree relative with documented VTE before the age 45 years)

Patients with recurrent thrombosis

Patients with thrombosis in unusual vascular beds

Patients with a history of warfarin-induced skin necrosis

Patients with arterial thrombosis

*VTE*, venous thromboembolism.

value of positive hypercoagulable state test and their role on the recurrence of VTE.

For sure, an effective anticoagulation therapy is the most important factor in reducing the rate of recurrent thrombosis. Of note, VTE recurrence while on anticoagulation treatment is uncommon and the rate is approximately 2.6% in the era of novel oral anticoagulation (NOAC) therapy.[74] Apart from poor compliance, aggravation of chronic condition (e.g., intermittent leg swelling during the course of postthrombotic syndrome) should not be mistaken, and true treatment failure should be meticulously investigated.[75]

## Postthrombotic Syndrome

Chronic venous insufficiency followed by DVT is called postthrombotic syndrome (PTS). The situation is practically common and affects 20%–50% of patients with DVTs, could be quite disabling and costly.[76] Although PTS is a clinical diagnosis, several clinical scoring systems have been designed, which the Villalta Score is recommended by most of the guidelines for both diagnosis and assessment of PTS severity (Table 34.10). Each criterion were graded from 0 to 3 points and score ≥15, score between 5 and 14, and score ≤4 were categorized as severe, mild to moderate, and absent, respectively. Of note patient referred with ulcer is also categorized as severe.[77]

Residual thrombosis forms the acute event and partially obstructed veins cause venous hypertension. This in conjunction with vascular remodeling creates the insufficient venous system and result in PTS.[78] Older age, obesity, DVT localization, primary varicose vein, smoking before pregnancy, poor INR control, ipsilateral DVT recurrence, and residual venous thrombosis are listed as strong risk factors in association with PTS.[78]

Effective anticoagulation is the main preventive strategy against the occurrence of PTS. Thrombolytic therapy and invasive endovascular therapies (CDT and thrombus removal) at the acute event in proximal DVTs might decrease the clot burden and consequently reducing the risk of PTS, but it is not still clear that this morbidity benefit outfits the potential risk.[79] Once an important strategy, compression therapy with stocking as a preventive strategy for PTS has lost its early enthusiasm.[78]

Once the diagnosis of PTS has been established, effective compression therapy accompanied by physical therapy is the cornerstone of management.[78] Several novel pharmacological treatments have been introduced, which still need to be validated by further studies. Also emerging endovascular treatment and venous stenting have shown promising results in patients with severe PTS.[19]

### Chronic Thromboembolic Pulmonary Hypertension

One of the chronic complications of PE is chronic thromboembolic pulmonary hypertension (CTEPH). The estimated incidence is between 0.9% and 4% and its median survival in patients with PAP >35 mmHg is less than 2 years.[78] The condition is explained in full detail in elsewhere.

### Post-PE Syndrome

As explained in the previous section, a small number of patients with PE will suffer from CTEPH. However, studies showed that a larger number of patients reported a reduced functional capacity in their daily activity after an episode of acute PE.[80] This group of patients are not classified as CTEPH; and although their prognosis is better and the severity of their symptoms is certainly less, the condition could be quite disabling. In a study on 109 previous healthy subjected suffered from recent episodes of acute PE, 41% showed poor exercise tolerance on their 6 months follow-up.[81] With PTS in mind, these observations have led researchers to defined this mid-term consequence as "post-PE syndrome."[82] Theoretically, venous hypertension created by partially obstructed pulmonary vasculature and vascular remodeling, increased the RV afterload which will develop into chamber failure in following years. Still, there is no consensus if more invasive therapies (i.e., systemic thrombolytics, pharmacomechanical treatment, or surgical embolectomy) will decrease the long-term outcome, but small clinical trials showed promising results.[80]

## TREATMENT

In this section, we review the major topics in the treatment of VTE in three categories of anticoagulation, thrombolytics, and invasive therapies. For the management of VTE several guidelines have been published by different societies.[61] Focusing on the entire guidelines is out of the scope of the present chapter, but the highlights of guidelines and their most practical points are summarized in Table 34.11.

### Anticoagulation

From early in the management of VTE, anticoagulation therapy is the cornerstone of the treatment. Although anticoagulation agents have a lesser role in dissolving the generated thrombosis, they do certainly affect the propagation (i.e., embolization) and generation of new thrombosis, and consequently, improve significantly the early and late survival of patients, and also

**TABLE 34.10**
**Villalta Score**

| Subjective Symptoms | Objective Sign |
| --- | --- |
| Heaviness | Pretibial edema |
| Pain | Induration of the skin |
| Cramps | Hyperpigmentation |
| Pruritus | New venous ectasia |
| Paresthesia | Redness |
| | Pain during calf compression |
| | Ulceration of the skin |

| | Level of Evidence |
|---|---|
| Anticoagulation therapy for PE and proximal DVT | ACCP: In patients with proximal DVT or PE, we recommend long-term (3 months) anticoagulant therapy over no such therapy (Grade 1B)<br><br>ACCP: For patients with DVT of the leg or PE and no cancer who are not treated with dabigatran, rivaroxaban, apixaban, or edoxaban, we suggest VKA therapy over LMWH (Grade 2C)<br><br>ACCP: In patients with DVT of the leg or PE and no cancer, as long-term (first 3 months) anticoagulant therapy, we suggest dabigatran, rivaroxaban, apixaban, or edoxaban over vitamin K antagonist (VKA) therapy (Grade 2B)<br><br>ESC: Anticoagulation should be started immediately, is recommended in patients with high or intermediate clinical probability of PE, while diagnostic workup is in progress (Class IC)<br><br>ESC: In patients intermediate- or low-risk pulmonary embolism, NOAC (apixaban, dabigatran, edoxaban, or rivaroxaban), is preferred to warfarin in eligible patients candidate for oral anticoagulation (Class IA)<br><br>ECS: In patients intermediate- or low-risk pulmonary embolism, LMWH or fondaparinux are preferred over UFH (Class IA)<br><br>ESC: For high-risk patients intravenous UFH should be started without delay (Class IC)<br><br>ESC: INR should be 2.5 (2–3) in patients treated with warfarin (Class IA)<br><br>ESC: Use of NOAC in patients with severe renal impairment, pregnancy, and antiphospholipid antibody syndrome is not recommended (Class IIIC) |
| Anticoagulation for distal DVT | ACCP: In patients with an isolated distal DVT of the leg provoked by surgery or by a nonsurgical transient risk factor, we suggest treatment with anticoagulation for 3 months over treatment of a shorter period (Grade 2C)<br><br>ESC: For patients with high risk for recurrence, 3-month full-dose anticoagulation is recommended. In patients with low-risk recurrence, 4–6 weeks anticoagulation (with full or lower dose) or venous surveillance is recommended |
| Anticoagulation in patients with VTE and cancer | ACCP: In patients with DVT of the leg or PE and cancer ("cancer-associated thrombosis"), as long-term (first 3 months) anticoagulant therapy, we suggest LMWH over VKA therapy (Grade 2C), dabigatran (Grade 2C), rivaroxaban (Grade 2C), apixaban (Grade 2C), or edoxaban (Grade 2C)<br><br>ACCP: In patients with DVT of the leg or PE and active cancer ("cancer-associated thrombosis") and who (i) do not have a high bleeding risk, we recommend extended anticoagulant therapy (no scheduled stop date) over 3 months of therapy (Grade 1B), or (ii) have a high bleeding risk, we suggest extended anticoagulant therapy (no scheduled stop date) over 3 months of therapy (Grade 2B)<br><br>ESC: In patients with cancer, weight-adjusted subcutaneous LMWH is preferred to warfarin (Class IIa)<br><br>ESC: In patients with cancer, edoxaban and rivaroxaban are alternative to LMWH except in gastrointestinal malignancies |
| Provoked vs unprovoked VTE (ACCP), major transient or reversible factors vs nonidentifiable risk factors (ESC) | ACCP: In patients with a provoked proximal DVT of the leg or PE, we recommend treatment with anticoagulation for 3 months over (i) treatment of a shorter period (Grade 1B), (ii) treatment of a longer time-limited period (e.g., 6, 12, or 24 months) (Grade 1B), or (iii) extended therapy (no scheduled stop date) (Grade 1B)<br><br>ACCP: In patients with an unprovoked DVT of the leg (isolated distal or proximal) or PE, we recommend treatment with anticoagulation for at least 3 months over treatment of a shorter duration (Grade 1B), and we recommend treatment with anticoagulation for 3 months over treatment of a longer time-limited period (e.g., 6, 12, or 24 months) (Grade 1B)<br><br>ACCP: In patients with a first VTE that is an unprovoked proximal DVT of the leg or PE and who have a (i) low or moderate bleeding risk (see text), we suggest extended anticoagulant therapy (no scheduled stop date) over 3 months of therapy (Grade 2B), and (ii) high bleeding risk (see text), we recommend 3 months of anticoagulation therapy over extended therapy (no scheduled stop date) (Grade 1B)<br><br>ACCP: In patients with a first VTE that is an unprovoked proximal DVT of the leg or PE and who have a (i) low or moderate bleeding risk |

Continued

| | Level of Evidence |
|---|---|
| | (see text), we suggest extended anticoagulant therapy (no scheduled stop date) over 3 months of therapy (Grade 2B), and (ii) high bleeding risk (see text), we recommend 3 months of anticoagulant therapy over extended therapy (no scheduled stop date) (Grade 1B) ACCP: In patients with a second unprovoked VTE and who have a (i) low bleeding risk (see text), we recommend extended anticoagulant therapy (no scheduled stop date) over 3 months of therapy (Grade 1B); (ii) moderate bleeding risk (see text), we suggest extended anticoagulant therapy over 3 months of therapy (Grade 2B); or (iii) high bleeding risk (see text), we suggest 3 months of anticoagulant therapy over extended therapy (no scheduled stop date) (Grade 2B) ESC: Anticoagulation ≥3 months is recommended in all VTE patients (Class IA) ESC: In patients with VTE due to major transient/reversible risk factor, anticoagulation should be stopped after 3 months (Class IB) ESC: Oral anticoagulation beyond 3 months is recommended in patients experienced recurrent VTE (i.e., with history of one or more episode(s) of VTE) not related to a major transient or reversible risk factor (Class IB) ESC: "Extended oral anticoagulation" beyond 3 months, is recommended after first episode of VTE, in patients with no or minimal transient/reversible risk factor. Persistent risk factor (excluding antiphospholipid antibody syndrome) can also be considered (Class IIa) ESC: Approved anticoagulation regimens of "extended oral anticoagulation" are apixaban (2.5 mg twice daily) or rivaroxaban (10 mg daily) (Class IIa) |
| Systemic thrombolytic therapy | ACCP: In patients with acute PE associated with hypotension (e.g., systolic BP <90 mmHg) who do not have a high bleeding risk, we suggest systemically administered thrombolytic therapy over no such therapy (Grade 2B) ACCP: In most patients with acute PE not associated with hypotension, we recommend against systemically administered thrombolytic therapy (Grade 1B) ACCP: In patients with acute PE who are treated with a thrombolytic agent, we suggest systemic thrombolytic therapy using a peripheral vein over CDT (Grade 2C) ESC: In patients with high-risk acute PE, systemic thrombolytic therapy is recommended (Class IB) ESC: In patient with acute PE without hypotension and shock, routine use of thrombolytic therapy is not recommended (Class III) ESC: In patients with low- to intermediate-risk PE on anticoagulation therapy, rescue thrombolytic therapy is recommended in hemodynamic deterioration (Class IB) |
| Catheter-directed thrombolysis (CDT) | ACCP: In patients with acute proximal DVT of the leg, we suggest anticoagulant therapy alone over CDT (Grade 2C) ACCP: In patients with acute PE associated with hypotension and who have (i) a high bleeding risk, (ii) failed systemic thrombolysis, or (iii) shock that is likely to cause death before systemic thrombolysis can take effect (e.g., within hours), if appropriate expertise and resources are available, we suggest catheter-assisted thrombus removal over no such intervention (Grade 2C) ESC: In patients with acute PE and shock or hypotension, CDT should be considered in patients whom systemic thrombolytic is contraindicated or failed (Class IIa) ESC: In patients with low- to intermediate-risk PE on anticoagulation therapy, CDT is recommended in hemodynamic deterioration (Class IIa) |

| Surgical embolectomy for PE | ESC: In patients with acute PE and shock or hypotension, surgical embolectomy is recommended in patients whom systemic thrombolytic is contraindicated or failed (Class IC)<br><br>ESC: In patients with low- to intermediate-risk PE on anticoagulation therapy, surgical embolectomy is recommended in hemodynamic deterioration (Class IIa) |
|---|---|
| Inferior vena cava filter | ACCP: In patients with acute DVT or PE who are treated with anticoagulants, we recommend against the use of an inferior vena cava (IVC) filter (Grade 1B)<br><br>ESC: IVC filter is recommended in patients with absolute contraindication to anticoagulation or recurrence despite therapeutic anticoagulation (Class IIa)<br><br>ESC: Routine deployment of IVC filter is not recommended (Class III) |
| Outpatient management of VTE | ACCP: In patients with low-risk PE and whose home circumstances are adequate, we suggest treatment at home or early discharge over standard discharge (e.g., after the first 5 days of treatment) (Grade 2B)<br><br>ESC: "Carefully selected patients with low-risk PE should be considered for early discharge and continuation of treatment at home, if proper outpatient care and anticoagulant treatment can be provided" (Class IIa) |
| Recurrent VTE | ACCP: In patients who have recurrent VTE on VKA therapy (in the therapeutic range) or on dabigatran, rivaroxaban, apixaban, or edoxaban (and are believed to be compliant), we suggest switching to treatment with LMWH at least temporarily (Grade 2C)<br><br>ACCP: In patients who have recurrent VTE on long-term LMWH (and are believed to be compliant), we suggest increasing the dose of LMWH by about one-quarter to one-third (Grade 2C) |

Three guidelines: American College of Chest Physician,[62] American Heart Association,[61] and European Society of Cardiology (ESC)[63] are the most popular guidelines in the field of VTE. The first two focused on both pulmonary emboli and deep venous thrombosis, and the ESC guideline focused only on PE. *ACCP*, American College of Cardiology; *AHA*, American Heart Association; *CDT*, catheter-directed thrombolysis; *DVT*, deep venous thrombosis; *ESC*, European Society of Cardiology; *IFDVT*, iliofemoral deep venous thrombosis; *IVC*, inferior vena cava; *LMWH*, low-molecular-weight heparin; *NOAC*, novel oral anticoagulation; *PE*, pulmonary emboli; *RV*, right ventricle; *UFH*, unfractionated heparin; *VKA*, vitamin K antagonist; *VTE*, venous thromboembolism.

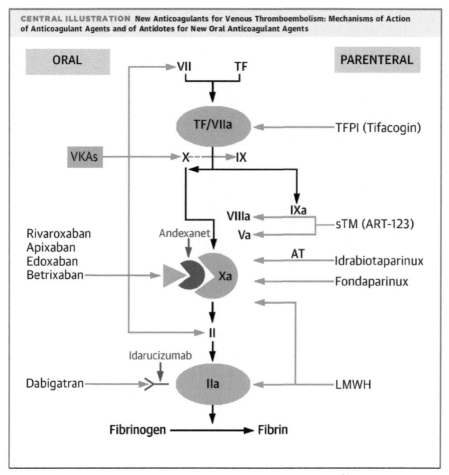

CENTRAL ILLUSTRATION New Anticoagulants for Venous Thromboembolism: Mechanisms of Action of Anticoagulant Agents and of Antidotes for New Oral Anticoagulant Agents

FIG. 34.8 Targets of various oral anticoagulation therapies and their antidotes.[84] (Reproduced with permission from Becattini C, Agnelli G. Treatment of venous thromboembolism with new anticoagulant agents. *J Am Coll Cardiol.* 2016;67(16):1941–1955.)

reduce their morbidity. The anticoagulation treatment should be started as soon as the diagnosis is established.[83] Three major issues exist on the anticoagulation therapies: How to start the therapy? How to continue the therapy? And finally, when the therapy should be discontinued?

### How to start the anticoagulation therapy?

Warfarin is the oldest oral anticoagulation agent prescribed in the treatment of VTE. Today we have some approved NOAC agents—dabigatran, rivaroxaban, apixaban, and edoxaban—with similar efficacy while potentially easier to use than the famous warfarin in the treatment of venous thrombosis.[84] According to ACCP guideline, the use of NOACs in patients with VTE was superior to warfarin in those without contraindications.[62]

The targets of various oral anticoagulation agents are summarized in Fig. 34.8. The important point is that apart from rivaroxaban and apixaban, all the other oral anticoagulation need prior treatment with parenteral anticoagulation (Fig. 34.9).[84] Actually, we have three approaches in the treatment of VTE, overlapping, switching, and oral monotherapy. For warfarin, the approach is overlapping which means we need to administer warfarin with unfractionated heparin (UFH), or low-molecular-weight heparin (LMWH) for 5 days and two consecutive days of international normalized ratio (INR) in the therapeutic range (i.e., 2–3). The second approach which is switching is used for dabigatran and edoxaban which means after 5 days of LMWH administration, it should be discontinued and treatment with these agents would be initiated. Finally, the last approach is monotherapy which is used

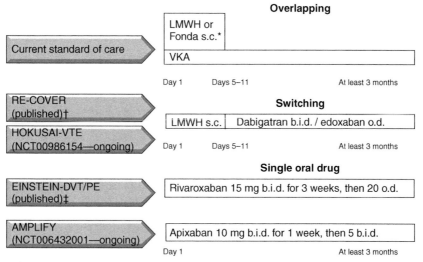

FIG. 34.9 Overlapping oral anticoagulation agents through parental therapy. (Modified from Konstantinides S, Goldhaber SZ. Pulmonary embolism: risk assessment and management. *Eur Heart J.* 2012;33(24):3014–3022.)

for apixaban and rivaroxaban that does not require any initial treatment with parenteral agents (Fig. 34.9).[84]

UFH, LMWH, and fondaparinux are the three major parenteral anticoagulation used in VTE. LMWH and fondaparinux are preferred over UFH due to their more predictable dose–response and longer half time. These features have omitted the need for a constant laboratory test for dose adjustment and permit weight-based dosing for both agents, and more importantly, have revolutionized the management of acute VTE by earlier discharge and possible outpatient management.[83] In addition, the risk of heparin-induced thrombocytopenia with LMWH and fondaparinux is significantly less than UFH.[85] Of note, UFH is preferred in patients with severe renal impairment, severe obesity, and patients who are candidate for primary reperfusion therapy or placement of inferior vena cava (IVC) filter.[63] Dosage of parenteral agents is summarized in Table 34.12.

Warfarin is a vitamin K antagonist and has been the gold standard anticoagulation therapy for more than 50 years. The classic starting dosage of warfarin is 5 mg and it is now recommended to be started on the first day. It has been also suggested that warfarin might be started at a dose of 10 mg in young (<60 years) and otherwise healthy patients.[63]

The pharmacological characteristics and clinical applicability of NOAC agents are summarized in Table 34.13. In patients with CrCl <30 (for apixaban CrCl <25 mL/min), pregnant patients, during lactation, patients with obesity which is defined as weight more

than 120 kg or BMI more than 40 kg/m$^2$ and patients with active gastroesophageal cancer the use of NOAC is not approved.[84] Furthermore, there are some significant drug–drug interactions that should be considered in this population. Importantly, the use of antiepileptics, rifampin, protease inhibitors, and azoles is not recommended with NOACs.[92]

**TABLE 34.12**
**Parenteral Anticoagulation in Venous Thromboembolism**

| Drug | Dosage |
| --- | --- |
| Unfractionated heparin | Intravenous bolus of 80 U/kg followed by 18 U/kg/h aPTT between 1.5 and 2.5 times the control value (60–80 s) |
| Enoxaparin | 1 mg/kg twice daily Or 1.5 mg/kg once daily |
| Dalteparin | 100 U/kg twice daily Or 200 U/kg once daily |
| Tinzaparin | 175 U/kg once daily |
| Fondaparinux | 5 mg (body weight <50) 7.5 mg (body weight <50–100) 10-mg (body weight 100<) Once daily |

**TABLE 34.13**
**Pharmacological Characteristics and Clinical Applications of Novel Oral Anticoagulation**

|  | Target | Prodrug | Half Life (h) | Time to Peak (h) | Dosage | Pivotal Study |
|---|---|---|---|---|---|---|
| Dabigatran etexilate | IIa | Yes | 12–17 | 2 | 150 mg twice daily (dose reduction in patients at increased risk of bleeding including patients ≥75 years with ≥1 risk factors for bleeding) | RE-COVER[86] and RE-MEDY[87] |
| Rivaroxaban | Xa | No | 9 | 3 | 15 mg twice daily for 3 weeks followed by 20 mg once daily | EINSTEIN-DVT[88] and EINSTEIN-PE[89] |
| Apixaban | Xa | No | 9–14 | 3 | 10 mg twice daily for 7 days followed by 5 mg twice daily | AMPLIFY[90] |
| Edoxaban | Xa | No | 10–14 | 1–2 | 60 mg once daily | HOKUSAI-VTE[91] |

**TABLE 34.14**
**Anticoagulation Therapy in Special Population**

| Condition | Preferred Agents |
|---|---|
| Malignancy | LMWH |
| Liver disease and coagulopathy | LMWH |
| Renal disease and CrCl <30 | Warfarin |
| Pregnancy | LMWH |
| Planned systemic thrombolytic or invasive therapies | UFH |
| HIT | Argatroban, bivalirudin |

*HIT*, heparin-induced thrombocytopenia; *LMWH*, low-molecular-weight heparin; *UFH*, unfractionated heparin.

Based on ESC guideline rivaroxaban and edoxaban can be considered for VTE in patients with cancer other than gastroesophageal who are not at high risk of bleeding.[27]

According to the latest National Comprehensive Cancer Network (NCCN) guideline 2020 for the treatment of cancer-associated VTE, apixaban can also be considered in this population (category 1 of recommendation).[93]

Some group of patients might need special consideration for choosing the best anticoagulation treatment; these considerations are summarized in Table 34.14.

### How to continue the anticoagulation therapy?

For patients on warfarin, monitoring is "both art and medicine."[83] After reaching the therapeutic INR level on two consecutive days in the acute setting, patients should be monitored closely in the following several weeks. The proposed interval between each INR test is debated and varied among population. An interval of 3–5 days has been suggested for otherwise healthy patients. When reaching a stable INR, the test can be prescribed every 4–6 weeks. Several protocols have been proposed for how to adjust warfarin dosage and INR, but it should always bear in mind that the monitoring of patients on warfarin should be individualized and the mentioned interval and protocols are arbitrary. The important point is that the prognosis of these patients is directly related to the time in therapeutic range (TTR) (i.e., the mean time in INR therapeutic range); a TTR of less than 60% of the time is associated with worse prognosis.[94] Various clinical scenario (e.g., worsening renal or hepatic function), dietary regimen (e.g., green leafy vegetables lowers INR), and drugs might affect the therapeutic level of warfarin, and consequently, a strong patient–physician relationship is needed for this group of patients. Self-monitoring test/device might help in this regards.[95] In addition, the use of pharmacogenetic testing might increase the accuracy of warfarin adjustment in a certain group of patients.[96]

One of the revolutionary characteristics of the NOAC is their simpler way of monitoring. Patients do not need monitoring tests in most circumstances and the medications have a fixed dose. This advantage has the potential to reduce bleeding complications and results in a more stable anticoagulation therapeutic level in patients treated for VTE. For sure in this group of medications also, various clinical scenario and drug interaction influence their pharmacokinetics.[84]

In some instance, patients on anticoagulation therapy might need temporary discontinuation of their treatment due to invasive diagnostic or surgical procedures. For patients on warfarin and a diagnosis of VTE within 3 months, overlapping parenteral anticoagulation is needed after stopping the medication. Due to their short half-life, NOAC agents can be simply stopped before the elective procedure without a need for bridging therapy. However, the present approach should be validated by further studies. It should be noted for some procedures with low bleeding risk (e.g., cataract surgery, dental cleaning, or tooth extraction) the discontinuation of anticoagulation is unnecessary.

### When anticoagulation therapy should be discontinued?

The optimal duration of anticoagulation therapy is still debated. Apparently one of the best characteristics which might have a great influence on the duration of anticoagulation is whether the VTE was developed due to any transient or reversible risk factor. "Provoked" vs "unprovoked" is no longer used in the guidelines, as this terminology could not be applied for decision-making on anticoagulation duration in patients with VTE.[27] The general agreement between guidelines is that 3 months of anticoagulation may be enough for those with reversible or transient risk factors, while for VTEs developed by a persistent risk factor or unknown reason we need a much longer time. An indefinite duration of anticoagulation therapy for the latter has also been suggested by some experts. According to ESC guideline, all patients with VTE should receive at least 3 months of anticoagulation. Furthermore, although extended anticoagulation could reduce VTE recurrence risk by approximately 90%, this benefit is counterbalanced by the risk of bleeding. Patients presenting with recurrent VTE not related to a major transient or reversible risk factor are candidates for the anticoagulation treatment of indefinite duration. VKA treatment for an indefinite period is recommended for patients with antiphospholipid antibody syndrome. For special population like patients with cancer, the approach must be individualized and an extended duration of anticoagulation might be needed. In patients with cancer, there is a higher risk for recurrence; therefore, it is advisable to administer indefinite anticoagulation after a first episode of VTE in this population. Apixaban 2.5 mg twice daily and rivaroxaban 10 mg daily after 6 months of therapeutic anticoagulation could be considered for those candidates for extended treatment. If the patient could not tolerate any forms of anticoagulation, aspirin or sulodexide can be considered. The highlights of the guideline on the duration of anticoagulation are summarized in Table 34.11.

### Bleeding risk and bleeding complication of anticoagulation therapies

The decision to start and continue anticoagulation for treatment of VTE should always be weighed against the patient bleeding risk. Most experts believe that patients with low bleeding risk should start/continue the anticoagulation therapy, while high bleeding risk patients should be prohibited. For a patient with moderate risk of bleeding the approach must be individualized. Several calculators (e.g., HAS-BLED) are available for evaluating the bleeding risk, but none of them has been validated for patients with VTE, and thus should be used cautiously.[96] Patients with contraindication for receiving anticoagulation might benefit from the use of IVC filter. It should be noted that those with IVC filter need to receive anticoagulation when the contraindication to the use of these agents had been resolved.

For patients suffering from life-threatening bleeding reversal agents for different anticoagulation therapies are summarized in Table 34.15. For NOAC, the proposed antidote needs to be validated by further studies.

### Systemic Thrombolytic Therapy in Patients With VTE

The suggested thrombolytic regimens and their contraindications are listed in Table 34.16. Alteplase is the approved agent by the FDA for use in VTE. The highlights of recommendations regarding thrombolytic therapy stated by various guidelines are summarized in Table 34.11.

### DVT

The only widely accepted indication for the use of systemic thrombolytic agents in patients with acute DVT

**TABLE 34.15**
**Reversal Agents for Anticoagulation Therapy**

| Anticoagulation Medication | Reversal Agents |
| --- | --- |
| UFH, LMWH | Protamine sulfate |
| Fondaparinux | PCC and rFVIIa |
| Warfarin | Vitamin K, FFP, PCC, and rFVIIa |
| Dabigatran etexilate | Idarucizumab[a], PCC |
| Rivaroxaban, apixaban, and edoxaban | Andexanet[a], PCC |

[a]Need to be validated by further studies.[90,97]
*FFP*, fresh frozen plasma; *LMWH*, low-molecular-weight heparin; *PCC*, prothrombin complex concentration; *rFVIIa*, recombinant factor VIIa; *UFH*, unfractionated heparin.

---

**TABLE 34.16**

**Thrombolytic Regimens and Absolute and Relative Contraindications[83]**

| Agents and Regimens | Contraindications |
|---|---|
| Streptokinase | **Absolute** |
| • 250,000 U as a loading dose over 30 min followed by 100,000 U/h over 12–24 h <br> • Accelerated regimen 1.5 million U over 2 h | • History of hemorrhagic stroke or stroke of unknown origin <br> • Ischemic stroke in previous 6 months <br> • Central nervous system neoplasms <br> • Major trauma, surgery, or head injury in previous 3 weeks |
| Urokinase | |
| • 4400 U per kg of body weight as a loading dose over 10 min, followed by 4400 U/kg/h over 12–24 h <br> • Accelerated regimen: 3 million U over 2 h | |
| Alteplasea | **Relative** |
| • 100 mg over 2 h <br> • Accelerated regimen: 0.6 mg/kg for 15 min | • Transient ischemic attack in previous 6 months <br> • Oral anticoagulation |
| Reteplase | • Pregnancy or first postpartum week |
| Two bolus injections of 10 U 30 min apart | • Noncompressible puncture sites <br> • Traumatic resuscitation |
| Tenecteplase | • Refractory hypertension (systolic blood pressure >180 mmHg) |
| 30–50 mg bolus for 5–10 s adjusted for body weight <br> • <60 kg: 30 mg <br> • ≥60 to <70 kg: 35 mg <br> • ≥70 to <80 kg: 40 mg <br> • ≥80 to <90 kg: 45 mg <br> • ≥90 kg: 50 mg | • Advanced liver disease <br> • Infective endocarditis <br> • Active peptic ulcer |

is extensive proximal DVT or iliofemoral DVT with severe symptomatic swelling or limb-threatening ischemia. In patients with low risk of bleeding and especially in the younger population, the clinical results of systemic thrombolytic are promising.[98]

## PE

Although the use of thrombolytic therapy in DVT is reserved for special condition, fibrinolytics are the Class I recommendation for patients presenting with massive PE unless they have a contraindication. A meta-analysis reviewing the latest studies performed on the use of thrombolytics in massive PE report a significant mortality reduction. Also, the thrombolytic therapy might decrease the recurrent VTE episodes, improve the RV function and consequently the functional capacity.[99] The practical point is that unlike in ST elevation myocardial infarction in which the time window for using fibrinolytic is narrow, patients with PE might benefit from these agents in a period of 14 days after the beginning of the symptoms.[83] In spite of clear clinical benefit of thrombolytic agents in the treatment of massive PE,

the potential bleeding risk and intracranial hemorrhage (0.9% in RCTs and 2%–3% in real world) have prevented the widespread use of this effective treatment. An integrated approach with a realistic bleeding risk estimation might help to identify the appropriate candidate for thrombolytic therapy.

The success of the thrombolytic therapy in massive PE has led investigators to evaluate the possible use of this therapy in submassive PE. The PIETHO trial is the largest trial evaluating the role of systemic thrombolytic in intermediate-risk pulmonary emboli. Although thrombolytics trend to improve the primary outcome, the bleeding complications were significantly greater in the thrombolytic therapy group.[100] Based on PIETHO trial and other evidences, guidelines are still cautioning about using this strategy in patients with submassive PE.

## Pharmacomechanical Catheter-Directed Therapies

The potential risk for major bleeding complication and especially ICH has prevented clinicians from using systemic thrombolytic therapy. CDT by local delivery of thrombolytic agents might improve the drug delivery and therapeutic action of these agents and consequently might decrease the total thrombolytic dosage needed for treatment of VTE. Combining this method with mechanical thrombus removal device, the clinical success might even be better.[80]

There is a paucity of data comparing the systemic vs CDT and the clinical success of endovascular methods was majorly approved by clinical trials with small sample size. Thus, the level of evidence given by the guidelines is still weaker than full-dose systemic thrombolytic therapy (Table 34.11).

Of note, a potentially better adverse risk profile of CDT might open room for a more invasive approach toward patients with intermediate risk (e.g., submassive PE).

### Surgical Management

Surgery has limited applicability in DVT and surgical thrombectomy should be considered in patients with symptomatic iliofemoral DVT unless the systemic/catheter-directed methods were not possible.

On contrary, the role of surgical embolectomy in PE patients is crucial. In massive PE surgical embolectomy offers a low operative mortality. The majority of guidelines reserved the use of surgical embolectomy for patients with contraindication or refractory to thrombolytics (Table 34.16) but, the treatment might be lifesaving even in patients with unstable hemodynamics and severe RV dysfunction as a first-line strategy. The potential indications of surgical embolectomy are listed in Table 34.17. Of note like systemic thrombolytic, surgical procedures are also underused.[101]

### SPECIAL THERAPEUTIC CONSIDERATION FOR PATIENTS WITH VTE

#### Ambulation in Patients With DVT

Despite prior recommendation regarding the restricted activity in patients presenting with acute DVT, early ambulation is now safe and should be even supported.

#### Inferior Vena Cava Filters

The suggested recommendation for the use of IVC filter is summarized in Table 34.11. Studies which have analyzed the routine deployment of IVC filters in DVT population showed that the rate of PE was decreased but on the other hand DVT rate was increased. No mortality benefit was reported.[102] Consequently, the routine IVC filters implantation should not be advised. The main indication is for patients with absolute contraindication to anticoagulation therapy (e.g., high bleeding risk, recent surgery, and hemorrhagic stroke).

#### Outpatient Management

As explained before, with the widespread use of LMWH, the possibility for outpatient management for VTE has been suggested. For patients who decided to manage with warfarin can receive their first dose of parenteral anticoagulation in the hospital and continue their treatment as outpatients. Warfarin can be started on the same day. This outpatient strategy can also be tailored for patients on NOAC. Eventually, close observation and a strong patient–physician relationship are mandatory. The Hestia exclusion criteria suggest a checklist if which one or more criteria are positive, the patient will not be suitable for outpatient management (Table 34.18).[104]

#### Multidisciplinary Pulmonary Embolism Response Team

Management of PE needs a mutual collaboration between various expertise and importantly most of the time a decision must be taken immediately. Therefore, with the help of heart team experience in coronary artery disease, some centers have started a genuine project and established a multidisciplinary pulmonary embolism response team (PERT) for improving the care of patients presenting with acute PE. Specially PERT team can offer a better risk stratification for patients who might benefit from more invasive management.[105]

### PREVENTION

VTE is one of the most common and at the same time preventable causes of morbidity and mortality in

| TABLE 34.17 Proposed Indication for Surgical Embolectomy in Pulmonary Emboli[101] |
| --- |
| Contraindication to fibrinolytic therapy |
| Active bleeding |
| Failed systemic fibrinolysis or catheter-directed thrombolysis |
| Clot-in-transit |
| Large patent foramen ovale |

**TABLE 34.18**
**The Hestia exclusion criteria[103]**

| Criterion |
| --- |
| Unstable hemodynamically |
| Reperfusion therapy or invasive management necessary |
| Ongoing or history of major bleeding |
| Need for more than 24 h of oxygen therapy for maintaining oxygen saturation >90% |
| PE occurrence while on anticoagulation |
| Parenteral pain management for more than 24 h? |
| Existed medical or social condition for treatment in the hospital for >24 h |
| CrCl of <30 mL/min |
| Severe liver impairment? |
| Pregnancy |
| History of heparin-induced thrombocytopenia? |

*CrCl*, creatinine clearance; *PE*, pulmonary embolism.

**TABLE 34.19**
**Common Regimens for Venous Thromboembolism Prevention**

| Condition | Prophylaxis |
| --- | --- |
| Hospitalization with medical illness | Unfractionated heparin 5000 U SC bid or tid or enoxaparin 2500 or 5000 U SC qd or fondaparinux 2.5 mg SC qd with normal renal function (in patients with heparin allergy such as heparin-induced thrombocytopenia) or graduated compression stockings or intermittent pneumatic compression for patients with contraindications to anticoagulation consider combination pharmacologic and mechanical prophylaxis for high-risk patients |
| General surgery | Unfractionated heparin 5000 U SC bid or tid or enoxaparin 40 mg SC qd or dalteparin 2500 or 5000 U SC qd |
| Major orthopedic surgery | Warfarin (target INR 2–3) or enoxaparin 30 mg SC bid or enoxaparin 40 mg SC qd or dalteparin 2500 or 5000 U SC qd or fondaparinux 2.5 mg SC qd or rivaroxaban 10 mg qd or aspirin 81 mg qd or dabigatran 220 mg qd (not in US) or apixaban 2.5 mg twice daily (not in the US) or intermittent pneumatic compression (with or without pharmacologic prophylaxis) |

hospitalized patients. There are several approved and effective prevention protocols. In some chronic diseases prone to VTE also prophylaxis may be useful. It is notoriously underused and lives can be saved by sticking to the approved protocols.[106,107] Fortunately, several drug regimens and some nondrug methods are safe and effective depending on the situation (Table 34.19).

**Inhospital Risk Factors for VTE and Bleeding**

One of the best risk scoring systems is the Padua Prediction Score (Table 34.20). A score of equal or more than 4 defines high-risk group (about 11% risk of VTE). Risk of bleeding must also be assessed and decision on prophylaxis be based on the relative weight of VTE vs bleeding.

One easy evidence-based way of finding patients high risk for bleeding is to exclude patients having active ulcer in their GI tract, bleeding 3 months or less before hospitalization or platelet count of less than 50,000.[108]

Another model of predicting VTE risk in patients hospitalized for medical purposes is designed by Intermountain Medical Center in Utah. Based on this model the patient is high risk if he has at least one of these four conditions: (1) history of VTE; (2) prolonged bed rest; (3) a peripherally inserted central venous catheter; or (4) cancer.[109]

**Inhospital Prophylaxis**

Simple low-dose anticoagulation has been shown to decrease the rate of VTE by half in patients hospitalized because of medical conditions without affecting major bleeding. Enoxaparin 40 mg, dalteparin 5000 U, and fondaparinux 2.5 mg (single daily dose) are all safe and effective.[110] Rivaroxaban 10 mg daily for 39 days obtained FDA approval as of October 2019 for those without contraindications based on MAGELLAN study results.[111]

**Mechanical Prophylaxis**

This type of prophylaxis mainly consists of intermittent pneumatic compression and graduated compression stocking. As its efficacy is not robust and some complications like skin damage are of concern, they must be

**TABLE 34.20**
**PADUA Prediction Score for Identification of Hospitalized Patients at Risk for Venous Thromboembolism**

| Risk Factor | Scoring |
| --- | --- |
| Cancer | 3 |
| Previous VTE | 3 |
| Immobility | 3 |
| Thrombophilia | 3 |
| Trauma/surgery | 2 |
| Age ≥70 years | 1 |
| Heart/respiratory failure | 1 |
| Acute MI or stroke | 1 |
| Infection/rheumatologic disorder | 1 |
| Obesity | 1 |
| Hormonal treatment | 1 |
| High risk for developing PE is defined as 4 score points or greater | |

reserved for patients with strong contraindications for anticoagulation.[110]

## Prophylaxis in Major Orthopedic Surgery

Many antiplatelet and anticoagulant drugs including aspirin and novel anticoagulants have been shown to be safe and effective in patients undergoing major orthopedic surgery. So, aspirin, LMWH, low-dose heparin, warfarin (target INR 2–2.5), dabigatran, fondaparinux, rivaroxaban, and apixaban all can be used in this regard for at least 14 days.[112] The duration of anticoagulation depends on the type of surgery. As with total knee replacement surgery, at least 10 days is recommended, whereas, for total hip replacement or fracture surgery, 4–6 weeks of treatment is suggested. For knee replacement surgery rivaroxaban (10 mg daily, 6–10 h after surgery) and apixaban (2.5 mg twice daily, 12–24 h after surgery) are recommended among DOACs. For hip replacement surgery dabigatran can also be used at the dose of 110 mg 1–4 h after surgery then 220 mg daily.[113]

## REFERENCES

1. Goldhaber SZ. Venous thromboembolism: epidemiology and magnitude of the problem. *Best Pract Res Clin Haematol.* 2012; 25(3):235–242.
2. Heit JA. Epidemiology of venous thromboembolism. *Nat Rev Cardiol.* 2015; 12(8):464–474.
3. Heit JA, Spencer FA, White RH. The epidemiology of venous thromboembolism. *J Thromb Thrombolysis.* 2016; 41(1):3–14.
4. Silverstein MD, Heit JA, Mohr DN, Petterson TM, O'Fallon WM, Melton LJ. Trends in the incidence of deep vein thrombosis and pulmonary embolism: a 25-year population-based study. *Arch Intern Med.* 1998; 158(6):585–593.
5. Geerts WH, Bergqvist D, Pineo GF, et al. Prevention of venous thromboembolism: American College of Chest Physicians evidence-based clinical practice guidelines. *Chest J.* 2008; 133(6 suppl):381S–453S.
6. Anderson FA, Zayaruzny M, Heit JA, Fidan D, Cohen AT. Estimated annual numbers of US acute-care hospital patients at risk for venous thromboembolism. *Am J Hematol.* 2007; 82(9):777–782.
7. Barsoum MK, Heit JA, Ashrani AA, Leibson CL, Petterson TM, Bailey KR. Is progestin an independent risk factor for incident venous thromboembolism? A population-based case-control study. *Thromb Res.* 2010; 126(5):373–378.
8. Noboa S, Mottier D, Oger E. Estimation of a potentially preventable fraction of venous thromboembolism: a community-based prospective study. *J Thromb Haemost.* 2006; 4(12):2720–2722.
9. Samama MM, Combe S, Conard J, Horellou M-H. Risk assessment models for thromboprophylaxis of medical patients. *Thromb Res.* 2012; 129(2):127–132.
10. Heit JA, O'Fallon WM, Petterson TM, et al. Relative impact of risk factors for deep vein thrombosis and pulmonary embolism: a population-based study. *Arch Intern Med.* 2002; 162(11):1245–1248.
11. Blom J, Vanderschoot J, Oostindier M, Osanto S, Van Der Meer F, Rosendaal F. Incidence of venous thrombosis in a large cohort of 66 329 cancer patients: results of a record linkage study. *J Thromb Haemost.* 2006; 4(3):529–535.
12. Gomes MP, Deitcher SR. Risk of venous thromboembolic disease associated with hormonal contraceptives and hormone replacement therapy: a clinical review. *Arch Intern Med.* 2004; 164(18):1965–1976.
13. Grady D, Wenger NK, Herrington D, et al. Postmenopausal hormone therapy increases risk for venous thromboembolic disease: the Heart and Estrogen/progestin Replacement Study. *Ann Intern Med.* 2000; 132(9):689–696.
14. Lidegaard Ø, Nielsen LH, Skovlund CW, Skjeldestad FE, Løkkegaard E. Risk of venous thromboembolism from use of oral contraceptives containing different progestogens and oestrogen doses: Danish cohort study, 2001–9. *BMJ.* 2011; 343:d6423.
15. Heit JA, Kobbervig CE, James AH, Petterson TM, Bailey KR, Melton LJ. Trends in the incidence of venous thromboembolism during pregnancy or postpartum: a 30-year population-based study. *Ann Intern Med.* 2005; 143(10):697–706.

16. Sultan AA, Tata LJ, West J, et al. Risk factors for first venous thromboembolism around pregnancy: a population-based cohort study from the United Kingdom. *Blood.* 2013; 121(19):3953–3961.

17. May R, Thurner J. The cause of the predominantly sinistral occurrence of thrombosis of the pelvic veins. *Angiology.* 1957; 8(5):419–427.

18. Kibbe MR, Ujiki M, Goodwin AL, Eskandari M, Yao J, Matsumura J. Iliac vein compression in an asymptomatic patient population. *J Vasc Surg.* 2004; 39(5):937–943.

19. Neglén P, Tackett TP, Raju S. Venous stenting across the inguinal ligament. *J Vasc Surg.* 2008; 48(5):1255–1261.

20. Corral J, Roldán V, Vicente V. Deep venous thrombosis or pulmonary embolism and factor V Leiden: enigma or paradox. *Haematologica.* 2010; 95(6):863–866.

21. Piazza G, Goldhaber SZ. Venous thromboembolism and atherothrombosis: an integrated approach. *Circulation.* 2010; 121(19):2146–2150.

22. Ageno W, Becattini C, Brighton T, Selby R, Kamphuisen PW. Cardiovascular risk factors and venous thromboembolism: a meta-analysis. *Circulation.* 2008; 117(1):93–102.

23. Glynn RJ, Danielson E, Fonseca FA, et al. A randomized trial of rosuvastatin in the prevention of venous thromboembolism. *N Engl J Med.* 2009; 360(18): 1851–1861.

24. Schwartz GG, Steg PG, Szarek M, et al. Peripheral artery disease and venous thromboembolic events after acute coronary syndrome: role of lipoprotein(a) and modification by alirocumab: prespecified analysis of the ODYSSEY OUTCOMES randomized clinical trial. *Circulation.* 2020; 141(20):1608–1617.

25. Baglin T, Bauer K, Douketis J, Buller H, Srivastava A, Johnson G. Duration of anticoagulant therapy after a first episode of an unprovoked pulmonary embolus or deep vein thrombosis: guidance from the SSC of the ISTH. *J Thromb Haemost.* 2012; 10(4):698–702.

26. Iorio A, Kearon C, Filippucci E, et al. Risk of recurrence after a first episode of symptomatic venous thromboembolism provoked by a transient risk factor: a systematic review. *Arch Intern Med.* 2010; 170(19): 1710–1716.

27. Konstantinides SV, Meyer G, Becattini C, et al. 2019 ESC Guidelines for the diagnosis and management of acute pulmonary embolism developed in collaboration with the European Respiratory Society (ERS). *Eur Heart J.* 2020; 41(4):543–603.

28. Mann DL, Zipes DP, Libby P, Bonow RO. *Braunwald's Heart Disease: A Textbook of Cardiovascular Medicine.* Elsevier Health Sciences; 2014.

29. McIntyre KM, Sasahara AA. The hemodynamic response to pulmonary embolism in patients without prior cardiopulmonary disease. *Am J Cardiol.* 1971; 28(3): 288–294.

30. Lankhaar J-W, Westerhof N, Faes TJ, et al. Quantification of right ventricular afterload in patients with and without pulmonary hypertension. *Am J Physiol Heart Circ Physiol.* 2006; 291(4):H1731–H1737.

31. Molloy WD, Lee K, Girling L, Schick U, Prewitt RM. Treatment of shock in a canine model of pulmonary embolism. *Am Rev Respir Dis.* 1984; 130(5):870–874.

32. Begieneman MP, van de Goot FR, van der Bilt IA, et al. Pulmonary embolism causes endomyocarditis in the human heart. *Heart.* 2008; 94(4):450–456.

33. Hull RD, Raskob GE, Hirsh J, et al. Continuous intravenous heparin compared with intermittent subcutaneous heparin in the initial treatment of proximal-vein thrombosis. *N Engl J Med.* 1986; 315 (18): 1109–1114.

34. Lankeit M, Jiménez D, Kostrubiec M, et al. Predictive value of the high-sensitivity troponin T assay and the simplified Pulmonary Embolism Severity Index in hemodynamically stable patients with acute pulmonary embolism: a prospective validation study. *Circulation.* 2011; 124(24):2716–2724.

35. Burrowes K, Clark A, Tawhai M. Blood flow redistribution and ventilation-perfusion mismatch during embolic pulmonary arterial occlusion. *Blood.* 2011; 1(3):365–376.

36. Qaseem A, Snow V, Barry P, et al. Current diagnosis of venous thromboembolism in primary care: a clinical practice guideline from the American Academy of Family Physicians and the American College of Physicians. *Ann Intern Med.* 2007; 146(6):454–458.

37. Scarvelis D, Wells PS. Diagnosis and treatment of deep-vein thrombosis. *Can Med Assoc J.* 2006; 175(9): 1087–1092.

38. Suwanabol PA, Tefera G, Schwarze ML. Syndromes associated with the deep veins: phlegmasia cerulea dolens, May-Thurner syndrome, and nutcracker syndrome. *Perspect Vasc Surg Endovasc Ther.* 2010; 22(4): 223–230.

39. Hull R, Hirsh J, Sackett DL, et al. Clinical validity of a negative venogram in patients with clinically suspected venous thrombosis. *Circulation.* 1981; 64(3):622–625.

40. Hirsh J, Lee AY. How we diagnose and treat deep vein thrombosis. *Blood.* 2002; 99(9):3102–3110.

41. Subramaniam RM, Snyder B, Heath R, Tawse F, Sleigh J. Diagnosis of lower limb deep venous thrombosis in emergency department patients: performance of Hamilton and modified Wells scores. *Ann Emerg Med.* 2006; 48(6):678–685.

42. Wells PS, Anderson DR, Bormanis J, et al. Value of assessment of pretest probability of deep-vein thrombosis in clinical management. *Lancet.* 1997; 350 (9094):1795–1798.

43. Tamariz LJ, Eng J, Segal JB, et al. Usefulness of clinical prediction rules for the diagnosis of venous thromboembolism: a systematic review. *Am J Med.* 2004; 117(9):676–684.

44. Righini M, Perrier A, De Moerloose P, Bounameaux H. D-Dimer for venous thromboembolism diagnosis: 20 years later. *J Thromb Haemost.* 2008; 6(7):1059–1071.

45. Bounameaux H, De Moerloose P, Perrier A, Reber G. Plasma measurement of D-dimer as diagnostic aid in suspected venous thromboembolism: an overview. *Thromb Haemost.* 1994; 71(1):1–6.

46. Farrell S, Hayes T, Shaw M. A negative SimpliRED D-dimer assay result does not exclude the diagnosis of deep vein thrombosis or pulmonary embolus in emergency department patients. *Ann Emerg Med.* 2000; 35(2):121–125.

47. Righini M, Van Es J, Den Exter PL, et al. Age-adjusted D-dimer cutoff levels to rule out pulmonary embolism: the ADJUST-PE study. *JAMA.* 2014; 311(11):1117–1124.

48. Schellong SM, Schwarz T, Halbritter K, et al. Complete compression ultrasonography of the leg veins as a single test for the diagnosis of deep vein thrombosis. *Thromb Haemost.* 2003; 89(2):228–234.

49. Mazzolai L, Aboyans V, Ageno W, et al. Diagnosis and management of acute deep vein thrombosis: a joint consensus document from the European Society of Cardiology working groups of aorta and peripheral vascular diseases and pulmonary circulation and right ventricular function. *Eur Heart J.* 2018; 39(47): 4208–4218.

50. Goodacre S, Sampson F, Thomas S, van Beek E, Sutton A. Systematic review and meta-analysis of the diagnostic accuracy of ultrasonography for deep vein thrombosis. *BMC Med Imaging.* 2005; 5:6.

51. Birdwell BG, Raskob GE, Whitsett TL, et al. The clinical validity of normal compression ultrasonography in outpatients suspected of having deep venous thrombosis. *Ann Intern Med.* 1998; 128(1):1–7.

52. Fraser DG, Moody AR, Morgan PS, Martel AL, Davidson I. Diagnosis of lower-limb deep venous thrombosis: a prospective blinded study of magnetic resonance direct thrombus imaging. *Ann Intern Med.* 2002; 136(2):89–98.

53. Lensing A, Büller H, Prandoni P, et al. Contrast venography, the gold standard for the diagnosis of deep-vein thrombosis: improvement in observer agreement. *Thromb Haemost.* 1992; 67(1):8–12.

54. Bates SM, Jaeschke R, Stevens SM, et al. Diagnosis of DVT: antithrombotic therapy and prevention of thrombosis: American College of Chest Physicians evidence-based clinical practice guidelines. *Chest J.* 2012; 141(2 suppl): e351S–e418S.

55. Lucassen W, Geersing G-J, Erkens PM, et al. Clinical decision rules for excluding pulmonary embolism: a meta-analysis. *Ann Intern Med.* 2011; 155(7):448–460.

56. Hunsaker AR, Lu MT, Goldhaber SZ, Rybicki FJ. Imaging in acute pulmonary embolism with special clinical scenarios. *Circ Cardiovasc Imaging.* 2010; 3(4):491–500.

57. Klok FA, Mos IC, Nijkeuter M, et al. Simplification of the revised Geneva score for assessing clinical probability of pulmonary embolism. *Arch Intern Med.* 2008; 168(19): 2131–2136.

58. Vanni S, Polidori G, Vergara R, et al. Prognostic value of ECG among patients with acute pulmonary embolism and normal blood pressure. *Am J Med.* 2009; 122(3): 257–264.

59. Kang DK, Ramos-Duran L, Schoepf UJ, et al. Reproducibility of CT signs of right ventricular dysfunction in acute pulmonary embolism. *Am J Roentgenol.* 2010; 194(6):1500–1506.

60. Revel M, Sanchez O, Couchon S, et al. Diagnostic accuracy of magnetic resonance imaging for an acute pulmonary embolism: results of the 'IRM-EP' study. *J Thromb Haemost.* 2012; 10(5):743–750.

61. Jaff MR, McMurtry MS, Archer SL, et al. Management of massive and submassive pulmonary embolism, iliofemoral deep vein thrombosis, and chronic thromboembolic pulmonary hypertension a scientific statement from the American Heart Association. *Circulation.* 2011; 123(16):1788–1830.

62. Kearon C, Akl EA, Ornelas J, et al. Antithrombotic therapy for VTE disease: CHEST guideline and expert panel report. *Chest J.* 2016; 149(2):315–352.

63. Konstantinides S, Torbicki A, Agnelli G, et al. 2014 ESC guidelines on the diagnosis and management of acute pulmonary embolism. *Eur Heart J.* 2014; 35(43): 3033–3069 3069a–3069k.

64. Murphy N, Broadhurst DI, Khashan AS, Gilligan O, Kenny LC, O'Donoghue K. Gestation-specific D-dimer reference ranges: a cross-sectional study. *BJOG.* 2015; 122(3):395–400.

65. Righini M, Robert-Ebadi H, Elias A, et al. Diagnosis of pulmonary embolism during pregnancy: a multicenter prospective management outcome study. *Ann Intern Med.* 2018; 169(11):766–773.

66. van der Pol LM, Tromeur C, Bistervels IM, et al. Pregnancy-adapted YEARS algorithm for diagnosis of suspected pulmonary embolism. *N Engl J Med.* 2019; 380(12):1139–1149.

67. Coppens M, Reijnders JH, Middeldorp S, Doggen CJ, Rosendaal FR. Testing for inherited thrombophilia does not reduce the recurrence of venous thrombosis. *J Thromb Haemost.* 2008; 6(9):1474–1477.

68. Christiansen SC, Cannegieter SC, Koster T, Vandenbroucke JP, Rosendaal FR. Thrombophilia, clinical factors, and recurrent venous thrombotic events. *JAMA.* 2005; 293(19):2352–2361.

69. Kearon C, Julian JA, Kovacs MJ, et al. Influence of thrombophilia on risk of recurrent venous thromboembolism while on warfarin: results from a randomized trial. *Blood.* 2008; 112(12):4432–4436.

70. Carrier M, Le Gal G, Wells PS, Fergusson D, Ramsay T, Rodger MA. Systematic review: the Trousseau syndrome revisited: should we screen extensively for cancer in patients with venous thromboembolism? *Ann Intern Med.* 2008; 149(5):323–333.

71. Schulman S, Lindmarker P, Holmström M, et al. Post-thrombotic syndrome, recurrence, and death 10 years after the first episode of venous thromboembolism treated with warfarin for 6 weeks or 6 months. *J Thromb Haemost.* 2006; 4(4):734–742.

72. Eichinger S, Weltermann A, Minar E, et al. Symptomatic pulmonary embolism and the risk of recurrent venous thromboembolism. *Arch Intern Med.* 2004; 164(1):92–96.

73. Kyrle PA, Minar E, Bialonczyk C, Hirschl M, Weltermann A, Eichinger S. The risk of recurrent venous thromboembolism in men and women. *N Engl J Med.* 2004; 350(25):2558–2563.

74. van Es J, Cheung YW, van Es N, et al. Short-term prognosis of breakthrough venous thromboembolism in anticoagulated patients. *Thromb Res.* 2020; 187:125–130.

75. Rodger MA, Miranda S, Delluc A, Carrier M. Management of suspected and confirmed recurrent venous thrombosis while on anticoagulant therapy. What next? *Thromb Res.* 2019; 180:105–109.

76. Deitelzweig S, Johnson B, Lin J, Schulman K. Prevalence of clinical venous thromboembolism in the USA: current trends and future projections. *Am J Hematol.* 2011; 86(2):217–220.

77. Kahn S, Partsch H, Vedantham S, Prandoni P, Kearon C. Definition of post-thrombotic syndrome of the leg for use in clinical investigations: a recommendation for standardization. *J Thromb Haemost.* 2009; 7(5):879–883.

78. Pesavento R, Prandoni P. Prevention and treatment of the post-thrombotic syndrome and of the chronic thromboembolic pulmonary hypertension. *Expert Rev Cardiovasc Ther.* 2015; 13(2):193–207.

79. Kahn SR, Shrier I, Julian JA, et al. Determinants and time course of the postthrombotic syndrome after acute deep venous thrombosis. *Ann Intern Med.* 2008; 149(10): 698–707.

80. Sista AK, Horowitz JM, Goldhaber SZ. Four key questions surrounding thrombolytic therapy for submassive pulmonary embolism. *Vasc Med.* 2016; 21(1):47–52.

81. Stevinson BG, Hernandez-Nino J, Rose G, Kline JA. Echocardiographic and functional cardiopulmonary problems 6 months after first-time pulmonary embolism in previously healthy patients. *Eur Heart J.* 2007; 28(20):2517–2524.

82. Klok F, Van der Hulle T, Den Exter P, Lankeit M, Huisman M, Konstantinides S. The post-PE syndrome: a new concept for chronic complications of pulmonary embolism. *Blood Rev.* 2014; 28(6):221–226.

83. Konstantinides S, Goldhaber SZ. Pulmonary embolism: risk assessment and management. *Eur Heart J.* 2012; 33(24):3014–3022.

84. Becattini C, Agnelli G. Treatment of venous thromboembolism with new anticoagulant agents. *J Am Coll Cardiol.* 2016; 67(16):1941–1955.

85. Stein PD, Hull RD, Matta F, Yaekoub AY, Liang J. Incidence of thrombocytopenia in hospitalized patients with venous thromboembolism. *Am J Med.* 2009; 122(10):919–930.

86. Schulman S, Kearon C, Kakkar AK, et al. Dabigatran versus warfarin in the treatment of acute venous thromboembolism. *N Engl J Med.* 2009; 361(24): 2342–2352.

87. Schulman S, Kearon C, Kakkar AK, et al. Extended use of dabigatran, warfarin, or placebo in venous thromboembolism. *N Engl J Med.* 2013; 368(8):709–718.

88. EINSTEIN Investigators. Oral rivaroxaban for symptomatic venous thromboembolism. *N Engl J Med.* 2010; 2010(363):2499–2510.

89. EINSTEIN–PE Investigators. Oral rivaroxaban for the treatment of symptomatic pulmonary embolism. *N Engl J Med.* 2012; 2012(366):1287–1297.

90. Connolly SJ, Milling Jr. TJ, Eikelboom JW, et al. Andexanet Alfa for acute major bleeding associated with factor Xa inhibitors. *N Engl J Med.* 2016; 375(12): 1131–1141.

91. Hokusai-VTE Investigators. Edoxaban versus warfarin for the treatment of symptomatic venous thromboembolism. *N Engl J Med.* 2013; 2013(369):1406–1415.

92. Steffel J, Verhamme P, Potpara TS, et al. The 2018 European Heart Rhythm Association Practical Guide on the use of non-vitamin K antagonist oral anticoagulants in patients with atrial fibrillation. *Eur Heart J.* 2018; 39(16):1330–1393.

93. National Comprehensive Cancer Network. NCCN Clinical Practice Guideline in Oncology. Cancer-Associated Venous Thromboembolic Diseases. April. Available from:(2020). https://www.nccn.org/store/login/login.aspx?ReturnURL=https://www.nccn.org/professionals/physician_gls/pdf/vte.pdf; 2020.

94. Dlott JS, George RA, Huang X, et al. A national assessment of warfarin anticoagulation therapy for stroke prevention in atrial fibrillation. *Circulation.* 2014; 129(13):1407–1414. https://doi.org/10.1161/CIRCULATIONAHA.113.002601.

95. Heneghan C, Alonso-Coello P, Garcia-Alamino J, Perera R, Meats E, Glasziou P. Self-monitoring of oral anticoagulation: a systematic review and meta-analysis. *Lancet.* 2006; 367(9508):404–411.

96. Epstein RS, Moyer TP, Aubert RE, et al. Warfarin genotyping reduces hospitalization rates: results from the MM-WES (Medco-Mayo Warfarin Effectiveness Study). *J Am Coll Cardiol.* 2010; 55(25):2804–2812.

97. Pollack Jr. CV, Reilly PA, Eikelboom J, et al. Idarucizumab for dabigatran reversal. *N Engl J Med.* 2015; 373(6):511–520.

98. Laiho M, Oinonen A, Sugano N, et al. Preservation of venous valve function after catheter-directed and systemic thrombolysis for deep venous thrombosis. *Eur J Vasc Endovasc Surg.* 2004; 28(4):391–396.

99. Chatterjee S, Chakraborty A, Weinberg I, et al. Thrombolysis for pulmonary embolism and risk of all-cause mortality, major bleeding, and intracranial hemorrhage: a meta-analysis. *JAMA.* 2014; 311(23):2414–2421.

100. Meyer G, Vicaut E, Danays T, et al. Fibrinolysis for patients with intermediate-risk pulmonary embolism. *N Engl J Med.* 2014; 370(15):1402–1411.

101. Poterucha TJ, Bergmark B, Aranki S, Kaneko T, Piazza G. Surgical pulmonary embolectomy. *Circulation.* 2015; 132(12):1146–1151.

102. PREPIC Study Group. Eight-year follow-up of patients with permanent vena cava filters in the prevention of pulmonary embolism the PREPIC (prévention du risque d'embolie pulmonaire par interruption cave) randomized study. *Circulation.* 2005; 112(3):416–422.

103. Zondag W, Hiddinga BI, Crobach MJ, et al. Hestia criteria can discriminate high- from low-risk patients with pulmonary embolism. *Eur Respir J.* 2013; 41(3):588–592.

104. Zondag W, Mos IC, Creemers-Schild D, et al. Outpatient treatment in patients with acute pulmonary embolism: the Hestia Study. *J Thromb Haemost.* 2011; 9(8): 1500–1507.

105. Dudzinski DM, Piazza G. Multidisciplinary pulmonary embolism response teams. *Circulation.* 2016; 133(1): 98–103.
106. Kakkar AK, Cohen AT, Tapson VF, et al. Venous thromboembolism risk and prophylaxis in the acute care hospital setting (ENDORSE survey): findings in surgical patients. *Ann Surg.* 2010; 251(2):330–338.
107. Anderson FA, Goldhaber SZ, Tapson VF, et al. Improving practices in US hospitals to prevent venous thromboembolism: lessons from ENDORSE. *Am J Med.* 2010; 123(12):1099–106. e8.
108. Decousus H, Tapson VF, Bergmann J-F, et al. Factors at admission associated with bleeding risk in medical patients: findings from the IMPROVE investigators. *Chest J.* 2011; 139(1):69–79.
109. Woller SC, Stevens SM, Jones JP, et al. Derivation and validation of a simple model to identify venous thromboembolism risk in medical patients. *Am J Med.* 2011; 124(10) 947–954.e2.
110. Qaseem A, Chou R, Humphrey LL, Starkey M, Shekelle P. Venous thromboembolism prophylaxis in hospitalized patients: a clinical practice guideline from the American College of Physicians. *Ann Intern Med.* 2011; 155(9): 625–632.
111. Spyropoulos AC, Lipardi C, Xu J, et al. Improved benefit risk profile of rivaroxaban in a subpopulation of the MAGELLAN study. *Clin Appl Thromb Hemost.* 2019; 25 1076029619886022.
112. Sobieraj DM, Lee S, Coleman CI, et al. Prolonged versus standard-duration venous thromboprophylaxis in major orthopedic surgery: a systematic review. *Ann Intern Med.* 2012; 156(10):720–727.
113. Falck-Ytter Y, Francis CW, Johanson NA, et al. Prevention of VTE in orthopedic surgery patients: Antithrombotic Therapy and Prevention of Thrombosis, 9th ed: American College of Chest Physicians evidence-based clinical practice guidelines. *Chest.* 2012; 141(2 suppl): e278S–e325S.

# CHAPTER 35

# Genetics of Cardiovascular Disease and Applications of Genetic Testing

NEJAT MAHDIEH[a,b] • BAHAREH RABBANI[c] • MAJID MALEKI[c]
[a]Cardiogenetic Research Center, Rajaie Cardiovascular, Medical & Research Center, Iran University of Medical Sciences, Tehran, Iran, [b]Growth and Development Research Center, Tehran University of Medical Sciences, Tehran, Iran, [c]Rajaie Cardiovascular, Medical & Research Center, Iran University of Medical Sciences, Tehran, Iran

## KEY POINTS

- Genetic diagnoses especially using single-gene and/or NGS tests are available for inherited cardiovascular diseases.
- NGS technologies have revolutionized our understanding of the molecular mechanisms of cardiovascular disorders and provide insights on potential therapies.
- Cascade screening is recommended when a pathogenic variant is identified in a patient.
- In the genetic evaluation of a child with a congenital heart defect (CHD), it is a critical step to determine if it is syndromic or isolated CHD.
- Approximately 30%–50% and 80% of DCM and HCM patients, respectively, have a genetic etiology.
- Genetic testing in patients with arrhythmias and cardiomyopathies is usually used for confirmation of diagnosis as well as for risk stratification and patient management.

## INTRODUCTION

Human cells include the nuclear genome composed of 20,000–25,000 genes and the mitochondrial genome (composed of 37 genes). The human nuclear genome consists of two sets of 23 chromosomes (pairs 1–22 are autosomes and the $23^{rd}$ pair is the sex chromosomes, i.e., X and Y); each set received from each parent is estimated to be $3.2 \times 109$ base pairs.[1] The hereditary material, DNA, is a polymer of four organic bases: adenine (A), thymine (T), cytosine (C), and guanine (G). A gene, a sequence of nitrogenous bases, located on a chromosome expresses a functional product whether an RNA molecule or subsequently a peptide. An allele, a variant form of a gene, is positioned on a locus, the specific location of a gene on a chromosome. Coding regions (exons) of a gene are interrupted by noncoding parts (introns). The flow of genetic information is required for cell division, survival, and reproduction; it consists of replication (DNA generates DNA); transcription (DNA produces RNA); RNA processing (capping, splicing, poly A tailing, and RNA translocation to cytoplasm); translation (RNA encodes protein); and protein processing, folding, transport, and incorporation. A mutation, alteration of the sequence of the genome, may cause disruption or affect one of these phases (Fig. 35.1). Mutations are classified according to their size, effect, location, and mode of inheritance (Table 35.1).[2] Three major classes of genetic diseases are single-gene (caused by mutation in a single gene), chromosomal (caused by chromosomal aberrations), and multifactorial or complex (caused by gene–environment interactions) disorders.

Unraveling the mechanism of diseases provides promising insights on potential therapies. Emergence of new technologies for mutation detection is helpful to find out the cause of diseases. Traditionally, two groups of tests—molecular and cytogenetic tests—have been used to detect mutations. Small-scale mutations are usually identified by polymerase chain reaction (PCR)/restriction fragment length polymorphism (RFLP) and direct sequencing, and large-scale mutations are checked by karyotyping (chromosome analysis).

As the primary cause of mortality and morbidity around the world, inherited cardiovascular diseases (CVD) have a genetic etiology. Familial clustering of CVD, especially in countries with traditional cultures, suggests the prominent role of genetic elements as its major etiology. Thus, cardiologists should be aware of

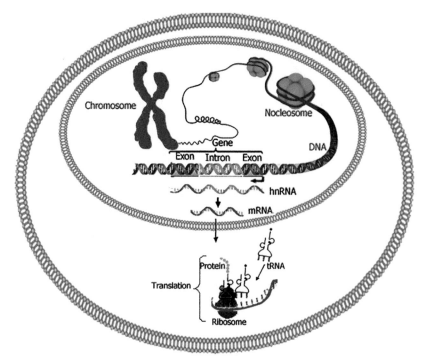

FIG. 35.1 Cell, chromosome, and gene expression (replication, transcription, and translation). *hnRNA*, heterogeneous nuclear RNA; *mRNA*, messenger RNA; *tRNA*, transfer RNA.

**TABLE 35.1**
**Classification of Mutations**

| Mutation | Definition | Example (Gene) | Technique for Detection | Disease |
|---|---|---|---|---|
| Small-scale mutation | Affects a gene, e.g., small insertion/deletions (indels), duplication (dup), point mutations (base substitutions like A>G purine to purine, T>C pyrimidine to pyrimidine) | c.920_923dupTCAG (*LDLR*), c.3524insA (*FBN1*) | ARMS, RFLP, MLPA, PCR, Sequencing | Familial hypercholesterolemia Marfan syndrome |
| **SIZE** | | | | |
| Large-scale mutation | Affects chromosomes, includes structural and numerical aberrations | | Karyotype, FISH, CGH, MLPA | |
| **STRUCTURAL** | | | | |
| Deletion | A part of the chromosome is deleted | 46,XX, del(22) (q11.21–q11.23) | FISH, array CGH, MLPA | DiGeorge syndrome |
| Duplication | A part of the chromosome is duplicated | 46,XX,dup(22q11.2) | Array-CGH, MLPA | Cat-eye syndrome |

*Continued*

**TABLE 35.1**
**Classification of Mutations—cont'd**

| Mutation | Definition | Example (Gene) | Technique for Detection | Disease |
|---|---|---|---|---|
| Translocation | An interchange of genetic material between nonhomologous chromosomes includes reciprocal (between two chromosomes) or Robertsonian translocation (fusion of the long arms of two acrocentric chromosomes and loss of their short arms) | 46,XY,t(2;13)(q22; q34)mat | FISH | Congenital heart disease |
| Inversion | A part of the chromosome is inverted; includes pericentric (between two arms) or paracentric (located on one arm) | 46,XX,inv. (9) (p11q13) | Karyotype | Normal |
| Ring | Both arms of the chromosome are fused to form a ring | 46,Xr(X) | Karyotype | Turner syndrome |
| Isochromosome | A chromosome with two identical arms | 46,Xi(Xq) | Karyotype | Turner syndrome |
| Dicentric chromosome | A chromosome with two centromeres | 46,X,psu dic(Y) (pter → q11.2:: q11.2 → pter) | Karyotype | Azoospermia |
| **NUMERICAL** | | | | |
| Aneuploidy | An abnormal number of chromosomes caused by an error in cell division | $2n + 1$; $2n - 1$ | Karyotype | |
| Monosomy | Only one of two homologous chromosomes exists ($2n - 1$) | 45,X | Karyotype | Turner syndrome |
| Uniparental disomy | Two pairs of a homologous chromosome are inherited from one parent and no copy from the other parent | 46,XX,upd(15)mat | MS-PCR, MS-MLPA | Prader–Willi syndrome |
| Trisomy | Three copies of a homologous chromosome ($2n + 1$) | 47,XX,+21 | Karyotype | Down syndrome |
| Tetrasomy | Four copies of a homologous chromosome ($2n + 2$) | 48,XXXX | Karyotype | X tetrasomy |
| Monoploidy | Having a single (nonhomologous) set of chromosomes ($n$) | 23X | Karyotype | |
| Triploidy | Having three sets of chromosomes ($3n$) | 69,XXX | Karyotype | Abortion hydatidiform mole |
| **EFFECT ON FUNCTION** | | | | |
| Loss of function (haploinsufficiency) | Results in reduced or abolished protein function; the reduced dosage is not adequate for a normal phenotype | p.A302V (*KCNQ1*) | ARMS, RFLP, PCR, sequencing | Early-onset lone AF |
| Gain of function | Gives new or enhanced activity to a protein | p.R420Q (*RyR2*) | ARMS, RFLP, PCR, sequencing | CPVT |

*Continued*

**TABLE 35.1**

**Classification of Mutations—cont'd**

| Mutation | Definition | Example (Gene) | Technique for Detection | Disease |
|---|---|---|---|---|
| Dominant negative | Its product interferes with the product of normal allele | c.G211T (*KCNJ2*) | ARMS, RFLP, PCR, sequencing | Andersen–Tawil syndrome |
| **EFFECT ON PROTEIN SEQUENCE** | | | | |
| Frameshift | Caused by insertion or deletion of a number of nucleotides nondivisible by three from the coding region | p.E20963KfsX10 (*TTN*) | ARMS, RFLP, PCR, sequencing | DCM |
| Missense (nonsynonymous) | Leads to a codon that codes for a different amino acid | p.G60A (*PTPN11*) | ARMS, RFLP, PCR, sequencing | Noonan syndrome |
| Nonsense | Leads to a premature stop codon | p.W4X | ARMS, RFLP, PCR, sequencing | Familial hypercholesterolemia |
| Synonymous | Leads a codon that codes an amino acid with similar properties, e.g., lysine to arginine | p.V153I (*GJB2*) | ARMS, RFLP, PCR, sequencing | Normal |
| Silent | (Usually in the third position of the codon) no change in amino acid sequences, e.g., GCT, GCC, GCA, and GCG all codes for alanine | p.I69I (*GJB2*) | ARMS, RFLP, PCR, sequencing | Normal |
| Neutral | A single nucleotide that does not have any harmful or beneficial effect on the organism; it usually occurs at noncoding DNA regions | | | |
| **INHERITANCE** | | | | |
| Somatic nutation | A mutation in somatic cells that is not usually transmitted to descendants | | | |
| Germline nutation | Mutation in reproductive cells could be transmitted to descendants or de novo | | | |
| Hereditary | Inherited from parents | | | |
| Dominant mutation | One mutant allele leads to an abnormal phenotype | | | |
| Recessive mutation | Both alleles must carry the mutation to produce the diseased phenotype | | | |
| De novo | A mutation that is present for the first time in one family member as a result of a mutation in a germ cell | | | |
| **OTHER** | | | | |
| Splice mutation | A sequence change in the site splicing of an intron; it may result in one or more introns remaining in mature mRNA | IVS2 + 1G>A ARMS, RFLP, PCR, sequencing | | Jervell and Lange-Nielsen syndrome (*KCNQ1*) |
| Dynamic mutation | An unstable mutation that the copies of a sequence are changed during meiosis division, e.g., trinucleotide expansion | (CGG)$n$ > 200 (*FMR1*) Southern blot, triple-repeat PCR | | Fragile X syndrome |

*ARMS*, amplification-refractory mutation system, a procedure developed for the analysis of single-nucleotide polymorphisms using allele-specific primers in two different tubes; *array CHG*, array comparative genomic hybridization, a molecular cytogenetic technique used for detecting chromosomal copy number variations on a genome-wide scale; *FISH*, fluorescence in situ hybridization, a molecular cytogenetic technique for identifying the positions of genes on chromosomes and chromosomal abnormalities; *MLPA*, multiplex ligation-dependent probe amplification, a multiplex polymerase chain reaction method detecting abnormal copy numbers of up to 50 different genomic DNA or RNA sequences; *MS-PCR*, methylation-specific polymerase chain reaction, a method for analysis of DNA methylation patterns; *PCR*, polymerase chain reaction, a technique for amplifying a piece of DNA sequence to millions of copies; *RFLP*, restriction fragment length polymorphism, on the basis of endonuclease enzyme digestion of polymerase chain reaction-amplified DNA at specific positions.

Data from Mahdieh N. *A Comprehensive Review on Genetics*. Baraye Farda Publisher; 2010:27–75.

the genetic aspects of cardiac diseases and the role of genetic testing in CVD. The approach to cardiogenetic evaluation should include an accurate clinical diagnosis in the proband, a detailed family history consistent with familial forms of CVD, awareness of the nature of genetic testing, and the need for genetic counseling.[3] In this chapter, a brief summary of cardiovascular genetics is presented to make cardiologists familiar with applications of genetic testing, the molecular basis of cardiovascular disorders, and applications of state-of-the art technologies.

## GENETIC TESTING AND VARIANT INTERPRETATION

Specific genetic testing is recommended for known syndromes with specific causes such as the Ullrich–Turner syndrome (X monosomy), 1p36 deletion syndrome, CHARGE syndrome (due to *CHD7* gene mutations), Cri du chat syndrome (5p deletion), Ellis–van Creveld syndrome (*EVC1* and *2* genes), Holt–Oram syndrome, Marfan syndrome (heterozygous *FBN1* mutations) microdeletion syndrome 22q11.2, Noonan syndrome (*PTPN11* mutations), trisomies 13, 18, and 21, VACTERL association, Williams (Beuren) syndrome, and Wolf–Hirschhorn syndrome. Single-gene analyses are applied to disorders having a monogenic cause with an accurate clinical diagnosis; next-generation sequencing (NGS) including gene-panel-based NGS and whole exome sequencing (WES) is used to detect causal variants in heterogeneous disorders. The vast majority of cardiac diseases have a highly genetic heterogeneity. Panel-based NGS/WES is preferred to single-gene testing in such disorders. After establishing the clinical diagnosis, genetic counseling, and taking informed consent, genetic testing is performed in the proband at the first step. If a variant(s) is identified it is categorized based on ACMG recommendations to a pathogenic variant(s), likely pathogenic, a variant with uncertain clinical significance (VUS), likely benign or benign variant. Usually in genetic testing reports, the likelihood of pathogenicity of the identified variant is made using literature searching (for "previously reported mutations") or in silico analyses. When a VUS is reported, its pathogenicity should be confirmed by segregation analysis (checking the variant in other family members and investigating if the variant is found only in healthy members of the family), population study (low frequency of the pathogenic variant) in silico analyses (using software tools), and functional analysis in human cells and animal models. In genetic reports, mutations are usually named at a DNA or protein level; for example, c.654–655delCA (deletion of two nucleotides CA at positions 654–655) in the *PKP2* gene ("c." designated for coding sequences) is a frameshift

mutation that causes a truncated protein (p. H218Qfs*9), or as another example, p.Gly2595Ser (p. G295S) in *FBN1* (Marfan syndrome) indicates a missense mutation at position 295 of the protein ("p." for the amino acid sequence of the protein), c.920_923dupTCAG in *LDLR* (hypercholesterolemia) is due to duplication of a unit of four nucleotides.

Genetic testing in adults needs informed consent, but in children, it is performed if a medical benefit exists. However, in the clinic, genetic testing is used to confirm the diagnosis of diseases with a similar clinical presentation (HCM may be due to *MYBPC3* and/or *MYH7* mutations, *TTR* amyloidosis or Fabry disease), to facilitate cascade screening and to target therapies of patients, e.g., targeted therapies using gene editing, silencing technologies and antibody-based therapeutics are being applied or developed for diseases such as *TTR* amyloidosis, Fabry disease, DMD and LQTS; likewise, surgical intervention may be considered at a smaller aortic aneurysm diameter if variants of *ACTA2*, *MYH11*, or *TGFBR2* genes are detected in a patient.[4] If a pathogenic variant is identified in the proband, it is recommended to screen asymptomatic first-degree relatives within the family (predictive genetic testing/cascade screening).

### Molecular Genetic Tests
#### Polymerase chain reaction
PCR is a method to amplify a small specific segment of the DNA (up to 2–3 kilo bases) to make millions to billions of copies, a large amount of DNA required to study in detail. PCR is based on the ability of DNA polymerase to synthesize a new strand of DNA using a pair of primers that provide the 3′OH group. Briefly, using high temperatures, the double-stranded DNA is denatured, the primers anneal to their targets and then the DNA polymerase (Taq polymerase is thermostable and has an optimum temperature of 72°C) adds the nucleotides to the 3′OH group based on the DNA template.[2]

#### Sanger sequencing
As the first generation of sequencing methods, Sanger sequencing (chain-termination or dideoxy technique) is used to determine the nucleotide sequence of a targeted DNA. Briefly, amplification is linearly performed using one primer, DNA polymerase, DNA sequence of interest, deoxynucleotides, and a labeled dideoxynucleotide. The growing strand is stopped when a dideoxynucleotide is added. The label is excited using a laser at the end of each sequence.[2] This method is used as the "gold standard" for clinical research sequencing, especially for single-gene disorders such as the Jervell and Lange-Nielsen syndrome, and to validate the variants found by NGS.

### Next-generation sequencing

NGS is based on simultaneous sequencing of a huge amount of DNA fragments, known as massive parallel sequencing. Briefly, the extracted DNA is digested to small fragments (up to 200–300 base); these fragments are sequenced in a massively parallel manner. In panel-based NGS and WES, targeted fragments are captured and sequenced. The sequence data, then, are compared with public databases such as ExAc and 1000 Genomes Project to exclude high prevalent and normal variants. A collection of software tools is applied to identify a candidate variant as a pathogenic or a likely pathogenic variant.

NGS has been used to detect novel causative variants of a single gene and common disorders of the cardiovascular system including familial hypercholesterolemia, different types of cardiomyopathies, long QT syndrome, CHD, and thoracic aortic aneurysms and dissections (TAAD). Different gene panels are available for HCM, DCM, LQT, and other inherited CVDs.[5]

## MONOGENIC FORMS OF CONGENITAL HEART DEFECTS

CHDs affect approximately 1%–3% newborns in the world.[6] CHDs may occur as presentation of some genetic syndromes or may be nonsyndromic. Thus, when a child has CHD it is crucial to determine if it is syndromic or nonsyndromic CHD. Genetic counseling is helpful in finding out the pattern of inheritance (Fig. 35.2) and estimating the recurrence risk. Because of phenotypic variability in many syndromes, diagnostic evaluation should be performed. Aneuploidies, such as trisomy 21 or Turner syndrome, are diagnosed by karyotyping, and chromosomal microdeletion syndromes are detected using array comparative genome hybridization (aCGH), fluorescence in situ hybridization (FISH), or multiplex ligation-dependent probe amplification (MLPA).

Particular gene(s), if suspected, should be analyzed using molecular techniques such as PCR for sequencing. An increasing number of single genes such as PTPN11 (Noonan syndrome) have been reported for nonsyndromic CHDs in addition to complex types.[6] Mutations in *Nkx2–5*, *GATA4*, and *NOTCH1* genes have been reported in Iranian CHD patients and in other parts of the world.[7–9] Mutation analysis using NGS tests may be ordered to confirm the clinical diagnosis. Genetic diagnosis provides an accurate counseling on the prognosis, causality, and recurrence risk for parents and their children. Unfortunately for isolated CHD, there is not much information, and the recurrent risk is assessed based on empiric recurrence data.

## INHERITED CARDIOMYOPATHIES

Cardiomyopathies include dilated cardiomyopathy (DCM), hypertrophic cardiomyopathy (HCM), restrictive cardiomyopathy (RCM), arrhythmogenic ventricular cardiomyopathy (AVC or previously named ARVC/D), and left ventricular noncompaction cardiomyopathy (LVNC).[10]

### Dilated cardiomyopathy

DCM accounts for approximately 55% of cardiomyopathies, and 30%–50% of them are caused by a genetic etiology with predominantly autosomal dominant inheritance and less commonly X-linked, autosomal recessive, and mitochondrial inheritance.[11–13] Involved genes in DCM encode for a number of cellular components, such as the nuclear envelope proteins; transcription factors; calcium handling proteins; and the sarcomere, cytoskeleton, and sarcolemmal proteins. Gene testing in DCM determines the disease-causing mutations only in about 30% of cases.[14] The *TTN* gene encodes titin, a giant protein acting as a molecular ruler for structural integrity and diastolic tension. *TTN* mutations are responsible for 25% of familial and 18% of sporadic forms of DCM.[15] Mutations in a nuclear envelope protein lamin A/C (*LMNA*) and dystrophin genes account for 10%–15% of all cases of DCM; *LMNA* is responsible for 30% of cases of DCM with conduction system disease and early life-threatening ventricular arrhythmia.[16,17] The use of NGS technology has helped to identify an increased number of involved genes in DCM.

### Hypertrophic Cardiomyopathy

To date, mutations in more than 20 genes have been identified to be involved in developing HCM, which affects 1 in 500 young adults. Nearly 80% of causal mutations occur in *MYH7* and *MYBPC3* genes,[18] but they are responsible for less than 50% in Iran (our unpublished data). *MYBPC3* mutations including missense, splice site, and deletion and insertion mutations account for about 45% of all cases of HCM.[19–21] Although recent clinical guidelines recommend testing of five genes (*MYBPC3*, *MYH7*, *TNNI3*, *TNNT2*, and *TPM1*) for finding the genetic causality of HCM, panel-based NGS provides widely available facilities to check known involved genes.

### Restrictive Cardiomyopathy

Mutations in a few genes have been described to cause RCM or a mixed RCM-HCM phenotype. These genes include *TNNI3*, *TNNT2*, *MYH7*, *ACTC1*, *TPM1*, *MYL3*, *MYL* and *MYPN*, *TTN*, and *Bag3*.[3,10,22,23]

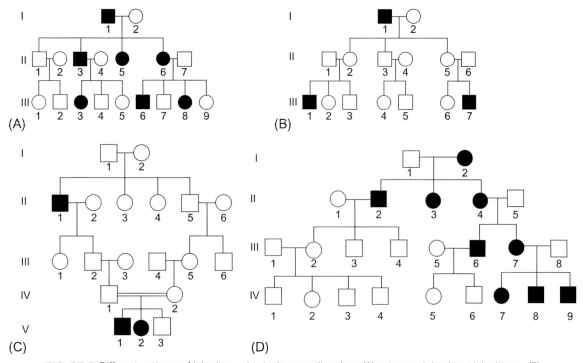

**FIG. 35.2** Different patterns of inheritance in single-gene disorders: (A) autosomal dominant inheritance, (B) autosomal recessive inheritance, (C) X-linked inheritance, and (D) mitochondrial inheritance.

## LEFT VENTRICULAR NONCOMPACTION CARDIOMYOPATHY

LVNC shows an autosomal dominant pattern in 70% and an X-linked inheritance pattern in 30% of cases.[24] Mutations in the X-linked *TAZ* gene can cause LVNC and Barth syndrome.[25] Multiple genes have been identified to cause autosomal dominant LVNC associated with CHD: α-Dystrobrevin mutations cause HLHS and LVNC, *NKX2.5* mutations lead to LVNC and atrial septal defect (ASD), and *MYH7* mutations are observed in patients with LVNC and Ebstein anomaly. In addition, mutations in the *Z*-line protein-encoding *ZASP/LDB3* gene and the sarcomere-encoding genes are responsible for more than 20% of cases of LVNC without CHD.[26]

### Arrhythmogenic Ventricular Cardiomyopathy

ARVC/D is familial in up to 50% of cases and mostly inherited as an autosomal dominant disease. At least 15 genes have been described for AVC, and plakophilin 2 (*PKP2*) mutations account for up to 40% of cases.[26] Mutation analysis of the *PKP2* gene in Iranian patients with AVC showed that this gene is responsible for approximately 25% of cases (our unpublished data).

Metabolic, mitochondrial, and secondary cardiomyopathies should be considered in the patient as a whole, not merely from the cardiac perspective, and therefore, an accurate test for finding the genetic causality should be ordered.

## CARDIAC ELECTROPHYSIOLOGY

As a heterogeneous group of cardiac diseases, primary electrical heart disorders affect the myocyte transmembrane ion channels (Na, K) including long QT syndrome (LQTS), short QT syndrome (SQTS), Brugada syndrome (BrS), and catecholaminergic polymorphic ventricular tachycardia (CPVT).

### Long QT Syndrome

Congenital LQTS affects 1 in 2000 worldwide.[27] Fifteen genes have been reported to involve in LQTS with predominant roles of *KCNQ1* (potassium voltage-gated channel subfamily Q member 1), *KCNH2* (potassium voltage-gated channel subfamily H member 2), and *SCN5A* (sodium voltage-gated channel alpha subunit 5). Dominant-negative or loss-of-function mutations in

*KCNQ1* lead to LQT1, and gain-of-function mutations in *KCNQ1* cause familial atrial fibrillation. Defining the type of the involved gene and location of the mutation could be used to interpret discrepancies in the clinical picture of patients and to select an appropriate therapeutic approach. Genetic testing in LQTS patients for at least the *KCNQ1*, *KCNH2*, and *SCN5A* genes is usually used for confirmation of diagnosis as well as risk stratification and patient management.[3] Genetic testing of these genes in Iranian LQT patients showed that they are responsible for less than 40% of cases.[28] Genetic testing is ordered in the following scenarios:

1. There is a strong suspicion for LQTS based on clinical examination.
2. The patient shows asymptomatic QT prolongation without other clinical conditions that may prolong the QT interval.
3. Asymptomatic patients with QTc values of more than 460 ms (prepuberty) or more than 480 ms (adults) on serial 12-lead electrocardiograms (ECGs) should be tested for gene mutations.
4. There is an index case with mutation; the patient's family members are recommended to check for the mutation.

## Short QT Syndrome

Mutations in *KCNH2*, *KCNQ1*, and *KCNJ2* genes have been reported to cause SQTS. Genetic testing in 18%–40% of patients with SQTS shows gene mutation.[29,30]

## Catecholaminergic Polymorphic Ventricular Tachycardia

In all, 60% of individuals with CPVT have a single mutation in ryanodine receptor (*RyR2*). Loss-of-function mutations in calsequestrin 2 (CASQ2), calmodulin 1 (*CALM1*), and triadin (*TRDN*) genes can cause autosomal recessive CPVT. Genetic testing is recommended when exercise-induced bidirectional ventricular tachycardia (VT), polymorphic VT, or emotional stress-induced arrhythmia is documented in a patient.[3] *TRDN* mutations can cause LQT and/or CPVT depending on patients' age in the same and/or different patients.[36]

## Brugada Syndrome

*SCN5A* mutation is the most common cause of BrS.[31] BrS is diagnosed by clinical history and ECG findings. Multiple-gene testing could find causal variants. One of the most common cardiac conduction disorders is progressive cardiac conduction defect (PCCD), representing the main cause of pacemaker implantation. *SCN5A* mutations are also found in PCCD patients.

# PHARMACOGENOMICS AND POLYMORPHISMS

## Warfarin Dosing and Clopidogrel Resistance

Genetic testing may be used to investigate drug dosing, i.e., susceptibility to sensitivity and resistance to drug response, e.g., some individuals are resistant or show sensitivity to warfarin or resistance to clopidogrel because of variations in *CYP2C9* (*2 and *3 variants) and *VKORC1* ($-1639G > A$) and *CYP2C19* (*2, *3, and *17 variants) genes, respectively.[32] However, their clinical use is still limited.

## Coagulation and Fibrinolysis

Thrombotic disorders, including venous and arterial thrombosis, may occur due to an abnormality in hemostasis. High levels of plasma factor VIII (FVIII) and von Willebrand factor (vWF) are associated with an increased risk for vascular disease. A single SNP (single-nucleotide polymorphism) (p.D1241E) in FVIII is associated with plasma FVIII concentration. Variations of other genes, including FVII, FV (p.Arg506Gln), prothrombin (G20210A), fibrinogen ($c.-455G > A$), and FXIII (p.Val34Leu) are involved in thrombotic disorders. The thrombomodulin (*THBD*) gene may have a protective role in thrombosis mediated by the activation of protein C. Variations in the *PROC* (protein C), *EPCR* (or PROCR, endothelial protein C receptor), *PROS1* (protein S), *SERPINC1* (antithrombin), and *TFPI* (tissue factor pathway inhibitor) genes have been reported to influence the coagulation cascade. A 4G/5G insertion/deletion at $-675$ position of PAI-1 (plasminogen activator inhibitor-1) has been described to cause high levels of PAI-1 ($\approx 25\%$ higher levels in the homozygous state of the 4G compared with the 5G allele).[33] However, as a controversial issue, there is no consensus on how this information should be used in clinics for patients.

# FUTURE PERSPECTIVES

Recently, some studies on epigenetic biomarkers, small and long noncoding RNAs (sncRNA and lncRNA), and extracellular or cell-free DNA (cfDNA) have been published to understand the mechanisms of CVDs. In addition, iPSCs (induced pluripotent stem cells) can provide a system for testing personalized therapeutics on patients' cells. Studies have shown that silencing a long ncRNA, cardiac regeneration-related long noncoding ribonucleic acid (CAREL) improves heart function and regeneration in mice. Inhibition of another noncoding RNA, AZIN2-sv, enhances the proliferation rate of cardiomyocytes. Several ncRNA molecules have been shown to perturb miRNA and/or directly bind to proteins and may involve in cardiomyocyte proliferation.[34]

Besides, the molecular therapeutic approach on CVD is widely welcomed; somatic genome editing using the CRISPR–Cas9 technology has been applied to target loss of function mutations in Pcsk9 in embryonic mouse liver to lower the postnatal serum level of total cholesterol. In the same way, the efficacy of CRISPR-Cas9 in humans has been checked in familial hypertrophic cardiomyopathy due to *MYBPC3* mutations.[35] Unraveling the molecular mechanisms of CVDs sheds light on the role of therapy and provides molecular therapeutic approaches for CVDs.

## REFERENCES

1. International Human Genome Sequencing C. Finishing the euchromatic sequence of the human genome. *Nature.* 2004;431(7011):931–945.
2. Mahdieh N. *A Comprehensive Review on Genetics.* 4th ed. Tehran: Baraye Farda Publisher; 2019.
3. Ackerman MJ, Priori SG, Willems S, et al. HRS/EHRA expert consensus statement on the state of genetic testing for the channelopathies and cardiomyopathies: this document was developed as a partnership between the Heart Rhythm Society (HRS) and the European Heart Rhythm Association (EHRA). *Europace.* 2011;13(8):1077–1109.
4. Dainis AM, Ashley EA. Cardiovascular precision medicine in the genomics era. *JACC Basic Transl Sci.* 2018;3(2): 313–326.
5. Kalayinia S, Goodarzynejad H, Maleki M, Mahdieh N. Next generation sequencing applications for cardiovascular disease. *Ann Med.* 2018;50(2):91–109.
6. Reuter MS, Chaturvedi RR, Liston E, et al. The cardiac genome clinic: implementing genome sequencing in pediatric heart disease. *Genet Med.* 2020;22:1015–1024.
7. Kalayinia S, Ghasemi S, Mahdieh N. A comprehensive in silico analysis, distribution and frequency of human Nkx2-5 mutations; a critical gene in congenital heart disease. *J Cardiovasc Thorac Res.* 2019;11(4):287–299.
8. Kalayinia S, Maleki M, Mahdavi M, Mahdieh N. A novel de novo dominant mutation of NOTCH1 gene in an Iranian family with non-syndromic congenital heart disease. *J Clin Lab Anal.* 2020;34:e23147.
9. Kalayinia S, Maleki M, Rokni-Zadeh H, et al. GATA4 screening in Iranian patients of various ethnicities affected with congenital heart disease: co-occurrence of a novel de novo translocation (5;7) and a likely pathogenic heterozygous GATA4 mutation in a family with autosomal dominant congenital heart disease. *J Clin Lab Anal.* 2019;33(7):e22923.
10. Maron BJ, Towbin JA, Thiene G, et al. Contemporary definitions and classification of the cardiomyopathies: an American heart association scientific statement from the council on clinical cardiology, heart failure and transplantation committee; quality of care and outcomes

11. Fatkin D. Guidelines for the diagnosis and management of familial dilated cardiomyopathy. *Heart Lung Circ.* 2011; 20(11):691–693.
12. Givertz MM, Mann DL. Epidemiology and natural history of recovery of left ventricular function in recent onset dilated cardiomyopathies. *Curr Heart Fail Rep.* 2013;10(4): 321–330.
13. Dec GW, Fuster V. Idiopathic dilated cardiomyopathy. *N Engl J Med.* 1994;331(23):1564–1575.
14. Leviner DB, Hochhauser E, Arad M. Inherited cardiomyopathies—novel therapies. *Pharmacol Ther.* 2015;155:36–48.
15. Herman DS, Lam L, Taylor MR, et al. Truncations of titin causing dilated cardiomyopathy. *N Engl J Med.* 2012;366 (7):619–628.
16. van Rijsingen IA, Arbustini E, Elliott PM, et al. Risk factors for malignant ventricular arrhythmias in lamin a/c mutation carriers a European cohort study. *J Am Coll Cardiol.* 2012;59(5):493–500.
17. Diegoli M, Grasso M, Favalli V, et al. Diagnostic work-up and risk stratification in X-linked dilated cardiomyopathies caused by dystrophin defects. *J Am Coll Cardiol.* 2011;58(9): 925–934.
18. Maron BJ, Maron MS. Hypertrophic cardiomyopathy. *Lancet.* 2013;381(9862):242–255.
19. Saltzman AJ, Mancini-DiNardo D, Li C, et al. Short communication: the cardiac myosin binding protein C Arg502Trp mutation: a common cause of hypertrophic cardiomyopathy. *Circ Res.* 2010;106(9):1549–1552.
20. Dhandapany PS, Sadayappan S, Xue Y, et al. A common MYBPC3 (cardiac myosin binding protein C) variant associated with cardiomyopathies in South Asia. *Nat Genet.* 2009;41(2):187–191.
21. Richard P, Charron P, Carrier L, et al. Hypertrophic cardiomyopathy: distribution of disease genes, spectrum of mutations, and implications for a molecular diagnosis strategy. *Circulation.* 2003;107(17):2227–2232.
22. Caleshu C, Sakhuja R, Nussbaum RL, et al. Furthering the link between the sarcomere and primary cardiomyopathies: restrictive cardiomyopathy associated with multiple mutations in genes previously associated with hypertrophic or dilated cardiomyopathy. *Am J Med Genet A.* 2011;155a(9):2229–2235.
23. Sen-Chowdhry S, Syrris P, McKenna WJ. Genetics of restrictive cardiomyopathy. *Heart Fail Clin.* 2010;6(2): 179–186.
24. Ichida F, Hamamichi Y, Miyawaki T, et al. Clinical features of isolated noncompaction of the ventricular myocardium: long-term clinical course, hemodynamic properties, and genetic background. *J Am Coll Cardiol.* 1999;34(1):233–240.
25. Bleyl SB, Mumford BR, Brown-Harrison MC, et al. Xq28-linked noncompaction of the left ventricular myocardium: prenatal diagnosis and pathologic analysis of affected individuals. *Am J Med Genet.* 1997;72 (3):257–265.

26. Towbin JA. Inherited cardiomyopathies. *Circ J.* 2014;78 (10):2347–2356.

27. Schwartz PJ, Stramba-Badiale M, Crotti L, et al. Prevalence of the congenital long-QT syndrome. *Circulation.* 2009;120 (18):1761–1767.

28. Mahdieh N, Khorgami M, Soveizi M, et al. Genetic homozygosity in a diverse population: An experience of long QT syndrome. *Int J Cardiol.* 2020;316:117–124.

29. Giustetto C, Schimpf R, Mazzanti A, et al. Long-term follow-up of patients with short QT syndrome. *J Am Coll Cardiol.* 2011;58(6):587–595.

30. Gollob MH, Redpath CJ, Roberts JD. The short QT syndrome: proposed diagnostic criteria. *J Am Coll Cardiol.* 2011;57(7):802–812.

31. Kapplinger JD, Tester DJ, Alders M, et al. An international compendium of mutations in the SCN5A-encoded cardiac sodium channel in patients referred for Brugada syndrome genetic testing. *Heart Rhythm.* 2010;7(1): 33–46.

32. Mahdieh N, Rabbani A, Firouzi A, et al. Clopidogrel pharmacogenetics in Iranian patients undergoing percutaneous coronary intervention. *Cardiovasc Toxicol.* 2018;18(5):482–491.

33. Ossei-Gerning N, Mansfield MW, Stickland MH, Wilson IJ, Grant PJ. Plasminogen activator inhibitor-1 promoter 4G/5G genotype and plasma levels in relation to a history of myocardial infarction in patients characterized by coronary angiography. *Arterioscler Thromb Vasc Biol.* 1997;17(1):33–37.

34. Gurha P. Noncoding RNAs in cardiovascular diseases. *Curr Opin Cardiol.* 2019;34(3):241–245.

35. Ma H, Marti-Gutierrez N, Park SW, et al. Correction of a pathogenic gene mutation in human embryos. *Nature.* 2017;548(7668):413–419.

36. Rabbani B, Khorgami MR, Dalili M, Zamani N, Mahdieh N, Gollob M. Novel cases of sudden cardiac death secondary to TRDN mutations presenting as LQT syndrome at rest and CPVT during exercise: The TRDN arrhythmia syndrome. Submitted.

# CHAPTER 36

# Renal Disorders and Cardiovascular Disease

SAMIRA TABIBAN • NASIM NADERI
Rajaie Cardiovascular, Medical & Research Center, Iran University of Medical Sciences, Tehran, Iran

---

### KEY POINTS

- Regulation of pH and acid-base homeostasis is vitally important for cellular function, its metabolism, and normal human physiology. Both kidneys and lungs regulate acid-base balance, although the brain and liver have some regulatory functions. The first part of this chapter provides comprehensive information on acid-base balance and describes associated disorders. The interconnection between electrolytes and their neutrality are major concepts to be applied in the diagnosis of acid-base imbalance and its disorders.
- The second part of this chapter provides practical information regarding the cardiorenal syndrome which is a term used to define the disorders of the kidneys and heart whereby acute or chronic dysfunction in one organ may induce acute or chronic dysfunction of the other.

---

## HOMEOSTASIS[1–22]

### General Considerations

The normal pH of the extracellular fluid (ECF) has a narrow range of $7.4 \pm 0.03$. Any deviation in this range can be shown in the ratio of bicarbonate to $pCO_2$. This ratio is described by an equation named the Henderson–Hasselbalch equation. According to this equation, pH can be measured as follows:

$$pH = 6.1 + \log\{[HCO_3^-] \div (pCO_2 \times 0.3)\}$$

Normal cellular function needs maintenance and stabilization of pH. There are general mechanisms that keep the pH within this narrow range, such as chemical buffering, handling of renal hydrogen ($H^+$), and alveolar ventilation.

- In ECF, bicarbonate, within the normal range of $24 \pm 2$ mEq/L, mediates chemical buffering; in the intracellular fluid, phosphate and protein buffers do it.
- Adaptation of kidneys to the changing acid–base status is done by bicarbonate reabsorption and excretion of acids such as the dihydrogen phosphate ion ($H_2PO_4^-$) and ammonium ions ($NH_4^+$). This **renal $H^+$ handling** can stabilize pH.
- Variation in pH can be minimized by **alveolar ventilation.** Alveolar ventilation alters the partial pressure of carbon dioxide within the normal range of $40 \pm 5$ mmHg.

## CLASSIFICATIONS AND DEFINITIONS[3–5]

To simplify the condition, acid–base disorders can be divided into acidosis and alkalosis. Acidosis can be classified into metabolic and respiratory. Alkalosis also has two subtypes, metabolic and respiratory.

According to the above discussion, if arterial pH is less than 7.35, the patient has acidemia, and if the pH is more than 7.45, the patient has alkalemia.

Also, as a primary abnormality, if arterial blood gas (ABG) shows a bicarbonate level of less than 22 mEq/L, the patient has metabolic acidosis, and if this amount is higher than 26 mEq/L, the patient is in a metabolic alkalosis condition. Conversely, in a primary abnormal condition, if ABG shows a $pCO_2$ of less than 35 mmHg, the patient is in respiratory alkalosis state, and if it shows a $pCO_2$ of more than 45 mmHg, the patient has respiratory acidosis.

There are two types of compensation:

- **Respiratory compensation:** If there is abnormal $pCO_2$ in a primary abnormal metabolic process, a rapid response has occurred to compensate for the situation.
- **Metabolic compensation:** In a primary abnormal respiratory condition, the bicarbonate level becomes slowly abnormal (in 3–5 days) to compensate for the situation.

## DIAGNOSIS

In an analysis of acid–base disorders, the first step is measuring pH, $pCO_2$, and bicarbonate. The next step is differentiating primary abnormalities from compensatory conditions. The final steps include finding the cause and managing the condition. Accordingly, there are five steps in the approach to acid–base imbalance:

1. Checking ABG

$$\text{Acidosis (acidemia): } pH < 7.37 \text{ vs alkalemia (alkalosis)}$$
$$: pH > 7.43$$

2. Finding the primary abnormalities

By looking at the shift of deviation, the process that causes a shift to that side is considered the primary abnormality. So, in acidosis, there is either elevated $pCO_2$ (respiratory acidosis) or decreased bicarbonate level (metabolic acidosis), and in alkalosis, there is either lowered $pCO_2$ (respiratory alkalosis) or increased bicarbonate level (metabolic alkalosis). There is also a **combined disturbance** when both $pCO_2$ and bicarbonate are abnormal but the pH is normal. However, it is important to know that the body does not fully compensate for primary acid–base disturbances.

3. Evaluating the compensatory process

The compensatory process is an adaptation mechanism to normalize pH. It is reemphasized that the compensatory effect is not complete and just in the way of attenuation, and a combined disorder shows inappropriate compensation.

4. Calculating the anion gap (AG)

In normal conditions, the balance of total serum cations is maintained by the total serum anions. However, routine laboratory tests cannot measure all types of ions, and most of these unmeasured ions are anions. This is why this value is named the AG. Both anions and cations have two measured and unmeasured parts.

The measured part of cations in daily practice is $Na^+$ alone, and the unmeasured parts are $Mg^{2+}$, $Ca^{2+}$, $K^+$, and a few serum proteins.

The measured parts of anions $Cl^-$ and $HCO_3$ and the unmeasured parts of anions consist of sulfates and serum proteins (mostly albumin). In *daily practice*, AG (within the normal range of $12 \pm 2$ mEq/L) can be calculated with the formula

$$AG = [Na^+] - ([Cl^-] + [HCO_3^-])$$

As can be seen, in the cation part of this formula potassium is not used, and in the anion part, there is no place for $PO_4^{3-}$ ions. In some forms of acidosis, there is an increase in the amount of unmeasured anion. Because serum albumin is the major part of unmeasured anions, AG can be corrected in the presence of gross changes in serum albumin levels. The formula for this calculation is

$$AG_{correct} = AG + \{(4 - [albumin]) \times 2.5\}$$

If the amount of AG is more than 20 mEq/L, there is primary metabolic acidosis regardless of the level of $HCO_3$ and pH, and it should be mentioned that the body in a primary disorder does not produce a large AG for compensation. In metabolic acidosis with increased circulating anions, there is an elevated AG.

Another important calculation is *excess AG*. It is the difference between total AG and normal AG, that is, 12 mEq/L. If this amount is more than normal serum $HCO_3$ (i.e., >30 mEq/L), one encounters an underlying metabolic alkalosis; in contrast, if that amount is less than normal serum bicarbonate (i.e., <23 mEq/L), one encounters non-AG metabolic acidosis.

5. Delta gap evaluation

In the assessment of metabolic acidosis with high AG, it is useful to assess delta gap or, more correctly, the delta ratio. This assessment is useful in mixed acid–base disorders. The delta ratio can be measured with the formula

$$\text{Delta ratio} = \Delta AG / \Delta [HCO_3^-]$$

or

$$\uparrow AG / \uparrow [HCO_3^-]$$

This measurement can also be shown by the formula

$$\text{Delta ratio} = \frac{\text{Measured anion gap} - \text{Normal anion gap}}{\text{Normal } [HCO_3^-] - \text{Measured } [HCO_3^-]}$$

$$= \frac{(AG - 12)}{(24 - [HCO_3^-])}$$

Theoretically, with the addition of each molecule of metabolic acid into the ECF, one ion of hydrogen is released, and with the reaction between this ion and one ion of bicarbonate, two molecules of $H_2O$ and $CO_2$ are produced. So with omission of one ion of bicarbonate, one ion from the other serum (unmeasured) anion increases, and the net result is increasing AG (buffering process).

On the basis of the above observation, four different delta gaps can be estimated:

a. If all buffering processes are completed by bicarbonate ions, the increase in AG will be equal to the decrease in bicarbonate, and the delta ratio should be 1:1. For example, this ratio in ketoacidosis is 1:1.

**TABLE 36.1**
**Delta Gap Types and Ratios**

| Delta Ratio | Assessment Guidelines |
|---|---|
| <0.4 | Hypochloremic normal AG acidosis |
| <1 | High AG and normal AG acidosis |
| 1–2 | Pure AG acidosis<br>Lactic acidosis: average value, 1.6 DKA more likely to have a ratio closer to 1 because of urine ketone loss |
| >2 | High AG acidosis and a concurrent metabolic alkalosis or a preexisting compensating respiratory acidosis |

*AG*, anion gap; *DKA*, diabetic ketoacidosis.[5,9]

b. Because more than 50% of excess acid is buffered in an intracellular process and some other parts are buffered in the bone, extracellular buffering is not done by bicarbonate ions solely. A few excess ions remain in the ECF, and they do not have the ability to pass the lipid layer of the cell membrane. As a result, an increase in AG is usually more than the decrease in bicarbonate ions. So the net result will be a delta ratio of more than 1. For example, in lactic acidosis, the delta ratio is approximately 1.6:1.

c. In mixed metabolic acidosis, we face a delta ratio of less than 1:1. In this form, there is a greater fall in bicarbonate ions more than the expected increase in AG. For instance, in lactic acidosis that has been complicated with severe diarrhea, there is an additional decrease in bicarbonate that is not in combination with the change in AG.

d. A delta ratio of more than 2:1 indicates a lesser fall in bicarbonate ions more than the expected change in AG. This can occur in concurrent metabolic alkalosis. Besides, in chronic respiratory acidosis, there is a preexisting high level of bicarbonate ions.

As presented in Table 36.1, theoretically, the delta gap can have different types and ratios.

## RESPIRATORY ACIDOSIS[3-5]

In respiratory acidosis, there are two subtypes:

* In acute respiratory acidosis, the pH is around 7.25, $pCO_2$ is about 60 mmHg, and the bicarbonate level is within the normal average range (i.e., 26 mEq/L). In such a medical emergency situation that needs intubation and medical ventilation, there is no metabolic compensation. The major causes are:

* Respiratory center depression caused by drugs or cerebrovascular accident
* Lung edema and lung infection (pneumonia)
* Pneumothorax and hemothorax
* Increased airway resistance (e.g., laryngospasm, bronchospasm, acute airway obstruction)
* Neuromuscular disorders: myopathies and neuropathies
* Flail chest
* Ventilator dysfunction
* In the chronic subtype, the pH is around 7.34, which means acidemia, but the other measurements are high and in opposite directions to compensate for this condition. The $pCO_2$ is around 60 mmHg, and the bicarbonate level is high at around 31 mEq/L. The metabolic compensation shows chronicity of the clinical situation. The major causes are:
* Chronic obstructive or restrictive pulmonary disease
* Increased lung dead space
* Chronic neuromuscular diseases
* Chronic pulmonary central depression or central hypoventilation

Symptoms of this condition result from a decrease in cerebrospinal fluid (CSF) pH. In the early period, these symptoms might include headache and fidgetiness, and they may progress to general hyperreflexia and finally coma.

The treatment is aimed toward the underlying disorder and to improve the ventilation. It is recommended *not* to administer $NaHCO_3$ in *pure* respiratory acidosis because it may inversely decrease pH by producing extra $CO_2$ and water in the tissues. This event increases $pCO_2$ and can cause worsening of hypercapnia.

## RESPIRATORY ALKALOSIS[3-5]

In this condition, the pH is around 7.50, $pCO_2$ is around 29 mmHg, and $HCO_3^-$ is nearly equal to 22 mEq/L. The primary disturbance in this situation is the low level of $pCO_2$. Similar to respiratory acidosis, this condition has two subtypes:

* **Acute form:** This is caused by a rise in CSF pH in association with a significant reduction in the brain blood flow that leads to decreased consciousness. From the acid–base perspective, this means normal $HCO_3^-$ level or no metabolic compensation. The major causes are related to hyperventilation and can be classified as:
* Central nervous system diseases
* Anxiety

- Drug overdose (e.g., salicylates, progesterone, catecholamines)
- Pregnancy
- Hypoxemia
- Mechanical ventilation (common finding)
- Sepsis or septicemia
- Hepatic encephalopathy
- **Chronic form:** Again, from an acid–base perspective, $pCO_2$ is less than the normal limit with a near-normal pH level. In chronic conditions, for each 10-mmHg decrease in $pCO_2$, the bicarbonate level decreases by 2 mEq/L. Using another formula, the change in $pH = 0.017 \times (40 - pCO_2)$. However, in the acute form, the change in $pH = 0.008 \times (40 - pCO_2)$.

The chronic subtype is usually symptom free because pH has been well compensated.

An increase in pH can cause hypocalcemia and a decrease in serum potassium level; so in the management of this condition, it is important to pay attention to $Ca^{2+}$ and $K^+$ and to treat the underlying causes. For instance, changing the setting of the ventilator in intensive care unit patients is absolutely important to control respiratory alkalosis.

A study by Park et al. has shown, "In patients with high-risk acute heart failure (AHF), respiratory alkalosis is the most frequent acid-base imbalance but *not* the most significant risk factor for mortality."

## METABOLIC ACIDOSIS[1–22]

This is the most common condition among acid–base disorders, and in this condition, the pH is about 7.20, $pCO_2$ is around 21 mmHg, and the bicarbonate level decreases to 8 mEq/L. Because of acidosis, $HCO_3^-$ as the primary abnormality is very low, and respiratory compensation is visible. This entity can be classified as "with AG" and "without AG." As mentioned before, in the calculation of AG, since the potassium value makes little contribution to the extracellular electrolyte pool, it has been excluded, and just the three elements of sodium, chloride, and bicarbonate have been used in its formula. Again, the normal level of AG is $12 \pm 2$ mEq/L.

- Metabolic acidosis with AG. The most common causes of this condition are:
  - Diabetes, alcoholic ketoacidosis, or starvation
  - Lactic acidosis (e.g., shock)
  - Kidney failure
  - Profound trauma and rhabdomyolysis
  - Drug exposures (e.g., methanol, salicylates)
- Metabolic acidosis without AG. The most common causes are:
  - All causes of gastrointestinal bicarbonate loss (e.g., severe diarrhea)

- Renal bicarbonate loss is nearly common in diseases such as:
  - Early renal failure
  - Renal tubular acidosis (RTA)
  - Carbonic anhydrase inhibitors
  - Aldosterone inhibitors
- Posthypercapnia
- HCl administration

RTA is failure of the kidneys to acidify urine appropriately, and the result of this inability is acidosis. Other functions of kidney in this disease are in the normal range. In this disorder, metabolic acidosis results from either reabsorption of enough bicarbonate in proximal tubules or insufficient secretion of $H^+$ ions into distal portions of nephrons (i.e., distal tubules). RTA produces metabolic acidosis with normal AG. This disease is classified into four subtypes:

Type 1: distal RTA

Type 2: proximal RTA

Type 3: combined proximal and distal RTA

Type 4: RTA (hyperkalemic RTA)

In type 1 or distal RTA, there is impaired secretion of $H^+$. This impairment can be seen in a variety of autoimmune diseases such as rheumatoid arthritis, systemic lupus erythematosus, and Sjögren syndrome. This impairment is caused by increased membrane permeability of distal tubules. Amphotericin B can also cause this impairment.

In type 2 or proximal RTA, there is impaired reabsorption of bicarbonate from proximal tubules. This problem can be observed in diseases such as Wilson disease, multiple myeloma, some autoimmune disorders, acetazolamide use, and toxins (e.g., heavy metals).

Finally, in type 3 RTA, because of either hypoaldosteronism or aldosterone resistance, the resulting hyperkalemia lowers the generation of urinary buffer $NH_3$. This ionic buffer cannot control the situation, and the net result is acidosis. This problem can be seen in patients with diabetes and patients taking certain drugs such as nonsteroidal antiinflammatory drugs (NSAIDs), cyclosporine, and beta blockers.

Diagnostic tools in metabolic acidosis are:

1. Preparing a detailed clinical history (e.g., alcohol ingestion).
2. Measurement of AG (gastrointestinal [GI] type can be differentiated from urine AG)
3. Serum $K^+$ and urine pH (to distinguish subtypes of RTA).
   a. In types 1 and 2 RTA, there is hypokalemia, but in type 4, the patient has hyperkalemia.
   b. In type 4 RTA, there is low urine pH ($<5.3$), and it is because of a deficit in generating $NH_3$ buffer. On the contrary, urine pH is high in RTA type 1

(>5.3) and in type 2, urine pH measurement is variable.
4. Serum lactate and ketone bodies
5. Measuring the osmolal gap in clinical suspicion of alcohol poisoning.

The gap can be calculated by subtracting the measured osmolality from the calculated serum osmolality:

$$[Osm]_{meas} - \{([Na^+] \times 2) + ([glucose] \div 18) + ([BUN] \div 2.8)\}$$

Management of metabolic acidosis is toward treating the underlying conditions:
1. Ketoacidosis due to causes other than diabetes such as starvation or ethanol overdose can be managed through oral feeding or dextrose solutions (or both) and by compensating for volume depletion.
2. Managing lactic acidosis can be done by treatment of underlying diseases; for instance, aggressive maneuvers for the treatment of shock is one of these approaches. It must be emphasized that administration of bicarbonate or other alkali substances may lead to rebound alkalosis.
3. Treatment of metabolic acidosis with normal AG is administration of $NaHCO_3$. The amount of deficit can be calculated with a formula; however, this medication can be given orally as a 650-mg tablet (equals 7 mEq of bicarbonate) four times a day or an intravenous (IV) injection of one ampule of this component that equals 50 mEq. Parenteral administration may cause pulmonary edema, hypokalemia, and hypocalcemia, so it must be used cautiously.
4. Management of RTA depends on the subtypes of this disorder.
   a. In type 1, oral bicarbonate replacement (1–2 mEq/kg/day) or sodium citrate is mandatory. In the case of accompanying hypokalemia, potassium citrate may be a good substitute.
   b. In type 2, a higher amount of alkali should be administered (10–15 mEq/kg/day). Potassium salts can control hypokalemia.
   c. For the management of type 4, treatment of high potassium levels is important. It is important to administer a loop diuretic to control high potassium levels. Oral mineralocorticoids such as fludrocortisone 50–200 mcg/day should be given to patients with primary adrenal insufficiency or hypoaldosteronism.

## METABOLIC ALKALOSIS[1–22]

In this condition, the pH is around 7.50, $pCO_2$ is about 48 mmHg, and the $HCO_3^-$ level is 36 mEq/L. The primary abnormality is increased levels of bicarbonate. It

is usually combined with respiratory compensation (i.e., a modest increase in $pCO_2$ level). If the increase in $pCO_2$ level reaches 55 mmHg, it is not solely compensation, and the nephrologist should pay attention to concomitant primary respiratory abnormalities.

Causes of this entity can be divided according to "urinary chloride level." In other words, it can be classified on the basis of extracellular volume.
• Low urinary chloride level:
  • Posthypercapnia
  • Vomiting
  • Nasogastric suction of GI secretion
  • Past use of diuretics
• Normal or high urinary chloride level:
  • Current or recent use of diuretics
  • High mineralocorticoid level or activity
    • Cushing syndrome
    • Exogenous steroid use
    • Licorice ingestion
    • High renin level
    • Bartter syndrome
    • Conn syndrome
  • High alkali administration

It should be emphasized that measuring urinary sodium concentration might be unreliable because even in a volume-depleted patient, renal threshold for bicarbonate might be high, and sodium may be added, as a cation, to bicarbonate. Thus, the best method of assessing renal response to circulating volume in metabolic alkalosis is measuring urine chloride levels.

Another way to describe metabolic alkalosis is defining both the initial cause and maintenance or persistent weakening of the renal compensatory response.
• Generation causes may be due to either high $H^+$ loss (loss of upper GI secretions) or excessive $HCO_3^-$ gain (alkali administration).
• Maintenance causes are related to a concomitant problem in the ability of the kidneys to excrete bicarbonate. This impairment might be related to decreased glomerular filtration rate or increased reabsorption of bicarbonate from renal tubulointerstitial system. The latter can occur because of extracellular volume contraction, chloride depletion, and hypokalemia.

Diagnosis of metabolic alkalosis is based on the patient's history (e.g., vomiting, diuretics) and clinical manifestations (e.g., volume depletion). Occasionally, excessive use of mineralocorticoids may enhance the ECF mildly, and the patient might be hypertensive.

As it has been explained in the above paragraphs, the most important diagnostic test of this form of acid–base balance is measuring the urinary level of chloride. If the patient has urine $Cl^-$ of less than

20 mEq/L, it is "chloride-responsive" metabolic alkalosis, and if urine $Cl^-$ is more than 20 mEq/L, the patient has "chloride-unresponsive" metabolic alkalosis. The second important diagnostic test is the serum potassium level. In metabolic alkalosis, hypokalemia is often seen. It contributes to tubular secretion of $H^+$ and waste of $Cl^-$ in alkalosis, and it is caused by transcellular shift.

Treatment in a "chloride-responsive" state is toward euvolemia by administration of saline solution. In other words, chloride load improves the renal handling of bicarbonate.

In a "chloride-unresponsive" state, saline administration may cause expansion of ECF volume and is not suitable. Management of this situation can be summarized as:

1. Treatment of hypokalemia with repletion of its deficit and administration of potassium-sparing diuretics such as spironolactone, eplerenone, and amiloride.
2. Discontinuation of excessive alkali administration to improve alkalosis if it has been assumed that kidney function is normal.
3. Although acetazolamide (Diamox) enhances potassium loss, it promotes renal bicarbonate excretion. It is especially useful in volume overload situations. The dosage of acetazolamide is one 250-mg tablet every 6 h. Treatment with this medication can be started with one 500-mg tablet as a single dose as well.
4. In severe alkalosis (pH >7.70) with volume overload or renal failure, isotonic HCl (150 mEq/L) can be administered via a central vein line. Calculation of the amount can be done on the basis of the formula

$$\{(0.5 \times \text{lean weight in kg}) \times ([HCO_3{}^-] - 24)\}$$

## CARDIORENAL SYNDROME

The heart and kidneys are interrelated, and the close relationship between these two organs makes them susceptible to the development and progression of dysfunction. Cardiorenal syndrome (CRS) is a setting in which acute or chronic heart or renal dysfunction leads to the development and worsening of the other organ's failure.[23–26]

CRS traditionally was classified info five types:

Type 1: Acute cardiorenal syndrome; worsening renal function (WRF) in acute decompensated heart failure patients

Type 2: Chronic CRS; WRF in chronic heart failure patients

Type 3: Acute renocardiac syndrome; development of signs and symptoms of heart failure in patients with primary and abrupt worsening of kidney function such as acute kidney injury (AKI), ischemia, or glomerulonephritis

Type 4: Chronic renocardiac syndrome; development of signs and symptoms of heart failure in patients with chronic or end-stage renal failure

Type 5: Secondary CRS; conditions in which a systemic disorder leads to heart and kidney dysfunction concomitantly

## Practical Points in Cardiorenal Syndrome Type 1[23–30]

WRF in acute decompensated heart failure (ADHF) may be caused by volume overload and congestion, low cardiac output, or both.

Sometimes patients may be volume depleted.

The typical form of CRS-1 is a patient with increased serum blood urea nitrogen (BUN) and creatinine level, suboptimal urinary output, and diuretic resistance in the course of AHF treatment.

If the patient is too "wet," then poor renal perfusion is caused by high central venous pressure (CVP). Diuretics are often held because of WRF and a misguided idea of "intravascular volume depletion."

In patients with marked congestion and volume overload who have elevated CVP, the first step in the treatment of diuretic resistance should be the increase in the diuretic dose and adding the second or third diuretic. With increasing diuresis, renal function may improve.

In patients who show inadequate response to increasing the diuretic dose or combined diuretic therapy adding an inotropic agent may be required.

Using hypertonic saline accompanied with high-dose diuretic is another therapeutic approach to diuretic resistance.

Assessing the hemodynamic condition of the patient by right heart catheterization may be very helpful in treatment and management of these patients.

If adequate diuresis cannot be achieved and volume overload persists, then the mechanical fluid removal (ultrafiltration, hemodialysis) should be considered.

In patients who have severe ascites, paracentesis may be useful if there is an increase in intra-abdominal pressure (>8 mmHg). The kidney perfusion and diuresis may improve after decreasing intra-abdominal pressure by paracentesis.

The other heart failure medications (angiotensin-converting enzyme [ACE] inhibitors, angiotensin II receptor blockers [ARBs], beta blockers, mineralocorticoid receptor antagonists [MRAs]) should be adjusted in the setting of CRS-1.

The nephrotoxic agents such as NSAIDs should be avoided in CRS-1, and the dosage of antibiotics with renal elimination should be appropriately adjusted.

Nutritional supports, particularly in patients with protein-energy wasting (in chronic advanced heart failure patients), and treatment of iron deficiency and anemia are usually helpful in kidney recovery.

If during treatment of AHF, the clinical condition of the patient improves and serum creatinine increases, this is pseudo WRF. With continuing treatment and improvement of the congestion, renal function will return to baseline.

The patients with pseudo WRF do not have poor outcome.

Vasopressin receptor antagonists (aquaretics) may have benefit in selected patients with CRS-1.

Aquaretics produce water diuresis, and not salt diuresis, and can be used in patients with dilutional hyponatremia.

Aquaretics had no effect on mortality and hospitalization of heart failure patients in clinical trials, but they improved dyspnea and edema and increased urinary output and serum sodium.

It has not yet been shown that adenosine A1 receptor antagonists such as rolofylline have any benefit in CRS-1 patients.

## Clinical Scenarios for Cardiorenal Syndrome Type 1

A 48-year-old woman is in the cardiac care unit with a diagnosis of AHF. She has shortness of breath at rest and fatigue. On physical examination, she has crackles on both lungs and 2+ pitting edema up to her knees and a palpable liver. On the second day of admission, she has still dyspnea, and despite 120 mg of IV furosemide, her urinary output is up to 50 cc in the past hour. She has also an increase in her baseline creatinine (from 1.4 to 2.3). A pulmonary artery catheter is placed for her.

### First scenario

Right atrial pressure (RAP) = 25 mmHg, pulmonary artery Pressure (PAP) = 60/30 mmHg, pulmonary capillary wedge Pressure (PCWP) = 35 mmHg, blood pressure (BP) 100/70 mmHg, heart rate (HR) = 90 beats/min
Cardiac output (CO) = 4.2 L/min
Cardiac index (CI) = 2.5 L/min/m$^2$
Stroke volume (SV) = 46 cc

On the basis of these measurements, which show a marked increase in filling pressures, the IV diuretic dose is increased to 200 mg/day, and one 2.5-mg dose of oral metolazone is given to the patient. Her urinary output increased 6 h later, and after 2 days, her edema improved, and creatinine returned to baseline.

This example demonstrates that in patients with WRF who are in an overload state, increasing the diuretic dose or adding another diuretic results in increasing the urinary output, decreasing renal congestion, and improvement in renal function.

### Second scenario

RAP = 25 mmHg, PAP = 60/30 mmHg
PCWP = 35 mmHg, SBP = 80/60 mmHg
HR = 110 beats/min, CO = 2.9 L/min
CI = 1.8 L/min/m$^2$, SV = 26 cc

This measurement demonstrates a low CO state with high filling pressures. The IV diuretic dose is increased, and the patient was also administered milrinone. After 3 h, she had an urinary output of 300 cc, her symptoms of shortness of breath improved, and her lung sounds were clear.

In this case, the filling pressures are markedly elevated, and in the presence of low CO, preload reduction alone will not be useful, and another treatment modality should be tried, such as an inotrope.

### Third scenario

For a 76-year-old man with a history of severe heart failure and recent pneumonia, a PAC is placed because of oliguria and a rise in urea and creatinine after IV diuretic therapy for AHF treatment. The following hemodynamic values are measured:

RAP = 5 mmHg, PAP = 25/12 mmHg, PCWP = 9 mmHg
BP = 85/60 mmHg, HR = 120 beats/min, CO = 3.6 L/min
CI = 2.1 L/min/m$^2$

After 200 cc of IV fluid therapy over 20 min:

RAP = 9 mmHg, PAP = 30/15 mmHg, PCWP = 12 mmHg
BP = 90/70 mmHg, HR = 100 beats/min, CO = 3.8 L/min
CI = 2.2 L/min/m$^2$

This hemodynamic assessment demonstrates volume depletion as a cause of WRF. Overdiuresis or intercurrent illness may result in volume loss and renal dysfunction in AHF patients. The increase in filling pressure and CI after fluid therapy shows that volume depletion could be considered as cause of oliguria, and IV fluid therapy should be the first treatment approach.

## Practical Points in Cardiorenal Syndrome Type 2[23–30]

The main issue in chronic heart failure patients with increasing the serum creatinine (CRS-2) is continuing standard guidelines recommended heart failure medical therapies, particularly ACE inhibitor and ARBs.

ACE inhibitor/ARB is recommended in heart failure reduced ejection fraction (HFrEF) patients with stage

3 chronic kidney disease (CKD) and might be considered in patients in stage 4 or 5 CKD with careful monitoring of serum electrolytes and kidney function.

Beta blockers are recommended in HFrEF patients with stage 3 CKD and should be considered in stages 4 and 5 CKD.

MRAs can be used in HFrEF patients with stage 3 CKD but should not be used in stage 4 or 5 CKD.

WRF after ACE inhibitor/ARB is more prevalent in patients who have an underlying kidney dysfunction. Thus these patients should be carefully monitored.

Isosorbide dinitrate/hydralazine may be considered as an alternative to ACE inhibitor/ARB.

Fig. 36.1 shows an algorithmic approach to heart failure patients with WRF.

## Cardiorenal Syndrome Type 3: Acute Renocardiac Syndrome[23-30]

AKI is a frequent disorder in hospital and intensive care unit patients. The mechanisms of cardiac dysfunction and heart failure include the following:

- Fluid overload predisposes patients to the development of pulmonary edema.
- Electrolyte imbalance, particularly hyperkalemia, contributes to cardiac arrhythmias and arrest.
- Acidosis has negative inotropic effects and causes pulmonary vasoconstriction and right-sided heart failure.
- Uremia and accumulation of myocardial depressant factors decrease myocardial contractility, and untreated uremia can cause pericarditis.
- Renal ischemia may activate inflammatory processes and precipitate apoptosis at the cardiac level.

### Practical points in cardiorenal syndrome Type 3

Specific management for the underlying cause is the mainstay of treatment of these patients.

Cardiac biomarkers, including troponins and natriuretic peptides, correlate with outcomes in these patients.

The standard treatment for heart failure should be performed for patients.

Nephrotoxic drugs should be stopped; however, ACE inhibitors and ARBs can be feasibly continued unless kidney function fails to stabilize or other dangerous situations arise (i.e., hypotension, hyperkalemia).

In severe AKI, renal replacement therapy should be considered.

In the setting of heart failure, continuous techniques of renal replacement in which the cardiovascular instability caused by rapid fluid and electrolyte shifts is less seems to be physiologically safer and more logical.

## Cardiorenal Syndrome Type 4: Chronic Renocardiac Syndrome[23-30]

In these patients, a primary CKD contributes to ventricular hypertrophy and impaired systolic and diastolic cardiac function. The risk of adverse cardiovascular events is very high in these groups of patients.

Mechanisms for cardiac dysfunction include:
- Chronic inflammation
- Accelerated atherosclerosis
- Heart–kidney interactions
- Subclinical infections

### Practical points in cardiorenal syndrome Type 4

Patients with CKD who have ischemic heart disease should be treated as patients with normal kidney, and specific treatments should not be excluded because of the concern of a worsening kidney function.

Therapeutic choices may be particularly challenging because of lack of data about the effects of specific treatments in the CKD population.

Ischemic heart disease should be managed according to guidelines.

Nephrology consultation is necessary before angiography using contrast agents.

A combination of aspirin, beta blockers, ACE inhibitors, and statins should be considered for CKD patients with acute myocardial infarction.

Medications necessary for the management of complications of advanced CKD, including phosphate binders, vitamins, calcium supplements, and erythropoiesis-stimulating agents, are generally safe with concomitant cardiac disease.

Heart failure should be treated according to guidelines.

In heart failure patients with overload symptoms, diuretics may be useless, and intensification of renal replacement therapy is recommended.

MRAs should be prescribed cautiously, and patients with more than moderate CKD should be excluded.

## Cardiorenal Syndrome Type 5 (Secondary CRS)[23-30]

In this group of patients, systemic conditions such as diabetes mellitus, sepsis, anaphylactic reactions, connective tissue diseases, or some storage diseases such

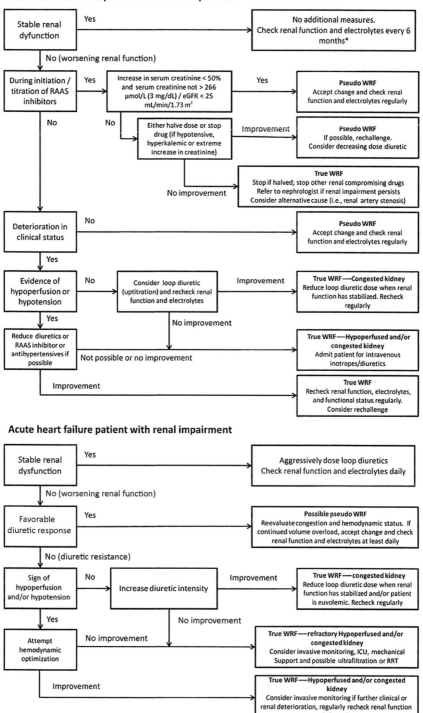

**Chronic heart failure patient with renal impairment**

Stable renal dysfunction — **Yes** → No additional measures. Check renal function and electrolytes every 6 months*

**No (worsening renal function)**

During initiation / titration of RAAS inhibitors — **Yes** → Increase in serum creatinine < 50% and serum creatinine not > 266 μmol/L (3 mg/dL) / eGFR < 25 mL/min/1.73 m² — **Yes** → **Pseudo WRF** Accept change and check renal function and electrolytes regularly

**No** → Either halve dose or stop drug (if hypotensive, hyperkalemic or extreme increase in creatinine) — **Improvement** → **Pseudo WRF** If possible, rechallenge. Consider decreasing dose diuretic

**No improvement** → **True WRF** Stop if halved; stop other renal compromising drugs Refer to nephrologist if renal impairment persists Consider alternative cause (i.e., renal artery stenosis)

Deterioration in clinical status — **No** → **Pseudo WRF** Accept change and check renal function and electrolytes regularly

**Yes**

Evidence of hypoperfusion or hypotension — **No** → Consider loop diuretic (uptitration) and recheck renal function and electrolytes — **Improvement** → **True WRF—Congested kidney** Reduce loop diuretic dose when renal function has stabilized. Recheck regularly

**No improvement** → **No**

**Yes**

Reduce diuretics or RAAS inhibitor or antihypertensives if possible — Not possible or no improvement → **True WRF—Hypoperfused and/or congested kidney** Admit patient for intravenous inotropes/diuretics

**Improvement** → **True WRF** Recheck renal function, electrolytes, and functional status regularly. Consider rechallenge

**Acute heart failure patient with renal impairment**

Stable renal dysfunction — **Yes** → Aggressively dose loop diuretics Check renal function and electrolytes daily

**No (worsening renal function)**

Favorable diuretic response — **Yes** → **Possible pseudo WRF** Reevaluate congestion and hemodynamic status. If continued volume overload, accept change and check renal function and electrolytes at least daily

**No (diuretic resistance)**

Sign of hypoperfusion and/or hypotension — **No** → Increase diuretic intensity — **Improvement** → **True WRF—congested kidney** Reduce loop diuretic dose when renal function has stabilized and/or patient is euvolemic. Recheck regularly

**No improvement**

**Yes**

Attempt hemodynamic optimization — No improvement → **True WRF—refractory Hypoperfused and/or congested kidney** Consider invasive monitoring, ICU, mechanical Support and possible ultrafiltration or RRT

**Improvement** → **True WRF—Hypoperfused and/or congested kidney** Consider invasive monitoring if further clinical or renal deterioration, regularly recheck renal function and electrolytes

FIG. 36.1 Approach to heart failure patients with worsening renal function (WRF). *eGFR*, estimated glomerular filtration rate; *ICU*, intensive care unit; *RAAS*, renin–angiotensin–aldosterone system; *RRT*, renal replacement therapy. *At least every 6 months, can be individually determined. (From Damman K, Testani JM. The kidney in heart failure: an update. *Eur Heart J.* 2015;36(23):1437–1444; with permission.)

as amyloidosis and sarcoidosis cause both cardiac and renal dysfunction.

These patients should be managed according to the cause, and all the principles discussed for other types of CRS apply.

## REFERENCES

1. Goldring RM, Cannon PF, Heinemann HO, Fischman AP. Respiratory adjustment to chronic metabolic alkalosis in man. *J Clin Invest.* 1968; 47:188–202.
2. de Strihou VY, Frans A. The respiratory response to chronic metabolic alkalosis and acidosis in disease. *Clin Sci Mol Med.* 1973; 45:439–448.
3. Narins RG, Emmett M. Simple and mixed acid-base disorders: a practical approach. *Medicine (Baltimore).* 1980; 59:161–187.
4. Winter SD, Pearson R, Gabow PA, Schultz AL, Lepoff RB. The fall of the serum anion gap. *Arch Intern Med.* 1990; 150:311–313.
5. Arbus GS. An in vivo acid-base nomogram for clinical use. *Can Med Assoc J.* 1973; 109:291–293.
6. Gennari FJ, Goldstein MB, Schwartz WB. The nature of the renal adaptation to chronic hypocapnia. *J Clin Invest.* 1972; 51:1722–1730.
7. Adrogue HJ, Brensilver J, Madias NE. Changes in the plasma anion gap during chronic metabolic acid-base disturbances. *Am J Phys.* 1978; 235:291–297.
8. Madias NE, Ayus JC, Adrogue HJ. Increased anion gap in metabolic alkalosis: the role of plasma-protein equivalency. *N Engl J Med.* 1979; 300:1421–1423.
9. Gabow PA, Kaehny WD, Fennessey PV, Goodman SI, Gross PA, Schrier RW. Diagnostic importance of an increased serum anion gap. *N Engl J Med.* 1980; 303:854–858.
10. Narins RG, Bastl CP, Rudnick MR. Anion gap and serum bicarbonate (letter). *N Engl J Med.* 1980; 303:161.
11. Osnes JB, Hermansen L. Acid-base balance after maximal exercise of short duration. *J Appl Physiol.* 1972; 32:59–63.
12. Fulop M, Horowitz M, Aberman A, Jaffe ER. Lactic acidosis in pulmonary edema due to left ventricular failure. *Ann Intern Med.* 1973; 79:180–186.
13. Assan R, Heuclin C, Girard JR, LeMaire F, Attali JR. Phenformin-induced lactic acidosis in diabetic patients. *Diabetes.* 1975; 24:791–800.
14. Orringer CE, Eustace JC, Wunsch CD, Gardner LB. Natural history of lactic acidosis after grand-mal seizures—a model for the study of an anion-gap acidosis not associated with hyperkalemia. *N Engl J Med.* 1977; 297:796–799.
15. Oh MS, Carroll HJ, Goldstein DA, Fein IA. Hyperchloremic acidosis during the recovery phase of diabetic ketosis. *Ann Intern Med.* 1978; 89:925–927.
16. Oh MS, Banerji MA, Carroll HJ. The mechanism of hyperchloremic acidosis during the recovery phase of diabetic ketoacidosis. *Diabetes.* 1981; 30:310–313.
17. Adrogue HJ, Wilson H, Boyd 3d AE, Suki WN, Eknoyan G. Plasma acid-base patterns in diabetic ketoacidosis. *N Engl J Med.* 1982; 307:1603–1610.
18. Gabow PA, Clay K, Sullivan JB, Lepoff R. Organic acids in ethylene glycol intoxication. *Ann Intern Med.* 1986; 105:16–20.
19. Fulop M, Hoberman HD. Diabetic ketoacidosis and alcoholic ketosis (letter). *Ann Intern Med.* 1979; 91:796–797.
20. Levy U, Duga J, Girgis M, Gordon EE. Ketoacidosis associated with alcoholism in nondiabetic subjects. *Ann Intern Med.* 1973; 78:213–219.
21. Goodkin DA, Krishna GG, Narins RG. The role of the anion gap in detecting and managing mixed metabolic acid-base disorders. *Clin Endocrinol Metab.* 1984; 13:333–349.
22. Proudfoot AT, Brown SS. Acidaemia and salicylate poisoning in adults. *Br Med J.* 1969; 2:547–550.
23. Kulkarni M. Cardio renal syndrome. *J Nephrol Ther.* 2016; 6 (233) 2161–0959.1000.
24. Hatamizadeh P, Fonarow GC, Budoff MJ, Darabian S, Kovesdy CP, Kalantar-Zadeh K. Cardiorenal syndrome: pathophysiology and potential targets for clinical management. *Nat Rev Nephrol.* 2013; 9(2):99–111.
25. Obi Y, Kim T, Kovesdy CP, Amin AN, Kalantar-Zadeh K. Current and potential therapeutic strategies for hemodynamic cardiorenal syndrome. *Cardiorenal Med.* 2015; 6(2):83–98.
26. Damman K, Testani JM. The kidney in heart failure: an update. *Eur Heart J.* 2015; 36(23):1437–1444.
27. Ter Maaten JM, Valente MA, Damman K, Hillege HL, Navis G, Voors AA. Diuretic response in acute heart failure—pathophysiology, evaluation, and therapy. *Nat Rev Cardiol.* 2015; 12(3):184–192.
28. Valente MAE, Voors AA, Damman K, et al. Diuretic response in acute heart failure: clinical characteristics and prognostic significance. *Eur Heart J.* 2014; 35(19):1284–1293.
29. Verbrugge FH, Grieten L, Mullens W. Management of the cardiorenal syndrome in decompensated heart failure. *Cardiorenal Med.* 2014; 4(3–4):176–188.
30. Ronco C, Haapio M, House AA, Anavekar N, Bellomo R. Cardiorenal syndrome. *J Am Coll Cardiol.* 2008; 52 (19):1527–1539.

# CHAPTER 37

# Endocrine Disorders and the Cardiovascular System

ZAHRA GHAEMMAGHAMI
Rajaie Cardiovascular, Medical & Research Center, Iran University of Medical Sciences, Tehran, Iran

---

**KEY POINTS**

- Endocrine disorders are common in the community and can affect the cardiovascular system. A cardiologist should be familiar with this disorder for early detection and refer to an endocrinologist to prevent complication.
- Growth hormone deficiency has a different metabolic complication that can predispose patient to atherosclerosis disease and replacement therapy can prevent this complication.
- Early detection and treatment of acromegaly can prevent of heart failure and other cardiovascular complications of disease.
- Thyroid dysfunction is common and can cause different cardiac manifestation ranging from simple tachycardia to advanced cardiac problem if it is not diagnosed and treated appropriately.
- Amiodarone can affect thyroid function and regular evaluation of thyroid function test is recommended for patient who take amiodarone.
- In the evaluation of secondary hypertension, attention to endocrine cause is essential and many endocrine causes of hypertension are curable with the treatment of endocrine disease that causes hypertension.
- Vitamin D deficiency is associated with cardiovascular disorders and when detected, appropriate treatment is indicated.

---

Normal function of endocrine system is essential for cardiovascular health[1]; many disorders of the endocrine system can affect different aspects of function of cardiovascular system. This chapter briefly reviews cardiovascular manifestation of some endocrine disorders.

## GROWTH HORMONE

Among the six hormones secreted by the anterior pituitary, we focus to the disorder of growth hormone that has more known cardiovascular manifestation. The growth hormone is the most abundant hormone in the adult pituitary gland, and it plays an important role in maintaining the metabolic process.[2] It is synthesized, stored, and secreted by somatotroph cells. That is located predominantly in the anterior pituitary gland and comprises between 35% and 45% of pituitary cells.[2] The cellular effects of hGH are exerted through two major pathways. The first is binding the hormone to specific hGH receptors on target cells that have been identified in the heart, skeletal muscle, fat, liver, and kidneys, as well as in many cells throughout fetal development. The second effect of hGH has done by stimulation of the synthesis of insulin-like growth factor type I (IGF-I). This protein is synthesized primarily in the liver, but other cell types can produce IGF-I under the influence of hGH. IGH-I acts as a second messenger and mediates most actions of hGH. The clinical activity of[3] disease in patients with an excess of hGH (acromegaly) correlates better with serum levels of IGF-I than with hGH levels.[3] GH enhances lipolysis and fatty acid oxidation and increases clearance of low-density lipoprotein (LDL) by activating expression of hepatic LDL receptors.[4,5] In GH deficiency, the atherogenic profile of lipoproteins increases and reduces by GH therapy.[6] Disorder-related GH mainly is divided into two categories: GH deficiency and GH excess (acromegaly).

## ADULT GH DEFICIENCY

GH deficiency in adults is categorized into three groups: patients with prior childhood GH deficiency, those with acquired GH deficiency secondary to structural lesions or trauma, and finally those with idiopathic GH deficiency.[7]

## GH Deficiency and Cardiovascular Risk Factor[8]

Low-density lipoprotein (LDL) and triglycerides increase in both sexes, whereas decreased high-density lipoprotein (HDL) has been observed only in women.[8] The prevalence of MetS is increased in GH Deficiency patients.[9] CRP increases in both lean and obese subjects with GH Deficiency four- to fivefold.[10] Increased IL-6 levels have been documented in patients with GH Deficiency independently of BMI or obesity; in addition, GH replacement was able to effectively reduce IL-6 production from monocytes.[11] In patients with GH Deficiency, a reduced protein's activity that was normalized after GH replacement was recently documented.[12] Most adult patients with GH Deficiency have impaired LV performance at peak exercise and report exercise intolerance. GH replacement therapy improves cardiac performance and increases LV mass, LV end-diastolic volume (LVEDV), and stroke volume.[13,14] Diagnostic test is to check serum IGF-I levels and some provocative test including insulin-induced hypoglycemia, combination of arginine and GH-releasing hormone (GHRH), which are potent stimuli for GH secretion. A subnormal increase in the serum GH concentration after stimulation test confirms the diagnosis of GH deficiency. Treatment of GH deficiency is hormone replacement therapy and follow-up of patient by laboratory tests and clinical examinations. Replacement in GH Deficiency patients leads to significant decrease in total cholesterol and LDL and an increase in HDL.[15–18]

## ACROMEGALY

GH hypersecretion in adults leads to acromegaly that is associated with increased morbidity and mortality, primarily from cardiovascular disease and cancer.[19] Acromegaly is a rare disease with prevalence ranging from 36 to 40 cases per million population.[20] Pituitary tumors arising from somatotroph cells is the most common cause. Diagnosis is suspected with clinical signs and symptoms and elevated of IGF-I level and confirmed by measuring growth hormone levels during a 2-h period after a standard 75-g oral glucose.

### Cardiovascular System and Acromegaly

The cardiovascular involvement of acromegaly varies from asymptomatic myocardial involvement in early stage to congestive heart failure in long-term untreated patients.[21,22] Some cardiovascular risk factors increase in acromegaly about 20%–50% of patients who have hypertension and diabetes mellitus is more common in patient with acromegaly about 15%–37%.[20] The prevalence of valvular heart disease has also increased in acromegaly.[23] ECG changes at rest are left axis deviation, increased QT intervals, septal Q-waves, and ST-T wave depression.[24] Dysrhythmias are seen in acromegaly, including atrial and ventricular ectopic beats, sick sinus syndrome, and supraventricular and ventricular tachycardia.[25] Transsphenoidal surgery and resection of the adenoma are the procedures of choice for initial management. If hGH and/or IGF-I levels remain elevated, radiotherapy in older patients or dopamine or somatostatin receptor agonists in younger patients can restore normal serum hGH and IGF-I levels.

## THYROID AND CARDIOVASCULAR SYSTEM

There is a close link between thyroid hormones and different component of cardiovascular system.[26] So it is not surprising that thyroid disease affects cardiovascular function. Both clinical and subclinical hypo- and hyperthyroidism can present with signs and symptoms related to the cardiovascular system in this section. We briefly review the cardiovascular presentation and complication of thyroid disorders.

### Thyrotoxicosis

Thyrotoxicosis is defined as the elevated level of free thyroid hormone in serum (from any source) and suppression of TSH. If it is caused by overproduction and secretion from thyroid gland, then it is called hyperthyroidism. If TSH is suppressed but thyroid hormone level is normal, then it is called subclinical hyperthyroidism.[27]

### Clinical and Hemodynamic Manifestation

Symptoms and signs are anxiety, emotional lability, weakness, tremor, palpitations, heat intolerance, increased perspiration, diarrhea, weight loss, disturbed sleep,[28] exercise intolerance, dyspnea on exertion, systolic hypertension,[29] and if untreated in long term, cardiac hypertrophy and diastolic dysfunction may be developed.[29–31] Hemodynamic effects of hyperthyroidism are decreased systemic vascular resistance (SVR), increased heart rate, increased cardiac preload, and finally increased cardiac output.[32,33] Sinus tachycardia occurs in approximately 40% of cases of overt hyperthyroidism.[34] The second common arrhythmia that seen in hyperthyroidism is atrial fibrillation and its prevalence increases with age.[35]

Treatments consist of symptomatic therapy with beta blocker and treatment for hyperthyroidism that should be done with any of the following modalities: radioactive iodine therapy, antithyroid drugs (methimazole or propylthiouracil), or thyroidectomy that choose by patient and physician based on, benefits, expected speed of recovery, potential side effects, and costs.[27]

## HYPOTHYROIDISM

Overt hypothyroidism is defined as elevated TSH, usually above 10 mIU/L, in combination with a subnormal free T4. Subclinical hypothyroidism is characterized by a serum TSH above the upper reference limit in combination with normal free thyroxine (T4).[36] Symptoms vary between patients but generally include fatigue, cold intolerance, dry skin, constipation, vocal changes, and muscle ache, slow movement, coarse hair and skin, and puffy facies. Hemodynamic and cardiovascular effects of hypothyroidism include bradycardia, systemic hypertension with decreased pulse pressure, increased SVR, exercise impairment, decreased cardiac output, and pericardial effusions. Treatment of hypothyroid patients with the restoration of a euthyroid state resolves these changes.[37] Hyperlipidemia, hyperhomocysteinemia, increased creactive protein levels, and altered coagulation parameters were also seen in hypothyroidism.[38] ECG includes sinus bradycardia, low-voltage complexes, prolonged PR and QT intervals, and flattened or inverted T waves.[39] Treatment of hypothyroidism is thyroid hormone replacement and with treatment metabolic and cardiovascular changes return to normal.

## THYROID AND AMIODARONE

Amiodarone is a class III antiarrhythmic drug with a similar structure to human thyroid hormone—thyroxine (T4).[40] Amiodarone is a potent drug used in the treatment of various heart arrhythmias such as paroxysmal supraventricular dysrhythmias, including atrial fibrillation (AF) and flutter and some ventricular dysrhythmias. Also, it is a good choice in the maintenance of sinus rhythm after electrical cardioversion of atrial fibrillation.[41] Amiodarone has complex effects on thyroid physiology. In about 20% of patients, this drug leads to development of amiodarone-induced hypothyroidism (AIH) or thyrotoxicosis (AIT).[42] For early detection and management of this disorder, TFT (TSH, free T4, T3) should be evaluated at baseline and every 6 months during amiodarone therapy.[41] Prevalence of amiodarone-induced thyroid dysfunction varies from 15% to 30% and is influenced by the environmental iodine supply, dosing, and duration of treatment.[43,44] Clinical and subclinical hypothyroidism develops in 5% and 25% of patients receiving amiodarone, respectively,[45] and is more prevalent among (1) inhabitants of

iodine-replete areas, (2) women (M:F = 1.0:1.5), and (3) the elderly.[46] TPO-Ab and female gender confer a relative risk (RR) of AIH of 7.3 and 7.9, respectively.[46,47] Diagnosis is confirmed by a persistently elevated TSH concentration (10 mU/L) in combination with low normal or low-free T4.

## TREATMENT

Management is discontinuation of the amiodarone therapy if possible, and in patients in whom discontinuation of amiodarone is not feasible, more reliable and safer option is thyroid hormone replacement therapy, starting with 25–50 µg of levothyroxine (LT4) daily, and increasing at intervals of 4–6 weeks until the symptoms have resolved and TSH has normalized.[48]

### Amiodarone-Induced Thyrotoxicosis

Epidemiological data indicate that AIT is more common in (1) regions with insufficient iodine intake and in (2) men (M:F = 3.2:1).[46] There are two types of AIT. Type 1 results in increased thyroid hormone synthesis and release in autonomous thyroid tissue and occurs in patients with an underlying thyroid condition (e.g., nodular goiter, Graves' disease).[48] Type 2 develops in patients without underlying thyroid pathology and is a result of a direct toxic effect of amiodarone leading to subacute, destructive thyroiditis. Distinction between the two types can often be challenging. The onset of symptoms in AIT is rapid including cardiac dysrhythmias that have been controlled with amiodarone and may recur (e.g., atrial fibrillation, supraventricular, or ventricular tachycardia) and symptoms of thyrotoxicosis are weight loss, sweating, palpitations, hyperkinesia, restlessness, muscle weakness, heat intolerance, low-grade fever, diarrhea, or an enlarging goiter.[46,49]

### Diagnosis

Usual lab tests are (a) elevated T4 and free T4 concentrations, (b) normal to high T3 and free T3 concentrations, and (c) markedly suppressed TSH concentration.

### Treatment

A significant increase of major adverse cardiovascular events in AIT immediate treatment is critical.[48,50] Discontinuation of amiodarone is usually required in AIT type 1 and the choice of treatment is antithyroid drugs.[43,51] Type 2 AIT is usually transient and may manage with amiodarone discontinuation and high-dose steroids, e.g., prednisone 40–60 mg daily, especially when amiodarone is continued. Many patients become euthyroid 3–5 months after stopping amiodarone.[43,48]

## ENDOCRINE HYPERTENSION

Secondary hypertension is defined as increased systemic blood pressure (BP) by an identifiable cause and consists 5%–10% of hypertensive patients.[52] The etiology of secondary hypertension is categorized into two group: renal and endocrine causes. There are at least 14 endocrine disorders for which hypertension may be the initial clinical presentation.[2] In this section, we review three important endocrine diseases that can present with secondary hypertension which includes primary aldosteronism, pheochromocytoma, and Cushing syndrome.

Primary aldosteronism is defined as aldosterone hypersecretion independent to the renin angiotensin system and has two main subtypes such as aldosterone-producing adenomas (APAs) and bilateral adrenal hyperplasia. Cardiovascular complication of hyperaldosteronism is disproportional to hypertension per se and it seems that aldosterone itself has an adverse effect on myocardium and blood vessels,[53] so diagnosis and treatment is very important. Treatment of APA is surgery, whereas treatment of bilateral adrenal hyperplasia is medical therapy with aldosterone receptor antagonist. Another endocrine disease that can present with HTN and cardiovascular complication is pheochromocytoma.

Pheochromocytomas are catecholamine-secreting tumors that arise from chromaffin cells of the adrenal medulla and the sympathetic ganglia, the second form also named as paraganglioma or extraadrenal pheochromocytoma.[2] Pheochromocytoma is a rare disease but it is serious and potentially fatal complication of its suspicion and at the time referring the patient to endocrinologist, it is crucial for cardiologist patient with pheochromocytoma that may be asymptomatic and tumor detect incidentally by imaging study or may have signs and symptoms that suspect by physician to this tumor. Patients may present with hypertension (episodic or sustained), cardiomyopathy and congestive heart failure, arrhythmia, and episodic symptoms that occur in spells and include dizziness, headache, flushing, forceful heartbeat, pallor tremor, and diaphoresis.[2] Hypertension is seen in more than 50% of patients. Hypertension is more variable in pheochromocytoma compared to essential hypertension.[54] Cardiomyopathy is a serious complication of pheochromocytoma that presents as hypertrophic or dilated and may be unrecognized by clinicians and can be reversible by early detection and treatment of pheochromocytoma. Diagnosis of pheochromocytoma is biochemically by measuring catecholamines and their metabolites in urine and serum and followed by localizing the tumor by imaging study. Treatment is surgical resection of the tumor.

## CUSHING SYNDROME

Cushing syndrome is a complex of symptoms and signs due to enhanced cortisol action and can be categorized into endogenous and exogenous. Endogenous Cushing syndrome is divided into ACTH dependent and nondependent, and exogenous Cushing syndrome is caused by supraphysiologic corticosteroid administration and is more common than endogenous form.[2] The excess of glucocorticoid in Cushing syndrome affects the cardiac, liver, and fat tissue and induces some metabolic abnormality such as hypertension, abdominal obesity, insulin resistance, dyslipidemia, and thrombotic diathesis which leads to accelerated atherosclerosis and cardiovascular complication.[55] In addition to above-mentioned complication, some cardiac structural changes are associated with reduced midwall systolic performance, LVH, and diastolic dysfunction observed in patients with Cushing syndrome that may contribute to the enhanced risk of cardiovascular events in these patients.[56] This structural changes may be reversible with normalization of hypercortisolism.[57] Hypertension is observed in up to 75% of cases[2] and depends on the duration of disease.[58] Several mechanisms have a role in hypertension that include: (1) activation of mineralocorticoid receptors by cortisol, (2) activation of the renin–angiotensin system (RAS), (3) increases in cardiovascular reactivity to vasoconstrictors, (4) suppression of vasodilatory systems, and (5) sleep apnea. All of these mechanisms act by three main pathophysiologic mechanisms including regulating plasma volume, peripheral vascular resistance, and cardiac output, all of them are increased in Cushing syndrome.[58] After exclusion of exogenous Cushing syndrome, the diagnosis of Cushing syndrome is made by demonstration of increased cortisol secretion with at least two tests, including 24-h urinary-free cortisol, late-night salivary free cortisol, and assessment of midnight plasma cortisol or 48-h low dose dexamethasone suppression test.[59] The choice of treatment would depend on underlying cause of hypercortisolism. For exogenous Cushing syndrome, glucocorticoid is tapered, and for endogenous Cushing syndrome, treatment modalities include transsphenoidal surgery for ACTH-producing pituitary adenoma radiotherapy, for refractory or recurrent adenoma, unilateral or bilateral adrenalectomy in cortisol-producing adrenal adenoma, and finally medical therapy if the patient is not suitable for surgery. The goals of treatment in Cushing syndrome are normalization of the cortisol level.[60] Clinical features of Cushing syndrome usually disappear over a period of 2–12 months after successful treatment. Hypertension improves, but, as with other secondary causes, it may not resolve completely and a significant proportion of patients require antihypertensive medication.[2]

## VITAMIN D AND CARDIOVASCULAR SYSTEM

Vitamin D is a prohormone that plays a significant role in intestinal calcium absorption for bone mineralization. It acts by binding to the vitamin D receptor, which is present in many cells in the body, including cardiomyocytes, vascular smooth muscle cells, and endothelial cells.[61] Several observational and prospective investigations have demonstrated that vitamin D deficiency is associated with a higher risk of hypertension, myocardial infarction, coronary artery disease, cardiomyopathy, congestive heart failure, peripheral arterial diseases, stroke, and diabetes.[62–65] This deficiency is also an independent risk factor for CVD.[66,67] Despite this evidence, however, randomized clinical trials have conflicting results concerning the efficacy of vitamin D supplementation in reducing CVD.[62,68] Finally, the bulk of available data suggest that normalizing the levels of the body's vitamin D stores not only confers significantly positive health outcomes but also lowers costs and assists in the control of the incidence and prevalence of CVD.[61]

## REFERENCES

1. Rhee SS, Pearce EN. The endocrine system and the heart: a review. *Rev Esp Cardiol (Engl Ed)*. 2011;64(3):220–231.
2. Melmed S, Polonsky KS, Larsen PR, Kronenberg HM. *Williams Textbook of Endocrinology*. Elsevier Health Sciences; 2015.
3. Klein I, Biondi B. Endocrine disorders and cardiovascular disease. In: Zipes DP, Libby P, Bonow RO, Mann DL, Tomaselli GF, eds. *Braunwald's Heart Disease: A Textbook of Cardiovascular Medicine*. 11th ed. Philadelphia: Elsevier Health Sciences; 2019:1807–1821.
4. Rudling M, Norstedt G, Olivecrona H, Reihnér E, Gustafsson J-A, Angelin B. Importance of growth hormone for the induction of hepatic low density lipoprotein receptors. *Proc Natl Acad Sci USA*. 1992;89(15):6983–6987.
5. Rudling M, Olivecrona H, Eggertsen G, Angelin B. Regulation of rat hepatic low density lipoprotein receptors. In vivo stimulation by growth hormone is not mediated by insulin-like growth factor I. *J Clin Invest*. 1996;97(2):292.
6. Maison P, Griffin S, Nicoue-Beglah M, Haddad N, Balkau B, Chanson P. Impact of growth hormone (GH) treatment on cardiovascular risk factors in GH-deficient adults: a metaanalysis of blinded, randomized, placebo-controlled trials. *J Clin Endocrinol Metab*. 2004;89(5):2192–2199.
7. Molitch ME, Clemmons DR, Malozowski S, Merriam GR, Vance ML. Evaluation and treatment of adult growth hormone deficiency: an Endocrine Society clinical practice guideline. *J Clin Endocrinol Metab*. 2011;96(6):1587–1609.
8. Abdu TA, Neary R, Elhadd TA, Akber M, Clayton RN. Coronary risk in growth hormone deficient hypopituitary adults: increased predicted risk is due largely to lipid profile abnormalities. *Clin Endocrinol*. 2001;55(2):209–216.
9. van der Klaauw AA, Biermasz NR, Feskens EJ, et al. The prevalence of the metabolic syndrome is increased in patients with GH deficiency, irrespective of long-term substitution with recombinant human GH. *Eur J Endocrinol*. 2007;156(4):455–462.
10. Ukropec J, Penesová A, Skopkova M, et al. Adipokine protein expression pattern in growth hormone deficiency predisposes to the increased fat cell size and the whole body metabolic derangements. *J Clin Endocrinol Metab*. 2008;93(6):2255–2262.
11. Serri O, St-Jacques P, Sartippour M, Renier GV. Alterations of monocyte function in patients with growth hormone (GH) deficiency: effect of substitutive GH therapy 1. *J Clin Endocrinol Metab*. 1999;84(1):58–63.
12. Cakir I, Tanriverdi F, Karaca Z, et al. Evaluation of coagulation and fibrinolytic parameters in adult onset GH deficiency and the effects of GH replacement therapy: a placebo controlled study. *Growth Hormon IGF Res*. 2012;22(1):17–21.
13. Colao A, di Somma C, Cuocolo A, et al. Improved cardiovascular risk factors and cardiac performance after 12 months of growth hormone (GH) replacement in young adult patients with GH deficiency 1. *J Clin Endocrinol Metab*. 2001;86(5):1874–1881.
14. Maison P, Chanson P. Cardiac effects of growth hormone in adults with growth hormone deficiency: a meta-analysis. *Circulation*. 2003;108(21):2648–2652.
15. Svensson J, Fowelin J, Landin K, Bengtsson B-A, Johansson J-O. Effects of seven years of GH-replacement therapy on insulin sensitivity in GH-deficient adults. *J Clin Endocrinol Metab*. 2002;87(5):2121–2127.
16. Van der Klaauw A, Romijn J, Biermasz N, et al. Sustained effects of recombinant GH replacement after 7 years of treatment in adults with GH deficiency. *Eur J Endocrinol*. 2006;155(5):701–708.
17. Gotherstrom G, Svensson J, Koranyi J, et al. A prospective study of 5 years of GH replacement therapy in GH-deficient adults: sustained effects on body composition, bone mass, and metabolic indices. *J Clin Endocrinol Metab*. 2001;86(10):4657–4665.

18. Colson A, Brooke A, Walker D, et al. Growth hormone deficiency and replacement in patients with treated Cushing's disease, prolactinomas and non-functioning pituitary adenomas: effects on body composition, glucose metabolism, lipid status and bone mineral density. *Horm Res Paediatr.* 2006;66(6):257–267.
19. Kauppinen-Mäkelin R, Sane T, Reunanen A, et al. A nationwide survey of mortality in acromegaly. *J Clin Endocrinol Metab.* 2005;90(7):4081–4086.
20. Mestrón A, Webb SM, Astorga R, et al. Epidemiology, clinical characteristics, outcome, morbidity and mortality in acromegaly based on the Spanish Acromegaly Registry (Registro Espanol de Acromegalia, REA). *Eur J Endocrinol.* 2004;151(4):439–446.
21. Bruch C, Herrmann B, Schmermund A, Bartel T, Mann K, Erbel R. Impact of disease activity on left ventricular performance in patients with acromegaly. *Am Heart J.* 2002;144(3):538–543.
22. Vitale G, Pivonello R, Auriemma RS, et al. Hypertension in acromegaly and in the normal population: prevalence and determinants. *Clin Endocrinol.* 2005;63(4):470–476.
23. Pereira AM, Van Thiel SW, Lindner JR, et al. Increased prevalence of regurgitant valvular heart disease in acromegaly. *J Clin Endocrinol Metab.* 2004;89(1):71–75.
24. Rodrigues EA, Caruana MP, Lahiri A, Nabarro J, Jacobs H, Raftery E. Subclinical cardiac dysfunction in acromegaly: evidence for a specific disease of heart muscle. *Br Heart J.* 1989;62(3):185–194.
25. Clayton R. Cardiovascular function in acromegaly. *Endocr Rev.* 2003;24(3):272–277.
26. Grais IM, Sowers JR. Thyroid and the heart. *Am J Med.* 2014;127(8):691–698.
27. Ross DS, Burch HB, Cooper DS, et al. American Thyroid Association guidelines for diagnosis and management of hyperthyroidism and other causes of thyrotoxicosis. *Thyroid.* 2016;26(10):1343–1421.
28. Goichot B, Caron P, Landron F, Bouée S. Clinical presentation of hyperthyroidism in a large representative sample of outpatients in France: relationships with age, aetiology and hormonal parameters. *Clin Endocrinol.* 2016;84(3):445–451.
29. Danzi S, Klein I. Thyroid hormone and blood pressure regulation. *Curr Hypertens Rep.* 2003;5(6):513–520.
30. Petretta M, Bonaduce D, Spinelli L, et al. Cardiovascular haemodynamics and cardiac autonomic control in patients with subclinical and overt hyperthyroidism. *Eur J Endocrinol.* 2001;145(6):691–696.
31. Mintz G, Pizzarello R, Klein I. Enhanced left ventricular diastolic function in hyperthyroidism: noninvasive assessment and response to treatment. *J Clin Endocrinol Metab.* 1991;73(1):146–150.
32. Kahaly GJ, Dillmann WH. Thyroid hormone action in the heart. *Endocr Rev.* 2005;26(5):704–728.
33. Davis PJ, Davis FB. Nongenomic actions of thyroid hormone on the heart. *Thyroid.* 2002;12(6):459–466.
34. Northcote R, MacFarlane P, Kesson C, Ballantyne D. Continuous 24 hour electrocardiography in thyrotoxicosis, before and after treatment. *Clin Sci.* 1987;72(s16):18P.
35. Osman F, Gammage MD, Sheppard MC, Franklyn JA. Cardiac dysrhythmias and thyroid dysfunction—the hidden menace? *J Clin Endocrinol Metab.* 2002;87(3):963–967.
36. Garber JR, Cobin RH, Gharib H, et al. Clinical practice guidelines for hypothyroidism in adults: cosponsored by the American Association of Clinical Endocrinologists and the American Thyroid Association. *Thyroid.* 2012;22(12):1200–1235.
37. Mann DL, Zipes DP, Libby P, Bonow RO, Braunwald E. *Braunwald's Heart Disease.* Elsevier Saunders; 2015.
38. Biondi B, Klein I. Hypothyroidism as a risk factor for cardiovascular disease. *Endocrine.* 2004;24(1):1–13.
39. Wald DA. ECG manifestations of selected metabolic and endocrine disorders. *Emerg Med Clin North Am.* 2006;24(1):145–157.
40. Rao R, McCready V, Spathis G. Iodine kinetic studies during amiodarone treatment. *J Clin Endocrinol Metab.* 1986;62(3):563–568.
41. Goldschlager N, Epstein AE, Naccarelli GV, et al. A practical guide for clinicians who treat patients with amiodarone: 2007. *Heart Rhythm.* 2007;4(9):1250–1259.
42. Newman C, Price A, Davies D, Gray T, Weetman A. Amiodarone and the thyroid: a practical guide to the management of thyroid dysfunction induced by amiodarone therapy. *Heart.* 1998;79(2):121–127.
43. Bogazzi F, Tomisti L, Bartalena L, Aghini-Lombardi F, Martino E. Amiodarone and the thyroid: a 2012 update. *J Endocrinol Investig.* 2012;35(3):340–348.
44. Preedy VR, Burrow GN, Watson RR. *Comprehensive Handbook of Iodine: Nutritional, Biochemical, Pathological and Therapeutic Aspects.* Academic Press; 2009.
45. Batcher EL, Tang XC, Singh BN, et al. Thyroid function abnormalities during amiodarone therapy for persistent atrial fibrillation. *Am J Med.* 2007;120(10):880–885.
46. Eskes SA, Wiersinga WM. Amiodarone and thyroid. *Best Pract Res Clin Endocrinol Metab.* 2009;23(6):735–751.
47. Trip MD, Wiersinga W, Plomp TA. Incidence, predictability, and pathogenesis of amiodarone-induced thyrotoxicosis and hypothyroidism. *Am J Med.* 1991;91(5):507–511.
48. Narayana SK, Woods DR, Boos CJ. The management of amiodarone-related thyroid problems. *Ther Adv Endocrinol Metab.* 2011;2:115–126. https://doi.org/10.1177/2042018811398516.
49. Cardenas GA, Cabral JM, Leslie CA. Amiodarone induced thyrotoxicosis: diagnostic and therapeutic strategies. *Cleve Clin J Med.* 2003;70(7):624–626. 628–631.
50. Yiu K-H, Jim M-H, Siu C-W, et al. Amiodarone-induced thyrotoxicosis is a predictor of adverse cardiovascular outcome. *J Clin Endocrinol Metab.* 2009;94(1):109–114.
51. Bogazzi F, Bartalena L, Martino E. Approach to the patient with amiodarone-induced thyrotoxicosis. *J Clin Endocrinol Metab.* 2010;95(6):2529–2535.
52. Mancia G, Fagard R, Narkiewicz K, et al. 2013 ESH/ESC Guidelines for the management of arterial hypertension:

the Task Force for the management of arterial hypertension of the European Society of Hypertension (ESH) and of the European Society of Cardiology (ESC). *Blood Press.* 2013;22(4):193–278.

53. Milliez P, Girerd X, Plouin P-F, Blacher J, Safar ME, Mourad J-J. Evidence for an increased rate of cardiovascular events in patients with primary aldosteronism. *J Am Coll Cardiol.* 2005;45(8):1243–1248.

54. Galetta F, Franzoni F, Bernini G, et al. Cardiovascular complications in patients with pheochromocytoma: a mini-review. *Biomed Pharmacother.* 2010;64(7):505–509.

55. Pivonello R, De Martino MC, De Leo M, Lombardi G, Colao A. Cushing's syndrome. *Endocrinol Metab Clin N Am.* 2008;37(1):135–149.

56. Muiesan ML, Lupia M, Salvetti M, et al. Left ventricular structural and functional characteristics in Cushing's syndrome. *J Am Coll Cardiol.* 2003;41(12):2275–2279.

57. Pereira AM, Delgado V, Romijn JA, Smit JW, Bax JJ, Feelders RA. Cardiac dysfunction is reversed upon successful treatment of Cushing's syndrome. *Eur J Endocrinol.* 2010;162(2):331–340.

58. Magiakou MA, Smyrnaki P, Chrousos GP. Hypertension in Cushing's syndrome. *Best Pract Res Clin Endocrinol Metab.* 2006;20(3):467–482.

59. Nieman LK, Biller BM, Findling JW, et al. The diagnosis of Cushing's syndrome: an endocrine society clinical practice guideline. *J Clin Endocrinol Metab.* 2008;93(5):1526–1540.

60. Stewart PM, Petersenn S. 3 Rationale for treatment and therapeutic options in Cushing's disease. *Best Pract Res Clin Endocrinol Metab.* 2009;23:S15–S22.

61. Vacek JL, Vanga SR, Good M, Lai SM, Lakkireddy D, Howard PA. Vitamin D deficiency and supplementation and relation to cardiovascular health. *Am J Cardiol.* 2012;109(3):359–363.

62. Vacek JL, Vanga SR, Good M, Lai SM, Lakkireddy D, Howard PA. Vitamin D deficiency and supplementation and relation to cardiovascular health. *Am J Cardiol.* 2012;109(3):359–363.

63. Mithal A, Wahl DA, Bonjour J-P, et al. Global vitamin D status and determinants of hypovitaminosis D. *Osteoporos Int.* 2009;20(11):1807–1820.

64. Giovannucci E, Liu Y, Hollis BW, Rimm EB. 25-hydroxyvitamin D and risk of myocardial infarction in men: a prospective study. *Arch Intern Med.* 2008;168 (11):1174–1180.

65. Forman JP, Giovannucci E, Holmes MD, et al. Plasma 25-hydroxyvitamin D levels and risk of incident hypertension. *Hypertension.* 2007;49(5):1063–1069.

66. Mandarino NR, Júnior FdCM, Salgado JVL, Lages JS, Salgado Filho N. Is vitamin D deficiency a new risk factor for cardiovascular disease? *Open Cardiovasc Med J.* 2015;9:40.

67. Perna L, Schöttker B, Holleczek B, Brenner H. Serum 25-hydroxyvitamin D and incidence of fatal and nonfatal cardiovascular events: a prospective study with repeated measurements. *J Clin Endocrinol Metab.* 2013;98 (12):4908–4915.

68. Manson JE, Cook NR, Lee I-M, et al. Vitamin D supplements and prevention of cancer and cardiovascular disease. *N Engl J Med.* 2019;380(1):33–44.

# CHAPTER 38

# The Heart and Pulmonary Diseases

HASAN ALLAH SADEGHI
[a]Rajaie Cardiovascular, Medical & Research Center

---

**KEY POINTS**

- Malfunction of heart or lung may lead to malfunction of cardiopulmonary pump and other organs in consequence.
- Chronic respiratory diseases (CRDs) are the leading cause of hypoxic or hypercapnic respiratory failure resulting in right heart dilation or failure.
- All CRDs cause abnormality of gas exchange; hypoxia, hypercapnia, or both; and increased pulmonary vascular resistance and PH that lead to RV hypertrophy, dilation, dysfunction, and finally RV failure. It is distinctly uncommon for CRD to cause right heart dilation or failure without concomitant hypoxemia and/or hypercapnia.
- Many kinds of systemic diseases with systemic manifestations may affect heart and lungs directly or indirectly. Remote effects of cancer secretion from the lung or other parts may induce cardiac arrhythmia.
- In practice, most often we find heart failure, pericarditis, and arrhythmia caused by cancer chemotherapy or radiotherapy.

---

## INTRODUCTION

The cardiopulmonary pump is designed to deliver $O_2$ to body organs and clean $CO_2$. The heart pumps blood with high $O_2$ and low $CO_2$ from the left ventricle to the systemic circulation and receives low $O_2$ and high $CO_2$ to the right heart, pumps it again into the low-pressure and high-compliance pulmonary vasculature system and distributes it in the pulmonary capillary system at the vicinity of the respiratory membrane. The lungs exchange gases between the inspired air and blood through the thin-walled alveolar-capillary membrane. It provides a large surface for the transfer of gases through which received blood gets rid of $CO_2$ and absorbs $O_2$ to maintain the pressures of $O_2$ and $CO_2$ in the arterial blood near 100 and 40 mmHg, respectively, at sea level. In addition, the lungs help in the filtration of blood flowing to the systemic circulation and metabolism of some active peptides because of their special structure and function. The lungs have a dual arterial blood supply from the pulmonary and bronchial arteries and dual venous drainage. The pulmonary circulation receives the right cardiac output plus some part of the bronchial artery circulation, estimated at about 1%–3% of systemic blood flow, and admixes them to make a major part of physiologic shunt of pulmonary system.

There is a wide anastomosis between the pulmonary and bronchial circulation. In comparison with the systemic circulation, the pulmonary vasculature is a low-pressure and high-compliant system, designed for the perfect exchange of respiratory gases. The distraction of this vascular system because of lung diseases or disorder imposes high resistance on the right ventricle (RV) and leads to a change in the structure and function and finally failure of it. The infectious diseases often present with systemic manifestations, and the lungs may also be affected directly or indirectly. A number of non-infectious systemic disorders may involve both the heart and lungs as a part of the total clinical picture. Pulmonary and cardiac manifestations are encountered in endocrine diseases (thyroid disorders, diabetes mellitus, and obesity), renal failure, or neurologic diseases that simultaneously may involve the heart. Sometimes the cardiac manifestations may arise as a result of treatment of pulmonary diseases. Pulmonary function tests, laboratory evaluation, and imaging studies, especially computed tomography scanning with high-resolution technique (HRCT), help in diagnosis, assessment of severity, obtaining disease activity, and evaluation of treatment efficacy. Cardiac involvement and dysfunction may happen with different lung diseases or disorders. The next section focuses on cardiac dysfunction in patients with primary lung diseases or systemic diseases with concomitant lung and cardiac involvement.

## HEART DYSFUNCTION CAUSED BY CHRONIC RESPIRATORY DISEASE

Chronic respiratory diseases (CRDs) are the leading cause of chronic respiratory failure (Box 38.1). They

**693**

include chronic obstructive pulmonary disease (COPD), sleep apnea syndrome (SAS), interstitial lung disease (ILD), and other restrictive lung diseases (neuromuscular disease, kyphoscoliosis, lung distraction). All of those diseases and disorders have a common pathway for affecting right heart function and leading to RV failure. The prevalence of COPD and ILD are increasing every year because of increasing industrialization, air pollution, smoking, and occupational exposure. Cardiac disease in patients with CRD portends a poor prognosis. Pulmonary hypertension (PH) and cor pulmonale are the best described cardiac consequences of respiratory diseases. Treatment in these patients should be directed at the underlying specific lung disorder and then right heart failure.

*Chronic obstructive pulmonary disease* is the fourth leading cause of death in the world and accounts for 3 million deaths every year (Box 38.2).[1] COPD as a mostly expiratory disease, is associated with the destruction of airways, pulmonary parenchyma, and vasculature,

and make prominent ventilation and perfusion mismatch, hypoxia, hypercapnia, and increased pulmonary vascular resistance and leads to PH, right heart (RV) dysfunction, and finally RV failure. Cardiac and pulmonary function and dysfunction are tightly connected to each other. Today with increasing rates of COPD and coronary artery disease (CAD), it is common to see patients with both CAD and COPD in all general and tertiary hospitals' routine practice.[2] COPD exacerbation may deteriorate cardiac function and vice versa, and management of the first may improve the second.

Clinically, patients with COPD may have dyspnea on exertion, paroxysmal nocturnal dyspnea, fatigue, edema, and other symptoms and signs similar to heart failure, and the disorders may exacerbate or obscure the symptoms and signs of each other. It is common to see chest radiographs with a normal size heart without obvious significant pulmonary congestion in a patient with severe symptomatic heart failure caused by normalization of an overinflated lung and decreased vasculature in a patient with advanced emphysema. Recent evidence[1,2] suggests that in COPD, inflammation is present in all classes of disease. Numerous systemic inflammatory markers that present in patients with COPD may also be found in some cardiovascular diseases. Patients with more frequent or severe exacerbations exhibit particularly robust endogenous proinflammatory responses.[2] Elevated C-reactive protein levels are said to be correlated with the presence of COPD exacerbations, the severity of lung function, and risk for hospitalization and death.[2]

### Interstitial Lung Diseases or Diffuse Parenchymal Lung Diseases

ILDs are a heterogeneous group of diseases that involve interstitial tissue of the lung with somewhat similar clinical, radiographic, and pathophysiologic presentations and often lead to parenchymal and structural distraction and decreased alveolar and capillary surfaces of the lung. Lung distraction leads to hypoxia, increased pulmonary vascular resistance, and PH. Environmental exposure, occupational and habitual hazards, drugs, and radiation are some causes of ILDs, and the causes of many of them remain unknown. The prevalence of PH varies from as low as 8% to as high as 84%. As in COPD, the diagnostic modality and criteria contribute to the variability among studies, with prevalence tending to be higher when echocardiography was used.[2]

### Sleep Apnea and Hypoventilation Syndrome

Sleep-disordered breathing (SDB) includes several disorders characterized by abnormal respiratory patterns or ventilation during sleep time. SAS is characterized by the presence of five or more apnea or hypopnea episodes per hour of sleep. Sleep apnea–hypopnea index (AHI) per hour is defined on polysomnography (PSG) and categorized into obstructive sleep apnea (OSA), central sleep apnea (CSA), or mixed based on the pattern of observed apnea in PSG report (Box 38.3). The most common SAS type is OSA, with an estimated reported overall prevalence of 9.1% in men and 4% in women and 2% and 4% of middle-aged women and men, respectively.[3] The prevalence of SDB is not necessarily associated with subjective complaints, but it is five to six times higher in symptomatic patients. SDBs are particularly more prevalent in obese and elderly populations. One in 3 elderly men has OSA, and 1 in 10 has moderate or severe SAS.[4] SAS is a closely linked to cardiac diseases, especially heart failure, hypertension, and arrhythmia. Increased pharyngeal mucosal fluids and edema, sleep apnea, desaturation, hypoxia, and sometimes hypercapnia during sleep are consequences of pathophysiologic changes that lead to volume retention, increased pulmonary resistance, PH, and finally right heart failure.

Although most patients with OSA do not have obesity hypoventilation syndrome (OHS), most patients with OHS have OSA. Patients with OHS frequently demonstrate both OSA and daytime hypoventilation, likely secondary to a combination of increased work of breathing and a decreased respiratory drive. OSA is frequently cited as a cause of secondary PH, and chronic daytime hypoxemia clearly leads to PH, RV failure, and cor pulmonale. OSA alone may cause mild PH, but

coexisting daytime hypoxia is typically required for the diagnosis of OSA. Some studies have suggested that OSA may be associated with an overall increased risk of death and sudden death at certain times.[5]

OSA may be associated with systemic hypertension, and an independent relationship exists between PSG-defined OSA and hypertension. Approximately 50% of patients with OSA have systemic hypertension. Continuous positive airway pressure (CPAP) treatment reduces sympathetic activity associated with OSA during sleep and systemic hypertension. OSA and CSA are common among patients with heart failure secondary to systolic dysfunction and may coexist in the same individual. Mechanisms potentially involved in the development of heart failure in patients with OSA include cardiac disorders, chronic hypoxia, sympathetic overactivation, and fluid retention.[6]

*Chest Bellows Disorder and Lung Distraction* may result from neuromuscular diseases such as muscular dystrophy, poliomyelitis, myasthenia gravis, or other factors affecting chest wall expansion such as severe obesity and kyphoscoliosis. These are diverse categories of diseases, and the exact prevalence of cor pulmonale in each is not well known. Respiratory muscle weakness, abnormalities in the lung parenchyma, and reduced chest wall compliance lead to prominent reductions in vital capacity and may result in hypoxemia, hypercapnia, and respiratory acidosis. Patients with advanced disease may need noninvasive mechanical ventilation before the development of true respiratory failure. However, it is believed that the risk for right heart failure is increased by a high prevalence of SDB, specifically nocturnal hypoventilation, in this patient population. Before daytime respiratory failure becomes apparent, nocturnal hypoventilation may be noted. We must be aware of patient complaints of morning headache, fatigue, daytime sleepiness, and lethargy or impaired concentration that may signal sleep disruption and nocturnal hypoventilation. Respiratory muscle weakness contributes to REM (rapid eye movement)-associated nocturnal hypoventilation and $O_2$ desaturation, and the severity of diaphragmatic dysfunction has been shown to correlate with the extent of REM-associated nocturnal $O_2$ desaturation.

Nocturnal $O_2$ desaturation is less frequent without concomitant daytime hypercapnia. In patients with neuromuscular disease and restrictive lung disease, pulmonary arterial pressure (PAP) increases with alveolar hypoventilation during sleep, and a correlation between the severity of SDB and cor pulmonale has been made in several studies.[3,5] $O_2$ therapy alone, however, does not correct the hypoventilation that causes hypoxemia and may actually worsen preexisting hypercapnia. Frequently, therapy with nocturnal ventilation, either via tracheostomy and intermittent positive-pressure ventilation or via noninvasive ventilation, may alleviate the symptoms of respiratory failure and correct hypercapnia, hypoxemia, and acidosis. Patients should be considered for nocturnal ventilation if their daytime $PaCO_2$ exceeds or equals 45 mmHg or if nocturnal hypoventilation with sustained $O_2$ desaturation and symptoms of sleep disturbance is present.[5,6]

## PATHOPHYSIOLOGY

All CRDs cause abnormality of gas exchange; hypoxia, hypercapnia, or both; and increased pulmonary vascular resistance and PH that transfer to the RV and lead to RV hypertrophy, dilation, dysfunction, and finally RV failure. It is distinctly uncommon for CRD to cause right heart dilation or failure without concomitant hypoxemia and/or hypercapnia. In addition, some of the CRDs may cause distraction of parenchyma and microvasculature and lead to increased vascular resistance and PH. These kinds of PH are classified as class 3 of PH in the international classification of PH, but there are additional mechanisms for chronic thromboembolic PH (CTEPH) that are caused by mechanical obstruction of the major pulmonary artery without the involvement of the microvasculature. In idiopathic PH (class 1 of the international classification), involvement of small pulmonary artery and capillary system may be caused by endothelial dysfunction. A minority of patients with CRD may have PH that is not proportionate with lung involvement and cannot be explained by disease per se. In these patients, treatment with medications used in class 1 PH is accepted.

Some evidence suggests that[6] in recumbent patients with heart failure, the development of edema in the upper airway tract can lead to narrowing of the pharynx and be a predisposing factor for pharyngeal collapsibility and OSA. In addition, in patients with heart failure, Cheyne–Stokes breathing, and CSA are seen more often in patients with more severe disease and lower blood $CO_2$ (<38 mmHg). At the start of sleep, lower $PCO_2$ gives less input to the respiratory center and causes apnea to increase $CO_2$ and regulate PH. Prolonged circulation time leads to delayed transfer of increased $PCO_2$ to the respiratory center, creating a notable lag for corrective response and leading to the phasic pattern of respiration seen in these patients. This phasic breathing may have prolonged apnea and hypoxia and explains the pattern of breathing in patients with severe heart failure.

## CLINICAL PRESENTATION AND DIAGNOSIS

In patients with advanced pulmonary disease, hypoxemia, and hypercapnia, it is common to see some degree of edema of the lower extremities without right heart dysfunction caused by higher intrathoracic pressure. The presence of disproportionate edema, fatigue, and generalized weakness must be followed with a more precise examination of the heart and echocardiography looking for signs of right heart dysfunction and PH. Right heart failure is relatively common in these patients, but generally, it is mild to moderate in severity. Dyspnea is a prevalent symptom, but it is not helpful because it is so common in these patients. An increase in dyspnea or the development of symptoms such as increased fatigue, lightheadedness, syncope, chest pain, or lower extremity edema may prompt further evaluation. In patients with excessive daytime somnolence, obesity, hypertension, the neck circumference of equal or more than 16 in. in a woman or 17 in. in a man, history of habitual snoring, or observed reports of nocturnal choking or gasping, sleep apnea should be suspected.[4]

In patients with COPD, barrel chest, overinflation of the lung, and noisy breathing may mask RV heave, the loud pulmonic component of the second heart sound, tricuspid regurgitant murmur, and S4 of the right heart, and these sign may not be found on clinical examination. Severe RV failure may also lead to ascites and peripheral edema. Some COPD patients with severe air trapping and hypercapnia may develop lower extremity edema in the absence of RV failure. Hypoxemia itself may also lead to renal vasoconstriction, thus reducing urinary sodium excretion and leading to edema.

These data suggest that in patients with COPD, a low B-type natriuretic peptide (BNP) (100 pg/mL) can be very helpful in ruling out significant heart failure, and a very high BNP (500 pg/mL) can be helpful in ruling in heart failure. Values between 100 and 500 pg/mL must be interpreted with caution and in the context of the entire clinical picture.[4]

Several electrocardiogram (ECG) findings reflective of cor pulmonale have been reported, including rightward P-wave axis deviation; an S1, S2, S3 pattern; an S1, Q3 pattern; evidence of RV hypertrophy; and right bundle branch block. Low-voltage QRS has also been reported, more frequently seen in cor pulmonale associated with COPD than other pulmonary diseases. Unfortunately, ECG findings are insensitive for the detection of PH. ECG abnormalities suggestive of RV hypertrophy can be helpful if present, but if the clinical picture is still suggestive of cor pulmonale, further testing should be persuaded.[1]

Chest radiography may give useful information. Underlying lung disease may obscure the usual findings of PH and ventricular failure. Because of overinflation, enlargement of the proximal pulmonary arteries and reduction in retrosternal air space may not be prominent. Pulmonary artery prominence may be noted on posteroanterior chest radiographs. Increased cardiothoracic ratio is a usual finding but may be less prominent in emphysematous patients. Reticular, reticulonodular shadows or honeycombing are indicators of ILDs.

Although echocardiography is the first step of evaluation for most forms of PH, its utility is more limited in patients with airway disease because of more prevalence of suboptimal images and poor windows. In a recent study of 374 lung transplant candidates, Doppler echocardiography and right heart catheterization were performed within a 72-h period.[7] The correlation between PAPs made by echocardiography vs catheterization is low, especially in mild PH. The overall sensitivity was 85%, and specificity was 55%. Given that sensitivity is better than specificity, a normal echocardiogram can help exclude significant cor pulmonale, but an elevated estimated RV systolic pressure must be interpreted with caution. Right heart catheterization is required to make a definitive diagnosis of PH.[8] We do echocardiography first to evaluate heart and pulmonary pressure because it is easy to do, not so expensive, and available in most centers.

If echocardiography has poor windows or shows normal pressure of the right side despite high clinical suspicion, right heart catheterization may be indicated. Magnetic resonance imaging may be used in some patients, but it probably cannot give more data than echocardiography and cannot replace the right heart catheterization.

PSG remains the gold-standard diagnostic test for OSA. OHS is characterized by hypersomnolence, dyspnea, and resting hypoxemia, leading to PH in patients with extreme obesity. Arterial blood gas testing is required to confirm daytime high serum bicarbonate, hypercapnia and typically demonstrates hypoxemia and a compensated respiratory acidosis. Laboratory testing sometimes reveals polycythemia caused by chronic hypoxemia.

## TREATMENT

In patients with right heart failure caused by CRDs, the primary focus of treatment must be on the underlying lung diseases. Treatment of COPD, ILD, SAS, and neuromuscular problems may improve right heart failure and cor pulmonale. If there is no treatment for primary lung diseases, treatment of consecutive problems, such as hypoxia and hypercapnia by $O_2$ therapy or noninvasive ventilator support, is the cornerstone. Reduction of afterload of the RV and RV pressure and improve contractility with inotropes and pulmonary-selective antihypertensive medications is probably a useful accompanying treatment.

Oxygen is the only therapy for COPD patients that has been shown to improve PAP and/or cor pulmonale and is one of the few noninvasive therapies for COPD that improves mortality rates. Neither anticholinergic medications such as tiotropium bromide nor beta$_2$ agonists that improve symptoms of COPD patients has proven effects on the survival of patients or reduction of PAP. Long-term $O_2$ therapy (LTOT) does appear to be associated with modest decreases in PAPs. However, the interruption of daily $O_2$ is followed by an increase in pulmonary vascular resistance. LTOT is recommended to maintain the oxygen saturation ($SpO_2$) above 90% if it is below 85% or below 90% with the clinical presentation of cor pulmonale. There are limited data regarding the role of vasodilators to ameliorate PH in patients with COPD.

CPAP treatment may reduce the incidence of death from cardiovascular diseases in patients with OSA, but no significant differences are seen in the incidence of new cases of systemic hypertension, cardiac disorders, or stroke.

Noninvasive ventilation (NIV) has been documented in patients with neuromuscular and chest wall diseases to improve nocturnal alveolar hypoventilation, dyspnea, and symptoms associated with SDB. In chest wall diseases, NIV (but not LTOT) improves dyspnea and symptoms associated with sleep disturbance. Corrective surgery of the spine is an option for patients in early childhood or adolescence.[8]

Several case reports have suggested that cor pulmonale can be at least partially reversed and PH improves with the initiation of NIV in patients with restrictive lung disease, although no prospective studies have specifically addressed this issue.

Treatment of right heart failure with attention to the reduction of RV afterload with a phosphodiesterase inhibitor (sildenafil), an endothelin receptor antagonist (bosentan), and prostaglandin was used by several researchers and had controversial effects. At present, there is no recommendation for it except for patients with nonproportionate PH. Losartan and nifedipine led to the little beneficial result in patients with COPD. Whether statins may have some benefit or improve survival in patients with COPD needs to be proved.

## SYSTEMIC DISEASES WITH CONCOMITANT LUNG AND HEART INVOLVEMENT

*Infectious diseases* often present with systemic manifestations. The heart and lungs may also be affected directly or indirectly. Nowadays, the best example of this kind of lung and heart involvement by infectious disease is COVID-19. This RNA virus involves lung as a primary organ, but heart and other organs may also be involved. Involvement of heart especially in ICU make confusing clinical and radiological sign and symptom. And in some cases, it would be very difficult to differentiate heart failure and pulmonary edema from ARDS in a critically ill patient. Cardiac involvement is a prominent feature in COVID-19 and makes worse prognosis. Brain-type natriuretic peptide levels were also elevated among patients admitted in ICU and appeared more universal than troponin elevations. Furthermore, myocardial damage and heart failure contributed to 40% of deaths, in some studies, either exclusively or associated with respiratory failure. Those with elevated circulating biomarkers of cardiac injury were at significantly higher risk of death. Mortality risk associated with acute cardiac injury has been more significant than age, diabetes mellitus, chronic pulmonary disease, or prior history of cardiovascular disease. Thus, cardiac involvement is both prevalent and, apparently, prognostic in COVID-19. The mechanisms of cardiac injury are likely related to increased cardiac stress due to respiratory failure and hypoxemia, direct myocardial infection by SARS-CoV-2, indirect injury from the systemic inflammatory response, or a combination of all three factors.[9]

Granulomatous diseases (tuberculosis and sarcoidosis); connective tissue disorders such as rheumatoid arthritis, systemic lupus erythematosus, and systemic sclerosis; Churg–Strauss syndrome; Wegener granulomatosis (now classed as granulomatosis with polyangiitis); Goodpasture syndrome; and other rare diseases, including tuberous sclerosis, lymphangioleiomyomatosis, histiocytosis X, and lymphoma, may involve both lung and heart at the same time.[10]

The cause of sarcoidosis is not well understood, but it probably results from an immune response after exposure to an as-yet-unknown substance. Viruses, bacteria, and organic and inorganic particles may be involved in triggering the immune response. It is not obvious why sarcoidosis affects the heart and other organs in some patients but not in others.

The involvement of the heart in sarcoidosis, so-called sarcoid heart disease (SHD), is a grave finding. All parts of the heart, including the myocardium, pericardium, valves (especially mitral) and conductive system, and

nodes may be involved. Cardiac granulomas are found in 25% of patients with sarcoidosis on autopsy, but SHD is clinically apparent in only 5% of sarcoid patients. The left ventricular free wall and the intraventricular septum, the most muscular parts of heart, are the most common locations for granulomas and scars, and the conducting system may be involved.[11] SHD presents clinically as cardiomyopathy with either systolic or diastolic dysfunction and failure or with tachyarrhythmia or bradyarrhythmias, including complete heart block and sudden death. Sudden death may be the first sign of SHD.[11,12]

Currently, cardiac magnetic resonance imaging (CMR) is the technique of choice in the evaluation of sarcoidosis. Sensitivity has been shown to be higher than with radionucleotide methods. CMR uses T2-weighted imaging and early gadolinium images to detect acute inflammation (edema). T1-weighted imaging illustrates wall motion abnormalities, hypertrophy caused by possible infiltrative disease, wall thinning, or heart failure. Late (delayed) gadolinium enhancement assesses fibrosis or scar and may represent chronic inactive disease.[12,13] The diagnostic yield of endomyocardial biopsy is low ($\approx$20%); therefore, a negative study cannot rule out the disease. Steroid therapy is generally reserved for patients with symptomatic SHD, including signs of cardiomyopathy and conduction abnormalities. The data regarding the impact of steroids on the survival of patients with SHD are limited, and add-on cytotoxic agents are rarely used. Cardiac transplantation may be considered in young patients with refractory heart failure or arrhythmia.[14]

Pulmonary manifestations are encountered in endocrine diseases (thyroid disorders, diabetes mellitus, and obesity), renal failure, or neurologic diseases that simultaneously may involve the heart and need separate discussion.

### Malignant Lung Diseases and the Heart

Primary lung cancer is the leading cause of death from cancer. The lungs are the destination of cancer cells from all parts of the body. Primary or metastatic lung cancer may affect the heart in different ways. One of the most common indications of heart and pericardium involvement is the local extension of lung cancer. Cardiac involvement through the pulmonary veins and lymphatics is possible. Extension of lung cancer through the pulmonary vein may involve the left atrium or even the left ventricle in rare cases (Fig. 38.1). Besides direct invasion, the heart may be affected by remote effects of cancer secretion from the lung or other parts and may induce cardiac arrhythmia. In practice, most often we

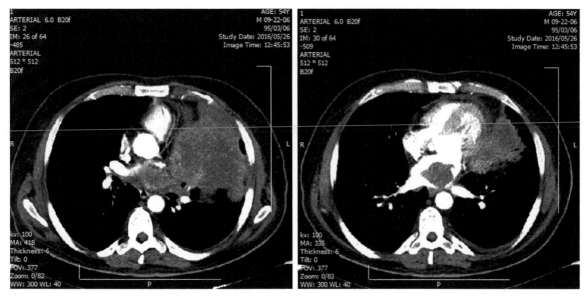

FIG. 38.1 Lung cancer in a 56-year-old man with local extension through the pulmonary vein into the left atrium and ventricle.

find heart failure, pericarditis, and arrhythmia caused by cancer chemotherapy or radiotherapy. Alkylating agents (cyclophosphamide, cisplatin), taxanes (paclitaxel, docetaxel), Herceptin, anthracyclines and related compounds (doxorubicin, daunorubicin, idarubicin, epirubicin, and the anthraquinone mitoxantrone), and other chemotherapy medications may have different impacts on cardiac function. Arrhythmias, myocardial necrosis causing a dilated cardiomyopathy, vasospasm or vaso-occlusion resulting in angina or myocardial infarction, and pericardial disease are serious complications of chemotherapy.[15]

Carcinoid heart disease is a typical example of cardiac involvement caused by tumor secretion and is characterized by pathognomonic plaque-like deposits of fibrous tissue that occur most commonly on the endocardium of the valvular cusps of the right heart, the cardiac chambers, and occasionally on the intima of the pulmonary arteries or aorta. Inactivation of humoral substances by the lung protects the left heart. Therefore, the involvement of valves and the endocardium of the right heart is more common.[9–16]

## REFERENCES

1. Lusuardi M, Garuti G, Massobrio M, Spagnolatti L, Bendinelli S. Heart and lungs in COPD. Close friends in real life—separate in daily medical practice? *Monaldi Arch Chest Dis.* 2008; 69(1):11–17.
2. Rutten FH, Cramer M-JM, Lammers J-WJ, Grobbee DE, Hoes AW. Heart failure and chronic obstructive pulmonary disease: an ignored combination. *Eur J Heart Fail.* 2006; 8:706–711.
3. Lavie P, Lavie L. Cardiovascular morbidity and mortality in obstructive sleep apnea. *Curr Pharm Des.* 2008; 14:3466–3473.
4. Han MK, McLaughlin VV, Criner GJ, Martinez FJ. Pulmonary diseases and the heart. *Circulation.* 2007; 116:2992–3005.
5. Machado MC, Vollmer WM, Togeiro SM, et al. CPAP and survival in moderate-to-severe obstructive sleep apnoea syndrome and hypoxaemic COPD. *Eur Respir J.* 2010; 35:132–137.
6. Butt M, Dwivedi G, Kheir O, Lip Gregory YH. *Obstructive Sleep Apnea and Cardiovascular Disease.* Elsevier; 2009 e journal.
7. Arcasoy SM, Christie JD, Ferrari VA, et al. Echocardiographic assessment of pulmonary hypertension in patients with advanced lung disease. *Am J Respir Crit Care Med.* 2003; 167:735–740.
8. Hasan-Allah S, Mehdi ZM, Ehteshami AA, Nazita P. Lung function after correction of scoliosis angle. *Tanaffos.* 2008; 7(4):27–31.
9. Akhmerov A, Marbán E. Covid-19 and the heart. *Circ Res.* 2020; 126(10):1443–1455.
10. McGoon M, Gutterman D, Steen V, et al. Screening, early detection, and diagnosis of pulmonary arterial

hypertension: ACCP evidence-based clinical practice guidelines. *Chest.* 2004; 126(suppl):14S–34S.

11. Froehlich W, Bogun FM, Crawford TC. Cardiac sarcoidosis. *Circulation.* 2015; 132:e137–e138.

12. Chapelon-Abric C. Cardiac sarcoidosis. *Curr Opin Pulm Med.* 2013; 19:493–502.

13. Sharma S. Cardiac imaging in myocardial sarcoidosis and other cardiomyopathies. *Curr Opin Pulm Med.* 2009; 15:507.

14. Bredy P-L, Prasad A, Frishman WH. Cardiac manifestations of sarcoidosis and therapeutic options. *Cardiol Rev.* 2009; 17:153–158.

15. Floyd JD, Nguyen DT, Lobins RL, et al. Cardiotoxicity of cancer therapy. *J Clin Oncol.* 2005; 23(30):76–85.

16. Modlin IM, Kidd M, Latich I, et al. Current status of gastrointestinal carcinoids. *Gastroenterology.* 2005; 128 (6):1717–1751.

# CHAPTER 39

# Cardiovascular Drugs and Hemostasis

BAHRAM FARIBORZ FARSAD • HANIEH SALEHI
Shaheed Rajaei Cardiovascular, Medical & Research Center, Iran University of Medical Sciences, Tehran, Iran

---

**KEY POINTS**

- Antiplatelet medications divide into oral and parenteral agents.
- Oral agents subdivide further based on the mechanism of action.
- Aspirin was the first antiplatelet medication and is a cyclooxygenase inhibitor.
- Other oral antiplatelet agents include clopidogrel, ticagrelor, prasugrel, pentoxifylline, cilostazol, and dipyridamole.
- Glycoprotein IIb/IIIa inhibitors such as tirofiban, eptifibatide are only available as parenteral agents and used in acute coronary syndrome (ACS).

---

## CONTRAST MEDIA

### Key Points

- Iodinated contrast media agents are used to facilitate visualization of the coronary vasculature.
- Common adverse effects of contrast media include bradycardia, hypotension, vasovagal reaction, direct negative inotropic effect on the myocardium, vasodilation, and nephropathy.
- Use of contrast media may induce immediate or delayed hypersensitivity reactions.
- Prednisone, methylprednisolone, and diphenhydramine are possible medications used as prophylaxis for immediate hypersensitivity reactions.

## INTRODUCTION

Coronary angiography uses contrast agents that allow for the visualization of the coronary vasculature. Currently available contrast agents contain iodine that more readily absorbs X-rays compared with the surrounding tissue. This differential absorption of radiation results in the ability of the contrast agents to provide contrast and visualization of the coronary arteries. Contrast agents are divided into three groups based on their osmolality (high, low, and isosmolar) (Table 39.1). The majority of contrast agents used in the current practice are low osmolar or isosmolar because high-osmolar agents have been found to have more hypotension, myocardial depression, heart failure, and electrical abnormalities (bradycardia, QRS and QT-interval prolongation, and ventricular fibrillation).[1]

### Cardiovascular Reactions

Iodinated contrast media (ICM) can cause hypotension and bradycardia. Vasovagal reactions, a direct negative inotropic effect on the myocardium, and peripheral vasodilatation probably contribute to these effects. The latter two effects may represent the actions of cardioactive and vasoactive substances that are released after the anaphylactic reaction to the ICM. This effect is generally self-limiting, but it can also be an indicator of a more severe, evolving reaction.

ICM can lower the ventricular arrhythmia threshold and precipitate cardiac arrhythmias and cardiac arrest. Fluid shifts caused by an infusion of hyperosmolar intravascular fluid can produce an intravascular hypervolemic state, systemic hypertension, and pulmonary edema. Also, ICM can precipitate angina.

The similarity of the cardiovascular and anaphylactic reactions to ICM can create confusion in identifying the true nature of the type and severity of an adverse reaction; this confusion can lead to the overtreatment or undertreatment of symptoms.[2]

### Nephropathy

Contrast agent-related nephropathy [or contrast-induced nephropathy (CIN)] is an elevation of the serum creatinine level that is more than 0.5 mg% or more than 50% of the baseline level at 1–3 days after the ICM injection. The elevation peaks by 3–7 days, and the creatinine level usually returns to baseline in 10–14 days. The incidence of contrast agent-related nephropathy in the general population is estimated to

**TABLE 39.1**
**Classification of Commonly Used Contrast Agents**

| Class | Trade Name | Genetic Name | Iodine (mg/mL) | Osmolarity (mOsm/kg) | Sodium (mEq L) |
|---|---|---|---|---|---|
| *Ionic* | | | | | |
| High osmolar | MD76 R | Sodium diatrizoate | 370 | 2140 | 190 |
| | Angiovist 370 | Sodium diatrizoate | 370 | 2076 | 150 |
| | Hypaque | Sodium diatrizoate | 370 | 2076 | 160 |
| Low osmolar | Hexabrix | Ioxaglate | 320 | 600 | 157 |
| *Nonionic* | | | | | |
| Low osmolar | Omnipaque | Iohexol | 350 | 844 | Trace |
| | Optiray 320 | Ioversol | 320 | 702 | Trace |
| | Oxilan 350 | Ioxilan | 350 | 695 | Trace |
| | Isovue 200 | Iopidamol | 200 | 413 | Trace |
| Isosmolar | Visipaque 320 | Iodixanol | 320 | 290 | Trace |

be 2%–7%. As many as 25% of patients with this nephropathy have a sustained reduction in renal function, most commonly when the nephropathy is oliguric.[3,4] The mechanism of this type of nephropathy is thought to be a combination of preexisting hemodynamic alterations; renal vasoconstriction, possibly through mediators such as endothelin and adenosine; and direct ICM cellular toxicity.[5]

Risk markers for the development of CIN, according to the correctable or not correctable, can be divided into two categories. The first group is nonmodifiable risk factors and the second group is modifiable risk factors.

Nonmodifiable categories include advanced age (>65 years), female sex, diabetes mellitus, hypertension, renal impairment, congestive cardiac failure, compromised left ventricle systolic performance, multiple myeloma, peripheral vascular disease, albuminuria, sepsis, and renal transplant.

Modifiable categories include anemia, hypovolemia, nephrotoxic drugs, hypoalbuminemia, and concomitant use of angiotensin-converting enzyme inhibitors or angiotensin II receptor blockers.[6]

## STRATEGY FOR PREVENTING RADIOCONTRAST-INDUCED NEPHROPATHY

1. Follow inpatients at risk of CIN is monitoring renal function by measuring serum creatinine and calculating the estimated glomerular filtration rate before and once daily for 5 days after the radiographic procedure.
2. Potentially nephrotoxic medications, such as aminoglycosides, vancomycin, amphotericin B, metformin,

and nonsteroidal antiinflammatory drugs, should be discontinued before contrast media administration. If the use of aminoglycosides is absolutely necessary, avoid using more than one shot of aminoglycosides for the treatment of infections.
3. In the choice of the contrast agent, either isosmolar (IOCM) or low osmolar (LOCM) is preferred.
4. Use the lowest dosage of contrast media.
5. Fluid intake should be encouraged, for example, 500 mL of water or soft drinks (tea and mineral water) orally before and 2500 mL for 24 h after contrast administration. High-risk patients should be administered 0.9% saline by intravenous (IV) infusion at a rate of approximately 1 mL/kg/h beginning 6–12 h before the procedure and continuing for up to 12–24 h after the radiographic examination, if diuresis is appropriate and the cardiovascular condition allows it.
6. In high-risk patients, *N*-acetylcysteine may also be given with an oral dose of 600 mg twice daily on the day before and the day of procedure. For patients unable to take it orally, IV doses of 150 mg/kg more than half an hour before the procedure or 50 mg/kg administered over 4 h may be used.[7]

## HYPERSENSITIVITY REACTIONS TO RADIOGRAPHIC CONTRAST MEDIA

Hypersensitivity reactions to radiocontrast are idiosyncratic and largely independent of dose and infusion rate. They can occur in response to minute amounts of contrast agent. These reactions can be further subdivided into immediate and delayed:

- Immediate hypersensitivity reactions develop within 1 h of administration.

- Delayed hypersensitivity reactions develop from 1 h to several days after administration. This category includes mild to moderate cutaneous eruptions; urticaria or angioedema; and various uncommon reactions, including erythema multiforme minor, fixed drug eruption, Stevens–Johnson syndrome, flexural exanthema, and vasculitis.

## PREMEDICATION REGIMEN IN IMMEDIATE HYPERSENSITIVITY REACTION

- Prednisone, given orally 13, 7, and 1 h before (in adults, 50 mg per dose and in children, 0.5–0.7 mg/kg per dose, up to 50 mg per dose). If oral administration is not feasible, methylprednisolone may be administered IV at the same time intervals (in adults, 40 mg and in children, 0.5 mg/kg up to a maximum of 40 mg per dose).
- Diphenhydramine, orally or parenterally, given 1 h before (in adults, 50 mg and in children, 1.25 mg/kg, up to 50 mg).[8]

## ANTIPLATELET THERAPY IN PERCUTANEOUS CORONARY INTERVENTION

### Key Points

- The goal of antiplatelet therapy for patients with acute coronary syndromes (ACSs) undergoing percutaneous coronary intervention (PCI) is to reduce the risk of ischemic events without increasing the risk of bleeding.
- Dual antiplatelet therapy (DAPT), the combination of aspirin and a $P2Y_{12}$-receptor inhibitor, is the basis of treatment of patients with ACS and of those undergoing PCI.
- The optimal duration of DAPT with aspirin and a thienopyridine after bare-metal stenting is at least 1 year and in patients after DES implantation. The optimal duration is for the patient's lifetime.
- Prasugrel should not be administered to patients with a prior history of stroke or transient ischemic attack.

## INTRODUCTION

The goal of antiplatelet therapy for patients with ACSs undergoing PCI is to reduce the risk of ischemic events without increasing the risk of bleeding.[9] Intracoronary thrombosis and the attendant risk of myocardial ischemia or infarction may occur soon after PCI with stent implantation. Stent thrombosis can occur acutely (within 24 h), subacutely (within 30 days), or as late as 1 year

(late) or more (very late) after stent placement. Stent thrombosis within the first year appears to occur with similar frequency in patients with bare-metal stents (BMS) or drug-eluting stents (DESs), as long as patients are treated with DAPT (aspirin plus a platelet $P2Y_{12}$ receptor blocker) for the recommended duration. The period of risk requiring DAPT is longer with DES, at least partly because of delayed neointimal coverage (Fig. 39.1).[10]

Aspirin, the most widely used antiplatelet agent, is effective, safe, and inexpensive and is recommended for all patients undergoing PCI. Clopidogrel, a thienopyridine agent, has been shown to reduce the rates of adverse cardiac events and mortality when given in a loading dose before PCI and in a maintenance dose thereafter. Questions remain as to the optimal loading and maintenance doses of clopidogrel, timing of administration before PCI, and duration of therapy after placement of BMS or DESs. All antiplatelet agents carry a risk of bleeding, which may significantly affect clinical outcomes.[9]

## ASPIRIN THERAPY

Aspirin (class IIa recommendation; level of evidence: A), the most widely used antiplatelet agent, is effective, safe, and inexpensive and is recommended for all patients undergoing PCI.

Aspirin irreversibly inhibits the cyclooxygenase enzyme, thus inhibiting thromboxane $A_2$ and prostaglandin $I_2$ synthesis for the life of the platelet.[11]

Aspirin was approved for use by the Food and Drug Administration (FDA) in patients with ACS undergoing PCI. For patients not receiving long-term aspirin, we pretreat with 300–325 mg, preferably given at least 2 h and preferably 24 h before PCI. In addition, this dose and time are used for those taking a maintenance dose of less than 325 mg.[11]

Aspirin-naïve patients should receive 300–325 mg of aspirin. A postprocedural maintenance dose of aspirin is also controversial, but the current guidelines recommend 162–325 mg for 1 month after BMS,[12] 3 months after sirolimus-eluting stents, and 6 months after paclitaxel-eluting stents. Thereafter, a maintenance dose of 75–162 mg/day is recommended indefinitely.[13]

For aspirin-allergic patients, we usually recommend desensitization therapy before the stent procedure. Patients who cannot tolerate long-term aspirin are usually treated with clopidogrel.[14]

## THIENOPYRIDINE THERAPY

Thienopyridines block the adenosine diphosphate (ADP) $P2Y_{12}$ receptor. They inhibit ADP-induced

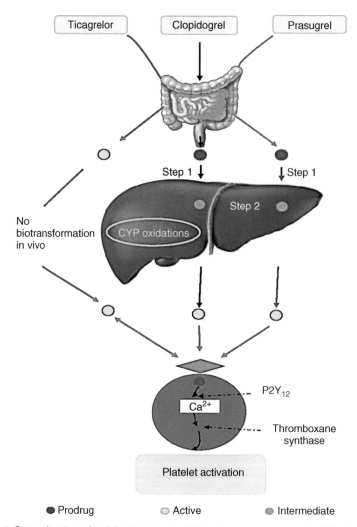

FIG. 39.1 Sites of action of antiplatelet agents. *ADP*, adenosine diphosphate; *GP*, glycoprotein.

platelet-fibrinogen binding, thus inhibiting platelet aggregation. Currently available agents in this class are ticlopidine, clopidogrel, and prasugrel.[15]

## TICLOPIDINE

Ticlopidine was the first widely used thienopyridine for the prevention of stent thrombosis. Ticlopidine was approved for use by the FDA in patients undergoing PCI. It significantly lowers the risk of stent thrombosis in patients receiving BMSs at 30 days when given with aspirin. In coronary artery stenting, the recommended adult dose of ticlopidine (class IIa recommendation; level of evidence: B) is a 500-mg loading dose, and

the maintenance dose is 250 mg twice daily taken with antiplatelet doses of aspirin for up to 30 days poststenting.[16] Ticlopidine should be administered with food.[17]

## LIMITATIONS OF USE

However, hematologic side effects, such as neutropenia (2.4%) and thrombotic thrombocytopenia purpura and hemolytic uremic syndrome (2.2%), limit its use.[16] Because of ticlopidine's hematologic side effects and only small incremental ischemic event benefit compared with aspirin, the latter remained the standard of therapy during POBA (plain old balloon angioplasty).[18]

# CLOPIDOGREL

Clopidogrel is also used with a loading dose in the PCI setting. Clopidogrel is a prodrug that must be converted in the liver to its active thiol derivative.[19] Clopidogrel was approved for use by the FDA in patients undergoing PCI. Clopidogrel (class I recommendation; level of evidence: A) is the preferred platelet $P2Y_{12}$ receptor blocker in patients with stable coronary artery disease undergoing PCI.[11]

We suggest pretreatment (before PCI) with clopidogrel for stable patients whose coronary anatomy is known from a recent diagnostic coronary angiogram. Both 300- and 600-mg loading doses of clopidogrel have been studied.[3,20] A 300-mg loading dose is required as long as 15–24 h to achieve its maximal clinical benefit. A 600-mg loading dose requires at least 2 h to achieve maximal clinical benefit. Clopidogrel's half-life is approximately 8 h.[19] The maintenance dose is generally 75 mg/day, but some data suggest this dose may be inadequate in patients with elevated body mass index or with intrinsic resistance as measured by the vasodilator-stimulated phosphoprotein index (VASP index).[21] For stable patients whose coronary anatomy is not known and who are scheduled for diagnostic coronary angiography with possible PCI, we suggest withholding the drug until after diagnostic coronary angiography is done because many patients will either not have disease that needs revascularization or will have disease that requires coronary artery bypass graft (CABG) surgery. In these situations, the patient will have been unnecessarily exposed to clopidogrel if it is given before angiography.[22]

## Limitations of use

An occasional stable patient may need CABG soon after catheterization. The 2011 American College of Cardiology Foundation/American Heart Association (ACC/AHA) guideline on CABG recommended that clopidogrel should be discontinued for at least 5 days before CABG, based on the recognition of an increase in perioperative bleeding in patients taking clopidogrel.[23] Clopidogrel is also metabolized in the liver and must be used with caution in patients with severe liver impairment.[24]

The optimal duration of DAPT with aspirin and a thienopyridine after bare-metal stenting has evolved. When high-pressure stent deployment was performed with or without intravascular ultrasound confirmation of excellent stent expansion and apposition, observational studies demonstrated very low stent thrombosis and major bleeding rates. Stent thrombosis rates of

approximately 1% were documented with 2–4 weeks of ticlopidine or clopidogrel added to aspirin.[25] Stent thrombosis more than 30 days after BMS implantation was an extraordinarily rare event. Major bleeding events were less than 2% in randomized trials and large observational series.[26]

Given the Clopidogrel for the Reduction of Events During Observation (CREDO) trial demonstration of reduced major adverse cardiovascular events unrelated to stent thrombosis when postprocedural DAPT with clopidogrel was extended to 12 months in patients receiving BMSs.[27]

With the development and widespread use of DES, a new issue, late (30 days to 1-year postimplant) and very late stent thrombosis (>1 year after implant), has developed. The pathophysiologic basis of this phenomenon has been recognition of incomplete endothelialization of many of these stent implants.[4] This has led to the recommendation of at least 1 year of DAPT with aspirin and clopidogrel. Many authorities recommend lifetime DAPT after DES implantation.[28]

# PRASUGREL

Prasugrel is a $P2Y_{12}$ platelet inhibitor and an ADP receptor antagonist indicated for the reduction of thrombotic cardiovascular events, including stent thrombosis (class I recommendation; level of evidence: A), in patients with ACS [e.g., unstable angina, non-ST-segment-elevation myocardial infarction (MI), or ST-segment elevation (STEMI)] who are to be managed with PCI.[11] Prasugrel was recently approved for use by the FDA as an alternative to clopidogrel in patients with ACS undergoing PCI.[29] Prasugrel 10-mg/day dose plus aspirin may be a sensible choice for patients with coronary syndrome who are undergoing PCI or diagnosed with stent thrombosis while taking clopidogrel and diagnosed with stent thrombosis who have completed the minimum recommended course of clopidogrel, have no risk factors for bleeding, and get to the hospital early enough for doctors to determine whether they might need bypass surgery instead (grade 2C).[4]

## Limitations of use

The use of prasugrel in patients 75 years or older is generally not recommended except in high-risk situations (i.e., with diabetes or history of MI) because of an increased risk of bleeding and uncertain efficacy, and patients with a history of stroke or transient ischemic attack (TIA) are at a higher risk of bleeding complications when prasugrel is used in combination with aspirin. People with active bleeding should avoid both drugs. Those who need bypass surgery should not take prasugrel or, if they have already started, should stop taking it at least 1 week before their operation.[30]

### Direct-Acting P2Y$_{12}$ Inhibitors

The newer, direct-acting P2Y$_{12}$ inhibitors (cangrelor and ticagrelor) change the conformation of the P2Y$_{12}$ receptor, resulting in reversible, concentration-dependent inhibition of the receptor.[31]

### Ticagrelor

In patients with ACS treated with DAPT after BMS or DES implantation, P2Y$_{12}$ inhibitor therapy (clopidogrel, prasugrel, or ticagrelor) should be given for at least 12 months and may continue beyond 12 months in select patients; discontinuation may be considered after 6 months in patients with newer generation DES and high bleeding risk. The FDA approved ticagrelor to demonstrate superior reductions in cardiovascular death and reduces the rate of stent thrombosis in patients who have been stented for the treatment of ACS. The maintenance dose of ticagrelor is 90 mg orally twice daily for 1 year after an ACS event and after that 60 mg twice daily; it should be used with aspirin 75–100 mg orally once daily.[11] Ticagrelor (class I recommendation; level of evidence: B) is also used with a loading dose in the PCI setting (load 500 mg; then 250 mg every 12 h for at least 10–14 days after successful stent placement). Treatment with ticagrelor 90 mg twice daily, compared with clopidogrel 75 mg once daily, resulted in fewer ischemic complications and stent thromboses but more frequent non-CABG-related bleeding events.[11]

### *Limitations of use*

Clinicians should suspect bleeding in any patient who is hypotensive and has recently undergone coronary angiography, PCI, CABG, or other surgical procedures, even if the patient does not have any signs of bleeding. However, in patients with severe hepatic impairment, ticagrelor is contraindicated.[32]

### Other Oral Antiplatelet Agents
### *Cilostazol*

For patients intolerant of aspirin or thienopyridines, the intracellular phosphodiesterase inhibitor cilostazol is effective as a second-line antiplatelet agent. Although the mechanism of action is not fully elucidated, cilostazol has a potent inhibitory effect on platelet aggregation.[3] Lee et al.[32] compared 1415 patients treated with triple antiplatelet therapy (aspirin, clopidogrel or ticlopidine, cilostazol) with 1597 patients treated with DAPT (aspirin, clopidogrel, or ticlopidine) after stenting.[33]

Stent thrombosis was reduced in the triple antiplatelet therapy group, with a strong trend in reduced major adverse cardiovascular events at 30 days. There was no significant increase in major bleeding or significant hematologic side effects: 1.8% in the dual therapy group and 2.6% ($P = 0.104$) in the triple therapy group. Although triple therapy has not been broadly adopted, cilostazol (class IIb recommendation; level of evidence: B) is a potentially useful alternative agent in aspirin- or thienopyridine-intolerant patients.[34]

**Limitations of Use.** The findings support the safety of triple antiplatelet therapy because the adverse effect profile of the triple antiplatelet therapy group was not significantly different from that of the DAPT group (major bleeding: 0.2% in the cilostazol group vs 0.4% in the dual therapy group). Patients who benefited the most from triple therapy were women, patients aged older than 65 years, and patients with diabetes.[35]

### *Dipyridamole*

Dipyridamole's antiplatelet activity is mediated by various mechanisms. Dipyridamole activates the nitric oxide-cyclic GMP signaling pathway that enhances platelet inhibition by amplifying the signaling of the nitric oxide donor sodium nitroprusside.[36] Dipyridamole alone or in combination with aspirin is not a currently used antiplatelet regimen during PCI.

### Parenteral Antiplatelet Agents

The platelet glycoprotein (GP) IIb/IIIa receptor became a target for therapeutic intervention to prevent thrombosis. The monoclonal antibody ultimately named abciximab (ReoPro) was developed to irreversibly bind and inhibit the IIb/IIIa receptor.[37] The IIb/IIIa receptor is the final common pathway to platelet aggregation because it mediates cross-linking of activated platelets with fibrinogen and von Willebrand factor. Hence, IIb/IIIa agents remain the most potent available antiplatelet agents.

Reversible small molecule antagonists, including eptifibatide (Integrilin) and tirofiban (Aggrastat), were subsequently developed. All three agents have demonstrated efficacy in the reduction of ischemic complications, particularly postprocedural myonecrosis, in balloon angioplasty and stenting. Meta-analysis of the PCI trials not including STEMI patients demonstrates a 38% reduction in death and MI at 30 days.[38] The individual properties of these agents and several of the pivotal trials that influence their current use in PCI are listed in Table 39.2.[41]

**TABLE 39.2**
**Comparison of Antiplatelet Categories**

| Class | Aspirin Nonsteroidal Antiinflammatory Agent | Clopidogrel Thienopyridine (Prodrug) | Prasugrel Thienopyridine (Prodrug) | Ticlopidine Cyto-pentyl-triazolopyridine | GP IIb/IIIa | PDE₃ Inhibitors |
|---|---|---|---|---|---|---|
| Drug | ASA | Clopidogrel (Plavix) (second generation) | Prasugrel (Effient) (third generation) | Ticagrelor (Brilinta) | Abciximab (ReoPro) | Cilostazol (Pletal) |
| Other drugs in this category | — | Ticlopidine (first generation) | — | Cangrelor | Eptifibatide (Integrilin) Tirofiban (Aggrastat) | — |
| Indications | • First- and second-degree prevention of stroke and MI<br>• ACS<br>• PCI with stent<br>• PVD | • ASA intolerance or failure<br>• First- and second-degree prevention of stroke and MI (±ASA)<br>• ACS (+ASA)<br>• PCI (+ASA)<br>• PVD | • With ASA, for treatment of ACS in patients treated with PCI<br>• Contraindicated if age >75 years or weight <60 kg or history of stroke<br>• Nonformulary | • With ASA, for treatment of ACS<br>• See BCHA restrictions below | • UA<br>• Adjunct to PCI<br>• Cardiogenic shock<br>• Adjunctive therapy during thrombolysis (off-label use) | Intermittent claudication, PAD, PCI |
| Dose and duration | Load: 160–325 mg Maintenance: 80 or 81 mg/day Duration: indefinite | Load: 300–600 mg Maintenance: 75 mg daily Duration:<br>• ACS: ≤1 year<br>• BMS: minimum 30 days<br>• DES: minimum 1 year | Load: 60 mg Maintenance: 10 mg daily Duration: ≤1 year | Load: 180 mg Maintenance: 90 mg BID Duration: ≤1 year | Start within 24 h before PCI, 0.25 mg/kg IV bolus followed by an IV infusion of 10 µg/min for 18–24 h, concluding 1 h after the PCI | 100 mg orally BID in place of ASA or clopidogrel in patients with an allergy or intolerance to either drug receiving dual antiplatelet therapy after BMS or DES placement |
| Peak effect | 1–3 h | 6 h (after load) | 4 h (after load) | 2 h (after load) | ~30 min (platelet inhibition) | ~2–4 weeks |

*Continued*

**TABLE 39.2**
**Comparison of Antiplatelet Categories—cont'd**

| Class | Aspirin Nonsteroidal Antiinflammatory Agent | Clopidogrel Thienopyridine (Prodrug) | Prasugrel Thienopyridine (Prodrug) | Ticlopidine Cyto-pentyl-triazolopyridine | GP IIb/IIa | PDE$_3$ Inhibitors |
|---|---|---|---|---|---|---|
| Half-life (active metabolite) | 3 h (salicylate) | 0.5 h | 7 h (range, 2–15 h) | 9 h (range, 6.7–9.1 h) | 30 min | 11–13 h |
| Elimination | Hydrolyzed by esterases; hepatic conjugation | Esterases; metabolism by CYP-450 enzymes | Esterases; metabolism by CYP-450 enzymes, CYP2B6 | Metabolism by CYP-450 enzymes | Through proteolytic cleavage | Urine (74%), feces (20%), CYP3A4 (major), CYP2C19 |
| When to hold dose before surgery | 7 days (optional) | 5–7 days | 7 days | 5 days | 36–48 h | 7 days |
| FDA approval | Adult: yes Pediatric: no | Adult: yes Pediatric: no | Adult: yes Pediatric: no | Adult: yes Pediatric: no | Adult: yes Pediatric: no | No |
| Place in therapy | Class IIa | Class I | Class I | Class I | Class IIa | Class IIb |

[a]Ticagrelor restricted to patients on or before admission or those on aspirin (ASA) with an acute coronary syndrome (ACS), that is, ST-segment-elevation myocardial infarction (STEMI), non-STEMI, unstable angina (UA) and one of the following: failure on optimal doses of clopidogrel and ASA therapy or recurrent ACS after revascularization with percutaneous coronary intervention (PCI) or STEMI and undergoing revascularization via PCI or non-STEMI or UA and high-risk angiographic anatomy and undergoing revascularization via PCI.
*ADP*, adenosine diphosphate; *BCHA*, *BID*, twice a day; *BMS*, bare-metal stent; *DES*, drug-eluting stent; *GP*, glycoprotein; *IV*, intravenous; *PAD*, peripheral artery disease; *PDE*, phosphodiesterase; *PVD*, peripheral vascular disease.
Information from Refs. 10, 11, 16, 30, 32, 35, 39, 40, and.

**TABLE 39.3**
Properties of the Parenteral Glycoprotein IIb/IIIa Receptor Antagonist

| Drug Name | Abciximab | Eptifibatide | Tirofiban |
|---|---|---|---|
| Type of agent | Monoclonal antibody | Small molecule (KGD sequence) | Small molecule (RGD sequence) |
| Plasma half-life | ~10 to 15 min | ~2.5 h | ~1.8 h |
| Platelet-bound half-life | Hours | Seconds | Seconds |
| Platelet transfusion | Yes | No | No |
| Reversibility without platelet transfusion | ~24 h | ~4 h[a] | ~4 h[a] |
| % of dose in initial bolus | ~75 | ~5 | ~5 |
| Renal dose adjustment | No | Yes | Yes |

[a]Assumes normal renal function.

When (100 U/kg) doses of IV unfractionated heparin (UFH) were coadministered in the EPIC trial.[26] In the Evaluation of PTCA to Improve Long-term Outcome by c7E3 GP IIb/IIIa Receptor Blockade (EPILOG) trial, abciximab had equal efficacy to prevent ischemic complications with a lower dose of IV UFH (70 U/kg) compared with higher doses (100 U/kg). Major bleeding with abciximab and lower dose heparin (1.1%) was identical to high-dose heparin (1.1%) alone.[39] Heparin doses of 50–60 U/kg are generally recommended when administered with IIb/IIIa therapy for a target activated clotting time (ACT) of 200–250 s.

The ISAR-REACT trial demonstrated no benefit of abciximab in low-risk patients undergoing PCI (A Clinical Trial of Abciximab in Elective Percutaneous Coronary Intervention after Pretreatment with Clopidogrel) with a stent who had been pretreated with 600 mg of clopidogrel as well as aspirin at least 2 h before intervention.[40] The ISAR-REACT 2 trial, however, demonstrated benefit of abciximab in unstable angina and NSTEMI-ACS patients undergoing PCI (Table 39.3).[40]

## ANTICOAGULANT THERAPY
### Key Points
- The goals of treatment for venous thromboembolism (VTE) are to prevent extension, propagation, or embolization and recurrence of thrombosis; preserve valve function; prevent the postthrombotic syndrome (PTS); and prevent chronic thromboembolic pulmonary hypertension (CTPH) and right ventricular dysfunction in individuals with pulmonary embolism (PE).
- Anticoagulant therapies can be classified according to their route of administration (parenteral or oral).
- The American College of Chest Physicians (ACCP) guidelines suggest low-molecular-weight heparin (LMWH) or fondaparinux or UFH for patients with acute deep vein thrombosis (DVT) of the leg, acute upper extremity DVT involving axillary or more proximal veins, or acute PE.
- The latest ACCP guidelines recommend at least 3 months of therapy with warfarin for patients with an idiopathic or unprovoked VTE and suggest that indefinite therapy is considered if the patient is at low risk for bleeding.

## INTRODUCTION
VTE is a common disease that includes both PE and DVT. The Iranian population is very young; however, with increasing age of the Iranian population, VTE will become a growing public health problem.[42]

The goals of treatment for VTE are to prevent extension, propagation, or embolization and recurrence of thrombosis. Treatment is also aimed at preserving valve function and preventing PTS in patients with DVT and to prevent CTPH and right ventricular dysfunction in individuals with PE. Initial inpatient management should begin with weight-adjusted UFH, a weight-based LMWH preparation, or the anti-Xa inhibitor fondaparinux. A vitamin K antagonist (VKA) should be started as soon as possible, overlapping for a minimum of 5 days with one of the above-listed anticoagulants until the international normalized ratio (INR) is stable and 2.0 or above for at least 24 h.

## ANTICOAGULANT THERAPY: CLASSIFICATION

The classification of anticoagulant agents is based primarily on the target-specific steps in the process, inhibiting a single coagulation factor or mimicking natural coagulation inhibitors. Most clinically available anticoagulant therapies block factor FII or thrombin and FX. Each class of inhibitors blocking a specific target can then be classified according to its mechanism of action to exert its inhibitory effects as direct or indirect, based on the need of a cofactor without which these agents would provide minimal or null effects (Fig. 39.2). Finally, anticoagulant therapies can be classified according to their route of administration (parenteral or oral). In the setting of ACS and PCI, parenteral agents are used and include a variety of thrombin inhibitors (direct and indirect). Anti-X inhibitors are also used in ACS patients, mostly medically managed, although to a lesser extent than thrombin inhibitors, and currently only an indirect anti-X inhibitor for parenteral use is clinically available.[43]

## PARENTERAL

### Unfractionated Heparin

Guidelines from the ACCP suggest LMWH or fondaparinux over IV or subcutaneous UFH for patients with acute DVT of the leg, acute upper extremity DVT involving axillary or more proximal veins, or acute PE.[44]

UFH is approved by the FDA for the treatment of DVT or PE and for reduction of the risk of recurrent DVT and PE. UFH (class IIa recommendation; level of evidence: B) is generally administered IV, although it can also be effective when given subcutaneously. Dosing is generally determined from a weight-based nomogram, and a bolus of 80 U/kg followed by 18 U/kg/h is commonly recommended for most adult patients. Subsequent dose adjustments are made based on the results of either an activated partial thromboplastin time (aPTT) or an anti-Xa assay using an amidolytic assay.[44]

Heparin has a number of drawbacks. It has a variable anticoagulant response among patients; a relatively short half-life; and adverse effects of bleeding, osteoporosis, and heparin-induced thrombocytopenia (HIT).

HIT (an immune-mediated disorder that typically occurs 4–11 days after exposure to heparin products) is reported to occur in as many as 3%–5% of all patients receiving UFH but occurs much less frequently in patients receiving any of the LMWH preparations, so for treatment, heparin should not be used. Treatment options are focused on inhibiting thrombin formation or direct thrombin inhibition.

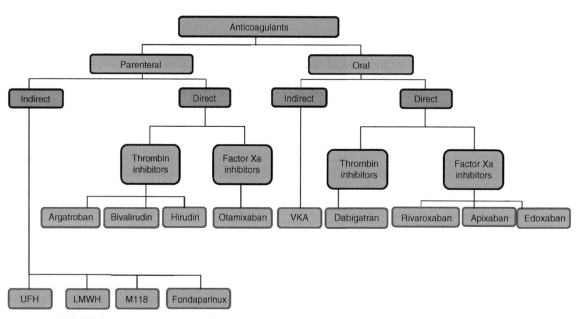

FIG. 39.2 Anticoagulant categories according to their mode of action and route of administration and place in therapy. *LMWH*, low-molecular-weight heparin; *UFH*, unfractionated heparin; *VKA*, vitamin K antagonist.

HIT can result in significant morbidity and mortality, with life- and limb-threatening thrombotic complications including the loss of a limb, stroke, MI, DVT, or PE. Treatment revolves around immediate cessation of UFH or LMWH and replacement with an alternative antithrombotic agent [direct thrombin inhibitor (DTI)]. Currently, two DTIs are approved by the FDA for the treatment of HIT: argatroban, a small synthetic molecule, and a hirudin derivative (lepirudin).

### Low-Molecular-Weight Heparin

Depolymerization of UFH by chemical or enzymatic cleavage of its polysaccharide chains yields a mixture of heparin fragments known as LMWH that have a mean molecular weight of approximately 5000 Da.[45] This reduction in molecular weight leads to more predictable pharmacokinetics and a greater bioavailability than with UFH. The UFDA approved the use of enoxaparin as low LMWH to treat DVT and PE and to reduce the risk of recurrent DVT and PE after initial treatment.[46] A subcutaneous administered LMWH (class IIa recommendation; level of evidence: B) is the preferred anticoagulant for most hemodynamically stable patients.[47]

Advantages of the LMWHs include:
- Once- or twice-daily subcutaneous injections
- Easy administration
- Dose by a weight-base adjusted regimen
- No monitoring necessary for most patients
- Outpatient administration
- Lower incidence of HIT
- Less osteoclast activation and lower incidence of osteoporosis

Although laboratory monitoring is generally not necessary, it is recommended in patients who are morbidly obese or who have significant renal disease and in pediatric or pregnant patients. In these individuals, a 4-h postinjection anti-Xa level using LMWH as the standard is recommended. Therapeutic levels are 0.6–1.0 IU/mL for twice-daily injections and 1.0–2.0 IU/mL for once-a-day administration.[48] LMWH preparations require dose adjustment for patients with a creatinine clearance of 30 mL/min or less and are contraindicated in patients on hemodialysis.
- LMWH is as efficient as UFH.
  Advantages over UFH include:
- Greater bioavailability
- More predictable dosing
- Subcutaneous delivery, usually without the need for monitoring
- Lower risk of HIT

Heparin should still be the first line of therapy in certain cases:
- Persistent hypotension caused by PE (massive PE)
- Increased risk of bleeding
- Concern about subcutaneous absorption (morbid obesity and anasarca)
- When thrombolysis is being considered
- Patients with end-stage renal disease (ESRD)

### Fondaparinux

Fondaparinux (Arixtra) (class IIa recommendation; level of evidence: B) is the only synthetic pentasaccharide that has been approved by the FDA for the treatment of acute DVT and PE.[44] It is administered subcutaneously once daily and is almost 100% bioavailable. Dosing is weight based; 5 mg is recommended for individuals weighing less than 50 kg, 7.5 mg for those who weigh 50–100 kg, and 10 mg for individuals who weigh more than 100 kg. Fondaparinux does not require dose adjustment or monitoring, but caution should be exercised while using this drug because of its long half-life and the lack of an antidote.[49] Warfarin should be started concurrently and continued for at least 5 days until a therapeutic INR is attained. Fondaparinux is contraindicated in patients with renal insufficiency defined as a creatinine clearance less than 30 mL/min and in patients on hemodialysis.

### Bivalirudin

Bivalirudin is indicated for patients with, or at risk of, HIT or HIT and thrombosis syndrome undergoing PCI; it is intended for use with aspirin (class IIa recommendation; level of evidence: B).[50]

#### Limitations of use

Safety and effectiveness have not been established in patients with ACSs who are not undergoing PTCA or PCI.[50]

### ORAL
#### Vitamin K Antagonists

Warfarin is the only VKA available for long-term management of VTE in the United States and currently remains the mainstay of therapy for long-term treatment of VTE and PE (class I recommendation; level of evidence: A).[51]

Despite its use for many decades, two areas often remain confusing and controversial to physicians. One is the optimal dose for initiating therapy; the other revolves around duration of anticoagulation. Two trials compared different initiating doses of warfarin (5 vs

10 mg). Both studies reported that 5 mg reduced the likelihood of excessive early anticoagulation, avoided rapid drops in the level of protein C, and did not appear to prolong the time required to achieve a therapeutic INR.[45,52] In contrast, a more recent study performed in the outpatient setting demonstrated that higher initial doses (10 mg) of warfarin were superior to lower doses (5 mg).[53] In this study, patients reached a target INR on average 1.4 days earlier, without an increase in recurrent events or major bleeding. In general, the dose should be tailored to each individual patient. Lower doses are often recommended for elderly patients and for those who have comorbid conditions such as recent surgery, hypertension, stroke, CHF, renal or liver disease, anemia, diabetes, cancer, or a history of bleeding. Genotype-based dosing is a tool that has gained much attention in managing warfarin. The FDA has approved labeling changes for warfarin, recommending lower initiation doses for patients with genetic variations in VKORC1 and CYP2C9 enzymes. However, clinical evidence for the clinical utility and cost-effectiveness of this approach is lacking.[54]

There is controversy about the optimal length of treatment. Most patients require 3 months of therapy if an underlying precipitating event (surgery, trauma, medical condition) has been identified and resolved; longer therapy is recommended if no underlying cause can be found (idiopathic or unprovoked) or if the precipitating factor cannot be rectified.

The ACCP guidelines recommend at least 3 months of therapy (class IIa recommendation; level of evidence: B) for patients with an idiopathic or unprovoked VTE and suggest that indefinite therapy is considered if the patient is at low risk for bleeding.[51]

Patients with the antiphospholipid antibody syndrome, individuals who are homozygous for factor V Leiden, patients who are deficient in antithrombin, and individuals with two or more hereditary thrombophilia conditions should also be considered for long-term anticoagulation, although no specific recommendations were addressed for these conditions in the latest ACCP guidelines. For patients with VTE and cancer, LMWH is recommended for the first 3–6 months of treatment. This patient population should receive indefinite anticoagulation or until the cancer is deemed cured.[51]

### Bridging Unfractionated Heparin, Low-Molecular-Weight Heparin, or Fondaparinux to Warfarin

In the treatment of VTE and PE, the parenteral anticoagulant should be overlapped with warfarin for a minimum of 5 days. In most cases, warfarin can be initiated on day 1, after the first dose of the parenteral agent has been given. Warfarin should not be initiated alone, and the parenteral anticoagulant should not be discontinued until the INR is in the therapeutic range for 2 consecutive days.

Depending on the patient's risk of thromboembolism and bleeding, bridging should occur when a patient's oral anticoagulation therapy needs to be interrupted (Table 39.4). Interruption is common in patients undergoing surgery. For most persons who are not having a minor procedure, warfarin will be stopped approximately 5 days before surgery and restarted 12–24 h postoperatively. LMWH should be restarted approximately 24 h after the procedure, and it may be prudent to wait 48–72 h before resuming the medication for patients at high risk of bleeding or who are undergoing major surgery. Fondaparinux is not recommended for this indication.[55]

For all warfarin indications, perioperative bridging is not indicated in patients at low risk of thromboembolism. For patients with a high risk of thromboembolism, bridging with a therapeutic dose of UFH or LMWH is indicated. The ACCP guidelines are less clear about how patients with a moderate risk of thromboembolism should be treated. Clinicians need to balance the individual's risk of thromboembolism, based on the medical history and surgical procedure, and risk of bleeding when determining what is optimal in persons in this moderate-risk category.[44]

### Most Common Warfarin Interactions

Warfarin is subject to many drug–drug, drug–food, and drug–disease state interactions. Table 39.5 lists selected drug–drug interactions that are considered highly likely to potentiate or inhibit the effects of warfarin.

Some medications, such as amiodarone and rifampin, can impact a patient's INR long after the medication is discontinued.[42–80] A patient taking a medication with higher interaction potential, such as metronidazole, should be monitored more frequently.[81] Depending on the patient and the medication, a prophylactic reduction in warfarin dosage may also be advised.

Foods with high vitamin K concentrations, such as leafy green vegetables, have the potential to partially reverse the anticoagulation effects of warfarin.[80] A consistent diet is more important than limiting dietary vitamin K.[56]

Medical conditions such as diarrhea, heart failure, fever, hyperthyroidism, and liver disease can potentiate warfarin's effects. Conversely, conditions such as hypothyroidism can decrease the expected effects of warfarin.[56] Genetic factors can predispose patients to reduced warfarin requirements, as well as warfarin

**TABLE 39.4**
**Warfarin Indications**

| Mechanical Heart Valve | Chronic Atrial Fibrillation | VTE | Risk Level for VTE | Bleeding Risk Category | Recommendation |
|---|---|---|---|---|---|
| At least one of the following:<br>• Aortic valve prosthesis (caged-ball or tilting-disk)<br>• Mitral valve prosthesis (any)<br>• Stroke or TIA within past 6 months<br>May also include:<br>• Patients with a history of stroke or TIA >3 months before surgery and a CHADS$_2$ score <5<br>• Patients undergoing surgeries with high risk of thromboembolism | At least one of the following:<br>• CHADS$_2$ score of 5 or 6<br>• Rheumatic mitral valve disease<br>• Stroke or TIA within past 3 months<br>May also include:<br>• Patients with a history of stroke or TIA >3 months before surgery and a CHADS$_2$ score <5<br>• Patients undergoing surgeries with high risk of thromboembolism | At least one of the following:<br>• Severe thrombophilia[a]<br>• VTE within past 3 months<br>May also include:<br>• Previous thromboembolism during temporary vitamin K antagonist interruption<br>• Patients undergoing surgeries with high risk of thromboembolism | High (>10% annual risk) | Very low (minor procedures) | Dental: continue warfarin with an oral prohemostatic agent or stop warfarin 2–3 days before procedure<br>Dermatologic: continue warfarin and optimize local hemostasis<br>Cataract: continue warfarin |
| | | | | Low | Stop warfarin 5 days before surgery and restart 12–24 h postoperatively<br>VTE prophylaxis *and*<br>Therapeutic dose of LMWH before the procedure[b] and beginning ≈24 h after the procedure |
| | | | | High[c,d,e] | Stop warfarin 5 days before surgery and restart 12–24 h postoperatively<br>VTE prophylaxis *and* ischemic stroke using UFH 5000 U SC q 8_12 h<br>Therapeutic dose of LMWH before the procedure[b] and beginning 48–72 h after the procedure |
| Aortic valve prosthesis (bileaflet) and at least one of the following:<br>• Age older than 75 years<br>• Atrial fibrillation<br>• Congestive heart failure<br>• Diabetes mellitus<br>• Hypertension<br>• Prior stroke or TIA | CHADS$_2$ score of 3 or 4 | At least one of the following:<br>• Active cancer[d]<br>• Nonsevere thrombophilic condition[e]<br>• Recurrent VTE<br>• VTE within past 3–12 months | Moderate (5%–10% annual risk) | Very low (minor procedures) | Dental: continue warfarin with an oral prohemostatic agent or stop warfarin 2–3 days before procedure<br>Dermatologic: continue warfarin and optimize local hemostasis<br>Cataract: continue warfarin |
| | | | | Low (base bridging on patient- and surgery-related factors[g]) | Stop warfarin 5 days before surgery and restart 12–24 h postoperatively<br>Therapeutic dose of LMWH before the procedure[b] and beginning ≈24 h after the procedure |
| | | | | High (base bridging on patient- and | Stop warfarin 5 days before surgery and restart 12–24 h postoperatively<br>Therapeutic dose of LMWH before the |

*Continued*

**TABLE 39.4**
**Warfarin Indications—cont'd**

| Mechanical Heart Valve | Chronic Atrial Fibrillation | VTE | Risk Level for VTE | Bleeding Risk Category (surgery-related factors[c]) | Recommendation |
|---|---|---|---|---|---|
| | | | | | procedure[b] and beginning 48–72 h after the procedure |
| Aortic valve prosthesis (bileaflet) without atrial fibrillation and no other stroke risk factors | No prior stroke or TIA and CHADS₂ score ≤2 | Single VTE that occurred >12 months ago and no other risk factors | Low (<5% annual risk) | Very low (minor procedures) | Dental: continue warfarin with an oral prohemostatic agent or stop warfarin 2–3 days before procedure<br>Dermatologic: continue warfarin and optimize local hemostasis<br>Cataract: continue warfarin |
| | | | | Low | Stop warfarin 5 days before surgery and restart 12–24 h postoperatively<br>Do not bridge |
| | | | | High[c] | Stop warfarin 5 days before surgery and restart 12–24 h postoperatively<br>Do not bridge |

*CHADS₂*, congestive heart failure, hypertension, age ≥75 years, diabetes mellitus, prior ischemic stroke or TIA (doubled); *TIA*, transient ischemic attack; *VTE*, venous thromboembolism.
[a]Such as protein C or S deficiency, antiphospholipid antibodies, or antithrombin deficiency.
[b]Stop subcutaneous low-molecular-weight heparin (LMWH) 24 h before surgery.
[c]Surgeries with a higher risk of bleeding include urologic surgeries, large colon polyp resection, and surgeries that involve vascular organs or have extensive tissue injury potential. Bleeding risk in hospitalized patients has been linked to multiple factors, including active gastric or duodenal ulcer, bleeding within 3 months before admission, and thrombocytopenia.
[d]Defined as cancer treated within 6 months or palliative.
[e]Such as heterozygous factor V Leiden mutation.

**TABLE 39.5**
**Most Common Warfarin Major Drug Interactions**

| Drug | Direction and Severity of Effect on INR | Mechanism | Anticipated Onset | Anticipated Offset (t½)[a] | Suggested Management |
|------|------------------------------------------|-----------|-------------------|-----------------------------|----------------------|
| ASA | No effect at doses <6 g/day, increased risk of bleeding Major | Irreversible inhibition of platelet function | 1–3 days | 5–7 days (inhibitory effects of ASA on platelets last for lifetime of each platelet) | Use lowest effective dose of ASA; use enteric-coated formulation; monitor for bleeding |
| Celecoxib | Increased INR Major (especially in elderly patients) | Celecoxib is metabolized by CYP2C9 but does not inhibit or induce this isozyme | 2–5 days | NR (t½ = 11 h) | Monitor INR closely when starting or stopping celecoxib; monitor for bleeding; AMS considers empiric 0%–15% warfarin dose reduction |
| Fenofibrate | Increased INR Major | Unknown | 5–10 days | Delayed (t½ = 20–22 h) | Monitor INR closely (i.e., weekly) when starting or stopping fenofibrate; AMS considers initial empiric 10%–15% warfarin dose reduction, in anticipation of eventual reduction of up to 40% |
| Metronidazole | Increased INR Major | Decrease in warfarin metabolism (through CYP2C9 inhibition) | 3–5 days | ~2 days (t½ = 8 h) | Monitor INR closely when starting or stopping metronidazole; AMS considers empiric 25%–40% warfarin dose reduction |
| Moxifloxacin | Increased INR Major | Unknown; possible inhibition of CYP1A2; clinically significant interaction more common among older patients | 2–5 days | 2–3 days (t½ = ~12.7 h) | Monitor INR closely when starting or stopping moxifloxacin; INR is affected by severity of illness; AMS considers 0%–25% warfarin dose reduction |
| Naproxen | No effect on INR; increased risk of bleeding | Inhibition of platelet aggregation and production of gastroprotective prostaglandins | 2–5 days | 3–7 days (t½ = 12–15 h) | Monitor closely for bleeding (especially GI); avoid or minimize concurrent use; take with food |
| Voriconazole | Increased INR Major | Inhibition of CYP2C9-mediated metabolism of S-warfarin | 3–7 days | NR (t½ = 6 h) | Monitor INR carefully when starting or stopping voriconazole; AMS considers empiric 25%–30% warfarin dose reduction |

*AMS*, *ASA*, aspirin; *GI*, gastrointestinal; *INR*, international normalized ratio; *NR*, *t½*, half-life.
[a]All the interactions included in this table are of major clinical significance.

resistance. Although there is a small subset of patients who may have unexpected responses to warfarin, it is not currently recommended that patients undergo genetic testing.[56]

## New Oral Anticoagulants

Until recently, warfarin was the only available oral anticoagulant for the treatment of VTE. Multiple new oral agents, with different mechanisms of action, have been evaluated in phase III clinical trials and have become available in the markets outside the United States. These new anticoagulants are poised to replace warfarin and potentially change completely the way patients with VTE are being managed. The agents that are most advanced in their development are the oral DTI (dabigatran etexilate) and oral direct factor Xa inhibitors (e.g., apixaban and rivaroxaban). In contrast to warfarin, these new oral anticoagulants in general have a more rapid onset of action that may obviate the need for parenteral anticoagulation in the initial treatment of VTE. Also, because these agents have stable pharmacodynamics, unlike warfarin, routine monitoring is not required, which makes them more ideal agents for long-term anticoagulation. Currently, there are no antidotes for these agents.[55]

## Oral Direct Thrombin Inhibitors

The effectiveness of warfarin is well established; however, it is a suboptimal anticoagulant because it requires frequent monitoring and dosage adjustments and because of its potential for multiple drug–drug, drug–food, and drug–disease state interactions. It has a lengthy half-life and a delayed anticoagulant effect, and it often requires bridging therapy.[55]

Since the approval of warfarin in 1954, no other oral option existed for patients who needed long-term anticoagulation therapy. This changed in 2010 with the FDA approval of the oral DTI dabigatran (Pradaxa), in 2011 with the FDA approval of the oral direct factor Xa inhibitor rivaroxaban (Xarelto), and again in 2012 with the FDA approval of the oral factor Xa inhibitor apixaban (Eliquis).[55]

## Oral Direct Factor Xa Inhibitors
### Dabigatran etexilate

Dabigatran etexilate, a prodrug, has been shown to be not inferior to subcutaneous enoxaparin in the prevention of VTE after total knee or total hip arthroplasty with similar bleeding risks.[42–46,48,50,51,53,54,66–94] Dabigatran does not require monitoring, dosage adjustments, or overlap with injectable anticoagulants such as heparin.

Without applicable laboratory monitoring, there is no mechanism to establish if a patient's INR is subtherapeutic or supratherapeutic.[90] Dabigatran is approved by the FDA for prevention and treatment of DVT, after parenteral therapy (class IIb recommendation; level of evidence: B).[89] When reversal of the anticoagulant effects of dabigatran is needed for emergency surgery or urgent procedures or in life-threatening or uncontrolled bleeding, idarucizumab is indicated for patients treated with dabigatran etexilate.[85]

**Limitation of use.** Dabigatran requires dose adjustments for patients with a creatinine clearance of 15–30 mL/min and is not recommended if the creatinine clearance is 15 mL/min or less.[44]

### Rivaroxaban

Rivaroxaban is an oral direct factor Xa inhibitor with a relatively short half-life of 5–9 h and rapid onset of action of 2.5–4 h. Rivaroxaban (class IIa recommendation; level of evidence: B) is indicated for prevention of DVT in patients undergoing knee or hip replacement surgery, for the treatment of DVT and PE, for reducing the risk of recurrent DVT and PE after initial treatment, and for prevention of systemic embolism in patients with nonvalvular atrial fibrillation (AF) (class IIb recommendation; level of evidence: B).[44–49,51,58–74] It is expected to prolong the aPTT and increase antifactor Xa levels; however, the usefulness of monitoring has not been established. In four trials evaluating the role of rivaroxaban in the prevention of VTE in patients undergoing orthopedic surgery, rivaroxaban significantly reduced the primary outcome (total VTE and all-cause mortality) compared with enoxaparin without significantly increasing bleeding risk.[42,44–46,48,51,53,65–80,82]

**Limitation of use.** Rivaroxaban should not be used in patients with severe renal insufficiency or significant hepatic impairment.[44]

### Apixaban

Apixaban is another oral direct factor Xa inhibitor with promising data. Apixaban is found comparable to warfarin in a small phase II trial for the treatment of DVT.[60] In two phase III trials,[78,79] apixaban is superior to enoxaparin when given using the European regimen (40 mg/day starting on the evening before surgery) in preventing VTE after knee and hip arthroplasty. However, in another study,[78] apixaban failed to meet the noninferiority standards for the prevention of VTE after knee arthroplasty when compared with enoxaparin (given in the North American regimen of 30 mg every 12 h starting 12–24 h after surgery). Other direct factor Xa inhibitors in development include betrixaban, razaxaban, and otamixaban.[44]

## PREGNANCY AND VENOUS THROMBOEMBOLISM

The risk of thromboembolism is increased in women during pregnancy and in the postpartum period. The risk of a first episode of DVT is five times higher in postpartum than pregnancy. The risk of PE is 15 times higher in postpartum than pregnancy.[83]

For women on hormonal therapy use, low-dose oral contraceptives increase the risk of thromboembolism by a factor of 2–5. Hormonal replacement increases the risk of thromboembolism by a factor of 2–4.[72]

The diagnosis of DVT or PE is the same in pregnant and nonpregnant patients, and if necessary, imaging should be used. The treatment for DVT and PE is similar in the acute stage and includes parenteral anticoagulation, inferior vena cava filter, embolectomy, or thrombolytic therapy. Long-term anticoagulation is different in pregnant patients, and the recommendation is to use LMWH because warfarin is teratogenic.[83]

## ANTICOAGULANT THERAPY TO PREVENT EMBOLIZATION IN ATRIAL FIBRILLATION

AF is the most common cardiac arrhythmia. It impairs cardiac function and increases the risk of stroke.[68]

Development and subsequent embolization of atrial thrombi can occur with any form (e.g., paroxysmal, persistent, or permanent) of AF. Although ischemic stroke is the most frequent clinical manifestation of embolization associated with AF, embolization to other locations in the systemic and pulmonary circulations also occurs but is less commonly recognized.[61]

As a result of embolic risk, chronic oral anticoagulation is recommended for most AF patients. However, such therapy is associated with an increased risk of bleeding, and recommendations for its use must take both benefit and risk into account.[69]

Anticoagulation therapy is needed with rate control and rhythm control to prevent stroke. Warfarin is superior to aspirin and clopidogrel in preventing stroke despite its narrow therapeutic range and increased risk of bleeding. Tools that predict the risk of stroke {e.g., $CHADS_2$ [congestive heart failure, hypertension, age $\geq 75$ years, diabetes mellitus, stroke (double weight)]} and the risk of bleeding (e.g., Outpatient Bleeding Risk Index) are helpful in making decisions about anticoagulation therapy (Table 39.6).[70]

## ANTICOAGULATION THERAPY IN ATRIAL FIBRILLATION

In patients with AF, the estimated risk of stroke without anticoagulation therapy is 5% per year.[88] Paroxysmal and chronic AF, treated by rate or rhythm control, requires long-term anticoagulation therapy unless the risks of anticoagulation use exceed the benefits.[69,91]

The ACC/AHA/European Society of Cardiology recommend that patients with nonvalvular AF who are at low risk of stroke be treated with 81–325 mg of aspirin per day, but patients at higher risk should be treated with warfarin (at a dosage necessary to achieve a target INR of 2–3).[69,91] There is general agreement that

---

**TABLE 39.6**
**Novel Oral Anticoagulants vs Warfarin for Stroke Prevention in Atrial Fibrillation and Treatment of Deep Vein Thrombosis and Pulmonary Embolism**

| | STROKE PREVENTION IN ATRIAL FIBRILLATION | | TREATMENT OF DVT/PE | |
| --- | --- | --- | --- | --- |
| NOAC | Prevention of Stroke vs Warfarin | Major Bleeding vs Warfarin | Prevention of Recurrent DVT/PE vs Warfarin | Major Bleeding vs Warfarin in DVT/PE |
| Dabigatran | ↓ | ↔ | ↔ | ↔ |
| Rivaroxaban | ↔ | ↔ | ↔ | ↓ |
| Apixaban | ↓ | ↓ | ↔ | ↓ |
| Edoxaban | ↔ | ↓ | ↔ | ↓ |

*DVT*, deep vein thrombosis; *NOAC*, novel oral anticoagulant; *PE*, pulmonary embolism.

**TABLE 39.7**
CHADS$_2$ Risk Prediction for Nonvalvular Atrial Fibrillation[a]

| Risk Factor | Points | CHADS$_2$ Score | Stroke Risk (%/year) | Anticoagulation Recommendation |
|---|---|---|---|---|
| Congestive heart failure | 1 | 0 | 1.9 (low) | ASA 81–325 mg OD |
| Hypertension | 1 | 1 | 2.8 (low to moderate) | Oral anticoagulants[b] |
| Age >75 year | 1 | 2–3 | 4.0–5.9 (moderate) | Oral anticoagulants[b] |
| Diabetes | 1 | 4–6 | 8.5–18.2 (high) | Oral anticoagulants[b] |
| Stroke or TIA (prior) | 2 | | | |

Also refer to American Heart Association/American College of Cardiology/Heart Rhythm Society (HRS) atrial fibrillation guidelines.
[a]Recent Canadian Cardiovascular Society (CCS) update recommends oral anticoagulants if age ≥65 years or age <65 years with at least one risk factor. *ASA*, aspirin; *CHADS₂*, congestive heart failure, hypertension, age ≥75 years, diabetes mellitus, prior ischemic stroke or transient ischemic attack (TIA) (doubled); *OD*, oral dose.
[b]Oral anticoagulants currently include warfarin international normalized ratio (2–3) and direct oral anticoagulants, e.g., apixaban, dabigatran, rivaroxaban.
Data from Gage BF, Waterman AD, Shannon W, et al. Validation of clinical classification schemes for predicting stroke: results from the National Registry of Atrial Fibrillation. *JAMA*. 2001;285:2864–2870; and Verma A, Cairns JA, Mitchell LB, et al. 2014 Focused update of the Canadian Cardiovascular Society Guidelines for the management of atrial fibrillation. *Can J Cardiol*. 2014;30(10):1114–1130.

warfarin should be recommended in patients with AF and a CHADS$_2$ score of 2 or greater (Table 39.7).

Decisions about the use of warfarin vs aspirin can be challenging in older patients and in those at risk of bleeding. The Outpatient Bleeding Risk Index is a validated tool used to predict the risk of bleeding in patients taking warfarin.[57,93] The Outpatient Bleeding Risk Index includes four risk factors, each counting as one point: (1) age older than 65 years; (2) history of stroke; (3) history of gastrointestinal bleeding; and (4) one or more of the following: recent MI, severe anemia (hematocrit level <30%), diabetes, or renal impairment (serum creatinine level >1.5 mg/dL (132.6 µmol/L)).[57] A score of 0 is considered low risk, a score of 1 or 2 is intermediate risk, and a score of 3 or 4 is high risk.[93] One study evaluating the Outpatient Bleeding Risk Index found that the risks of major bleeding after 1 year in low-, intermediate-, and high-risk patients were 3%, 12%, and 48%, respectively.[59]

The anticoagulation agent dabigatran (Pradaxa), a DTI, was recently approved by the FDA for the prevention of stroke and systemic embolism with AF. In a randomized trial, 150 mg of dabigatran twice per day was shown to be superior to warfarin in decreasing the incidence of ischemic and hemorrhagic strokes. Patients assigned to dabigatran had a higher incidence of MI than those assigned to warfarin, but the difference was not statistically significant.[62,63]

## UNFRACTIONATED HEPARIN IN ATRIAL FIBRILLATION

UFH is the FDA approved for the treatment of AF and disseminated intravascular coagulation (class IIa recommendation; level of evidence: B). It is used as a prophylaxis for PE, thrombosis, venous catheter occlusion, and VTE.

Patients with AF with a duration of less than 48 h undergoing cardioversion receive anticoagulation with full therapeutic-dose heparin (80 U/kg IV bolus followed by infusion of 18 U/kg/h or fixed-dose 5000 U IV bolus followed by 1000 U/h) at presentation, and unstable patients with AF undergoing urgent cardioversion be initiated on full therapeutic-dose heparin before the procedure if possible.[95]

### Dabigatran in AF

In patients with AF, dabigatran is better than warfarin at preventing stroke and lowered the risk of bleeding in and around the brain (one of the most dangerous complications of anticoagulants). Dabigatran is approved by the FDA for stroke prevention in AF. The dose of dabigatran is 150 mg twice daily. Because the kidneys eliminate dabigatran from the body, poor kidney function can result in higher levels of dabigatran and increased bleeding risk. Therefore, for stroke prevention in AF, the FDA approved a reduced kidney dose of dabigatran, provided in a 75-mg capsule taken twice daily.[62,64]

### Rivaroxaban in Atrial Fibrillation

Rivaroxaban is the FDA approved and is a reasonable option for secondary prophylaxis of stroke in patients with nonvalvular AF and a history of an ischemic stroke or TIA (class IIb recommendation; level of evidence: B). For stroke prevention in AF, rivaroxaban (20 mg orally once daily in the evening) is similarly effective as warfarin but reduces the risk of bleeding in and around the brain.[74]

### Limitation of use

For stroke prevention in AF, rivaroxaban requires dose adjustments for patients with a creatinine clearance for patients with chronic kidney disease.[76]

### Apixaban in Atrial Fibrillation

In December 2012, the FDA approved apixaban (Eliquis) to reduce the risk of stroke and blood clots for secondary stroke prophylaxis in patients with non-valvular AF (paroxysmal or persistent) (class IIa recommendation; level of evidence: A).[74]

The advantage of this drug when compared with other drugs in this category is that no dose adjustment is recommended for patients with renal impairment alone.[84]

### Limitation of use

In patients with ESRD (creatinine clearance <15 mL/min), the dosing recommendations are based on pharmacokinetic and pharmacodynamic (antifactor Xa activity) data in subjects with ESRD maintained on dialysis.[85]

### Edoxaban in Atrial Fibrillation

The FDA has approved the anticlotting drug edoxaban tablets (Savaysa) to reduce the risk of stroke and dangerous blood clots (systemic embolism) in patients with AF that is not caused by a heart valve problem (class IIb recommendation; level of evidence: B). The usual dose of edoxaban is 60 mg orally once daily.[86]

### Limitation of use

Edoxaban is less effective in patients with AF with a creatinine clearance greater than 95 mL/min.[86]

## ANTICOAGULATION BEFORE CARDIOVERSION FOR ATRIAL FIBRILLATION TREATMENT

It is generally recommended that anticoagulation be instituted for 3 weeks before cardioversion is attempted in patients with AF with a duration of more than 2 days.

To minimize thromboembolic complications, anticoagulants should be continued for 4 weeks after cardioversion. This period is required for recovery of atrial mechanical contractility after conversion to a sinus rhythm (Table 39.8).[96]

## HEMOSTASIS MANAGEMENT OF CARDIAC SURGICAL HEMORRHAGE

### Key Points

- Mechanisms of bleeding common to virtually all patients after heart surgery are platelet dysfunction, enhanced fibrinolysis, dilution of all components of the coagulation system, and the presence of heparin and protamine.
- The use of warfarin is increasing in patients with heart disease requiring surgery.
- Individualized heparin and protamine dosing, antifibrinolytic drug administration, minimization of blood loss and dilution, and minimal time on cardiopulmonary bypass (CPB) are basic adjuncts to meticulous surgical hemostasis.
- When bleeding is observed in the postoperative period, initial therapy should be given according to the laboratory test results. Treatment options include fresh-frozen plasma (FFP), prothrombin complex concentrates (PCCs), cryoprecipitate, fibrinogen concentrate, tranexamic acid (TXA), epsilon aminocaproic acid (EACA), desmopressin, recombinant factor VIIa, activated PCC, factor XIII, and platelets.

## INTRODUCTION

In Iran, 10,000 cases of this surgery are performed every year.[97] Each year, in cardiac surgery, 90% of blood products are used by only 10% of patients, and over the past 25 years, much innovation and research have gone into improving perioperative diagnosis and therapy for these patients.[98]

Viscoelastic tests performed at the bedside, with modifications to allow direct quantification of fibrinogen levels, are probably the biggest advancement. There is no clear advantage of thromboelastometry over thromboelastography, and the published literature remains scarce. Viscoelastic testing has recently been coupled with the systematic replacement of clotting factors by means of factor concentrates, with objective improvement in terms of blood loss, red blood cell (RBC) usage, and surgical reexploration.[98]

Viscoelastic assays, such as ThromboElastoGraphy (TEG) and ROtational ThromboElastoMetry (ROTEM) (TEM International, Munich, Germany) and TEG alone

**TABLE 39.8**
**Comparison of Oral Anticoagulants**

| Drug Name | Warfarin | Dabigatran | Rivaroxaban | Apixaban | Edoxaban |
|---|---|---|---|---|---|
| Dosing regimen | Depends on INR | Twice daily | Twice daily | Once daily | Once daily |
| Approved indications | 1. AF: thromboembolic disorder and prophylaxis<br>2. MI prophylaxis<br>3. Prosthetic cardiac valve component embolism and prophylaxis<br>4. VTE | 1. Approved for VTE prevention after elective hip or knee replacement in adults<br>2. Stroke prevention and systemic embolization in nonvalvular AF | 1. Approved for VTE prevention after elective hip or knee replacement in adults<br>2. Stroke prevention and systemic embolization in nonvalvular AF | 1. Approved for VTE prevention after elective hip or knee replacement in adults<br>2. Stroke and systemic embolism in patients with nonvalvular AF<br>3. For treatment of acute DVT and prevention of VTE recurrence | 1. Approved in Japan for VTE prophylaxis joint replacement<br>2. For the treatment of DVT, PE, and risk of stroke and embolism caused by AF; approved January 2015 |
| Typical effective dose | Maintain a target INR of range 2–3 | 150 or 220 mg once daily (VTE prophylaxis)<br>75 or 150 mg twice daily (AF) | 2.5 BID (VTE prophylaxis) | 10 mg once daily (VTE prophylaxis)<br>15 mg twice daily (1–21) followed by 20 mg once daily (DVT treatment or prevention of recurrent VTE)<br>20 mg once daily (AF) | 30 mg (VTE prophylaxis) |
| Food interaction | Yes | No | No | No | NR |
| Postoperative resumption of new oral anticoagulants | — | Low bleeding risk surgery: resume on day after surgery, 150 mg twice daily<br>High bleeding risk surgery: resume 2–3 days after surgery, 150 mg twice daily | Low bleeding risk surgery: resume on day after surgery, 20 mg once daily<br>High bleeding risk surgery: resume 2–3 days after surgery, 20 mg once daily | Low bleeding risk surgery: resume on day after surgery, 5 mg twice daily<br>High bleeding risk surgery: resume 2–3 days after surgery, 5 mg twice daily | Can be restarted after the surgical or other procedure as soon as adequate hemostasis has been established, noting that the time to onset of pharmacodynamic effect is 1–2 h |
| PPI/H2 B absorption | Increased INR and potentiation of anticoagulant effects | –12% to 30% | Not affected | Not affected | Not affected |
| Antidote | Vitamin K | Idarucizumab | ANNEXA-R | Andexanet alfa | Andexanet alfa |

*AF,* atrial fibrillation; *BID,* twice a day; *DVT,* deep vein thrombosis; *INR,* international normalized ratio; *PE,* pulmonary embolism; *PPI,* proton pump inhibitor; *VTE,* venous thromboembolism.

**TABLE 39.9**
**Relative Factor Content and Cost of Current Hemostatic Treatment**

| Drug Name | Factor Content of Therapeutic Plasma Replacement Dose for 70-kg Patient | Fibrinogen Content | Volume | Donor Exposures (Estimated) | Place in Therapy |
|---|---|---|---|---|---|
| FFP | 1000 U | 2 g | 1000 mL | 4 | 2C[a] |
| PCC | 1000 U (higher if reversing warfarin) | NA | 40 | >20,000 | 1D |
| Cryoprecipitate | 240 U | 2 g | 100 | 10 | 1C |
| Fibrinogen concentrate | NA | 1 g | 50 | >20,000 | 1C |

*FFP*, fresh-frozen plasma; *NA*, not applicable; *PCC*, prothrombin complex concentrate.
[a]Place in therapy according to British Committee for Standards in Hematology guideline.

(Haemonetics, Braintree, MA), have evolved from the simple addition of heparinase to allow hemostatic assessment during CPB while the patient is fully heparinized.[99] Available clotting factor concentrates, their relative factor content, and cost are compared in Table 39.9.

## FIBRINOGEN

Replacing fibrinogen if levels are low has taken center stage with regard to the relative importance of coagulation factor replacement in major bleeding, and after CPB in particular. In the 2004 British Committee for Standards in Hematology (BCSH) guidelines,[100] a target of 1 was suggested in recognition of the changes in major bleeding management. A new guideline is due to be published, and this is likely to set a trigger for giving fibrinogen (in the form of cryoprecipitate) at 1.5–2.0 g L$^{-1}$. The American and Japanese guidelines state a minimum target of 0.8 g L$^{-1}$, and German and Austrian/European trauma guidelines suggest 2 g L$^{-1}$.[101,102] Indeed, clot firmness improves up until fibrinogen greater than 3 g L$^{-1}$, with clot formation rate highest at 2 g L$^{-1}$.[103] Although there is no evidence of harm, raising the transfusion threshold increases the number of eligible patients, and given that factor concentrates expose the patient to 20,000 donations or more, this could be potentially hazardous. The manufacturers quote the resultant extreme dilution of individual donations as an advantage, but history has proven that, depending on the pathogen, this may or may not be true. Although data on overall survival benefit are not available, caution should be exercised, particularly given the cost difference between cryoprecipitate and fibrinogen concentrate on a gram-for-gram basis and the lack of data on risk–benefit and cost-effectiveness.[98]

The choice between cryoprecipitate and fibrinogen concentrate varies from country to country, partially because of availability. Non-heat-treated fibrinogen concentrate was withdrawn in the United States and replaced with cryoprecipitate to reduce the risk of transmission of non-A and non-B hepatitis, which affected up to 5% of batches in the late 1970s, with a number of countries following suit. Fibrinogen concentrate is now heat treated, but this has not led to a reintroduction of this product in all countries where the license had been previously withdrawn. Cryoprecipitate itself was not originally designed as a treatment for hypofibrinogenemia but was intended as a treatment for hemophilia A and von Willebrand disease and was subsequently found to also be rich in fibrinogen and factor XIII.[104] Interestingly, the National Institute for Health and Care Excellence (NICE) guideline on viscoelastic testing does not refer to cryoprecipitate at all and recommends fibrinogen concentrate instead, despite the absence of a UK license for the treatment of acquired coagulopathy.[105]

## FRESH-FROZEN PLASMA

FFP has been the component of choice to manage the coagulopathy of bleeding, but there is limited evidence for the therapeutic benefit of FFP in postoperative coagulopathy.

FFP should be a part of initial resuscitation in major hemorrhage in at least a 1 unit:2 unit ratio with RBCs until results from coagulation monitoring are available. When bleeding is under control, further FFP should be guided by abnormalities in laboratory tests with transfusion trigger of prothrombin time and/or aPTT more than 1.5 times normal for a standard dose [e.g., 15–20 mL/kg (class 2C recommendation)]. If laboratory results are not available and bleeding continues, further FFP may be transfused in at least a 1:2 ratio with

RBCs before moving on to blood product use guided by laboratory results (class 2C recommendation).[106]

A dose of 30 mL/kg of FFP has been quoted as potentially a more effective therapeutic alternative. Although this dose makes sense from a coagulation point of view, the major setback is the large volume of administration (2.25 L for a 75-kg patient), which could potentially nearly double the circulating plasma volume. This could be detrimental in patients exhibiting a degree of myocardial stunning or cardiac failure after cardiac surgery.[107]

## PROTHROMBIN COMPLEX CONCENTRATES
### Drug Action Reversal and Vitamin K Antagonists for Urgent Surgery or Invasive Procedures

PCC for IV use, lyophilized powder for the urgent reversal of acquired coagulation factor deficiency induced by VKA (e.g., warfarin) (class IIa recommendation; level of evidence: B) therapy in adult patients with acute major bleeding. It was approved by the FDA in 2013. PCC is not indicated for urgent reversal of VKA anticoagulation in patients without acute major bleeding.[108]

Four-factor PCC (containing protein C and S, as well as factors VII, IX, X, and II and traces of heparin) was noninferior and superior to plasma with regard to effective hemostasis (90% vs 75%) and rapid INR reduction (55% vs 10%) in an open-label, randomized trial ($n = 168$) of patients needing rapid VKA reversal for urgent surgical or invasive interventions. Patients with an INR of 2 or higher were enrolled. An INR of 1.3 or lower 1 h after start of infusion was achieved by significantly more patients who received prothrombin complex compared with plasma (54% vs 0%); additionally, plasma levels of vitamin K-dependent coagulation factors and proteins C and S were significantly higher with prothrombin complex at 0.5, 1, 3, and 6 h after start of infusion. There were no significant differences between groups in number of patients who received RBC transfusions or mean number of transfusions. Fluid overload or similar cardiac events were significantly lower with prothrombin complex (3% vs 13%), but there was no significant difference in thromboembolic adverse events (7% vs 8%).[109]

A dose equivalent in vitamin K-dependent clotting factor activity to (between 10 and 30 mL/kg) 15 mL/kg FFP. At these therapeutic doses, a 70-kg patient might receive between 700 and 2100 mL of fluid as opposed to more than 11 mL in the case of FFP. However, there are few data as yet comparing PCC with FFP for the treatment of acute perioperative hemorrhage, let alone in the cardiac surgical setting. The main benefit is the speed of administration, reliable effect, and small treatment volume; however, further research is awaited.[101,106,107,109–128]

## PLATELETS

Thrombocytopenia is considered as a late event in massive hemorrhage, typically seen only after a loss of at least 1.5 blood volumes. Outside trauma and in major hemorrhage other than after CPB, there is little evidence to inform optimal use of platelet transfusion. Increasing numbers of patients take antiplatelet medications, and there is the uncertain contributory role of platelet function defects in patients with major bleeding. The specific role of platelets in major hemorrhage in trauma is discussed later.

Platelet transfusion should be given as one adult therapeutic dose (one apheresis pack or 4-pooled units) when the platelet count falls below $50 \times 10^9$/L. Many hospitals do not keep a stock of platelets, and therefore the transfusion laboratory will need to order platelets from the blood transfusion center early in major hemorrhage (e.g., when the platelet count has fallen below $100 \times 10^9$/L). Practical guidance on the provision of platelets when the patient blood group is not known is described later.

### Recommendation

In major hemorrhage, aim to keep platelets at above $50 \times 10^9$/L (class 1B recommendation); we suggest that platelets should be requested if there is ongoing bleeding and the platelet count has fallen below $100 \times 10^9$/L (class 2C recommendation).[106]

## ANTIFIBRINOLYTIC DRUGS

Although excessive bleeding is widely recognized as a common complication of cardiac surgery, the recent success of antifibrinolytic drugs as prophylactic hemostatic agents has received little attention outside the surgical literature. The etiology of the coagulopathy after cardiac surgery is clearly multifactorial; however, the success of antifibrinolytic drugs (e.g., EACA and TXA) as hemostatic agents suggests that fibrinolysis contributes to bleeding in this setting. This may help to avoid the use of blood products such as FFP with its associated risks of infections or anaphylactic reactions. Increasingly widespread administration of these drugs necessitates increased awareness of the risks and benefits posed by perioperative antifibrinolytic therapy.[127]

TXA, used almost ubiquitously in cardiac surgical practice, and EACA, are synthetic lysine analogs that reversibly block the lysine binding site of plasminogen, which inhibits the lysis of polymerized fibrin. They have a plasma half-life of around 2 h and are excreted in the urine in high concentrations.[128] The optimum dose of TXA is unknown despite its widespread international use, with a 10 mg/kg[1] bolus followed by 1 mg/kg[1]/h[1] as a continuous infusion being the most commonly used regimen, with little evidence for higher doses.[129] Seizures are the main reported adverse event with TXA, but thrombotic events after its use have not been reported. Both agents have been shown to reduce blood loss when used prophylactically in cardiac surgery.[129]

### Tranexamic Acid

The optimal dosage regimen of TXA in prevention of hemorrhagic complications after heart surgery (class IIb recommendation; level of evidence: B) has not been established. But in study dosing, the following has been used: 10 mg/kg IV bolus followed by a 1-mg/kg/h infusion with 1 mg/kg added to priming solution (low-dose) or a 30-mg/kg IV bolus followed by a 16-mg/kg/h infusion with 2 mg/kg added to the priming solution (high-dose) or 15 mg/kg IV before initiating coronary bypass followed by 1-mg/kg/h IV infusion for 5–6 h or 10 g IV preoperatively or 100 mg/kg IV preoperatively followed by 50 mg/kg IV postoperatively or 2.5 g IV before skin incision with 2.5 g added to the bypass priming solution.[130]

### Epsilon Aminocaproic Acid

The synthetic lysine analogs EACA (class IIb recommendation; level of evidence: B) was first described in 1957 by Okamoto. The plasma half-life is about 2 h, and the drugs are excreted unchanged into the urine, which typically continues for up to 36 h.[112,131]

### Desmopressin

Desmopressin (DDAVP), a synthetic vasopressin derivative, has been used in patients with bleeding after cardiac surgery to reduce postoperative blood loss and transfusion requirements. This reaction is exhaustible, and the drug is typically administered no more frequently than once in 24 h. It is most often used in patients with mild hemophilia A, von Willebrand disease, and platelet disorders, and it is also a useful adjunct in uremic and cirrhotic bleeding. Rapid administration can lead to hypotension, and the antidiuretic hormone-like effect can lead to fluid retention.[132] The evidence for the use of DDAVP in cardiac surgery comes from two trials showing that in small cohorts of patients undergoing complex cardiac surgery, DDAVP administration led to a reduction in mean 24-h blood loss compared with placebo, and patients with the lowest von Willebrand factor levels benefitted the most.[118,133] Subsequent trials have failed to show a reduction in blood loss after DDAVP administration. Horrow et al.[119] were able to show that coadministration of TXA was necessary in a small group of patients to reduce blood loss, which the authors attributed to concomitant tissue plasminogen activator release.

### Recombinant Factor VIIa

Pharmacologic doses of recombinant factor VIIa (rVIIa) concentrate should only be used as a last resort because of the excess of prothrombotic events and lack of evidence for a reduction in overall mortality.[115] Recombinant factor VIIa contains factor levels in excess of 4 logs of the physiologic concentration of VIIa, which are able to activate factor Xa in the presence of activated platelet surfaces. A recent meta-analysis included 4468 patients and showed that rVIIa increased the risk of arterial thrombosis (5.5% vs 3.3%), especially in older adults, but the risk of VTE remained unchanged.[118] When rVIIa is used, coagulopathy must be addressed first because there is a greatly reduced effect in the presence of hypothermia, hypocalcemia, hypofibrinogenemia, or major coagulopathy.

## ACTIVATED PROTHROMBIN COMPLEX CONCENTRATE

Activated prothrombin complex is plasma derived and contains similar quantities of factor VII, IX, and X compared with (nonactivated) four-factor PCC. In addition, small quantities of factor VIIa and Xa are present. It has been shown to be effective in small cohorts of patients but also produced thrombosis in unusual sites as a side effect, and its use should be restricted in a similar way to rVIIa.[134]

### Factor XIII

Factor XIII concentration is reduced during CPB, consistent with other clotting factors. Over the past 20 years, there have been a few small studies with conflicting results regarding the link between low factor XIII plasma levels and excessive bleeding after cardiac surgery. In a randomized controlled trial of recombinant factor XIII vs placebo, there was no therapeutic benefit on transfusion avoidance, transfusion requirements, or operative revision despite an observed correction of factor XIII levels. Factor XIII administration outside clinical trials should, therefore, be discouraged.[100–102,105,106,108,117–129,132–136]

## TOPICAL SEALANTS

The first use of human plasma as a topical hemostatic agent was documented in 1909.[111] There are a number of situations considered amenable to topical hemostatic agents, including diffuse raw surface bleeding or oozing, venous-type bleeds, bone bleeding, and needle-hole bleeding. As a rule of thumb, low-flow situations are most amenable to topical hemostatic agents, meaning that the best time to apply them may be before weaning from CPB, while there is low flow in the wound bed. However, this is suboptimal because the unselective use of these agents is undesirable. Moreover, the surgeon has to weigh the risks and benefits carefully before their application because some of these topical agents may be inadvertently aspirated by the cell saver or cardiotomy sucker and, therefore, reinfused to the patient intravascularly. In addition, leakage of these agents through incompletely sealed wounds into the surgical site and embolization have been described.[114] Topical hemostatic agents rely on the patients' native platelets and hemostatic system to provide a framework for platelet or clot adhesion. They are mostly isolated or combined animal-, human-, or plasma-derived clotting proteins; recombinant clotting proteins; or other polymers. Broadly, four types of topical agents are in use, even though the nomenclature is somewhat confusing, given the heterogeneity of the components.[98]

### Mechanical

Mechanical hemostatic agents (microporous polysaccharide, chitin or chitosan based, collagen, gelatin, and cellulose) provide a framework for platelet or red cell adhesion, with little alteration in hemostasis. Examples include Surgicel (Johnson & Johnson Medical Inc., Arlington, TX) and Oxycel (Oxycel, Pershore, UK).[98]

### Flowable

Flowable agents are also based on gelatin from various animal sources, but some, such as Surgiflo (Ethicon, Livingston, UK) or FloSeal (Baxter, Compton Newbury, UK), contain plasma-derived human thrombin.[98]

## FIBRIN, ALBUMIN, AND SYNTHETIC SEALANTS

Fibrin or synthetic sealants are based on the dual action of fibrinogen and thrombin and contain human pooled thrombin and fibrinogen. Examples include Tisseel (Baxter) or Evicel/Quixil (Ethicon). Synthetic alternatives function by a similar mechanism but do not contain human or animal plasma derivatives. Examples include cyanoacrylate (Omnex; Ethicon) and CoSeal (Proseal, Macclesfield, UK). Tisseel contains a fibrinolysis inhibitor, bovine aprotinin, and Quixil contains TXA. The sealant Bioglue (Cryolife, Kennesaw, GA) contains bovine serum albumin and glutaraldehyde, making it difficult to categorize as it contains albumin rather than fibrin or synthetic sealant but does not rely on the action of added thrombin.[98]

### Active

Active topical hemostatic agents are based on bovine (Thrombin-JMI; Pfizer, Walton Oaks, UK), human (Evithrom; Ethicon), or recombinant thrombin (Recothrom; The Medicines Company, Parsippany, NJ). A completely synthetic tissue sealant consisting of recombinant fibrinogen, thrombin, and factor XIII has recently been described.[104] Evidence for the use of these products is limited, and most of the studies have a considerable risk of bias due to sponsorship by manufacturers.[137] Also, the criteria for determining a response are difficult to standardize, and there are often clinical confounding factors.

Those products that are based on bovine thrombin are associated with a risk of inducing antihuman factor V antibodies due to bovine prothrombin cross reacting with human factor V (Thrombin-JMI; Pfizer, New York).[97,98,107,110–113,137,138]

Since their first inception in 1943, the purity of the products has improved substantially. The incidence of factor V inhibitor with the currently available bovine thrombin product (Thrombin-JMI), which contains less bovine thrombin product, remains unknown.[135] Patients who refuse blood products would have to be specifically consented with regard to the preferred topical sealant, making particular reference to the biosource of the components. The benefit of these agents is likely twofold: reduction in allogeneic blood use, which is not clinically significant in many cases because the agents are not applied in low-flow situations, and a reduction in time to chest closure and subsequent transfer to the intensive care unit.[114,137]

Patient blood management is a multidisciplinary, evidence-based approach to reduce avoidable blood transfusion as much as possible. A patient blood management program should include patient and clinician education and intervention, a review of the frequency and volume of blood testing, use of near patient hemoglobin testing, adherence to approved indications and transfusion triggers when requesting blood, optimization of preoperative anemia, and reversal of preoperative anticoagulant therapy by using agreed-upon protocols.

The optimal transfusion support of the bleeding patient after cardiothoracic surgery remains to be established. A "state-of-the-art" transfusion algorithm should include indicators for residual heparin, measures of hemodilution or coagulation factor consumption, an indicator specific for hypofibrinogenemia, and a platelet count. The tests should be rapidly available, and clinicians should be familiar with their interpretation and limitations. The routine use of platelet function tests cannot currently be recommended. More evidence, particularly from randomized controlled trials, is required to identify the hemostatic agents that are most appropriate to treat postoperative hemorrhage and to identify the optimum postoperative treatment algorithm, including differentiated point-of-care testing. This will allow a more tailored transfusion strategy, with minimal turnaround times in patients with postoperative hemorrhage after cardiac surgery.[98]

## REFERENCES

1. BP Griffin, SR Kapadia The Cleveland Clinic Cardiology Board Review (2nd ed.), Lippincott, Williams & Wilkins.
2. Siddiqi NH. *Contrast Medium Reactions 2016*; 2016. Updated Jun 2. Available from: http://emedicine.medscape.com/article/422855-overview.
3. Cuisset T, Frere C, Quilici J, et al. Benefit of a 600-mg loading dose of clopidogrel on platelet reactivity and clinical outcomes in patients with non-ST-segment elevation acute coronary syndrome undergoing coronary stenting. *J Am Coll Cardiol*. 2006;48(7):1339–1345.
4. Dasbiswas A, Rao MS, Babu PR, et al. A comparative evaluation of prasugrel and clopidogrel in patients with acute coronary syndrome undergoing percutaneous coronary intervention. *J Assoc Physicians India*. 2013;61(2):114–116, 126.
5. Bansal R. *Contrast-Induced Nephropathy*; 2016. Updated Jan 18. Available from: http://emedicine.medscape.com/article/246751-overview.
6. Mullasari A, Victor SM. Update on contrast induced nephropathy, ESC clinical practice guidelines—European Society of Cardiology. *Eur J Cardiol Pract*. 2014;13:738–756.
7. Lewington A, MacTier R, Hoefield R. *Prevention of Contrast Induced Acute Kidney Injury (CI-AKI) in Adult Patients*. The Renal Association, British Cardiovascular Intervention Society and The Royal College of Radiologists; 2013. Publication in August.
8. Reactions to Radiocontrast Media and Its Management. Drug Information Center. Available from: http://www.just.edu.jo/DIC/Manuals/Reactions%20to%20radiocontrast%20media%20and%20its%20managment/2012.
9. Bode C, Huber K. Antiplatelet therapy in percutaneous coronary intervention. *Eur Heart J Suppl*. 2008;A13–A20. First published online.
10. Levine GN, Bates ER, Bittl JA, et al. *Focused Update on Duration of Dual Antiplatelet Therapy in Patients With Coronary Artery Disease*. ACC/AHA Guideline; 2016.
11. Llau JV, Ferrandis R, Sierra P, et al. Prevention of the renarrowing of coronary arteries using drug-eluting stents in the perioperative period: an update. *Vasc Health Risk Manag*. 2010;6:855–867. https://doi.org/10.2147/VHRM.S7402. Published online 2010 Oct 5.
12. Yu J, Mehran R, Dangas GD, et al. Safety and efficacy of high- versus low-dose aspirin after primary percutaneous coronary intervention in ST-segment elevation myocardial infarction. *J Am Coll Cardiol*. 2012;5(12):1231–1238.
13. Krumholz HM, Anderson JL, Bachelder BL, et al. ACC/AHA 2008 performance measures for adults with ST-elevation and non-ST-elevation myocardial infarction. A report of the American College of Cardiology/American Heart Association Task Force on Performance Measures. *J Am Coll Cardiol*. 2008;52:2046–2099.
14. Ramanuja S, Breall JA, Kalaria VG. Approach to "aspirin allergy" in cardiovascular patients. *Circulation*. 2004;110(1):e1–e4.
15. Godard P, Zini R, Metay A, et al. The fate of ticlopidine in the organism. II. Distribution and elimination of ticlopidine 14C after a single oral administration in the rat. *Eur J Drug Metab Pharmacokinet*. 1979;4:133–138.
16. Product Information. *Ticlid(R), ticlopidine hydrochloride tablets*. Roche Laboratories Inc: Nutley, NJ; 2001.
17. Product Information. *Ticlopidine hydrochloride oral tablet*. Spring Valley, NY: Par Pharmaceutical Inc; 2002.
18. Schwartz L, Bourassa MG, Lesperance J, et al. Aspirin and dipyridamole in the prevention of restenosis after percutaneous transluminal coronary angioplasty. *N Engl J Med*. 1988;318:1714–1719.
19. Savi P, Pereillo JM, Uzabiaga MF, et al. Identification and biological activity of the active metabolite of clopidogrel. *Thromb Haemost*. 2000;84:891–896.
20. Taubert D, Kastrati A, Harlfinger S, et al. Pharmacokinetics of clopidogrel after administration of a high loading dose. *Thromb Haemost*. 2004;92:311–316.
21. Frere C, Cuisset T, Quilici J, et al. ADP-induced platelet aggregation and platelet reactivity index VASP are good predictive markers for clinical outcomes in non-ST elevation acute coronary syndrome. *Thromb Haemost*. 2007;98:838–843.
22. Ferraris VA, Brown JR, Despotis GJ, et al. 2011 update to the society of thoracic surgeons and the society of cardiovascular anesthesiologists blood conservation clinical practice guidelines. *Ann Thorac Surg*. 2011;91:944–982.
23. 2011 American College of Cardiology Foundation/American Heart Association guideline on CABG.
24. Harder S, Klinkhardt U. Thrombolytics: drug interactions of clinical significance. *Drug Saf*. 2000;23:391–399.
25. Colombo A, Hall P, Nakamura S, et al. Intracoronary stenting without anticoagulation accomplished with

intravascular ultrasound guidance. *Circulation.* 1995; 91:1676–1688.

26. EPISTENT Investigators. Randomised placebo-controlled and balloon-angioplasty controlled trial to assess safety of coronary stenting with use of platelet glycoprotein-IIb/IIIa blockade. *Lancet.* 1998;352:87–92.

27. Steinhubl SR, Berger PB, Mann 3rd JT, et al. Early and sustained dual oral antiplatelet therapy following percutaneous coronary intervention: a randomized controlled trial. *JAMA.* 2002;288:2411–2420.

28. King 3rd SB, Smith Jr SC, Hirshfeld Jr JW, et al. Focused update of the ACC/AHA/SCAI 2005 guideline update for percutaneous coronary intervention: a report of the American College of Cardiology/American Heart Association Task Force on Practice Guidelines. *J Am Coll Cardiol.* 2008;51:172–209.

29. Wiviott SD, Braunwald E. Prasugrel versus clopidogrel in patients with acute coronary syndromes. *N Engl J Med.* 2007;357:2001–2015.

30. Product Information. *EFFIENT(TM) oral tablets, prasugrel oral tablets.* Indianapolis, IN: Eli Lilly; 2009.

31. Wallentin L. P2Y$_{12}$ inhibitors: differences in properties and mechanisms of action and potential consequences for clinical use. *Eur Heart J.* 2009;30:1964–1977. First published online: 24 July. Product Information: BRILINTA(R) oral tablets, ticagrelor oral tablets. AstraZeneca (per Manufacturer), Wilmington, DE; 2015.

32. Lee SW, Park SW, Kim YH, et al. Comparison of triple versus dual antiplatelet therapy after drug-eluting stent implantation (from the DECLARE-Long trial). *Am J Cardiol.* 2007;100:1103–1108.

33. Vandvik PO, Lincoff AM, Gore JM, et al. Primary and secondary prevention of cardiovascular disease: antithrombotic therapy and prevention of thrombosis, 9th ed: American College of Chest Physicians Evidence-Based Clinical Practice Guidelines. *Chest.* 2012;141 (suppl. 2):e637S–e668S.

34. Smith Andrew J, Wilczynska P. Pharmacology Consult, Triple antiplatelet therapy after PCI with aspirin, clopidogrel and cilostazol. *Cardiology Today.* 2010. February.

35. Meadows TA, Bhatt DL. Clinical aspects of platelet inhibitors and thrombus formation. *Circ Res.* 2007; 100:1261–1275.

36. Coller BS. GPIIb/IIIa antagonists: pathophysiologic and therapeutic insights from studies of c7E3 Fab. *Thromb Haemost.* 1997;78:730–735.

37. Labinaz M, Ho C, Banerjee S, et al. Meta-analysis of clinical efficacy and bleeding risk with intravenous glycoprotein IIb/IIIa antagonists for percutaneous coronary intervention. *Can J Cardiol.* 2007;23:963–970.

38. Kereiakes DJ. Adjunctive pharmacotherapy before percutaneous coronary intervention in non-ST-elevation acute coronary syndromes: the role of modulating inflammation. *Circulation.* 2003;108:III22–III27.

39. Kastrati A, Mehilli J, Schuhlen H, et al. A clinical trial of abciximab in elective percutaneous coronary intervention

after pretreatment with clopidogrel. *N Engl J Med.* 2004; 350:232–238.

40. Kastrati A, Mehilli J, Neumann FJ, et al. Abciximab in patients with acute coronary syndromes undergoing percutaneous coronary intervention after clopidogrel pretreatment: the ISAR-REACT 2 randomized trial. *JAMA.* 2006;295:1531–1538.

41. The EPIC Investigators. Use of a monoclonal antibody directed against the platelet glycoprotein IIb/IIIa receptor in high-risk coronary angioplasty. *N Engl J Med.* 1994; 330:956–961.

42. Nikparvar Fard M, Zahed Pour Anaraki M. Pulmonary embolism and deep vein thrombosis in northern Iran. *Arch Iran Med.* 1999;2(2):17–23.

43. Avanzas P, Clemmensen P, eds. Chapter 3. Anticoagulation therapy. In: *Pharmacological Treatment of Acute Coronary Syndromes.* London: Springer-Verlag; 2014. Kaski JC, Series ed. http://www.springer.com/la/book/978144 7154235.

44. Kearon C, Akl EA, Comerota AJ, et al. Antithrombotic therapy for VTE disease: antithrombotic therapy and prevention of thrombosis, 9th ed: American College of Chest Physicians Evidence-Based Clinical Practice Guidelines. *Chest.* 2012;141(suppl. 2):e419S–e494.

45. Harish J. Low-molecular-weight heparin: a review of the results of recent studies of the treatment of venous thromboembolism and unstable angina. *Circulation.* 1998;98(15):1575–1582.

46. Merli GJ, Groce JB. Pharmacological and clinical differences between low-molecular-weight heparins implications for prescribing practice and therapeutic interchange. *P T.* 2010;35(2):95–105.

47. Braunwald E, Elliott M, et al. *Report of the American College of Cardiology/American Heart Association Task Force on Practice Guidelines.* (Committee on the Management of Patients With Unstable Angina), Sep 5, 2000.

48. Hirsh J, Lee AY. How we diagnose and treat deep vein thrombosis. *Blood.* 2002;99:3102–3110.

49. Buller HR, Davidson BL, Decousus H, et al. Fondaparinux or enoxaparin for the initial treatment of symptomatic deep venous thrombosis: a randomized trial. *Ann Intern Med.* 2004;140(11):867–873.

50. Product Information. *ANGIOMAX(R) intravenous injection, bivalirudin intravenous injection.* Parsippany, NJ: The Medicines Company (per FDA); 2016.

51. Kearon C, Akl EA, Ornelas J, et al. Antithrombotic therapy for VTE disease: CHEST Guideline and Expert Panel Report. *Chest.* 2016;149(2):315–352.

52. Crowther MA, Ginsberg JB, Kearon C, et al. A randomized trial comparing 5-mg and 10-mg warfarin loading doses. *Arch Intern Med.* 1999;159:46–48.

53. Kovacs MJ, Rodger M, Anderson DR, et al. Comparison of 10-mg and 5-mg warfarin initiation nomograms together with low-molecular-weight heparin for outpatient treatment of acute venous thromboembolism. A randomized, double-blind, controlled trial. *Ann Intern Med.* 2003;138:714–719.

54. Schwarz UI, Ritchie MD, Bradford Y, et al. Genetic determinants of response to warfarin during initial anticoagulation. *N Engl J Med.* 2008;358:999–1008.

55. Wigle P, Hein B, et al. Updated guidelines on outpatient anticoagulation. *Am Fam Physician.* 2013;87(8):556–566.

56. Holbrook A, Schulman S, Witt DM, et al. Antithrombotic therapy and prevention of thrombosis, 9th ed: American College of Chest Physicians Evidence-Based Clinical Practice Guidelines. *Chest.* 2012; 141(suppl. 2): e152S–e184S.

57. Aspinall SL, DeSanzo BE, Trilli LE, Good CB. Bleeding Risk Index in an anticoagulation clinic. Assessment by indication and implications for care. *J Gen Intern Med.* 2005;20(11):1008–1013.

58. Bauersachs R, Berkowitz SD, Brenner B, et al. Oral rivaroxaban for symptomatic venous thromboembolism. *N Engl J Med.* 2010;363:2499–2510.

59. Beyth RJ, Quinn LM, Landefeld CS. Prospective evaluation of an index for predicting the risk of major bleeding in outpatients treated with warfarin. *Am J Med.* 1998;105 (2):91–99.

60. Buller H, Deitchman D, Prins M, et al. Efficacy and safety of the oral direct factor Xa inhibitor apixaban for symptomatic deep vein thrombosis. The Botticelli DVT dose-ranging study. *J Thromb Haemost.* 2008;6 (8):1313–1318.

61. Chen-Scarabelli C, Scarabelli TM, et al. Device-detected atrial fibrillation: what to do with asymptomatic patients? *J Am Coll Cardiol.* 2015;65(3):281–294.

62. Connolly SJ, Ezekowitz MD, Yusuf S, et al. RE-LY Steering Committee and Investigators published correction appears in N Engl J Med. 2010;363(19):1877. Dabigatran versus warfarin in patients with atrial fibrillation. *N Engl J Med.* 2009;361(12):1139–1151.

63. Connolly SJ, Ezekowitz MD, Yusuf, et al. Randomized evaluation of long-term anticoagulation therapy investigators. Newly identified events in the RE-LY trial. *N Engl J Med.* 2010;363(19):1875–1876.

64. Davis EM, Packard KA, Knezevich JT, Campbell JA. New and emerging anticoagulant therapy for atrial fibrillation and acute coronary syndrome. *Pharmacotherapy.* 2011;31 (10):975–1016.

65. Eriksson BI, Borris LC, Friedman RJ, et al. Rivaroxaban versus enoxaparin for thromboprophylaxis after hip arthroplasty. *N Engl J Med.* 2008;358(26):2765–2775.

66. Eriksson BI, Dahl OE, Büller HR, et al. A new oral direct thrombin inhibitor, dabigatran etexilate, compared with enoxaparin for prevention of thromboembolic events following total hip or knee replacement: the BISTRO II randomized trial. *J Thromb Haemost.* 2005;3:103.

67. Eriksson BI, Dahl OE, Rosencher N, et al. Dabigatran etexilate versus enoxaparin for prevention of venous thromboembolism after total hip replacement: a randomised, double-blind, noninferiority trial. *Lancet.* 2007;370:949.

68. Falk RH. Atrial fibrillation. *N Engl J Med.* 2001; 344:1067–1078.

69. Fuster V, Rydén LE, Cannom DS, et al. ACC/AHA/ESC 2006 Guidelines for the Management of Patients with Atrial Fibrillation: a report of the American College of Cardiology/American Heart Association Task Force on Practice Guidelines and the European Society of Cardiology Committee for Practice Guidelines (Writing Committee to Revise the 2001 Guidelines for the Management of Patients With Atrial Fibrillation): developed in collaboration with the European Heart Rhythm Association and the Heart Rhythm Society. *Cardiology.* 2006;114:e257–e354.

70. Gutierrez C, Blanchard DG. Atrial fibrillation: diagnosis and treatment. *Am Fam Physician.* 2011;83(1):61–68.

71. Harrison L, Johnston M, Massicotte MP, et al. Comparison of 5-mg and 10-mg loading doses in initiation of warfarin therapy. *Ann Intern Med.* 1997;126:133–136.

72. Heit JA, Kobbervig CE, et al. Trends in the incidence of venous thromboembolism during pregnancy or postpartum: a 30-year population-based study. *Ann Intern Med.* 2005;143(10):697–706.

73. Kakkar AK, Brenner B, Dahl OE, et al. Extended duration rivaroxaban versus short-term enoxaparin for the prevention of venous thromboembolism after total hip arthroplasty: a double-blind, randomised controlled trial. *Lancet.* 2008;372(9632):31–39.

74. Kernan WN, Ovbiagele B, Black HR, et al. Guidelines for the prevention of stroke in patients with stroke and transient ischemic attack: a guideline for healthcare professionals from the American Heart Association/ American Stroke Association. *Stroke.* 2014;45 (7):2160–2236.

75. Krajewski KC. Inability to achieve a therapeutic INR value while on concurrent warfarin and rifampin. *J Clin Pharmacol.* 2010;50(6):710–713.

76. Kubitza D, Becka M, et al. Effects of renal impairment on the pharmacokinetics, pharmacodynamics and safety of rivaroxaban, an oral, direct factor Xa inhibitor. *Br J Clin Pharmacol.* 2010;70:703–712.

77. Lassen MR, Ageno W, Borris LC, et al. Rivaroxaban versus enoxaparin for thromboprophylaxis after total knee arthroplasty. *N Engl J Med.* 2008;358(26):2776–2786.

78. Lassen MR, Raskob GE, Gallus A, et al. Apixaban or enoxaparin for thromboprophylaxis after knee replacement. *N Engl J Med.* 2009;361:594–604.

79. Lassen MR, Raskob GE, Gallus A, et al. Apixaban versus enoxaparin for thromboprophylaxis after knee replacement: a randomized double-blind trial. *Lancet.* 2010;375:807–815.

80. Nutescu E, Chuatrisorn I, Hellenbart E. Drug and dietary interactions of warfarin and novel oral anticoagulants: an update. *J Thromb Thrombolysis.* 2011;31(3):326–343.

81. Thi L, Shaw D, Bird J. Warfarin potentiation: a review of the "FAB-4" significant drug interactions. *Consult Pharm.* 2009; 24(3):227–230.

82. Patel MR, Mahaffey KW, Garg J, et al. Rivaroxaban versus warfarin in nonvalvular atrial fibrillation. *N Engl J Med.* 2011;365(10):883–891.

83. Pomp ER, Lenselink AM, et al. Pregnancy, the postpartum period and prothrombotic defects: risk of venous thrombosis in the MEGA study. *J Thromb Haemost.* 2008; 6(4):632–637.

84. Product Information. *ELIQUIS(R) oral tablets, apixaban oral tablets.* Princeton, NJ: Bristol-Myers Squibb Company and Pfizer Inc (per FDA); 2016.

85. Product Information. *Praxbind (idarucizumab), specific reversal agent for Pradaxa (dabigatran etexilate).* Ingelheim, Germany: The Medicines Company (per FDA); 2015:19.

86. Product Information. *SAVAYSA(TM) oral tablets, edoxaban oral tablets.* Parsippany, NJ: Daiichi Sankyo, Inc. (per FDA); 2015.

87. RCOG. Reducing the risk of venous thromboembolism during pregnancy and the puerperium. In: *Green-top Guideline No. 37a, April,* 2015.

88. Risk factors for stroke and efficacy of antithrombotic therapy in atrial fibrillation. Analysis of pooled data from five randomized controlled trials published correction appears in Arch Intern Med. 1994;154 (19):2254. *Arch Intern Med.* 1994;154(13):1449–1457.

89. Schulman S, Kakkar AK, Goldhaber SZ, et al. Treatment of acute venous thromboembolism with dabigatran or warfarin and pooled analysis. *Circulation.* 2014;129 (7):764–772.

90. Schulman S, Kearon C, Kakkar AK, et al. Dabigatran versus warfarin in the treatment of acute venous thromboembolism. *N Engl J Med.* 2009;361:2342.

91. Snow V, Weiss KB, LeFevre M, et al. Management of newly detected atrial fibrillation: a clinical practice guideline from the American Academy of Family Physicians and the American College of Physicians. *Ann Intern Med.* 2003;139(12):1009–1017.

92. Turpie AG, Lassen MR, Davidson BL, et al. Rivaroxaban versus enoxaparin for thromboprophylaxis after total knee arthroplasty (RECORD4): a randomised trial. *Lancet.* 2009;373(9676):1673–1680.

93. Wells PS, et al. The Outpatient Bleeding Risk Index: validation of a tool for predicting bleeding rates in patients treated for deep venous thrombosis and pulmonary embolism. *Arch Intern Med.* 2003;163(8):917–920.

94. Wolowacz SE, Roskell NS, Plumb JM, et al. Efficacy and safety of dabigatran etexilate for the prevention of venous thromboembolism following total hip or knee arthroplasty. A meta-analysis. *Thromb Haemost.* 2009; 101:77.

95. You JJ, Singer DE, Howard PA, et al. Antithrombotic therapy for atrial fibrillation: antithrombotic therapy and prevention of thrombosis, 9th ed: American College of Chest Physicians Evidence-Based Clinical Practice Guidelines. *Chest.* 2012;141(suppl. 2):e531S–e575S.

96. Akhtar W, Reeves WC, Movahe A, et al. Indications for anticoagulation in atrial fibrillation. *Am Fam Physician.* 1998;58(1):130–136.

97. Branca P, McGaw P, Light R. Factors associated with prolonged mechanical ventilation following coronary artery bypass surgery. *Chest.* 2001;119(2):537–546.

98. Besser MW, Ortmann E, Klein AA. Haemostatic management of cardiac surgical hemorrhage. *Anesthesia.* 2015;70(suppl. 1):87–95. e29–e31. https://doi.org/10.1111/anae.12898.

99. Whiting D, DiNardo JA. TEG and ROTEM: technology and clinical applications. *Am J Hematol.* 2014;89(2):228–232.

100. O'Shaughnessy DF, Atterbury C, Bolton Maggs P, et al. Guidelines for the use of fresh-frozen plasma, cryoprecipitate and cryosupernatant. *Br J Haematol.* 2004;126:11–28.

101. Levy JH, Szlam F, Tanaka KA, Sniecinski RM. Fibrinogen and hemostasis: a primary hemostatic target for the management of acquired bleeding. *Anesth Analg.* 2012; 114:261–274.

102. Schlimp CJ, Schochl H. The role of fibrinogen in trauma-induced coagulopathy. *Hamostaseologie.* 2014;34:29–39.

103. Solomon C, Cadamuro J, Ziegler B, et al. A comparison of fibrinogen measurement methods with fibrin clot elasticity assessed by thromboelastometry, before and after administration of fibrinogen concentrate in cardiac surgery patients. *Transfusion.* 2011;51:1695–1706.

104. Sorensen B, Bevan D. A critical evaluation of cryoprecipitate for replacement of fibrinogen. *Br J Haematol.* 2010;149:834–843.

105. National Institute for Healthcare and Excellence (NICE). *Health Technologies Adoption Programme. NICE Diagnostic Support for Viscoelastometric Point-of-Care Testing;* 2014. http://guidance.nice.org.uk/htdg13. Accessed 1 September 2014.

106. Hunt BJ, Allard S, Keeling D, et al. A practical guideline for the haematological management of major haemorrhage. *Br J Haematol.* 2015;170(6):788–803.

107. Chowdary P, Saayman AG, Paulus U, Findlay GP, Collins PW. Efficacy of standard dose and 30 ml/kg fresh frozen plasma in correcting laboratory parameters of haemostasis in critically ill patients. *Br J Haematol.* 2004;125:69–73.

108. Morgenstern LB, Hemphill JC, Anderson C, et al. Guidelines for the management of spontaneous intracerebral hemorrhage: a guideline for healthcare professionals from the American Heart Association/American Stroke Association. *Stroke.* 2010;41(9):2108–2129.

109. Goldstein JN, Refaai MA, Milling Jr TJ, et al. Four-factor prothrombin complex concentrate versus plasma for rapid vitamin K antagonist reversal in patients needing urgent surgical or invasive interventions: a phase 3b, open-label, non-inferiority, randomised trial. *Lancet.* 2015;385(9982):2077–2087.

110. Bruce D, Nokes TJ. Prothrombin complex concentrate (Beriplex P/N) in severe bleeding: experience in a large tertiary hospital. *Crit Care.* 2008;12:R105.

111. Carlson MA, Calcaterra J, Johanning JM, Pipinos II, Cordes CM, Velander WH. A totally recombinant human fibrin sealant. *J Surg Res.* 2014;187:334–342.

112. Coleman R, Hirsch J, Marder V, Clowes A, George J. *Hemostasis and Thrombosis, Principles and Practice.* 4th ed. Philadelphia: Lippincott, Williams & Wilkins; 2000.

113. Dorion RP, Hamati HF, Landis B, Frey C, Heydt D, Carey D. Risk and clinical significance of developing antibodies induced by topical thrombin preparations. *Arch Pathol Lab Med.* 1998;122:887–894.

114. Forcillo J, Perrault LP. Armentarium of topical hemostatic products in cardiovascular surgery: an update. *Transfus Apher Sci.* 2014;50:26–31.

115. Gill R, Herbertson M, Vuylsteke A, et al. Safety and efficacy of recombinant activated factor VII: a randomized placebo-controlled trial in the setting of bleeding after cardiac surgery. *Circulation.* 2009; 120:21–27.

116. Godje O, Gallmeier U, Schelian M, Grunewald M, Mair H. Coagulation factor XIII reduces postoperative bleeding after coronary surgery with extracorporeal circulation. *Thorac Cardiovasc Surg.* 2006;54:26–33.

117. Grossmann E, Akyol D, Eder L, et al. Thromboelastometric detection of clotting factor XIII deficiency in cardiac surgery patients. *Transfus Med.* 2013;23:407–415.

118. Harker LA. Bleeding after cardiopulmonary bypass. *N Engl J Med.* 1986; 314:1446–1448.

119. Horrow JC, Van Riper DF, Strong MD, Brodsky I, Parmet JL. Hemostatic effects of tranexamic acid and desmopressin during cardiac surgery. *Circulation.* 1991; 84:2063–2070.

120. Karkouti K, von Heymann C, Jespersen CM, et al. Efficacy and safety of recombinant factor XIII on reducing blood transfusions in cardiac surgery: a randomized, placebo-controlled, multicenter clinical trial. *J Thorac Cardiovasc Surg.* 2013;146:927–939.

121. Knobl P, Lechner K. Acquired factor V inhibitors. *Baillieres Clin Haematol.* 1998;11:305–318.

122. Lawson JH, Lynn KA, Vanmatre RM, et al. Antihuman factor V antibodies after use of relatively pure bovine thrombin. *Ann Thorac Surg.* 2005;79:1037–1038.

123. Levi M, Levy JH, Andersen HF, Truloff D. Safety of recombinant activated factor VII in randomized clinical trials. *N Engl J Med.* 2010;363:1791–1800.

124. Levy JH, Gill R, Nussmeier NA, et al. Repletion of factor XIII following cardiopulmonary bypass using a recombinant A-subunit homodimer. A preliminary report. *J Thromb Haemost.* 2009;102:765–771.

125. Lin DM, Murphy LS, Tran MH. Use of prothrombin complex concentrates and fibrinogen concentrates in the perioperative setting: a systematic review. *Transfus Med Rev.* 2013;27:91–104.

126. Makris M. Optimisation of the prothrombin complex concentrate dose for warfarin reversal. *Thromb Res.* 2005;115:451–453.

127. Slaughter TF, Greenberg CS. Antifibrinolytic drugs and perioperative hemostasis. *Am J Hematol.* 1997; 56:32–36.

128. Ranucci M, Aronson S, Dietrich W, et al. Patient blood management during cardiac surgery: do we have enough evidence for clinical practice. *J Thorac Cardiovasc Surg.* 2011;142:e1–e32.

129. Ortmann E, Besser MW, Klein AA. Antifibrinolytic agents in current anaesthetic practice. *Br J Anaesth.* 2013; 111:549–563.

130. Sigaut S, Tremey B, Ouattara A, et al. Comparison of two doses of tranexamic acid in adults undergoing cardiac surgery with cardiopulmonary bypass. *Anesthesiology.* 2014;120(3):590–600.

131. Verstraete M. Clinical application of inhibitors of fibrinolysis. *Drugs.* 1985;29:236–261.

132. Ogawa S, Ohnishi T, Hosokawa K, Szlam F, Chen EP, Tanaka KA. Haemodilution-induced changes in coagulation and effects of haemostatic components under flow conditions. *Br J Anaesth.* 2013; 111:1013–1023.

133. Salzman EW, Weinstein MJ, Weintraub RM, et al. Treatment with desmopressin acetate to reduce blood loss after cardiac surgery. *N Engl J Med.* 1986; 314:1402–1406.

134. Negrier C, Dargaud Y, Bordet JC. Basic aspects of bypassing agents. *Haemophilia.* 2006; 12(suppl. 6):48–52.

135. Plesca D. A review of topical thrombin. *Cleve Clin Pharmacother Update.* 2009;XII:1–4.

136. Shainoff JR, Estafanous FG, Yared JP, DiBello PM, Kottke-Marchant K, Loop FD. Low factor XIIIA levels are associated with increased blood loss after coronary artery bypass grafting. *J Thorac Cardiovasc Surg.* 1994; 108:437–445.

137. Barnard J, Millner R. A review of topical hemostatic agents for use in cardiac surgery. *Ann Thorac Surg.* 2009; 88:1377–1383.

138. Banninger H, Hardegger T, Tobler A, et al. Fibrin glue in surgery: frequent development of inhibitors of bovine thrombin and human factor V. *Br J Haematol.* 1993; 85:528–532.

# CHAPTER 40

# COVID-19 Infection: A Novel Fatal Pandemic of the World in 2020

MAJID MALEKI[a] • ZEINAB NOROUZI[b] • ALIREZA MALEKI[c]

[a]Rajaie Cardiovascular, Medical & Research Center, Iran University of Medical Sciences, Tehran, Iran,
[b]Cardiac Rehabilitation Department, Rajaie Cardiovascular, Medical & Research Center, Tehran, Iran,
[c]Resident of Anesthesiology, Iran University of Medical Sciences, Tehran, Iran

## EPIDEMIOLOGY

A respiratory syndrome with a novel coronavirus called COVID-19 was diagnosed on November 17, 2019 for the first time in Wuhan, China[1] and it was reported to WHO (World Health Organization) on December 31, 2019.[2] In a short time, the infection with this virus spread and was reported from other countries; and in less than a few months a pandemic has happened and many countries were involved with the COVID-19 virus. Corona infection outbreak was reported from more than 210 countries[3] and most cases were reported from Europe and America although every part of the globe was involved too. According to the last updated report of WHO, the highest prevalence of the infection has occurred in several countries including the United States, India, Brazil, France, Russian Federation, Spain, United Kingdom, Argentina, Italy, and Colombia.[4]

According to the genetic data, it seems that the COVID-19 virus is related to two other viruses including Middle East Respiratory Syndrome coronavirus (MERS-CoV) and Severe Acute Respiratory Syndrome coronavirus (SARS-CoV).[5] The symptoms of these two viruses are more severe, but COVID-19 can spread faster and infect more patients in comparison with MERS-CoV and SARS-CoV.[6]

## SIGNS AND SYMPTOMS

The virus can infect the cells by using the receptors of the angiotensin-converting enzyme (ACE) that is connected with the renin–angiotensin–aldosterone system (RAAS).[7] The incubation period has a wide range, from 0 to 24 days and the average time is 3 days.[8]

COVID-19 infection may present large spectrum of signs and symptoms. On the one hand, it can occur as an asymptomatic infection, and on the other hand, severe life-threatening pneumonia may happen.[9]

Pneumonia is one of the first ominous findings in corona infection.[10] Fever and cough are the most common symptoms. Other common clinical manifestation includes fatigue, myalgia, and dyspnea. Some patients may experience pharyngalgia, headache, diarrhea, rhinorrhea, and sore throat.[11] Pneumonia can gradually become worse and the patient may suffer severe respiratory distress[8] and in the cases with severe hypoxia mechanical ventilator may be necessary although it is recommended not to use ventilator support as far as possible. Some studies showed that coronavirus infection can deteriorate faster in elderly patients and the time between the beginning of the disease until death is shorter in comparison with young patients.[12] Young patients may experience gastrointestinal symptoms or may even be completely asymptomatic[10] (Figs. 40.1 and 40.2).

In the first months of the pandemic, a Chest CT (computerized tomography) scan was used for screening COVID-19 infection in the suspected patients.[13,14] The findings of the CT scan include ground-glass opacity (GGO), consolidation, and interlobular septal thickening. In many CT scans, multiple lesions are seen.[15] With improvement in the experience of COVID-19 some data suggested that RT-PCR (reverse transcription polymerase chain reaction) is superior in comparison with chest CT scan.[16] However, several studies reported false-negative results from RT-PCR.[17] Although technology is improving, clinical judgment plays an important role in controlling the pandemic. Health-care providers should not rely on imaging or laboratory tests alone. Early diagnosis even with negative paraclinical data and quarantining the patients soon can effectively prevent the spreading of the disease[16] (Figs. 40.3 and 40.4).

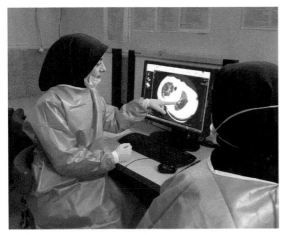

FIG. 40.1 Pneumonia is one of the first findings and is common in patients with COVID-19 infection.

## TREATMENT

The definite treatment for COVID-19 infection is not clear yet. In some studies, empirical therapy, Oseltamivir, Ganciclovir, and Lopinavir/ritonavir were used.[11,18,19] Several studies suggest interleukin-6 antibody blockers (e.g., Tocilizumab in severe disease), convalescent plasma transfusion, and stem cell therapy to control the cytokine storm of the infection.[20,21] Other studies suggested nucleoside analogs, HIV-protease inhibitors,[22] and remdesivir.[23] Several other drugs are under study and more clinical trials should be done for introducing an effective drug and also a vaccination for this pandemic life-threatening infection.

## COVID-19 AND CARDIOVASCULAR DISEASE

According to some unpublished research, COVID-19 may damage the heart in up to 20% of the patients. It is still unclear if the virus attacks the heart directly. Although concentration in the COVID-19 pandemic is on the respiratory system with providing good ventilation, many physicians in the front line are talking about its effects on the cardiovascular system and death due to cardiac arrest. There is much data from China, Italy, and other countries that show this disease can infect heart muscle with subsequent heart failure and death.

The risk of mortality and morbidity is higher in patients with underlying cardiovascular disease.[24,25] It is unclear if the virus or body response to virus injury may introduce cardiovascular disorders although it is difficult to conclude that the virus by itself can affect a

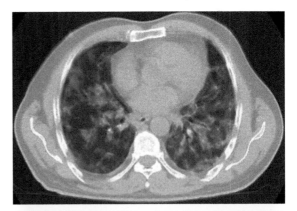

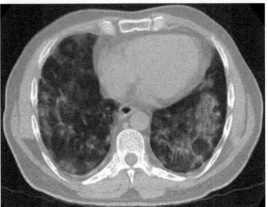

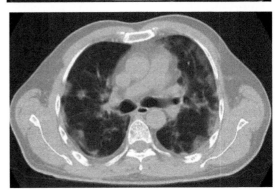

FIG. 40.2 The CT scan of a 67-year-old male who was presented with fatigue and cough, showed multifocal multilobar dense ground-glass opacities with peripheral extension. He was admitted in a COVID-19 center.

healthy heart. It is almost clear that preexisting heart problems can aggravate the disease with the acceleration of congestive heart failure. In addition, the infection causes some difficulties in heart transplants and the management of the patients after surgery.[24]

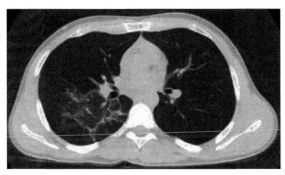

FIG. 40.3 The CT scan of a 31-year-old male showed a ground-glass opacity in the upper lobe of the right lung. He was treated with the diagnosis of COVID-19 infection.

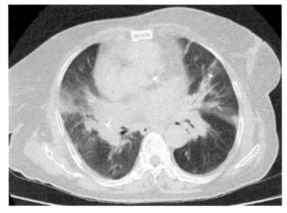

FIG. 40.4 A 76-year-old female with fever, dyspnea, and cough was admitted to the hospital. In the CT scan, bilateral subpleural ground-glass opacity with central extension was seen. She was treated with the diagnosis of COVID-19 infection.

As mentioned in the previous sections, the infection can occur by using ACE receptors by the virus. In addition, this receptor plays an important role in cardiovascular diseases, hypertension, and diabetes mellitus.[26] Inhibition of the RAAS by using ACE inhibitors or angiotensin-receptor blockers (ARB) can upregulate the ACE receptors and lead to severe infection.[27] Several studies revealed that the risk of infection with COVID-19 and also the severity of the disease is higher in the patients with hypertension, diabetes mellitus, coronary heart disease, and cerebrovascular disease who were under treatment with ACE inhibitors before the infection.[28–30] The corona virus attaches itself to some receptors in the lungs; the same happens in heart muscle as

well. According to some data that must be proved, if a patient is using these drugs, it is advisable to choose other antihypertensive drugs such as calcium channel blockers (CCB).[31]

In addition to ACE receptors, cytokine storm,[32,33] respiratory distress and hypoxia in COVID-19 infection can cause myocardial damage. In addition, the patients should be monitored for probable cardiovascular complications due to antiviral or antimicrobial drugs such as hydroxychloroquine which may cause malignant arrhythmia due to long QT arrhythmia; and also, they should be followed up for latent cardiovascular disease.[27] It must be pointed out that after hopeful termination of such a pandemic situation many patients may suffer heart problems as one of the worst late complications due to COVID-19 and cardiologists must prepare themselves for diagnosis, treatment, and follow up of these patients.

It is known that since many years ago and according to several studies, a condition like pneumonia and any kind of widespread inflammation in the body may damage the heart and even lead to plaques in the arteries or making them unstable with subsequent heart attacks. Furthermore, myocarditis and cardiomyopathies are among the results of these kinds of inflammations and perhaps COVID-19.

New protocols should be implemented in the patients with suspected COVID-19, especially in heart attacks, which may mimic acute ST-elevation or non-ST-elevation myocardial infarction to avoid an unnecessary rush to catheterization laboratory or providing facilities for primary PCI (percutaneous coronary intervention).

Interestingly, some reports show that the mortality rate from heart damage due to myocarditis in patients with a previous healthy heart is more than in patients with preexisting heart damage. It is also worth noting that the patients with preexisting heart problems had less mortality than the ones with normal cardiovascular disorders who developed myocarditis due to COVID-19. It will be valuable if a risk score can be developed for clinicians to help them better observe the patients, who may develop heart failure during the disease.

Some clinicians recommend daily electrocardiography, echocardiography, and measurement of biomarkers to identify patients at risk of developing cardiovascular disease due to corona infection as a part of a routine management of the disease. Although according to some data evaluating these patients may increase additional staff into the room and more exposure, especially in the era of limited masks or protective equipment.

It is emphasized that the physician must pay a lot of attention to the patients with COVID-19 infection who had a history of cardiovascular disease. This special group of the patients is at a higher risk of cardiac complications including cardiovascular events.[34]

Managing the patients with STEMI (ST-elevation myocardial infarction) is an issue. On the one hand, several studies suggested thrombolytic therapy during the corona pandemic[35-37] for preventing transmission of the virus. On the other hand, primary PCI is recommended for the patients with definite criteria for COVID-19 and STEMI. A study in a tertiary center for cardiovascular disease by Firouzi et al. showed that although corona infection is common due to the recent pandemic, primary PCI is still the gold standard for managing the patients with STEMI even in those who have definite criteria for COVID-19. Personal protective equipment is essential and is the first step to approach to these patients.[38] In addition, several studies showed that during the COVID-19 pandemic, the delay for the patients' referral and treatment was increased significantly.[39,40]

Asymptomatic carriers are one of the serious sources of the infection and can play an important role in spreading the infection for many people silently,[41] and evaluating the patients and health-care providers before any interventional procedures is essential.

In conclusion, there is not any specific treatment or vaccination for COVID-19 infection; so, prevention plays an important role in controlling the burden of the disease. Simple actions like isolating the patients, using suitable masks, better personal hygiene, and good ventilation can prevent the infection.[42]

It is emphasized that the health-care provider's role for controlling this pandemic is early diagnosis of the patients with COVID-19 infection. Getting a complete history of the symptoms and underlying diseases, careful physical examination with full protection for themselves and history of the recent exposure with other patients with corona infection plays an important role in early diagnosis. The suspected patients must be quarantined as soon as possible and the physicians should not postpone their management until doing the paraclinical evaluations. In addition, educating all the members of the society for self-care is essential in preventing this serious infection.

## ACKNOWLEDGMENT

We want to especially thank Dr. Zahra Aires, the resident of Radiology from Boali Hospital, Zahedan University of Medical Sciences (ZAUMS) in Iran, for her time and attention for preparing the photos of this chapter and the CT scans of the patients with the diagnosis of COVID-19 infection.

## REFERENCES

1. https://www.theguardian.com/world/2020/mar/13/first-covid-19-case-happened-in-november-china-government-records-show-report.
2. https://www.who.int/emergencies/diseases/novel-coronavirus-2019/events-as-they-happen.
3. https://www.who.int/emergencies/diseases/novel-coronavirus-2019.
4. https://covid19.who.int/.
5. Zhou P, Yang XL, Wang XG, Hu B, Zhang L, Zhang W. Discovery of a novel coronavirus associated with the recent pneumonia outbreak in humans and its potential bat origin. *Nature.* 2020; https://doi.org/10.1038/s41586-020-2012-7.
6. Kannan S, Ali PSS, Sheeza A, Hemalatha K. COVID-19 (novel coronavirus 2019)—recent trends. *Eur Rev Med Pharmacol Sci.* 2020; 24:2006–2011.
7. Vaduganathan M, Vardeny O, Michel T, McMurray JJV, Pfeffer MA, Solomon SD. Renin–angiotensin–aldosterone system inhibitors in patients with Covid-19. *N Engl J Med.* 2020; https://doi.org/10.1056/NEJMsr2005760.
8. Guan W, Ni Z, Yu H, et al. Clinical characteristics of 2019 novel coronavirus infection in China. *medRxiv.* 2020; 382:1708–1720. Preprint posted online on Feb. 9 https://doi.org/10.1101/2020.02.06.20020974.
9. Zhu N, Zhang D, Wang W, et al. A novel coronavirus from patients with pneumonia in China, 2019. *N Engl J Med.* 2020; 382:727–733. https://doi.org/10.1056/NEJMoa2001017 [Epub ahead of print].
10. Chan JF, Yuan S, Kok KH, et al. A familial cluster of pneumonia associated with the 2019 novel coronavirus indicating person-to-person transmission: a study of a family cluster. *Lancet.* 2020; 395:P514–P523. https://doi.org/10.1016/S0140-6736(20)30154-9.
11. Chen N, Zhou M, Dong X, et al. Epidemiological and clinical characteristics of 99 cases of 2019 novel coronavirus pneumonia in Wuhan, China: a descriptive study. *Lancet.* 2020; 395:507–513. https://doi.org/10.1016/S0140-6736(20)30211-7.
12. Sun P, Lu X, Xu C, Sun W, Pan B. Understanding of COVID-19 based on current evidence. *J Med Virol.* 2020; 92:1–4. https://doi.org/10.1002/jmv.257224.
13. Fang Y, Zhang H, Xie J, et al. The sensitivity of chest CT for COVID-19: comparison to RT-PCR. *Radiology.* 2020; 19: E115–E117.
14. Ai T, Yang Z, Hou H, et al. Correlation of chest CT and RT-PCR testing in coronavirus disease 2019 (COVID-19) in China: a report of 1014 cases. *Radiology.* 2020; 200642.
15. Wu J, Wu X, Zeng W, et al. Chest CT findings in patients with corona virus disease 2019 and its relationship with

clinical features. *Invest Radiol.* 2020; 55:257–261. https://doi.org/10.1097/RLI.0000000000000670.

16. Yang W, Yan F. Patients with RT-PCR-confirmed COVID-19 and normal chest CT. *Radiology.* 2020; 295. https://doi.org/10.1148/radiol.2020200702.

17. Xie X, Zhong Z, Zhao W, Zheng C, Wang F, Liu J. Chest CT for typical 2019-nCoV pneumonia: relationship to negative RT-PCR testing. *Radiology.* 2020; 2020:200343. https://doi.org/10.1148/radiol.2020200343PubMedGoogleScholar Published online February 12.

18. Huang C, Wang Y, Li X, et al. Clinical features of patients infected with 2019 novel coronavirus in Wuhan, China. *Lancet.* 2020; 395:497–506. https://doi.org/10.1016/S0140-6736(20)30183-5.

19. Wang D, Hu B, Hu C, et al. Clinical characteristics of 138 hospitalized patients with 2019 novel coronavirus-infected pneumonia in Wuhan, China. *JAMA.* 2020; 323:1061–1069. https://doi.org/10.1001/jama.2020.1585 [Epub ahead of print].

20. Chen C, Zhang XR, Ju ZY, He WF. Advances in the research of cytokine storm mechanism induced by Corona Virus Disease 2019 and the corresponding immunotherapies. *Zhonghua Shao Shang Za Zhi.* 2020; 36:E005. https://doi.org/10.3760/cma.j.cn501120-20200224-00088 Epub ahead of print.

21. Xu X, Han M, Li T, et al. n.d. Effective Treatment of Severe COVID-19 Patients With Tocilizumab, *Proc Natl Acad Sci U S A.* 2020 May 19;117(20):10970–10975. Published online 2020 Apr 29. https://doi.org/10.1073/pnas.2005615117.

22. Ren LL, Wang YM, Wu ZQ, et al. Identification of a novel coronavirus causing severe pneumonia in humans: a descriptive study. *Chin Med J.* 2020; 133:1015–1024. https://doi.org/10.1097/CM9.0000000000000722.

23. Wang M, Cao R, Zhang L, et al. Remdesivir and chloroquine effectively inhibit the recently emerged novel coronavirus (2019-nCoV) in vitro. *Cell Res.* 2020; 30:269–271.

24. Clerkin KJ, Fried JA, Raikhelkar J, et al. Coronavirus disease 2019 (COVID-19) and cardiovascular disease. *Circulation.* 2020; 141:1648–1655. https://doi.org/10.1161/CIRCULATIONAHA.120.046941.

25. Chen C, Yan JT, Zhou N, Zhao JP, Wang DW. Analysis of myocardial injury in patients with COVID-19 and association between concomitant cardiovascular diseases and severity of COVID-19. *Zhonghua Xin Xue Guan Bing Za Zhi.* 2020; 48:E008. https://doi.org/10.3760/cma.j.cn112148-20200225-00123.

26. Turner AJ, Hiscox JA, Hooper NM. ACE2: from vasopeptidase to SARS virus receptor. *Trends Pharmacol Sci.* 2004; 25:291–294.

27. Zheng Y-Y, Ma Y-T, Zhang J-Y, Xie X. COVID-19 and the cardiovascular system. *Nat Rev Cardiol.* 2020.

28. Yang X, Yu Y, Xu J, et al. Clinical course and outcomes of critically ill patients with SARS-CoV-2 pneumonia in Wuhan, China: a single-centered, retrospective, observational study. *Lancet Respir Med.* 2020; 8: P475–P481.  published online Feb 24https://doi.org/10.1016/S2213-2600(20)30079-5.

29. Guan W, Ni Z, Hu Y, et al. Clinical characteristics of coronavirus disease 2019 in China. *N Engl J Med.* 2020; 382:18. https://doi.org/10.1056/NEJMoa2002032 published online Feb 28.

30. Zhang JJ, Dong X, Cao YY, et al. Clinical characteristics of 140 patients infected by SARS-CoV-2 in Wuhan, China. *Allergy.* 2020; 75:1730–1741. https://doi.org/10.1111/all.14238 published online Feb 19.

31. Fang L, Karakiulakis G, Roth M. Are patients with hypertension and diabetes mellitus at increased risk for COVID-19 infection? *Lancet Respir Med.* 2020; 8(4):PE21. https://doi.org/10.1016/S2213-2600(20)30116-8.

32. Huang C, Wang Y, Li X, et al. Clinical features of patients infected with 2019 novel coronavirus in Wuha, China. *Lancet.* 2020; 395:497–506.

33. Wong CK, Lam CWK, Wu AKL, et al. Plasma inflammatory cytokines and chemokines in severe acute respiratory syndrome. *Clin Exp Immunol.* 2004; 136:95–103.

34. Alemzadeh-Ansari MJ. Coronavirus disease 2019 (COVID-19) and cardiovascular events. *Res Cardiovasc Med.* 2020; 9:1–2.

35. Zeng J, Huang J, Pan L. How to balance acute myocardial infarction and COVID-19: the protocols from Sichuan provincial People's hospital. *Intensive Care Med.* 2020; 46:1111–1113.

36. Welt FGP, Shah PB, Aronow HD, et al. Catheterization laboratory considerations during the coronavirus (COVID-19) pandemic: from ACC's Interventional Council and SCAI. *J Am Coll Cardiol.* 2020; 75:2372–2375.

37. Sadeghipour P, Talasaz AH, Eslami V, et al. Management of ST-segment-elevation myocardial infarction during the coronavirus disease 2019 (COVID-19) outbreak: Iranian "247" National Committee's position paper on primary percutaneous coronary intervention. *Catheter Cardiovasc Interv.* 2020; .

38. Firouzi A, et al. Effects of the COVID-19 pandemic on the management of patients with ST-elevation myocardial infarction in a Tertiary Cardiovascular Center. *Crit Pathw Cardiol.* 2020; https://doi.org/10.1097/HPC.0000000000000228 Volume Publish Ahead of Print—Issue.

39. Kirtane AJ, Bangalore S. Why fibrinolytic therapy for STEMI in the COVID-19. Pandemic is not your new best friend. *Circ Cardiovasc Qual Outcomes.* 2020; 13:e006885.

40. Tam CF, Cheung KS, Lam S, et al. Impact of coronavirus disease 2019 (COVID-19) outbreak on ST-segment-elevation myocardial infarction care in Hong Kong, China. *Circ Cardiovasc Qual Outcomes.* 2020; 13 Circoutcomes120006631.

41. Wang Y, Wang Y, Chen Y, Qin Q. Unique epidemiological and clinical features of the emerging 2019 novel coronavirus pneumonia (COVID-19) implicate special control measures. *J Med Virol.* 2020; 92:568–576.

42. Guan W, Ni Z, Hu Y, et al. Clinical characteristics of 2019 novel coronavirus infection in China. *medRxiv.* 2020; https://doi.org/10.1101/2020.02.06.2002097418.

# CHAPTER 41

# Cardiovascular Disease in the COVID-19 Era: Myocardial Injury and Thrombosis

AHMAD AMIN • PARHAM SADEGHIPOUR • MITRA CHITSAZAN
Rajaie Cardiovascular, Medical & Research Center, Iran University of Medical Sciences, Tehran, Iran

## KEY POINTS

- Acute cardiac injury occurs in approximately up to one-third of patients with Coronavirus disease-2019 (COVID-19), and it is associated with worse prognosis and higher mortality in these patients.
- Signs and symptoms of acute cardiac injury in COVID-19 might be nonspecific; however, laboratory tests show elevated cardiac troponin and natriuretic peptides. The ECG, chest X-ray, and echocardiography may help the physicians in detecting other cardiovascular problems, and/or complications of acute cardiac injury in COVID-19 patients.
- Acute myocardial injury may result in arrhythmias, heart failure, and cardiogenic shock.
- The COVID-19-associated coagulopathy is characterized by markedly elevated D-dimer concentration, a normal or relatively modest decrease in platelet count, and a prolongation of the prothrombin time.
- This hypercoagulable state along with prolonged bed rest and endothelial cell injury (endotheliitis) might increase the risk of thrombotic events (including pulmonary embolism) in patients with COVID-19.

## INTRODUCTION

The severe acute respiratory syndrome coronavirus 2 (SARS-CoV-2; first referred to as 2019-nCoV) emerged in Wuhan, China in late December 2019, and resulted in the Coronavirus disease-2019 (COVID-19) pandemic.[1,2]

Although the primary organ involved in COVID-19 appears to be the lungs, cardiac involvement can also occur. Acute myocardial injury has been linked to worse prognosis and higher mortality in patients with COVID-19.[3-7]

The definition of acute myocardial injury is nonspecific and differed in various studies. In most studies, acute cardiac injury was defined as cardiac troponin value above the 99th percentile upper reference limit (URL) or the occurrence of new abnormalities in electro-cardiography and echocardiography.[4,8] The frequency of myocardial injury has been reported to range from 7% to 28% among hospitalized patients with COVID-19.[3,5,8-10] However, data on the frequency of myocardial damage in outpatient setting is lacking.

According to the Fourth Universal Definition of Myocardial Infarction (2018), the 99th percentile URL is considered as the decision level for the diagnosis of myocardial injury[11]; however, this cutoff level includes all conditions causing "myocardial cell death" with subsequent elevation in cardiac troponin levels. Based on the data from case series and reports, putative causes of myocardial injury include:

- **Ischemic causes:**
  - Acute coronary syndrome caused by either plaque instability and rupture (type I myocardial infarction) or demand ischemia (type II myocardial infarction)
  - Endotheliitis[12] leading to endothelial dysfunction and microvascular damage
- **Nonischemic causes:**
  - Hypoxic injury
  - Stress cardiomyopathy (i.e., takotsubo cardiomyopathy)[13,14]
  - Profound systemic inflammatory response/cytokine storm leading to myocardial suppression
  - Right heart failure[15-17] (i.e., acute cor pulmonale), may result from pulmonary thromboembolism, pulmonary hypertension caused by ARDS (due to hypoxemic vasoconstriction, vascular remodeling, external compression of the vasculature by edema or fibrosis, and reduced pulmonary compliance), and high-pressure mechanical ventilation

SARS-CoV-2 uses transmembrane ACE2 receptors to enter the host cells. In addition to type-2 pneumocytes, the ACE2 receptors are expressed on cardiac myocytes, endothelial cells, and pericytes.[18,19] This might also contribute to the cardiac damage in SARS-CoV-2 infection, though the exact pathophysiologic mechanisms are still unclear.

Key cardiovascular manifestation of COVID-19 and suggested pathophysiologic mechanisms are summarized in Fig. 41.1.[20]

## Key Points

- Although the clinical presentation of myocarditis has been described in a few case reports in patients with COVID-19,[21,22] viral myocarditis caused by direct invasion of SARS-CoV-2 to myocardial tissue has not been definitively confirmed by histologic examinations and viral genome assays.
- Despite considerable incidence and prognostic implications of acute cardiac injury in hospitalized patients with COVID-19, there is insufficient evidence to recommend routine measurement of cardiac troponin to screen for acute myocardial injury in all COVID-19 patients.
- However, patients with history of prior coronary artery disease (CAD), structural heart disease, diabetes mellitus, hypertension, and chronic kidney disease tend to have more severe COVID-19 infection; and should be closely monitored for the occurrence of acute myocardial injury.

## DIAGNOSTIC APPROACH TO PATIENTS WITH ACUTE CARDIAC INJURY

Cardiac injury symptoms are nonspecific in COVID-19 and patients mostly present with the typical symptoms of SARS-CoV-2 infection, including fever, cough, dyspnea, or fatigue and a minority present with anginal chest pain and palpitations. A new-onset and/or unexplained dyspnea, orthopnea, peripheral edema, and jugular venous distension should raise clinical suspicious for cardiac involvement in patients with severe COVID-19 infection.

In clinically suspected patients, the diagnostic approach should include the following.

## Electrocardiogram

- A 12-lead electrocardiogram (ECG) should be obtained initially in all patients with suspected myocardial damage. The most common ECG abnormality reported in patients with acute cardiac injury was ST-segment elevation or depression, T-wave depression and inversion, and Q waves. The QT interval (and corrected QT interval) should also be assessed, in particular in patients on QT-prolonging therapies.

- Initial ECG may provide clues to specific diagnoses, which require a change in management.
  - QT prolongation of >500 ms or ventricular tachycardia in patients receiving certain medications (including chloroquine, hydroxychloroquine, lopinavir–ritonavir, azithromycin, etc.) may result in early discontinuation and replacement of the responsible medication.
  - New pathologic Q waves, ST-T changes, or arrhythmia would mandate further cardiac assessments such as echocardiography.
- Various tachy- or bradyarrhythmia would require close electrolyte assessments, QT measurement, inotrope/vasopressor change, or proper therapies (antiarrhythmics/cardioversion).

## Routine Laboratory Tests

- A complete blood count (with differential), blood glucose, blood urea nitrogen, creatinine, serum electrolytes, and liver function tests should be assessed in all patients.

## Chest X-ray

- Although bilateral chest infiltration from the underlying pneumonia and ARDS from COVID-19 infection may obscure abnormalities caused by cardiac dysfunction, a CXR may help in the detection of cardiomegaly and pleural effusions.

## Cardiac Troponins

- A cardiac troponin value above the 99th percentile upper reference limit is indicative of acute myocardial injury.[11] Since an elevated troponin level in patients with COVID-19 is nonspecific and multifactorial, the results should be interpreted based on the clinical presentation, ECG findings, and echocardiographic examination.

## Natriuretic Peptides (BNP or NT-proBNP)

- Natriuretic peptides are mainly released from the heart in response to increased myocardial wall stress. Several studies have demonstrated elevated BNP or NT-proBNP levels in COVID-19 patients, and an elevated NT-proBNP level has been associated with worse outcomes in patients with severe COVID-19.[23,24] However, it should be noted that elevated NT-proBNP level has been reported in patients with acute lung injury and acute respiratory distress syndrome from other causes,[25–30] even in the absence of clinical findings of heart failure; therefore, an elevated NT-proBNP level should be interpreted based on the whole clinical presentation.

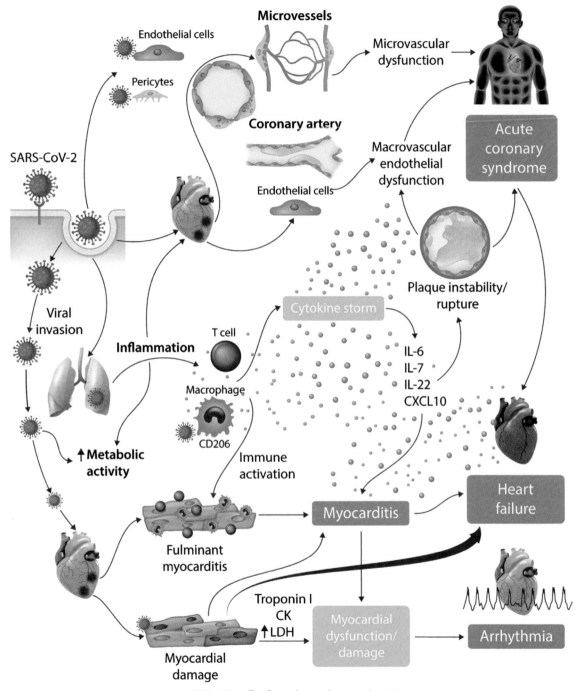

FIG. 41.1  For figure Legend see next page

*Continued*

FIG. 41.1, CONT'D Cardiovascular involvement in COVID-19—key manifestations and hypothetical mechanisms. SARS-CoV-2 anchors on transmembrane ACE2 to enter the host cells including type 2 pneumocytes, macrophages, endothelial cells, pericytes, and cardiac myocytes, leading to inflammation and multiorgan failure. In particular, the infection of endothelial cells or pericytes could lead to severe microvascular and macrovascular dysfunction. Furthermore, in conjunction with the immune over-reactivity, it can potentially destabilize atherosclerotic plaques and explain the development of the acute coronary syndromes. Infection of the respiratory tract, particularly of type 2 pneumocytes, by SARS-CoV-2 is manifested by the progression of systemic inflammation and immune cell overactivation, leading to a "cytokine storm," which results in an elevated level of cytokines such as IL-6, IL-7, IL-22, and CXCL10. Subsequently, it is possible that activated T cells and macrophages may infiltrate infected myocardium, resulting in the development of fulminant myocarditis and severe cardiac damage. This process could be further intensified by the cytokine storm. Similarly, the viral invasion could cause cardiac myocyte damage directly leading to myocardial dysfunction and contribute to the development of arrhythmia. (From Guzik TJ, Mohiddin SA, Dimarco A, et al. COVID-19 and the cardiovascular system: implications for risk assessment, diagnosis, and treatment options. Cardiovasc Res. 2020;116(10):1666–1687; with permission.)

## Echocardiography

- Currently, there is insufficient evidence to recommend routine echocardiography for all COVID-19 patients with suspected cardiac damage. Considering the limitations in personal protective equipment and the importance of social distancing, the echocardiographic examination can be tailored to the presentation of each individual patient.
- In selected cases, point-of-care ultrasonography (POCUS) and focused cardiac ultrasound study (FoCUS) could help in detecting gross abnormalities in cardiac structure and/or function. These bedside options may also be performed by the trained non-cardiologists who might already be in the room with these patients, thereby reducing the risk of cardiologists' exposure to the virus.

## COMPLICATIONS OF CARDIAC INJURY IN COVID-19

### Arrhythmias and Conduction Abnormalities

Although no specific arrhythmia has been linked to SARS-CoV-2 infection, both brady- and tachyarrhythmias, as well as sudden cardiac death have been reported in patients with COVID-19.[5,6,31-33]

Myocardial injury and damage to the conduction system, as well as hypoxia may be directly related to the development of arrhythmias in these patients. Arrhythmias can also occur as a complication of electrolyte abnormalities, acute heart failure, acute coronary syndrome, myocarditis, and cardiogenic and/or septic shock in patients with COVID-19.

In addition, QT-prolongation has been reported in COVID-19 patients, even though the majority

of cases seemed to be drug-induced, mostly related to chloroquine, hydroxychloroquine, and azithromycin.[34-36]

Epidemiologic studies also reported an increased incidence of out-of-hospital cardiac arrest during COVID-19 pandemic[37,38]; however, other factors such as increased stress during the pandemic, and unwillingness or delay in seeking medical care by patients with cardiac problems might also be responsible in addition to COVID-19 infection.

### Heart Failure

In patients with COVID-19, both de novo acute heart failure and acute decompensation of chronic heart failure might develop.

- In addition to heart failure with reduced ejection fraction (HFrEF), the occurrence of heart failure with preserved ejection fraction (HFpEF) should also be considered in COVID-19 patients failure.[39] Acute myocardial injury, cytokine-induced inflammatory state, comorbidities such as hypertension, side effects of medications, and vigorous intravenous fluid administration might impair myocardial relaxation, in particular in the elderly and those with underlying diastolic dysfunction, resulting in acute heart failure.
- The presence of potential precipitating factors for acute decompensation of chronic heart failure should be carefully assessed and monitored in COVID-19 patients.
- Patients with previous history of chronic heart are recommended to continue their previous guideline-directed medical therapy, including

beta-blockers, ACE inhibitors or angiotensin II receptor blockers, and mineralocorticoid receptor antagonists.[40]

- When administering intravenous fluids to these patients, attempt should be done to avoid both volume overload and circulatory failure.
- For the management of fever, nonsteroidal antiinflammatory drugs (NSAIDs) should be used with caution in these patients, considering their potential effect on water and sodium retention; thus, acetaminophen may be generally preferred in these patients.

### Cardiogenic Shock

In patients with COVID-19, cardiogenic shock may be caused by:
- Acute decompensated heart failure
- Myocardial infarction
- Myocarditis
- Sustained refractory arrhythmia

In critically ill patients with COVID-19, a combination of cardiogenic shock and septic shock (mixed shock) may contribute to hemodynamic deterioration and impaired end-organ perfusion.

## THROMBOSIS IN THE COVID-19 OUTBREAK

Since the early report from China, an unusual increased coagulopathy has been reported in COVID-19 population.[7] In several population-based studies, non-survived population had significantly higher levels of D-dimer and fibrin degradation products and longer prothrombin and activated partial thromboplastin times (aPTT), which also confirmed an important prognostic role for the coagulopathy.[41] Initially, the nature of this coagulopathy was related to the accompanied septic shock and disseminated intravascular coagulation (DIC).[7] In one of the early reports, Tang et al. observed that DIC occurred in 71.4% of the non-survivors vs 0.6% of the survivors during hospitalization.[41] However, as our knowledge grew, it became more apparent that a direct viral impact on the coagulation cascade may also play a role. For instance, in a report by Klok et al., none of the ICU patients with thrombotic complication developed DIC.[42]

### Venous Thromboembolism

The described coagulopathy, along with prolonged bed rest and concomitant therapeutic regimen, increase the risk of thrombotic events in COVID-19.[43] Depending on the screening methods, investigation sites (wards vs ICUs) and the use of thrombophylaxis, incidence of thrombotic events varies across studies between 7% and 85%.[31,42,44–49] Klok et al. observed a 31% (95% CI: 20%–41%) incidence of thrombotic complications in three academic/teaching hospitals in the Netherlands, the majority of which were venous thromboembolism (VTE).[42] High incidence (20.6%) of pulmonary embolism has also been reported by Poissy et al. at least two times higher than previous year during the same time interval.[44] In a report by Middeldorp et al., the incidence of VTE in ICU was significantly higher than ward [59% (95% CI: 42–72) vs 9.2% (95% CI: 2.6–21)].[46] In addition, several postmortem studies have frequently shown the presence of pulmonary micro- and macrothrombosis and deep vein thrombosis, at times as the cause of unexpected death.[50,51]

It should be noted that diagnosis of VTE might be very challenging in patients hospitalized for COVID-19: the inapplicability of D-dimer, issues with transferring to imaging wards, and difficulties in optimal patient positioning have left the diagnostic process of considerable numbers of patients, particularly the sickest, incomplete.[52] Although not definite, but some diagnostic measures like right ventricular enlargement/dysfunction in echocardiography or deep venous thrombosis in lower limb detected by ultrasound might be helpful toward the diagnosis of pulmonary embolism.[52] There is a clear controversy on the treatment of patients without definite diagnosis (i.e., incomplete diagnosis), and intermediate to full-dose anticoagulation have been suggested by some experts.[52]

The symptom overlap between pulmonary emboli and acute respiratory disease in COVID-19[53] and the mentioned challenges in diagnosis and treatment of pulmonary embolism call for an appropriate prophylaxis strategy. Tang et al. investigated the validity of the sepsis-induced coagulopathy score and the D-dimer level in the risk stratification of patients with COVID-19 with regard to VTE prophylaxis.[54] In their retrospective analysis on 449 hospitalized COVID-19 patients, no 28-day mortality benefit was observed among heparin (LMWH or UFH) users vs nonusers. However, in patients with a minimum sepsis-induced coagulopathy score of 4 or a D-dimer level of greater than 3.0 μg/mL, heparin prophylaxis significantly improved the 28-day mortality. Hence, Tang and colleagues recommended prophylaxis application based on risk stratification.[54] Other risk stratification tools (e.g., Caprini and IMPROVE) have also been suggested to be applied.[52] The International Society on Thrombosis and Haemostasis (ISTH) has offered a liberal recommendation suggesting the administration of LMWH in all patients hospitalized for COVID-19 (including those that are not critically ill) who do not have contraindications (platelet count ≤25,000/L or active bleeding).[55] This routine approach might be justified by the high incidence of VTE (27%) observed in hospitalized COVID-19 patients. Of note, mechanical prophylaxis has been suggested for patients with contraindication for pharmacological prophylaxis.[52]

Although the importance of VTE prophylaxis has been recognized since the early days of pandemic, it still seems to be overlooked. Wang et al. in their short report showed that more than 40% of the 1026 hospitalized patients with COVID-19 had a Padua Prediction Score ≥4 (i.e., high risk for[41] VTE), yet only 7% received appropriate treatment.[41]

## REFERENCES

1. World Health Organization. *Pneumonia of Unknown Cause—China;* 2020. https://www.who.int/csr/don/05-january-2020-pneumonia-of-unkown-cause-china/en/. Published January 5, Accessed April 4, 2020.
2. WHO. WHO Director-General's opening remarks at the media briefing on COVID-19—11 March 2020. https://www.who.int/dg/speeches/detail/who-director-general-s-opening-remarks-at-the-media-briefing-on-covid-19- - -11-march-2020. Published March 11, Accessed April 4, 2020.
3. Shi S, Qin M, Shen B, et al. Association of cardiac injury with mortality in hospitalized patients with COVID-19 in Wuhan, China. *JAMA Cardiol.* 2020;5:802–810.
4. Huang C, Wang Y, Li X, et al. Clinical features of patients infected with 2019 novel coronavirus in Wuhan, China. *Lancet.* 2020;395(10223):497–506.
5. Wang D, Hu B, Hu C, et al. Clinical characteristics of 138 hospitalized patients with 2019 novel coronavirus-infected pneumonia in Wuhan, China. *JAMA.* 2020;323:1061–1069.
6. Guo T, Fan Y, Chen M, et al. Cardiovascular implications of fatal outcomes of patients with coronavirus disease 2019 (COVID-19). *JAMA Cardiol.* 2020;5:811–818.
7. Guan WJ, Ni ZY, Hu Y, et al. Clinical characteristics of coronavirus disease 2019 in China. *N Engl J Med.* 2020;382(18):1708–1720.
8. Zhou F, Yu T, Du R, et al. Clinical course and risk factors for mortality of adult inpatients with COVID-19 in Wuhan, China: a retrospective cohort study. *Lancet.* 2020;395(10229):1054–1062.
9. Lippi G, Lavie CJ, Sanchis-Gomar F. Cardiac troponin I in patients with coronavirus disease 2019 (COVID-19): evidence from a meta-analysis. *Prog Cardiovasc Dis.* 2020;63:390–391.
10. Clerkin KJ, Fried JA, Raikhelkar J, et al. COVID-19 and cardiovascular disease. *Circulation.* 2020;141(20):1648–1655.
11. Thygesen K, Alpert JS, Jaffe AS, et al. Fourth universal definition of myocardial infarction (2018). *J Am Coll Cardiol.* 2018;72(18):2231–2264.
12. Pons S, Fodil S, Azoulay E, Zafrani L. The vascular endothelium: the cornerstone of organ dysfunction in severe SARS-CoV-2 infection. *Crit Care.* 2020;24(1):353.
13. Giustino G, Croft LB, Oates CP, et al. Takotsubo cardiomyopathy in COVID-19. *J Am Coll Cardiol.* 2020;76(5):628–629.
14. Minhas AS, Scheel P, Garibaldi B, et al. Takotsubo syndrome in the setting of COVID-19 infection. *JACC Case Rep.* 2020;2:1321–1325.
15. Creel-Bulos C, Hockstein M, Amin N, Melhem S, Truong A, Sharifpour M. Acute cor pulmonale in critically ill patients with COVID-19. *N Engl J Med.* 2020;382(21):e70.
16. Argulian E, Sud K, Vogel B, et al. Right ventricular dilation in hospitalized patients with COVID-19 infection. *JACC Cardiovasc Imaging.* 2020;13:2459–2461.
17. Pagnesi M, Baldetti L, Beneduce A, et al. Pulmonary hypertension and right ventricular involvement in hospitalised patients with COVID-19. *Heart.* 2020;106:1324–1331.
18. Chen L, Li X, Chen M, Feng Y, Xiong C. The ACE2 expression in human heart indicates new potential mechanism of heart injury among patients infected with SARS-CoV-2. *Cardiovasc Res.* 2020;116(6):1097–1100.
19. Nicin L, Abplanalp WT, Mellentin H, et al. Cell type-specific expression of the putative SARS-CoV-2 receptor ACE2 in human hearts. *Eur Heart J.* 2020;41(19):1804–1806.
20. Guzik TJ, Mohiddin SA, Dimarco A, et al. COVID-19 and the cardiovascular system: implications for risk assessment, diagnosis, and treatment options. *Cardiovasc Res.* 2020;116(10):1666–1687.
21. Chen C, Zhou Y, Wang DW. SARS-CoV-2: a potential novel etiology of fulminant myocarditis. *Herz.* 2020;45(3):230–232.
22. Inciardi RM, Lupi L, Zaccone G, et al. Cardiac involvement in a patient with coronavirus disease 2019 (COVID-19). *JAMA Cardiol.* 2020;5:819–824.
23. Gao L, Jiang D, Wen XS, et al. Prognostic value of NT-proBNP in patients with severe COVID-19. *Respir Res.* 2020;21(1):83.
24. Han H, Xie L, Liu R, et al. Analysis of heart injury laboratory parameters in 273 COVID-19 patients in one hospital in Wuhan, China. *J Med Virol.* 2020. https://doi.org/10.1002/jmv.25809 [Epub ahead of print].
25. Lai CC, Sung MI, Ho CH, et al. The prognostic value of N-terminal proB-type natriuretic peptide in patients with acute respiratory distress syndrome. *Sci Rep.* 2017;7:44784.
26. Determann RM, Royakkers AA, Schaefers J, et al. Serum levels of N-terminal proB-type natriuretic peptide in mechanically ventilated critically ill patients—relation to tidal volume size and development of acute respiratory distress syndrome. *BMC Pulm Med.* 2013;13:42.
27. Park BH, Park MS, Kim YS, et al. Prognostic utility of changes in N-terminal pro-brain natriuretic peptide combined with sequential organ failure assessment

scores in patients with acute lung injury/acute respiratory distress syndrome concomitant with septic shock. *Shock.* 2011;36(2):109–114.

28. Park BH, Kim YS, Chang J, et al. N-terminal pro-brain natriuretic peptide as a marker of right ventricular dysfunction after open-lung approach in patients with acute lung injury/acute respiratory distress syndrome. *J Crit Care.* 2011;26(3):241–248.

29. Karmpaliotis D, Kirtane AJ, Ruisi CP, et al. Diagnostic and prognostic utility of brain natriuretic peptide in subjects admitted to the ICU with hypoxic respiratory failure due to noncardiogenic and cardiogenic pulmonary edema. *Chest.* 2007;131(4):964–971.

30. Sun YZ, Gao YL, Yu QX, et al. Assessment of acute lung injury/acute respiratory distress syndrome using B-type brain natriuretic peptide. *J Int Med Res.* 2015;43(6):802–808.

31. Goyal P, Choi JJ, Pinheiro LC, et al. Clinical characteristics of Covid-19 in New York City. *N Engl J Med.* 2020;382(24):2372–2374.

32. Bhatla A, Mayer MM, Adusumalli S, et al. COVID-19 and cardiac arrhythmias. *Heart Rhythm.* 2020;17:1439–1444.

33. Shao F, Xu S, Ma X, et al. In-hospital cardiac arrest outcomes among patients with COVID-19 pneumonia in Wuhan, China. *Resuscitation.* 2020;151:18–23.

34. Voisin O, Lorc'h EL, Mahe A, et al. Acute QT interval modifications during hydroxychloroquine-azithromycin treatment in the context of COVID-19 infection. *Mayo Clin Proc.* 2020;95(8):1696–1700.

35. Cavalcanti AB, Zampieri FG, Rosa RG, et al. Hydroxychloroquine with or without azithromycin in mild-to-moderate Covid-19. *N Engl J Med.* 2020;383:2041–2052.

36. Moschini L, Loffi M, Regazzoni V, Di Tano G, Gherbesi E, Danzi GB. Effects on QT interval of hydroxychloroquine associated with ritonavir/darunavir or azithromycin in patients with SARS-CoV-2 infection. *Heart Vessel.* 2020. https://doi.org/10.1007/s00380-020-01671-4 [Epub ahead of print].

37. Baldi E, Sechi GM, Mare C, et al. Out-of-hospital cardiac arrest during the Covid-19 outbreak in Italy. *N Engl J Med.* 2020;383(5):496–498.

38. Lai PH, Lancet EA, Weiden MD, et al. Characteristics associated with out-of-hospital cardiac arrests and resuscitations during the novel coronavirus disease 2019 pandemic in New York City. *JAMA Cardiol.* 2020;5:1154–1163.

39. Mehra MR, Ruschitzka F. COVID-19 illness and heart failure: a missing link? *JACC Heart Fail.* 2020;8(6):512–514.

40. Cardiology. TESf. ESC Guidance for the Diagnosis and Management of CV Disease During the COVID-19 Pandemic; 2020. https://www.escardio.org/Education/COVID-19-and-Cardiology/ESCCOVID-19-Guidance. Updated Last update: 10 June. Accessed.

41. Tang N, Li D, Wang X, Sun Z. Abnormal coagulation parameters are associated with poor prognosis in patients with novel coronavirus pneumonia. *J Thromb Haemost.* 2020;18(4):844–847.

42. Klok FA, Kruip M, van der Meer NJM, et al. Incidence of thrombotic complications in critically ill ICU patients with COVID-19. *Thromb Res.* 2020;191:145–147.

43. Bikdeli B, Madhavan MV, Jimenez D, et al. COVID-19 and thrombotic or thromboembolic disease: implications for prevention, antithrombotic therapy, and follow-up: JACC state-of-the-art review. *J Am Coll Cardiol.* 2020;75(23):2950–2973.

44. Poissy J, Goutay J, Caplan M, et al. Pulmonary embolism in COVID-19 patients: awareness of an increased prevalence. *Circulation.* 2020;142:184–186.

45. Moores LK, Tritschler T, Brosnahan S, et al. Prevention, diagnosis, and treatment of VTE in patients with COVID-19: CHEST guideline and expert panel report. *Chest.* 2020;158:1143–1163.

46. Middeldorp S, Coppens M, van Haaps TF, et al. Incidence of venous thromboembolism in hospitalized patients with COVID-19. *J Thromb Haemost.* 2020;18:1995–2002.

47. Cui S, Chen S, Li X, Liu S, Wang F. Prevalence of venous thromboembolism in patients with severe novel coronavirus pneumonia. *J Thromb Haemost.* 2020;18(6):1421–1424.

48. Helms J, Tacquard C, Severac F, et al. High risk of thrombosis in patients with severe SARS-CoV-2 infection: a multicenter prospective cohort study. *Intensive Care Med.* 2020;46(6):1089–1098.

49. Lodigiani C, Iapichino G, Carenzo L, et al. Venous and arterial thromboembolic complications in COVID-19 patients admitted to an academic hospital in Milan, Italy. *Thromb Res.* 2020;191:9–14.

50. Wichmann D, Sperhake JP, Lütgehetmann M, et al. Autopsy findings and venous thromboembolism in patients with COVID-19. *Ann Intern Med.* 2020:M20-2003.

51. Ackermann M, Verleden SE, Kuehnel M, et al. Pulmonary vascular endothelialitis, thrombosis, and angiogenesis in Covid-19. *N Engl J Med.* 2020;383(2):120–128.

52. Bikdeli B, Madhavan MV, Jimenez D, et al. COVID-19 and thrombotic or thromboembolic disease: implications for prevention, antithrombotic therapy, and follow-up. *J Am Coll Cardiol.* 2020;75:2950–2973.

53. Danzi GB, Loffi M, Galeazzi G, Gherbesi E. Acute pulmonary embolism and COVID-19 pneumonia: a random association? *Eur Heart J.* 2020;41:1858.

54. Tang N, Bai H, Chen X, Gong J, Li D, Sun Z. Anticoagulant treatment is associated with decreased mortality in severe coronavirus disease 2019 patients with coagulopathy. *J Thromb Haemost.* 2020;18:1094–1099.

55. Thachil J, Tang N, Gando S, et al. ISTH interim guidance on recognition and management of coagulopathy in COVID-19. *J Thromb Haemost.* 2020;18:1023–1026.

# CHAPTER 42

# Cardio-Oncology

AZIN ALIZADEHASL

Cardio-Oncology Research Center, Rajaie Cardiovascular, Medical & Research Center, Iran University of Medical Sciences, Tehran, Iran

## INTRODUCTION

Cardiovascular disease and cancer are the two main causes of morbidity and mortality worldwide, for at least 70% of the medical causes for mortality across the world. Cancer patients frequently have multiple comorbidities like diabetes and hypertension that may intensely influence their cancer care and clinical outcomes.

A central aspect of caring for a patient undergoing hypothetically cardiotoxic anticancer therapy is interdisciplinary communication, especially between cardiology, oncology, and also hematology departments and, finally, primary-care providers. Particularly, the cardiologist must have a thorough understanding of the prognosis, intentional treatment plan, estimated benefit of the proposed treatment, cardiac and relevant noncardiac toxicities, and alternative treatment options. Contrariwise, oncologists should be informed of the patient's cardiovascular risk factors and the status of preexisting cardiovascular disease along with their prognosis.[1–5]

There is a high level of evidence that cardiac monitoring in certain anticancer settings helps limit the cardiovascular impact of a patient's cancer therapy. The cardiology consultation may be associated with better cardioprotection, therapy adherence, and survival in patients receiving anthracyclines and other cardiotoxic agents. The multidisciplinary team's goal must be a balanced approach to minimizing cardiovascular toxicity while also limiting reduction or termination of anticancer therapy (Figs. 42.1 and 42.2).

## SCREENING BEFORE ANTICANCER THERAPY

### Baseline Cardiovascular Risk Assessments (Pre-Anticancer Therapy)

While cardiovascular risk factors should be controlled in all patients with cancer, a thorough cardiovascular risk factor study is essential before the initiation of anticancer therapies, especially those therapies with known cardiovascular toxicities. A comprehensive assessment with proper initiation of risk reduction strategies might decrease the likelihood of developing cancer-related cardiovascular complications and outcomes.[2,5–8]

### Baseline Measurement of Cardiac Biomarkers

Various chemotherapy regimens are associated with a wide range of potential cardiovascular toxicities and in selected situations cardiac biomarkers might help identify or predict cardiovascular toxicities, mainly cardiomyopathy and heart failure. The exact role and the timing of biomarker measurement in each patient undergoing potentially cardiotoxic chemotherapy is yet to be determined. The specific timing of when to measure cardiac biomarkers in relation to chemotherapy has varied meaningfully in different clinical studies.

In selected high-risk cases, such as those with relapsed multiple myeloma, or those receiving high doses of cardiotoxic chemotherapy (predominantly anthracyclines), a baseline biomarker assessment before the initiation of chemotherapy must be considered, as this might identify individuals at greatest risk for developing cardiovascular dysfunction.[6–8]

### Baseline Electrocardiogram

The importance of drugs induced QTc prolongation as a key drug safety parameter is widely recognized. The QT interval is a surrogate marker for cardiac repolarization abnormalities, with important prolongation related with the development of potentially life-threatening ventricular arrhythmias such as torsade de pointes. While QT interval prolongation is common in cancer patients, clinical events are rare, but might be fatal. The QTc interval should be calculated by either of the five most standardized formulas:

$$Bazett : QTcB = QT/RR^{1/2}$$

$$Fridericia : QTcFri = QT/RR^{1/3}$$

$$Framingham : QTcFra = QT + 0.154 \, (1 - RR)$$

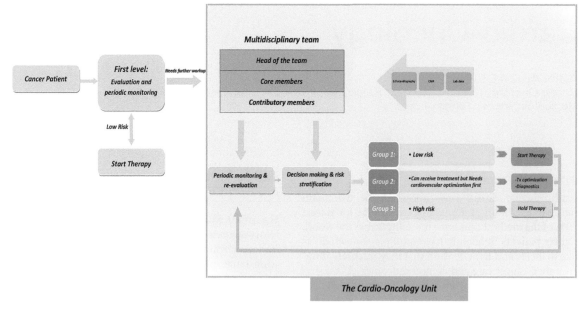

FIG. 42.1 Overview of the design and function of a cardio-oncology unit. After first-level evaluations, patients in need of further workup are referred to the cardio-oncology unit, where risk stratification based on imaging and laboratory data is performed and individualized treatments and monitoring programs of each patient are planned. *CMR*, cardiac magnetic resonance imaging; *LAB*, laboratory.[1]

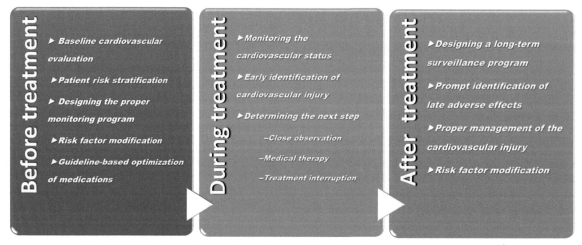

FIG. 42.2 Objectives of the cardio-oncology unit during the stages of cancer management.[1]

$$\text{Hodges}: \text{QTcH} = \text{QT} + 0.00175\,([60/\text{RR}] - 60)$$

$$\text{Rautaharju}: \text{QTcR} = \text{QT} - 0.185\,(\text{RR} - 1) \\ + k\,(k = +0.006\,s\text{ for men and } + 0\,s\text{ for women})$$

and the comparative measurements during treatment period must all utilize the same selected method.[5–9]

## Baseline Assessment of Left Ventricular Ejection Fraction

Presently, therapies related with a important risk of heart failure or left ventricular dysfunction contain, but are not limited to, anthracyclines, human epidermal growth factor receptor 2 (HER2) molecular-targeted therapies (such as trastuzumab or pertuzumab), vascular endothelial growth factor signaling pathway inhibitors (such as sarofenib, sunitinib, and bevacizumab), and some proteasome inhibitors (carfilzomib).

Quantitative evaluation of LV ejection fraction (LVEF) and diastolic function before the beginning of potentially cardiotoxic chemotherapy may help to recognize individuals at higher risk of future cardiovascular complications and to form a baseline, should symptoms suggestive of cardiovascular dysfunction happen during treatment.[6–8,10–12]

## PRIMARY PREVENTION THERAPY

Patients receiving anticancer therapies known to be related with cardiotoxicity must be considered as stage A heart failure patients (at risk of heart failure but without structural heart disease or symptoms of failure).

### Cardiovascular Therapeutics for Prevention

In patients with preexisting cardiovascular disease and risk factors who are receiving potentially cardiotoxic therapy (doxorubicin, trastuzumab, or both), there is often a measurable change in LVEF over the span of 3 years, and this is not limited to higher cardiovascular risk patients. Patients treated with these therapies are at higher risk for the development of subsequent heart failure and therapy directed at prevention of the progression of LV dysfunction is warranted. There are some studies to suggest that angiotensin-converting enzyme inhibitors (ACE-I), angiotensin receptor blockers (ARBs), or selected beta-blockers (BBs) such as carvedilol and nebivolol might be the preferred agents to reduce the risk of cardiotoxicity.

Based on the previous studies (but with small period of follow up), carvedilol did show improvement in diastolic function and protection from troponin elevations.

Patients with HER2-positive breast cancer demonstrated that trastuzumab-induced cardiotoxicity was more frequent in patients with prior exposure to anthracyclines compared with those without anthracycline exposure. Both lisinopril and carvedilol were effective in preventing cardiotoxicity in patients receiving trastuzumab with prior exposure to anthracycline. Also, in a separate therapeutic class, the aldosterone antagonist spironolactone has also been studied in the previous reports in breast cancer patients on anthracyclines, with improvement in LVEF compared with placebo.

Dexrazoxane is primarily an iron chelator and might reduce the production of free radicals formed at the time of anthracycline therapy. It also alters topoisomerase II to prevent its binding with anthracycline. This therapy

has been established to be effective in children and is approved in metastatic breast cancer when the total doxorubicin dose (or equivalent) is $>300$ mg/m$^2$. Though, this strategy does not address the challenge faced by patients with preexisting cardiomyopathy when they need anthracyclines.[8,10–13]

In addition to completely control of hypertension and diabetes before and during treatment, there are many evidences that hyperlipidemia has a contributing effect to inflammation in patients with cancer. Some reports found benefit to continuous statin treatment (compared with no or noncontinuous treatment) in patients with breast cancer treated with anthracyclines.

## SURVEILLANCE STRATEGIES DURING CANCER TREATMENT

Surveillance strategies to identify potential cardiovascular complications might allow early intervention that is likely to have potentially lifesaving implications.

Accurate, reproducible, measureable volumetric analyses are preferred. Three-dimensional (3D) echocardiography provides quantitative volumetric analysis with superior precision and serial reproducibility compared with two-dimensional (2D) echocardiography, mainly due to direct volume measurement without geometric assumptions.

Nonionizing radiation modalities might be most suitable due to concerns regarding cumulative radiation dose in cancer patients, as traditional MUGA scanning may expose patients to substantial radiation with each exam. It is also recognized that echocardiography provides substantial additional information on cardiac structure, valve function, hemodynamics, and also physiology not classically found with MUGA scanning. The use of CMR imaging is increasing; nonetheless, limitations in availability, cost, and expertise might impede a wide adoption of this technique. Quantitative 2D echocardiography using Simpson's biplane method is the most appropriate method when 3D echocardiography imaging is not regularly available; in addition echocardiographic contrast agents are useful when endocardial definition is inadequate with routine imaging. Of course, the most appropriate modality will vary with patient characteristics as well as center availability and also local expertise.

Myocardial deformation imaging might facilitate early detection of subclinical cardiac dysfunction, or provide reassurance when there are serial changes of LVEF potentially due to measurement variability rather than truly anticancer treatment emergent LV dysfunction (variation in LVEF of $<6\%$ with noncontrast 3D echocardiography and <10% with 2D echocardiography).

The incorporation of GLS assessment into the cardio-oncology echocardiographic protocol published by the ASE and EACVI demonstrates a major step toward wider acceptance of this useful modality. Contemporary myocardial deformation imaging for assessment of GLS is most commonly carried out with 2D speckle tracking echocardiography, which has well-known normal but vendor-specific ranges (18%–22%) and higher reproducibility (5.5%–9.5% variability) compared with conventional LVEF assessment (12%–15% variability).

Studies have consistently shown that abnormal GLS precedes diagnostic reductions of LVEF by about 3 months, which might provide a window of chance to initiate cardioprotective therapy aimed at preventing cardiotoxicity and the following interruption or discontinuation of potentially lifesaving anticancer treatment.

The risk of cardiotoxicity has been higher in metastatic patients compared with adjuvant patients, frequently with 10% experiencing heart failure and 25% suffering reduced LVEF while on therapy. This is likely related to higher prior cumulative doses of anthracycline, concomitant treatment, and relatively older patients with more comorbidities. Nonetheless, there was a marked survival advantage with trastuzumab in these trials, with a relatively low termination rate due to cardiotoxicity. The willingness to continue trastuzumab despite reduced LVEF likely reflects a shift in benefit/risk related to the poor survival in metastatic breast cancer (22% at 5 years) compared with early-stage disease (97% and 77%, respectively, in 5 years). It has been observed that breast cancer survivors are at a higher risk for cardiovascular-related mortality compared with age-matched counterparts without cancer, and these patients have closely twice the whole risk of mortality.[8,10–14]

### Asymptomatic Patients and LVEF Decrease

Cardiology consultation, if possible by a cardio-oncology specialist, has been related with better rates of cardioprotective medication adherence and better survival compared with patients without cardiology consultation in a retrospective study of patients with anthracycline cardiotoxicity. According to the previous study, patients with anthracycline-induced reduced LVEF have a 50% chance of partial LVEF recovery on ACE-I therapy, in combination with carvedilol if it is possible. Treatment is related with improved cardiac event-free survival, and the clinical benefit appears greatest if the medication is started early (within

6 months) vs late (more than 1 year). No specific trials have assessed the efficacy of ARB or BBs therapy alone in patients with anthracycline-induced reduced LVEF.

Patients with reduced LVEF (less than 50%) at baseline are high risk and must be treated with anthracyclines carefully due to the risk of recurrent or progressive and irreversible cardiotoxicity with further cumulative anthracycline dosing. If there are acceptable alternative anticancer drugs to anthracycline, these must be considered.

If anthracycline chemotherapy is essential, LVEF should be measured before at least every other cycle of chemotherapy. Multiple lines of high-level evidence prove the efficacy of reducing anthracycline cardiotoxicity with dexrazoxane, often with a threefold to fourfold or more reduction in LVD. However, concerns regarding reduced antitumor efficacy (with no definitive data) and significant myelosuppression have limited its clinical impact. Dexrazoxane might be appropriate in patients with the highest risk of cardiotoxicity, such as those with pretreatment reduced LVEF, provided that it is prescribed before each anthracycline dose. Though liposomal doxorubicin preparations might reduce anthracycline cardiotoxicity, its widespread use in patients at high risk is not presently supported by high-level evidence.[6,8,11–15]

### Asymptomatic Patients and LVEF Decrease Treated With Trastuzumab

FDA suggested cardiology consultation and discontinuing of trastuzumab for 4 weeks if the LVEF falls by 15% from baseline, or if LVEF falls 10% below the lower limit of normal. Of course, trastuzumab may be safely restarted if the LVEF returns to normal and within 15% of baseline. Though, more recently, some studies reported worsening in cardiac dysfunction in patients who were continued on trastuzumab therapy despite evidence of mild LV dysfunction during screening by transthoracic echocardiography (TTE) (LVEF >50%). The authors recommend considering continuing to treat patients with trastuzumab despite mild asymptomatic LV dysfunction by first beginning preventive and cardioprotective therapy (BBs and ACE-Is or ARBs) without discontinuing of trastuzumab.[8,10–13]

### Asymptomatic Patients With Normal LVEF but Reduction in Average GLS

There is early evidence that carvedilol might be helpful in improving GLS in patients undergoing chemotherapy, especially when it is reduced during treatment. Use of ACE-Is and ARBs in this setting is based on expert opinion and the established successful use in patients with depressed LVEF. It would be noted that the utility of advanced speckle tracking including GLS in the cardio-oncology population is helpful but needs further researches.

## Asymptomatic Patients and an Increase in Cardiac Troponin

Troponin elevation has been studied to allow for an early diagnosis of cardiac injury during cancer chemotherapy. It has been shown to predict the development of future ventricular dysfunction as well as its severity. This strategy might be particularly helpful and must be considered in high-risk patients. Early initiation of cardioprotective therapy with ACE-Is in patients with high TnI has been shown to prevent late cardiotoxicity in the form of cardiomyopathy and heart failure. For patients undergoing anthracycline-based chemotherapy, simultaneous dexrazoxane use might also be considered.

Though BBs, specially carvedilol in combination with ACEIs, have been shown to have a cardioprotective effect in preventing anthracycline-induced cardiomyopathy, when used for primary prevention, there are no specific data regarding the use of BBs with elevated TnI without LV dysfunction; however, it is clinically rational to use cardioprotective therapy in this setting.

Minor troponin elevation without substantial LV dysfunction does not necessarily warrant permanent discontinuation of anticancer therapy, but rather a careful assessment and the addition of cardioprotective therapy with close cardiac following should be considered.[6–8]

## Clinical Cardiac Dysfunction

The mortality rate of patients with clinical cardiac dysfunction with symptoms of heart failure induced by cancer therapy is worse than that of many cancers. In addition, essential antitumor therapy is interrupted in a significant number of patients due to heart failure. It is suggested that a close collaborative relationship be established between oncologists, radiotherapists, and cardiologists when anticancer therapy is discontinued due to heart failure, or when choices about anticancer therapy are meaningfully modified due to preexisting or coexistent cardiac disease. Symptomatic patients with significant reduction in LVEF are classified as stage C heart failure (structural heart disease with prior or current symptoms of heart failure) and must be treated with heart failure-specific medications in accordance with clinical practice guidelines. In many instances,

standard cardiac-based therapy might stabilize or correct abnormalities that would allow anticancer therapy to continue. However, these interventions are only likely to be effective when initiated early in the course of heart failure. Therefore, early recognition of the clinical signs and symptoms of heart failure is vital to simplify early intervention. Acute heart failure is a life threatening but remediable medical condition. If acute heart failure happens, the patient must be managed intensively in an emergency setting.

In principle, this would be constant with an AHA/ACC stage B patient who has evidence of structural heart damage. All such patients must be optimized, if possible, before beginning potentially cardiotoxic therapy. Patients with *LVEF <40%*. Due to the fact that moderate to severe LV dysfunction might progress, if not treated efficiently, and has a considerable impact on heart failure morbidity and mortality, patients with this degree of LV dysfunction must generally not be treated with anthracyclines. Regardless of the type of anticancer therapy contemplated, all patients with symptoms or signs suggesting heart failure must be assessed further, including an assessment of LVEF and other tests as needed, which might be extensive or limited in scope. Patients must be diagnosed quickly to ensure appropriate management of symptoms, decrease of recurrent events, and safe continuance and completion of anticancer therapy if it is possible (Figs. 42.3–42.5).[8,10–16]

## PATIENTS WITH A HISTORY OF MEDIASTINAL CHEST RADIATION

Rate of coronary artery disease happens at an increased rate beginning 2–4 years after treatment, and the degree of increased risk of cardiac events is proportional to the dose of radiation received. In breast cancer patients receiving >10 Gy of radiotherapy to the heart, there was a >100% increased relative risk of major cardiac events. In the same way, in patients with chest radiotherapy for lung cancer, there was a >10% chance of severe cardiac events, and that risk was higher with preexisting heart disease. Radiation-induced valvular disease is an increasingly recognized entity occurring late after mediastinal radiotherapy with a median time to diagnosis of 22 years. Radiotherapy induces thickening, fibrosis, retraction, and calcification of valvular tissue that continues for at least 20 years, unrelatedly of patient age and traditional risk factors. Regurgitation related to leaflet retraction predominates in the first decade, followed by progressive stenosis due to fibrosis and calcification in the second decade and later. The incidence of

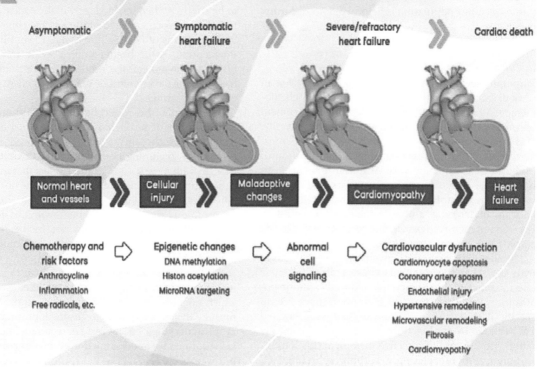

FIG. 42.3 Staging of heart failure in chemotherapy.

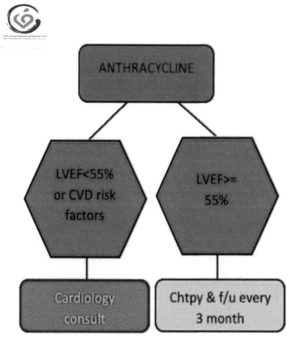

FIG. 42.4 LVEF in anthracycline therapy.

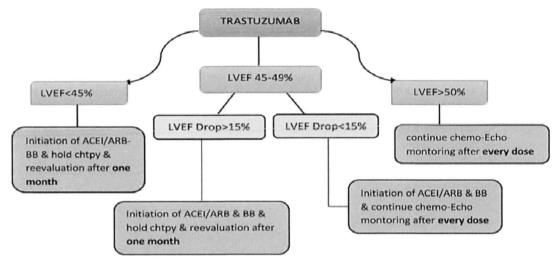

FIG. 42.5 Monitoring and management of trastuzumab-induced cardiotoxicity.

moderate or more valvular stenosis or regurgitation is 1% at 10 years, 4% at 15 years, 6% at 20 years, and 9% at 25 years. Left-sided lesions predominate, with the aortic valve the most commonly affected valve, followed by the mitral valve.

The ASE and the EACVI recommend a targeted yearly clinical history and physical examination with echocardiography for symptomatic patients. For asymptomatic patients, the ASE/EACVI recommends a screening transthoracic echocardiogram at 10 years post-radiotherapy and serial exams every 5 years afterward. The National Comprehensive Cancer Network (NCCN) has similar period recommendations for stress echocardiography. Specific transesophageal (specially 3D) and stress echocardiography may be considered for the assessment of radiotherapy-induced mitral valve disease and also dobutamine stress echocardiography for detection of low-flow aortic valve stenosis.[12–14]

## CONCLUSION

Concerns about potential cardiovascular damage resulting from anticancer therapies should be weighed against the potential benefits. Cardiovascular complications in patients with cancer are complex, and it is dominant that individual patient management is personalized. Though cancer treatment-related cardiotoxicity was initially observed as early as the 1970s, the current scene has changed intensely with the introduction of novel targeted therapies. The scope of cardio-oncology is wide and includes not just prevention, detection, monitoring, and treatment of cardiovascular toxicity related to anticancer therapy, however, also the development of future novel anticancer treatments that have minimal impact on cardiovascular health. Close association between oncologists, cardiologists, and allied health-care professionals will ensure delivery of optimal care for cancer patients, based on current best clinical practices, without compromising cardiovascular health. Precise and comprehensive researches will help describe best strategies for prevention, early detection, and also management of cardiovascular complications related to anticancer therapy. The integration of surveillance strategies in cancer survivors will help prevent the potential long-term cardiovascular morbidity and mortality related with oncological treatments. Education of health-care providers, mainly the next generation of cardiologists and oncologists, along with patients, on the importance of cardiovascular health and anticancer treatments should translate into better cancer and cardiovascular clinical outcomes.

## REFERENCES

1. Alizadehasl A, Amin A, Maleki M, Noohi F, Ghavamzadeh A, Farrashi M. Cardio-oncology discipline: focus on the necessities in developing countries. *ESC Heart Fail.* 2020;7:2175–2183. https://doi.org/10.1002/ehf2.12838.
2. Lenneman CG, Kimmick GG, Sawyer DB. Epidemiology of cardio-oncology. In: Kimmick GG, Lenihan DJ, Sawyer DB, Mayer EL, Hershman DL, eds, *Cardio-Oncology.* Springer; 2017:1–14.

3. Al-Kindi SG, Oliveira GH. Prevalence of preexisting cardiovascular disease in patients with different types of cancer: the unmet need for Onco-Cardiology. *Mayo Clin Proc.* 2016;91:81–83.

4. Patnaik JL, Byers T, DiGuiseppi C, Dabelea D, Denberg TD. Cardiovascular disease competes with breast cancer as the leading cause of death for older females diagnosed with breast cancer: a retrospective cohort study. *Breast Cancer Res.* 2011;13:R64.

5. Melloni C, Inohara T, Endo A. Unmet needs in managing myocardial infarction in patients with malignancy. *Front Cardiovasc Med.* 2019;6:57.

6. Fradley MG, Brown AC, Shields B, et al. Developing a comprehensive cardio-oncology program at a cancer institute: the Moffitt Cancer Center experience. *Oncol Rev.* 2017;11:340.

7. Nhola LF, Villarraga HR. Rationale for cardio-oncology units. *Rev Esp Cardiol (Engl Ed).* 2017;70:583–589.

8. Plana JC, Galderisi M, Barac A, et al. Expert consensus for multimodality imaging evaluation of adult patients during and after cancer therapy: a report from the American Society of Echocardiography and the European Association of Cardiovascular Imaging. *J Am Soc Echocardiogr.* 2014;27:911–939.

9. Quaresma M, Coleman MP, Rachet B. 40-Year trends in an index of survival for all cancers combined and survival adjusted for age and sex for each cancer in England and Wales, 1971–2011: a population-based study. *Lancet.* 2015;385:1206–1218.

10. Allemani C, Weir HK, Carreira H, et al. Global surveillance of cancer survival 1995–2009: analysis of individual data for 25,676,887 patients from 279 population-based registries in 67 countries (CONCORD-2). *Lancet.* 2015;385:977–1010.

11. Freeman AM, Herrmann J, Iliescu C, et al. Cardiovascular health of patients with cancer and cancer survivors: a roadmap to the next level. *J Am Coll Cardiol.* 2015;65: 2739–2746.

12. Alizadehasl A, Khorasani SH, Maleki M. Left ventricular dyssynchrony and chemotherapy-induced cardiotoxicity. *EC Cardiol.* 2020;SI.02:01–02.

13. Zohrian F, Alizadehasl A, Zahedi L, Ghaderian H, Anbiaee R, Azade P. Assessment of cardiac function by advanced echocardiography in breast cancer patients (HER2 positive vs HER2 negative). *Multidiscip Cardio Annal.* 2020;e103004.    https://doi.org/10.5812/mca.103004. Online ahead of Print.

14. Jaworski C, Mariani JA, Wheeler G, Kaye DM. Cardiac complications of thoracic irradiation. *J Am Coll Cardiol.* 2013;61:2319–2328.

15. Darby S, Ewertz M, McGale P, et al. Risk of ischemic heart disease in women after radiotherapy for breast cancer. *N Engl J Med.* 2013;368:987–998.

16. Witteles RM, Telli M. Underestimating cardiac toxicity in cancer trials: lessons learned. *J Clin Oncol.* 2012;30: 1916–1918.

# CHAPTER 43

# Anesthesia and Sedation in Cardiac Patients

RASOUL AZARFARIN
Rajaie Cardiovascular, Medical & Research Center, Iran University of Medical Sciences, Tehran, Iran

---

**KEY POINTS**

- Anesthetic management of patients includes preoperative evaluation of patients, intraoperative management, and postanesthesia care in the recovery room or intensive care unit; another name for anesthesiology is *perioperative medicine*.
- Cardiac anesthesia is a rapidly growing subspecialty that can be challenging for both trainees and practitioners.
- Cardiac anesthesiologists must understand pathophysiology, pharmacology, intensive care medicine, cardiology, and cardiac surgery. They must have comprehensive knowledge of and skill in airway management, respiratory care, and cardiopulmonary resuscitation and treatment of critically ill patients.

---

## INTRODUCTION

Anesthesiology can be defined as "intensive internal medicine," so an anesthesiologist must have the knowledge of an internist about the function of all organ systems such as cardiovascular, respiratory, gastrointestinal, renal, hematologic, and so on in critical situations. The anesthesiologist transfers the patient from a physiologic awake status to a nonphysiologic "anesthesia" status (anesthesia induction), maintains the patient in this controlled nonphysiologic status until the end of the surgery (or any invasive medical procedure), and then gradually returns the patient to his or her previous physiologic status (recovery from anesthesia and sedation). An anesthesiologist must maintain all organ system functions in physiologic normal limits during this special critical and intensive circumstance.

In addition to basic anesthesiologist knowledge and skills, a "cardiac anesthesiologist" must be extensively literate in cardiovascular diseases and adequately informed about various cardiovascular surgeries and interventional procedures. The cardiovascular field is a rapidly growing discipline, so each year, numerous novel drugs, procedures, and guidelines are introduced; as such, cardiologists and cardiac anesthesiologists must be up to date in all of these new findings and literature.

On the other hand, cardiologists routinely face numerous clinical scenarios when their patients require analgesia, sedation, and even full anesthesia. In acute coronary syndrome (ACS), patients need adequate pain management to reduce sympathetic activation and manage the oxygen supply and demand equation. Also, opioid (e.g., morphine) administration has a crucial role in the management of patients with pulmonary edema. Different imaging modalities such as cardiac magnetic resonance imaging and transesophageal echocardiography need patient sedation and analgesia to provide a calm situation and better cardiologist and patient satisfaction. Most diagnostic cardiac interventions and all therapeutic cardiac catheterizations require light to deep patient sedation and even total anesthesia (e.g., during transcatheter aortic valve implantation (TAVI), endovascular aneurysm repair, and endovascular aortic repair (EVAR)). Therefore, cardiologists must have adequate knowledge about various hypnotics and opioid and nonopioid analgesics and sedation techniques. Considering the risk of cardiorespiratory arrest in cardiac care units (CCUs) or catheterization laboratories, cardiologists should be trained enough to do cardiopulmonary resuscitation (CPR) procedures, including airway management (mask-bag ventilation or endotracheal intubation). On the other hand, sick patients in the CCU may require mechanical ventilation, so cardiologists should have basic knowledge and skills in the primary setting of mechanical ventilation machines. Thus, in training cardiology courses, these topics must be learned by cardiac anesthesiologists theoretically and in "skills labs."

Patients with coronary artery, valvular, and congenital heart diseases may undergo cardiovascular surgery for palliative or definitive treatment. Also, some cardiac patients may be candidates for different noncardiac surgeries. Risk assessment and preoperative preparation of such patients is the combined responsibility of anesthesiologists, cardiologists, and surgeons to schedule patients for surgery in the best medical condition.

## PREOPERATIVE ANESTHETIC ASSESSMENT OF PATIENTS FOR CARDIAC SURGERY

Nowadays, there is a trend toward the evaluation of elective cardiac surgery patients in "preadmission anesthesia clinics," usually 7–14 days before an operation. This approach permits most of the necessary laboratory and imaging tests to be ready before hospital admission, allowing enough time to organize supplementary patient medical workup without delaying surgery and allowing admission of the patient on the day of surgery.[1] With this strategy, hospital beds are saved for more surgical patients and patients' stressful waiting days before surgery have been shortened. Additionally, through careful examination of the patient's respiratory, endocrine, and other organ systems by an expert anesthesiologist, most of the routine (and unnecessary) consultations with pulmonologists, endocrinologists, and other specialists can be omitted, leading to significant savings of time and resources.

It is well known that coexisting risk factors have been related to higher mortality and morbidity in the perioperative period.[1] These consist of age older than 60 years, body mass below 20 or above 35 kg/m$^2$, diabetes, systemic and pulmonary hypertension,[2] heart failure, peripheral vascular disease, renal failure, ACS, chronic lung disease (COPD), neurologic disorders, and redo cardiac operations. In addition to taking cardiovascular drugs such as antianginal, antihypertensive, antiplatelet, anticoagulant, and diuretic drugs, it is common that patients are also receiving bronchodilator, oral hypoglycemic (or even insulin), proton pump inhibitor, corticosteroid, or psychological drugs. It is very important to ask the patient whether he or she has recently used drugs that have an effect on the coagulation system such as aspirin, warfarin, heparin (unfractionated or enoxaparin), nonsteroidal antiinflammatory drugs, clopidogrel, or thrombolytic drugs and to clearly ask the time interval since cessation of the drug.[1] In addition to the usual laboratory tests of coagulation (prothrombin

time, partial thromboplastin time, international normalized ratio, or platelet count),[3] it is crucial to assess platelet aggregometry and rotational thromboelastography (ROTEM) in patients who have taken clopidogrel recently (<3–5 days) and candidates for coronary bypass grafting surgery (CABG) as soon as possible.

Mahla et al.[4] assessed the role of platelet function testing by thromboelastography in clopidogrel-treated patients who were candidates for CABG. They measured maximal clot firmness (MCF) in thromboelastography and concluded that the patients have reduced postoperative bleeding and blood transfusion if CABG was done within 1 day when MCF is greater than 50 mm and within 3–5 days if MCF was 35–50 mm and that surgery should be postponed for more than 5 days if MCF is less than 35 mm![4] Unfortunately, anemia is a common finding in cardiac patients, especially those with heart failure.[5]

## RISK ASSESSMENT OF PATIENTS FOR CARDIAC SURGERY

Despite improvements in surgical and anesthetic methods, cardiac surgery potentially has a limited risk of mortality and morbidity. It is the shared responsibility of the cardiologist, anesthesiologist, and cardiac surgeon to assist the patient to weigh the risks and benefits of surgery against medical or interventional therapy. Therefore, it is crucial that the cardiologist understand how risk is evaluated in a specific patient who is referred to the cardiology clinic and in candidates for cardiac surgery. In 1989, Parsonnet et al.[6] recognized 14 independent risk factors for death after cardiac surgery. The so-called Parsonnet score (Table 43.1) was accepted by many centers around the globe and is still in use.

However, with the development of the European System for Cardiac Operative Risk Evaluation (EuroSCORE)[7] in 1999, most surgeons replaced the Parsonnet score by EuroSCORE. The EuroSCORE offers a tougher risk assessment, which similar to its ancestor, can be easily calculated at the bedside of patients in clinics and has been shown to be having a good predictive value regarding major complications, duration of intensive care unit (ICU) stay, and resource consumption (Table 43.2). For high-risk patients, the new logistic EuroSCORE II (http://www.euroscore.org/calc.html) delivers a more precise prediction than the previous additive score. It must be kept in mind that each community has its own characteristics of population and pattern of cardiovascular risk factors that should be considered by the community's practitioners.[8]

For example, a 60-year-old man presenting with asymptomatic severe left main stem coronary artery

## TABLE 43.1
## The Parsonnet Additive Risk Stratification Model for Cardiac Surgery

| Factor | Points |
|---|---|
| **AGE (YEAR)** | |
| 70–74 | 7 |
| 74–79 | 12 |
| >84 | 20 |
| Diabetes mellitus | 3 |
| Hypertension | 3 |
| Morbid obesity | 3 |
| Female | 1 |
| Dialysis dependent | 10 |
| Catheter laboratory complication | 10 |
| "Catastrophic state" | 10–50 |
| "Rare conditions" | 2–10 |
| **LV FUNCTION** | |
| Good (LVEF ≥50%) | 0 |
| Moderate (LVEF 30%–49%) | 2 |
| Poor (LVEF <30%) | 4 |
| LV aneurysm | 5 |
| *Redo procedure* | |
| First | 5 |
| Second or subsequent | 10 |
| Preoperative IABP | 2 |
| Mitral valve surgery | 5 |
| Pulmonary artery pressure ≤60 mmHg | 3 |
| Aortic valve surgery | 5 |
| Aortic valve gradient >120 mmHg | 2 |
| Valve + CABG surgery | 2 |

*CABG*, Coronary artery bypass graft; *IABP*, intraaortic balloon pump; *LV*, left ventricular; *LVEF*, left ventricular ejection fraction.
From Parsonnet V, Dean D, Bernstein AD. A method of uniform stratification of risk for evaluating the results of surgery in acquired adult heart disease. *Circulation*. 1989;79:I3-I12; with permission.

stenosis and normal left ventricular ejection fraction (LVEF) who is a candidate for elective isolated CABG surgery has a EuroSCORE II predicted mortality of 0.94%. On the other hand, a 75-year-old woman with LVEF less than 30%, chronic lung disease, and class IV angina scheduled for emergency CABG has a predicted mortality of 38.74% (see http://www.euroscore.org/calc.html).

At the end of the preoperative evaluation, the cardiac anesthetist should explain what the patient can anticipate on the day of surgery—for example, the fasting period, premedication with anxiolytics, transfer time to the operating room, and placement of intravenous (IV) or arterial access before anesthesia induction. The anesthesiologist can explain the situation of the immediate postoperative period, including having an endotracheal tube in place during transfer to the ICU and the gradual awakening of the patient some hours later. The patient can receive enough information about the course of weaning from mechanical ventilation, assurance about the provision of analgesia, adequate warming, and prevention of nausea and vomiting. Also, common anesthetic minor sequelae (e.g., bruising in IV access sites, peripheral vein phlebitis, hoarseness, sore throat, and nausea and vomiting) should also be discussed with the patient.

## PRINCIPLES OF CARDIAC ANESTHESIA

Regarding the complexity of cardiovascular diseases, including a long list of anesthetic and cardiovascular drugs and techniques, as well as various monitoring systems and management guidelines, *cardiac anesthesia* is a rapidly expanding subspecialty that is challenging for both trainees and everyday practitioners. Cardiac anesthesiologists are required to understand physiology, pathology, pharmacology, internal medicine, intensive care medicine, cardiology, and cardiac surgery perform to their extensive duties. Cardiac anesthesiologists must have comprehensive knowledge and skills on airway management, mechanical ventilation, respiratory care, and CPR (including postresuscitation care). They should be able to manage critically ill cardiac patients in cardiogenic shock who may require advanced support systems such as intra-aortic balloon pumps, left ventricular assist devices, and extracorporeal membrane oxygenation (ECMO).

By establishing a multidisciplinary approach—including a cardiac anesthesiologist, cardiologist, and cardiac surgeon—cardiac surgery outcomes have constantly improved despite the increasing complexity of procedures and comorbid sicker patients. Nowadays sophisticated and high-technologic monitoring techniques (invasive systemic, pulmonary and central venous pressure measurement, peripheral pulse, cerebral and regional oximetry, bispectral index (BIS), intraoperative transesophageal echocardiography (TEE, both two and three dimensional), capnography, nerve stimulator,

**TABLE 43.2**
**EuroSCORE: The European System for Cardiac Operative Risk Evaluation Additive Risk Stratification Model**

| Factor | | Points | β |
|---|---|---|---|
| Age | Per 5 year or part there of more than 60 year | 1 | 0.0666354 |
| Sex | Female | 1 | 0.3304052 |
| Chronic pulmonary disease | Long-term use of bronchodilators or steroids for lung disease | 1 | 0.4931341 |
| Extracardiac arteriopathy | *Any one or more of the following:* claudication, carotid occlusion or >50% stenosis, previous or planned intervention on the abdominal aorta, limb arteries, or carotids | 2 | 0.6558917 |
| Neurologic dysfunction | Severely affecting ambulation or day-to-day functioning | 2 | 0.841626 |
| Previous cardiac surgery | Requiring opening of the pericardium | 3 | 1.002625 |
| Serum creatinine | >200 μmol/L before operation | 2 | 0.6521653 |
| Active endocarditis | Patient still under antibiotic treatment for endocarditis at the time of surgery | 3 | 1.101265 |
| Critical preoperative state | *Any one or more of the following:* VT or VF or aborted sudden death, preoperative cardiac massage, preoperative ventilation before arrival in the anesthetic room, preoperative inotropic support, IABP, or preoperative acute renal failure (anuria or oliguria <10 mL/h) | 2 | 0.9058132 |
| Unstable angina | Rest angina requiring IV nitrates until arrival in the anesthetic room | 2 | 0.5677075 |
| LV dysfunction | Moderate (LVEF 30%–50%)<br>Poor (LVEF <30%) | 1<br>3 | 0.4191643<br>1.094443 |
| Recent myocardial infarct | Within 90 days | 2 | 0.5460218 |
| Pulmonary hypertension | Systolic pulmonary artery pressure >60 mmHg | 2 | 0.7676924 |
| Emergency operation | Carried out on referral before the beginning of the next working day | 2 | 0.7127953 |
| Other than isolated CABG | Major cardiac procedure other than or in addition to CABG | 2 | 0.5420364 |
| Surgery on thoracic aorta | For disorder of ascending arch or descending arch | 3 | 1.159787 |
| Postinfarct septal rupture | | 4 | 1.462009 |

*CABG*, coronary artery bypass graft; *IABP*, intraaortic balloon pump; *LV*, left ventricular; *LVEF*, left ventricular ejection fraction; *VF*, ventricular fibrillation; *VT*, ventricular tachycardia.
From Nashef SA, Roques F, Michel P, et al. European system for cardiac operative risk evaluation (EuroSCORE). *Eur J Cardiothorac Surg*. 1999;16:9–13; with permission.

point-of-care coagulation and blood gas analyses, and various noninvasive measurements of numerous hemodynamic parameters) have come into practice to ensure the best patient safety. So, the mortality rate completely attributable to anesthesia becomes very rare. The anesthesia-related death rate was 1.1 per million

population per year, with the rate for males almost twice the rate for females (1.45 vs 0.77). In an epidemiologic study of anesthesia-related deaths in the United States, Guohua et al.[9] reported that the death rate was 1.1 per 1 million population per year. The death rate for men is nearly twice the rate for women (1.45 vs 0.77). The mortality rate was different with age. The lowest rate was seen in children aged 5–14 years, and the highest rate was observed in those aged 85 years of age or older.[9]

## CARDIAC ANESTHESIA DRUGS AND TECHNIQUES

A wide range of drugs is used for induction and maintenance of general anesthesia. Currently, there is not a single universally recognized drug or drug combination or technique for anesthetic management in cardiac surgery. Balanced general anesthesia, by definition, consists of four principal components: hypnosis (loss of consciousness), amnesia, analgesia, and muscle relaxation.[10] Generally, the single or various combinations of anesthetic drugs used are based on the pathophysiologic condition of the cardiac patient and the individual preference and experience of the cardiac anesthesiologist.

The main goals of cardiac anesthesiologists are to provide balanced general anesthesia while maintaining stable hemodynamics, preserving myocardial (and other organs') function, providing acceptable cardiac output, and preventing myocardial ischemia. To achieve these goals, most anesthesiologists consider the opioids a core component of "cardiac anesthesia" to provide intense analgesia to adequately suppress sympathetic stimulation to noxious stimuli. They also use appropriate doses of hypnotics (inhalational or IV) to reach a complete loss of consciousness and administer some doses of muscle relaxants to immobilize the patient. For high-risk cardiac patients with ventricular

dysfunction, monitoring of depth of anesthesia (by BIS) or neuromuscular blockade (by nerve stimulator) allows anesthesiologists to use minimum acceptable doses of hypnotics and muscle relaxant drugs to maintain stable hemodynamics and rapid recovery from anesthesia after surgery. Table 43.3 summarizes the effect of commonly used anesthetic drugs on four components of general anesthesia.

Some anesthesiologists use spinal or epidural[11] anesthesia, especially in noncardiac surgery (NCS) in cardiac patients. Bupivacaine and lidocaine with or without combination with opioids, epinephrine, or corticosteroids are commonly used for this reason.[12]

### Inhalational Anesthetics

Three volatile inhalational agents—isoflurane, sevoflurane, and desflurane—are commonly used in cardiac anesthesia. Nitrous oxide is not used in open heart surgery because of the risk of bubble formation and embolization. The potency of inhalational agents is defined as the minimal alveolar concentration (MAC). MAC denotes the alveolar concentration of vapor at which 50% of patients do not move in response to a painful surgical stimulus. MAC is also used to compare the potency of inhaled anesthetics. For the determination of MAC, the skin incision was used as a stimulus. At a level of $1.3 \times$ MAC, nearly all (95%) patients do not respond to painful stimuli.[12] The rate of anesthesia induction, variations in anesthetic depth, and recovery from inhalational anesthetics depend on the blood: gas solubility ratio. The higher the blood:gas solubility

**TABLE 43.3**
**Anesthesia-Related Effects of Specific Drugs**

| Drug | Hypnosis | Analgesia | Amnesia | Muscle Relaxation[a] |
|---|---|---|---|---|
| Volatile anesthetics | ↑ | ↑ | ↑ | ↑ |
| Barbiturates | ↑↑ | NC | ↑ | NC |
| Ketamine | ↑↑ | ↑ | ↑↑ | NC |
| Propofol | ↑↑ | ↑ | ↑ | ↑ |
| Etomidate | ↑↑ | ↑ | NC | NC |
| Benzodiazepines | ↑↑ | NC | ↑↑ | NC |
| Opioids | ↑ | ↑↑ | NC | ↓ |
| Succinylcholine | NC | NC | NC | ↑↑ |
| Non-depolarizing neuromuscular blockers | NC | NC | NC | ↑↑ |

NC, no change.
[a]Arrows indicate degree of increase or decrease.
From Alwardt CM, Redford D, Larson DF. General anesthesia in cardiac surgery: a review of drugs and practices. J Extra Corpor Technol. 2005;37 (2):227–235; with permission.

ratio, the slower the reaction (induction or recovery) to inhalational anesthetics.

*Isoflurane* is the most commonly used inhalational anesthetic in cardiac surgery. Its acceptance is partly related to its minimal cardiovascular effects compared with the older volatile anesthetics halothane and enflurane. Because of airway irritation and pungency, isoflurane is not a good volatile agent for inhalational induction (especially in pediatric patients). Isoflurane decreases systemic vascular resistance in higher degrees than other agents. However, cardiac output is preserved because of an active "carotid baroreceptor reflex" and reduced afterload. The chemical structure and clinical characteristics of desflurane are very similar to those of isoflurane.

*Sevoflurane* is the volatile anesthetic that is commonly used because of its nonpungency and relatively fast increases in alveolar concentration (low solubility). Also, sevoflurane has myocardial protective effects and can preserve ventricular function. However, unlike with isoflurane and desflurane, cardiac output is not maintained in higher concentrations of sevoflurane. A benefit of sevoflurane over isoflurane is that there is no coronary steal effect. Also, sevoflurane has some bronchodilatory effects that are valuable in preventing bronchospasm, similar to isoflurane and other inhaled anesthetics.

*Thiopental sodium* is the barbiturate used for IV induction of anesthesia in cardiac surgery. It is the only ultrashort-acting drug that is used for induction. This short duration of action is caused mainly by rapid redistribution and not by elimination. Barbiturates have neuroprotective and anticonvulsive effects and are used to protect the central nervous system (CNS) during cardiopulmonary bypass (CPB) with deep hypothermic circulatory arrest.

*Propofol* is a lipid-soluble agent that rapidly crosses the blood–brain barrier and has a fast onset of action, so induction of anesthesia occurs within 40 s. Propofol is a common choice among anesthesiologists because of rapid induction and emergence from anesthesia that enable early extubation because of its fast metabolism. Propofol decreases blood pressure, heart rate, and myocardial function dose-dependently. Heart rate and blood pressure decrease; although this is transient with propofol, it may be significant and can be dangerous in a patient with reduced cardiovascular reserve. Propofol also has a dose-dependent respiratory depressant effect and rapidly causes apnea in induction doses. It has some bronchodilator effect. Propofol should not be used by nonanesthesiologists.

*Etomidate* is commonly used for induction of general anesthesia. Its injection into peripheral veins sometimes causes pain. Etomidate is unique in its cardiovascular and respiratory effects that are almost negligible, with mild reductions in blood pressure and ventilation. Although etomidate leads to nearly no cardiac depression in healthy individuals, it can cause indirect cardiac depression in compromised and critically ill patients. Etomidate induction can induce myoclonic movements in some patients. But pretreatment with midazolam or sufentanil may decrease myoclonus. Etomidate also has a potential of temporary adrenal suppression even with a single induction dose.

*Midazolam* is the most commonly used benzodiazepine for induction of anesthesia in cardiac surgery. Also, midazolam has amnestic and anxiolytic effects and could be a good agent for premedication. Compared with barbiturates, benzodiazepines have fewer cardiorespiratory effects, including a mild reduction in blood pressure and cardiac output. These effects are more prominent when used in combination with opioids. Generally, benzodiazepines seem to be safer than barbiturates in patients with cardiac disease. Respiratory suppression with midazolam is often mild, but it could be severe even with small doses in older adults and when used with narcotics.

Narcotics are the essential components of cardiac anesthesia. The most frequently used narcotics in cardiac surgery are *sufentanil*, *fentanyl*, and *remifentanil*. High-dose narcotic anesthesia has the benefit of hemodynamic stability without myocardial depression, but because of prolonged respiratory depression, mechanical ventilation is required after surgery. Although narcotics can certainly cause patient unconsciousness, obviously, they cannot induce complete general anesthesia. Narcotics can decrease the MAC of inhalational agents. In general, opioids must be used in combination with other hypnotic drugs. Most opioids are metabolized by the liver, and their metabolites are mainly excreted by the kidneys. Remifentanil has an ultrashort duration of action mainly because of its metabolism by nonspecific esterase enzymes. The most common side effect of opioids is respiratory depression; some patients may experience muscle rigidity. The effects of opioids can be reversed by an opioid antagonist, naloxone. Reversal of opioid effect in cardiac patients must be done with caution because this drug also antagonizes analgesic effects and can cause severe tachycardia, hypertension, and myocardial ischemia.

The neuromuscular blocking agents such as *vecuronium* and *cisatracurium* are nondepolarizing drugs that competitively antagonize acetylcholine in the nicotinic acetylcholine receptor at the neuromuscular junction. Vecuronium and cisatracurium have nearly no cardiovascular side effects, but *atracurium* causes some degrees of hypotension caused by histamine release. Muscle relaxants can be administered as multiple bolus doses or continuous infusion during surgery.[13] *Pancuronium* has an atropine-like structure and can cause tachycardia that is detrimental in ischemic patients and those with stenotic valvular lesions. Pancuronium could be an attractive muscle relaxant in pediatric patients who need an increased heart rate to have better cardiac output. Induction and maintenance doses of anesthetic drugs are summarized in Table 43.4.

Anesthetic management during cardiac surgery is not limited to the administration of anesthetic drugs; in fact, maintaining the patient's organ system functions in physiologic ranges is the main anesthesiologist responsibility. While the cardiac surgeon focuses on the operative field, the anesthesiologist must maintain normal hemodynamics and artificial (mechanical) respiratory function. He or she should preserve fluids and electrolytes within normal limits. Also, monitoring of the coagulation system and management of bleeding during CPB, particularly in complex cases, is the duty of the cardiac anesthesiologist. In addition, monitoring the nervous system (BIS or cerebral oximetry), glycemic control, temperature control, and assessing the urine output of anesthetized patients all are within the responsibility of the anesthesiologist. Hyperglycemia is a common finding during cardiac surgery both in diabetic and nondiabetic patients.[14–16] Glycemic control should be considered in both pediatric and adult patients during and after cardiac surgery.[17]

## Cardiopulmonary Bypass

In open heart surgery, CPB is needed to stop the heart from beating and open the cardiac chambers to surgically correct the defect, replace a valve, or bypass the coronary artery. CPB is a system that temporarily performs the function of the heart and lungs while the heart is arrested and ventilation is stopped during surgery. CPB circulates the blood through the body and supplies the oxygen requirements of the patient. The heparinized blood enters the reservoir via venous cannulation from the atria. Then blood passes through the membrane oxygenator while delivering $CO_2$ and getting $O_2$ (e.g., a lung). A ruler pump drives the oxygenated blood to the patient's aorta via an arterial cannula. Cardiac arrest for surgery is done by cardioplegia, which is a high-potassium solution injected into the coronary system from the aortic root. CPB is a shock-like state in which all body blood exits the body and enters an artificial tubing system. Severe inflammatory system activation occurs, and platelet activation and widespread adhesion lead to decrease in platelet count and function. Lack of pulsatile blood flow, change in osmotic pressure, and inflammation make the patient susceptible to generalized edema and multiorgan dysfunction. Coagulation system monitoring by activated clotting time (ACT) and blood component therapy is needed during and after CPB.

## NONCARDIAC SURGERY IN CARDIAC PATIENTS

Recent recommendations and guidelines for perioperative cardiovascular assessment and management for noncardiac operations are based mostly on clinical expert opinion; observational research; and in the best situation, prospective randomized clinical trials. The use of American College of Cardiology/American Heart Association or European Society of Cardiology (ESC)/ European Society of Anaesthesiology (ESA) practice guidelines to do appropriate preoperative laboratory tests, diagnostic imaging, and complementary treatments of coexisting diseases improves patient outcomes and decreases costs.[18,19] Preoperative evaluation of cardiac patients for noncardiac surgeries includes history

## TABLE 43.4
### Induction and Maintenance Dose of Commonly Used Anesthetic Drugs

| Drug | Initial (Induction) Dose | Maintenance (Infusion) Dose |
|---|---|---|
| Thiopental sodium[a] | 3–4 mg/kg | 10–120 µg/kg/h |
| Midazolam[a] | 0.05–0.2 mg/kg | 1–2 µg/kg/min |
| Propofol[a] | 1–2.5 mg/kg | 50–150 µg/kg/min |
| Etomidate[a] | 0.2–0.6 mg/kg | 0.2–0.7 µg/kg/h |
| Fentanyl[b] | 2–10 µg/kg | 0.5–5 µg/kg/h |
| Sufentanil[b] | 0.25–2 µg/kg | 0.2–2 µg/kg/h |
| Remifentanil[b] | 0.25–1 µg/kg | 0.1–1 µg/kg/min |
| Cisatracurium[c] | 0.1–0.2 mg/kg | 1–2 µg/kg/min |
| Atracurium[c] | 0.3–0.6 mg/kg | 2–10 µg/kg/min |
| Vecuronium[c] | 0.08–0.1 mg/kg | 0.8–1.2 µg/kg/min |
| Pancuronium[c] | 0.05–0.1 mg/kg | 0.1 mg/kg/h |

[a]Hypnotic.
[b]Opioid.
[c]Muscle relaxant.

taking; physical examination; and taking 12-lead electrocardiogram (ECG), exercise test, echocardiography, nuclear imaging test, and coronary angiography for assessing left ventricular function and evaluating cardiopulmonary function (Table 43.5).

Performing percutaneous coronary intervention or coronary artery bypass grafting before NCS should only be considered in patients with high-risk anatomic features and unstable coronary artery disease.[20] Most of the cardiovascular medication should be continued

**TABLE 43.5**
**Summary of Recommendations for Supplemental Preoperative Evaluation**

| Recommendations | COR | LOE |
|---|---|---|
| **THE 12-LEAD ECG** | | |
| Preoperative resting 12-lead ECG is reasonable for patients with known coronary heart disease or other significant structural heart disease, except for low-risk surgery | IIa | B |
| Preoperative resting 12-lead ECG may be considered for asymptomatic patients, except for low-risk surgery | IIb | B |
| Routine preoperative resting 12-lead ECG is not useful for asymptomatic patients undergoing low-risk surgery | III: no benefit | B |
| **ASSESSMENT OF LV FUNCTION** | | |
| It is reasonable for patients with dyspnea of unknown origin to undergo preoperative evaluation of LV function | IIa | C |
| It is reasonable for patients with HF with worsening dyspnea or other change in clinical status to undergo preoperative evaluation of LV function | IIa | C |
| Reassessment of LV function in clinically stable patients may be considered | IIb | C |
| Routine preoperative evaluation of LV function is not recommended | III: no benefit | B |
| **EXERCISE STRESS TESTING FOR MYOCARDIAL ISCHEMIA AND FUNCTIONAL CAPACITY** | | |
| For patients with elevated risk and excellent functional capacity, it is reasonable to forgo further exercise testing and proceed to surgery | IIa | B |
| For patients with elevated risk and unknown functional capacity, it may be reasonable to assess for functional capacity if it will change management | IIb | B |
| For patients with elevated risk and moderate to good functional capacity, it may be reasonable to forgo further exercise testing and proceed to surgery | IIb | B |
| For patients with elevated risk and poor or unknown functional capacity, it may be reasonable to perform exercise testing with cardiac imaging to assess for myocardial ischemia | IIb | C |
| Routine screening with noninvasive stress testing is not useful for low-risk noncardiac surgery | III: no benefit | B |
| **CARDIOPULMONARY EXERCISE TESTING** | | |
| Cardiopulmonary exercise testing may be considered for patients undergoing elevated risk procedures. | IIb | B |
| **NONINVASIVE PHARMACOLOGICAL STRESS TESTING BEFORE NONCARDIAC SURGERY** | | |
| It is reasonable for patients at elevated risk for noncardiac surgery with poor functional capacity to undergo either DSE or MPI if it will change management | IIa | B |
| Routine screening with noninvasive stress testing is not useful for low-risk noncardiac surgery | III: no benefit | B |
| **PREOPERATIVE CORONARY ANGIOGRAPHY** | | |
| Routine preoperative coronary angiography is not recommended | III: no benefit | C |

*COR,* class of recommendation; *DSE,* dobutamine stress echocardiogram; *ECG,* electrocardiogram; *HF,* heart failure; *LOE,* level of evidence; *LV,* left ventricular; *MPI,* myocardial perfusion imaging; *N/A,* not applicable.
From Parsonnet V, Dean D, Bernstein AD. A method of uniform stratification of risk for evaluating the results of surgery in acquired adult heart disease. *Circulation.* 1989;79:I3-I12; with permission.

before noncardiac operations. Clopidogrel can be continued before general surgeries with minimal risk of bleeding such as inguinal hernia repair and laparoscopic cholecystectomy.[21] It seems better to hold clopidogrel use 5–7 days before high-risk surgeries such as neurosurgical and major cancer or orthopedic operations. However, some studies recommended that the feasible time for clopidogrel discontinuation before NCSs is less than 5 days.[22] Platelet aggregometry or rotational ROTEM could be useful for precise assessment of platelet function before deciding to perform major noncardiac procedure, especially in emergency settings, to balance the risks and benefits of doing or delaying the surgery in

those taking clopidogrel (Tables 43.6 and 43.7 and Fig. 43.1).[23]

To apply the recommendations of perioperative practice guidelines, comprehensive perioperative teamwork is required. The perioperative team's work is aimed to include clinicians with related expertise to balance the benefits and risks of NCS. The team, by implementing evidence-based evaluation and considering the patient's preferences and values, makes the best decision. Members of this team should consist of the patient and his or her family along with the cardiologist, surgeon, anesthesiologist, an appropriate consultant, and the patient's primary care physician.

**TABLE 43.6**
**Summary of Recommendations for Anesthetic Consideration and Intraoperative Management**

| Recommendations | COR | LOE |
|---|---|---|
| **VOLATILE GENERAL ANESTHESIA VS TOTAL IV ANESTHESIA** | | |
| Use of either a volatile anesthetic agent or total IV anesthesia is reasonable for patients undergoing noncardiac surgery | IIa | A |
| **PERIOPERATIVE PAIN MANAGEMENT** | | |
| Neuraxial anesthesia for *postoperative* pain relief can be effective to reduce MI in patients undergoing abdominal aortic surgery | IIa | B |
| Preoperative epidural analgesia may be considered to decrease the incidence of *preoperative* cardiac events in patients with hip fracture | IIb | B |
| **PROPHYLACTIC INTRAOPERATIVE NITROGLYCERIN** | | |
| Prophylactic intraoperative nitroglycerin is not effective in reducing myocardial ischemia in patients undergoing noncardiac surgery | III: no benefit | B |
| **INTRAOPERATIVE MONITORING TECHNIQUES** | | |
| Emergency use of perioperative TEE in patients with hemodynamic instability is reasonable in patients undergoing noncardiac surgery if expertise is readily available | IIa | C |
| Routine use of perioperative TEE during noncardiac surgery is not recommended | III: no benefit | C |
| **MAINTENANCE OF BODY TEMPERATURE** | | |
| Maintenance of normothermia may be reasonable to reduce perioperative cardiac events | IIb | B |
| **HEMODYNAMIC ASSIST DEVICES** | | |
| Use of hemodynamic assist devices may be considered when urgent or emergency noncardiac surgery is required in the setting of acute severe cardiac dysfunction | IIb | C |
| **PERIOPERATIVE USE OF PULMONARY ARTERY CATHETERS** | | |
| Use of pulmonary artery catheterization may be considered when underlying medical conditions that significantly affect hemodynamics cannot be corrected before surgery | IIb | C |
| Routine use of pulmonary artery catheterization is not recommended | III: no benefit | A |

*COR*, class of recommendation; *LOE*, level of evidence; *IV*, intravenous; *MI*, myocardial infarction; *N/A*, not applicable; *TEE*, transesophageal echocardiogram.
From Velasco A, Reyes E, Hage FG. Guidelines in review: comparison of the 2014 ACC/AHA guidelines on perioperative cardiovascular evaluation and management of patients undergoing noncardiac surgery and the 2014 ESC/ESA guidelines on noncardiac surgery: cardiovascular assessment and management. *J Nucl Cardiol.* 2017;24(1):165–170; with permission.

**TABLE 43.7**

**Surgical Risk Estimate of 30-Day Cardiovascular Risk of Myocardial Infarction and Cardiovascular Death According to European Society of Cardiology (ESC)/European Society of Anaesthesiology (ESA) Guidelines**

| Low-Risk Surgery (<1%) | Intermediate-Risk Surgery (1%–5%) | High-Risk Surgery (>5%) |
| --- | --- | --- |
| Superficial surgery | Intraperitoneal | Pulmonary or liver transplant |
| Breast | Carotid, symptomatic | Total cystectomy |
| Dental | Intrathoracic minor | Aortic and major vascular surgery |
| Endocrine: thyroid | Peripheral arterial angioplasty | Duodenopancreatic surgery |
| Reconstructive | Endovascular aneurysm repair | Liver-resection bile duct surgery |
| Eye | Head and neck surgery | Esophagectomy |
| Carotid, symptomatic | Major orthopedic, neurologic, gynecologic, or urologic procedure | Repair of perforated bowel |
| Minor gynecologic | Renal transplant | Adrenal resection |
| Minor orthopedic | | Pneumonectomy |
| Minor urologic | | |

From Velasco A, Reyes E, Hage FG. Guidelines in review: comparison of the 2014 ACC/AHA guidelines on perioperative cardiovascular evaluation and management of patients undergoing noncardiac surgery and the 2014 ESC/ESA guidelines on noncardiac surgery: cardiovascular assessment and management. *J Nucl Cardiol.* 2017;24(1):165–170; with permission.

## SEDATION AND ANALGESIA FOR CARDIOVASCULAR PROCEDURES

An increasing number of various minimally invasive cardiovascular procedures are performed in millions of patients around the globe. These procedures range from different diagnostic or interventional angiographic catheterizations, TEE and other interventional imaging modalities, electrophysiology studies, and pacemaker implantation. All of these patients need local anesthesia and some degree of light to deep sedation and even full general anesthesia to make the procedure comfortable and safe for the patient and feasible for the practitioner. Usually, a moderate level of sedation is chosen. Moderate sedation and analgesia or conscious sedation is a drug-induced suppression of consciousness in which the patient responds to verbal commands, either alone or by a light tactile stimulation. No additional intervention is needed to maintain the patient's airway, and spontaneous breathing is adequate. Cardiovascular function and hemodynamic status are usually maintained within normal limits.

Preprocedural preparation and assessment are necessary for all patients planned for cardiovascular procedures. Careful history taking about previous experiences of anesthesia or sedation and any kind of drug or food allergy, cardiovascular and other drugs received by the patient, and any history of medical intervention is mandatory. It is well known that coexisting risk factors have been associated with higher mortality and morbidity in the periprocedural period.[1] The patient's American Society of Anesthesiologists (ASA) physical status class; New York Heart Association (NYHA) class; and other comorbidities such as obesity, systemic and pulmonary hypertension, heart failure, renal failure, ACSs, chronic lung disease, sleep apnea disorder, and neuropsychological disorders all are important to be considered. Airway assessment is an essential part of physical examination by the anesthesiologist or nonanesthesiologist provider of sedation.

Lidocaine usually is used for local anesthesia of the needle or catheter insertion site or the patient's pharynx in TEE examination. Lidocaine with 1%–2% concentration is used for cutaneous infiltration and local anesthesia. The maximum allowable dose of lidocaine is 4.5 mg/kg or 300 mg in normal healthy adults. Lidocaine must be administered only by trained clinicians who are well experienced in the diagnosis and management of the drug toxicity and other acute emergencies. Supplemental oxygen, CPR equipment, and drugs should be immediately available for proper management of toxic reactions and probable emergencies. Any delay in proper management of local anesthetic systemic toxicity, cardiac depression, or hypotension may rapidly progress to severe metabolic acidosis, cardiac arrest, and even the patient's death.

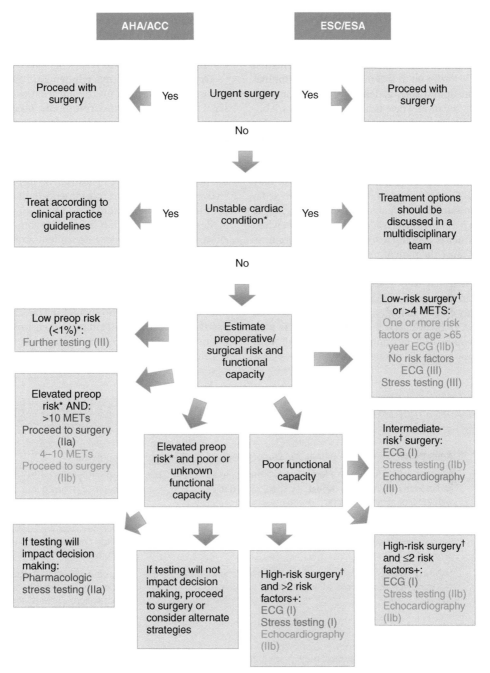

FIG. 43.1 Comparison of stepwise approach based on American College of Cardiology/American Heart Association and European Society of Cardiology/European Society of Anaesthesiology guidelines. *Asterisk* indicates unstable angina, acute heart failure, significant cardiac arrhythmia, symptomatic valvular heart disease, myocardial infarction within the past 30 days, and residual myocardial ischemia. †, *, and + are explained in Table 43.7. *ECG,* electrocardiogram; *MET,* metabolic equivalent. (Adapted from Fleisher LA, Fleischmann KE, Auerbach AD, et al. ACC/AHA guideline on perioperative cardiovascular evaluation and management of patients undergoing noncardiac surgery. A report of the American College of Cardiology/American Heart Association Task Force on Practice Guidelines. American College of Cardiology; American Heart Association. *J Am Coll Cardiol.* 2014;64(22):e77–e137; with permission.)

## DRUGS USED FOR PROCEDURAL SEDATION

*Midazolam* is the most commonly used benzodiazepine for procedural sedation. For normal adults, incremental doses of 0.01 mg/kg up to 2–3 mg alone or in combination with an opioid such as fentanyl provide smooth and pleasant sedation. There is high individual variability in patients' response to benzodiazepines, and this feature is unpredictable. Therefore, the best way to reach moderate sedation is titration of the drug and waiting 3–5 min to achieve peak effect of the drug, and if the patient is not adequately tranquilized, the dose may be repeated. One of the most common errors in sedation with midazolam or fentanyl (or other agents) is not waiting 3–5 min to reach adequate drug effect when the practitioner is in a hurry to initiate the procedure, which may cause the patient pain and discomfort.

An interventional procedure in an insufficiently sedated patient may lead to tachycardia and hypertension and can cause myocardial ischemia, arrhythmia, or pulmonary edema. In high-risk patients such as those who are ASA or NYHA class 3 or more and those with difficult airways, it is recommended to consult with an anesthesiologist to ensure better patient safety.

Midazolam dosage and some pharmacologic properties are summarized in Table 43.8. In the case of midazolam overdose or severe respiratory depression, flumazenil 0.2 mg IV can be used to reverse its effect.

*Opioids* such as fentanyl, remifentanil, and morphine are used frequently for procedural sedation and analgesia. Fentanyl is the most commonly used opioid for analgesia and is usually used in combination with other hypnotics such as midazolam. The onset of action of fentanyl is rapid (1–2 min), and peak effect is reached in 3–5 min (see Table 43.8) and lasts 30–60 min with a 2-µg/kg dose. Smaller doses (25–50 µg) have shorter recovery times and are recommended in conjunction with low-dose midazolam (0.5–1 mg).

Respiratory depression is the most common adverse effect of opioids. It is dose-dependent and is more frequent when used with other sedative drugs (midazolam or propofol), in patients with pulmonary diseases, and in older adults. Opioids in combination with other sedatives may cause hypotension. This effect can be more profound in patients who spend long fasting times with baseline hypovolemia. Fentanyl when used alone has minor hemodynamic effects even in the presence of ventricular or hepatorenal dysfunction.

**TABLE 43.8**
**Commonly Used Drugs for Procedural Sedation and Analgesia in Adults**

| Drug | Adult Dose | Onset of Action | Duration of Action[a] | Comments |
|---|---|---|---|---|
| Midazolam | 0.02–0.1 mg/kg IV initially; if further sedation is required, may repeat with 25% of initial dose after 3–5 min; not to exceed 2.5 mg/dose (1.5 mg for older adults) and 5-mg cumulative dose (3.5 mg for older adults) | 1–2 min (time to peak = 3–5 min) | 30–60 min | Respiratory depression or hypotension may occur, particularly when rapidly administered or combined with fentanyl (may need to decrease midazolam dose); does not provide analgesia; action reversed by flumazenil |
| Fentanyl | 1–2 mcg/kg slow IV push (over 1–2 min); may repeat dose after 30 min | 1–2 min (time to peak = 3–5 min) | 30–60 min | May cause chest wall rigidity, apnea, respiratory depression, or hypotension; elicits minimal cardiovascular depression; may cause dysphoria, nausea, vomiting; action reversed by naloxone |
| Propofol | 0.5–1 mg/kg IV loading dose; may repeat by 0.5–mg/kg increments every 3–5 min | <1 min | 3–10 min | Provides rapid onset and recovery phase and brief duration of action; can rapidly cause deepening sedation; causes cardiovascular depression and hypotension |

*IV*, Intravenous.
[a]Duration of action based on normal drug elimination (i.e., nonelderly adult with normal renal and hepatic function).
From Orlewicz MC, Schraga ED. Procedural sedation. http://emedicine.medscape.com/article/109695-overview#a7; with permission.

Morphine may cause some degrees of hypotension (caused by vasodilation and histamine release) and is not the first choice for procedural analgesia. However, it is the best analgesic agent in the ICU setting and in the postoperative period. Remifentanil is a short-acting opioid with a fast recovery time and thus is an attractive drug for outpatient settings. However, it must be kept in mind that this opioid agent, if used by nonanesthesiologists and nonskilled persons, may rapidly cause apnea and hypotension, and if the user cannot manage the airway and hemodynamics, it could lead to a catastrophic outcome and patient death.

In the case of significant respiratory depression or opium overdose, naloxone (0.4 mg IV) can be used for opium effect reversal. In patients with coronary artery disease or pulmonary hypertension, opioid effect must be reversed with caution to avoid myocardial ischemia or hypertension crisis.

*Propofol* is a short-acting hypnotic drug. It delivers hypnotic, sedative, amnestic properties without any analgesic effects. Propofol quickly crosses the blood–brain barrier, and its effects are mediated by positive modulation of GABA (γ-aminobutyric acid) receptors in the CNS. It seems that sedation with propofol has some advantages for TEE oversedation with a benzodiazepine-opioid combination regarding faster recovery and better physician and patient satisfaction. Also, propofol-sedated patients have better scores on psychomotor function, superior near memory, and mental status after sedation.

However, propofol has powerful cardiorespiratory depressant effects and should not be administered by nonanesthesiologists. Risk of hypotension or apnea by propofol is higher than with other hypnotics and analgesics and when used by a person who is not experienced in airway management and not able to maintain hemodynamics. Propofol loading dose for sedation is 0.5–1 mg/kg IV and can be continued by repeated doses of 0.5 mg/kg each 3–5 min (see Table 43.8) or continuous infusion of 25–75 µg/kg/min.

Ketamine is usually used in pediatric patients for procedural sedation. However, some physicians use it safely in adults. Ketamine has dissociative effects and causes amnesia and analgesia in patients. This combined sedative-analgesic activity is useful to administer is as a single agent for painful procedures. Ketamine may cause hypertension, tachycardia, and increases in intracranial pressure. Some patients may experience unusual dreams, hallucinations, excitation, physical combativeness, delirium, and nightmares after ketamine use, and for this reason, most anesthesiologists do not choose it as a first drug for sedation in adults.

Dexmedetomidine is a highly selective $\alpha_2$-adrenergic agonist with sedative, anxiolytic, and analgesic effects by activating presynaptic receptors. This drug has been successfully used for cardiovascular procedural sedation. Its starting dose is 1 µg/kg, which is administered over 10 min and then followed by 0.2–0.7 µg/kg/h. Generally, dexmedetomidine is similar to other sedatives in achieving sufficient levels of sedation with comparable rates of respiratory depression, oxygen desaturation, and hemodynamic instability.[24–26]

## MONITORING DURING PROCEDURAL SEDATION

The ASA guidelines recommend continuous ECG monitoring and noninvasive blood pressure measurement in patients with the cardiopulmonary disease during sedation.[27] In addition, all patients undergoing IV sedation should be monitored with continuous pulse oximetry monitoring efficiently diagnoses oxygen desaturation and hypoxemia. Pulse oximetry is partially insensitive to the early stages of respiratory depression because major changes in arterial partial pressure of oxygen (in ranges >60 mmHg) may happen with minimal changes in oxygen saturation. Therefore, observation of the patient's chest movements and ensuring an open airway during the TEE procedure is mandatory.

Capnography is a noninvasive measurement of end-tidal carbon dioxide and monitoring of real-time respiratory activity. It more readily detects respiratory depression than pulse oximetry and thereby helps in early recognition of hypoventilation to improve patient safety. The ASA guidelines recommend that capnography must be measured for all patients undergoing deep sedation and is useful during moderate sedation in patients whose ventilation cannot be observed directly.[27,28] The BIS index is an electroencephalographic-based technique of evaluating level of consciousness using an algorithm to create a weighted index.[29]

## SEDATION AND RESPIRATORY CARE IN CRITICALLY ILL CARDIAC CARE UNIT PATIENTS

Generally, cardiac patients are admitted to CCUs because of deteriorating cardiopulmonary conditions. Decompensated heart failure, worsening myocardial ischemia or myocardial infarction, cardiac arrhythmias, crisis of systemic and pulmonary hypertension, pulmonary edema, low cardiac output state, or cardiogenic shock are the main causes of CCU admission. Some cardiac patients have complications of deteriorating COPD or pneumonia, cerebrovascular accident, renal failure, or sepsis. Most CCU patients experience some degree of increased work of breathing and respiratory distress caused by pulmonary congestion, edema, or infection. Respiratory distress is an unpleasant sensation, and in addition to supplementary oxygen, they need some degrees of sedation to tolerate this situation. Also, low cardiac output state for any reason reduces cerebral blood flow and causes patients' agitation and restlessness. Thus, after treating the primary cause of cardiac or respiratory dysfunction, establishing and maintaining sufficient levels of sedation and analgesia in these critically ill patients are essential parts of CCU care.

Each cardiologist must have enough knowledge about basic clinical pharmacology of commonly used sedative drugs such as midazolam and propofol and also opioids (e.g., morphine and fentanyl) to be able to administer suitable doses of these drugs to achieve anticipated clinical effects while reducing the risk of unwarranted sedation and cardiorespiratory depression. Appropriate sedation and analgesia, in addition to providing patient comfort and satisfaction, reduce oxygen consumption and improve supply–demand balance in those with myocardial ischemia and heart failure.

Differential diagnoses of patient agitation and anxiety in CCUs, especially in those who are intubated and under mechanical ventilation, are hypoxemia, hypercapnia, hypotension, and reduced cerebral blood flow, urinary retention, an environment that is too cold or hot, hypoglycemia, acidosis, electrolyte abnormalities, and pain caused by tracheal intubation or other indwelling catheters and tubes. Thus, the cardiologist must have a high degree of suspicion about cardiovascular causes of patient agitation and correct them. Inappropriate patient sedation without correcting underlying causes of the distress and agitation may suppress compensatory sympathetic activity and mask warning signs of the deteriorating patient by inducing significant cardiac depression or vasodilation and may lead to cardiogenic shock and finally patient death.

It is strongly recommended that in all agitated and distressed CCU patients, laboratory tests of electrolytes, blood sugar, and arterial blood gas analyses are rapidly taken and echocardiography performed to rule out underlying causes. With this approach, most causes of patient restlessness can be diagnosed and treated. If the final diagnosis is that the cause of the agitation is pain and anxiety in a critical CCU patient with heart failure or myocardial ischemia, titrated small doses of a sedative drug such as midazolam (0.5–1 mg repeated every 3–5 min in a 70-kg adult patient) can be used to achieve an adequate sedation level. For analgesia, minimal doses of morphine (0.05 mg/kg) or fentanyl

(0.5–1 µg/kg) can be injected intravenously. If a practitioner wants to use a sedative drug with an opioid, the synergic cardiopulmonary depressant effects of this combination must be considered. An additive effect of fentanyl with propofol can cause cardiogenic shock in vulnerable patients.[30]

If a critically ill patient needs moderate to deep levels of sedation, anesthesiology consultation is necessary. Administration of moderate to high doses of hypnotic or opioid drugs in hemodynamically unstable patients is very dangerous and can lead to severe hypotension and shock state and rapidly progress to patient death. In patients with unstable rhythm or blood pressure or low oxygen saturation, it is recommended to use an indwelling arterial catheter to invasively and continuously monitor blood pressure and to take arterial blood gas periodically.

For moderate sedation, midazolam (0.01–0.03 mg/kg/h) or propofol (25–75 µg/kg/min) can be infused in intubated patients. Considering some degree of vasodilation by these drugs, infusing 200–300 mL of IV solution prevents hypotension. Regarding minimal hemodynamic adverse effects of fentanyl, infusion of this opioid is useful in intubated critically ill patients or those with myocardial dysfunction. A continuous infusion dose of fentanyl begins with 1 µg/kg/h and can be adjusted until there is appropriate patient comfort. Dexmedetomidine can be used for sedation in hemodynamically stable patients. Its starting dose is 1 µg/kg administered over 10 min followed by 0.2–0.7 µg/kg/h. There are some reports of cardiogenic shock with dexmedetomidine in susceptible patients that may relate to the presynaptic sympathetic blocking effect of the drug.[25,26] In a study on cardiac patients undergoing TEE Alizadeasl et al. fund longer time from the beginning of sedation in dexmedetomidine in comparison with propofol. Dexmedetomidine provides a satisfactory level of sedation (patient and physician satisfaction) and hemodynamic stability and shorter time to recovery.[31]

## REFERENCES

1. Cornelissen H, Arrowsmith JE. Preoperative assessment for cardiac surgery. *Contin Educ Anaesth Crit Care Pain.* 2006;6(3):109–113. https://doi.org/10.1093/bjaceaccp/mkl013.
2. Hakim H, Samadikhah J, Alizadehasl A, Azarfarin R. Chronobiological rhythms in onset of massive pulmonary embolism in Iranian population. *Middle East J Anaesthesiol.* 2009;20(3):369–375.
3. Yaghoubi A, Golmohamadi Z, Alizadehasl A, Azarfarin R. Role of platelet parameters and haematological indices in myocardial infarction and unstable angina. *J Pak Med Assoc.* 2013;63(9):1133–1137.

4. Mahla E, Suarez TA, Bliden KP, et al. Platelet function measurement-based strategy to reduce bleeding and waiting time in clopidogrel-treated patients undergoing coronary artery bypass graft surgery: the timing based on platelet function strategy to reduce clopidogrel-associated bleeding related to CABG (TARGET-CABG) study. *Circ Cardiovasc Interv*. 2012;5(2):261–269 [Epub 2012/03/08].

5. Alizadehasl A, Golmohammadi Z, Panjavi L, Mahmoodmoradi S, Azarfarin R. The incidence of anaemia in adult patients with cardiovascular diseases in Northwest Iran. *J Pak Med Assoc*. 2011;61(11):1091–1095.

6. Parsonnet V, Dean D, Bernstein AD. A method of uniform stratification of risk for evaluating the results of surgery in acquired adult heart disease. *Circulation*. 1989;79:I3–I12.

7. Nashef SA, Roques F, Michel P, Gauducheau E, Lemeshow S, Salamon R. European system for cardiac operative risk evaluation (EuroSCORE). *Eur J Cardiothorac Surg*. 1999;16:9–13.

8. Yaghoubi A, Safaie N, Azarfarin R, Alizadehasl A, Golzari SE. Evaluation of cardiovascular diseases and their risk factors in hospitalized patients in East Azerbaijan province, Northwest Iran: a review of 18323 cases. *J Tehran Heart Cent*. 2013;8(2):101–105.

9. Guohua L, Margaret Warner PH, Barbara H, Lang BS, Lin Huang MS, Lena SS. Epidemiology of anesthesia-related mortality in the United States, 1999–2005. *Anesthesiology*. 2009;110(4):759–765.

10. Alwardt CM, Redford D, Larson DF. General anesthesia in cardiac surgery: a review of drugs and practices. *J Extra Corpor Technol*. 2005;37(2):227–235.

11. Ziyaeifard M, Azarfarin R, Golzari SE. A review of current analgesic techniques in cardiac surgery. Is epidural worth it? *J Cardiovasc Thorac Res*. 2014;6(3):133–140.

12. Naghipour B, Aghamohamadi D, Azarfarin R, et al. Dexamethasone added to bupivacaine prolongs duration of epidural analgesia. *Middle East J Anaesthesiol*. 2013;22(1):53–57.

13. Mirinejad M, Azarfarin R, Asl AA. Cisatracurium in cardiac surgery–continuous infusion vs. bolus administration. *Middle East J Anaesthesiol*. 2007;19(3):563–572.

14. Faritous Z, Ardeshiri M, Yazdanian F, Jalali A, Totonchi Z, Azarfarin R. Hyperglycemia or high hemoglobin A1C: which one is more associated with morbidity and mortality after coronary artery bypass graft surgery? *Ann Thorac Cardiovasc Surg*. 2014;20(3):223–228.

15. Azarfarin R, Sheikhzadeh D, Mirinazhad M, Bilehjani E, Alizadehasl A. Do nondiabetic patients undergoing coronary artery bypass grafting surgery require intraoperative management of hyperglycemia? *Acta Anaesthesiol Taiwan*. 2011;49(2):41–45.

16. Azarfarin R, Alizadeh AA. Prevalence and intensity of hyperglycemia in non-diabetic patients undergoing coronary artery bypass graft surgery with and without cardiopulmonary bypass. *Saudi Med J*. 2008;29(9):1294–1298.

17. Alaei F, Davari PN, Alaei M, Azarfarin R, Soleymani E. Postoperative outcome for hyperglycemic pediatric cardiac surgery patients. *Pediatr Cardiol*. 2012;33(1):21–26.

18. Fleisher LA, Fleischmann KE, Auerbach AD, et al. 2014 ACC/AHA guideline on perioperative cardiovascular evaluation and management of patients undergoing noncardiac surgery. A report of the American College of Cardiology/American Heart Association Task Force on Practice Guidelines. American College of Cardiology; American Heart Association. *J Am Coll Cardiol*. 2014;64(22):e77–e137. https://doi.org/10.1016/j.jacc.2014.07.944.

19. Velasco A, Reyes E, Hage FG. Guidelines in review: comparison of the 2014 ACC/AHA guidelines on perioperative cardiovascular evaluation and management of patients undergoing noncardiac surgery and the 2014 ESC/ESA guidelines on noncardiac surgery: cardiovascular assessment and management. *J Nucl Cardiol*. 2017;24(1):165–170.

20. Schulman-Marcus J, Pashun RA, Feldman DN, Swaminathan RV. Coronary angiography and revascularization prior to noncardiac surgery. *Curr Treat Options Cardiovasc Med*. 2016;18(1):3.

21. Chu EW, Chernoguz A, Divino CM. The evaluation of clopidogrel use in perioperative general surgery patients: a prospective randomized controlled trial. *Am J Surg*. 2016;211(6):1019–1025.

22. Joo MS, Ahn BM, Kim HJ, et al. Evaluation of feasible timing of elective noncardiac procedure after antiplatelet discontinuation in patients treated with antiplatelet agents. *J Investig Med*. 2014;62(5):808–812.

23. Orlewicz MC, Schraga ED. Procedural Sedation. (2016). http://emedicine.medscape.com/article/109695-overview #a7; Available on November 14, 2016.

24. Cooper L, Candiotti K, Gallagher C, Grenier E, Arheart KL, Barron ME. A randomized, controlled trial on dexmedetomidine for providing adequate sedation and hemodynamic control for awake, diagnostic transesophageal echocardiography. *J Cardiothorac Vasc Anesth*. 2011;25(2):233–237.

25. Sichrovsky TC, Mittal S, Steinberg JS. Dexmedetomidine sedation leading to refractory cardiogenic shock. *Anesth Analg*. 2008;106(6):1784–1786.

26. Fischer GW, Silverstein JH. Dexmedetomidine and refractory cardiogenic shock. *Anesth Analg*. 2009;108(1):380.

27. American Society of Anesthesiologists Task Force on Sedation and Analgesia by Non-Anesthesiologists. Practice guidelines for sedation and analgesia by non-anesthesiologists. *Anesthesiology*. 2002;96(4):1004–1017.

28. Ziyaeifard M, Azarfarin R. Efficacy and safety of sedation in cardiac imaging. *Arch Cardiovasc Imaging*. 2014;2(1): e17357. https://doi.org/10.5812/acvi.17357.

29. Drake LM, Chen SC, Rex DK. Efficacy of bispectral monitoring as an adjunct to nurse-administered propofol

sedation for colonoscopy: a randomized controlled trial. *Am J Gastroenterol.* 2006;101:2003–2007.

30. Prabhakaran AJ. Additive effect of propofol and fentanyl precipitating cardiogenic shock. *J Pharmacol Pharmacother.* 2013;4(3):217–219.

31. Alizadehasl A, Sadeghpour A, Totonchi Z, Azarfarin R, Rahimi S, Hendiani A. Comparison of sedation between dexmedetomidine and propofol during transesophageal echocardiography: a randomized controlled trial. *Ann Card Anaesth.* 2019;22(3):285–290.

# CHAPTER 44

# Principles of Cardiovascular Surgery

SAEID HOSSEINI[a] • ALIREZA ALIZADEH GHAVIDEL[b]

[a]Heart Valve Disease Research Center, Rajaie Cardiovascular, Medical & Research Center, Iran University of Medical Science, Tehran, Iran, [b]Rajaie Cardiovascular, Medical & Research Center, Iran University of Medical Sciences, Tehran, Iran

## KEY POINTS

- Deep hypothermic circulatory arrest with selective cerebral perfusion provides a safe, bloodless surgical field in selected cardiac surgeries, including aortic arch replacement and pulmonary thromboendarterectomy.
- A postoperative hemoglobin (Hgb) level greater than 8 g/L is usually considered sufficient, but for higher risk patients such as older adults or patients with chronic obstructive pulmonary disease or congestive heart failure, higher Hgb levels are useful.
- Patients with heart valve replacement on sinus rhythm and good ejection fraction do not require anticoagulation immediately after surgery.
- Therapeutic levels of international normalized ratio for patients with mechanical valve replacement are 2–3 for aortic valve replacement, 2.5–3.5 for mitral valve replacement, and 3–4 for eight-sided heart valves.
- Because the platelet depletion is consumptive, patients with heparin-induced thrombocytopenia (HIT) usually present with intra-arterial or intravenous thrombosis instead of bleeding.
- Using heparin in patients with a history of HIT for more than 3 months, normal platelet count, and negative antiplatelet factor 4 who need percutaneous coronary intervention or cardiac surgery may be safe.
- Patient–prosthesis mismatch is a challenging issue in aortic valve surgery that can be managed by aortic root enlargement techniques (Manougian and Konno-Rastan procedures), aortic root replacement, low-profile new-generation valves, or sutureless tissue valves.
- Moderate degrees of tricuspid insufficiency would require tricuspid valve repair if the maximum end-systolic diameter is greater than 40 mm or larger than 21 mm/m$^2$ in preoperative echocardiography or over 70 mm in the surgical field of an arrested heart.
- Minimally invasive valve surgeries have similar or even better outcomes when performing by well-trained surgeons for selected patients.
- Special considerations need for preoperative and postoperative assessments during COVID-19 outbreak and afterward.

## EXTRACORPOREAL CIRCULATION

Before the invention of the cardiopulmonary bypass (CPB) machine, heart surgery was limited and sporadic. However, this particular invention and its application brought along dramatic advancements, improved outcomes of heart surgery, and established a surprisingly upward trend in the number of cardiac operations. The uniqueness of heart surgery is mainly attributable to the nature of the extracorporeal circulation while using the CPB machine. Also, adding the word "open" in conjunction with heart surgery means that CBP has been used in the course of heart surgery. The machine consists of four or five consoles of roller pumps, one of which is designed to create and provide systemic blood circulation. Sometimes because of safety considerations and higher efficiency, a centrifugal pump is externally attached to the machine, which replaces a roller pump. Two of the other mentioned roller pumps are for sucking out the blood and returning it to the CPB system (Fig. 44.1). One or two of the remaining roller pumps are used for infusion of cardioplegia solutions and myocardial protection.

For promoting CPB system performance, a number of single-use and disposable materials are also consumed, which include oxygenator cannula and corresponding lines and arterial, venous, and cardioplegia cannulas. In fact, the oxygenator is responsible for the function of the lungs during CPB operations. At the beginning, the oxygenator was of the bubble type, and because of its various complications, it became obsolete and was later replaced with membrane oxygenators, which are still in use. This system is designed to exchange gases, remove $CO_2$, and add oxygen to the blood. It consists of very fine hollow fibers made of polypropylene or silicon rubber with a diameter of about 0.3–0.8 μm, all of which have tiny pores for gas exchange. Because blood and gas are somehow in contact with the oxygenator and because of plasma leakage through this membrane, the maximum safe operational time is limited to no more than several hours.

Because of the nature of extracorporeal blood flow in CPB, activation of the coagulation system is to be expected. For this reason, before using a cannula and CPB, a high dose of heparin is administered for anticoagulation. The initial heparin dose for injection should be 3–4 mg/kg. To monitor heparinization efficacy, two tests, the activated clotting time (ACT) and Hepcon (measuring the concentration of heparin in the blood), are in use. ACT test is more popular and is usually done 3 min after heparin injection, when heparinization has taken full effect. When the elapsed time approaches 480 s, CPB can be started. During CPB operation, the test is repeated every half hour to every hour, and if the result is lower than expected, more heparin is injected. At the end of surgery and by the end of CPB operation and removal of the cannula, the effect of heparin is neutralized by protamine injection. Recently, as a new technology, manufacturers added disposable CPB materials with heparin-coated parts to reduce the chances of thrombosis and clot formation in CPB, especially the oxygenator.

It should be noted that before starting the machine, the CPB reservoir should be primed with crystalloids or colloid solutions, which result in hemodilution. In any case, however, during CPB operation, a hematocrit of about 20%–25% is acceptable. With the start of CPB operation, natural pulsatile circulation, which was generated by the heart and maintained by the body vessels, temporarily ceases to function and is replaced with CPB continuous flow. This change in the blood circulation model, which is accompanied by lower than normal average blood pressure, affects organs' perfusion. To overcome the resulting complications during CPB operation, the patient's body temperature is lowered, and the patient is in a state of hypothermia. In the early years of heart surgery, patients were operated on at much lower temperatures, and until a few years ago, cardiac surgeries were practiced at temperatures between 25 and 28°C. However, in the recent years, a temperature of about 30–32°C is more desirable for heart surgeons.

Cardiopulmonary bypass blood flow is based on the patient's body surface area (BSA) and, of course, adjusted according to the body temperature. Usually, a body temperature of 30–32°C can be called mild hypothermia. The blood flow rate is adjusted to 2.5 $L/m^2$ of BSA. So accordingly, lower blood flow is possible with lower body temperatures. During CPB operation, the adequacy of blood flow is regulated by monitoring various factors, including urine output and blood gas analysis. At the end of the surgery, when the required procedures have all been accomplished and the patient is being warmed up and ready for weaning from the CPB, it is crucial that it is all done slowly and that its adequacy is determined by different methods of monitoring, including heart transesophageal echocardiography (TEE).

## DEEP HYPOTHERMIA AND CIRCULATORY ARREST

In a number of cardiac surgeries, we have to take the patient to a deep hypothermia condition (down to about 18°C) to be able to completely stop the CPB blood flow and to operate on the patient in total circulatory arrest (TCA). This group of surgeries is among the surgical procedures in which, because of their nature, blood flow in the body must be cut off (e.g., surgeries on the aortic arch, especially in aortic dissection or the procedures in which the field of operation must be completely free of blood, as in pulmonary endarterectomy or some complex congenital surgeries).[1–3] In normal temperatures, the brain can tolerance ischemia for up to 5 min maximum, which is definitely not enough time to do these types of procedures. Therefore, to increase this time, we have to cool down the patient's body. For this purpose, the patient's body is cooled down to about 18°C, in which organs and especially the brain can tolerate the circulatory arrest more safely.

There are a few points to be considered for a safe outcome. The minimum time required from the start of CPB to reach deep hypothermic circulatory arrest should

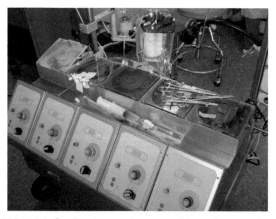

FIG. 44.1 Cardiopulmonary bypass machine and accessories.

be 30 min to ensure the patient's body is uniformly cooled down to the desired temperature. However, we are more likely to achieve this goal if this time is extended up to 60 min. The temperature gradient difference between heater-cooler device and the patient's body should be a maximum of 10°C. Brain arteries can selectively be perfused, which can be through either antegrade or retrograde methods. Of course, the antegrade method is more acceptable.

## MYOCARDIAL PROTECTION

During heart surgery, to be able to perform surgery on a silent heart or take action on the cardiac chambers, particularly, inside them, the heart must be in an arrested condition. For this purpose, the ascending aorta is clamped, and cardioplegia solution is infused into the aortic root to perfuse the coronary arteries. The main ingredient of this solution is potassium, with a concentration of about 20 mEq/L, as an initial dose for induction to arrest the heart. And for the subsequent doses, the usual potassium concentration is considered to be about 10 mEq/L.

The volume of cardioplegia solution for induction in adults is around 750–900 cc in a 3-min period; this amount is more for enlarged and hypertrophied hearts with perfusion pressure of 30 mmHg. Subsequent doses should be 250 cc within a 1-min period. The safest interval time between doses of cardioplegia solutions is usually about 20 min. However, this period has been increased to more than 1 h with the new cardioplegia HTK solutions.

Even though crystalloid solution was primarily used as cardioplegia, in the recent years, the most widely used new solution is blood cardioplegia. In terms of optimum temperature, cardioplegia solution used to be applied cold at the beginning of cardiac arrest induction; however, considering that the enzymatic activity of the heart is stopped in cold temperatures yet myocardial cooling does not significantly affect the amount of myocardial oxygen consumption, most cardiac surgeons apply warm to tepid cardioplegic solution.

Another delivery method of cardioplegia is retrograde cardioplegia infused through the coronary sinus, which is performed by embedding a special cannula. This method contributes a great deal to heart protection, and it is not usually used as an initial dose of cardiac arrest induction, but it is used in subsequent doses. The injection pressure of the cardioplegic solution must definitely be checked in this method. The acceptable pressure is 20–40 mmHg. A possible complication of this method is a lack of appropriate protection for the right ventricle.

## POSTOPERATIVE CARE

Because hemodynamic instability, postoperative bleeding, electrolyte abnormalities, and arrhythmia are common after cardiac surgeries, such patients are usually transferred to the intensive care unit (ICU) under intravenous sedation and intubation for safe postoperative care. Proper circulation must be ensured immediately after the patient is transferred to the ICU bed. Setting up multiple monitors, all intubation and fusion pumps for the patient's medications by the nursing group can take some time. Natural color and warmth of patient's feet along with the normal dorsalis pedis and posterior tibialis artery pulses, consistent with the arterial line pressure, can ensure the patient's sufficient circulation. A low-output state with hypotension is one of the most important early complications after open-heart surgery that could have various cardiac and noncardiac causes.

## INSUFFICIENT PRELOAD

Vasodilatation secondary to the anesthetics and vasodilators such as nitroglycerin nitroprusside is a common complication. However, hypovolemia is the common cause of low preload after cardiac surgery. Fluid sequestration after open-heart surgery, excessive diuresis caused by diuretics, increased insensible loss caused by mechanical ventilation, and subtle or obvious bleeding are the most important causes of hypovolemia. Surgical bleeding has always been one of the challenges for cardiac surgeons. A decrease in the patient's hematocrit level without evident bleeding maybe secondary to the tamponade or clotted hemothorax and gastrointestinal or retroperitoneal bleeding.

The patient's general appearance and chest bottles should be checked. When the patient is pale and the chest bottle is filled with significant bloody drainage, prompt surgical management should be started. Otherwise if there's no obvious bleeding and the patient's hypotension is assured, we need to check for other possible causes. Make sure the administered doses of vasodilator were not excessive. Check the central venous pressure (CVP) and the patient's hematocrit level, and control the trend of hematocrit level changes. Compensate volume depletion by administrating colloid and crystalloid solutions, and then seek the cause of bleeding, compensate for anemia, and control the bleeding. Low-risk patients do not need blood transfusion when the hemoglobin (Hgb) level is more than 8 g/L. For younger patients, we can even wait up to 7 g/L of Hgb. However, an Hgb level higher than 8 g/L is necessary for high-risk patients, such as older adults or patients with congestive heart failure or chronic obstructive pulmonary disease.

Unnecessary transfusions may increase the mortality and morbidity rates.[4] While compensating for anemia, the origin of the bleeding must also be determined. Check the coagulation tests and patient's coagulation status with rotational thromboelastometry (ROTEM) if available, and compensate for coagulation factor deficiency exclusively (target therapy). ROTEM can contribute to proper management of postoperative bleeding.[5,6]

If there is no important coagulopathy but postoperative blood drainage continues, mediastinal reexploration must be performed after hemodynamic stabilization and resuscitation. There is no reason to continue with conservative management, if the patient has more than 200 cc/h of drainage or the total bleeding volume is more than 1000 cc (10–15 cc/kg of valves) within the first hours after surgery. For a pale patient who has a sudden drainage of more than 400 cc and hemodynamic instability, no further time should be wasted on the possibility of coagulopathy or other causes. These patients usually have a life-threatening surgical bleeding. Therefore, while resuscitation is done with blood and crystalloid solution, the patient should be transferred to the operating room along with the surgical and anesthetics teams. It should be noted that unusual doses of inotropes without enough resuscitation are not effective.

In hypotensive patients with elevated CVP, cardiac tamponade is the most important differential diagnosis. Oliguria can be considered diagnostic for cardiac tamponade in the presence of high CVP, low blood pressure, and tachycardia. Several other factors such as having a Swan-Ganz catheter and bedside echocardiography can also be helpful for the diagnosis of cardiac tamponade. In suspicious cases, chest radiography findings may be useful; a wider or denser mediastinum shadow in comparison with the preoperative chest radiographs may reflect clot formation in the pericardial sac and tamponade. Echocardiographic findings (transthoracic echocardiography, TEE) can be very helpful to differentiate among the various causes of hypotension.

Diagnostic delays may result in prolonged hypotension, cardiac arrest, or irreversible organ damage. Therefore, when there is a high suspicion for tamponade clinically, do not wait for imaging. If the patient is in shock and does not have adequate perfusion pressure, emergent opening of the sternum would be lifesaving secondary to immediate mediastinal pressure removal and venous return improvement. In selected cases, sternal wire removal in the ICU may result in a quick recovery of the patient's pressure and allows the patient to be transferred to the operating room in a more stable and safer condition.

## CARDIAC CAUSES

Low cardiac output syndrome and residual cardiac pathologies are two important causes of postoperative hypotension. Incomplete revascularization, a suboptimal valve repair result, and residual intracardiac shunt may reduce cardiac performance in the postoperative period. Poor myocardial protection during open-heart surgeries plays a major role in low-output states. Inappropriate cardioplegic solution dose, content, or infusion route may permanently damage myocytes during the ischemic cardiac arrest period. Temporary functional myocyte damage is more common, so-called stunning that may continue from a few minutes to a few hours, leading to a low-output state in patients. It is a self-limiting condition; however, impaired tissue perfusion requires life support measures and the use of an inotrope or even an intra-aortic balloon pump (IABP).

Perioperative myocardial infarction (MI) or poor myocardial management during open-heart surgery may cause postoperative left ventricular (LV) failure. Incomplete revascularization, coronary embolization or thrombosis of the graft, postaortic valve replacement (AVR) damage or functional stenosis of coronary artery ostia, coronary artery damage during other valve surgeries, and severe perioperative hypotension during induction of anesthesia or during surgery are all of the known causes of postoperative MI.

## INCREASED VENTRICULAR AFTERLOAD

Increased ventricular afterload is the other cause of postoperative hypotension. Hypoxia, restlessness, or even aggressive suctioning of the endotracheal tube can easily cause increased LV afterload. These are generally well tolerated by the patients; however, in patients with low cardiac reserve, it can be dangerous. Ventricular septal defect closure or even mitral valve repair (MVr) in patients with severe mitral regurgitation (MR) can increase LV afterload and result in low cardiac output, especially in patients with significant LV dysfunction. Increased right ventricular afterload during a hypertension crisis or pulmonary embolism, in addition to causing hypoxia through the displacement of ventricular septum and reduced LV preload, can lead to a low-output state and hypotension.

## APPROACH TO A LOW-OUTPUT STATE

Approaches for dealing with the cases in which reduced preload causes hypotension were explained in the previous pages. Hypotension caused by stunning manifests itself from the very beginning when the CPB machine detachment is done. These types of patients are infused with low to moderate doses of inotrope before being transferred from the operating room to the ICU. Postoperative MI is one of the most important causes of low-output syndrome. MI can manifest itself in a variety of ways after open-heart surgery. Unstable hemodynamics or ventricular tachyarrhythmia may be the main clinical presentation of early postoperative MI. The practitioner should check for ST-T changes and other new findings in postoperative electrocardiogram; check the patient's cardiac enzymes (troponin); and perform bedside echocardiography for the presence of LV dysfunction, wall motion abnormality, or any other internal cardiac pathologies such as MR. If these three diagnostic tools confirm postoperative MI, the patient's surgeon should be consulted for a further possible surgical procedure (graft revision or additional graft), insertion of a balloon pump, or even insertion of assist devices.

During the first hours after coronary artery bypass graft (CABG), MI may be caused by graft thrombosis, poor myocardial protection, technical problems such as shortness of the graft, graft under tension, a long graft or kinking of the graft, a twisted graft, spasm or dissection on arterial conduits, or air or small particle embolism. Early diagnosis and proper management can prevent transmural Q-wave MI. Urgent post-CABG coronary angiography may be helpful and diagnostic in selected stable cases. In this situation, if there is no doubt in doing complete revascularization without any complication, performing emergency angiography and possible intervention can prevent severe myocardial damage, particularly in cases where anatomy of the coronary arteries for CABG is satisfactory.

When the patient's hemodynamics are unstable and there is high suspicion for graft failure, emergent mediastinal reexploration, intraoperative TEE, graft revisions, and a possible additional procedure such as a new graft may be useful in patient management. Additional graft anastomosis and insertion of an IABP can be beneficial in early postoperative graft failure to save the myocardium and prevent obvious LV dysfunction. However, if the patient has diffused atherosclerotic changes and poor coronary artery runoff, conservative management and IABP insertion to reduce afterload and myocardial oxygen demand would be the best options.

Sometimes the global ischemia or postoperative MI of the patient is so severe that the conservative or even interventional measures mentioned are not enough. In this case, for patients who have a long-life expectancy and if their end organs are not seriously damaged and particularly have no severe brain injury, it is advisable

to consult with the patient's surgeon about the usefulness of using assist devices or extracorporeal membrane oxygenation (ECMO). Considering the availability of assist devices, they can be properly used as a bridge to recovery, or even the bridge to transplant, based on the patient's condition and the ruling scientific criteria. It must be noted that surgical intervention for hypotension and low cardiac state is only indicated in a small number of patients, and the majority of patients can be managed by supportive measures, including adequate oxygenation, appropriate intravascular volume, enough doses of inotropes, proper acid–base and electrolyte status, appropriate heart rate and rhythm, and even IABP insertion.

## ANTICOAGULATION

Postoperative prophylactic heparin can significantly reduce the risk of thromboembolic events in patients undergoing cardiac surgeries similar to other major surgeries. For patients undergoing nonvalvular surgeries, the use of low-molecular-weight heparin (LMWH) is recommended postoperatively, but the administration of 5000–7500 units of unfractionated heparin (UFH) has its own advocates. The concomitant use of mechanical prophylaxis has been demonstrated.[6]

In patients undergoing CABG, the use of heparin prophylaxis during the first postoperative 48 h can prevent thromboembolic complications in patients with new-onset atrial fibrillation (AF). If postoperative AF is transient, some surgeons recommend carefully continuing anticoagulation for 6–12 months postoperatively.

### Mitral Valve Repair

Patients on sinus rhythm with good ejection fraction do not require heparin immediately after surgery. Heparin can be started on the first day after surgery. Oral anticoagulation for 6–8 weeks in high-risk patients with thromboembolic complications can be useful, and international normalized ratio (INR) ranging from 2 to 2.5 is sufficient.[7–9] Then, aspirin 80–100 mg/day should be continued for 1 year. The use of a single antiplatelet can be an acceptable alternative for low-risk patients.[7,9–11]

### Mitral Valve Replacement

Heparin should be administered during the first 24 h after surgery in patients with a history of valve thrombosis, deep vein thrombosis, and previous thromboembolic events, LV dysfunction, and large left atrium (LA). Moreover, warfarin is prescribed with 5–7.5 mg/day on the second postoperative day and is adjusted based on INR checking. The therapeutic range of INR in patients undergoing mechanical mitral valve replacement (MVR) without severe LV dysfunction and a lack of abovementioned risk factors is 2.5–3.5. It is better to consider INR ranges 0.5 above these values in patients with old-generation mechanical valves such as Starr-Edwards valves, having a large LA, or having a low ejection fraction.[6–9] In patients with a biologic mitral valve, warfarin is used for 3 months after surgery.[9,10] The therapeutic INR range for high-risk patients is considered 2.5–3. In patients with contraindications of warfarin use, an antiplatelet is an acceptable alternative.

### Aortic Valve Replacement

Patients undergoing aortic valve replacement (AVR) do not need an immediate postoperative anticoagulation during the first 24 h unless it is for other indications such as AF. If the patient does not have a risk of bleeding, warfarin can be begun on the second postoperative day. The therapeutic range of INR for a mechanical aortic valve is usually recommended to be 2–3. If a patient has old-generation mechanical aortic valves, the range of INR should be higher than these values (2.5–3.5). Patients with biologic valves in the aortic position do not usually need oral anticoagulation, and using an antiplatelet is sufficient.[7–9] Also, patients with aortic valve repair or aortic valve-sparing surgeries have no need for anticoagulation, and use of an antiplatelet is sufficient.[9]

### Pulmonary and Tricuspid Valves

The use of warfarin for tissue valves in pulmonary or tricuspid positions is reasonable for 3 months. Mechanical valves in the right side of the heart need higher INR values because of lower pressures and a high probability of thrombosis, and it should range from 3 to 4. Mechanical valve dysfunction secondary to thrombosis usually leads to critical clinical conditions because the lower pressure gradient beyond these valves prevents opening of limited motion of valve leaflets.[8,9]

## HEPARIN-INDUCED THROMBOCYTOPENIA

Heparin-induced thrombocytopenia (HIT) is a life-threatening adverse event that results from immune system activation caused by the heparin molecule and leads to platelet activation. HIT has two types. In type I, the immune system is not involved, and it is caused by interaction between heparin and platelets, leading to platelet sequestration and aggregation. It is also called *heparin-associated thrombocytopenia*. This event develops in 10% of patients, and the platelet count decreases by 30%–50%. In type I, the platelet count usually falls below 100,000 mm[3]. However, it returns to normal ranges a few days after heparin discontinuation.[12,13]

Type II HIT develops as a result of antiplatelet factor 4 in the presence of heparin, and it is dangerous, leading to systemic intra-arterial or intravenous thrombosis. It should be considered that bleeding is not common in HIT, and thrombocytopenia is consumptive. This type is referred to as the immunologic type. About 10% of patients receiving heparin may develop HIT antibody, but only 1%–5% of them develop HIT, and 30% of these patients will have life-threatening thrombotic complications. The probability of HIT is higher in patients receiving UFH than in those receiving LMWH (about 10 times higher). In a study, it has been shown that 1.2% of patients receiving heparin for more than 4 days develop HIT. In any patient receiving heparin, the possibility of HIT should be kept in mind, and the platelet count should be checked every 2–3 days. If the platelet count decreases more than 50%, especially 5–14 days after heparin administration, and there is no reason for thrombocytopenia such as sepsis, HIT should be strongly suspected.[12,13]

Systemic arterial or venous thrombosis may be the first clinical presentation of HIT. In such situations, the heparin infusion should be stopped, and another anticoagulation agent should be started along with a test for antiplatelet factor 4 in serum. Argatroban, danaparoid, and bivalirudin are direct thrombin inhibitors that may be used as an alternative to heparin. The US Food and Drug Administration (FDA) has not approved dabigatran for use in patients with HIT. Bivalirudin infusion (0.15 mg/kg/h) should be started and adjusted so that the activated partial thromboplastin time ranges 1.5–2.5 times higher than normal ranges. It should be kept in mind that the use of warfarin in patients with HIT can result in microthrombosis and consequent skin necrosis and fingertip gangrene caused by lower levels of protein C. Therefore, it is necessary to wait for some days until the platelet count is above 150,000/mm[3] before warfarin therapy is started. Intravenous vitamin K should be used if the patient is already taking warfarin when diagnosed with HIT.[13] Warfarin should be initiated with a dosage of less than 5 mg/day. Alternative anticoagulation should be continued for the first 3–5 days. If a patient with HIT has a thrombotic complication, it is better to use argatroban because it is approved by the FDA for such cases. The usual dose of this agent is 2 mcg/kg/min, but it should be adjusted for patients with liver failure or heart failure and after cardiac surgeries (0.5–1.2 mcg/kg/min). For patients with HIT after percutaneous coronary intervention (PCI) or patients with HIT requiring cardiac surgery or a cardiopulmonary pump, bivalirudin is the drug of choice.[13] In patients with HIT 3 months ago and normal platelet count and negative anti-platelet factor 4 who need PCI or cardiac surgery, the use of UFH may not be problematic.

## Mitral Valve Surgery

The standard approach for mitral valve (MV) surgery is via midsternotomy. After CPB and arresting the heart with cardioplegic solution, the LA is opened longitudinally through the entrance of the right pulmonary veins. A transseptal approach is another option to expose the MV through an iatrogenic atrial septal defect. This option can be used in patients with concomitant tricuspid surgery or redo mitral surgeries. The third technique for exposing the MV is incision in the roof of the LA [between the ascending aorta and superior vena cava (SVC)] that gives good exposure to the MV. The use of less invasive procedures for the MV is increasing in daily practice. There are two main techniques of minimally invasive procedures, including da Vinci robot and video thoracoscopic access. A right mini-thoracotomy and peripheral arterial cannulation (i.e., femoral vein and artery) is used in both techniques for CPB establishment and valve surgery.

MVr and MVR are the two main and common procedures for MV disease. MVR is generally limited for patients with dominant mitral stenosis in which thickened, calcified, and inflexible leaflets prevent the surgeon from doing an appropriate MVr. During an MVR procedure in rheumatic MV with high scores, both leaflets and thickened chordae are resected completely, and papillary muscles remain intact. However, for MVR in a patient with degenerative mitral valve pathology and failed MVr during an MVR for degenerative MR, it is better to save both leaflets or at least posterior leaflets along with the corresponding chordae, and then the prosthetic valve is placed in the native valve and sutured to the annulus of the native valve (valve-in-valve technique). The latter technique better saves LV function and decreases atrioventricular groove rupture. It has been also demonstrated that saving the subvalvular apparatus does not lead to an increase in thromboembolic events.[14]

Continuous and interrupted suturing are the two main techniques used for suturing the prosthetic valve to the annulus of the native valve; however, there is no superiority of one technique over another, and they are selected based on surgeon's preference and experience. The selection of valve type is based on the patient's age, sex, background of diseases, life expectancy and survival, pregnancy, valve position, and socioeconomic status. Obviously, the final decision should be made after the patient and family members have gone through a complete description and are enlightened regarding the advantages and disadvantages of their choices (Table 44.1). MVr is the standard operation for degenerative diseases of the MV and some congenital MV diseases. Selection of the MVr technique is based on the Carpenter classification (Table 44.2). Generally, type II cases, which are MV prolapse caused by elongated or ruptured chordae of at least one scallop of the MV, are generally repaired by neochordae. The neochorda is usually a polytetrafluoroethylene (PTFE) suture that comes from papillary muscle to the free edge of the prolaptic leaflet to create good coaptation depth between two mitral leaflets. Resection or plication of the prolaptic scallop of the MV is another technique that is generally used for a prolaptic posterior leaflet. An annuloplasty ring with a complete ring or band is a part of the MVr that is chosen by the surgeon's preference and the pathology of the MV. In type I MR, the repair technique is mainly focused on minimizing and repairing the annulus, which is usually performed by complete and rigid rings. MVr in type III is more complex and may include different techniques and a combination of augmentation by a pericardial patch, resection of secondary chordae, and papillary muscle approximation.

## Aortic Valve Surgery

Patient–prosthesis mismatch (PPM) remains a challenging issue in aortic surgery and is defined as indexed

| TABLE 44.1 Different Types Prosthetic Heart Valves |||
|---|---|---|
| **Type of Prosthesis** | **Group** | **Brand (Examples)** |
| Mechanical valve | Caged-ball<br>Tilting disc<br>(mono-leaflet)<br>Bileaflet | Starr-Edwards<br>Bjork-Shiely<br>Medtronic-Hall<br>St. Jude<br>On-X<br>Sorin (Carbomedics) |
| Tissue valves | Stented | Carpentier-Edwards<br>Edwards-Perimount<br>Edwards-Magna<br>Pericarbon More<br>St. Jude Trifecta<br>Biocore (Epic) |
| | Stentless<br>(only for aortic position) | FreeStyle<br>Toronto SPV |
| | Sutureless<br>(only for aortic position) | Sorin (Perceval)<br>Medtronic (3F Enable)<br>Edwards (Intuity Elite) |

**TABLE 44.2**
**Carpentier Mitral Regurgitation Classification**

| Classification | Type I | Type II | Type IIIa | Type IIIb |
|---|---|---|---|---|
| Leaflet motion status | Normal | Increased | Restricted systolic and diastolic | Restricted in systole and tattered in diastole |
| Pathology | Annular dilatation Leaflet cleft or perforation | Leaflet prolapse Chorda or PM rupture | Commissural fusion Thickened/calcified leaflet ± subvalvular apparatus | PM displacement and chorda tattering |
| Clinical diagnosis | FMR Endocarditis Congenital MV cleft | Degenerative MR Barlow disease Flail MV | Rheumatic disease | IMR LV aneurysm |
| Schematic MR jet mechanism | | | | |

*FMR,* functional mitral regurgitation; *IMR,* ischemic mitral regurgitation; *LV,* left ventricular; *MR,* mitral regurgitation; *MV,* mitral valve; *PM,* papillary muscle.

effective orifice area (iEOA/BSA) less than 0.85. When the iEOA is less than 0.75, the PPM is severe, and the patient is usually symptomatic.[15,16] Despite new-generation prostheses with good EOA, some patients still need aortic root enlargement. A posterior root enlargement (Manougian procedure) technique is widely used and is effective with good surgical outcomes.[17] In this method, the aortotomy incision is extended toward the aortic annulus and anterior mitral leaflet, and the aortic annulus is enlarged by reconstruction, creating a gap using an autologous pericardial or synthetic Dacron patch (Fig. 44.2).

An anterior root enlargement technique (Kono-Rastan procedure) is used on complex congenital LV outflow tract obstruction with higher mortality and morbidity rates. In this technique, the aortotomy incision is extended in the right side or right coronary artery orifice toward the ventricular septum and the RV outflow tract. Then, defect repair is done with two separate patches.[18] Sutureless tissue valves are a good alternative for older patients with calcified aortic stenosis and a small aortic root. These valves (Perceval/Sorin, Intuity/Edwards, 3f enable/Medtronic) can be implanted by minimally invasive approaches (Fig. 44.3).

Surgery of the aortic root aneurysm is the other challenging issue in cardiac surgery (Fig. 44.4).

Because it is performed in a high-pressure area and the patients usually have underlying connective tissue disorders or old ages, the high probability of postoperative bleeding and its consequent problems may affect the patient outcome.[19]

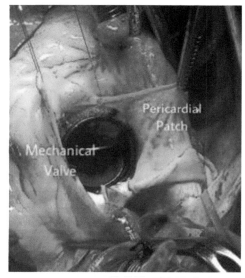

FIG. 44.2 Aortic valve replacement with aortic root enlargement with the Manougian technique using autologous pericardial patch.

The Bentall operation is a well-known procedure for some patients with ascending aorta aneurysm or type A aortic dissection, in which the entire aortic valve and aneurysmal tissues are resected and coronary ostia are prepared as a button. Then, a suitable size of composite graft (prosthetic valve plus Dacron tube graft) is implanted and end-to-side anastomosis is done for

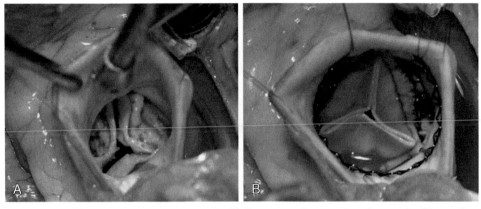

FIG. 44.3 (A) Calcified aortic valve stenosis. (B) Placement of a sutureless tissue valve (Perceval).

both coronary artery buttons on the proper side of the composite grafts (Fig. 44.5).

Valve-preserving methods (David and Yacoub operation) are usually used for patients who have normal aortic leaflets and aortic annulus size of less than 30 mm. In the David operation, the diseased aortic wall, including the Valsalva sinuses, is resected and the coronary artery buttons prepared. Then, the preserved native aortic valve is reimplanted inside a cylindrical Dacron tube graft, and coronary buttons are implanted the same as for the Bentall procedure. In the Yacoub technique,

the aortic resection and coronary ostia implantation are the same, but instead of valve resuspension, the rim of the remnants of the native Valsalva sinuses is anastomosed to a prefashioned cylindrical Dacron graft to create new Valsalva sinuses (Fig. 44.6).

These techniques can be used for type A aortic dissection; however, because of various extensions of dissection, the distal-end anastomosis of the Dacron graft maybe different. If the side branches of the aortic arch are intact and the dissection flap only involves the lesser curvature of the arch, the diseased aortic wall is resected,

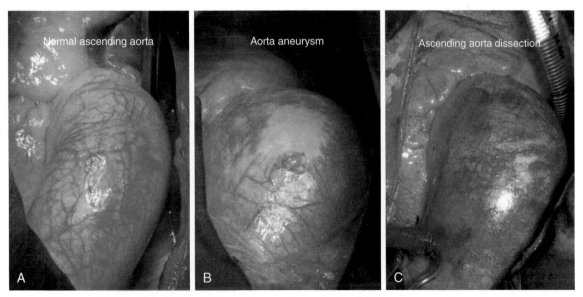

FIG. 44.4 Surgical views of different forms of ascending aorta disease. (A) Normal ascending aorta. (B) Aortic aneurysm. (C) Ascending aorta dissection.

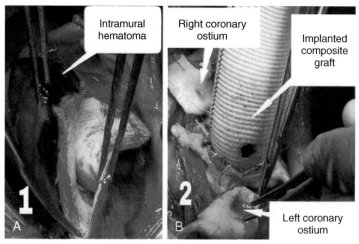

FIG. 44.5 (A) and (B) Bentall procedure with a composite graft.

and the distal end of the tube graft is tailored into a beveled shape and anastomosed to the arch remnant (hemiarch techniques). If the aortic arch branches are involved with dissection, each branch can be interposed with a smaller Dacron graft, or different anastomosis techniques can be specialized for each case. TCA is mandatory for arch replacement, and the antegrade (exclusive cerebral perfusion via the arterial route) or retrograde (exclusive cerebral perfusion via the SVC route) techniques may improve brain protection and increase the safe circulatory arrest time.

### Tricuspid Valve Surgery

Functional tricuspid regurgitation (TR) is the main cause of tricuspid valve (TV) involvement that is secondary to left-sided heart valve diseases.

During the surgical treatment of MV, when there is severe TR or moderate TR associated with a dilated annulus (i.e., maximum end-systolic diameter >40 mm or >21 mm/m$^2$), TV repair is strongly recommended.[20] Suture annuloplasty and ring annuloplasty are the two main TV repair techniques. In suture annuloplasty, the diameter of the TV annulus is minimized

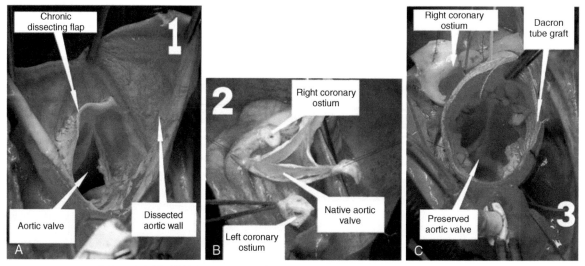

FIG. 44.6 (A)–(C) Valve-sparing aortic root reconstruction with the David technique.

using a two-layered suture thread. The well-known technique of suture annuloplasty is the De-vega technique, during which the suture thread is passed through the periphery of the annulus except for half of the septal leaflet that is close to the conductive pathway.

In ring annuloplasty, a specialized incomplete ring for TV is used to minimize and stabilize the TV annulus (Fig. 44.7). This technique is more common nowadays. TV rings have three types similar to MV rings, including flexible (e.g., Cosgrove band), semirigid (e.g., classic Carpentier Edwards), and rigid (e.g., Edwards/MC3). Acceptable results have been reported using all ring types. There are acceptable outcomes of three types for repairing the TV. The repair of TV cannot be always performed by only applying a ring, and it sometimes needs to use neochordae, patch augmentation, resection, and plication.

In cases with thickened and calcified TV leaflets such as rheumatic diseases and when the repair's result is undesirable, the TV should be replaced by a large-sized prosthetic valve. There are some controversies regarding the selection of valve type. Advocates of biologic valves believe that the pace of degeneration is lower in the right side because of lower pressures, and when the valve destructs, it is not an emergent situation, and there is enough time to make an intervention; however, thrombosis in right-sided mechanical valves is an emergent condition. Another benefit of biologic valves is that another biologic valve can be implanted percutaneously with the "valve-in-valve" technique.

On one hand, advocates of mechanical valves believe that most patients requiring TV replacement have undergone MV or aortic valve replacements by mechanical valves, and they need to take warfarin. On the other hand, right-sided mechanical valve thrombosis, either

of the tricuspid or pulmonary valve, can be treated with thrombotic agents.[21,22] Isolated TV surgery is done in rare cases of endocarditis or Ebstein anomaly.

## Atrial Fibrillation Surgery

In this surgery, the aberrant pathways are blocked to restore sinus rhythm. James Cox has innovated this technique by implementing incision and suturing of these incisions in the LA and right atrium. The development of fibrosis in the location of cut and sew leads to the blockage of pathologic aberrant pathways.

Because this technique requires experience and proficiency and the incisions are located in potentially hazardous parts such as adjacent to the MV and coronary sinus, there have been some modifications of incision number and energy source for this technique. Nowadays, during MV surgeries that require ablation of the AF, a combination of cut and sew, radiofrequency, and cryoablation is used so that in addition to desirable outcomes, the incidence of complications and bleeding is decreased. Pulmonary vein isolation is a technique limited to the pulmonary vein orifices and does not need cutting. It can be performed in some minutes using different sources of energies, and according to our experience, its success rate to restore sinus rhythm is about 65%.[23] Given the minimally invasive surgeries, AF can be performed as an isolated and an off-pump surgery with acceptable results.

## Pericardium Surgery

Subxiphoid pericardial drainage along with pericardial window creation by a left thoracotomy are two usual approaches to massive pericardial effusion or tamponade. Radical pericardiotomy, when possible, is the classic surgical management of constrictive pericarditis (CP). The major part of the thickened (or even calcified) parietal pericardium should be resected using an off- or on-pump technique. It is also important that the thickened epicardium is removed as much as possible. Two stripes of pericardium adjacent to the phrenic nerves should be preserved on each side to prevent diaphragmatic paresis. Total pericardiectomy is not possible in some cases of postoperative or tuberculosis CP because of dense adherence of diseased pericardium to the epicardium in critical locations such as the atrioventricular groove, vena cava, or coronary artery course. Despite the technical difficulties and surgical complications such as bleeding myocardial damages or even perforation of the fragile portion of the heart, patients' late survival outcomes are usually good after total pericardiectomy.[24]

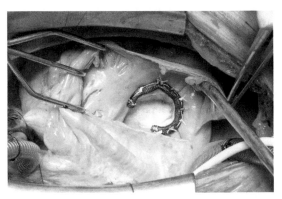

FIG. 44.7 Tricuspid valve ring annuloplasty with a rigid ring.

## CORONARY ARTERY BYPASS GRAFT

The routine approach for CABG is midsternotomy, which is performed in most cardiac surgery centers. Thereafter, the left internal mammary artery (LIMA) is routinely, and almost as an essential component of CABG, harvested. LIMA harvest is recommended in the form of skeletonization because it provides more length while at the same time causing less impaired blood supply to the sternum and thereby increasing the probability of mediastinitis. Care must be taken to harvest the LIMA carefully because even an intimal injury decreases the longevity of this graft. If desired, the right internal mammary artery is used immediately after LIMA harvest is finished. If more conduits, such as the saphenous vein or radial artery, are required simultaneously with midsternotomy and LIMA harvesting, they are also open or endoscopically harvested.

However, in certain cases, if the patient only has single-vessel coronary artery disease, particularly of the left anterior descending coronary artery (LAD), a small left anterior thoracotomy incision is used, which is known as minimally invasive direct coronary artery bypass (MIDCAB). In certain cases, a left lateral thoracotomy incision is used, especially in redo surgeries in which the previous LIMA graft opens into the LAD and the patient needs a graft on the obtuse marginal branch.

After the conduit harvest, heparinization, and cannulation, the patient is placed on CPB. Subsequently, based on the diseased coronary artery, suitable sites for graft are reviewed and preferably marked with a knife superficially. The main strategy for complete revascularization, which means graft bypassing all coronary arteries with a diameter of more than 1 mm and a constriction of more than 50%. After clamping the aorta and cardioplegic arrest, the prepared conduits are anastomosed to the selected targets.

A suitable segment that is free of atheroma should be chosen for grafting. An incision of about 5 mm is made. Then, for saphenous vein graft (SVG) or radial artery anastomosis, 7–0 polypropylene sutures are used. For LIMA anastomosis, 8–0 sutures of the same suture material are used. In the sequential bypass method, one conduit is anastomosed to more than one coronary artery. In this method, after finishing with distal anastomosis, the aortic clamp is released, and the proximal end(s) is anastomosed on the ascending aorta with a side clamp. In some patients with extensive atherosclerotic involvement, endothelium must be removed along with atheroma tissues (coronary endarterectomy) in order to create an appropriate lumen for anastomosis. Usually the longevity of this type of anastomosis is less than grafts on vessels without endarterectomy.[25] Thus, endarterectomy is usually avoided in our surgeries unless for poor runoff targets or when the coronary artery is opened in an inappropriate segment and there are no lumens for anastomosis.

To perform endarterectomy, an incision of approximately 6–8 mm is made on a completely occluded coronary artery, and then with the help of an endarterectomy probe, the atheroma tissue on the opened section of vessel is removed from the adjacent walls. Maximum precision is applied to completely remove the atheroma tissue distal to the anastomosis position. To perform this, it is usually sufficient to separate the anterior part of atheroma from the remaining wall of the vessel with the help of an endarterectomy probe. Complete and precise endarterectomy may lead to better graft patency.

## OFF-PUMP CORONARY ARTERY BYPASS GRAFT

With the introduction of off-pump coronary artery bypass (OPCAB), to avoid the complications of CPB, many cardiac surgeons favored this method. However, after gaining experience, they noticed the possibility of incomplete revascularization, and perhaps the quality of the anastomosis is not as desirable as with the on-pump method. Also, the complications of CPB are not significant. Most surgeons are returning to the on-pump method, and presently, only about one-fifth of surgeons routinely perform the OPCAB technique, with associated good results.[26]

## MINIMALLY INVASIVE CARDIAC SURGERY

Postoperative mediastinal bleeding and mediastinitis are the nightmares of cardiac surgeons that adversely affect patient outcomes. On the other hand, patients are usually concerned about sternotomy and the long incision scar. Minimally invasive cardiac surgery (MICS) has been a rapidly improving technique in the last decade that aimed at reducing surgical trauma with a small-sized incision. Besides the small incision and scar, MICS procedure is very important for the patients as there are several clinically important advantages for this surgical approach including reduced rates of bleeding, blood product transfusion, postoperative atrial fibrillation, sternal wound infection, ventilation time, ICU stay, hospital length of stay, and time to return to normal activity. Thoracoscopic direct vision approach, video-assisted port access method, and robotic surgeries are different methods for less invasive cardiac surgeries. All these techniques follow the same surgical principles with different instruments. These surgical techniques are usually time consuming and more complex than the standard approaches that have a steep learning curve, therefore, many centers still have a low volume of MICSs.[27] Prolonged cardiopulmonary bypass and aortic cross-clamp times are the two major weaknesses of the minimal invasive approaches, however, the recent studies have shown that the surgical results are usually comparable or even better than the standard median sternotomy regarding the long-term outcome.[28] A study by Mariscalco et al. demonstrates that the thoracotomy approach could be a good alternative for heart valve surgeries without increasing mortality and morbidity.[29]

There are different choices for incision, cannulation, and myocardial protection during MICS that are selected based on the type of procedure, patient characteristics, and surgeon's preference and experience. Mostly a 4–6 cm right lateral thoracotomy in the fourth intercostal space is performed for mitral and tricuspid valve surgeries and also for atrial septal defect (ASD) repair. The femoral artery and vein cannulation is usually used for the establishment of the CPB (Fig. 44.8).

Minimally invasive aortic valve surgery is usually carried out by upper mini-sternotomy or a small right anterior thoracotomy (RAT). Both peripheral and central cannulation could be used for CPB establishment. More complex aortic surgeries like Bentall or David operations, aortic root enlargement, and septal myectomy could also be performed using these small incisions. Implanting a sutureless tissue valve may simplify minimally invasive AVR and diminish the operation time. This technique is a good option for high-risk elderly patient with aortic stenosis.

Minimally invasive techniques play a limited role in coronary artery diseases and can only be performed for one or two grafts on the left coronary systems by a small left thoracotomy incision with dedicated instruments. This method is usually performed as a beating heart LIMA to LAD anastomosis named minimally invasive direct coronary artery bypass (MIDCAB).

Although the minimal access surgeries are more technically challenging in obese patients, the risk of bleeding, wound infection, and hospital stay are less than standard approaches. In addition, these techniques may be safer in patients with poorly controlled diabetes mellitus and severe osteoporosis.[27] There are some limitations and concerns about the safety and efficacy of minimally invasive valve surgeries in patients with concomitant coronary artery disease, LV dysfunction, severe pulmonary hypertension, severe mitral annulus calcification, severe chest deformities, previous thoracotomy and pulmonary adhesion, and peripheral vascular disease. These surgeries can also be performed in selected

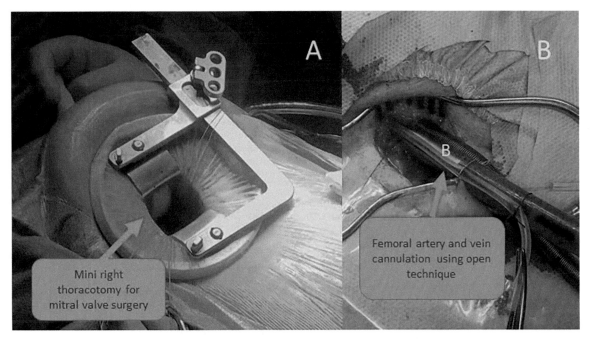

FIG. 44.8 (A) and (B) Minimally invasive approach for mitral valve surgery.

cases of redo valve operation by well-experienced surgeons. Intraoperative TEE plays an important role for patient's cannulation, planning the surgical strategy, and assessment of surgical results.[27]

Overall, MICS should be considered as routine valve surgery in selected patients as a multidisciplinary approach in most referral centers with well-trained cardiac surgeons because they have less pain, less bleeding, shorter ICU and hospital stay, comparable results, and finally better cosmetic results and patients' satisfaction.

## CARDIAC SURGERY AND COVID-19

COVID-19 pandemic affects all aspects of life including cardiac surgery programs. Special programs should be considered for achieving good surgical outcomes and protecting the medical team during this outbreak and afterwards. During the crisis of this pandemic, cardiac surgery should be limited for lifesaving operations while considering all aspects of personal protection principles. Extracorporeal membrane oxygenation (ECMO) may play a role in high-risk COVID-19 patients, however, some reports are discouraging.[30]

For preoperative evaluation of elective surgeries in this pandemic, it is recommended for all candidates to be carefully checked for a history of unprotected contact with COVID-19 patients and suspicious clinical symptoms like fever, cough, and shortness of breath during the last 2 weeks. Besides the usual laboratory tests, all candidates for elective surgeries should be evaluated twice by more specific COVID-19 tests like PCR within 24 h prior to surgery. Although chest CT scan is not recommended as a routine screening method, some centers use this diagnostic tool because of the high false negative results of the PCR tests. For elective surgeries in patients with a recent history of COVID-19 infection, two negative PCR tests and also good respiratory and functional capacity should be achieved.

We should keep in mind that the postcardiac surgery problems like atelectasis, pulmonary infection, pulmonary or pericardial effusion, pump failure, and pulmonary thromboembolic may mimic those of COVID-19 infection symptoms.[30]

## REFERENCES

1. Pouard P, Bojan M. Neonatal cardiopulmonary bypass. *Semin Thorac Cardiovasc Surg Pediatr Card Surg Annu.* 2013; 16(1):59–61.
2. Rice RD, Sandhu HK, Leake SS, et al. Is total arch replacement associated with worse outcomes during repair of acute type A aortic dissection? *Ann Thorac Surg.* 2015; 100(6):2159–2165.
3. Kim NH, Delcroix M, Jenkins DP, et al. Chronic thromboembolic pulmonary hypertension. *J Am Coll Cardiol.* 2013; 62(suppl. 25).
4. Murphy Gavin J, Reeves Barnaby C, Rogers Chris A, Rizvi Syed IA, Culliford L, Angelini GD. Increased mortality, postoperative morbidity, and cost after red blood cell transfusion in patients having cardiac surgery. *Circulation.* 2007; 116:2544–2552. (2007). https://doi.org/10.1161/CIRCULATIONAHA.107.698977 Originally published online Nov 12, 2007.
5. Alizadeh Ghavidel A, Toutounchi Z, Shahandashti FJ, Mirmesdagh Y. Rotational thromboelastometry in prediction of bleeding after cardiac surgery. *Asian Cardiovasc Thorac Ann.* 2015; 23(5):525–529. (2015). https://doi.org/10.1177/0218492314566330.
6. Jamieson WR, Cartier CP, Allard M. Surgical management of valvular heart disease. *Can J Cardiol.* 2004; 20(suppl. E): 7–120.
7. Dunninga J, Versteeghb M, Fabbric A, et al. Guideline on antiplatelet and anticoagulation management in cardiac surgery. *Eur J Cardiothorac Surg.* 2008; 34(1):73–92.
8. Vahanian A, Alfieri O, Andreotti F, et al. Guidelines on the management of valvular heart disease (version 2012). *Eur Heart J.* 2012; 33:2451–2496. (2012). https://doi.org/10.1093/eurheartj/ehs109.
9. Nishimura RA, Otto CM, Bonow RO, et al. American College of Cardiology/American Heart Association Task Force on Practice Guidelines. 2014 AHA/ACC guideline for the management of patients with valvular heart disease: a report of the American College of Cardiology/American Heart Association Task Force on Practice Guidelines. *J Am Coll Cardiol.* 2014; 63(22):e57–e185. (2014). https://doi.org/10.1016/j.jacc.2014.02.536 [Epub 2014 Mar 3].
10. El-Husseiny M, Salhiyyah K, Raja SG, Dunning J. Should warfarin be routinely prescribed for the first three months after a bioprosthetic valve replacement? *Interact Cardiovasc Thorac Surg.* 2006; 5:616–623.
11. Asopa S, Patel A, Dunning J. Is short term anticoagulation necessary after mitral valve repair? *Interact Cardiovasc Thorac Surg.* 2006; 5:761–765.
12. Watson H, Davidson S, Keeling D. Haemostasis and Thrombosis Task Force of the British Committee for Standards in Haematology. Guidelines on the diagnosis and management of heparin-induced thrombocytopenia: second edition. *Br J Haematol.* 2012; 159(5):528–540. (2012). https://doi.org/10.1111/bjh.12059 [Epub 2012 Oct 9].
13. Ahmed I, Majeed A, Powell R. Heparin induced thrombocytopenia: diagnosis and management update. *Postgrad Med J.* 2007; 83:575–582. (2007). https://doi.org/10.1136/pgmj.2007.059188.
14. Alizadeh Ghavidel A, Mirmesdagh Y, Harifi M, Sadeghpour AN, Nakhaeizadeh R, Omrani G. The impact of sub-valvular apparatus preservation on prosthetic valve dysfunction during mitral valve replacement. *Res Cardiovasc Med.* 2012; 1(2):55–61.
15. Alizadeh-Ghavidel A, Azarfarin R, Alizadehasl A, Sadeghpour-Tabaei A, Totonchi Z. Moderate patient-prosthesis mismatch

has no negative effect on patients' functional status after aortic valve replacement with CarboMedics prosthesis. *Res Cardiovasc Med.* 2016; 5(2):e29038.

16. Alizadeh GA. Surgical management of small aortic root (review article). *Iran J Cardiac Surg.* 2007; 3:15–22.

17. Alizadeh Ghavidel A, Omrani G, Chitsazan M, Totonchi Z, Givtaj N. Long-term results of aortic valve replacement with posterior root enlargement. *Asian Cardiovasc Thorac Ann.* 2014; 22:1059. (2014). https://doi.org/10.1177/0218492314528923.

18. Tabatabaie MB, Alizadeh Ghavidel A, Yousefnia MA, Hoseini S, Javadpour SH, Raesi K. Classic konno-rastan procedure: indications and results in the current era. *Asian Cardiovasc Thorac Ann.* 2006; 14(5):377–381.

19. Alizadeh Ghavidel A, Tabatabaei MB, Yousefnia MA, Omrani GR, Givtaj N, Raesi K. Mortality and morbidity after aortic root replacement: 10-year experience. *Asian Cardiovasc Thorac Ann.* 2006; 14(6):462–466.

20. Dreyfus GD, Martin RP, Chan K, Dulguerov F, Alexandrescu C. Functional tricuspid regurgitation: a need to revise our understanding. *J Am Coll Cardiol.* 2015; 65(21):2331–2336. (2015). https://doi.org/10.1016/j.jacc.2015.04.011.

21. Khajali Z, Mohammadzadeh S, Maleki M, et al. Fibrinolytic therapy for mechanical pulmonary valve thrombosis. *Pediatr Cardiol.* 2014; 36:171–176 101007/00246-014.

22. Dehaki MG, Alizadeh Ghavidel A, Omrani G, Javadikasgari H. Long-term outcome of mechanical pulmonary valve replacement in 121 patients with congenital heart disease. *Thorac Cardiovasc Surg.* 2015; 63(5):367–372. (2015). http://dxdoiorg/101055/s-0034-1387129 Epub 2014 Sep.

23. Alizadeh Ghavidel A, Javadpour H, Shafiee M, Tabatabaie MB, Raiesi K, Hosseini S. Cryoablation for surgical treatment of chronic atrial fibrillation combined with mitral valve surgery: a clinical observation. *Eur J Cardiothorac Surg.* 2008; 33(6):1043–1048.

24. Alizadeh Ghavidel A, Gholampour M, Kyavar M, Mirmesdagh Y, Tabatabaie MB. Constrictive pericarditis treated by surgery. *Tex Heart Inst J.* 2012; 39(2):199–205.

25. Wang J, Gu C, Yu W. Short- and long-term patient outcomes from combined coronary endarterectomy and coronary artery bypass grafting: a meta-analysis of 63,730 patients (PRISMA). *Medicine (Baltimore).* 2015; 94(41):e1781.

26. Polomsky M, He X, O'Brien SM, et al. Outcomes of off-pump versus on-pump coronary artery bypass grafting: impact of preoperative risk. *J Thorac Cardiovasc Surg.* 2013; 145(5):1193–1198.

27. Alizadeh Ghavidel A. Minimally invasive mitral valve surgery: when & why? In: *Oral Presentation, Caspian Meeting, Mashad, Iran 4–7 December 2018*; 2018.

28. Mkalaluh S, Szczechowicz M, Dib B, et al. Early and long-term results of minimally invasive mitral valve surgery through a right mini-thoracotomy approach: a retrospective propensity-score matched analysis. *PeerJ.* 2018; 6:e4810. Published 2018 May 28(2018). https://doi.org/10.7717/peerj.4810.

29. Mariscalco G, Musumeci F. The minithoracotomy approach: a safe and effective alternative for heart valve surgery. *Ann Thorac Surg.* 2014; 97(1):356–364. https://doi.org/10.1016/j.athoracsur.2013.09.090.

30. Asdaghpour E, Baghaei R, Jalilifar N, Radmehr H. Iranian society of cardiac surgeons position statement for the treatment of patients in need of cardiac surgery in the COVID-19 pandemic period (Version I). *Multidiscip Cardiovasc Ann.* 2020; 11(1):e104296https://doi.org/10.5812/mca.104296.

# Index

Note: Page numbers followed by *f* indicate figures, *t* indicate tables, and *b* indicate boxes.

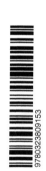